COMMUNITY HEALTH NURSING
Process and Practice for
Promoting Health

SECOND EDITION

COMMUNITY HEALTH NURSING

Process and Practice for Promoting Health

Marcia Stanhope, RN, DSN

Associate Professor and Director,
Division of Community Health Nursing and Administration,
College of Nursing, University of Kentucky,
Lexington, Kentucky

Jeanette Lancaster, RN, MSN, PhD, FAAN

Dean and Professor,
Wright State University–Miami Valley School of Nursing,
Dayton, Ohio

with 199 illustrations

THE C. V. MOSBY COMPANY
St. Louis • Toronto • Washington, D.C. 1988

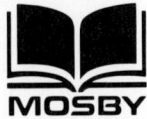

MOSBY

A TRADITION OF PUBLISHING EXCELLENCE

Editor: **Tom Lochhaas**
Assistant editor: **Laurie Sparks**
Developmental editor: **Mark Spann**
Project manager: **Mark Spann**
Designer: **Susan E. Lane**

Previous edition copyrighted 1984

Printed in the United States of America

The C.V. Mosby Company
11830 Westline Industrial Drive, St. Louis, Missouri 63146

Library of Congress Cataloging-in-Publication Data

Community health nursing.

   Includes bibliographies and index.
   1. Community health nursing.   I. Stanhope, Marcia.
II. Lancaster, Jeanette.   [DNLM: 1. Community Health
Nursing—United States. W Y 106 C7356]
RT98.C6562   1988   362.1'73   87-20431
ISBN 0-8016-4966-8

CONTRIBUTORS

Rena Alford, RN, MN, PNP
Director of Nurses
Pee Dee District 1
South Carolina Department of
Health and Environmental Control
Florence, South Carolina

Sandra Anderson, RN, PhD
Nurse Educator
World Health Organization
Kathmandu, Nepal

Ellen Bailey, RN, MSN, FNP
Nurse Practitioner/Manager
Spencer County Rural Health Clinic
Taylorsville, Kentucky

Julia W. Balzer, RN, MN
Staff Instructor
Training and Development
Baptist Medical Center
Jacksonville, Florida

Eleanor Bauwens, RN, PhD, FAAN
Associate Dean
Baccalaureate Program
University of Arizona
Tucson, Arizona

Marjorie Glaser Bindner, Artist
(Marjorie B. Glaser RN, MA)
Continuing Education Consultant
Kentucky Nurses Association
Louisville, Kentucky

Kathleen Beckman Blomquist, RN, PhD
Assistant Professor
Division of Community Health
Nursing and Administration
College of Nursing
University of Kentucky
Lexington, Kentucky

Carol Loveland-Cherry, RN, PhD
Assistant Professor
Community Health Nursing
The University of Michigan
School of Nursing
Ann Arbor, Michigan

Marcia Kaplan Cowan, RN, MSN, PNP
Clinical Nurse Specialist
Perinatal Nursing Division
University Hospital
Birmingham, Alabama

Nancy Dickenson-Hazard RN, MSN, CPNP
Executive Director,
National Board of Pediatric Nurse Practitioners and Associates,
Rockville, Maryland

Beverly C. Flynn, RN, PhD, FAAN
Professor and Chairperson
Department of Community Health
Nursing, Graduate Program, School
of Nursing, Indiana University,
Indianapolis, Indiana

Sara T. Fry, RN, PhD
Assistant Professor
University of Virginia
School of Nursing
Charlottesville, Virginia

Eileen Garvey, RN, MSN
Executive Director
Home Health Incorporated
Birmingham, Alabama

Jean Goeppinger, RN, PhD
Professor
University of Virginia
School of Nursing
Charlottesville, Virginia

Phyllis Graves, RN, DSN
formerly Professor and Head of Baccalaureate Program
College of Nursing
Northwestern State University of Louisiana,
Shreveport, Louisiana

Rosemary Johnson, RN, MPH
Professor
College of Nursing
Arizona State University,
Tempe, Arizona

Marjorie Keller, RN, DNS
Associate Professor
Coordinator, Community/Mental Health Nursing,
    School of Nursing
The University of Southern Mississippi
Hattiesburg, Mississippi

David Kerschner, RN, MSN
Community Health/Family Nurse Clinician
US Public Health Service
Division of Indian Health
Pendleton, Oregon

Karen T. Labuhn, RN, PhD
Assistant Professor
University of Virginia
School of Nursing
Charlottesville, Virginia

Jeanette Lancaster, RN, PhD, FAAN
Dean and Professor
Wright State University/Miami Valley School of
   Nursing
Dayton, Ohio

Wade Lancaster, PhD
Associate Professor, Marketing
   College of Business and Administration
Wright State University
Dayton, Ohio

Peggye Lassiter, RN, MSN
Assistant Professor
University of Virginia
School of Nursing
Charlottesville, Virginia

Roberta K. Lee, RN, DrPH
Associate Professor
School of Nursing
University of Texas Medical Branch
Galveston, Texas

Gwendolen Lee, RN, Ed D
Associate Professor and Director
Division of Parent Child Nursing
College of Nursing
University of Kentucky
Lexington, Kentucky

Jacquelyne Huebel Logue, RN, BS
Director of Community Affairs
Home Health Incorporated
Birmingham, Alabama

Margaret Millsap, RN, Ed D
Chairman, Department of Nursing
Birmingham Southern College
Birmingham, Alabama

Cynthia E. Northrop, RN, MS, JD
Nurse Attorney
Member of Maryland Bar
New York, New York

Charlene Ossler, RN, MSN
Associate Professor, School of Nursing
University of Wisconsin
Milwaukee, Wisconsin

Paula Pointer, MA, CASE
Pointer Associates, Human
Resources Development
Birmingham, Alabama

Cynthia Selleck, RN, DSN, FNP
Assistant Professor
School of Nursing
The University of Alabama at Birmingham
Birmingham, Alabama

George F. Shuster III, RN, DNSc
Assistant Professor
University of Virginia
School of Nursing
Charlottesville, Virginia

Sharon Sheahan, RN, MSN, CFNP
Associate Professor
Division of Community Health
Nursing and Administration
College of Nursing
University of Kentucky
Lexington, Kentucky

Ann Sirles, RN, DSN, FNP
Associate Professor
School of Nursing
University of Alabama at Birmingham
Birmingham, Alabama

Delois H. Skipwith, RN, DSN
Professor, School of Nursing
The University of Alabama at Birmingham
Birmingham, Alabama

Rebecca Sloan, RN, MSN, CRNP
Nurse Researcher
Infant Growth Project,
Department of Pediatrics
University of Alabama at Birmingham
Birmingham, Alabama

Marcia K. Stanhope, RN, DSN
Associate Professor and Director
Division of Community Health Nursing and
   Administration
College of Nursing
University of Kentucky
Lexington, Kentucky

Patricia Starck, RN, DSN
Dean and Professor
School of Nursing
University of Texas
Health Science Center at Houston
Houston, Texas

Joan Turner, RN, DSN
Associate Professor
School of Nursing
The University of Alabama at Birmingham
Birmingham, Alabama

Barbara Valanis, RN, DrPH, FAAN
Senior Investigator
Center for Health Research
Kaiser Permanente
Portland, Oregon

Carolyn A. Williams, RN, PhD, FAAN
Dean and Professor
College of Nursing
University of Kentucky
Lexington, Kentucky

Cora Withrow RN, DSN
Chairperson
Nursing Department
Berea College
Berea, Kentucky

This book is dedicated to the fond memories of the past, the joys of the present, and the dreams of the future. In remembrance of my parents, Loretta and Clark Stanhope, whose love of family spurred them to struggle for a life quality and quantity that often seemed unattainable. The humility and patience they exhibited in their pursuit to conquer health problems of unquestionable magnitude will serve as a constant reminder of the obstacles confronted and the need for a health care system that is more responsive to client needs and concerns. A special dedication to Pete, Maggi, Josie, and Sophie who were great little companions. To my brother Gerald who keeps my thoughts in perspective and my Aunt Betty who offers friendship, understanding, and support as I attempt to manage my rigorous schedule. Finally to those friends who give me joy; and to Jeanette who served as my mentor in the beginning of this endeavor and tolerated my procrastinations.

Marcia Stanhope

Without the support, encouragement, and loving kindness of six people, my contributions to this book would not have been possible. My parents, Glada and Howard Miller, have always encouraged me to reach for higher levels of accomplishment. My husband Wade has continuously raised issues and questions and urged me to think more critically and carefully about many life pursuits, including writing. My daughters, Melinda and Jennifer, have been patient while I spent hours working on this project. With my dear friend, Marcia, I have enjoyed many hours of both hard work and fun as we have revised the first edition of our text.

Jeanette Lancaster

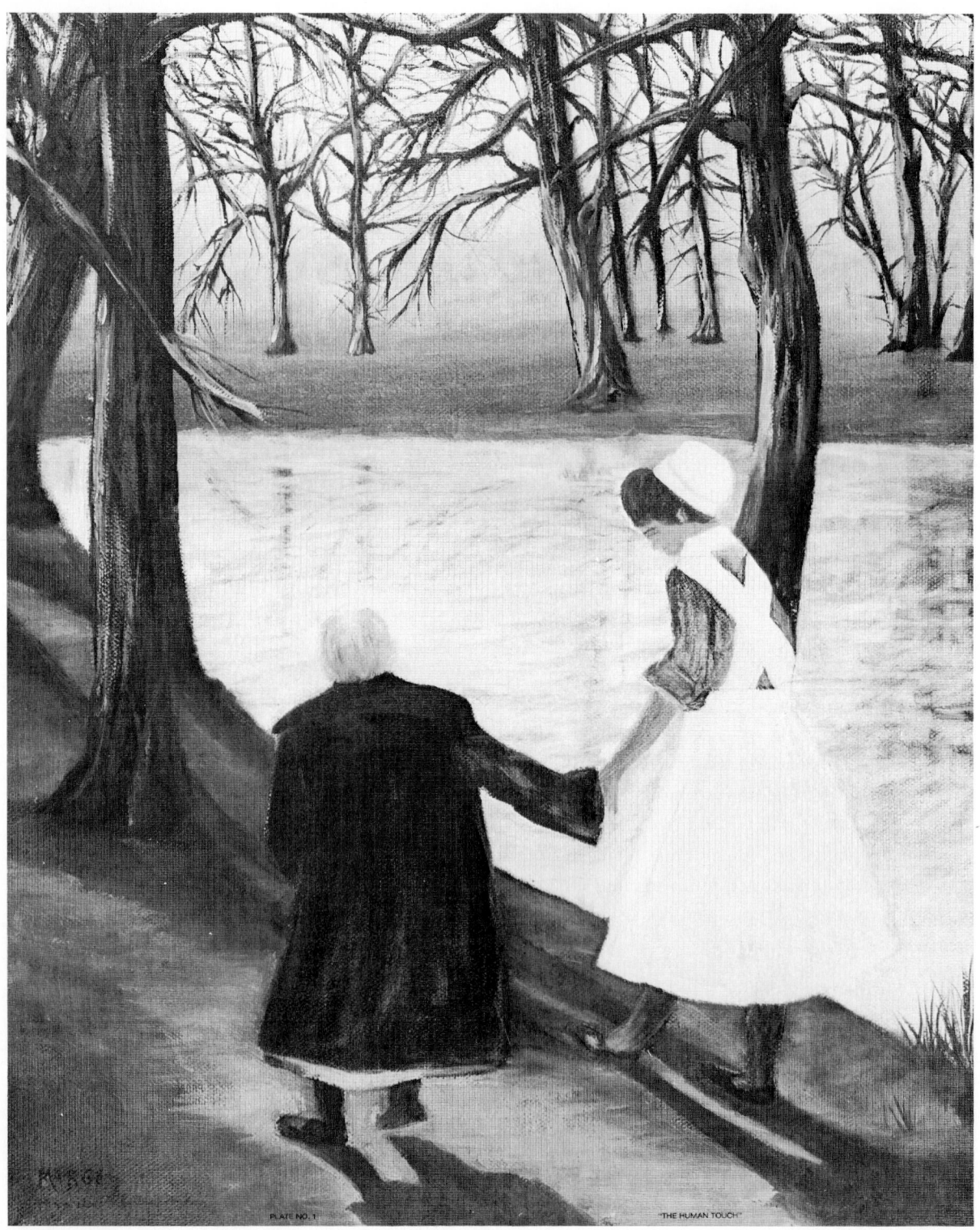

The Human Touch by Marjorie Glaser Bindner
Copyright 1980

Limited Edition
Full-color Print

FOREWORD

The challenge for today's nursing educator is to provide meaningful learning opportunities for the practitioners and leaders of tomorrow. Such responsibility entails a number of significant decisions, and the choice of key texts and reference materials is particularly important. Those trying to design and develop materials that will address the educator's need to speak to students of the present and yet stretch their thinking in ways that will prepare them for the future also have a formidable task. While it may be generally understood and accepted that a first-rate text should encompass the central concepts and principles of a given field, illustrate the application of the basic concepts in ways that have current relevance yet stand the "test of time," challenge the readers' analytical abilities, be clear, be interesting, and above all be affordable, it is not easy to produce such a virtuous volume. This is especially the case in the diverse and dynamic field of community health nursing. Yet, Stanhope and Lancaster have again provided educators with a compelling choice.

This second edition of *Community Health Nursing: Process and Practice for Promoting Health* maintains strengths of the first but includes new, expanded, and reorganized material in several key areas. Particularly notable are the sections on community as client and the developmental approach to the individual and family as client.

For some time basic content in community health nursing has been seen by nursing educators as fundamental to the preparation of the professional nurse. Never before, however, has it been more important to focus attention on developing professionals who have a solid grounding in the synthesis of concepts from nursing science and the public health sciences. It is this synthesis that sets community health nursing apart from other arenas of nursing, and it is this synthesis that provides a meaningful framework for understanding and action in the fast-paced world of health care delivery. Stanhope and Lancaster's second edition presents an unusually sound, useful, and appealing introduction to this world from a perspective that shouldn't be missed.

Carolyn A. Williams, RN, PhD, FAAN
Professor and Dean
College of Nursing
University of Kentucky
Lexington, Kentucky

PREFACE

Current health problems increasingly illustrate that human progress has been purchased at a great cost. Indeed, the accounting mechanisms of history may never accurately document the price that has been paid for urbanization, technological advances, and human comforts, since not all societal changes have served to promote health. At present the most well-fed and affluent society in history can document serious signs of health disruption in the form of a severely damaged environment, crumbling and loss of influence of many traditional social institutions, mortality and morbidity statistics that reflect the effects of unhealthy life-styles on health, and an alarming amount of mental illness and crime. People are not effectively responding to the rapidly changing times; the onslaught of societal stimulation and change has affected both physical and emotional coping mechanisms.

Recent estimates indicate that as much as one half of the mortality from the ten leading causes of death is attributed to an unhealthy life-style. Health care funds have historically been allocated to the treatment of disease rather than to prevention. In an era of economic constraints, attention turns to prevention as a cost-saving measure.

A public health revolution has begun to recast the nation's health strategy to emphasize disease prevention. The nation's first public health revolution dealt with infectious diseases via major sanitary reforms, the development of effective vaccines, and mass immunization. By the middle of the twentieth century, major health problems were no longer related to the communicable diseases of childhood or those resulting from crowding and poor sanitation, but rather morbidity and mortality resulted from the chronic diseases of the middle and later years.

By and large, medical practices have not markedly influenced the overall decline in mortality in the United States since the early 1900s. In fact, despite the vast amount of money spent on health care, the United States still lags behind several of the industrialized nations, which is readily noted when one compares mortality and morbidity statistics.

Individual health practices such as maintenance of desirable weight, eating and drinking in moderation, and getting adequate rest have been demonstrated to be inversely related to mortality. The solution to life-style–induced health problems involves both individual and social commitment to the faciliation of health promotion choices. People must understand the need for changes in personal health-related practices; society, and especially health care providers, must provide support including education, alterations in health policy priorities, changes in financing, and research to demonstrate the benefits of health promotion.

What does this mean for nurses? Nursing as a caring and helping profession exists because people are not always healthy and self-sufficient. Nursing's challenge is to become the central unifying figure in the health care system. Community health nursing is a practice that is continuing and comprehensive, is directed toward all age groups, takes place in a wide variety of settings, and includes health education, maintenance, coordination, and evaluation for individuals, families, groups, and communities.

Society, the health care system, nursing, and health status indicators are all in a state of continuous change. To meet the demands of a constantly changing environment, nursing must become increasingly futuristic in developing roles and practice areas. Such a view encompasses the importance of several key variables, including a knowledge of public health tradition and principles, the current and evolving characteristics of the health care system with a keen awareness of the role and responsibilities of nurses, the constraints and facilitators of a health promotion orientation, and the necessity for consumer responsibility for health.

This text was written to provide nursing students and practitioners with a comprehensive source book that provides a foundation for designing community health nursing strategies for individuals, families, and communities. The unifying *theme* for the book is the integration of health promotion concepts into the multifaceted role of the community health nurse. Such a preventive focus emphasizes traditional public health practice with increased attention directed toward the effect of the environment (both internal and external) and life-style–induced health problems.

To achieve this goal, the text is divided into seven

sections: (1) an introduction to the contemporary health care delivery system that describes the historical and current status of the health care system, including a variety of factors that can promote or constrain the provision of community health nursing services; (2) the conceptual foundations for community health nursing, which describes selected conceptual models for nursing care as well as specific skills inherent in the community health nursing role; (3) the community as client, which describes the aggregate concept, the influence of groups in communities, and the extent to which environment affects the health of the community; (4) major community health problems from a developmental approach from birth through senescence; (5) the tools and techniques used in promoting health; (6) ways to intervene in major community health problems and (7) diversity in the role of community health nurses, which describes the changing roles, functions, and practice settings.

We wish to take this opportunity to express sincere appreciation to our families and friends who supported and encouraged us through this herculean task and to the administration and staff of the University of Kentucky College of Nursing and to the staff at Wright State University—Miami Valley School of Nursing who generously contributed their time, effort, and support to this endeavor. In addition we wish to thank Glenn Blomquist, Ph.D., Associate Professor, Economics and Public Administration, University of Kentucky; Mary Albrecht, R.N., M.S.N., Assistant Professor, Elmhurst College, Elmhurst, Illinois; Barbara K. Andersen, R.N., Ed.D., Associate Professor, University of Tennessee at Chattanooga; Marjorie A. Muecke, C.R.N., Ph.D., Associate Professor, School of Nursing, University of Washington; Anne Whetzell Saletta, R.N., M.S.N.; and Karen A. Wolfe, R.N., M.S., Assistant Professor, Department of Community Nursing, Southeastern Massachusetts University, North Dartmouth, Massachusetts for their time and effort in assisting with the refinement of this text.

The attitudes of cooperation and commitment to quality evidenced by the Mosby staff members who worked with us on this project are greatly appreciated. A special thanks to Alison Miller and Suzi Epstein for their attention to our project, and to Tom Lochhaas, Laurie Sparks, and Mark Spann for sticking with us through the second edition.

Marcia Stanhope
Jeanette Lancaster

CONTENTS

APPENDIXES

PHOTOGRAPHY CREDITS

COMMUNITY HEALTH NURSING
Process and Practice for
Promoting Health

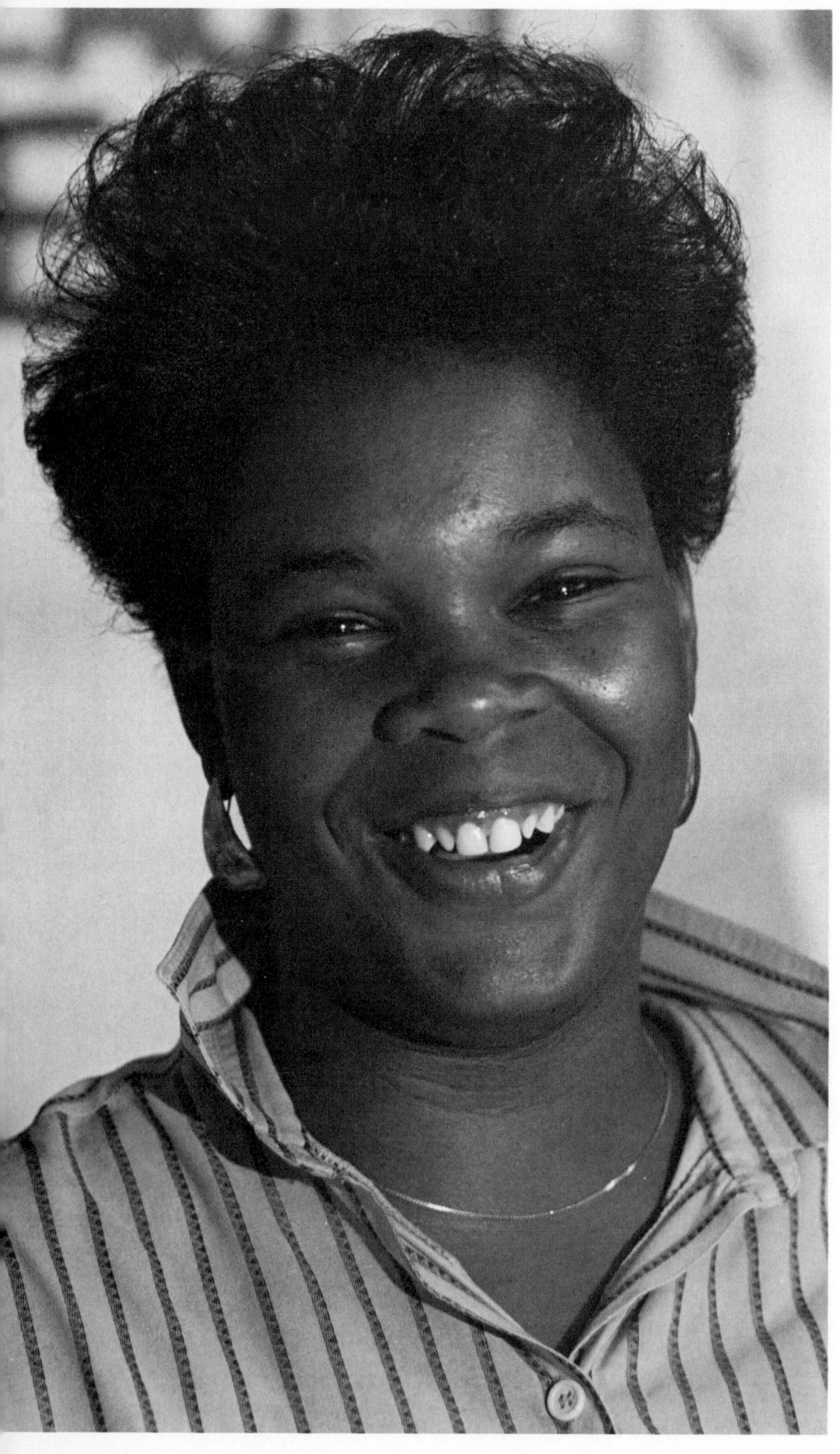

CONTEMPORARY HEALTH CARE DELIVERY SYSTEM AND COMMUNITY HEALTH NURSING

Community health nurses have been leaders in improving the quality of health care for people since the late 1800s. Over the decades community health nurses have been instrumental forces for change; they have courageously tried many new approaches designed to improve the overall health status of their communities. Early nursing leaders recognized the need for specific preparation for community health nurses and the influence of legal, economic, social, ethical, and political forces on their practice. However, despite many contributions to health care, the system for delivery continues to need major changes to be entirely responsive to the needs of Americans.

Health care providers and consumers have accelerated their demands for a reorientation of the American health care system. In fact, some critics say that there is no system but rather a loosely connected and often fragmented array of providers and facilities that make up a nonsystem. Health care is criticized as being inconsistent in accessibility, affordability, and quality. Simultaneously, the most common causes of death continue to be heart disease, cancer, strokes, and accidents. Each of these killers has been associated with personal behaviors.

Even though the United States spends a larger portion of its gross national product on health than any other nation, it does not rank in the top 10 countries of the world in terms of overall health status of residents.

If community health nurses are to be effective and be vital forces for promoting the health of Americans, it is necessary to understand the history of community health nursing as well as the current status of the health care system. Too often we fail to learn from our predecessors because we do not appreciate that history often repeats itself. The challenges currently facing community health nursing are similar to those facing nurses in earlier times. The approaches that have proved successful in the past often can be modified and implemented to deal with contemporary challenges.

Similarly, effective strategies for community health nurses must be designed so that they are consistent with the total mosaic of health care delivery. The professional must understand the scope and nature of change and the future directions of the health care system to plan effective nursing approaches. The status of the health care system as described in Chapter 2 is determined by a wide range of variables, including the organization for practice, providers, and available resources. Three major influences on the health care system are emphasized in Part One because of their paramount role in influencing the system. Chapters 3, 4, 5, and 6, respectively, describe how economics, ethics, social, cultural, political and governmental forces influence health care.

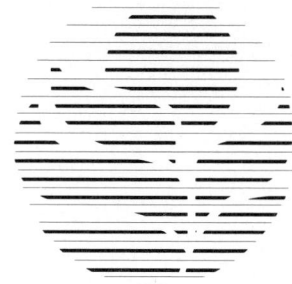

Health care has become big business in the United States, and various groups volley for control of the fiscal picture. To date hospitals account for the largest single portion of health care funds. Whether or not this pattern will change as health promotion is increasingly encouraged is a question that is as yet unanswered. The economics of health care are heavily influenced by ethics and governmental regulations. As fiscal resources for health care decrease, more questions are raised about how money should be spent, and ethical dilemmas continue to cloud the picture of who gets what resources.

Though the govenment neither owns nor solely finances health care, its influence is felt in all sectors. Currently, governmental funds provide a wide range of direct and indirect health care services. As in all other situations in life, this form of the golden rule applies: "He who has the gold, rules." That is, the government, along with providing funds, has a history of issuing many regulations about the use of the funds. Frequently, only agencies meeting certain standards and following selected guidelines are given governmental funds. Community health nurses must clearly understand the health care system in which they function and recognize the constraints and facilitators of their practice.

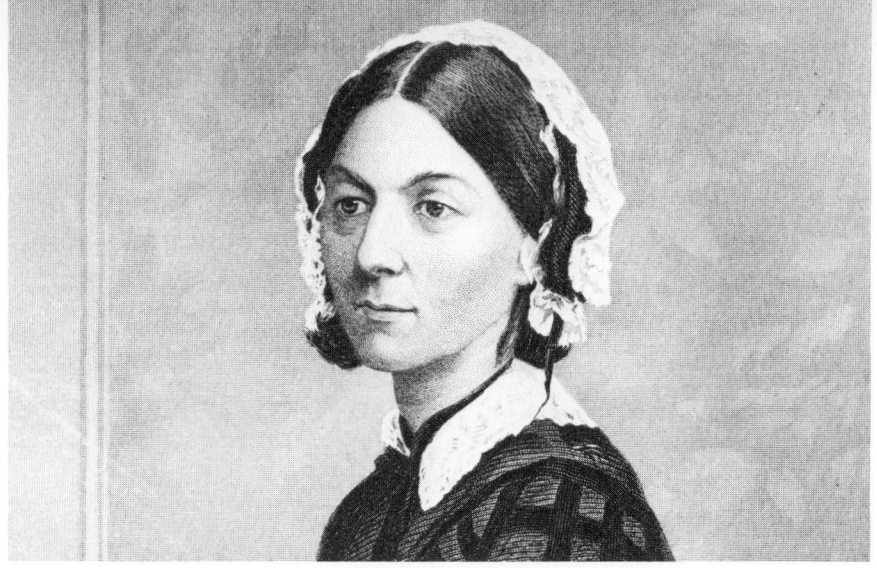

Jeanette Lancaster

1

HISTORY OF COMMUNITY HEALTH AND COMMUNITY HEALTH NURSING

OBJECTIVES

After reading this chapter, the student should be able to:

Trace current community health practices from the pre-Christian era. Describe one leader in nursing who had a profound impact on community health nursing practice.

Identify two famous reports of the early twentieth century, which called attention to conditions in medical education and public health.

Discuss the work of one voluntary agency by describing its purpose, programs or services offered, criteria for eligibility for services, and source of funding.

Describe the purpose and activities of three agencies devoted to improving international health.

Discuss the evolution of the first two nursing organizations in the United States.

Summarize the history of home health care beginning with the Sisters of Charity in Paris.

Analyze three historical events that have influenced the contemporary definition of community health nursing.

KEY TERMS

American Nurses' Association

American Public Health Association

American Red Cross

child welfare movement

Children's Bureau

Food and Drug Administration

home health care

humanism

Industrial Revolution

instructive district nursing

Lillian Wald

National League for Nursing Education

Notes on Nursing

public health

Shattuck Report

The House on Henry Street

The Report of the Committee for Study of Nursing Education

United Nations Children's Fund

United States Public Health Service

voluntary agencies

World Health Organization

Historically the term *public health* was used more often than community health. In this chapter the terms will be used interchangeably as the development of this area of health care is traced. Early definitions of public health focused on sanitation and community health hazards. Today these problems are under much better control and require less attention, thereby allowing public health providers the opportunity to emphasize health promotion as well as eradication of disease. Hanlon and Pickett (1984, p. 5) described public health as being "dedicated to the common attainment of the highest level of physical, mental, and social well-being and longevity consistent with available knowledge and resources at a given time and place."

This chapter traces the historical development of health care from the pre-Christian era to the present and incorporates the evolution of nursing, particularly public health nursing throughout each era.

HISTORICAL REVIEW

An understanding of the dominant cultural ideas of each era since early recorded history is useful in understanding the antecedents of the current community health care system. The patterns of health care in previous eras influence and in turn are influenced by the prevalent patterns of medical and nursing practice.

Pre-Christian Era

People have always been concerned with the events surrounding birth, death, and illness. With few exceptions primitive tribes had a certain amount of group spirit and a sense of hygiene. In their struggles to exist, early people tried to understand disease to devise ways to cope with disease-producing agents. They based health practices on magic and superstition rather than on facts about the cause and effect of certain events and actions on health. Shamans, or medicine men, cared for both health and religious needs and were highly esteemed.

Rudiments of community health can be traced to the earliest recorded civilizations. Excavations from the Middle Kingdom (2100-1700 BC) reflect community health practices in ancient Egypt. Two thousand years before the Christian era, securing an adequate supply of drinking water was a major concern. In Babylonia the "notion persisted that illness was caused by sin and displeasures of the gods; that

disease was inflicted as a punishment for sinning" (Dolan, 1978, p. 10). Sick people were seen as unclean and in need of purification, and temples became the seat of medical care. Sick people were often taken to a busy market where passersby could offer suggestions for treatment. In spite of their primitive practices, both the Babylonians and Egyptians emphasized hygiene and possessed some medical skills.

The Egyptians of about 1000 BC, the healthiest of all early civilizations, used principles based on observation and empirical knowledge rather than on magic. They also developed a variety of pharmaceutical preparations and constructed earth closets and public drainage systems. From their observations of the decay of organic matter, the Egyptians developed complex explanations of the causes of disease. They believed disease resulted from absorption of noxious substances back into the intestine. Based on these beliefs, they developed treatment approaches using cathartics, enemas, purges, bloodletting, and opening of abscesses. Their custom of embalming led them to a knowledge of the structure of the human body (Griffin and Griffin, 1973).

The Mosaic health code of the Hebrews which is clearly reflected in the Old Testament, discussed many aspects of individual, family, and community hygiene and provided a sound basis for practices to maintain health and prolong life. Also, Hebrew nurses participated in carefully planned programs of visiting the sick in their homes and caring for them by bringing physical and spiritual refreshment for the sick person and the family.

Greek Era

The early Greeks viewed people as part of nature and believed health resulted from a harmonious relationship with nature. Kalisch and Kalisch (1986, p. 5) said "The notion most persistent and most damaging to the practice and theory of medicine was the doctrine of the four humors, first elaborated by Empedocles of Acragas (494-433 BC)." The four humors—yellow and black bile, blood, and phlegm—corresponded to the four elements of the world: fire, air, water, and earth. Health resulted from the equilibrium of the humors; medical care sought to achieve balance. For example, if a person had fever (i.e., was hot) he needed cold; if he had a chill, he needed heat. Because these beliefs had no basis in physiology, their application was largely useless.

The Greeks saw health care delivery as a responsibility of civilized man, and the medical ethics established in Greece guided contemporary medical practice. The Greeks also paid attention to personal cleanliness, exercise, diet, and sanitation. Despite their many farsighted practices, the Greeks ignored or destroyed the weak, sick, and crippled.

Aristotle (384-433 BC) was influential in the development of Greek science during this era. Although he demonstrated that the hearts of animals were the source of blood vessels, religious bans prohibited the application of this knowledge to the study of humans.

Additionally, the first notation of women being associated with healing is found in connection with the Greek mythological character of Aesculapius, who eventually became deified as the god of healing. One of his five children, Hygeia, became the goddess of health and another, Panacea, the restorer of health. In later Greek civilizations, healing largely occurred in shrines where patients congregated and were looked after by attendants called "basket healers" (Deloughery, 1977).

The first clear-cut evidence of acute communicable disease is recorded in classical Greek literature. There are numerous references to severe sore throats that often ended in death. The Greek work *Kynanche* mentioned acute inflammatory processes of the throat and larynx and probably referred to what is now known as diphtheria. In ancient Greece, medicine was an itinerant vocation, with practitioners going from town to town, knocking on doors and offering their services. Larger cities appointed physicians and paid for their services from funds; these probably were the earliest community physicians.

Roman Empire

The Roman view of health shared many concepts with the Greeks yet focused much more on pragmatic application of ideas rather than astute observation and a continual search for new knowledge. The Roman Empire is remembered for its administrative and engineering efforts. According to Pellegrino (1963), Romans viewed medicine from a community health and social medicine perspective. They emphasized regulation of medical practice, punishment for negligence, drainage of swamps, provision of pure water, establishment of sewage systems, and supervision of street cleaning and public food preparation. They also made substantial efforts at census taking. This civilization established laws that provided for the registration of slaves and other citizens as well as the periodic collection of census information.

The Roman censor Appius Claudius Crassus Caecus, who built the first great Roman road, the Appian Way, was responsible for bringing a supply of water to Rome by means of an aqueduct (Rosen, 1958, p. 39). To monitor the purity of water, settling basins were established at points along the aqueduct to allow sediment to deposit. When the water reached Rome, it was received in large reservoirs from which emerged smaller reservoirs so that water could be segregated according to its purpose. The Romans not only valued pure water but also had sewage systems in major cities. The Romans developed community health services with an ef-

fective and systematic organization, which continued to function as the Empire disintegrated. Additionally, at the peak of the Roman Empire women visited and cared for the sick. Special hospitals were established when it became impractical to shelter patients in the bishop's houses.

Middle Ages

The decline of the Greco-Roman era led to both a decay of urban culture and a disintegration of community health organization and practice (Rosen, 1958, p. 50). The period between 500 and 1500 AD is referred to as the Middle Ages and represents a heterogeneous phase in history during which superstitions dominated thinking yet advances such as the development of health care facilities originated. As cities grew, they built great walls to protect their inhabitants against invasions by hostile groups. These encircling walls, while necessary for safety and protection, also led to considerable crowding and poor sanitary and hygienic conditions. Clean water supplies and freedom from excessive accumulations of refuse in the streets were difficult to ensure.

With the dawn of the Christian era, a new conceptualization of man influenced health practices. The early Christian church believed that the Roman and Grecian ways pampered the body at the expense of the soul. Disease was seen as punishment for sin.

During this era thinking reverted to mysticism and superstition, and there was religious persecution of those who tried to introduce new ideas. Progress in medicine came to a halt. People considered it immoral to look at their own bodies, hence bathing was an infrequent practice and people often wore dirty clothes. Sanitation was not appreciated, and refuse and body waste were allowed to accumulate near dwellings. However, despite this reversal in thinking about health, hospitals for the poor and neglected were developed.

The progress made in medicine and hygiene during this period is attributed to the terrible plagues that swept the land. During the seventh century, with the emergence of Islam and the subsequent death of the religion's leader, Mohammed, it became a custom among Moslems to journey to Mecca, the place of Mohammed's birth. During each pilgrimage cholera spread rapidly and was ultimately carried to the homelands of the pilgrims (Hanlon and Pickett, 1984).

Leprosy also spread across Egypt, Asia Minor, and Europe during this period assisted by the Crusades, which were a series of religious wars between Turks and Christians, and other vast migrations. Because of the disfiguring nature of leprosy, lepers terrified people. Laws regulated the activities of lepers, and many were declared legally dead and isolated from others by being forced to wear identifying clothes and to warn of their approach with a bell or horn. Although inhumane, these measures were successful in reducing the incidence of this dreaded disease because lepers often died from hunger, exposure, and lack of treatment (Rosen, 1958).

No sooner did leprosy wane as a major European epidemic than an even deadlier menace, bubonic plague, spread as a result of increased trade between Europe, the Near East, and Asia. No other disease has paralleled the plague in its destruction of the human species. During the 1340s more than 13 million Chinese died from the disease. India was nearly depopulated, and Europe was ravaged by plague in 1348; an estimated 25 million Europeans died of the plague. Clearly, the label "Black Death" was appropriate for bubonic plague.

The rise of monasteries and convents as places for caring for the sick led to the early existence of nursing activities, since care at that time included meeting both physical and spiritual needs. Between 1091 and 1291, early male and female nurses joined military orders during the Crusades. As the early Christian church developed, those who had devoted their lives to Christian service cared for the poor, fatherless, and sick. Initially they cared for all three groups under the same roof. However, the knowledge the Crusaders gained from the Arabs led to the establishment of hospitals. Early hospitals were known as a *Hôtel-Dieu,* with the best known being in Paris. During this era several orders of nuns provided simple nursing care directed primarily toward meeting the patient's physiological needs (Griffin and Griffin, 1973).

Health education and personal hygiene knowledge also increased during the Middle Ages, yielding books on healthful living and emphasizing moderation in diet. Three recommended procedures for maintaining health were purging (cleansing the bowels through the use of a purgative medicine), cupping (applying a glass vessel devoid of air to the skin to draw blood to the surface), and bleeding (process used in ancient times for emitting blood to relieve people of disease). Barbers and bath attendants carried out these procedures (Rosen, 1958, p. 79).

Renaissance

The great epidemics of the Middle Ages led to attitudes of fatalism and a general depressed orientation toward health. However, during the Renaissance people started opening their minds to new ideas, and between 1500 and 1700 medicine began to advance. In general, the Renaissance was characterized by achievements in the arts and scholarly efforts as well as by a rise in commerce and industry. Belief in humanism developed. Human dignity and worth began to influence health practices.

The Renaissance ushered in a new period of history during which community health as currently known was begun (Rosen, 1958). The many technological advances designed to cure the epidemics of the Middle Ages provided the impetus and resources necessary for the changes that took place in the Renaissance. These changes, while not directly influencing community health, supplemented the foundation of modern community health.

A matter of serious debate during the Renaissance was whether diseases prominent at the time—including scarlet fever, rickets, scurvy, syphilis, smallpox, and malaria—were caused by contagion or constitution. The invention of the microscope by Anton van Leeuwenhoek in the late seventeenth century supported the contagion view by permitting the observation of microorganisms in soil and water.

Although establishment of a systematic national health policy in Europe failed, health problems began to be analyzed and proposals for national action were set forth (Rosen, 1958). William Perry contributed significantly with his belief that communicable disease control would save infant lives and improve the lot of the people. Although this idea made sense, there was no way of enforcing it, since local authorities had no jurisdiction outside their boundaries and ships frequently brought contagious diseases into the ports.

During this time residents supposedly kept the streets clean. They had no system of sewage disposal, and private enterprises supplied water. Towns provided assistance for the sick and lame. Hospitals during this period became places not only to care for the sick but also to study and teach medicine. These advances were forerunners of later scientific discoveries and gains.

One of the most versatile figures of the Renaissance was Leonardo da Vinci (1452-1519). da Vinci was a sculptor, inventor, mathematician, architect and engineer. His greatest contribution was the dissection of the human body with the subsequent recording of his work in anatomical sketches. Other significant contributions were made by Andreas Vesalius of Brussels and an Englishman, William Harvey. Vesalius (1513-1564) is credited with the scientific development of anatomy through his work in scientific dissection and the correction of previous inaccuracies in anatomy. Harvey (1578-1657) was the major contributor to the field of physiology. In 1628 he announced his discovery of the circulation of blood.

Industrial Revolution

The Industrial Revolution, with its emphasis on power and profits, reversed many of the gains of the Renaissance. Also, as urban populations grew because of the emphasis on industry and production, the number of people needing health care outpaced the voluntary and often piecemeal efforts to provide services. The 80 years between 1750 and 1830 influenced the future determination of community health because of the upheaval and change prevalent at that time.

Population increased dramatically. Major problems included a high infant mortality rate, neglect and often murder of illegitimate infants, poor working conditions, diseases of certain occupations, and the growing incidence of mental illness. During the eighteenth century people with mental illness were locked in jails, workhouses, or madhouses. An early defender of the mentally ill, Vincenzo Chiarugi, brought about major reforms at St. Bonifacio in Florence, Italy, where in 1788 he established a system in which properly trained nurses cared for mentally ill people under the direct supervision of a physician. Likewise, the work of William Tuke at York Retreat in England and Philippe Pinel at Le Bicetre Hospital in Paris brought about major advances for mentally ill people. Kindness, physical exercise, good food, and fresh air characterized the care at each asylum.

The growth of hospitals paralleled the development of asylums. In 1731 Blockley Hospital, which later became known as Philadelphia General, was established to receive the sick, poor, insane, prisoners, and orphans. This hospital was also connected to a poorhouse. In 1737 Charity Hospital was established in New Orleans, based on a legacy left in 1736 when a sailor, Jean Louis, died in New Orleans leaving money to be used to found a hospital to care for the sick of that city. In 1751, through the efforts of Benjamin Franklin and Dr. Thomas Bond, Pennsylvania Hospital was founded in Philadelphia to admit acutely ill or injured people. Interestingly, the seal of that institution was that of the Good Samaritan and the motto was "Take care of him and I will repay thee" (Dolan, 1978, p. 111).

Most early U.S. hospitals were begun on the Northeast coast, following the pattern of settlement in the United States. In 1770 Eastern State Hospital, known as the "Lunatick Hospital" was established in Williamsburg, Virginia. This is one of the first American state hospitals for the mentally ill. Community minded citizens established New York Hospital in 1771, and the Philadelphia Dispensary opened in 1786 thanks to work of the Quakers. (Dolan, 1978, p. 111).

At the turn of the eighteenth century few hospitals existed in England other than in London. Recognizing the population growth, laymen and physicians worked together to establish many new general hospitals. By 1797, seven general hospitals in London had 1970 beds (Rosen, 1958). Also, by the middle of the century specialty hospitals cared for such groups as seamen and their families; obstetrical patients; children; and patients with special conditions such as eye, chest, and orthopedic disease.

Around the turn of the century urban living conditions improved in England, and in 1764 a group of medical police began to create a medical policy regulated by the government. This group advanced the belief that people were responsible for their own health. Health education efforts, largely directed toward the middle and upper classes, grew.

The Industrial Revolution witnessed tremendous advances in transportation, communication, and other forms of technology. Modern public health efforts began in England, the first modern industrial nation. However, to understand how these efforts came into being it is necessary to consider the primary social problem of that era—caring for the poor. The Elizabethan Poor Law of 1601 guaranteed medical and nursing care to the blind, lame, and poor. Table 1-1 chronicles significant community health events beginning with the Elizabethan Poor Law. The Poor Law Amendment Act of 1834 ushered in a new era of social welfare and community health (Rosen, 1958). This act set up a Commission of Inquiry on the Poor Laws, which was administered by Edwin Chadwick.

Chadwick, educated as a lawyer, devoted his career to helping the poor. In a laissez-faire era characterized by a belief that the state should not interfere with the lives of people, Chadwick attempted to make immediate changes to ensure freedom for all. Two primary points in the Poor Law Amendment Act affected community health. First, the act had established an administrative system based on "unions of parishes run by boards of guardians under a central Poor Law Commission. Each union was to have a medical officer; there would also be medical inspectors" (Swinson, 1965, p. 27). Secondly, this act purported that most pauperism was voluntary. However, Chadwick vigorously campaigned that poverty was a social, not an individual problem and that bad housing, sanitation, and poor water supplies should be corrected to prevent disease. The poor should not be punished for poverty but rather educated to help themselves. He believed that the report of the commission would be enthusiastically received in a Christian country like England. However, the report, which included statements by physicians of the amount of child labor occurring in unhealthy mines, was received as an exaggeration.

TABLE 1-1

Milestones in the history of community health and community health nursing: 1600-1866

1601	Elizabethan Poor Law written
1617	Sisterhood of the Dames de Charite organized in France by St. Vincent de Paul
1765	First American medical school started in Philadelphia
1789	Marine Service Hospital and Baltimore Health Department established
1797	Seven general hospitals in service in London
1812	Sisters of Mercy established in Dublin where nuns visited the poor
1813	Ladies' Benevolent Society of Charleston, South Carolina founded
1834	Poor Law Amendment in England sets up a Commission of Inquiry on the Poor Laws administered by Edwin Chadwick
1836	Modern order of Lutheran Deaconesses created by Pastor Fliedner at Kaiserwerth
1845	National Institute established
1847	American Medical Association (AMA) established
1848	Hygiene committee formed by the AMA
1850	Shattuck Report prepared on the status of medical education
1851	Florence Nightingale goes to Kaiserwerth; first International Sanitary Conference in Paris
1855	Quarantine Board established in New Orleans; beginning of tuberculosis campaign in the United States
1859	District nursing established in Liverpool by William Rathbone
1860	Florence Nightingale Training School for Nurses established at St. Thomas Hospital in London; nursing program started at New England Hospital
1864	Factory Act of 1864 passed to control treatment of children in industries; Treaty of Geneva; inauguration of Red Cross
1866	New York Metropolitan Board of Health established

Several bills were introduced into Parliament during the first half of the nineteenth century to regulate the working hours of children; however, they were defeated because the millowners exerted more power in Parliament than the proponents of safe working conditions for children. Also, while Chadwick was vigorously campaigning to secure aid to remedy unsanitary conditions, Poor Relief funds were designated to only treat poor people not to remedy social and environmental conditions. Chadwick pointed out that unlimited funds were being spent on treating a filthy, destructive epidemic whereas prevention would be much less costly.

Finally an investigation was approved to study the extent to which typhus was present. It took 2 years to complete the study, which Chadwick detailed in a document entitled "Report on the Sanitary Condition of the Labouring Population." The commission refused to publish Chadwick's report when they saw how the measures suggested would influence landowners. The report, published under Chadwick's name, became a major social document by emphasizing the destructive effects of filth in the cities, including poor sewage systems and lack of waste disposal facilities. In his report Chadwick established four main conclusions: (1) health depended on sanitation, (2) sanitation was an engineering matter, (3) in each area one authority should administer all sanitary matters, and (4) expert engineering and medical advisers were essential (Swinson, 1965, p. 36). The government reacted to Chadwick's report by establishing a Health of Towns Commission to determine how Chadwick's recommendations could be put into actions.

As mentioned, during the Renaissance women visited the homes and cared for the sick. Early forerunners of community health nursing are found when one reviews the work of nursing orders in the British Isles. Mary Aikenhead (Sister Mary Augustine) started the Irish Sisters of Charity. In 1812 she and a friend went to the Convent of the Blessed Virgin Mary at York where they observed nuns visiting among the poor. They subsequently began a similar work in Dublin. The Sisters of Mercy were a similar order who founded a home for destitute girls and visited the sick in their homes. These were the first nursing orders in the British Isles.

During the latter part of the Industrial Revolution women performing nursing functions changed from a caring group of women largely supported by a religious order to a group often referred to as the "dregs of the community: dirty, drunken, and dishonest" (Swinson, 1965, p. 22). Charles Dickens (1975) in *Martin Chuzzlewit* provided a lasting impression of nursing in the eighteenth century with his description of Sairy Gamp, a drunk, untrained servant who reportedly provided a semblance of nursing care. However, not all nurses were Sairy Gamps.

Colonial Period

While changes described in discussion of the Industrial Revolution were occurring in Europe, other events influential in determining the course of community health were taking place in the English colonies later to become the United States. Epidemics, especially smallpox, characterized the early years of North American settlement. Possibly the colonists were able to settle in North America because the diseases they brought in were fatal to natives who lacked immunity to them.

Interestingly, the early New England settlers carried on the census-taking activities so highly valued by the Roman Empire. Early Colonial community health efforts included the collection of vital statistics, improved sanitation, and the avoidance of exotic diseases brought in from trade routes. However, they lacked a continuing and organized mechanism for ensuring that community health efforts would be supported and enforced (Rosen, 1958).

Because of the pressure to establish a federation of states, community health received little attention before the American Revolution. Following the American Revolution, the threat of a variety of diseases, especially yellow fever, led to considerable interest in the establishment of official boards of health. By the end of the eighteenth century New York City, with a population of 75,000, had established a public health committee for monitoring water quality, sewer construction, drainage of marshes, planting of trees and vegetables, construction of a masonry wall along the water front, and interment of the dead (Rosen, 1958).

In July 1798 Congress created a Marine Service Hospital to provide care for sick and disabled seamen. This service was significant for at least three reasons: (1) it served as the stimulus for what later became the United States Public Health Service; (2) it supplied an organized effort to bring about national quarantine efforts and prevent dreaded diseases from entering the United States at its seaports; and (3) it was one of the first recorded examples of prepaid medical insurance, because for twenty cents monthly, merchant seamen were guaranteed medical and hospital care.

Nineteenth Century America

Although the United States grew tremendously between 1800 and 1850, community health efforts by no means kept pace. During this period threats to health escalated as epidemics of smallpox, yellow fever, cholera , typhoid, and typhus entered the country along with the influx of migrants from many parts of the world. By 1850 the living conditions and the average life span in the older American settlements were worse than in London, which at that time was well known for its deprived living conditions.

The quality of medical care reflected the inadequacies of this period. There had been no medical education until 1765 in Philadelphia when John Morgan patterned the first school after the British model. However, until publication of the Flexner Report in 1910 medical education was taught in a haphazard way with facilities limited both in quality and quantity. Before Abraham Flexner's historical report, many physicians were self-taught with no formal educational or practical experiences. The impact of the movement to reform medical education had far-reaching implications following Flexner's Carnegie Foundation study of medical schools (Schudson, 1974).

At this time medical education followed the pattern originally established by law schools of having lectures and no clinical work in the curriculum. Any applicant who could pay was accepted, and an apprenticeship followed the lecture

FLORENCE NIGHTINGALE
Founder of Modern Nursing

During the nineteenth century early training schools began to develop in hospitals. The dominant figure in organizing nursing was Florence Nightingale (1820-1910). Her greatest accomplishments were her efforts to reform the British military health-care system, establish training schools for nurses, develop professional standards of practice, and advance nursing into a profession viewed with pride rather than scorn (Cohen, 1984). The legacy of Florence Nightingale is especially significant in light of the social conditions of the 19th century. To fully understand her, it is important to remember that she came from a wealthy, well-educated family. Her parents were opposed to her burning desire to be a nurse because of the image of nursing and their desire for their daughter to have a gentle life. She deferred to her family's wishes for several years but finally entered nurses' training with Pastor Fliedner at Kaiserwerth in Germany. She was 33 years old when her dream of becoming a nurse was realized. Her first position, as the unpaid superintendent of an "establishment for gentle women during illness" (Cohen, 1984, p. 128) lasted one year. In September, 1854, British and French troops invaded the Crimea on the north coast of the Black Sea. Seeing this as a golden opportunity, Nightingale wrote to her longtime friend, Sidney Herbert, the Secretary at War, asking if she might volunteer her services. Amidst deplorable conditions, she launched a reform of British military health care. Using her own funds and contributions she raised and fighting the military officers every step of the way she began her campaign by establishing a laundry, installing extra kitchens, supplying things such as socks, shirts, knives, forks, spoons, tin baths, operating tables, cabbage, carrots, precipitate for destroying lice, scissors, bed pans, and stump pillows. Half a year after her arrival at Scutari, mortality in the hospital dropped from 42.7% to 2.2%.

After the Crimean War, she set out to establish a commission to study military health care. She decided that the most compelling argument she could make would be through the use of statistics. Her methods of calculating mortality dramatized both the impact of disease and the effects of improved sanitary conditions. She summarized her work in 1856 in Notes in Matters Affecting the Health, Efficiency and Hospital Administration of the British Army. In ensuing years people sought her out for advice on hospital administration and construction; she was elected a member of the statistical society for developing a method of uniformly naming and classifying diseases and worked vigorously to reform nursing.

Her many accomplishments cannot be given adequate treatment here; entire books have been written describing the far-reaching and insightful accomplishments of this legend in modern nursing. However, it should be noted that she established the first modern training school for nurses at St. Thomas Hospital in 1850. This hospital served as an example for Bellevue Hospital, established in New York City in 1873. Her insistence on trained nurses is detailed in *Notes on Nursing* (Nightingale, 1858) in which she describes assessment, intervention, and evaluation as nursing activities.

Her interest extended beyond nursing. She was also a social worker in that she worked to improve the life of soldiers' wives by establishing reading rooms, games, and other entertainment to keep soldiers interested in wholesome activities and away from the "dramshop and loose living" (Griffin and Griffin, 1973, p. 69). She also established a savings bank through which soldiers could forward money to their families in England. (See Table 1-1 for additional details about Nightingale.)

---

series. The prestige of medical education reached its lowest ebb; practitioners were disorganized and split by the array of healing philosophies and cults (Schudson, 1974).

At the same time hospitals were generally unsanitary places, staffed by poorly trained workers and with the purpose of providing a place where people, especially the poor, could come to die. Surgery, conducted under highly unsanitary conditions, caused many to develop infections and subsequently die from their treatment.

Just as American cities began establishing community health efforts, an influx of immigrants poured in from the troubled European countries. These immigrants taxed the stability of cities, especially those on the Eastern coast. Housing and sanitation became major problems. As urban communities grew and their sanitary conditions deteriorated, major conflict arose between those wanting health reforms and those wishing to maintain the status quo. A number of voluntary health associations developed to create a base for the mobilization of forces for the community.

From the 1840s on, attention focused on attacking community health problems and improving urban living conditions. The National Institute, a distinguished scientific body, was formed in Washington, D.C., in 1845. Founded in 1847, the American Medical Association (AMA) responded to pressure to form a hygiene committee to carry out sanitary surveys and develop a system for collecting vital statistics. Such a committee established this mechanism in 1848 to secure sanitary surveys for all parts of the country.

Concurrently efforts were being carried out in Massachusetts which produced the famous Shattuck Report. This report, published in 1850 by the Massachusetts Sanitary Commission, was the result of massive work by Lemuel Shattuck, a bookseller and publisher. Originally a teacher in Detroit, he became an active member of the school committee in Concord, Massachusetts, and reorganized the public school system of the city. Through an interest in genealogy, Shattuck recognized the need for vital statistics and established statewide registration of vital statistics, which became a model for other states (Rosen, 1957).

Although the Shattuck Report now receives credit as a noteworthy and farsighted document, it was virtually ignored in its own time. Implementation of the actions recommended by the report came 19 years after its publication. Major recommendations called for the establishment of a state health department and local health boards in every town; sanitary surveys; varying kinds of vital statistics; environmental sanitation, food, drug, and communicable disease control; well-child care including immunizations and health education; and proposals on smoke and alcohol control, town planning, and the teaching of preventive medicine in medical schools. Perhaps his greatest accomplishment was to adapt the ideas and practices of both his predecessors and contemporaries to the needs of America in the 1850s. In the tracing of community health history the themes Shattuck mentioned were also reflected in the sanitary efforts of the Babylonians, the holistic views of the Greeks, the system for health care of the Romans, the social assistance for illness and the development of hospitals in the Middle Ages, the advances in health policy of the Renaissance, and the efforts made to improve sanitary conditions during the Industrial Revolution.

The repeated introduction of yellow fever and other epidemics brought about the inception of a quarantine board in New Orleans in 1855. In determining its range of activities, the New Orleans quarantine board decided to limit its activities to hygiene education efforts, housing, preventable diseases, slaughtering of animals, sale of poisons, and general living conditions of the large population of poor people (Rosen, 1958). This first quarantine board also requested information from local boards about their duties and powers as well as about the leading causes of death within their jurisdiction.

Some claim that Louisiana's quarantine board was the first state health department. However, Massachusetts established the first truely operational state board of health in 1869. The power of this first board was limited to investigation and advice, and the board had a budget of $5000, no trained personnel to carry out its activities and no models in the country on which to draw for experience (Rosenkrantz, 1972). Other boards of health came on line as follows: Baltimore in 1798; Charleston, South Carolina in 1815 and Philadelphia in 1818, thereby establishing the first three full-time local health departments (Hanlon and Pickett, 1984). By the end of the nineteeth century, 38 states had health boards.

Between 1857 and 1864 several major cities held National Quarantine and Sanitary Conventions, which prepared the way for the American Public Health Association in 1872. In 1866 the New York Metropolitan Board of Health came into existence. This marked a turning point in community health history in New York as well as in the entire country. The foundation was now established for stable community health advancement.

Development of Controls on Infectious Disease

It was Louis Pasteur (1822-1895) in 1860 who confirmed the presence of airborne bacteria. Through a series of experiments he learned that bacteria could be killed with heat. Joseph Lister (1827-1912) was the first to apply Pasteur's discoveries to the field of surgery. Shocked and horrified at the contagious nature of infection associated with open wounds and with the postsurgical death rate, he introduced a carbolic spray to kill germs in the air and also made students wash and scrub their hands thoroughly before sur-

gery (Swinson, 1965). Robert Koch (1843-1910) was a brillant German physician who demonstrated that every infectious disease was caused by a specific organism.

In 1878 Congress passed the National Quarantine Act, creating the National Board of Health. This body existed until 1883. The passage of this act reflected national interest in the prevention of epidemic diseases. This law gave authority for investigating the origin and causes of epidemic diseases and for preventing their introduction and spread.

Medical Education

Simultaneous with the advancements in community health, medical education improved in quality and a medical school was established in 1893 at Johns Hopkins University. The Flexner Report provided a boost for medical education when it urged schools to improve the quality of their education through more stringent admission criteria and the closing of financially insolvent schools. Essentially, the Flexner Report is indirectly credited with the elimination of diploma mills and their replacement with approximately 100 medical schools.

These early reforms in medical education of the 1900s also influenced the development of hospitals. Specialization in medical practice existed as early as 485 to 425 BC, as reflected in Herodotus' statement that "every physician is for one disease and not for several, and the whole country is full of physicians; for there are physicians for the eyes, others of the head, others of the teeth, others of the belly, others of the obscure diseases" (Rees, 1968).

By the late 1880s Johns Hopkins University had medical specialties, and the French concept of "interne" was introduced in 1897. By the 1930s it became customary for almost all medical graduates to take a year of internship before beginning a practice. Also, as these new highly educated physicians moved across the United States, the need for hospitals grew. In 1873 there were only 178 nongovernmental U.S. hospitals compared with 4359 in 1909 (Weinstein, 1968). Poor people who had no other place to go and no one else to care for them typically used the early hospitals. Interestingly, the Phillips House at Massachusetts General Hospital in Boston was that city's first hospital solely designed to care for affluent patients (Freymann, 1977). However, it was not until the 1930s that patients used these hospitals for anything besides surgery.

Evolution of Nursing Education: Late 19th and Early 20th Centuries

Dr. Marie Zakrzewska, professor of obstetrics at the New England Female Medical College in Boston, began teaching nurses in 1860. However, her efforts were unsuccessful until she introduced the graded course system based on the Kaiserwerth method in 1872. Linda Richards successfully completed this one year course in 1873, becoming America's first trained nurse (Dock and Stewart, 1938).

Three other training schools for nurses were established in the United States in 1873 at Bellevue Hospital in New York, New Haven Hospital in Connecticut, and Massachusetts General Hospital in Boston. Each of these hospitals used the model developed by Florence Nightingale. However, lack of funds led each to be controlled by the hospital rather than being an autonomous educational unit as Nightingale had advocated. Each school grew and developed in its own individual manner with long classes, no standard curriculum, military-type discipline, and full obedience to physicians.

The first nursing program associated with a university began in 1909 at the University of Minnesota. Simultaneously, several hospitals started to affiliate with colleges for the education of nurses. In addition, Teachers College in New York developed college courses for graduate nurses.

Initially community health nursing required special education. Debate ensued as to whether community health nurses needed a basic nursing education or just special training in home care. Nursing leaders decided that all nurses needed some community health content, hence basic undergraduate courses began to include the topic of community health, with Boston leading the way with the first undergraduate community health course.

As community health nursing grew as a specialized and respected area of nursing, it became apparent that the inclusion of this content in basic curricula was insufficient. In 1914 Mary Adelaide Nutting offered the first postgraduate nursing course in community health at Teachers College in affiliation with the Henry Street Settlement (Deloughery, 1977). When this turned out to be successful, Boston began a special training program for community health nurses, which developed into an 8-month course affiliated with Simmons College (Figure 1-1).

In 1918 during World War I the Vassar Camp School for nurses started as a unique and patriotic aspect of nursing education. The American Red Cross and the Council of National Defense jointly supported this novel program, which proposed that nursing education could be shortened from 3 years to 2 years for college graduates. The Vassar

Camp School, modeled after the Plattsburg Military Camp in New York, gave intensive training to college graduates so they could become army reserve officers and meet urgent wartime needs. A total of 435 graduates of this program represented many colleges across the country. The program ended when peace was declared.

Nursing education profited from the landmark study published in 1923 as *The Report of the Committee for Study of Nursing Education.* This study, directed by Josephine Goldmark, led to the Rockefeller Foundation's endowment of the School of Nursing at Yale University. During this same year, the financial support of Frances Payne Bolton, a wealthy Cleveland citizen, established the School of Nursing at Western Reserve University. She had become interested in nursing education on reading the Goldmark report and subsequently contributed significantly to nursing education.

Schools of nursing proliferated during the 1920s amid turmoil and change. In 1925 the three major nursing organizations (National League for Nursing, American Nurses' Association, and National Organization for Public Health Nursing) authorized a program for grading schools, and in 1926 the Committee on the Grading of Nursing Schools began with 21 members. The committee had three major goals: to study the supply and demand for nursing service, to complete a job analysis of nurses, and to grade nursing schools. Grading began in 1929 and was repeated again in 1932, leading to the closing of several hundred weak schools.

Collegiate programs increasingly included content in community health nursing. The first basic program in nursing was accredited in 1944 and included sufficient community health content so that graduates did not need additional training courses in order to practice community health nursing (National Organization for Public Health Nursing, 1944, p. 371).

Over the next 30 years several major changes in nursing education occurred, including the development and rapid expansion of practical nursing programs and the establishment in 1953, with Mildred Montag's doctoral dissertation at Teachers College in New York City, of associate degree nursing programs. Moreover, starting in 1963 the National League for Nursing required baccalaureate programs to include public health nursing in order to be eligible for accreditation. Additionally, a major conceptual change in nursing resulted from the 1965 American Nurses' Association position paper on nursing practice which proposed that the education of nurses should take place in institutions of higher learning. In recent decades nursing has advanced as a scholarly profession characterized by increased research among practitioners and the development of a conceptual basis for practice.

Organizations for Nursing Education and Practice

By 1893, with 225 schools of nursing in operation, it became necessary to establish some form of standards (Shyrock, 1959). Isabel Hampton Robb assumed the leadership role in establishing the Society of Superintendents of Training Schools of Nurses in the United States and Canada in 1893. This new society sought to establish training stan-

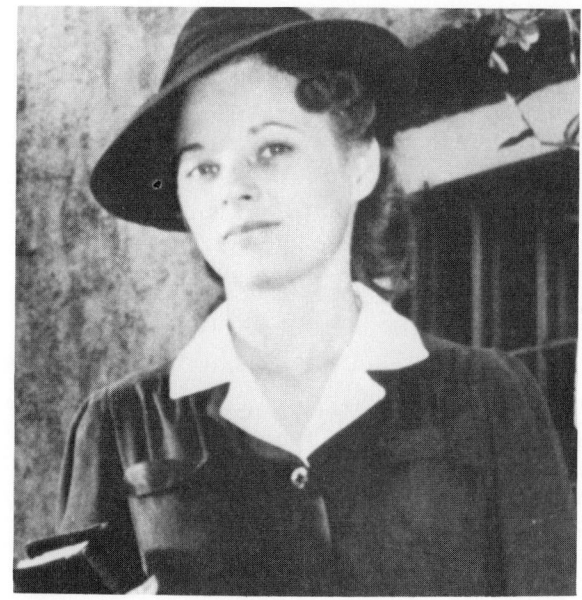

FIGURE 1-1

Early public health nurse. (Donated by the Jefferson County Department of Health, Birmingham, Ala., Myra Downs, Director, Bureau of Public Health Nursing.)

dards and promote colleagueship among nurses. This organization later became the National League for Nursing. Two years later the Nurses' Associated Alumnae of the United States and Canada was organized. This group later became the American Nurses' Association with the original purpose of strengthening the union of nursing organizations, elaborating nursing education, and promoting ethical standards.

Initially the American Society of Superintendents of Training Schools limited its membership to the heads of the larger schools. However, it soon became apparent that it would be beneficial to expand the membership. The first wave of expansion included the superintendents of smaller schools, and later membership became available to all people interested in nursing education.

In 1911 a joint committee was appointed, composed of representatives of the American Nurses' Association and the American Society of Superintendents of Training Schools to standardize nurses' services outside the hospital. Lillian Wald chaired the committee, and Mary Gardner served as secretary. The committee recommended that a new organization be formed to meet the needs of community health nurses. They subsequently invited 800 agencies known to be involved in community health nursing activities to send delegates to an organizational meeting in Chicago in June 1912. A heated debate commenced as to the name and purpose of this organization; however at noon on June 7, 1912 the delegates unanimously voted the National Organization for Public Health Nursing into existence with Lillian Wald as its first president.

The new organization sought "to standardize public health nursing activities on a high level and coordinate all efforts in the field" (Deloughery, 1977, p. 116). Although primarily a nursing organization, all people interested in community health nursing could be members. Because of its willingness to cooperate with other groups with similar interests, the organization grew rapidly and remained in existence until the American Public Health Association came into being.

Also during 1912 the American Society for Superintendents of Training Schools became the National League for Nursing Education. This new group immediately formed a committee to study the products of nursing education and to identify ways to standardize educational programs. The first major step toward this goal occurred in 1917 with the publication of the Standard Curriculum for Nursing Schools, which established the National League for Nursing Education as the source of information on nursing education.

EVOLUTION OF COMMUNITY HEALTH NURSING

Many of the early accomplishments of community health nurses have been discussed in the preceding sections. However, this section traces the efforts of community health nurses from the first records of visiting nursing sponsored in 1683 by St. Vincent de Paul in Paris and carried out by the Sisterhood of the Dames de Charité. Tables 1-1 and 1-2 chronicle the milestones in community health nursing.

St. Francis De Sales (1567-1662) conceived a voluntary association of friendly visitors to go to the homes of the poor and care for the sick. The ensuing organization, supported in time and money by influential women, was an early form of visiting nursing. "The cofounder and director of the association, the Order of the Visitation of Mary, was Madame de Chantal. She and the members of her group visited the sick in their homes, cleaned and dressed their

---

TABLE 1-2

Milestones in the history of community health and community health nursing: 1866-1986

1872	American Public Health Association established
1873	Training schools established at Bellevue Hospital, New Haven Hospital, and Massachusetts General Hospital; Linda Richards becomes first nurse to graduate in the United States
1877	Women's Board of the New York Mission hires Frances Root to visit the sick poor
1878	National Quarantine Act passed by Congress
1879	New York Ethical Society places trained nurses in dispensaries
1880	Division of Child Hygiene established in New York Health Department
1885	District Nursing Association in Buffalo established
1886	First visiting nursing society in Philadelphia provides home health care; instructive district nursing begins in Boston
1889	Chicago Visiting Nursing Association established
1892	School nursing first undertaken in London
1893	Visiting nursing service for the poor in New York organized by Lillian Wald and Mary Brewster; American Society of Superintendents of Training Schools for Nurses organized (became National League for Nursing Education in 1912)
1895	Industrial nursing program initiated at Vermont Marble Works
1896	Nurses' Associated Alumnae of United States and Canada organized (became ANA in 1911)
1898	Public health nurses hired by Los Angeles Health Department; Detroit Visiting Nurse Association formed
1899	International Council of Nurses organized; university education for nurses introduced at Teachers College, New York.
1900	*American Journal of Nursing* begins publication
1901	58 organizations providing public health nursing (about 130 nurses)
1902	School nursing started in New York (Lina Rogers)
1903	First nurse practice acts; tuberculosis nursing in Baltimore
1905	200 organizations providing public health nursing (about 440 nurses)

TABLE 1-2

Milestones in the history of community health and community health nursing: 1866-1986—cont'd

1906	First post graduate course in district nursing offered by the Instructive District Nursing Association (Boston)
1907	Alabama law permitting employment of public health nurses passed
1908	Detroit Health Department hires public health nurses
1909	The Visiting Nurse Quarterly first published in Cleveland (in 1918 became a monthly, *The Public Health Nurse,* and in 1931 name changed to *Public Health Nursing*); first nursing program affiliated with a university (Minnesota) inaugurated; 566 organizations providing 1413 public health nurses; Metropolitan Life Insurance initiates offer of home nursing to its industrial policy holders
1910	Public health nursing program instituted at Teachers College, New York
1911	First state public health nursing laws passed
1912	National Organization for Public Health Nursing formed with Lillian Wald as first president; Rural Nursing Service of American Red Cross established; National League for Nursing Education started
1913	Division of Public Health Nursing, New York State Department of Public Health, organized
1914	First undergraduate nursing education course in public health offered by Adelaide Nutting at Teachers College
1916	1922 organizations providing 5,152 public health nurses
1917	Publication of the Standard Curriculum for Nursing Schools
1918	Vassar Camp School for Nurses organized; USPHS establishes division of public health nursing to work in extracantonment zones
1919	*Public Health Nursing* written by Mary S. Gardner
1920	NOPHN approves university programs in public health nursing; passage of Sheppard-Towner Act
1922	4040 public health agencies providing 11,548 nurses
1923	Report issued by Committee for Study of Nursing Education (Goldmark Report)
1024	U.S. Indian Bureau Nursing Service established
1925	Frontier Nursing Service using nurse-midwives organized (Mary Breckenridge); first NOPHN statement of qualifications for public health nurses; John Hancock Mutual Life Insurance Company starts Visiting Nurse Service
1926	Committee on Grading of Nursing Schools begins studies
1931	4,255 public health organizations providing 15,865 nurses
1933	Pearl McIver becomes first nurse employed by USPHS
1934	*Survey of Public Health Nursing* published by NOPHN
1935	*Facts about Nursing* first published by ANA; Passage of Social Security Act
1942	American Association of Industrial Nurses established
1943	Bolton-Bailey Act for nursing education and Cadet Nurse Program passed; Division of Nursing Education started by USPHS (Lucille Petry appointed)
1944	First basic program in nursing accredited as including sufficient public health content
1946	Nurses classified as professionals by U.S. Civil Service Commission; Hill Burton approved; passage of National Mental Health Act
1948	NLN establishes accrediting service
1949	National Federation of Licensed Practical Nurses organized
1950	25,091 nurses employed in public health field
1951	NLN recommends collegiate basic nursing education include content in public health nursing; National Association of Colored Graduate Nurses merges with ANA
1952	Six nursing organizations merge into two: ANA and NLN; associate degree nursing started; Boston University begins program in general nursing approved for preparation of public health nurses
1953	*Nursing Outlook* published
1955	27,112 nurses employed in public health field
1959	NLN votes that no new specialized baccalaureate program be accredited (move toward general education in nursing); after 1963 only baccalaureate programs including public health nursing to be eligible for accreditation
1960	NLN establishes criteria for evaluation of educational programs in nursing that lead to baccalaureate and master's degrees
1964	Nurse Training Act passed
1965	Position paper of ANA proposes that education for nurses take place in institutions of higher learning
1970	National Commission on Nursing and Nursing Education offers Abstract for Action
1971	Nurse Training Act expanded
1972	Health Maintenance Organization Act became law
1974	Nurses Coalition for Action in Politics (N-CAP) formed; first certification exams for excellence in clinical practice offered by ANA
1975	Health Services, Health Revenue Sharing and Nurse Training Acts passed
1977	Passage of Rural Health Clinic Services Act, which provides indirect reimbursement for nurse practitioners in rural health clinics
1978	President Carter vetoes Nurse Training Act
1980	Medicaid amendment to the Social Security Act for direct reimbursement for nurse practitioners in rural health clinics
1983	Advent of prospective payment for the Medicare program, that is, diagnostic-related groups (DRG's)

wounds, made their beds, gave them clothes . . ." (Dolan, 1978, p. 90).

St. Vincent De Paul (1576-1669) is a prominent figure in the history of nursing and social welfare. In 1617 he organized the Sisterhood of the Dames de Charite, which systematically introduced the modern principles of visiting nursing and social welfare. His aim was to help people learn to help themselves. The Sisterhood comprised a group of women who went from cottage to cottage, much like the plan used by de Sales, to provide home care. As their numbers increased and the demands for their services rose, Mademoiselle Le Gras was appointed as supervisor. The work of the sisterhood conveyed the belief that home nursing could best be carried out if based on sound principles rather than just kindness and intuition and that nurses needed supervision in their activities. They based their work on a belief in teaching nurses as well as the people they visited how to help themselves (Maynard, 1939).

Home Health Care

The next significant era for community health nursing is traced to William Rathbone in Liverpool, England. Because of the outstanding care provided to his dying wife, Rathbone in 1859 led in establishing a district nursing service. Based on his experience, Rathbone concluded that many people with long-term illnesses could be better cared for in their own homes than in a hospital. He urged his wife's nurse, Mary Robinson, to begin a program of home nursing care for poor people. Subsequently, at Rathbone's urging the Liverpool Relief Society divided the city into nursing districts, and assigned a committee of "Friendly Visitors" to each district to provide health care to needy people (Kalisch and Kalisch, 1978).

Based on the Liverpool experience, Rathbone wrote a book entitled *Social Organization of Effort in Works of Benevolence and Public Charity by a Man of Business* in which he outlined a philosophy for home health care (Dolan, 1978). England became a forerunner in home health care, and Rathbone's work spurred Florence Nightingale to publish a pamphlet on nursing entitled *Suggestions for Improving Nursing Service,* which recommended steps for nursing care in the home. Rathbone ultimately founded the Metropolitan Nursing Association to provide home health nursing (Bullough and Bullough, 1964). During this time the largest religious organization in London, the Bible and Domestic Mission, sent women into the slums to read the Bible and in 1868 added nursing care to their program (Dolan, 1973).

In 19th century America, the first visiting nurse society began in Philadelphia in 1886 to provide home health care to the sick. Earlier efforts had been noted in New Amsterdam (New York) in the works of the *Krankenbezoekers* (seekers out of sick) and *Ziskentroosters* (ones who gives comfort to the sick). Following the War of 1812, a Ladies Benevolent Society was organized to aid sick and impoverished people. In 1877, the Women's Board of the New York Mission hired Frances Root, a graduate of Bellevue Hospital's first nursing class, to visit the sick poor and provide nursing care and religious instruction (Bullough and Bullough, 1964).

Nurses at the first visiting nursing society in Philadelphia strictly followed physician's orders, gave selected treatments, and kept temperature and pulse records. Since their visits were brief, the nurses soon recognized the need to teach family members basic elements of care. Thus from the very beginning community health nursing included teaching and prevention.

In 1886 two women in Boston approached the Women's Education Association to seek support for district nursing. They used the term *instructive district nursing* to emphasize the relationship to education and to increase their likelihood of receiving support from this group. They then met with representatives of the Boston Dispensary, which was providing free medical care to the poor according to the dispensary district in which they lived. In February 1886 the first district nurse was hired in Boston. As the number of district nurses increased, they worked closely with physicians to carry out medical orders. Patients paid no fees, and initially two lay managers of the association supervised the nurses. In 1888 the Instructive District Nursing Association became incorporated as an independent voluntary agency to provide care to the sick poor under the direction of a trained physician and to instruct families to take better care of themselves and their neighbors by living a wholesome life (Brainard, 1922).

Settlement Houses

During this era wealthy people became interested in charitable activities and began to fund settlement houses in the poorer sections of many larger cities. These settlement houses offered a variety of services for members of the community. For example, in 1893 Lillian Wald and her friend Mary Brewster, both trained nurses and wealthy women, organized a visiting nursing service for the poor of New York.

Lillian Wald was an extremely far-sighted woman, who after graduating from New York Hospital's Training School in 1891 attended classes at a local medical college while simultaneously conducting classes in personal health care on New York's lower East side (Kalisch and Kalisch, 1978). Shocked by the neglect of a critically ill woman in a tenement, she conceived of the idea of a neighborhood nursing service for the sick poor in the area. She was fortunate in interesting two prominent and wealthy lay people, Mrs. Soloman Loeb and Joseph H. Schiff, in her plan. She also had the encouragement and support of a nursing classmate, Mary Brewster, in her efforts. Wald's concept was that the nurse's visit "should be like that of a very interested friend rather than that of an impersonal, paid visitor" (Dolan, 1978, p. 227). To be readily accessible to the recipients of their care, these women moved into the neighborhood they served and led in the establishment of the Henry Street Settlement. Although highly diversified, nursing remained at the center of Henry Street activities. Nurses at Henry Street visited patients being cared for by a large number of different physicians and charged for their services according to the patient's ability to pay. From the beginning nurses supervised nurses at Henry Street Settlement.

According to Christy (1970, p. 50), Wald was the predecessor of the modern public health nurse in the United States. Just as Nightingale chronicled much of her work, Wald wrote *The House on Henry Street*. Not only did she establish the Henry Street Settlement, but she led in the development of payment by insurance companies for nursing services. In 1909, along with Lee Fraskel, Lillian Wald established the first community health nursing program for workers at the Metropolitan Life Insurance Company. Believing that keeping workers healthier meant their productivity would increase, she urged that nurses at agencies such as Henry Street Settlement provide skilled nursing care to ensure healthier workers. Wald convinced the company that it would be more economical to use the services of community health nurses than to employ their own nurses and also that services could be available to anyone desiring them, with fees graduated according to the ability to pay. This project existed for 44 years and contributed several significant accomplishments to community health nursing, including the following:

1. Providing home nursing care on a fee-for-service basis
2. Establishing an effective cost-accounting system for visiting nurses
3. Using advertisements in both newspapers and the radio to recruit nurses
4. Reducing mortality rates from infectious diseases

Lillian Wald also believed that the nursing efforts at Henry Street Settlement should be aligned with an official health agency, and she arranged for nurses to wear an insignia that signified that they served under the auspices of the board of health. Also, she established rural health nursing services through the Red Cross to provide nursing care to rural people and thereby improve their quality of life. Her other accomplishments included helping to establish the Children's Bureau, fighting in New York City for better tenement living conditions, city recreation centers, parks, pure food laws, graded classes for mentally handicapped children, and assistance to immigrants (Figure 1-2).

At about this same time a group of women in Los Angeles established the College Settlement. They requested that the City Council give them a monthly allowance so a district nurse could visit the sick poor. In 1898 public funds paid the first nurse to provide nursing care in the home.

Health Departments and Community Health Nursing

Advances in community health nursing paralleled those in both nursing and community health. During the 1920s community health nursing recognized the relationship between health and economic security and began to assume responsibility for community health. By 1920 all states and most large cities had health departments with the majority of the staff being community health nurses. During this period community health nursing assumed a leadership role

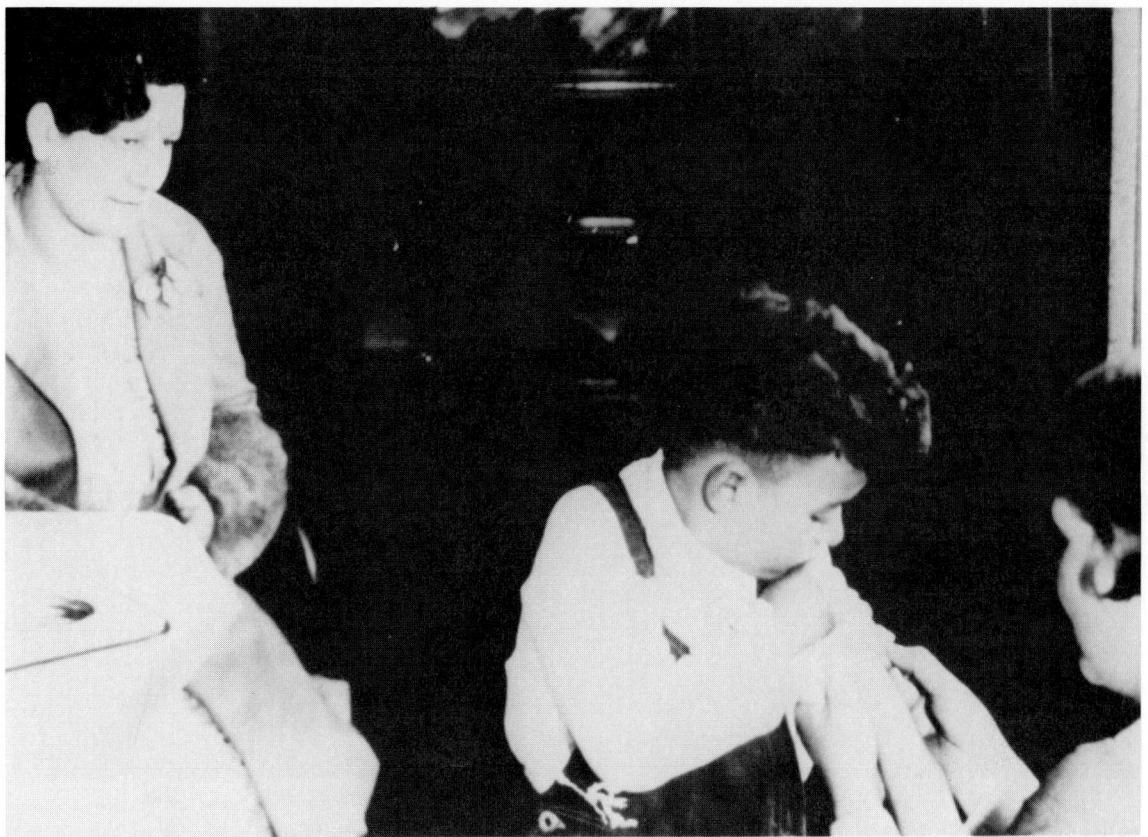

FIGURE 1-2

Clinic visit for immunization. (Donated by the Jefferson County Department of Health, Birmingham, Ala., Myra Downs, Director, Bureau of Public Health Nursing.)

in establishing standards for nursing practice. As mentioned earlier, community health nurses received advanced preparation and the major community health nursing organization provided for collaboration among citizens, nurses, and other health providers. All who desired community health nursing care received it regardless of their ability to pay. The type of nursing care provided in the community during this era serves as a prototype of contemporary community health nursing. During the early decades of the twentieth century the scope of community health nursing included disease prevention, health promotion, and family-oriented services.

Immunization

By the end of the nineteenth century people could become resistant to certain diseases by immunization of either live or extracted disease-producing organisms. Because of the German cholera epidemic of 1892, the New York City Health Department created a division of bacteriology and disinfection and made the first application of bacteriology to community health. The 1900s witnessed the disappearance of many infectious diseases. Active immunization of children began in New York City in 1920, and by 1940 an estimated 60% of this age group were protected.

Child Welfare Movement

The child welfare movement, similar in America and Europe, emphasized the need for clean milk, well-child clinics, and instruction to mothers. The child health movement profited from the establishment of a Division of Child Hygiene in the New York City Health Department in 1880. Led by Dr. Josephine Baker, this division demonstrated that infant deaths could be greatly reduced through prevention. In a congested area of New York's lower East Side community health nurses visited each mother and newborn on the day after birth to teach ways to keep the baby well, as shown in Figure 1-3 (Rosen, 1958). After 2 months 1200 fewer infant deaths in the district occurred than during the same period a year earlier. Simultaneously with the development of well-baby clinics, clean milk was provided by monitoring sources and by requiring pasteurization.

The New York City activities for improving child health spurred other states and provoked governmental action. In 1912 President Taft signed a bill creating the Children's Bureau to investigate and report "matters pertaining to the welfare of children and child life among all classes of our people" (Rosen, 1958, p. 360). The Children's Bureau was based on the belief that infant health depended on the protection of maternity. The idea for such a bureau came

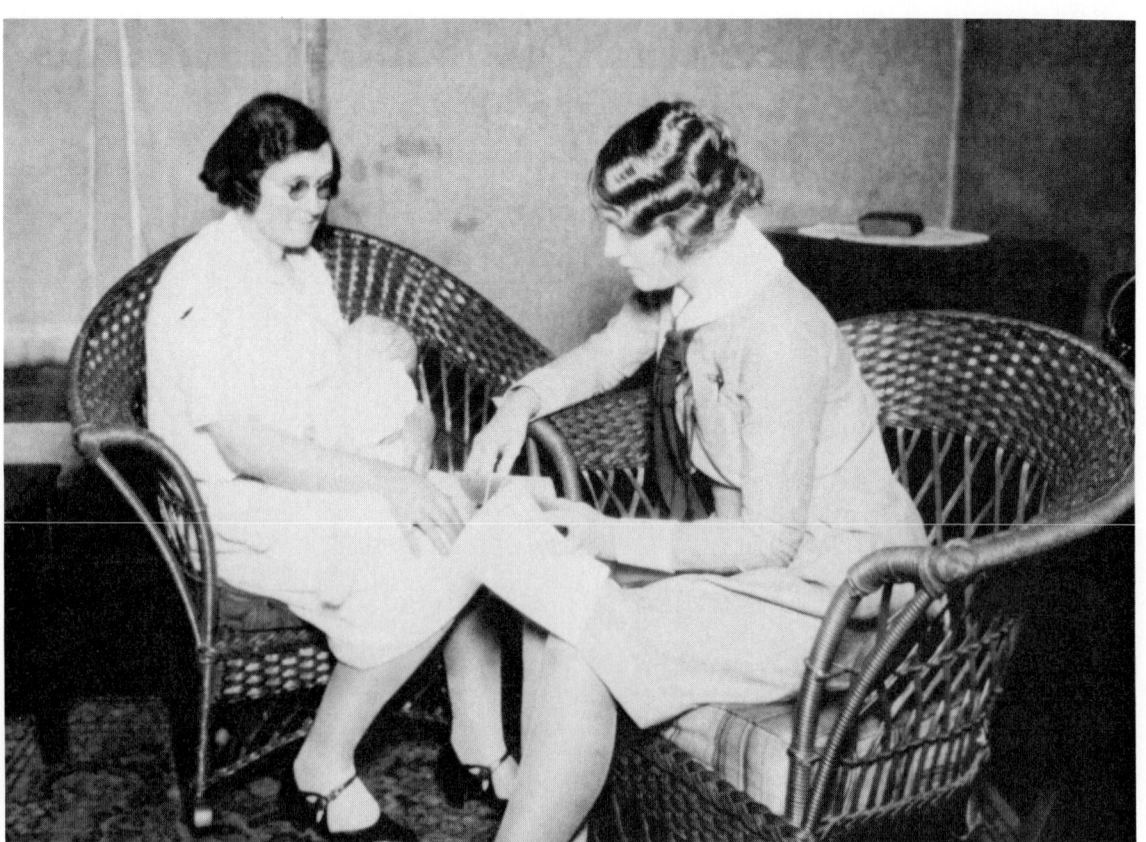

FIGURE 1-3

Early public health nurse making home visits to mother and newborn. (Donated by the Jefferson County Department of Health, Birmingham, Ala., Myra Downs, Director, Bureau of Public Health Nursing.)

from Florence Kelley and Lillian Wald. Kelley served as the first Chief Inspector of Factories of Illinois and later as General Secretary of the National Consumers League, and Wald founded community health nursing in America and established the Henry Street Settlement in New York. Figure 1-4 is an example of instruction in dietetics in a public school classroom in the early 1900s.

In 1908 the pediatric department of the New York Outdoor Medical Clinic began the first organized prenatal program. Visiting nurse services for pregnant women began in Boston in 1909 and in St. Louis in 1912. The Maternity and Infancy Act (Sheppard-Towner) in 1920 was heralded as landmark legislation and was the first measure to appropriate Federal funds for a health and social welfare program (Rosen, 1958). A successful program ensued for 7 years until funding was discontinued. However, in 1935 Title V of the Social Security Act reenacted the Children's Bureau.

Role of Government

The early twentieth century witnessed multiple improvements that both directly and indirectly affected health status. Organized community health efforts improved simultaneously with changes in medical care and the development of hospitals as treatment facilities for all people. In 1902 Congress renamed the Marine Hospital Service and gave it

an established organizational format under the direction of a surgeon general. The title was again broadened in 1912 to become the United States Public Health Service (USPHS). Tables 1-1 and 1-2 list several events in the history of community health in the United States.

Several significant events influenced the further development of community health efforts, including two major wars followed by an economic depression. In 1894, Louisiana recognized the need to care for people with leprosy. Money was raised to buy an abandoned sugar plantation in Carville to house lepers; a physician, Dr. L.A. Wailes, volunteered to take care of them. In 1917 Congress passed a law authorizing the purchase of this facility and named it the National Leprosarium.

In that same year the USPHS assumed responsibility for providing health examinations for all immigrants. In 1918 entry into World War I called attention to the need for prevention, detection, and treatment of sexually transmitted diseases, leading to the establishment of the Division of Venereal Diseases within the USPHS. This division cooperated with state health departments to control and prevent these diseases. Subsequently, in 1929 the Narcotics Division, later renamed the Division of Mental Hygiene, became responsible for the confinement and treatment of narcotic addicts.

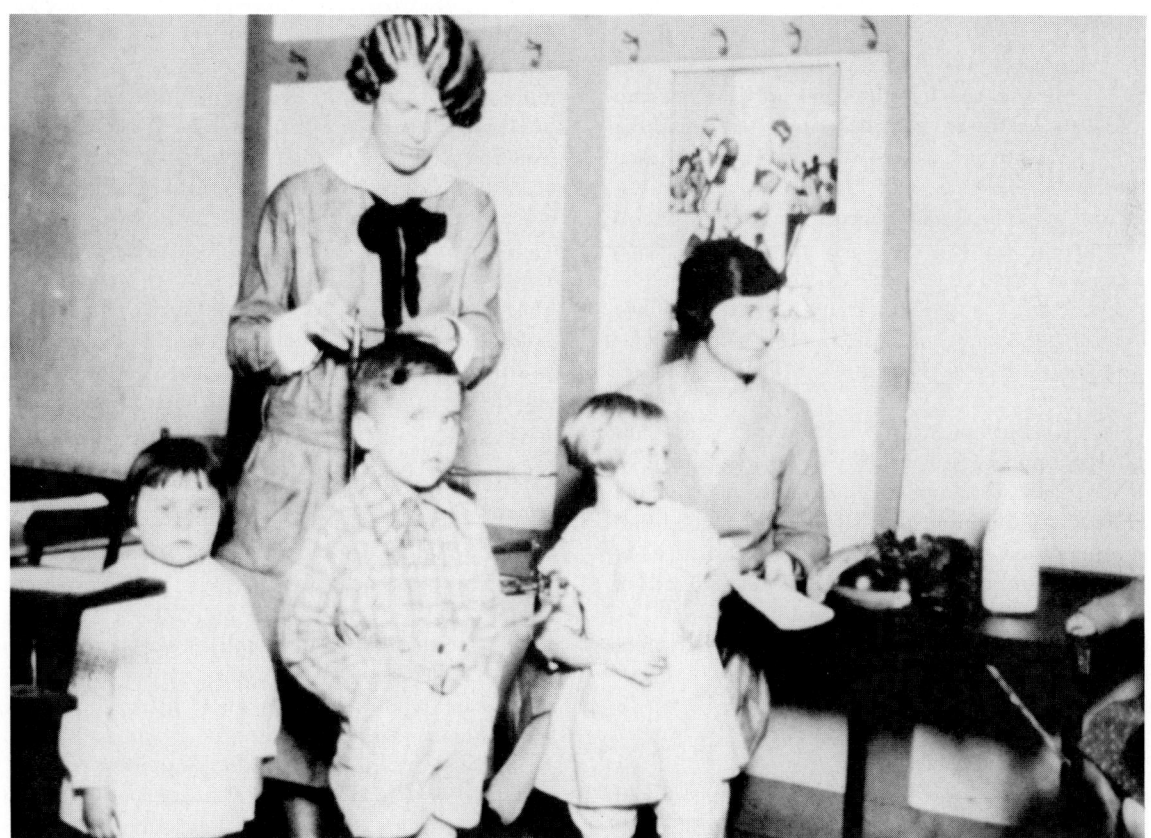

FIGURE 1-4

Instruction in dietetics in school in early 1900. (Donated by the Jefferson County Department of Health, Birmingham, Ala., Myra Downs, Director, Bureau of Public Health Nursing.)

During the next several decades substantial changes took place at the Federal level, which affected the structure of community health resources and included the Federal Social Security Act of 1935. Title VI of the act affected the scope of community health through its original mission to assist states and their subdivisions in the establishment and maintenance of adequate community health services including the training of personnel for both state and local health activities. Other influential developments included the passage in 1937 of the National Cancer Institute Act, which provided for research into the cause, diagnosis, and treatment of cancer.

Finally, in 1939 the Public Health Service relocated from the Treasury Department to the newly created Federal Security Agency, which President Roosevelt planned as a major effort to reorganize and consolidate federal services. The Public Health Services had undergone many changes in organization as well as alterations resulting from passage of several health-related acts such as the National Mental Health Act of 1946 and the establishment in 1948 of institutes in the four areas of heart, microbiology, experimental biology and medicine, and dental research.

In 1949 the Mental Hygiene Division moved from the Bureau of Medical Services to the National Institutes of Health to form the National Institute of Mental Health. Other major institutes formed in the ensuing years included the National Institute of Neurological Diseases and Blindness (1950) and the National Institute of Arthritis and Metabolic Diseases (1959); both the Division of General Medical Sciences and the Institute of Child Health and Human Development were established in 1962, and the Division of Environmental Health Sciences was established within the Public Health Service in 1966. When the Environmental Protection Agency opened in 1970, most of the environmental health activities of the Public Health Service were transferred to it. Additionally, for more effective service to states, the Public Health Service developed 10 regional offices located in Boston, New York, Philadelphia, Atlanta, Chicago, Kansas City, Dallas, Denver, San Francisco, and Seattle.

Both the Hill-Burton Act (1946) and the Children's Bureau (1912) influenced community health. Each will be discussed in a later section. Other federal agencies whose work influences community health include the Food and Drug Administration, agencies within the Departments of Agriculture and Interior, Office of International Health of the Public Health Service, Agency for International Development of the Department of State, and the Department of Health, Education, and Welfare (which on May 4, 1980, became the Department of Health and Human Services).

Food Control

The first efforts of the federal government to control and supervise the quality of food began in 1879 with a bill introduced into Congress to prohibit the adulteration of food and drink. It took 27 years for this goal to be realized, and ultimately the present Food and Drug Administration grew out of this aim. In 1906 President Theodore Roosevelt signed the Pure Food and Drugs Act; the present Federal Food, Drug, and Cosmetics Act was signed in 1938.

Within the Department of Agriculture several bureaus conduct community health activities. The Bureau of Animal Industry investigates the cause, prevention, and treatment of diseases of domestic animals which have implications for people. The Bureau of Dairy Industry is concerned with the sanitary regulation and handling of milk, and the Bureau of Human Nutrition and Home Economics has made considerable gains in the areas of rural health and nutrition.

World War I and Community Health Nursing

The great demand for nurses created by the onset of World War I in 1915 threatened the role of community health nurses, whose numbers were insufficient to meet the need. However, the American Red Cross helped to sustain community health nursing by establishing a roster of nurses who could be enlisted to supply health care. The Red Cross emphasized educational programs for the community as well as programs directed toward communicable diseases.

During the war the National Organization of Public Health Nurses loaned a nurse to the U.S. Public Health Service to establish a community health nursing program for military outposts, which led to the first community health nursing program sponsored by the federal government (Gardner, 1919, p. 44). After World War I many changes occurred that subsequently affected community health nursing. Despite the economic constraints of the depression, this era witnessed many advancements in community health nursing. Because of limited local and national resources many people volunteered to assist others, and these volunteers rapidly learned the value of community health nursing. Also, many federally funded relief projects utilized nurses, which led to the need for governmental consultation to the states. In 1934 Pearl McIver became the first nurse employed by the U.S. Public Health Service to provide consultation services to state health departments. Initially only a few states had budgeted community health nursing positions; by 1936 all states included some type of community health nursing consultation services in their budgets.

Community Health Nursing Between Two World Wars

As the Social Security Act of 1935 attempted to overcome the national setbacks of the depression, it expanded community health nursing. Title VI stipulated protection and health promotion for all people. Two major provisions of Title VI included (1) the appropriation of $8 million to assist states, counties, and medical districts to establish and maintain adequate health services as well as to train public health workers and (2) the allocation of $2 million for research and the investigation of disease and sanitation. This act also provided funds for the education and employment of public health nurses. Training for Nurses for National Defense, the GI Bill, the Nurse Training Act of 1943, and Public Health and Professional Nurse Traineeships provided additional educational funds (McNeil, 1967). The onset of

World War II in 1941 accelerated the need for nurses. The National Nursing Council, comprising six national nursing organizations and assisted by the U.S. Department of Education, received a million dollars to expand facilities for nursing education. The U.S. Public Health Service managed these nursing education funds. During this time community health nursing expanded its scope of practice. Community health nurses moved into rural areas, and many official agencies began to provide bedside nursing care.

In 1946 a committee of representatives for agencies interested in community health met to establish guidelines for this area of nursing (Public Health Nursing 1946, p. 387). These guidelines became necessary because community health nursing evolved in an unplanned fashion with sponsorship by many voluntary agencies, thereby leading to a great deal of overlap. The guidelines took into account the history of community health nursing and proposed that a population of 50,000 was required to support a community health program and that there should be one nurse for each 2000 people. Other principles addressed were that (1) the function of community health nursing includes health teaching, disease control, and care of the sick and (2) the community should adopt one of the following three organizational patterns (Public Health Nursing, 1946):

1. All community health nurse services administered by the local health department
2. Preventive health care provided by health departments and home health care by a cooperating voluntary agency
3. A combination service jointly administered and financed by official and voluntary agencies with all services provided by one group of community health nurses

By the early 1960s community health nursing began to assume a more active role in society. Practice in community health nursing became a requirement of all baccaleaurate programs in nursing. In 1964 the ANA defined a community health nurse as a graduate from a baccalaureate program in nursing accredited by the National League of Nursing.

In 1966 the American Public Health Association and the NLN jointly developed a program for accrediting community health nursing services. This was the first effort to accredit the delivery of nursing services and continues today as a vital and sought-after program.

Frontier Nursing Service

The Frontier Nursing Service (FNS) was influential in the development of community health programs and characterized by a unique pioneering spirit. Its historical development is detailed here because of its contributions from nurses to improve the health care of a rural and often inaccessible population. The FNS came into being from the commitment of a nurse, Mary Breckenridge, to provide care to isolated and needy people in Appalachian sections of Kentucky. Breckenridge came from a wealthy Southern family and devoted her life to the establishment of the FNS after the death of her first husband, the failure of her second marriage, and the loss of a 4-year-old son and a newborn daughter. The loss of her own children motivated her to devote her life to promoting the health care of disadvantaged women and children (Browne, 1966).

A graduate of St. Luke's hospital in New York, Mary Breckenridge organized community health nursing activities in France. Working with the American Committee for Devastated France, she saw the tremendous health needs of women and children. Based on her experiences in France, Breckenridge decided that people in rural areas of the United States would benefit from the service of nurse-midwives (Dolan, 1978).

To prepare herself for providing midwifery services in the Kentucky mountains, Breckenridge spent time auditing public health, statistics, and psychology courses at Teachers College in New York. In 1923 she went to England to obtain nurse-midwifery training. The Kentucky committee for Mothers and Babies was organized in 1925, and the name was changed to Frontier Nursing Service when the organization was incorporated in 1928. At the suggestion of a supportive physician, baseline data were obtained as to infant and maternal mortality rates before beginning services.

The reduced mortality rates following the inception of the FNS are especially remarkable considering the environmental conditions in which these rural Kentuckians lived. Many homes had no heat, electricity, or running water; often physicians were over 40 miles from their patients (Tirpak, 1975). During the 1930s nurses lived and saw patients from one of six outposts and often had to make their visits on horseback (Figure 1-5). However, on completion of the FNS hospital in Hyden, Kentucky, in 1928, physicians began entering service. Payment of fees ranged from labor and supplies to funds raised through annual

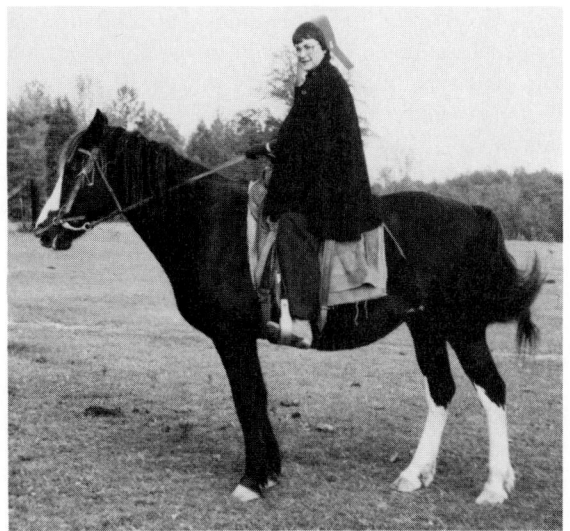

FIGURE 1-5

Nurses rode horseback in the Frontier Nursing Service. (Donated by K. Huttlinger, graduate of M.S.N. program at University of Alabama in Birmingham.)

family dues, philanthropy, and fund-raising efforts of Mary Breckenridge (Holloway, 1975). The inception of Medicaid and Medicare made available a more predictable source of revenue.

In 1939 Mrs. Breckenridge established the FNS School of Midwifery. Over the years deliveries increasingly took place in hospitals, thereby reducing the need for midwifery and accelerating the demand for family nursing. By 1975, with only 7% of nursing time devoted to midwifery, the 41 FNS nurses devoted their attention to meeting the primary care needs of the residents of Leslie County, Kentucky (Frontier Nursing Service, 1978). Once admitted to a nurse's district, clients are seen at least once a year until they die or move. This service continues today as a vital and creative mode for delivering public health services to rural families. The role of nurses, similar in many ways to the contemporary nursing role in the FNS, is discussed in detail in Chapter 39.

The Years Following World War II

During World War II many nurses joined the Army and Navy Nurse Corps. To provide sufficient nurses to meet wartime demands, the Bolton Act of 1943 established the Cadet Nurses Corps and authorized $60 million to recruit and educate 70,000 cadets in 1125 schools between 1944 and 1946. During this time these nurses constituted 90% of the enrollment in basic nursing programs. The chief of this program, Lucille Petry, provided leadership in nursing education during a particularly difficult time.

After the war the need for nurses continued and many utilized the GI Bill to further their education. Before its discontinuation in 1948, the National Nursing Council for War Service, comprising a variety of nursing organizations concerned about the future of nursing, launched what is known as the Brown Report (Brown, 1948). This report recommended that professional nursing education be carried out in institutions of higher learning, that nonprofessional nursing education be the responsibility of public vocational schools, and that inferior diploma schools be closed and good ones strengthened. Subsequently, Mildred Montag's dissertation in 1951 served as a model for the development of nursing education within junior colleges.

The year 1952 witnessed some major changes in professional nursing organizations. The American Nurses' Association (ANA) and the National League for Nursing (NLN) became the two major nursing organizations. The ANA set out to improve professional nursing practice, including economic and general welfare, and limited membership to registered nurses. In contrast, the NLN, open to both nurses and lay people, established a goal of providing cooperative relationships between nurses and friends of the profession to work together for quality education and practice. A coordinating council provided collaboration between the two groups. Also, during these years both the ANA and NLN aided in the establishment of the National Student Nurses' Association.

Over the years the NLN has focused on the quality of educational programs and mechanisms for their evaluation. In 1948 the NLN established an accrediting service to eval-uate all nursing programs in a systematic fashion. In contrast, the ANA has maintained a major interest in the economic welfare of nurses, certification and nursing practice.

At the end of World War II, President Truman requested that Congress address the following aspects of the health care system (Kalisch and Kalisch, 1977, p. 8):

1. Prepayment of medical costs with compulsory insurance and general revenues
2. Protection from loss of wages as a result of sickness
3. Government aid to medical schools for research
4. Increased construction of hospitals, clinics, and medical institutions

However, only the Hospital Survey and Construction (Hill-Burton) Act of 1946 enacted this last aspect and provided funds to assess the need for hospitals and, if need existed, the planning and construction of hospitals and public health centers. This program, which required state matching funds (two-thirds) and federal funds (one-third), accounted for the widespread development of hospitals in the United States.

Many changes after World War II subsequently affected community health nursing. These included a more prosperous economy, prohibition, and the increasing use of the automobile. Where community health nurses had previously made visits on foot, in horse-drawn buggies, or on bicycles, automobiles made it possible to see far more people. Additionally, wartime service called national attention to the poor health of young and middle-aged males. Approximately 29% of all men called up for military service were rejected because of poor and often preventable health conditions.

Following World War II, community health nurses were accused of being more interested in organizing their practice than in actually providing care to clients. The leadership and maverick spirit of early nursing leaders appeared to wane, and an era began when community health nursing became defensive rather than exhibiting leadership in health care. Some contend that this trend still exists.

DEPARTMENT OF HEALTH AND HUMAN SERVICES (HEALTH, EDUCATION, AND WELFARE)

The Department of Health, Education, and Welfare came into being on April 11, 1953, as part of President Eisenhower's reorganization of the executive branch of the government. The original purpose was to "bring into closer functional relationship and to improve the administration of the important health, education, welfare, and Social Security functions then being carried on by the federal government" (Hanlon and Pickett, 1979, p. 43). These functions have not entirely been attained, since the Department has traditionally been comprised of multiple separate subdepartments with their own goals and objectives. Unity of purpose has yet to be realized. However, on May 4, 1980, the Department of Health, Education, and Welfare was restructured to become the Department of Health and Human Services. A second agency, the Department of Education, was formed to handle selected activities.

VOLUNTARY ACTION FOR HEALTH

Although the government retains a major responsibility for the health and welfare of its citizens, voluntary organizations play key roles in community health. Rapid economic growth in the United States helped to create many of the problems attracting the attention of voluntary health agencies and also provided the resources and leisure time necessary for volunteers to start such organizations. By 1945 there were about 20,000 agencies with 300,000 volunteers in the United States. Currently, there are more than 100,000 voluntary, nongovernmental health and welfare agencies (Wilner et al., 1978). Appendix H describes health organizations used by community health nurses.

Voluntary agencies dealing with health fall into several categories. An important group includes those which are supported by citizen contributions and donations. Despite the diversity among these agencies they tend to fall into four general categories:

1. Those dealing with specific diseases such as cancer or diabetes. Examples include: American Cancer Society, the Cystic Fibrosis Foundation, the American Diabetes Association and many others.
2. Those involved with certain organs of the body, for example, The American Lung Association or the American Heart Association.
3. Those involved with the health and welfare of special groups such as the aged or children and including groups such as the National Council on Aging, or the National Society for Crippled Children.
4. Those dealing with health problems that affect the community as a whole, such as the National Safety Council and the Planned Parenthood Federation of America.

The second large group of voluntary organizations engaged in health activities is comprised of foundations established by private philanthropy. Leaders in this area include the Rockefeller Foundation, the W.K. Kellogg Foundation, the Carnegie Foundation, the Milbank Memorial Fund, the Mott Foundation, the Rosenwalk Fund, and the Markle Foundation (Hanlon and Pickett, 1984).

The third influential group of voluntary health agencies is made up of professional associations such as the American Public Health Association, the American Medical Association, the ANA, the NLN, and their state and local affiliates. These groups not only meet the needs of their professional members for meetings, dissemination of information but they also establish and improve standards for practice and education, encourage research, further health education and promote educational programs for professionals and consumers.

Competition is keen among voluntary agencies to secure donations and service of volunteers. The rapid growth of agencies and the number of individual fund-raising efforts led many cities to form community chests or united funds. These agencies carry out a single drive or appeal for funds and then divide the monies received among the participating organizations (Wilner, et al., 1978). The first united fund-raising effort began in 1949 in Detroit as the Torch Drive. Currently most larger cities have a combined fund-raising campaign, which lessens the number of requests made on people.

Although space does not permit a thorough discussion of the history of specific voluntary agencies, the progression and development of two major agencies is summarized here.

National Tuberculosis Association

The National Tuberculosis Association is the oldest agency of its type, and its development epitomizes the voluntary health movement. Initially tuberculosis was viewed as a hereditary disease, which could only be treated by a change in climate. However, Koch's discovery in 1882 of the tubercle bacillus dramatically changed this view.

The first tuberculosis dispensary was the Victoria Dispensary for Consumption, which was started in 1887 in Edinburgh. The National Association for the Prevention of Consumption and Other Forms of Tuberculosis developed in 1898 to educate people about disease prevention (Rosen, 1958, p. 386). In 1893 the Michigan State Board of Health voted to require the reporting of tuberculosis to local health departments, and similar efforts in Baltimore and Philadelphia followed. The Pennsylvania Society for the Prevention of Tuberculosis, organized by physician Lawrence Fleck, was a pioneer effort in many ways. This marked the first attempt to combine professionals and laymen in combating a specific disease. Secondly, this organization called for coordination among hospitals and boards of health to work toward prevention through community education. The National Association for the Study and Prevention of Tuberculosis was formed in Atlantic City in 1904 (its name was changed in 1918 to the National Tuberculosis Association). Because of financial problems, the Russell Sage Foundation supplemented funding for 10 years.

Red Cross

The Red Cross began accidentally in northern Italy in 1859. At that time, with 300,000 Italian and French soldiers actively fighting, deaths and injuries abounded. Hundreds died from lack of attention. This appalling situation attracted the attention of a Swiss tourist, Jean Henri Dunant, who assembled female volunteers from the town of Solferino, Italy, to care for the wounded. Inspired by Florence Nightingale's work in the Crimea he devoted his life to preventing the horrors he had seen in Solferino. Traveling from country to country he urged the establishment of bands of volunteers to treat wounded men. Finally in 1863 the Society of Public Utility of Geneva, Switzerland, convened with 36 representatives from 14 countries to study Dunant's proposal. This meeting established the basic principles of the Red Cross and developed plans to organize Red Cross societies in selected countries across the world.

Before it could be fully organized, the Red Cross was called into service to care for the wounded of the bloody war between Denmark and newly organized Prussia in 1863 to 1864. The Geneva Convention of 1864 established Dunant's original principles and made the Red Cross an official international group for caring for the wounded. Out of this Convention came the International Red Cross Committee, the coordinating committee of all the Red Cross committees. The international committee aids victims of war and disaster when the magnitude of the problem is greater than the scope of national committees.

During wars the National Red Cross Societies (component parts of the International Red Cross) assist by mobilizing nurses, nurses's aides, and volunteers to establish ambulance services, hospitals, hospital ships, canteens, libraries for soldiers, entertainment, occupational therapy, and so forth. It also aids war refugees and prisoners and may assist citizens in devastated cities. Aid may also extend to families of war victims and to providing housing for disabled men. Nurses have always played a major role in the Red Cross by directly carrying out many of the designated functions (Deloughery, 1977).

American Red Cross

The American Red Cross largely resulted from the tireless efforts of Clara Barton. She had undertaken the work of the Red Cross during the Franco-Prussian War. In 1881, she organized in Washington a Red Cross Committee and in 1882 persuaded the government to ratify the Geneva Convention and give the committee official standing.

The yellow fever epidemic of 1888 in Florida required that the Red Cross be called into action. Over the years an extensive organization developed with local committees and sections for selecting and training volunteer nurses who could, with little notice, be called into service. In the latter part of the nineteenth century the Red Cross sponsored a nurses' training program lasting two years and 3 months. This was discontinued as nursing education advanced and modern training schools were developed in hospitals.

In 1898 the Red Cross was officially recognized as the American National Red Cross Relief Committee. Lillian Wald recommended that community health nursing be a part of the Red Cross in 1903. Although these efforts originated in New York, they initially served rural areas. By 1913 the towns having populations as large as 25,000 received nursing care through the Red Cross. This activity, called the Town and Country Nursing Service, included "home hygiene and care of the sick, dietetics, public hygiene in rural areas and small towns, disaster nursing and instruction of nurses's aides" (Deloughery, 1977, p. 79) (Fig. 1-4).

Over the years the American Red Cross method of teaching instructors has been adapted to the needs of many countries. Since 1945 the Red Cross home nursing instruction has been part of the curriculum in many secondary schools where it can be taught not only by nurses but also by teachers and volunteers. The blood program began in 1947. Today the Red Cross boasts of nearly 4000 chapters in the United States, each with a voluntary board of directors and voluntary committees to direct its efforts. Chapters plan programs to meet the needs of specific communities, including needs for health education.

Voluntary health agencies accomplish a great deal through their persistent and at times pioneering efforts at research and demonstration projects as well as professional lay education. However, they have been under scrutiny in recent years because of questions about their expenditure of funds. Critics contend that too little of the money contributed goes to research, service, or education. Despite what may seem like shortcomings in the operation of some agencies, others devote a sizable portion of funds to carry out the specified aims of the agency and remain a potent and beneficial force in the health care system.

INTERNATIONAL HEALTH

The extent and nature of world health problems are related to such factors as population density, climate, biological factors, and social, economic, and political forces. Most preventable diseases to which humans are subject involve bacteria, viruses, protozoa, helminths, insects, and a climate conducive to the transmission of disease. The most widespread diseases in the world result from infection by human feces, such as infectious diarrheas, intestinal parasites, typhoid and paratyphoid bacillary and amoebic dysentery, infectious hepatitis, and cholera (Hanlon and Pickett, 1984, p. 72). A second prominent category of diseases results from vectors; malaria is the most prominent vector transmitted disease, with mosquitoes being a primary agent of transmission.

Four other diseases warrant attention: plague, leprosy, tuberculosis, and acquired immune deficiency syndrome (AIDS). Plague, while considered a disease of antiquity, continues to be present in at least 29 countries. Leprosy claims about 15 million victims annually. The areas most severely affected by leprosy are southern India, the People's Republic of China, many parts of Africa, southeast Asia, and some Latin American countries. Tuberculosis, considered a disease of poverty, claims at least 3.5 million new victims annually. More than half of these victims die of the disease (Hanlon and Pickett, 1984, p. 73). AIDS is described in Chapter 17. However, this disease is occurring worldwide, with an estimated 1 to 1.5 million persons having the causative virus in the U.S. alone.

One of the most serious aspects of the world's health problems is the shortage of health personnel in most parts of the world. This is especially true in the developing nations, which have the poorest living conditions and the greatest predisposition to disease. Where living conditions are inadequate, health care primitive or available only at a distant location, food in short supply, and educational levels low, the prospects for disease are great.

Organizations for International Health

International health cooperation began in Paris in 1851 with the establishment of the First International Sanitary Conference. Twelve countries participated, and each sent a physician and a diplomat. The objective of the first conference was limited to "harmonize and reduce to a safe minimum the conflicting, vexatious, and costly maritime quarantine requirements of different European nations, and especially those of Mediterranean parts" (Introducing WHO, 1976 p. 8). A series of conferences led to the establishment of a permanent international health agency known as the International Office of Public Health (d'Office International d'Hygiene Publique), which began in Paris in 1909. Known as the "Paris Office," the small full-time staff primarily gathered information, revised international regulations, and arbitrated differences (Wilner, Walkley, and O'Neill, 1978).

The League of Nations was established at the end of World War I. A health section came into being in 1923 and became known as the "Geneva Office." Functioning alongside the Paris Office, both dealt with international efforts to prevent and control disease. In addition, the Geneva Office developed an Epidemiological Intelligence Service, conducted studies of rural hygiene, housing, health of school children, health centers, and health insurance (Rosen, 1958). The technical studies of this agency facilitated international consensus on crucial areas such as the serological diagnosis of syphilis and the standardization of biological products employed therapeutically. Concurrently, the Pan American Sanitary Organization constituted a third international health organization. Consultation and cooperation existed among these three organizations.

World Health Organization

International health work practically came to a standstill with the outbreak of World War II. In 1945, a United Nations Conference on International Organizations meeting in San Francisco unanimously approved the establishment of an international conference on health. This conference, held in New York, led to the approval of the constitution of the World Health Organization in July, 1946.

The constitution of WHO defines the organization's objective as "the attainment by all peoples of the highest possible level of health" (WHO, Basic Documents, 36th edition, 1986). The constitution lists 22 functions by which this objective may be attained. WHOs main functions are: to act as the directing and coordinating authority on international health; to ensure valid and productive technical cooperation, and to promote research (Health for All, WHO, undated).

WHO is one of 14 specialized agencies that maintains working relationships with the United Nations and with one another. Three of these agencies are mentioned here: United Nation's Educational, Scientific and Cultural Organization (UNESCO), Pan-American Health Organization (PAHO), and United Nation's Children's Fund (UNICEF).

United Nation's Educational, Scientific and Cultural Organization

WHO and UNESCO, founded in 1946, collaborate on activities related to education and training of health professionals and health educators and some scientific projects. UNESCO was created as a specialized agency of the United Nations to work "for the unrestricted pursuit of objective truth and the free exchange of ideas and knowledge . . ." (Jordan, 1984, p.286).*

UNESCO's major focus is upon education including early childhood education and literacy training for girls, women,

---

*The United States has been at odds with UNESCO since the early 1970s. This dispute led to U.S. withdrawal from UNESCO. In 1970, UNESCO decided to change its focus from providing technical assistance to Third World news media to focus on the content of the information. Since 90 percent of the news to the Third World was provided by Western nations, the United States, the United Kingdom, and France, the United States resented the monitoring of its broadcasts. In both 1984 and 1885 UNESCO spent approximately $8 million in communications.

the handicapped, refugees and migrants (Jl. of Communication, 1985). Other aspects of UNESCO's function include their cultural programs which emphasize "preserving the cultural and natural heritage of mankind, promoting various levels of cultural identity, stimulating artistic and cultural development and promoting local cultural activities (Jl of Communication, 1985, p.12). Other foci include social science research and training and the General Information Program which provides an infrastructure for library and information programs and archives.

United Nations Children's Fund

This agency has worked closely with WHO since its inception at the end of World War II. Its initial purpose was to provide assistance to the war-torn countries. Over the years UNICEF has spent vast amounts of money on food and supplies to promote maternal and child welfare throughout the world. Often in partnership with WHO, UNICEF has carried out many programs of BCG vaccination and yaws and malaria control. In recent years family planning has been emphasized. Originally planned as a temporary emergency agency, UNICEF has filled such a void in international health, that in 1953 it was given permanent status and officially named the United Nations Children's Fund. A key effort has been the development of the International Children's Center, in the late 1940s to bring together and coordinate the efforts of many health disciplines concerned with physical, mental, and social development of children. The international activities of this group are fourfold: teaching about child welfare problems and methods, medical-social research, documentation and publications, and cooperation regarding child welfare (Hanlon and Pickett, 1984, p. 80).

Pan American Health Organization

The Pan American Health Organization (PAHO) originated in 1902 in Mexico City as the International Sanitary Bureau and was organized by a Pan-American Sanitary Conference. This organization, with headquarters in Washington, D.C., is the center of coordination of international public health information and activities in the Western Hemisphere. The Pan-American Health Organization became a regional office of WHO in 1949, although it still maintains its own organizational identity. It is supported by annual financial quotas contributed by each of the American republics. PAHO seeks to strengthen health education in Latin America and the Caribbean by fostering improved physical and mental health, lengthening life, and combatting major health problems of people in its member nations. PAHOs first priority is health for all by the year 2000. To attain this goal, PAHO collaborates with national health authorities to extend health services to the 40% of the population in member nations without access to health care (PAHO, 1985). To meet this goal, PAHO: (1) helps countries develop comprehensive health policies and the legislation to put these policies into effect; (2) cooperates with countries to establish and improve their health services and (3) improves the supply of health personnel.

Two additional international organizations not part of WHO have implications for community health nursing.

These are the Agency for International Development (AID) and the International Council of Nursing (ICN) which is discussed in a later section.

Agency for International Development

The Agency for International Development (AID) was organized in 1961 within the U.S. Department of State and promotes the work of the United States with other nations on a one-to-one basis. A major contribution of AID is in the training of health professionals. It provides fellowships for several thousand health workers to study health care in the United States; thousands more have been provided with short-term inservice health education. Critics of AID say that the agency at times fails to take into account the unique needs of the countries receiving the assistance; that is, the teacher tends to provide information suited to the sponsoring country and not carefully adapted to meet the needs of the recipient nation. AID is also accused of getting involved in local political issues, which is not part of its mission.

The United States is a major contributor to AID; however, Sweden, the United Kingdom, the Federal Republic of Germany, France, the Soviet Union, and the People's Republic of China also contribute to AID.

Nongovernmental Agencies

Although governmental agencies have played a major role in international health, substantial contributions have been made by a variety of nongovernmental agencies. Both churches and private philanthropic foundations have given vast amounts of money, time, and service to promote world health. Among the most notable of the religious groups to serve in international health are the foreign mission agencies of the Baptist, Methodist, and Seventh Day Adventist churches, the Unitarian Service Committee, the American Friend's Service Committee, a variety of Roman Catholic mission groups, and the American Bureau for Medical Aid to China.

Notable among the foundations involved in international health is the Rockefeller Foundation. For nearly seven decades, this foundation has been active in international health in such efforts as control of malaria and yellow fever, the financing of centers of learning in public health and medicine and the provision of a wide range of fellowships for health care study. Similarly, the W.K. Kellogg Foundation has demonstrated a long-standing interest in improving professional education in Latin American countries and in supporting health care personnel to study in the United States.

Nursing and International Health

Over 22,000 American nurses are employed overseas. Broadly defined, an international nurse is one who is involved in health work which concerns more than one nation (Henkle, 1979). Working in international health is typically a challenging career. (Expectations of what nursing will be may be vastly different than what the nurse grew to expect in school and while practicing in the United States.) The setting, people, customs, language, and style of life in an international setting may be remarkably different from that in the United States. Often the resources available to practice are less than adequate, necessitating creativity on the part of the nurse. Although certainly not an inclusive list, the following characteristics typically are useful qualities for a nurse working in an international site to possess: ability to communicate in the language of the people, flexibility, adaptability, superior problem-solving skills, ability to tolerate frustration and to wait for what may seem like an inordinate amount of time to get a task accomplished; and knowledge of the health characteristics of the population with whom the nurse is working. Working in international health can be a rewarding and exciting career, but it does demand special characteristics of the aspirant.

International Council of Nursing

The ICN is a nonpolitical organization of nurses from around the world. Initially the ICN had individual memberships because in its early days there were no national nursing organizations in many countries. In 1904 three national organizations from Great Britian, the United States, and Germany joined as charter members. Today, the ICN is a federation of national associations from 93 countries. To belong, the national association must "be an autonomous, self-directing and self-governing body, nonpolitical, nonsectarian, and participate in no form of discrimination" (Kelly, 1981, p. 596). The membership of the organization must be composed exclusively of nurses. The American Nurses' Association is the representative organization for the United States. The ICN headquarters is in Geneva, Switzerland. The purpose of this organization is to develop a means for nurses to share knowledge so that nursing practice around the world is strengthened and improved.

CURRENT STATE OF COMMUNITY HEALTH NURSING

The indecision about what constitutes community health nursing is consistent with the controversy and confusion present in the entire profession. Community health nursing has evolved into a focus on care of individuals, families, and communities. Although nurses in other areas work in the same domain as the public health nurses, the focus and orientation are different. The scope of practice is defined by the nature of community health nursing rather than being dominated solely by the setting. Providing nursing care in the community does not in itself constitute community health nursing. Community health nursing is a specific and specialized orientation to care that embodies principles of public health as guiding concepts. The key difference between community health nursing and the other areas of nursing is the emphasis on the personal and environmental health of the total population not just of selected individuals. Because several chapters provide more in-depth discussion on community health nursing, this section only highlights the current role to demonstrate how it has evolved from the early days of visiting nurses carried out first by religious orders and then by insightful and energetic leaders like Lillian Wald. Chapter 6 compares the ANA and APHA conceptual frameworks for community health nursing and supplements this brief review of the current status of community health nursing.

Primary health care is one aspect of community health nursing. Community health nursing focuses on the physical, biological, social, psychological, and environmental health of a population group, while primary care is a "coordinated system of personal health care, emphasizing first-contact care and continuity" (Ruth and Partridge, 1978, p. 625). Primary care emphasizes ambulatory care that is accessible and coordinated and that addresses total client needs both for curative as well as preventive services. Primary care generally focuses on the individual whereas community health nursing is population based.

Williams (1977, p. 251) has helped to clarify the focus and goals of community health nursing by emphasizing the unit of care as the health of population groups or aggregates of people "who have in common one or more personal or environmental characteristics." Aggregates may be defined at many levels: age, risk for certain health problems, race, and so on. A major factor differentiating community health nursing is the focus on promoting health-related behaviors as well as providing personal health services to members of populations or communities. Rather than serving only the subgroups who need care, community health nurses anticipate, estimate, and design measures to interrupt the onset of personal health problems. Such a focus may sound global or vague; however, it is specific, highly complex, and scientific. It takes considerable skill to estimate the potential onset of a health problem as a result of unsafe living conditions (such as polluted water supplies) and intervene before health problems ensue.

Community health nurses must understand the natural history of disease, recognize potential causative agents, and implement intervention as soon as possible. Inherent in a community health philosophy is attention to the influence of environmental factors (physical, biological, and sociocultural) on the health of populations, and priority is given to preventive and health maintenance strategies rather than curative strategies (Williams, 1977).

CLINICAL APPLICATION

The only certainty in community health comes from our history. The present as well as the future will continue to offer challenges, many of which stem from almost constant change and uncertainty. More than ever before, we need to rely on our historical antecedents. Few events in today's health care system are without predecessors. The content of change is different, but the past offers ideas for solving contemporary problems. As crises appear in home health care as a result of new reimbursement patterns, we can look to the visionary work of Lillian Wald and gain strength from pioneering nurses who managed to develop patterns of nursing care despite innumerable odds. At times change may come more rapidly than at other times, but it always comes. To resist is to fail to keep pace with current community health nursing. To deal with change constructively by looking to the history of nursing is to learn from others

ways to deal more effectively with contemporary challenges.

SUMMARY

The history of community health nursing can be traced to the earliest record of civilization. Throughout its development there have been numerous progressive campaigns often overshadowed by transient setbacks as health has been alternately given high priority and then ignored. Many of the advances in community health arose out of necessity. Epidemics and other devastating health conditions demanded resolutions that could not be postponed until a more propitious time.

Major social, economic, and political developments have influenced community health programs in the United States, with many advances made as a result of congressional action. Citizens have pressed their congressmen to work for better living and health conditions. Community health nursing has been at the forefront in developing and encouraging other groups to institute healthier living conditions and care for all people.

The history of the early Christian church is replete with examples of home health care. Of considerable importance was the work of St. Vincent de Paul and Mademoiselle Le Gras, who established what was probably the first actual community health nursing program. The life and work of Florence Nightingale influenced all nursing practices, including education, hospital development, and the actual delivery of nursing care. Likewise, it is difficult to imagine how one woman, Lillian Wald, could have been so farsighted, energetic, and resourceful in her development of varied and numerous community health nursing efforts. Lillian Wald organized visiting nursing in New York, established the unique program at the Henry Street Settlement, and was responsible for many improvements in living conditions in New York City. She also established the first program of nursing services provided by an insurance company. Had there been more women like Lillian Wald in both the history of nursing and community health nursing, one can imagine the gains that might have been made.

Expansion in nursing education progressed steadily from the first school to train nurses established in Boston at the New England Female Medical College. Only 1 year after this school was established, three additional ones began on the East Coast: Bellevue Hospital in New York City, New Haven Hospital in Connecticut, and Massachusetts General Hospital in Boston. By 1893, just 22 years later, there were 225 schools of nursing in the United States. These early schools were located in hospitals, and it was not until 1909 that the first basic nursing program associated with a university began at the University of Minnesota. The inclusion of community health nursing content was first provided in 1914 under the leadership of Mary Adelaide Nutting at Teachers College in New York. This trend continued and was supported by major nursing organizations. Two landmark studies pertaining to nursing education were completed by Josephine Goldmark and Mildred Montag. In their unique ways each study influenced the future development of nursing education.

Over the years community health nursing has evolved from a home care service characterized as being delivered by caring women who ministered to both the health and spiritual needs of individuals and families to a broadly based, population-focused discipline that considers individuals, families, groups, and communities as the scope of practice.

KEY CONCEPTS

An understanding of the dominant cultural ideas of each era since early recorded history is useful in understanding the antecedents of the current community health care system.

Rudiments of community health can be traced to the earliest civilizations.

With the dawn of the Christian era, a new conceptualization of man influenced health practices. The early Church believed that the Roman and Grecian ways pampered the body at the expense of the soul. Disease was viewed as a punishment for sin.

The Renaissance ushered in a new period of history during which community health as currently known was begun.

The history of the early Christian Church is replete with examples of home health care. Of considerable importance was the work of St. Vincent de Paul and Mademoiselle Le Gras, who established what was probably the first actual community health nursing program.

The Industrial Revolution witnessed tremendous advances in transportation, communication, and other forms of technology. Modern public health efforts began in England, the first modern industrial nation.

The Poor Law Amendment Act of 1834 ushered in a new era of social welfare and community health in England.

Lillian Wald organized visiting nursing in New York in the nineteenth century, established the unique program at the Henry Street Settlement, and was responsible for many improvements in living conditions in New York City.

The first visiting nurse society in America began in Philadelphia in 1886 to provide home health care to the sick.

The early twentieth century witnessed multiple improvements that both directly and indirectly affected health status.

Several significant events influenced the further development of community health efforts in the first half of the twentieth century, including two major wars and an economic depression.

As the Social Security Act of 1935 attempted to overcome the national setbacks of the depression, it expanded community health nursing.

The Frontier Nursing Service (FNS) was influential in the development of community health programs and was characterized by a unique pioneering spirit.

Although the government retains a major responsibility for the health and welfare of its citizens, voluntary organizations play key roles in community health.

A United Nations conference in 1945 led to the establishment of the World Health Organization (WHO). The objective of WHO is "the attainment by all peoples of the highest possible level of health."

An international nurse is one who is involved in health work that concerns more than one nation. Over 22,000 American nurses are employed overseas.

The indecision about what constitutes community health nursing is consistent with the controversy and confusion present in the entire profession.

Over the years community health nursing has evolved from a home care service characterized as being delivered by caring women who ministered to both the health and spiritual needs of individuals and families to a broadly based, population-focused discipline that considers individuals, families, groups, and communities as the scope of practice.

LEARNING ACTIVITIES

1. Write a summary of what you believe were Lillian Wald's greatest contributions to community health nursing.

2. If you were Lillian Wald and chose to devote your energy to critical forces affecting the health of Americans, what would be your three highest priority efforts?

3. Of the three efforts, take one and develop a realistic plan for (a) implementation and (b) evaluation.

4. Telephone or visit one voluntary agency in your community and describe its purpose, source of funding, major programs or services, and eligibility of recipients of services.

5. Interview three nurses employed in community health nursing to determine how they currently define their role.

BIBLIOGRAPHY

Brainard, A.M.: Evolution of public health nursing, Philadelphia, 1922, W.B. Saunders Co.

Brown, E.L.: Nursing for the future, New York, 1948, Russell Sage Foundation.

Browne, H.: A tribute to Mary Breckenridge, Nurs. Outlook 14:54-55, May 1966.

Bullough, V., and Bullough, B.: The emergence of modern nursing, New York, 1964, Macmillan Publishing Co.

Christy, T.: Portrait of a leader: Lillian Wald, Nurs. Outlook, 18:50-54, March 1970.

Cohen, I.B.: Florence Nightingale, Sci. Am. 250(3):128-137, 1984.

Deloughery, G.L.: History and trends of professional nursing, ed. 8, St. Louis, 1977, The C.V. Mosby Co.

Desirable organization for public health nursing for family service, Public Health Nurs. 38:387-389, Aug. 1946.

Dickens, C.: Martin Chuzzlewit, New York, 1975, Penguin Books (Edited by P.N. Furbank).

Dock, L., and Steward, I.: A short history of nursing, ed. 4, New York, 1938, G.P. Putnam's Sons.

Dolan, J.: History of nursing, ed. 14, Philadelphia, 1978, W.B. Saunders Co.

Freyman, J.G.: The American health care system: its genesis and trajectory, Huntington, N.Y., 1977, Robert Kreiger Publishing Co.

Frontier Nursing Service: FNS Q. Bull. 540(2):3-6, 1878.

Gardner, M.S.: Public health nursing, ed. 3, New York, 1919, Macmillan Publishing Co.

Griffin, G.J., and Griffin, J.K.: History and trends of professional nursing, ed. 7, St. Louis, 1973, The C.V. Mosby Co.

Hanlon, J.J., and Pickett, G.E.: Public health: administration and practice, ed. 7, St. Louis, 1979, The C.V. Mosby Co.

Hanlon, J.J., and Pickett, G.E.: Public health: administration and practice, ed. 8., St. Louis, 1984, The C.V. Mosby Co.

Health for all: one common goal, Geneva, Switzerland, undated, World Health Organization.

Henkle, J.O.: International nursing a specialty? Int. Nurs. Rev 26(6): 170-173, 1979.

Holloway, J.B.: Frontier Nursing Service 1925-1975, J. Ky. Med. Assoc. 13:491-492, Sept. 1975.

Introducing WHO, Geneva, Switzerland, 1976, World Health Organization.

Jordan, R.S.: Boycott diplomacy: the U.S., the U.N., and UNESCO, Public Admin. Review 44(4):283-291, 1984.

Kalisch, P., and Kalisch, B.J.: Nursing involvement in the health planning process, DHEW pub. no. HRA 78-25, Hyattsville, Md, 1977, U.S. Department of Health, Education and Welfare.

Kalisch, P., and Kalisch, B.J.: The advance of American nursing, ed. 2, Boston, 1986, Little, Brown & Co.

Kelly, L.: Dimensions of nursing practice, ed. 4, New York, 1981, Macmillan Publishing Co.

Maynard, T.: The apostle of charity: the life of St. Vincent de Paul, New York, 1939, Dial Press.

McNeil, E.E.: Transition in public health nursing, John Sundwall Lecture, University of Michigan, February 27, 1967.

National Organization for Public Health Nursing: approval of Skidmore College of Nursing as preparing students for public health nursing, Public Health Nurs. 36:371, July 1944.

Nightingale, F.: Notes on nursing, Philadelphia, 1946, J.B. Lippincott Co. Originally published in 1859.

Pan American Health Organization, Washington, D.C., 1985, Pan American Health Organization.

Pellegrino, E.D.: Medicine, history, and the idea of man, Ann. Am. Acad. Pol. Soc. Sci. 346:9-20, March 1963.

Rees, W.D.: Personal view: Herodotus, Br. Med. J. 4:182, Oct. 19, 1968.

Rosen, G.: A history of public health, New York, 1958, M. D. Publications.

Rosenkrantz, B.G.: Public health and the state: changing views in Massachusetts, 1842-1936, Cambridge, Mass., 1972, Harvard University Press.

Ruth, M.V., and Partridge, K.B.: Differences in perception of education and practice, Nurs. Outlook 26:622-629, Oct. 1978.

Schudson, M.: The Flexner Report and the Reed Report on the history of professional education in the United States, Soc. Sci. Q. 55:347-361, Sept. 1974.

Shyrock, H.: The history of nursing, Philadelphia, 1959, W.B. Saunders Co.

Swinson, A.: The history of public health, Exeter, England, 1965, A. Wheaton & Co.

Telecommunications development: The U.S. Effort, J. Comm. 35(2):10-13, Spring, 1985.

Tirpak, H.: The Frontier Nursing Service—fifty years in the mountains, Nurs. Outlook 33:308-310, May, 1975.

Weinstein, M.R.: The illness process, psychosocial hazards of disability programs, JAMA 20:209-213, April 1968.

Williams, C.A.: Community health nursing—what it is, Nurs. Outlook 25:251-254, April 1977.

Wilner, D.M., Walkey, R.P., and O'Neill, E.J.: Introduction to public health, ed. 7, New York, 1978, Macmillan Publishing Co.

Winslow, C.E.A.: The untitled field of public health, Mod. Med. 2:183, March 1920.

World Health Organization: Basic documents, ed. 36, Geneva, Switzerland, 1986, World Health Organization.

Jeanette Lancaster
Wade Lancaster

2

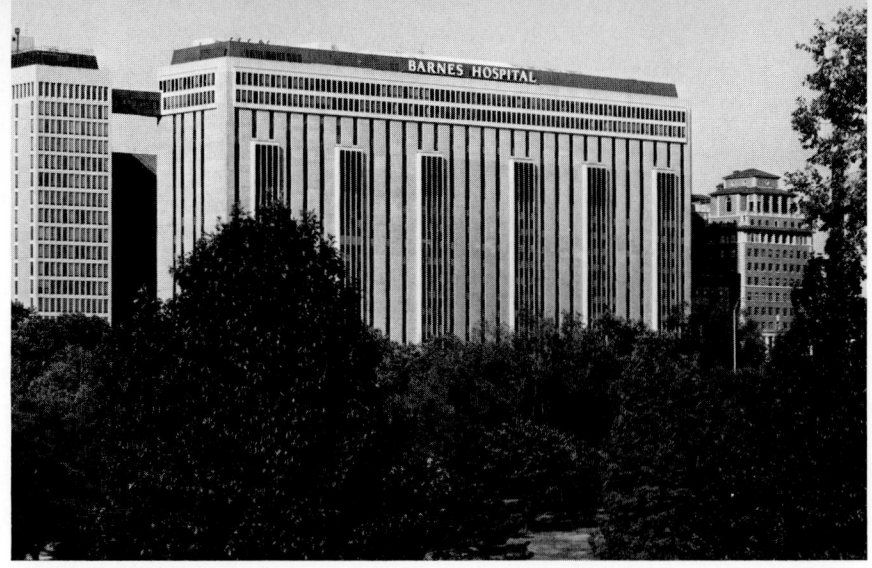

CURRENT STATUS OF THE HEALTH CARE SYSTEM

OBJECTIVES

After reading this chapter, the student should be able to:

Define health care.

Differentiate between health promotion and disease prevention.

Enumerate five advantages and five disadvantages of HMOs.

Analyze the concept of consumerism.

Evaluate three criticisms of the current health care system and document or refute their accuracy.

Discuss four economic trends affecting health care.

Describe three technological trends in health care.

Define *Preferred Provider Organization*.

KEY TERMS

alternate delivery system

ambulatory care centers

consumerism

demographic trends

dependent practitioners

deregulation

disease prevention

elementary model

health care services

health care system

health promotion

Health Maintenance Organizations (HMOs)

home health agency

hospice

independent practitioners

medical care

modified elementary model

nurse-midwives

Preferred Provider Organizations (PPOs)

private sector model

procompetition environment

professional model

Prospective Payment System (PPS)

public and private sector's model

Health is a topic of concern to all Americans, either directly or indirectly, individually or collectively, consciously or unconsciously. Health, inextricably linked with all aspects of daily living, is a prerequisite for living a productive and satisfying life. The concept of health is related to the notion of well-being; health is not an end in itself but represents on-going efforts to enrich one's level of well-being. Health is not just "feeling good," but instead is a broad concept embracing social, emotional, and physical aspects of life. It includes the cognitive, affective, and action domains of human behavior as it refers not only to individuals but also to the capabilities of families, communities, organizations, institutions, societies, and even nations. Health is a complex, multidimensional concept with biological, physical, personal, professional, technical, economic, legal, ethical, political, social, and cultural components. This chapter discusses the current health care system and the trends affecting it by examining the concept of health and describing the current structure of the system, including consumers, providers, and the current organizational arrangements for delivering services.

WHAT IS HEALTH AND HEALTH CARE?

The term *health* is defined in widely divergent ways. The World Health Organization defines health as "a state of complete physical, mental, and social well-being and not merely the absence of disease or infirmity" (WHO, 1986, p. 1). In contrast, a more contemporary definition of health is suggested by Brody and Sobel (1981, p. 30). They define health as "the ability of a system (for example, cell, organism, family, society) to respond adaptively to a wide variety of environmental challenges (for example, physical, chemical, infectious, psychological, social)." From this perspective health is seen as a positive process, not just the absence of symptoms. This definition also moves beyond the restriction of health as biological or mental well-being and includes a consideration of the surrounding environment.

One of our positions is that health promotion is a major responsibility of community health professionals. This stance is important because the current health care system has only recently begun moving away from focusing on repairing illness conditions to placing greater attention on health and promoting health-maintaining behaviors. To better understand the conceptual view of community health

as outlined in many of the following chapters, several additional terms are introduced below before turning our attention to describing the current health care system. A brief definition of each term is provided in Table 2-1.

The term *health care system* is used to denote all the resources a society distributes in the organization and delivery of *health services*. As such, the health care system is the organized local, state, or national effort designed to deliver services deemed essential to support the health of the residents.

Although the terms *medical care* and *health care* are often used interchangeably, they have distinct differences. *Medical care* is a generic term that describes the organization, financing, and delivery of health services that focus on individual or personal health needs. It encompasses the services and skills of a variety of providers, including physi-

TABLE 2-1

Selected health care definitions

Term	Definition
Health care system	The organization and distribution of all the resources a society allocates for the delivery of health services.
Health services	The performance by institutions and individuals of both personal and community or public service activities that have as their goal maintaining or restoring health.
Medical care	The delivery of personal or individually oriented health service activities.
Health care	The output of health service activities.
Health promotion	Activities which have as their goal developing human resources and behaviors that maintain or enhance well-being.
Disease prevention	Activities that have as their goal protecting people from actual or potential health threats and their harmful consequences.

cians, dentists, nurses, and various health therapists, as well as the provision of medications; orthopedic appliances; hospital, nursing home, and mental health care; and other care and resources from a variety of institutions. A major concern of medical care is the diagnosis and treatment of the disease process, which means that medical care is actually a subset of the broader concept of health care.

Health care includes not only the treatment of disease but also health promotion and disease prevention, and it is delivered through two vehicles: personal health services and community health services.

Two additional terms that are frequently used synonymously are *health promotion* and *disease prevention.* Although they appear to be similar, there are important conceptual differences between them. *Health promotion* focuses on maintenance or enhancement of well-being, whereas *disease prevention* focuses on protection from health threats. Both of these activities have a focus different from treatment of illness; therefore they often are not considered a legitimate part of the medical care system that focuses on diagnosis and treatment.

TRENDS AFFECTING THE HEALTH CARE SYSTEM

Revolution is changing the American health care system. Disgusted with years of accelerating costs, big purchasers of health care services—such as governments, corporations, and unions—are forcing changes in the ways physicians, hospitals, and other providers are used and paid (Califano, 1986).

The changes currently taking place in the health care system are unquestionably some of the most dramatic in the history of American health care. The impact of the trends now affecting our current health care system will undoubtedly influence the structure and functioning of the system that will accompany us into the twenty-first century. Several of the more significant trends affecting health care are demographical, social, economical, political, and technological.

Demographic Trends

The world's population is growing fast; it is expected to double in the next 30 years. Most of this explosive growth is occurring in Third World countries. In contrast, population growth in the United States has slowed dramatically. However, this doesn't mean that our population growth has stopped.

The Census Bureau predicts that the U.S. population will continue to grow at least until 2050, hitting a record high of 300 million before declining in the latter part of the next century. Interestingly, most of this future growth is expected to come from immigration. Let's take a look at some of these trends and what they mean to the health care system.

The U.S. birth rate has fluctuated greatly in the last 50 years. For 15 years following World War II, we witnessed a baby boom that lasted into the early 1960s. This was followed by the baby bust of the 1970s, which reached its low point in 1976. After 1976 the birth rate began rising again, but only slightly.

In addition to the modest increase in birth rates predicted for the population, there will be major changes in our society because of the continuing rise in the average age (ANA, 1985). One contributing factor is that for the last decade we have been experiencing declining mortality rates for both sexes in all age groups (Fagin, 1986). A more significant reason for the changing age distribution is that the baby boom produced about 20% of our present population.

At present, people over the age of 65 represent about 12% of the population (Fagin, 1986). Within this segment of the population is the group of people over 85; this group is growing at a rate of six times that of the general population. By 2025 the Census Bureau projects 60 million Americans—almost 20% of the population—will be over 65. This aging of the population will bring with it the four-generation society, in which it will be common to have two generations of the same family retired and receiving Social Security, Medicare, and nursing care (Califano, 1986).

Not only is there a rapidly increasing number of people in the over 65 age group, but the middle-age category will also continue increasing because nearly one-third of Americans were born between 1945 and 1960. As one sage observed, "It's like a pig passing through a boa constrictor."

Because older people tend to have more chronic diseases, they consume a larger portion of health care services than other age groups. This is becoming apparent as higher morbidity rates are noted for the middle (45 years) and older age groups. Although there appear to be fewer acute problems, more time is being devoted to caring for chronic problems such as hypertension, arthritis, and sinusitis (Fagin, 1986).

These changing demographic trends will dramatically affect the health care system. It is expected that hospital admissions will increase, with more of these admissions dealing with acute, intensive, and complicated illnesses (Andreoli and Musser, 1985). It is also anticipated that the aging population will require more home health care and nursing home services than previous generations because of their increasing longevity and the chronic nature of their illnesses. Chapter 3 explores the relationship of these demographic trends and health economics.

Social Trends

So far, we have been concerned with the size and changing age distribution of our population. It is obvious, however, that other factors also affect the health care system. Several noteworthy long-range social trends include changing lifestyles, a growing appreciation of quality of life, changing composition of families and living patterns, rising household incomes, and a new definition of quality health care.

During the 1960s and 1970s there was a major shift in American values and lifestyles (ANA, 1985). The post-World War II "American Dream" emphasized the work ethic—work hard, get a good education, and your life will be better than that of your parents. But for the past two decades, the drive to achieve these goals has diminished.

Replacing the work ethic is an increasing emphasis on an improved quality of life and fulfillment of personal goals.

This shift in values is reordering the relative importance of economic success and can be seen in a variety of behaviors, such as increased attention to leisure pursuits, self-help, fitness, and nutrition.

The self-help movement, for example, has emphasized the belief that people are responsible for their own health—and good health maintenance reduces the number of health disruptions. Increasingly, people are learning that health is a valuable asset and efforts should be taken to promote it. Centers for promoting all aspects of health are developing in response to this movement.

The nature of families has also changed in recent years. People are marrying at a later age, delaying child bearing, and having fewer children. Couples with no children under 18 now account for almost half of all families.

People are not staying together as long as they did in the past. About 4 of 10 marriages end in divorce (ANA, 1985). Also, because more people are marrying at a later age and because there is an increasing number of both divorced and never married people, more adults are living alone. In fact, about 20% of all households are single adult households.

Another factor that deserves attention is the growing number of women with paying jobs. Since 1950, the proportion of married women in the workforce has increased from less than 25% to a current rate of over 50%. It is estimated that by 1995, nearly two-thirds of all working-age women will be employed (ANA, 1985).

The increasing number of women in the workforce has obviously contributed to rising family incomes. However, there are a number of other factors that have also effected changes in family incomes.

Economic Trends
Consumer Income

Sixty years ago income was distributed in such a way that a relatively small proportion of elite households earned high incomes; a somewhat larger proportion of families were in the middle income range; and the largest proportion of households were bunched together at the low end of the income scale. But by the 1970s, household income had risen so much it was becoming more evenly distributed. This was a significant trend because it meant that more families had money to spend on major improvements in living standards.

The inflation-ridden 1970s also marked the end of the continuous rise—actually a temporary drop was recorded—of real median income. In contrast, predictions for the 1980s estimated a 20% increase in family incomes (ANA, 1985).

Although the distribution of income has dramatically changed over time, it is important to remember that higher-income groups are still important. They account for a very large share of total income—and an equally large share of increases in income. For example, the top 20% of the households receive more than 40% of total income. Well-to-do households—the top 5%—get more than 15% of total income.

At the lower end of the income scale, more than 12 million families—about 20% of the households—receive

only 5% of total income. Two-thirds of this group are below the poverty level. This means that a sizable proportion of Americans with low earned incomes will continue to rely on public support to maintain a minimum standard of living.

The emphasis on quality health care is diminishing as costs escalate. According to Stevens (1985, p.27), "Until recently, people sought to preserve life at all costs. But today, society twists and turns on subtle issues of life's quality." In a recent survey of 1000 experts in health care conducted by the American College of Hospital Administrators and Arthur Andersen and Company (1985), 98% of the respondents believed that a minimum level of health care was the right of all Americans, whereas only 12% believed that everyone is entitled to the same level of service. According to the survey, little change in the quality of health care is expected for people with private insurance, whereas uninsured people without the ability to pay will experience the greatest declines in health care services.

In short, health care providers confronted with financial constraints will influence decisions about the quality and accessibility of health care. At the same time, some consumers may have to readjust their expectations regarding these issues.

Economic Changes in the Health Care System

The American economy can be characterized as a service economy because the service sector accounts for a larger share of total employment than the manufacturing sector. This is not a relatively recent phenomenon; it began shortly after World War II. Today, the service sector accounts for over 60% of employment, and recent employment growth has been concentrated in communications, financial services, information processing, and health care (ANA, 1985).

Total employment in the health care field is expected to increase 48% from 1982 levels to about 10.3 million employed by 1995 (ANA, 1985). Concurrent with this growth is the expectation that some physician-specialty categories and some groups of allied health care workers will experience workforce surpluses.

It is projected that 700,000 physicians will be practicing in the United States by 2000, reflecting a 54% increase from 1980. In other words, the number of active physicians is projected to increase at an average annual rate of 2.7%—3 times the projected rate of population growth.

This rapid growth will not only produce a physician surplus, it will likely affect the roles of other health professionals and increase the cost of some health services. It is predicted that a physician surplus may cause some redistribution into underserved areas. For example, an increasing number of physicians may be attracted to inner city and rural areas, and also to multispecialty groups and health maintenance organizations. They may also begin offering services previously delivered by other health professionals (Andreoli and Musser, 1985).

Historically, nursing care has been provided in a variety of settings, with the hospital being the dominant setting. Currently, two-thirds of the registered-nurse workforce is employed in hospitals. It is predicted that as alternative health settings gain popularity, a redistribution of the nurse workforce will follow. For example, as health maintenance organization enrollments increase, the number of nurses employed by these organizations will increase.

Employment pattern predictions for nursing through the end of this century see nursing care being delivered in entirely new as well as existing settings. There will be an increasing need for nurses in nonhospital settings, such as outpatient clinics, health maintenance organizations, home health care, nursing homes, and joint and solo practice arrangements. By 2000, the need for nursing personnel is estimated to be about 1.8 million—a 65% increase from 1980. In contrast to the predicted physician surplus, a modest shortage of nurses is being forecast (ANA, 1985).

If current trends continue and no changes in the way we presently finance health care occur, national health expenditures will probably approach $760 billion by 1990. Approximately 57% will be private spending, and the other 43% will be public spending. By 1990, health care expenditures will consume almost 12% of the Gross National Product (GNP). This is approximately equivalent to $3000 per person for total health care, with almost half going for hospital care.

Of the $431 billion projected for total private spending, the proportion of personal health expenditures for hospital and nursing home care will increase to approximately 60%. Total public spending for health care is predicted to be $325 billion, of which the federal government will finance about 71%.

Political Trends

The federal government plays a major role in our health care system by establishing a national health care policy. Currently, three interrelated trends are changing the nature of the system and the roles of the various participants.

The first trend is the procompetition environment advocated by President Reagan and other supply-side–economics supporters. Proponents argue that deregulation of the health care sector lets marketplace forces control costs. Making price a supreme consideration in the purchase of medical care places providers at financial risk for their actions. Deregulation also stimulates increased nonprice competition, such as improved quality and greater substitution of products and services, expanded markets, and increasingly sophisticated marketing (Weil, 1985).

Another aspect of the procompetition trend focuses on the intensive competition developing between investor-owned hospitals and not-for-profit multihospital or multiinstitutional systems that have evolved through horizontal and vertical diversification. The anticipated outcome of this multihospital system growth is a more effective health care delivery system (Weil, 1985).

A goal of the procompetitive environment and a thrust of the second trend is reducing total health care expenditures by making significant reductions in the federal fiscal commitment to the Medicare and Medicaid programs (Weil, 1985). Evidence of this trend is the Prospective Payment System (PPS) that was devised as a new way to pay hospitals for the services they provide to Medicare patients (Fagin, 1986). In the 5-year period from 1981 through 1986, Medicare spending dropped $22 billion and federal Medicaid expenditures fell by $3.8 billion, with more cuts being proposed.

The general thrust of this federal fiscal policy is to shift an increasing burden for the payment of health care services onto nongovernment entities. Proponents argue that fiscal contraction of the health care/hospital system will enable providers to supply the same services by improved effectiveness and efficiency of their current operations. Thus more pressure will be placed on physicians to practice less expensive medicine (Weil, 1985).

The third trend is a shifting to the states of the responsibility of providing appropriate incentives when regulatory policies are enacted that will slow down the rise of health care costs, especially until the procompetition/supply-side economic policies are well in place (Weil, 1985).

Technological Trends

Changing technology is altering the health care system. Innovations have been introduced at an increasing rate over the last 10 years; and the rate of technological innovation continues to accelerate. Changes in technology not only include aspects such as computer hardware and software, instruments, and drugs, but also new ways of thinking about and performing diagnostic techniques and surgical procedures (Andreoli and Musser, 1985; and Stevens, 1985).

Technology has had various effects—both positive and negative—on our health care system. On the positive side, technological advances promise improving health care services and reducing care costs. Recent biomedical developments are reducing hospital days, cutting labor costs, decreasing the cost of care in both hospitals and patients' homes, and increasing the number of at-home procedures and techniques. For example, medical technology now makes it possible to shift a number of diagnostic and treatment services from the hospital to either the physician's office or the patient's home. Some of the high-technology services that can be delivered in nonhospital settings include chemotherapy, kidney dialysis, intravenous (hydration) therapies and feeding, insulin therapy, antibiotic therapy, apnea monitoring, parenteral and enteral nutritional support services, and biotelemetry (ANA, 1985).

Many of these advances in technology have contributed to the increasing number of people the health care system serves. The survival chances for many patients have also dramatically increased as a result of advances in medical technology. For example, computers are used to record and analyze vital signs and regulate medications; other machines that regulate themselves are used as intravenous regulatory pumps. In short, expanding and improved technology is contributing to an improved quality of life for many people (Andreoli and Musser, 1985; and Califano, 1986).

The negative side of this rapidly changing technological environment is its cost. One cost is associated with the accelerating obsolescence of knowledge and techniques that accompany technological advances. Another cost is more obvious: biomedical technology advances are expensive and have been indicted as a cause of escalating health care costs. Presently, no effective mechanisms exist to assess the cost and effectiveness or to control the diffusion of new technologies (ANA, 1985).

Unquestionably, advances in medical technology will continue. However, it is anticipated that the emphasis will shift away from expensive diagnostic and therapeutic technologies toward efforts to devise simpler, more mobile, less costly, less tertiary-care oriented tests and procedures that can be used in nonhospital settings.

As the adoption of prospective payment systems spreads among third-party payers, it is predicted that patients will be leaving the hospital in more acute stages of their illnesses. As a result, there will be a rise in demand for high-technology home care equipment and services.

ISSUES RELATED TO THE HEALTH CARE SYSTEM

Health care issues have attracted a considerable amount of attention in recent years. As we noted in the discussion of trends, a variety of factors are fueling a revolution in our health care system. Until recently, health care was commonly viewed as a public good that should be available to everyone in some form, regardless of their ability to pay. The marketplace is now challenging this notion as well as a number of other ideas about health and health care. Collectively, these challenges are not only forcing us to change the way we think about the delivery system, they are pushing rapid and dramatic changes. Of special interest is the rapid growth of alternative health care systems and providers, and the extraordinary growth in the for-profit sector in health care delivery. For the first time a spirited air of competition is swirling through the health industry.

A close examination of the contemporary health care system and some major criticisms of the system are the subjects of the remainder of this chapter.

Criticisms of the Health Care System

Criticisms of our health care system have never been in short supply. In fact, considerable debate has occurred over a variety of issues, running the gamut of ethical and philosophical issues such as, What is health and whose responsibility is it? to political and economic issues such as dealing with the provision, distribution, and cost of health care services. Our present concern is only with those criticisms of the health care system that focus on structural issues.

It is often said that no health care system exists in the United States. This criticism actually focuses on two separate issues. The first issue attacks our system for being primarily oriented toward illness care; health has been viewed as a renewable resource or commodity that can be repaired as the need arises. Health care professionals have largely ignored the issue of health maintenance, claiming that they are too busy taking care of the sick (Bruhn, 1981).

The second issue refers to the structure of the health care industry. The industry is dominated by several hundred thousand small, inefficient, uncoordinated, more or less independent enterprises (i.e., physicians, nurses, hospitals, clinics, nursing homes, and home health care agencies) that add up to a fragmented and wasteful industry. This lack of

effective planning and coordination has resulted in widespread duplication of costly facilities, equipment, and patient record-keeping systems. It has also spawned a serious maldistribution of resources, with a relative abundance of facilities in affluent urban areas and a corresponding lack of facilities in many rural and poorer urban areas.

ORGANIZATION OF THE HEALTH CARE SYSTEM

The health care system is composed of consumers, providers, and mechanisms for delivery of health services. Several factors distinguish health services and differentiate the patterns of delivery of health services from those of other services.

Characteristics of the Health Care System

From birth to death, everyone is part of the market potential for health care services. Thus the number of people needing to enter, and to remain in, the system is quite large. Also, consumers of health care often are unable to determine their need for specific services.

In addition, the consumer of health care services is a client, not a customer. In the purest sense of the marketing term, when customers purchase something they take title to it, and the seller has little or no control over its use. In contrast, clients, being in a more dependent position, place themselves in the hands of providers. The client can decide whether to buy the services and treatment offered, but in most instances the provider decides what should be purchased. The provider is a gatekeeper who determines when and how entry into the health care system shall occur. Without a physician or other licensed practitioner, such as a dentist or in some instances a nurse practitioner, clients cannot avail themselves of medication, diagnostic and treatment procedures, nursing care, or hospitalization.

Consumers tend to be less informed about health services than anything else they purchase (Lancaster, 1984). With most other products and services, people shop around to compare goods and services as to price, availability, and potential usefulness. People who switch physicians more than once are considered neurotics because the expectation is that clients select providers, not methods of treatment. In general, health consumers know what product they want—health—but they do not know what treatment will ensure this outcome. Most consumers do not know that for many forms of health disruption, certain behaviors, such as diet and exercise, are often as useful as expensive medications.

The health care system is unique because it is not a competitive market. For a market to be competitive it must consist of (1) well-informed buyers and sellers, no one of whom is powerful enough to influence price, (2) buyers and sellers who act independently, and (3) free entry for other buyers and sellers not currently in the market.

In contrast, the health care system violates the characteristics of a competitive market in a variety of ways. First, the notion of well-informed consumers—merits attention because it affects the health care system in several ways. In general, the only way people know if they need the services of a health care provider is by seeing one. Physician advertising is sparse, and in most states pharmacies continue to do minimal if any advertising on prescription items.

In the health care system sellers have tremendous control over price, because health is such a precious commodity to buyers, most are reluctant to ask health care providers for estimated costs (Lancaster, 1984). There are few incentives in the health care system to keep costs at a fixed level. Although insurers often establish price ceilings, physicians then bill clients for the portion of the bill not covered by a third party.

Restricted entry into the health care system is the final unique characteristic. On the one hand, compulsory licensure of providers restricts entry for sellers. On the other hand, many buyers are denied free entry. For example, the poor are typically limited as to which hospitals and providers they can use. Hospitals often require proof of third-party payment or personal ability to pay before admitting people. Similarly, most physicians require proof of insurance or payment at the time of treatment.

Models of Health Care Delivery

The four models presented here depict the organization of the current health care system. Local, state, and national components are only mentioned briefly in this chapter and in much greater depth in Chapter 6. The most *elementary model* of a health care system is depicted in Figure 2-1. Two constant and fundamental components of the system are the consumers and the providers. In this simplified model, consumers engage in exchange relationships with providers.

The organization of health care reflects a strange blend of private and public enterprise. The vast majority of providers are in private practice, which means that they can decide where they want to practice, who they will accept as patients, and how much they will charge. Also, an increasing number of medical care providers are labeled as specialists, which further complicates the point of entry. If clients do not know what is wrong with them, how can they know which specialist to choose? There is also a great deal of competition among providers. Many physicians are reluctant or refuse to acknowledge the value of other providers such as nurse practitioners.

The health care system is composed of two major groups, clients and providers, and is largely built on a fee-for-service basis. Until recently the prevalent mode of financing health services was personal payment. In recent years third-party payments have increased dramatically and affected the entire system. In Figure 2-2, the *modified elementary model,* third-party funding agencies are added to the elementary model. The bulk of health care services in the United States are paid for either directly or indirectly by the consumer. Although more Americans are covered by insurance than have been in previous years, a large proportion of all health care costs come directly out of the individual's pocket. As will be discussed in detail in Chapter 3, national health care expenditures have grown monumentally since the 1940s. As discussed earlier, much of the increase is caused by inflation, new and expensive technology, larger salaries for health care professionals, increased life span, and regulations. These factors, especially inflation, technology, and

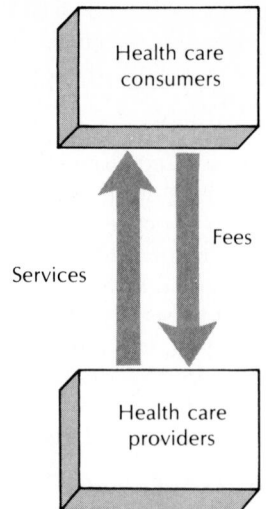

FIGURE 2-1

Elementary model of the health care delivery system.

changes in the characteristics of the population, are discussed in Chapter 3. Chapters 3 and 6 address the organization and financing of the health care system from the viewpoint of regulatory mechansims.

Figure 2-3 depicts the *private sector model* and illustrates an increasing level of complexity by the health care system. The illustration is initially broken down into three components: personnel, facilities, and suppliers. According to this model, providers include both personnel and facilities such as hospitals, clinics, ambulatory centers, health maintenance organizations, nursing homes, home care agencies, medical laboratories, and pharmacies. The final component is made up of companies that supply health products to providers and consumers, such as distributors of pharmaceutical supplies, medical equipment manufacturers, medical furnishing companies, and distributors of general supplies.

The existing health care system as depicted in Figure 2-3 is called the *professional model* because its most conspicuous ingredient is the physician. In contrast to many other American industries that have changed structurally to keep pace with technological and social advances, the health care industry has largely retained its pre-Industrial Revolution organizational structure. Consequently, it is often referred to as a "cottage industry," relying heavily on small, independent firms (Lancaster, 1982).

Figure 2-3 illustrates the central role of the physician as gatekeeper and, in many instances, navigator of the health care system. With few exceptions in the private sector, medication, nursing care, laboratory tests, hospitalization, treatments, and the use of specialists are determined by the physician.

The *public and private sectors model* is illustrated in Figure 2-4. Also shown is an alternate conceptual view of the private sector. As seen in the illustration, the public sector is composed of public health agencies, both voluntary and official, which operate at the federal, state, and local level. Voluntary agencies are nonprofit organizations that depend

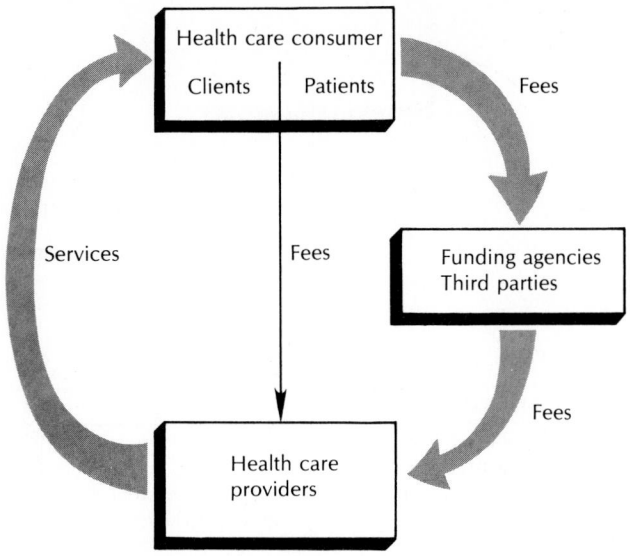

FIGURE 2-2

Modified model of the health care delivery system.

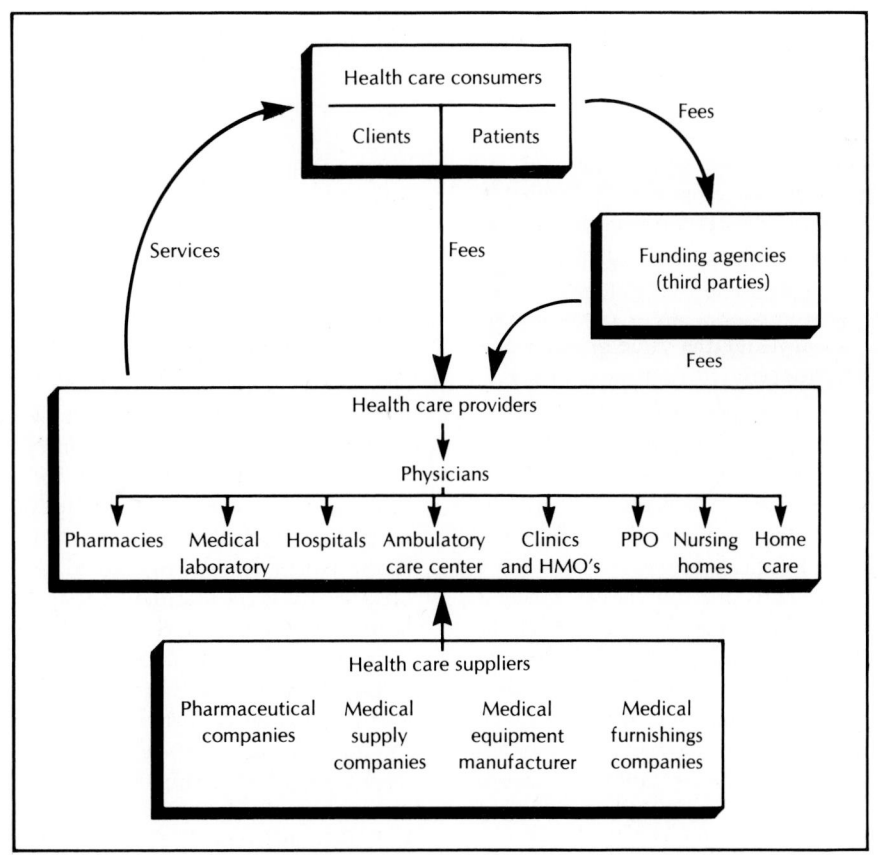

FIGURE 2-3

Health care delivery model: private sector.

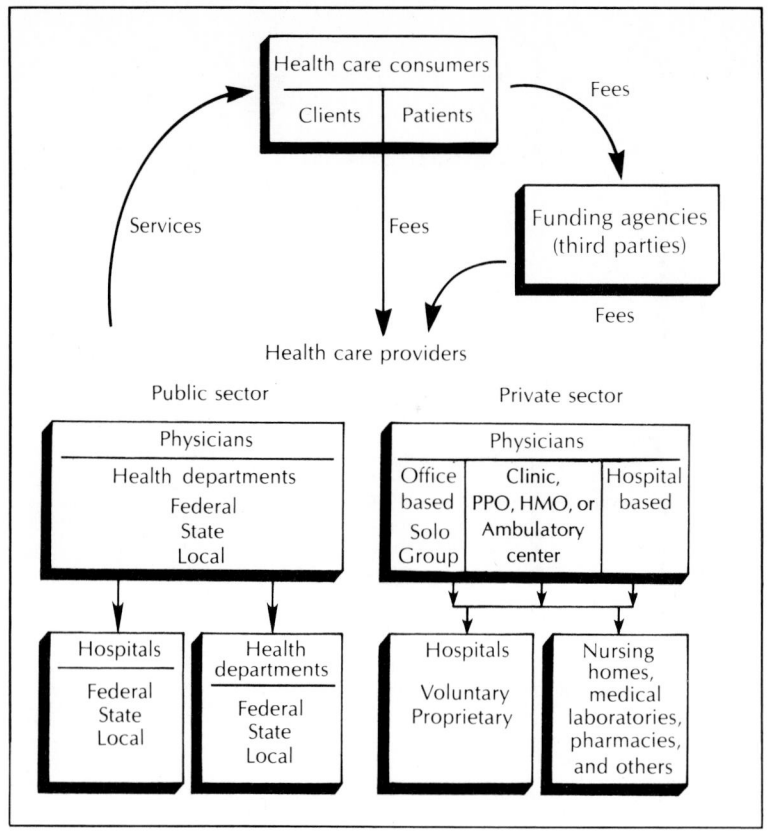

FIGURE 2-4

Health care delivery model: public and private sectors.

on donations, fees, membership dues, endowments, payments from insurance plans, and contracts. In contrast, official agencies are primarily tax supported. Voluntary agencies were briefly discussed in Chapter 1. Official agencies include the armed forces, Veterans Administration, the United States Public Health Service, and various state and local health departments that provide medical care, preventive services, and environmental control services directly to the public. Collectively, these agencies carry on a variety of tasks. Federal agencies deal with national and international health as well as the health of specific population groups, such as military personnel, veterans, Indians, the aged, and the economically deprived as well as people who are physically or mentally handicapped.

At the federal level, the basis of public health concerns lie in the United States Constitution. The authors of the Constitution used broad phrases such as "promote the general welfare," which influence the scope of public health. Additionally, several powers are granted to the federal government that influence health care activities. Further information on the organization of health care from a local, state, and national perspective is found in Chapter 6.

Mechanisms for Health Care Delivery

An enormous number and range of facilities make up the health care delivery system, including physician's offices,

dentists' offices, hospitals, HMOs, nursing homes and other related inpatient facilities, mental health centers, ambulatory care centers, rehabilitation centers, and local, state, and federal agencies.

Hospitals

Historically, hospitals began as institutions to house poor people who were seriously ill and had no family or other resources to care for them. Members of religious groups who saw their work as a missionary activity ran many of the early hospitals. The word *hospital* is derived from *hospice*, meaning guest room, and historically referred to a place of refuge for travelers or the unwanted to go to for care. The oldest North American hospital was erected in 1524 in Mexico City as the Hospital of Jesus of Nazareth. The oldest hospital in the United States still operates in New Orleans as the Charity Hospital (Shindell et al., 1976).

Generally, hospitals attempt to carry out no more than four major services: patient care, education, research, and community service. As shown in Figure 2-5, three predominant forms of ownership of nonfederal, short-term hospitals exist: (1) privately owned, nonprofit; (2) state and local; and (3) proprietary.

Before the late 1970s, the corporate structure in hospitals was reasonably simple, and most hospitals were privately owned, nonprofit facilities. As hospitals began to feel the

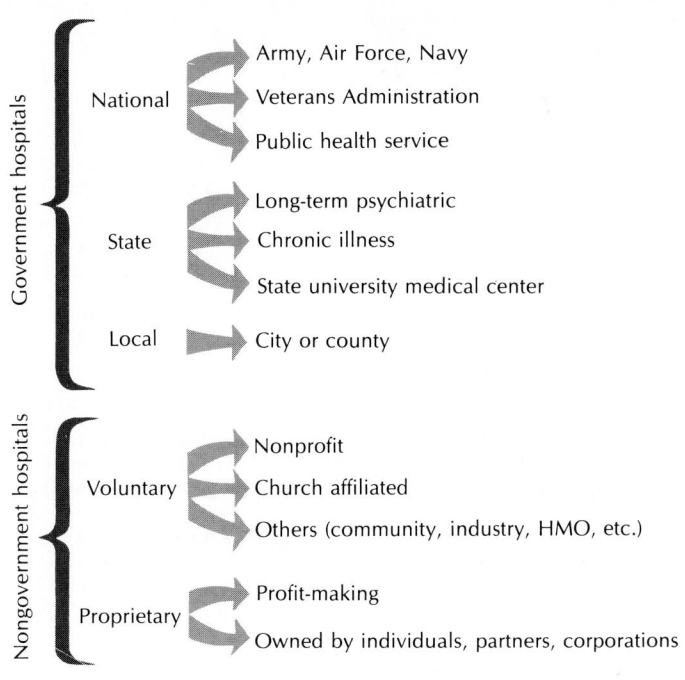

FIGURE 2-5

Types of hospitals in the United States.

effect of prospective payment it became essential to look at ways to cut costs, and new corporate structures emerged as a viable way to do so. "Multihospital systems were among the first to emerge because they offered a way of sharing expertise and services" (Andreoli and Musser, 1985, p. 30). It is anticipated that in the next decade greater consolidation of hospitals will occur as new systems emerge through mergers and acquisitions. It is predicted that by 1995 investor-owned hospitals will constitute 23% of the nation's hospitals, compared to 14% in 1982.

Government hospitals are expected to decrease by 6% to comprise 29% of the hospitals, and not-for-profit hospitals will decline by 3% to 48%, according to the Arthur Andersen survey (1985).

Alternative Delivery Systems

In recent years the term *alternative delivery systems* (ADSs) has come into being. The organizations grouped under this umbrella include Health Maintenance Organizations (HMOs) and Preferred Provider Organizations (PPOs). "Alternative delivery systems are no longer alternative; they are fast becoming the mainstream" (Ellwood, 1985, p. 1). A *health maintenance organization* is an "organized system of health care that guarantees to provide high-quality physician services, emergency and preventive treatment and hospital services to individuals who have agreed to obtain their medical care from the HMO for an extended period of time" (Ellwood and Herbert, 1973, p. 100). By December, 1984, enrollment in 337 HMOs reached 16.7 million. A record high of 3 million people joined HMOs in 1984 alone. The effect of HMOs on the health care system is far

reaching. By 1984, over 85,000 physicians were participating in HMOs.

The distinguishing characteristic of HMOs is that all care is provided for a fixed, prenegotiated fee paid periodically and in advance of need. The chief advantage lies in the economic incentive to keep costs under control. Prevention is emphasized to reduce the need for costly services. The greatest potential for savings from HMOs, reduction of the costs of unnecessary hospitalization, also accounts for the greatest fear: that providers will underuse necessary services to save money.

As a part of these services people receive complete and continuous care. Services are provided to all segments of society in exchange for prepayment, and prevention is emphasized.

A PPO may be generally defined as an organization of providers that contracts on a fee-for-service basis with third-party payers to provide comprehensive medical services to subscribers. The agreement between the PPO and the third-party payer allows subscribers to receive medical services at lower-than-usual rates by going through the PPO, which has contracted directly with providers (Roble, Knowlton and Rosenberg, 1984).

The PPO concept appears to offer a number of advantages to the traditional delivery system; however, at present our experience with them is too limited to make a full evaluation. There are several obvious disadvantages with PPOs. First, measuring the cost effectiveness of PPOs is difficult. This measurement problem is complicated because consumers are not obligated to use the PPO and may use both PPO and non-PPO services concurrently. Second, the third-party payer assumes a volume risk because there is no way to control subscriber use. Third, there is no way of evaluating whether a PPO physician's discounted fees are actually less expensive than those of non-PPO providers (NAQ Forum, 1985).

Other Health Care Delivery Organizations

As shown in the health care delivery models, there are a number of additional facilities and organizations that make up our contemporary health care system. The importance of many has been elevated as hospital use patterns have shifted in recent years.

For example, programs providing health care services in the home have become noteworthy. *Home health agency* is a term used to refer to an agency that participates in the Medicare and Medicaid programs and is eligible to receive federal funds. Home care programs are provided by a variety of organizations such as hospitals, health departments, visiting nurse associations, and independent agencies. Home health care is covered in detail in Chapter 42; however, it is important that the significant growth and shift in market share by these organizations be recognized here. The significance of this growth is that for years visiting nurse associations (VNAs) and public health departments provided high-quality, low-cost services, and commercial, for-profit organizations were relatively unsuccessful in this field. That has all changed. Proprietary home health organizations have successfully penetrated the market in the past few years and taken over half the market away from VNAs and public health departments (Fagin, 1986).

Recently, a popular European concept in health care, called *hospice care*, has gained popularity in the United States. It is a "humane alternative in health care delivery for terminally ill patients" (Andreoli, 1982, p. 318).

Another group of health care facilities, collectively known as *ambulatory centers,* represent additional settings for providing health care services. These facilities are either hospital or community based. Hospital-based services are provided in either ambulatory care units or clinics.

Community-based settings include neighborhood health centers, ambulatory care centers, and mental health centers. Neighborhood health centers provide a comprehensive array of health services to a defined geographic population; their major focus is on disease prevention and health maintenance and promotion. Ambulatory centers—variously known as urgicenters, emergicenters, medical care walk-in centers, and doc-in-a-box—are being established in many middle-class urban and suburban neighborhoods to provide services similar to those provided by physicians' offices and hospital-based programs (Fagin, 1986).

Community mental health centers provide comprehensive mental health services to defined geographic areas. The types of services available are often based on community needs. Chapter 32 provides an indepth discussion of these facilities.

With the increasingly aging population comes the need for facilities to care for the elderly. One type of organization dedicated to serving this need is the nursing home. These long-term care facilities can be classified according to the level of health care services they provide, which ranges from minimal to constant professional nursing services.

But nursing home care is expensive, and the costs continue to escalate as a result of environmental pressures such as inflation and increasing demand. One alternative currently being evaluated is to assign elderly people to case managers who can assess their health and social needs and design and implement a plan to meet those needs. Plans would include various alternatives, one being nursing home care (Federal Register, 1979).

Another group of alternatives includes board and care homes or personal care homes (*Health: United States,* 1980). It is estimated that at present there are over 200,000 state-certified beds in this type of home. Other options for providing long-term care include home health care, chronic disease hospitals, mental institutions, and community-based day care centers (*Health: United States,* 1981).

Health Work Force

Health care providers are shown in the models of the health care delivery system as both facilities and personnel. Thus far, we have focused on the various mechanisms available for delivering health care services. We now turn our attention to those who provide health care.

Health care providers can be divided into three separate groups: independent practitioners, dependent practitioners, and support staff.

Independent Practitioners

Independent practitioners include physicians, dentists, optometrists, chiropractors, and podiatrists. These practitioners are legally permitted to provide a specific range of services without relying on supervision from any other provider. All of these independent practitioners are called "doctor," and this can be confusing (Raffel, 1980). Therefore it might be helpful if we briefly describe each of them.

The most commonly known independent practitioner is the medical doctor (M.D.). On completion of a prescribed and approved program of premedical and medical school preparation, this person earns an M.D. degree. After medical school the doctor undertakes a one-year hospital-based internship. Many medical doctors follow up their internship with a 2 to 5 year residency, depending on the specialty selected. Of the more than 20 specialties, some of the more common ones include family practice, surgery, anesthesiology, obstetrics/gynecology, pediatrics, psychiatry, and neurology.

A similar type of doctor is the osteopathic physician (D.O.). Although their educational requirements parallel that of medical doctors, it also includes extra hours of osteopathic manipulation.

Dentists follow a program of study that is typically a minimum of 4 years of undergraduate study followed by 4 years of dental school. There are two equivalent dental degrees: doctor of dental medicine (D.M.D.) or doctor of dental surgery (D.D.S.).

Chiropractors (D.C.) also assume the title of doctor. Their education generally consists of 4 years of training beyond at least 2 years of college. They believe that many conditions are the result of misalignment (subluxated) vertebrae, and that cure can be effected by manipulation.

Optometrists (O.D.) are trained to examine eyes and prescribe and fit visual aids such as glasses and contact lenses. Schools of optometry are usually 4-year programs that follow 3 to 4 years of preoptometry course work.

Two additional types of doctor are podiatrists (D.P.M.) and chiropodists (D.S.C.). Both are specially trained to diagnose and treat foot conditions. The degrees for each of these doctors require a minimum of 2 years of college followed by 4 years of podiatry.

Dependent Practitioners

Dependent practitioners are allowed by law to deliver a specified range of services that must be performed under the supervision and authorization of independent practitioners. Dependent practitioners include nurses, psychologists, social workers, pharmacists, physicians' assistants, dental hygienists, and the various therapists such as occupational, physical, and speech. The line separating dependent and independent practitioners is becoming blurred as many groups, including nurses, strive for more autonomous forms of practice.

The federal government is actively trying to improve access to health care in physician-shortage areas by supporting the education and employment of health care providers who are not physicians. Two types making major contributions in primary care are nurse practitioners (NPs) and physician assistants (PAs). The primary distinction between these groups is that NPs perform functions previously considered within the domain of physicians along with their nursing role; in contrast, PAs assist or substitute for the physician in the performance of specific medical tasks. The best use of both NPs and PAs is not as a substitute for the physician but rather as members of a collaborative health care team. PAs and NPs perform the following basic functions (*Health: United States,* 1980, p. 83):

1. Take medical histories and do physical examinations to define health and medical problems.
2. Institute therapeutic regimens within established protocols and recognize when to refer the patient to a physician or other health care provider.
3. Provide counseling to individuals, families, and groups in the area of health promotion and maintenance.

The federal government has encouraged the increased preparation of NPs and PAs through substantial financial subsidies since 1969. In 1969 funds for NP and PA training programs was $1 million, whereas 1979 witnessed $21 million in federal funding (Congressional Budget Office, 1979). The first NP program began in 1965 at the University of Colorado to train pediatric nurse practitioners. During the same year, the first PA program was developed at Duke University. Initially, both programs were privately funded, with the first federal funding going to the MEDEX program at the University of Washington. This program trained PAs to work in underserved rural or urban areas under physician supervision.

In 1971 the President's Annual Message on Health endorsed the use of NPs and PAs to improve access to care

and contain costs (*Health: United States,* 1979). The Nurse Training Act (PL 94-63) of 1974 provided funds for increased training of NPs, while the Comprehensive Health Manpower Training Act (PL 92-157) provided funds for both NPs and PAs. Further, in 1977, the Health Profession's Educational Assistance Act of 1976 (PL 94-184) was amended by the Health Services Extension Act (PL 95-83) to fund programs to train NPs who both came from and would agree to practice in health personnel shortage areas. Additional support was given to NPs and PAs when the Rural Health Clinic Services Act of 1977 (PL 95-210) provided for Medicare and Medicaid coverage for medical services furnished by these two groups in certified clinics located in rural physician shortage areas.

Nurse-midwives, like NPs and PAs, emphasize the care of well rather than ill persons. The American College of Nurse Midwives (ACNM) defines nurse-midwifery as "the independent management and care of essentially normal newborns and women antepartally, intrapartally, postpartally, and or gynecologically, occurring within a health care system that provides for medical consultation, collaborative management, or referral . . ." (*Health: United States,* 1979, p. 50). The mother is the primary focus of care for the nurse-midwives, with the majority of their time spent on prenatal, labor and delivery, and postpartal care as well as family planning services.

Research findings have indicated that NPs, PAs, and nurse-midwives have a definite place in the health care delivery system. These providers have been judged capable of carrying out a substantial number of tasks previously reserved for physicians without compromising the quality of care. In general, services can be provided at considerable cost savings to consumers while maintaining quality and a high level of consumer acceptance and satisfaction. But in recent years, these groups have received considerable pressure to limit their practice so as to avoid infringing on what physicians perceive as their role.

Two factors significantly influence the geographical distribution and use of NPs and PAs. The first involves the restrictions placed on their practice by various professional practice acts and rules and regulations in the different states. In many states the acts and rules governing their practice are restrictive because of supervision requirements and the scope of practice permitted. For example, some states require direct (on the premises) supervision by a physician, whereas others allow NPs and PAs to practice in remote sites if on-site physician supervision is regular (usually weekly or biweekly) and telephone supervision is continuously available. In general, supervision requirements for NPs are not as strict as those for PAs. Both groups, however, are prohibited from prescribing drugs in most states.

The second restriction on the practice of PAs and NPs deals with the question of whether reimbursement is made for their services by third-party insurers, including Medicare and Medicaid. Traditionally, reimbursement from third-party payers has only been forthcoming when physicians were on-site and services were billed by them. The exception was established in 1977 by Public Law 95-210, which amended Titles XVIII and XIX of the Social Security Act.

This legislation provided for Medicare and Medicaid reimbursement for NP or PA services in certified clinics that lacked a full-time physician. An additional threat to the practice of these providers may be the rapidly increasing number of physicians in the United States. Chapter 39 provides detailed information on nurse practitioners.

Support Staff

Supporting staff members carry out work tasks authorized and often delegated by either independent or dependent practitioners. The work of members of this group is not always regulated by laws directly pertaining to them, in which case they work under the legal sanctions provided by their supervisors. Members of the supporting staff group include research assistants, various types of technicians, and clerical, maintenance, housekeeping, and food processing workers.

CONSUMERISM

The consumerism movement is built on the belief that people have both a right and a responsibility to be knowledgeable about and involved in the choices made about their health and illness care. This movement presupposes that consumers will take time to acquaint themselves with selected health-related information and that providers will make a concerted effort to disseminate such information in easily understood forms.

As mentioned in an earlier section of this chapter, consumers of health care differ from consumers of many other products and services. Health care consumers typically invest complete, unquestioning trust in health care providers, especially physicians. Few consumers devote as much time to researching the relative merits of a proposed medical treatment as they devote to choosing automobiles. Also, health care consumers are often hesitant to raise questions about costs or to do any sort of comparative shopping. Several reasons for the lack of informed health care consumers are discussed in this section.

The tendency to passively rely on health care providers to repair one's physical and emotional maladies has changed considerably in recent years. People increasingly recognize their personal responsibility for health and realize that many health problems can be avoided by proper care, including preventive maintenance such as health promotion. Advocates like Bess Myerson and Ralph Nader continue to diligently inform people of both their rights and responsibilities as consumers. People are encouraged to scrutinize both the products *and* services they purchase by reading about them, asking carefully formulated questions, and thinking critically about what is best for them.

Consumerism is not a new concept. Early consumer participation can be traced to medieval times (400 to 1400 AD) when guilds of workers in Europe joined together to protect their common interests. These guilds developed "sick chests" to provide funds for medical care needed for sickness or disability resulting from accidents. Hence, this early evidence of health insurance was devised by consumers. Likewise, in seventeenth century England, societies such as the Oddfellows or the Ancient Order of Foresters extended the "sick chest" idea to include people outside their guilds. The friendly society concept also developed in the colonies, and by 1867 more than 24,000 benevolent societies operated in the United States (Hamilton, 1982). Over the years the consumer movement has taken many forms, with the guiding aim being to secure health care that is accessible, effective, and reasonable in cost.

A major hurdle for consumers to overcome is their perceived or actual lack of power. According to Hamilton (1982, p. 14), "Power, or the lack of it, is at the root of all consumer issues." As mentioned earlier in this chapter, the power ratio is unevenly distributed in health care because physicians largely control entry into the system. Consumerism in health care discounts the basic notions held by economists about the role and influence of consumers. According to classic economic theory, consumers create mandates for producers, who then concede to consumer demands. In accordance with this view, in the 1800s W.H. Hutt coined the phrase "consumer sovereign" to describe the power held by consumers in determining the behavior of producers (Hutt, 1936).

For consumer sovereignty to occur the following four conditions must exist (Hamilton, 1982, p. 15):

1. Consumer demand must determine production of goods and provision of services.
2. Consumers must have the information necessary to judge the quality, utility, and safety of products and services.
3. Consumers must choose products and services that give the greatest utility for the lowest prices.
4. Both consumers and providers must have free access to the marketplace.

These conditions do not presently exist in health care. First, demand is not left up to consumers but rather is determined by providers, who decide what services and products are needed and in many instances prescribe them by specific company names. One reason providers retain such control is that consumers have not had sufficient information to make informed choices (the second condition for consumer sovereignty). Only recently have unbiased sources of information become available to consumers. In recent years the U.S. Food and Drug Administration (FDA) has taken an active role in informing consumers about the hazards of health care. Consumers now serve on FDA advisory panels and participate in the review of drugs, diagnostic and treatment devices, and radiological equipment (Hamilton, 1982).

In most other consumer-provider interactions advertising plays a much greater role than it does in health care. Advertising, although biased in many instances toward the product being discussed, does inform consumers about prices, the relative merits of products, and locations for purchase. Health care providers look down on advertising as being "below them." Although advertising would increase competitiveness for products such as eyeglasses and dentures, it probably would not solve the problem of poorly informed consumers. The third condition of consumer sovereignty, which is that consumers spend to get the greatest utility at the lowest price, does not hold true in health care. Because of the fear involved in illness and disability, people do not consistently seek second opinions, negotiate prices, or question the provider's rationale for selecting a proposed treatment. Erroneously, consumers equate quality with high prices. Similarly, because of the fear of a potential malpractice suit, some providers charge far greater fees than others. Consider the dramatically different fee accrued in one hour by a neurosurgeon compared to that of a psychiatrist. People are more willing to pay very high charges for brain surgery than for the examination of emotional problems. Hence, emotions play a significant role in determining health care costs.

The last condition of consumer sovereignty holds that consumers and providers have equal access to the marketplace. In the present health care system, access is largely influenced by physicians and third-party payers. Physicians prescribe and order services, many of which would be otherwise unavailable. In many instances consumer participation in hospital-sponsored health education provided by nurses must be prescribed by physicians. Further, insurance carriers and Medicare and Medicaid influence what services will be reimbursed and at what rate.

What can and should be done to alter the power ratio in health care? Should consumers become more involved in their care and, if so, how do they begin? If one believes in consumer involvement in health, the place to begin is with a recognition of consumer rights. There have been several attempts on the part of providers to draft documents setting forth patient rights. However, consumers *must* assume responsibility for their rights because they have the most to gain if their rights are acknowledged and respected and the most to lose if their rights are ignored or violated. Consumers are entitled to privacy, confidentiality, and self-determination of care as well as effective and compassionate care. Yet these rights are only realized when providers are sincerely committed to client-centered care.

To become participants in the health care system, consumers must become better informed and also gain more power. Consumers, individually and collectively, need to know what choices are available and what are the potential consequences of selecting one rather than the other. Nurses can play a key role in advancing the cause of consumerism by informing clients of their choices, encouraging them to seek additional information, and motivating them to become involved in consumer issues beyond their personal sphere. Consumers can organize groups to promote health care by approaching and enlisting the support of various power groups in the community.

CLINICAL APPLICATION

The goal of community health nursing is to promote and preserve the health of the population. The practice is general and comprehensive and is not limited to a particular age group. As a student or community health nurse it is important for you to guide and direct clients so they can seek the health care services best suited to their needs and resources.

During a well-child clinic you meet a young mother who has recently moved to your community. As you talk to the mother in preparation for giving her child the necessary immunizations for her age level, you learn that the woman's husband is employed by a local company and that his company provides good health care coverage. In fact, employees may choose whether they wish to belong to a well-established and respected HMO in the area or receive health care coverage through the company insurance plan. The insurer is also a large and well-established company. The mother came to the public health clinic because she knew her toddler needed to have the last in a series of immunizations. She did not know what an HMO was and was unable to choose which form of insurance coverage the family should select. She knows that her husband has to make a selection in the first 30 days of employment. Until that time the family is not covered by health insurance.

What factors will influence your nursing intervention with this young woman? Examples might include: 1. You would assess her level of intelligence by the questions she asks and your perception of how well she understands you. In this case, let us assume that the young woman is of average intelligence and able to understand your explanations with no difficulty. 2. You would assess her past experiences with health care providers. What has she liked and disliked previously? 3. You would provide a basic definition of an HMO so that she can make an informed choice. In doing this you would want to be objective and refrain from stating any opinions you may hold about her alternatives. If literature is available about HMOs you could give her a copy. 4. You would reinforce her seeking of health promotion behaviors and commend her for securing health care in a new city when she had little information about what is available. 5. If printed information is available about health services such as physician referrals, nurse practitioners, and hospitals, you might give her that form of assistance.

The aims of your interventions are to encourage the woman to continue in her questioning and data gathering about the health care services in the community; provide accurate, objective information; give the needed services for that visit (i.e., the correct immunization); provide support to a person who is actively seeking to promote the health of the family; and make any referrals that seem appropriate based on your assessment of the child.

SUMMARY

The health care system continues to be criticized for lack of access of services to all people at an affordable cost. Most writers who address the current dilemmas in the health care system contend that major sources of problems originate with cost, availability, and accessibility of services. In many sections of the country, health personnel and resources are poorly distributed. Some urban areas have an abundance of both providers and facilities, whereas people in many rural areas and some inner-city areas have virtually no services available within a reasonable commuting distance.

Critics state that major weaknesses in the health care system can only be overcome by a reshaping of national priorities regarding health care. Although there is no doubt that the United States possesses some of the finest hospitals, health care providers, and health care facilities in the world, there is no question that additional efforts are essential to reshape the system and move from a focus on restoration of health to one of promoting health. As discussed in Chapter 1, community health providers have consistently advocated that it is less costly to prevent illness than to provide adequate treatment once disruption has occurred. However, the study of the cost of preventive measures has been neglected in the past; therefore few statistics support the belief in the cost effectiveness of prevention. Nurses who work in preventive care are in a key position to contribute to research efforts in this much-needed area.

Additionally, changes in the health care system need to recognize that the community itself is a major determinant of the health of its residents. Clean water, adequate sewage disposal, food, heat, and proper personal health practices are major factors in determining the health of the residents. Nursing has a major role to play in the ultimate restructuring of the health care system by continuing to urge communities and other health care providers to focus on health, personal responsibility for health, and a view that takes into account the needs, sources of support, and resources in a given community.

≡ KEY CONCEPTS

Health is a concern of all Americans; it is inextricably linked with all aspects of daily living and is a prerequisite for living a healthy and productive life.

Medical care is a generic term describing the organization, financing, and delivery of health services to individuals; *health care* includes not only treatment of disease but also health promotion and disease prevention.

Health care is one of the largest industries in the United States.

Health promotion focuses on maintaining or enhancing well-being; disease prevention focuses on protection from health threats.

The changes now occurring in the health care system are some of the most dramatic changes in the history of American health care.

Several important trends affecting the health care system are demographical, social, economic, political, and technological trends.

The federal government plays a major role in our health care system by establishing a national health care policy.

Among the major issues related to the health care system are recent challenges to the notion that health care should be available to all regardless of their ability to pay, the rapid growth of health care systems and providers, and competition among for-profit health care providers.

The health care system is composed of consumers, providers, and mechanisms for delivery of health care services. However, the consumer of health care services is a client, not a customer.

Five models of the current health care system are the elementary model, the modified elementary model, the private sector model, the professional model, and the public and private sectors model.

Consumerism is a major movement affecting the health care industry.

Many critics of the present health care industry criticize its orientation toward illness care rather than health maintenance and its structure of several hundred thousand independent and uncoordinated enterprises. Many critics say these weaknesses can only be overcome through a reshaping of priorities regarding health care.

LEARNING ACTIVITIES

1. Describe three health promotion activities that community health nurses should include in their repertoire of skills.

2. If you were asked to plan a program designed for disease prevention in your community, what would you do? Describe a hypothetical process of program planning.

3. If there is an HMO in your community, interview three providers and three consumers to determine what each sees as the advantages and disadvantages of this type of care delivery system.

4. Debate whether consumerism should exist in health care as it exists in the distribution of other products and/or services.

5. Debate the following: The major problem with the health care system is (choose one of the following topics):
Escalating costs
Fragmentation
Inaccessibility

BIBLIOGRAPHY

Andreoli, K.G.: Future directions: organizational settings for practice. In Lancaster, J., and Lancaster, W.: Concepts for advanced nursing practice: the nurse as a change agent, St. Louis, 1982, The C.V. Mosby Co., pp. 316-333.

Andreoli, K.G., and Musser, L.A.: Trends that may affect nursing's future, Nurs. Health Care 6(1):47-51, 1985.

American Nurses' Association: Environmental assessment: factors affecting long-range planning for nursing and health care, Kansas City, Mo., 1985, American Nurses' Association.

Brody, H., and Sobel, D.S.: A systems view of health and disease. In Lee, P.R., Brown, N., and Red, L., editors: The nation's health, San Francisco, 1981, Boyd and Fraser Publishing Co., pp. 27-37.

Bruhn, J.: Personal health in a sustainable society, Appalachian Business Rev. 8(1):29-40, 1981.

Califano, J.A.: America's health care revolution, New York, 1986, Random House, Inc.

Congressional Budget Office: Physician extenders, their current and future role in medical care delivery, Congress of the United States, Washington, D.C., April 1979, U.S. Government Printing Office.

Ellwood, P.M.: Alternative delivery systems: health care on the move, J. Ambulatory Care Management 8(4):1-2, 1985.

Ellwood, P.M., and Herbert, M.E.: Health care: should industry buy or sell?, Harvard Business Rev. 51:99-107, July-Aug. 1973.

Fagin, C.M.: Opening the door on nursing's cost advantage, Nursing and Health Care. 7(7):352-357, 1986.

Federal Register 44:75720, Dec. 21, 1979.

Garfield, S.R.: The delivery of medical care, Sci. Am. 222:15-23, April 1970.

Hamilton, P.A.: Health care consumerism, St. Louis, 1982, The C.V. Mosby Co.

"Health Care in the 1990's: Trends and strategies: Chicago, 1985, Arthur Anderson and American College of Hospital Administrators.

Health: United States, 1979, DHEW Pub. No. (PHS) 80-1232, Washington, D.C., Dec. 1979, Department of Health, Education, and Welfare.

Health: United States, 1980, DHHS Pub. No. (PHS) 81-1232, Washington, D.C., Dec. 1980, Department of Health and Human Services.

Health: United States, 1981, DHHS Pub. No. (PHS) 82-1232, Washington, D.C., Dec. 1981, Department of Health and Human Services.

Hutt, W.H.: Economists and the public, London, 1936, Jonathan Cape Ltd.

Lancaster, W.: Health and health care delivery systems. In Lancaster, J., and Lancaster, W.: Concepts for advanced nursing practice: the nurse as a change agent, St. Louis, 1982, The C.V. Mosby Co. (pp. 175-199.)

Lancaster, W.: A study of primary care physician selection by geographically mobile families. In Smith, S., and Venkatesan, M.: Advances in health care research, Park City, Utah, 1984, Association for consumer research, Health care conference. (pp. 50-55.)

NAQ Forum, Trandel-Korenchuk, K., and Trandel-Korenchuk, D.: Alternative delivery systems, Nurs. Admin. Q. 10(1):61-64, 1985.

National League for Nursing: Health maintenance organization, New York, 1978, The League.

Raffel, M.W.: The U.S. health care system: origins and functions, New York, 1980, John Wiley & Sons.

Roble, D.T., Knowlton, W.A., and Rosenberg, G.A.: Hospital-sponsored preferred provider organizations, Law, Medicine Health Care 12(5):204-209, 1984.

Shindell, S., Salloway, J.C., and Obernabt, C.M.: A coursebook in health care delivery, New York, 1976, Appleton-Century-Crofts.

Stevens, B.J.: Tackling a changing society head on, Nurs. Health Care 6(1):27-30, 1985.

Weil, T.P.: Procompetition or more regulation? Health Care Manag. Rev. 10(3):27-35, 1985.

Wilner, D.M., Walkley, R.P., and O'Neill, E.J.: Introduction to public health, ed. 7, New York, 1978, Macmillan Publishing Co.

World Health Organization: Basic documents, Thirty-sixth edition, Geneva, 1986, WHO.

Marcia Stanhope

3

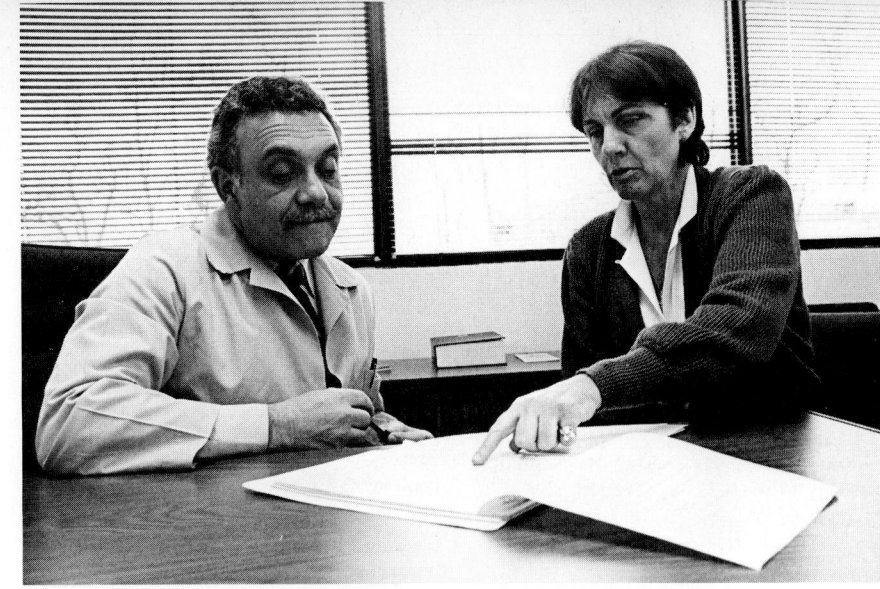

ECONOMICS OF HEALTH CARE DELIVERY

OBJECTIVES

After reading this chapter, the student should be able to:

Define health economics.

Trace the evolution of the components of health care services.

Identify the factors influencing health care economics.

Trace the involvement of government and other third-party payers in health care
financing.

Discuss national health care financing and direct service delivery plans.

Discuss proposed health care financing for the future.

Describe types of cost studies applied in health care delivery.

Analyze the impact of a primary prevention goal on health care economics.

Name the factors affecting health levels.

KEY TERMS

benefit schedule
cost-plus reimbursement
diagnosis-related groups
economics
enabling legislation
fee-screen system
gross national product
    (GNP)

health economics
Health Maintenance
    Organization Act
Medicaid Program
medical technology
medically indigent
Medicare Program
population demography

price inflation
prospective cost
    reimbursement
prospective payment
    system
retrospective cost
    reimbursement
third-party payments

The present health care delivery system, characterized by limited resources, regulatory restrictions, increased technological advances, increased competition, and more emphasis on health care delivery in the community, is unlike the health care delivery system of the 1960s and 1970s, which experienced vast expansions, unlimited financial resources, an open job market, and a nursing discipline that was expanding and broadening its responsibilities and influence.

Because of the present system characteristics, the concerns of the 1990s and the twenty-first century will focus on examining the economics of health care delivery, limiting the continuous growth of the largest employing industry in the United States, and organizing and assigning priorities to the use of available resources at the least cost. Nursing will be concerned with establishing its contribution to the health of the nation and ensuring its economic viability in the market structure as a major contributor in health care delivery.

This chapter provides an overview of the economic issues of the health care delivery system. Discussion focuses on factors influencing health care, schema for financing health care, economics of primary prevention, methods for evaluating health and nursing costs, and the value of human life in health care spending.

DEFINITIONS

To grasp the importance of the economics of health care and its significance to nursing, a basic understanding of key economic terms is essential.

Economics is the social science concerned with the problems of using or administering scarce resources in the most efficient way to attain maximum fulfillment of society's unlimited wants (Heider-Dorneich, 1978). *Health economics* is concerned with the problems of producing and distributing the health care resources of the nation in a way that will provide maximum benefit to the most people.

The *goal* of health economics is maximum benefit, or quality care, from the goods that are produced and supplied by health providers, and demanded and purchased by the consumer. The availability of health goods (services) requires money. The spending of money on health goods limits the benefits derived from other goods available in society, such as food, clothing, shelter, transportation, education, and recreation.

Society must begin to make tough decisions about the allocation of available resources. Today the nation allocates approximately one tenth of the gross national product for health goods. This one tenth represented $387 billion spent in 1984 for health care alone. Health care expenditures are projected to reach $690 billion, or 12% of the gross national product, by 1990.

The *gross national product* (GNP) is defined as the total value of all goods and services produced in the economy in one year (*Health: United States,* 1985; Dombusch and Fischer, 1981). The GNP is an important statistical measure because it is the most comprehensive measure of a nation's total output of goods and services. It is useful for comparing and contrasting expenditures on all of society's benefits, telling us on what we place the most value. The value, or price, of a service is determined by using a U.S. Bureau of Labor Statistics indicator, the consumer price index. The *consumer price index* is a shopping basket approach that compares prices of all consumed goods and services purchased by urban wage earners and clerical workers and their families on a monthly or quarterly basis. The medical care component of the consumer price index compares selected prices of hospital, dental, and pharmaceutical products and services (Health: United States, 1985).

HEALTH SERVICES COMPONENTS

From the 1800s to the 1980s, the U.S. health care delivery system experienced three developmental stages with differing emphasis on health care economics. The health services component framework is used to describe the system's evolution.

Three basic components provide the framework for health services delivery: labor (work force), facilities, and technology. Historically, changes in the three components have occurred as changes have occurred in morbidity, mortality, national health policy, and economic and social forces.

The *first developmental stage* of the health care delivery system occurred during the period 1800 to 1900. As mentioned in Chapter 1, the period was characterized by epidemics of infectious diseases, such as plague, cholera, typhoid, smallpox, influenza, malaria, yellow fever, and gastric disorders. The health problems of the period were related to contaminated food and water supplies, inadequate sewage disposal, and poor housing conditions (Hanlon and Pickett, 1984; Muscovice, 1984; Rushmer, 1984; Torrens, 1984).

Minimal technology was available to aid in disease control. The doctor's black bag contained the few medicines and tools available for health care in the era, and hospitals were characterized by overcrowding, disease, and lack of cleanliness. Since the sick, if cared for in a hospital, usually died because of hospital conditions, most people were cared for at home by family and friends (Lee, 1981; Rushmer, 1984).

During this period the labor force was composed of poorly trained physicians who attained their skills through apprenticeships with practicing physicians. Nurses were typically volunteers recruited from the lower social strata or from religious orders. Their primary focus was to assist the clients with activities of daily living. In 1867 the first nurse training school was established at the New England Hospital for Women and Children to provide formal preparation for nursing in the U.S.; by 1886 organized district nursing (home nursing) had been established (Aiken, 1981; Moscovice, 1984). In this first developmental phase the method of financing was private pay for those who could afford health care, bartering with the physicians, or care provided through charitable contributions from individuals and organizations.

The *second developmental stage* of the health care delivery system, dating from 1900 to 1945, was marked by the control of acute infectious diseases. Environmental conditions began to improve, with major advances in water purification, sanitary sewage disposal, milk and water quality, and urban housing quality. The health problems of the era changed from mass epidemics to individual acute infections or traumatic episodes (Hanlon and Pickett, 1984; Rushmer, 1984; Torrens, 1984).

The workers of the period were better educated. Physician education evolved from apprenticeships to scientifically based college education; the change occurred after the publication of the Flexner Report of 1910. Clinical medicine was in its "golden age" because of major advances in surgery and childbirth, identification of the cause of pernicious anemia, and such technological discoveries as insulin in 1922 for the control of diabetes, sulfa drugs in 1932 for treatment of infectious diseases, and antibiotics such as penicillin in the 1940s (Lee, 1981; Rushmer, 1984).

Nurses of the era were primarily trained in hospital schools of nursing whose goal was to educate nurses in the dependent function of following physicians' orders. Hospitals and health departments were growing in numbers and strength. The public health departments' major emphasis was on quarantine and case finding. These tasks were delegated to the public health nurse. Also, 225 visiting nurse organizations were offering skilled attendance and were focusing on the teaching of cleanliness and the proper care of the sick in the home. Thus health education was identified as a nursing function early in the development of the health care delivery system (Lee, 1981; Rushmer, 1984).

In addition to private and charitable financing of health care, city, county and state governments were beginning to contribute through the provision of hospitals and clinics for the poor, state mental institutions, and other specialized hospitals, such as tuberculosis hospitals.

The *third developmental stage,* from 1945 to 1984, has shown a shift away from acute infectious health problems and a shift toward chronic health problems such as heart disease, cancer, and stroke. Table 3-1 provides a comparison of the leading causes of mortality from 1900 to 1984. With decreasing infant mortality and increasing life expectancy, chronic illnesses resulting from environmental and lifestyle influences promise to be the major health threats of the twenty-first century.

Major technological advances of the era have included the development of chemotherapeutic agents, immunological prophylaxis, advances in anesthesia, advances in electrolyte and cardiopulmonary physiology, expansion of diagnostic laboratories and complex equipment such as the CT scan, organ and tissue transplants, radiation therapy,

TABLE 3-1

Leading causes of death in the United States, 1900 and 1984

Cause	Death rate per 100,000 population
1900	
Influenza and pneumonia	202.2
Tuberculosis	194.4
Diarrhea and enteritis	139.9
Heart disease	137.4
Cerebral hemorrhage	106.9
Nephritis	88.7
Accidents	72.3
Cancer	64.0
Diseases of early infancy	62.6
Diphtheria	40.3
Simple meningitis	33.8
Typhoid and paratyphoid	31.3
All causes	1719.1
1984	
Heart diseases	326.0
Malignant neoplasms	187.2
Cerebrovascular accidents	68.0
Accidents	40.6
Chronic obstructive pulmonary disease	25.8
Influenza and pneumonia	21.1
Diabetes mellitus	14.9
Suicide	12.2
Liver cirrhosis	11.9
Arteriosclerosis	11.6
Homicide	9.6
Diseases of early infancy	9.0
All causes	852.0

specialty units for critical care, coronary care, and intensive care. The numbers and kinds of health service facilities have increased; health care providers constitute more than 5% of the total U.S. work force. Table 3-2 shows the increase in the number of people employed in the health industry from 1970 through 1984. The three largest employers over the 14-year period have been hospitals, convalescent institutions, and physician's offices. Between 1970 and 1984 the number of persons employed in the health care industry grew by 90%, from 4.2 to 7.9 million. After a slight decline, the numbers of personnel employed in "other sites," such as the community, are on the increase.

Before 1940 there were fewer than 40 titles for health care providers; in 1985 the number of identifiable titles, as reported by the U.S. Department of Labor, had risen to more than 700. The increase in specialization has led to changes in certification, qualifications, education, and standards of care in each professional area. The combination of these factors has contributed to the increased number and kinds of providers to meet the demands of the health care system. As of 1985, there were approximately 500,000 physicians and 1.5 million nurses in the United States providing health care services to a population of 240 million. Of the practicing nurses, approximately 6.6% were employed in areas of community health. The total represents approximately 190 physicians per 100,000 population and 600 registered nurses per 100,000 population. Since 1970 the physician population has grown by 35% and the nurse population by 63%.

During this third developmental stage the system has appeared to have unlimited resources for growth and expansion. The period has been marked by the introduction of the health insurance industry and substantial growth of the federal government's role in financing health care.

Since 1984 the health care delivery system has been entering a *fourth developmental stage,* one of increasingly limited resources, restricted growth, and a reorganization of methods of financing and care delivery (Torrens, 1984). This stage is forcing health care providers to be more introspective, to look at alternatives and options to the unlimited resources, growth, and services of previous decades. With substantial federal health policy changes, emphasis in health care delivery is slowly moving toward increased health care delivery in the community and increased emphasis on preventive health care.

The health care provider must be aware of the possibility of a shift in types of health and illness problems in the fourth stage. A shift backward toward increases in communicable, infectious, and environmental illnesses may be the plight of the future.

FACTORS INFLUENCING THE ECONOMICS OF HEALTH CARE

Three major factors have been instrumental in influencing the growth of the health care delivery system throughout history: price inflation, technology, and changes in population demography.

Price Inflation

Price inflation was the major economic problem between 1960 and 1980. General inflation affected the prices of all goods and services in the nation, including health care costs,

---

TABLE 3-2

Persons employed in selected health service sites, according to place of employment in United States for selected years from 1970 to 1984*

Place of employment	Number of persons in thousands								
	1970†	1975	1978	1979	1980	1981	1982	1983	1984
Total	4,246	5,945	6,798	6,990	7,339	7,617	7,810	7,874	7,934
Offices of physicians	477	618	771	775	777	811	898	888	896
Offices of dentists	222	331	366	392	415	423	415	441	468
Offices of chiropractors‡	19	30	33	36	40	46	53	54	61
Hospitals	2,690	3,441	3,854	3,925	4,036	4,186	4,341	4,348	4,288
Convalescent institutions	509	891	1,020	1,048	1,199	1,230	1,217	1,342	1,362
Other health service sites	330	634	754	814	872	921	886	800	859

Data from U.S. Bureau of the Census: 1970 census of population, occupation by industry, Final report PC(2)-7C, Washington, D.C., 1972, U.S. Government Printing Office; U.S. Bureau of Labor Statistics: Labor force statistics derived from the current population survey: a databook, vol. 1, Washington, D.C., 1982, U.S. Government Printing Office; Employment and earnings, 31(1), 32(1), 1984, 1985, U.S. Government Printing Office; Unpublished data, American Chiropractic Association.

*Data are based on household interviews of a sample of the civilian noninstitutionalized population. Totals exclude persons in health-related occupations who are working in nonhealth industries, as classified by the U.S. Bureau of the Census, such as pharmacists employed in drugstores, school nurses, and nurses working in private households. Totals include federal, state, and county health workers.

†April 1, derived from decennial census; all other data years are annual averages from the Current Population Survey.

‡Data for 1978-1982 are from the American Chiropractic Association; data for the preceding years and 1983 and 1984 are from the U.S. Bureau of Labor Statistics.

TABLE 3-3

National health expenditures and percent distribution, according to type of expenditure, in United States for selected years from 1950 to 1984*

Type of expenditure	1950	1960	1965	1970	1975	1980	1982	1983	1984
AMOUNT IN BILLIONS									
Total	$12.7	$26.9	$41.9	$75.0	$132.7	$247.5	$321.2	$355.1	$387.4
PERCENT DISTRIBUTION									
All expenditures	100.0	100.0	100.0	100.0	100.0	100.0	100.0	100.0	100.0
Health services and supplies	92.4	93.6	91.6	92.8	93.7	95.2	95.6	95.7	95.9
Personal health care	86.0	88.0	85.5	87.1	88.3	88.5	88.7	88.8	88.2
Hospital care	30.4	33.8	33.3	37.3	39.5	40.9	41.9	41.9	40.8
Physician services	21.7	21.1	20.2	19.1	18.8	18.9	19.2	19.3	19.5
Dentist services	7.6	7.4	6.7	6.3	6.2	6.2	6.1	6.1	6.5
Nursing home care	1.5	2.0	4.9	6.3	7.6	8.2	8.4	8.3	8.3
Other professional services	3.1	3.2	2.5	2.1	2.0	2.3	2.2	2.3	2.3
Drugs and drug sundries	13.6	13.6	12.4	10.7	9.0	7.5	6.8	6.7	6.7
Eyeglasses and appliances	3.9	2.9	2.8	2.6	2.4	2.1	1.7	1.8	1.9
Other health services	4.2	4.0	2.7	2.8	2.8	2.4	2.4	2.4	2.4
Expenses for prepayment	3.6	4.1	4.2	3.8	3.0	3.7	4.0	4.1	4.9
Government public health activities	2.9	1.5	1.9	1.9	2.4	2.9	2.9	2.8	2.8
Research and construction	7.6	6.4	8.4	7.2	6.3	4.8	4.4	4.3	4.1
Research	0.9	2.5	3.6	2.6	2.5	2.2	1.8	1.7	1.8
Construction	6.7	3.9	4.8	4.6	3.8	2.6	2.6	2.6	2.3

From Levit, K.R., Lazanby, H., Waldo, D.R., and Davidoff, L.M.: National health expenditures, 1984, Health Care Financing Review, HCFA Pub. No. 03200, Washington, D.C., Fall 1985, U.S. Government Printing Office.

*The Health Care Financing Administration has made revisions in their health expenditure estimates. Data in this table may differ from those appearing in earlier volumes of *Health, United States.*

which increased approximately 12% faster than the consumer price index.

Table 3-3 depicts the changes in money spent for health care from 1950 to 1984. Note that Table 3-3 shows a rise in health care expenditures from $12.7 billion in 1950 to $387.4 billion in 1984. While the population has increased by 58% over this 34-year-period, health care costs have increased by 3000%. Health services and supplies accounted for 92% to 95% of the total costs, whereas construction costs decreased from 6.7% to 2.3%. Research costs accounted for a mere 0.9%, increasing to 2.2% in 1980 and dropping again to 1.8% in 1984.

In the early 1980s inflation began to decline. In 1984 with the decline in prices for other goods and services came the lowest annual increase in health care prices since 1960. Nevertheless, hospital services continued to increase at twice the overall inflation rate. During these years hospitals and physicians have been the two major recipients of health care expenditures, whereas government-sponsored public health programs have received less than 3% of the total health care dollars. Inflation in health care delivery remains the dominant factor in health economic issues today. While the slowdown in price increases, especially in hospital care, may be attributed to the new *prospective payment system* (see p. 54) a number of assumptions have been made regarding reasons for price inflation in health care delivery:

1. Rising income and the growth of insurance have increased use of the system and the demand for new services.
2. Expenditures are rising in response to increased hospital wages and lagging employee productivity in the hospital industry.
3. New and costlier methods of care force prices up.
4. Prices rise because of capital investment in costly, expensive-to-maintain facilities that already exist in sufficient supply.
5. Increases in supply, equipment, and salary expenditures have occurred with the growth and the number of insurance plans reimbursing at cost.
6. Changes in consumer lifestyles and environmental hazards have created a new set of health problems that require services.
7. Comprehensive health insurance encourages increased utilization.

8. Discontinuation of the federal Economic Stabilization Program resulted in increased prices as a way of making up for increases that may have been lost in the price controls of the 1970s (Health: United States, 1985; Joel, 1985; Richardson, 1984).

Although all factors mentioned have contributed to inflation in health care costs, some have had more effect than others. The availability of insurance to cover health care costs and the development of new and costlier methods of health care technology appear to be the major contributors to increased costs. To the extent that new categories of health care personnel have been introduced into the system, such as nurse practitioners, physician's assistants, and dental technicians, increased wages have contributed to increased costs. The increased numbers of health care facilities and the vast duplication of services offered have contributed to the need for more employees, supplies, and equipment, and thus to increased costs through the 34-year-period. However, some change is occurring. For example, although hospitals have been the single largest employer of health personnel in the United States, accounting for the largest increase in employment, in 1984 the number of hospital employees had declined. As changes in health care reimbursement schemes occur, shifts in personnel distribution from hospital to community may be expected. The effects of today's trends in health care delivery on price inflation remain to be seen.

Technology

Medical technology has been defined by the Congressional Office of Technology Assessment as "the set of techniques, drugs, equipment, and procedures used by health care professionals in delivering medical care to individuals and the system within which such care is delivered" (Health: United States, 1978). Included in any discussion of costs of technology is the cost of use of technology.

Health care professionals, such as physicians, have become dependent on technology for diagnosis and treatment and have become the principal purchasing agents of technology for the client. The population, with an increasing sophistication about health and health care needs, demands the use of laboratory, radiological, diagnostic, palliative, and therapeutic services for treatment.

One of the most significant examples of new technology contributing to increasing cost is renal dialysis. After a 1972 congressional amendment to the Social Security Act extended Medicare coverage to pay for renal dialysis, approximately 16,000 people received care under this program at a cost of $250 million. By 1979 costs had risen to $1 billion for 51,000 clients. Costs were projected to reach $2.8 billion by 1986.

As new and more complex technology is introduced into the system, the trend toward increasing use and cost is evident. For example, between 1979 and 1983 there was a 400% increase in CT scans performed on nonfederal short-stay hospital inpatients. The rate of ultrasound diagnostic procedures tripled, and intraocular lens transplants increased by 66% (Health: United States, 1985).

Renal dialysis programs and other new technology place a demand on institutions for personnel and investments in

---

EXAMPLES OF FEDERAL REGULATORY MECHANISMS CONTRIBUTING TO TECHNOLOGY COSTS/CONTROL

1906 Prescription drug regulation passes—Food, Drug, and Cosmetic Act

1938 Manufacturers required to prove drug safety—Food, Drug, and Cosmetic Act

1952 Hill-Burton Act provides construction monies and requires a specified volume of "free care" in exchange

1962 Manufacturers required to prove drug efficacy—Food, Drug, and Cosmetic Act

1965 Amendments to Social Security Act providing Medicare and Medicaid result in increased use of technologies

1972 Social Security Act amendments extending coverage for end-stage renal disease provide payment for use of treatment technologies

1972 Social Security Act amendments provide for Professional Standards Review Organizations to review appropriateness of hospital care for Medicare and Medicaid recipients

1974 Health Planning and Resources Development Act introduces certificate-of-need authority to limit major capital expenditures at local and state levels

1976 Medical Devices Amendments regulates safety and effectiveness of medical equipment, such as pacemakers

1978 Medicare End-Stage Renal Disease Amendment provides for home dialysis and for kidney transplantation

1978 Health Services Research, Health Statistics, and Health Care Technology Act establishes a national council on health care technology to develop standards, criteria, and norms for the use of particular medical technologies

1982 Tax Equity and Fiscal Responsibilities Act establishes prospective payment system providing lump sum payment for hospitalized medicare patients by DRG category.

---

equipment and facilities, and they add to administrative costs, especially when the federal government is involved in the financing and regulating of the technology. The boxed material on this page lists a few federal regulatory mechanisms that have contributed to the control and cost of technology.

Changes in Population Demography

The third major contributor to rising health care costs is the changing *population demography*. Table 3-4 depicts the present distribution of the three factors affecting increased costs of health care delivery from 1965 to 1984. One can see that population has been a significant third contributor after inflation and technology. In 1965 prices and intensity had similar effects on health care costs. In 1973 the effects of inflation began to outdistance all other factors influencing health care expenditures, and in 1984 prices contributed 76% to the growth of all health care expenditures.

Between 1970 and 1983 the number of people in the United States aged 15 and under began to decline, and the number of people aged 65 and over increased. These data suggest an aging population with increased health risks. Projections indicate that the population of the United States

TABLE 3-4

Average annual percent change in personal health care expenditures and percent distribution of factors affecting growth in United States from 1965 to 1984*

Period	Average annual percent change	Percent distribution of factors affecting growth			
		All factors	Prices	Population	Intensity†
1965-1984	12.6	100	61	8	31
1965-1966	10.6	100	45	12	43
1966-1967	12.2	100	54	8	38
1967-1968	13.1	100	44	8	48
1968-1969	13.4	100	41	8	51
1969-1970	14.5	100	47	8	45
1970-1971	10.4	100	59	12	29
1971-1972	11.6	100	38	9	53
1972-1973	10.5	100	42	9	49
1973-1974	14.0	100	66	6	28
1974-1975	15.4	100	71	6	23
1975-1976	13.4	100	67	7	26
1976-1977	12.3	100	67	8	25
1977-1978	12.2	100	68	9	23
1978-1979	13.3	100	72	8	20
1979-1980	15.6	100	73	8	19
1980-1981	15.6	100	75	6	19
1981-1982	12.4	100	78	7	15
1982-1983	10.1	100	67	9	24
1983-1984	8.5	100	76	11	13

*Data are compiled by the Health Care Financing Administration. The Health Care Financing Administration has made revisions in their health expenditure estimates. Data in this table may differ from those appearing in earlier volumes of *Health, United States.*
†Represents changes in use and/or kinds of services and supplies.

will increase to 260 million people by the year 2000 and that death rates will continue to decline. The population had already reached 240 million by 1984, and the crude death rate had declined from 963.8 per 100,000 people in 1950 to 866.8 per 100,000 people in 1984. Projected age-specific population data for the year 2000 suggest there will be a decrease in ages 0 to 24, a slight increase in the age groups 25 to 64, and 58% more people in the 65-plus age group than in 1970.

The population 75 years and older is projected to increase four times faster than the average annual rate for persons under 65 years of age. This is expected to lead to pressure to spend more money, especially for long-term care. Table 3-5 gives population data by age group from 1950 to 1983.

Data indicate the major increases have been in health care expenditures for the elderly population, whereas the least expenditures have been for people under 19 years of age. Since the Social Security Amendments of 1965, the rate of Medicare expenditures for health care for the elderly has been greater than the rate of increased expenditures for the remainder of the population. Reasons for the increased rate of expenditures are the rapid growth of the numbers

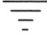

TABLE 3-5

Population data, in millions, for selected age groups from 1950 to 1983

Age (years)	1950	1970	1983
Under 15	40.4	57.9	51.6
15-24	22.0	35.4	40.7
25-44	45.2	47.9	69.5
45-64	30.8	41.9	44.6
65 and over	11.1	20.0	27.4

of elderly in the United States, the increased number of elderly women who are heavier users of health services than men, the decline in family social support requiring the elderly to seek care and assistance outside the family structure, the increase in surgery rates, the greater use of more complex medical and surgical services, and the increased ability of the elderly to pay for services received.

TABLE 3-6

Personal health care expenditures and percent distribution, according to source of payment in
United States for selected years from 1929 to 1984*

Year	Total in billions†	Per capita	All sources	Direct payment	Private health insurance	Philanthropy and industry	Government Total	Government Federal	Government State and local
1929	$ 3.2	$ 26	100.0	88.4‡	§	2.6	9.0	2.7	6.3
1935	2.7	21	100.0	82.4‡	§	2.8	14.7	3.4	11.3
1940	3.5	26	100.0	81.3‡	§	2.6	16.1	4.1	12.0
1950	10.9	70	100.0	65.5	9.1	2.9	22.4	10.4	12.0
1955	15.7	93	100.0	58.1	16.1	2.8	23.0	10.5	12.5
1960	23.7	129	100.0	54.9	21.1	2.3	21.8	9.3	12.5
1965	35.9	177	100.0	51.6	24.2	2.2	22.0	10.1	11.9
1970	65.4	305	100.0	40.5	23.4	1.7	34.3	22.2	12.1
1971	72.2	333	100.0	38.9	23.8	1.8	35.5	23.2	12.3
1972	80.5	368	100.0	38.0	23.6	2.5	35.8	23.5	12.3
1973	89.0	403	100.0	37.4	24.0	2.5	36.1	23.7	12.4
1974	101.3	455	100.0	35.7	24.8	1.5	38.0	25.4	12.6
1975	117.1	522	100.0	32.5	26.7	1.3	39.5	26.8	12.7
1976	132.8	586	100.0	31.6	28.3	1.4	38.7	27.2	11.5
1977	149.1	653	100.0	31.1	28.8	1.3	38.7	27.4	11.3
1978	167.4	725	100.0	30.3	29.3	1.2	39.2	27.7	11.5
1979	189.7	813	100.0	29.4	30.0	1.2	39.3	28.1	11.2
1980	219.1	929	100.0	28.5	30.7	1.2	39.6	28.5	11.1
1981	253.4	1,063	100.0	27.9	31.1	1.2	39.8	29.3	10.5
1082	284.9	1,184	100.0	27.1	31.9	1.2	39.8	29.5	10.3
1983	315.2	1,297	100.0	27.4	31.8	1.2	39.6	29.5	10.1
1984	341.8	1,394	100.0	27.9	31.3	1.2	39.6	29.6	10.0

From Levit, K.R., Lazanby, H., Waldo, D.R., and Davidoff, L.M.: National health expenditures, 1984, Health Care Financing Review, HCFA Pub. No. 03200, Washington, D.C., Fall 1985, U.S. Government Printing Office.
*Data are compiled by the Health Care Financing Administration. The Health Care Financing Administration has made revisions in their health expenditure estimates. Data in this table may differ from those appearing in earlier volumes of *Health, United States.*
†Includes all expenditures for health services and supplies other than expenses for prepayment and administration and government public health activities.
‡Includes any insurance benefits and expenses for prepayment (insurance premiums less insurance benefits).
§Figures are not separable from direct payment.

FINANCING OF HEALTH CARE

Health care financing has evolved through the twentieth century from a system primarily financed by the consumer to a system primarily financed by third-party payers. Table 3-6 shows changes in the percentage of financing for the consumer, the government, and private third-party payers from 1929 to 1984. From 1950 to 1984, direct consumer payment has decreased by 38%, philanthropic payments have decreased by 1.7%, and third-party governmental and private insurance payments have increased by 39%. The combined state and federal governments' contributions have been higher than those of private payers; the federal government's contribution has been similar to the contribution of the private payers. In 1984 all third-party payers contributed 72% toward the total cost of health care for the consumer.

Government Payments

The federal government became involved in health care financing for population segments early in U.S. history. As mentioned in Chapter 1, in 1798 the federal government created the Marine Hospital Service to provide medical service for sick and disabled sailors and to protect the nation's borders against importation of disease through the seaports. The Marine Hospital Service is considered the first national health insurance plan in the United States. The original plan cost each sailor 20¢ per month in a payroll deduction for illness care. The average monthly cost for private health insurance today is $70 per individual, and Medicare enrollees pay $19 per month.

The National Health Board was established in 1879. The board was later renamed the United States Public Health Service (USPHS). Under the aegis of the USPHS, the federal government developed a public health liaison with state and local health departments for the purpose of controlling communicable diseases and improving sanitation. Additional health programs were also developed to meet obligations to federal beneficiaries, including American Indians (Indian Health Service), the armed forces (Department of Defense), and veterans of wars (Veterans Administration).

Today the federal government is involved in health care research, training, financing, and delivery and provides money for four aspects of public health: (1) broad national health interests; (2) special groups, such as mothers, infants, and the aged; (3) special problems or programs, such as food and drugs; and (4) international health.

See Appendix G for an overview of the major historical events depicting the federal government's increasing involvement in financing health care delivery.

Third-Party Payments

Medical insurance in the private sector was first offered in 1847 by a commercial insurance company. The purpose of the insurance was to defray financial losses from disability attributable to accidents. Sickness benefits were later attached to the accident policies as cash payments for income losses caused by specific catastrophic communicable diseases, such as smallpox and scarlet fever.

A comprehensive study in the 1920s by the Committee on the Costs of Medical Care showed that a small portion of the population was paying most of the costs of medical care for the majority of the people. The Depression, rising medical costs, and the need to spread financial risk across communities spurred the development of the *third-party payment* system.

The system began as a major industry in the 1930s with the Blue Cross system, which initially provided prepayment for hospital care. It was modeled on the Baylor University prepayment plan to provide teachers with hospital coverage, established in 1929.

In 1939 Blue Shield plans to provide physician payment were started. The Blue Cross plans began as taxfree, nonprofit organizations established under special *enabling legislation* in various states. In the 1940s and 1950s major growth in inpatient hospital and medical-surgical coverage occurred. Employee group coverage appeared and profit-making commercial insurance underwriters began offering health insurance packages with competitive premiums.

The commercial insurance companies could offer lower premium rates because of the methods used to set rates. Whereas Blue Cross used a *community rate,* establishing a similar premium rate for all subscribers regardless of illness risk, the commercial companies used an *experience rate* in which the premium paid by a subscriber was based on an estimate of the risk of claims by the subscriber.

The premium competition, the popularity of health insurance packages as a fringe benefit, and the use of health insurance as a negotiable collective bargaining item led to increased numbers of covered benefits, payment of higher portions of inpatient and outpatient expenses, and increased employer-paid premiums. These factors led to higher premium costs, higher health care costs, and plans that could not economically cover high-risk segments of the population such as the aged, poor, and disabled.

Needs of the high-risk population segments led to passage of Medicare and Medicaid legislation to provide these groups with health care coverage. Medicare, Medicaid, and other national health programs were authorized for specific population segments. In addition to federal regulations, insurance companies' reimbursement methods are a contributing factor to increased technological costs. These methods discourage physicians, hospital managers, and clients from making cost-effective decisions regarding the use of medical technology. Three reimbursement methods have been commonly used to pay agencies for health goods and services:

1. *Cost-plus reimbursement:* an agency was reimbursed for actual costs plus added allowable costs, such as depreciation of facilities and equipment and administrative costs.
2. *Retrospective cost reimbursement:* an agency was reimbursed per unit of service, an agreed-on price usually predetermined by the state insurance departments or departments of health.
3. *Prospective cost reimbursement:* an attempt was made by agencies and insurance companies to predict, using previous experience and current rates, what an agency's cost would be for the coming year. The agency planned an annual budget with projected goals for service units. The insurance company reimbursed the agency before provision of service.

Positive and negative incentives were built into the reimbursement system. The cost-plus reimbursement scheme encouraged agencies to add depreciation and administrative costs that may inflate actual service costs for the budgetary period. The retrospective cost reimbursement method encouraged agencies to pad unit cost prices to cover unexpected cost increases for purchased goods and services during the budgetary period. The prospective cost reimbursement scheme encouraged agencies to stay within budget limits and added an incentive for providing less service units to contain or reduce costs. In 1983 the government instituted prospective reimbursement for the Medicare program. The new hospital payment scheme has reversed the financial incentives away from the provision of more care and the use of more technology to the provision of less hospital care.

Most public agencies operate on an annual budget and plan for costs by estimating salaries, expenses, and costs of inputs for a budgetary period. Public agencies receive primary funding from tax revenues with additional reimbursement for select goods and services through private third-party payers. As health care costs have increased and as cost reduction has become the key issue, prospective cost reimbursement and projected annual budgeting for the next fiscal year is the trend of the future for the private sector, as it is now for public agencies.

Along with agency reimbursement, physician reimbursement is a key factor in the use and cost of technology. The two primary methods for fee-for-service physician reimbursement are:

1. *Benefit schedule:* a list of physician services with monetary or unit values attached by third-party payers that specifies the amount third parties must pay for specific services.
2. *Fee screen system:* the usual, customary, and reasonable charge (UCR) that allows physicians to set their own reimbursement levels for units of service. The UCR is based on a regional evaluation of physician charges in all specialities. The evaluation provides for the establishing of a maximum reimbursement limit on units of service by third parties.

According to Lee (1981), the fee-for-service reimbursement schemes have been shown to be inflationary. The numbers and kinds of services provided a client are physician controlled, and as third-party reimbursement increases, physicians' fees increase. The consumer has the burden to cover the costs over and above the third-party coverage. Negative experience with fee-for-service physician reimbursement and the inflationary nature of the system may impede progress toward third-party reimbursement for other health care providers, such as nurses.

The third-party pay system is often blamed for rising health care costs. To summarize, many reasons are cited for the relationship between third-party payment system and increasing costs:

1. The cost-plus reimbursement scheme previously used to pay hospital care for Medicare-Medicaid and Blue Cross clients provided little incentive to hold costs down.
2. The third-party payers provided better coverage for the more expensive hospital services than for ambulatory care, home health care, or nursing home care, thus encouraging consumer use of hospitals.
3. Consumer demand for services has increased and incentives to use less costly services have been lacking since government or private insurers pay most hospital and physician bills.
4. The usual, customary, and reasonable (UCR) charge pay system provides physicians with incentive to charge all clients maximum fees so they can boost the UCR charge schedule.
5. The number of unnecessary operations and other tests performed and use of other technology increase because third parties will pay.

Health care costs have been rising faster than the cost of goods and services generally.

Consumer Payments

As previously indicated, direct out-of-pocket payment by the consumer had declined through 1983 with a slight increase for the years 1983 and 1984. Before 1930 and the beginning of Blue Cross, the consumer had more influence over health care costs because nearly all health bills were paid out-of-pocket.

However, the health care system has always been a sellers' market. In a sellers' market all goods and services are provided and controlled by the physician once the buyer, the client, makes the decision to enter the health care market. When the health care system was economically controlled by the consumer market, it restricted entrance into the system to those who could afford to pay or to those few who could find care financed by charitable and philanthropic organizations.

After 1930, with more third-party and government contributions to the health care bill, health care costs increased, quality of care efforts became greater, and consumer demand and availability of services increased. Today the consumer pays directly approximately 40% of all physician fees and 10% of all hospital bills. However, these figures do not reflect the amount of money the consumer pays in taxes to finance government-supported programs such as Medicare and Medicaid, the insurance premiums that come from wages and therefore decrease the size of paychecks, or the direct insurance premiums paid for supplemental insurance to plug the gaps in the primary health insurance policy and in Medicare.

Consumer demands have increased and strengthened benefits of private health insurance packages, the numbers of government programs available to the aged and poor, and the availability and accessibility of health care services. These consumer demands have contributed to health care inflation and are causing a financial drain on the economic potential of the individual.

NATIONAL HEALTH CARE PLANS

The *Medicare Program,* Title XVIII of the Social Security Act of 1965, provides hospital insurance, Part A, and medical insurance, Part B, to the elderly, to the permanently and totally disabled, and to people with end-stage renal disease (*Health: United States,* 1985).

The hospital insurance package, Part A, is available to the entire elderly population without cost if the individual has paid Social Security taxes. Part A of Medicare provides payment for hospital services, home health services, and extended care facilities. Part A includes an annual deductible that is based on a rate equal to a 1-day stay in the hospital. The deductible has increased over the years as daily hospital costs have increased; it was $520 in 1987. Estimates indicate that 98% of the elderly population are covered by Part A.

The medical insurance package, Part B, is available to all people who wish to pay a monthly premium for the coverage. The premium cost was $17.90 per month in 1987. Part B of Medicare provides coverage for other than hospital services, such as physician services, outpatient hospital care, outpatient physical therapy and speech therapy, home health care, laboratory services, ambulance transportation, prostheses, equipment, and some supplies. After a small deductible, up to 80% of reasonable charges are paid for these services. Part B resembles major medical insurance coverage of private insurance carriers. Approximately 96% of the elderly population are covered by Part B of Medicare. Table 3-7 shows the increasing cost of the Medicare program from 1967 to 1984.

Since the passage of the Medicare amendments to the Social Security Act in 1965, the cost of Medicare has increased dramatically. Hospital care continues to be the major factor contributing to Medicare costs and has prompted

TABLE 3-7

Medicare expenditures and percent distribution, according to type of service, in United States for selected years from 1967 to 1984*

Type of service	1967	1970	1975	1980	1982	1983	1984†
AMOUNT IN BILLIONS							
All expenditures	$4.5	$7.1	$15.6	$35.7	$51.1	$57.4	$63.1
PERCENT DISTRIBUTION							
All services	100.0	100.0	100.0	100.0	100.0	100.0	100.0
Hospital care	69.1	71.5	73.8	72.6	72.1	70.6	70.4
Physician services	24.7	22.8	21.6	22.1	22.3	23.3	23.1
Nursing home care	4.6	3.7	1.9	1.1	0.9	0.9	0.9
Other health services‡	1.6	1.9	2.8	4.1	4.7	5.2	5.6

*Data compiled by the Health Care Financing Administration.
†Preliminary estimates.
‡Other services include home health agencies, home health services, eyeglasses and appliances, and other professional services.

many debates about control of the spiraling costs of the program. As a result of the increasing costs, in 1983 Congress passed a law that radically changed Medicare's method of payment for hospital services. The Social Security amendments of 1983 (PL 98-21) mandated an end to cost-plus reimbursement by Medicare and instituted a 3-year transition to a *prospective payment system (PPS)* for inpatient hospital services. Reimbursement is based on a fixed price per case for clients in 468 *diagnosis-related groups (DRGs).* The objective of this system is to reduce hospital costs while maintaining an acceptable level of quality and health care access. Although this type of reimbursement is currently for hospitals only, debates continue about using prospective payment for physicians, home health, long-term care, and ambulatory care as well.

The *Medicaid program,* Title XIX of the Social Security Act of 1965, provides financial assistance to states and counties to pay for medical services to the aged poor, the blind, the disabled, and families with dependent children. The Medicaid program is jointly sponsored and financed with matching funds from the federal and state governments.

Full payment for four types of service was provided originally: (1) inpatient and outpatient hospital care; (2) laboratory and radiological services; (3) physician services; and (4) skilled nursing care, at home or in a nursing home, for people over 21. The 1972 Social Security Amendments added family planning to the list of full-pay services. Prescriptions, dental services, eyeglasses, intermediate facilities care, and coverage for the *medically indigent* are allowable program options. By law the medically indigent are required to pay a monthly premium.

Any state participating in the Medicaid program is required to provide the five basic services to participants who are below state poverty income levels. The optional programs are provided at the discretion of each state. Federal government reorganization of the Medicaid program in the 1980s may include a requirement for states to begin prospective payment systems in their Medicaid programs to reduce costs. Table 3-8 indicates the increased cost of the Medicaid program from 1967 to 1984. In contrast to Medicare, the major contributor to costs in the Medicaid program has been nursing home care; with hospital care, it accounts for 76% of all costs to the program. See Table 3-9 for a comparison of Medicare and Medicaid programs.

The *military medical care system* is another federal program providing health care and insurance to a population group—military personnel and their dependents. This program is described as a "well organized system of high-quality health care provided at no direct cost to the recipient" (Torrens, 1984, p. 23).

With Medicare and Medicaid, the federal government purchases goods and services for population segments through existing health care systems. With the military medical care system, the government is in the health care business, providing military personnel with health care wherever they are located. This health care system has several important characteristics: (1) the system is all-inclusive and ever-present; (2) coverage is effective at all times; (3) prevention, early case finding, and health promotion are emphasized; and (4) dependents and families are served by a subsystem that combines military and civilian health services (Torrens, 1984).

The Civilian Health and Medical Program of the Uniformed Services (CHAMPUS) allows families and dependents to purchase private sector care if service is unavailable in the military system. The program is provided, financed, and supervised by the military system. In 1981 the CHAMPUS Program began direct, independent reimbursement of nurse practitioners and physician assistants for services to military dependents.

The *Veterans Administration health care system,* linked to the military health care system, is operated within the United States for retired, disabled, and other specified categories of military service veterans. The system has a hospital orientation. The system, comprising 171 hospitals and more than 200 outpatient departments, is one part of a benefit package received by veterans. Eligibility for health care is often tied to other financial benefits within the system structure.

TABLE 3-8

Medicaid expenditures and percent distribution, according to type of service, in United States for selected years from 1967 to 1984*

Type of Service	1967	1970	1975	1980	1982	1983	1984†
AMOUNT IN BILLIONS							
All expenditures	$2.9	$5.2	$13.5	$25.2	$31.3	$34.0	$36.7
PERCENT DISTRIBUTION							
All services	100.0	100.0	100.0	100.0	100.0	100.0	100.0
Hospital care	42.3	42.9	35.3	38.1	37.6	38.0	38.3
Physician services	10.9	13.3	13.9	9.7	8.9	8.6	8.4
Dentist services	4.4	3.2	2.7	2.0	1.5	1.4	1.3
Other professional services	0.9	1.4	1.8	2.2	2.1	2.2	2.3
Drugs and drug sundries	7.2	7.9	6.6	5.5	5.4	5.5	5.6
Nursing home care	31.7	27.2	35.6	38.8	39.5	38.4	37.9
Other health services‡	2.6	4.1	4.1	3.7	5.0	5.9	6.3

From Levit, K.R., Lazanby, H., Waldo, D.R., and Davidoff, L.M.: National health expenditures, 1984, Health Care Financing Review, HCFA Pub. No. 03200, Washington, D.C., Fall 1985, U.S. Government Printing Office.
*Data compiled from state and federal government sources. Medicaid expenditures from federal, state, and local funds under Medicaid. Includes per capita payments for Part B of Medicare and excludes administrative costs.
†Preliminary estimates.
‡Other services include laboratory and radiological services, home health, and family planning services.

TABLE 3-9

Comparison of Medicare and Medicaid programs

Feature	Medicare	Medicaid
Obtain information	Social Security Office	Welfare Office
Recipients	Persons aged 65 + ; disabled under 65 eligible after 2 years	Needy and low income, persons aged 65 +, blind, disabled, families with dependent children, some other children
Type of program	Insurance	Assistance
Government affiliation	Federal	Federal/state partnership
Availability	All states	All states
Hospital insurance	Financed by working persons' payroll contributions	Financed by federal and state government
Medical insurance	Monthly premiums paid by recipients (25%) and federal government (75%)	Federal and state government
Types of coverage	Inpatient and outpatient hospital care Posthospital skilled nursing facility Home health care Physician services Medical services and supplies Hospice care	Inpatient and outpatient hospital care Skilled nursing facilities Home health care Physician services Other laboratory and x-ray services Screening, diagnosis, and treatment of children under 21 Family planning Rural health clinic services Supplements Medicare payments

Modified from Medicaid/Medicare: which is which? USDHHS Pub. No. 02129, Washington, D.C., 1984, National Health Care Financing Administration.

To spur the development of a comprehensive health care system for the entire U.S. population, the *Health Maintenance Organization Act* became law in 1972. As discussed in Chapter 2, health maintenance organizations (HMOs) are prepaid systems providing comprehensive health care services to participants for a basic monthly premium. Prepaid group practice plans existing in the United States since the 1940s served as models for the HMO Act.

HMO plans usually provide more coverage to an enrollee without copayment or deductible than is typical of other health insurance schemes. Federal and state governments continue to encourage the development of HMOs by providing grants and loans for planning and operation, and some states are requiring employers to offer HMOs as health insurance options in benefit packages. There are more than 300 HMOs in the United States with 13 million enrollees and 126 independent provider associations with 8 million enrollees, thereby offering a competitive system to other health insurance schemes. The intent of HMOs was to prevent costly hospitalization and to educate consumers in illness prevention and health maintenance. A degree of success has been realized, as shown by a 30% reduction in hospital utilization for HMO clients (Quinn, 1984; Booth, 1985).

◆   ◆   ◆

Since 1847 health care coverage by governmental and private third-party payers has greatly increased. By 1984 estimates indicated that 50% of the U.S. population were covered by a health insurance plan. Approximately 60% of those persons had group health insurance plans as a result of their employment. Approximately 98% of the elderly had Medicare hospital insurance coverage and 96% had Medicare medical insurance. Over 22 million American poor were covered by Medicaid; over 1 million veterans obtained health care through the Veterans Administration system, 10 million military personnel had access to care through the military system; and 21 million people were enrolled in HMOs and IPAs. The population groups finding health care inaccessible were the working poor, low-income childless couples, low-income families with an unemployed father present, and the medically indigent (persons who have money to buy the necessities of life, but who cannot afford an acute illness crisis or catastrophic illness). These groups constituted 15% of the total population.

FUTURE HEALTH CARE FINANCING PLANS

While there is no definitive answer to the questions of cost containment and cost reduction, a number of plans for future payment of health care are being considered. To solve the problems of rising health care costs several things are occurring:

1. New financing mechanisms are being introduced in an effort to reduce the use of health care resources.
2. Competition is being introduced into health care delivery, allowing providers and agencies to advertise and market health care services.
3. Alternative health care delivery mechanisms are proliferating.

The Medicare PPS is expected to be used for Medicaid payment and to be adopted by private insurers. This new system of financing may pose certain problems relative to the quality of care the clients receive and access to hospital services and necessary technology. It may also alter employment patterns in the health care system, may result in layoffs of health care personnel, and may affect medical and nursing education. While hospital employment may be reduced, community employment opportunities are expected to increase.

Competition in health care delivery has resulted in the introduction of marketing and advertising of health care services, in incentives between agencies to reduce costs to the consumer, and in an increase in for-profit multihospital corporations. To become more cost-effective, hospitals are consolidating their services, and fewer facilities are offering more costly services such as obstetrics, pediatrics, and complex care (high-technology surgery and specialty care units).

Although consumers are provided with more options in hospital care and hospitals are becoming more responsive to consumer needs, this competition reduces access to certain services and limits access by certain population groups like the uninsured poor. Competition and prospective payment systems have also resulted in the closing of smaller or less efficient community hospitals that cannot compete.

New financing mechanisms for in-hospital care and competition in the system have provided an incentive for the development of alternative health care delivery mechanisms.

The development of HMOs, preferred provider organizations (PPOs), and independent provider associations (IPAs) allows the consumer, primarily through an employer, to purchase a package of health services on a prepaid fee basis. The intent of such organizations is to instill price competition between providers, thereby reducing costs. Costs are reduced to the HMO, PPO, or IPA through consumer education in disease prevention and health maintenance and a reduction in the use of costly unnecessary hospitalization. While consumer costs are limited and a comprehensive health care service is offered, access and quantity of service are limited by the organization.

In addition to the comprehensive health care organizations, other alternative health care delivery services are emerging or expanding: alcohol and drug abuse centers, ambulatory care centers, ambulatory surgical centers, birthing centers, diagnostic imaging centers, freestanding emergency centers, hospices, mammography centers, oncology centers, pain management centers, psychiatric centers, rehabilitation centers, wellness centers, home health agencies, and skilled nursing facilities. These services represent a major change in the structure and pattern for delivering health care and reflect the increasing emphasis on direct out-of-pocket payment for health care services. While the development of such health care alternatives provide ready access to a number of services to those who can pay, it encourages fragmentation of care.

Since the new financing mechanisms, competition, and alternative delivery services limit access to those who are employed and have health insurance, those who can pay out-of-pocket, and the population covered by Medicare and

Medicaid, it has been suggested that the only way to provide health care for all is to declare a three-tiered health care system (Reinhardt, 1986, Thurow, 1985).

The first tier would provide a publicly financed health care program, financed primarily by a competitively bid, prepaid capitation plan with rationing of health care services. Social Security taxes, general taxation for all people, or taxation of employer health insurance contributions and health insurance benefits may be used to finance this health care program. The government would pay health care providers a fixed fee to provide a minimal level of health care to the uninsured, poor, and elderly.

The second tier would be established by private industry and would depend on the level of health care they are willing to provide their employees. Corporations would likely establish a self-insurance program and purchase a package of services for a fixed price through HMOs, PPOs, or IPAs. The traditional private insurance fee-for-service system would continue to be an option.

The third tier would be a free market, individual system where health care could be purchased in excess of that provided by employers or government. Care would be limited only by the amount of money a person was willing to pay.

The implications of the three-tiered system are many. The quality of care is of major concern. Quality of care in the first tier would depend largely on the ethics and expertise of the health care providers. If providers who are motivated by the need to help others are in this system, quality care may be enhanced from present-day care often offered to these population groups. If only those providers are employed who cannot find positions in the second and third tier, quality may become an issue. Access to care would be made more equitable across population groups by such a system, while costs and use would be controlled by the buyers of service—the government and corporation in the first and second level, and the consumer in the third level.

As changes in health care financing occur, nurses must plan for the future so we can be a part of it. Nurses must be able to show the cost of nursing services and become more knowledgeable about economics and finance, develop new interventions or methods of care that provide efficient quality care, take advantage of the opportunities to play a leading role in the new alternative delivery systems, and assume a greater role in decision making and evaluating client care and nurse performance.

COST STUDIES APPLIED TO HEALTH CARE DELIVERY

Excessive and inefficient use of goods and services in health care delivery have been viewed by many as the major causes of rising costs in health care delivery. For this reason Congress established in 1978 the Center for National Health Care Technology and mandated the center to define the safety, efficacy, efficiency, and cost effectiveness of medical procedures. Recent studies released by the center present a strong argument for the cost effectiveness of nurse practitioners (LeRoy and Solkowitz, 1981; Nurse practitioners, 1986).

Many studies appear in the literature about the cost effectiveness of nurse practitioners and cost benefit, effi-

ciency, efficacy, and effectiveness of medical procedures and programs; however, minimal data are available about the cost benefit, efficiency, and effectiveness of nurses generally.

A recent statement issued by the American Nurses' Association indicates that nurses should receive third-party reimbursement and that nursing care should become a separate budget item in all organizations so that cost studies can show the efficiency and effectiveness of the nursing profession. Presently hospitals include nursing care costs in daily patient hotel costs (room charges), whereas other agencies, such as home health care agencies, include administrative costs, supplies, and equipment costs with nursing care costs. Major efforts are underway that can be used by nurses to show actual costs of nursing care in most places where nurses are employed and their contributions to the system (Grimaldi et al., 1982; McKibbon et al., 1985; Reitz, 1985; Thompson, 1984).

At present a movement exists in the United States to provide third-party reimbursement for nurses. Medicare and Medicaid provide *indirect nurse reimbursement* to agencies offering home health care services. The Rural Health Clinic Services Act of 1977 provides for indirect reimbursement for the services of nurse practitioners in rural health clinics; and a 1980 Medicaid amendment to the Social Security Act provides for *direct reimbursement* of nurse-midwives. Currently a bill is being considered in Congress to establish community nursing centers to provide direct reimbursement for ambulatory nursing and related care to defined community populations. In 1978 Maryland was the first state to provide direct reimbursement for nurse practitioners and nurse-midwives; Maryland extended the legislation in 1979 to provide direct reimbursement for "any duly licensed health care providers" for services within their lawful scope of practice. Presently there are 13 states providing direct reimbursement for nurse practitioner or nurse-midwifery services and many others are pursuing reimbursement legislation. Such a trend will provide impetus for separating general nursing care costs from other program costs and give an adequate environment for performing cost studies in nursing.

The four major types of cost studies primarily applied in the health care industry are cost accounting, cost benefit, cost efficiency, and cost effectiveness. A discussion of types of cost studies is presented to give the reader an idea about the types of questions that can be answered with such studies. Nurses must be willing to supply answers to these questions to help show the actual costs of nursing care delivery.

Cost Accounting

Cost accounting studies are performed to find the actual budgetary cost of a program, procedure, or technique. A question answered by this method could be, "What is the cost of providing a family planning program in Anytown, U.S.A.?" To answer the question, the total costs of equipment, facilities (rental), personnel (salaries and benefits), and supplies are figured. The total program costs are divided by the number of clients participating in the clinic for a set time period; the total program cost per client is the end product. Thus a cost accounting study can provide data about total program costs and about total cost per client. A simple example of cost accounting is what one does each month in balancing a checkbook. One looks at the costs of providing food, shelter, and clothing for a family versus the income for the family.

Cost Benefit

Cost benefit studies are a way of assessing the desirability of a program, procedure, technique, or intervention by placing a specific quantifiable value, a dollar amount, on all costs and all benefits. If benefits outweigh the costs, then the program is said to have a net positive impact. The major problem with cost benefit analysis is placing a quantifiable value on all benefits of a program. The question is, Can a dollar value be placed on human life, on safety, on the relief of pain and suffering, or on prevention of illness? If an attempt is made to perform cost benefit analysis of a hospice program, can a quantifiable value be placed on the family and client support and comfort provided or on the relief of pain of the terminally ill? Can such benefits be weighed against costs to justify continuing the program?

Theoretically, it is recognized that public health programs have net positive impacts, or high cost benefit ratios, because preventing morbidity with illness prevention programs, such as hypertensive screening, averts or reduces the future cost of chronic long-term illness from stroke or cardiovascular disease. Yet the cost benefit of investments in such programs can only be shown with multiple longitudinal research studies and time. To initiate a cost benefit study for a program, it must be decided which costs and which benefits are to be included, how the costs and benefits are to be valued, and what constraints are to be considered— legal, ethical, social, and economic. For instance, if the length of a client's life or the disease incidence after program participation are considered benefits, will client morbidity or mortality during or after the program be considered negative impacts on the program, and will placing values on these benefits favor higher socioeconomic groups over lower ones, men over women, those of working age over those younger and older? (LoGerfo and Brook, 1980.) For example, in a home health care program funded by the state health department to offer care to AIDS clients, the mortality rate would continue to be high because a cure is not available. Would the program be considered to have a low cost benefit ratio (negative impact) because the clients cannot be cured? The program would be considered to have a high cost benefit ratio (positive net impact) if the cost of home health care services were less expensive than providing similar care in the hospital. The benefits of the program would include the reduction in costs to client and reduction in need for hospital services (Rossi and Freeman, 1985).

Cost Efficiency

Cost efficiency analysis for purposes of this discussion is the analysis of actual costs to perform a number of services at different volumes if the same standards are applied. Volume implies numbers of clients. To determine cost efficiency of

a program or procedure, productivity must be analyzed. Productivity is the relationship between the output and the input of a process. The concept of nurse productivity encompasses the effectiveness, the quality, and the efficiency of nursing care (nursing output with minimal resource waste, for example the number of clients served at the least cost).

To determine the nursing input for a given output (clients served) in a cost efficiency analysis, one is primarily concerned with a nurse's workload, including direct client care and indirect care activities such as charting, phone calls, client care conferences, and travel. The functions are then related to the client load, client need, nursing organizational structure, and staff mix.

Figure 3-1 shows an example of the cost efficiency of a home health agency. The graph indicates that as the number of client visits per year increases, the cost per client visit decreases. The graph assumes that there are the same number of nurses from the beginning to the end of the time period, that the nurses' workloads were essential to provide home health services, that caseloads were assigned based on staff mix and client need, and that organizational structure was conducive to maximize nursing input to produce identified output.

Cost Effectiveness

Cost effectiveness analysis, a measure of the quality of a program, procedure, technique, or intervention as it relates to cost, is the most frequently used analysis in nursing. Cost effectiveness is a subset of cost benefit analysis and is designed to provide an estimate of costs incurred in achieving a given outcome. A cost effectiveness study can answer several questions: Did the program meet its objectives? Were the clients and the nurses satisfied with the effects of the interventions? Are things better as a result of the interventions? (Kaluzny and Veney, 1984). In cost benefit analysis both costs and outcomes are quantitative, whereas

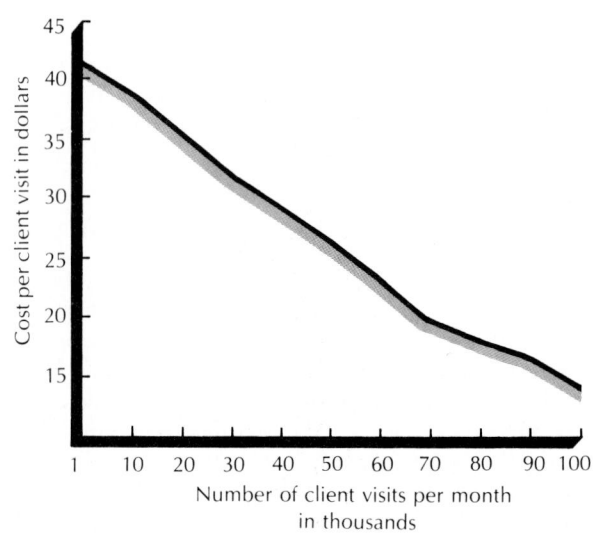

FIGURE 3-1

Cost per client visit at home health agency.

in cost effectiveness analysis the outcomes are qualitative. Outcome measures addressed by cost effectiveness studies might be increased client knowledge after health teaching, changes in client's condition after treatment, differences in graduates of two nursing programs with similar goals, and the ability of two hearing screening programs to detect hearing loss.

The boxed material below shows the procedure for completing a cost effectiveness study. A cost effectiveness study requires collection of baseline data on clients before implementing the study and the testing or evaluation at a predetermined time after the study is completed.

There are several potential outcomes of a cost effectiveness study. For example, a community health nurse is interested in comparing two methods for teaching diabetic clients self-care techniques. The nurse chooses self-teaching modules and a group formal instruction program for comparison. There are nine potential outcomes the nurse may find in comparing the two teaching methods. One teaching method may be (1) less costly and less effective than the other, (2) less costly and equally as effective, (3) less costly and more effective, (4) equal in cost but less effective, (5) equal in cost and equally effective, (6) equal in cost and more effective, (7) more costly and less effective, (8) more costly and equally effective, or (9) more costly and more effective than the other. Of the nine potential outcomes in a cost effectiveness study, the program of choice would be the most effective teaching method for the least cost (outcome 3), unless the most costly program demonstrates superior effectiveness (outcome 9) or the least costly program demonstrates less quality (outcome 1).

All of the cost studies have three major tasks: financial, research, and statistical. The financial tasks involve identifying total program costs and breaking them down into smaller parts. To identify the costs of a nurse's participation in a teaching program, the costs for facilities, equipment, supplies, and salaries would have to be examined. All costs associated with the teaching program, such as nurse's time and use of facilities, equipment, and supplies, should be compared to the total program costs. The statistical tasks involve the identification of appropriate quantifiable measures for analyzing data, and the research tasks involve setting up an appropriate study design to answer the questions of benefit, efficiency, or effectiveness.

Nurses of all educational preparation may be involved in cost studies with the assistance of people knowledgeable in research statistics and accounting techniques. Nurses with undergraduate preparation may be involved in the actual implementation of a cost study, whereas nurses with graduate preparation may be involved in planning, designing, implementing, analyzing, and evaluating study results.

Although cost studies are essential to show the worth of nursing in the marketplace of the future, nurses must be ready to provide input so that sound decisions may be made from the study results. Nurses must be ready to identify appropriate program outcomes, client outcomes, total dimensions of roles of graduates, and total dimensions of nursing procedures so that appropriate decisions about nursing services delivery will be made using adequate information.

PREVENTION

An area in the health care delivery system that needs to show cost effectiveness is the area of primary prevention. *Primary prevention*, distinguished from secondary and tertiary prevention, consists of activities that prevent a disease from occurring. Primary prevention has three major aspects: personal health services, such as immunization against infectious diseases; environmental services, such as adequate water and sewage treatment to prevent parasitic diseases or water fluoridation to prevent dental caries; and health behavior practices, such as nonsmoking programs to prevent lung cancer, use of seat belts to prevent accident fatalities, and good nutrition to prevent obesity and ensuing complications.

Secondary prevention consists of activities designed to detect disease and provide early treatment (early case-finding). Secondary prevention consists primarily of screening for disease before complaint of symptoms, such as hypertensive screening, hearing and vision testing, glaucoma screening, and Pap tests and breast examinations for cancer. *Tertiary prevention* is the activity engaged in by most health providers, that is, the treatment, care, and rehabilitation of people with acute and chronic illnesses (Hanlon and Pickett, 1984).

Although estimates indicate that 97% of the health care dollars are spent on secondary and tertiary prevention, the major causes of morbidity and mortality in our adult population have shown little net decline. Several assumptions can be made about the causes of the slight decline in morbidity and mortality in the past decade: The slight decline in heart disease mortality rates, about 2% per year, may be caused by changes in smoking habits, diet, increased awareness of health risks, increased exercise, and the greater avail-

---

STEPS IN COST EFFECTIVENESS ANALYSIS

Step I   Identify the treatment goals or client outcome to be achieved.

Step II   Identify at least two alternative means of achieving the desired outcomes.

Step III Determine client's pretreatment level on desired outcomes.

Step IV   Determine the costs associated with each treatment.

Step V   Determine amount of treatment given to each group of clients.

Step VI   Determine the posttreatment level on desired outcome variables.

Step VII Combine the costs (Step IV), amount of treatment (Step V), and outcome information (Step VI) to express costs relative to outcomes of treatment.

Step VIII Compare cost outcome information for each treatment type to present cost effectiveness analysis.

From Prescott, P.: Nurs. Outlook. 29(11):722-728, Nov. 1979. Copyright, American Journal of Nursing Co.

ability of coronary care units and advances in medical and surgical treatment. The 2% decline in strokes may be attributed to better control of hypertension, better methods of diagnosis, and improved management and rehabilitation. Slight declines in stomach cancer may be related to nutritional factors and extensive use of refrigeration, which reduces the need for certain food preservatives.

Injuries from auto accidents, reduced by 20% since 1973, may be due to seat belts, lower speed limits, and higher gasoline prices. Decreases in infant and maternal mortality rates may result from declining birth weights, prenatal care, and family planning. Most of the reasons cited for declining problems are primary preventive measures.

Given that primary preventive measures could reduce the risk of early death, disease, disability, and discomfort from disease, why then have the federal and private third-party payers not provided coverage for such measures? The answer is in the following discussion. In addition to the benefit of improved health status of the population, a focus on prevention could mean a reduction in the need for and use of medical, dental, hospital, and health provider services. This would mean for the largest employer in the United States that the market would be reduced in size and become more controlled by the consumer of goods and services than by the seller of these services. Medicare, Medicaid, and private insurance carriers have encouraged a sickness-oriented system. Although there are existing data to indicate that primary preventive care is cost effective, most of our dollars continue to be spent for secondary and tertiary prevention. With the increasing costs of health care, consumer demand, and changes in financing mechanisms, there may be a trend toward financing more preventive care services.

The goal of public health is to provide activities to improve and protect the well-being and health of the nation. Preventive community health services include health planning, disease prevention and control, consumer safety, and occupational safety and health. National health priorities are set by the federal government, and financial support through block grants is provided to the 55 state and territorial health agencies and to the over 3000 local health departments. These health departments use funds to provide direct community services such as public health nursing, home health care, immunizations, venereal disease control, chronic disease screening, and consumer protection.

Expenditures for public health activities have increased from $2.0 billion in 1972 to $8.6 billion in 1982 with projected increases to $18 billion in 1990. The possible increases in communicable diseases and increased awareness of measures to prevent chronic diseases, mental illness, suicide, accidents, substance abuse, homicide, and sexually transmitted diseases may influence the resources allocated to public health activities (Freeland and Schendler, 1984).

In 1979 the Surgeon General of the United States published a report entitled *Healthy People.* The report called for a renewed preventive health care commitment through the identification of priorities and specific goals. The central theme of the report was that the health of the nation could be significantly improved through actions taken by individuals and by policy makers to promote a safer, healthier environment for all at home, at work, and at play.

The report suggested that most people could improve their personal health by observing the following practices:

- Elimination of cigarette smoking
- Reduction of alcohol abuse
- Moderate dietary changes to reduce intake of excess calories, fat, salt, and sugar
- Moderate exercise
- Periodic screening for major causes of morbidity and mortality, such as blood pressure and cancer
- Adherence to speed laws and use of seat belts

The report also emphasized the link between physical and mental health and the need to maintain strong family ties, assistance of supportive friends, and use of community support systems.

For the policy makers, the report suggested a need to recognize the relationship between health and the physical environment, which could lead to the reduction of morbidity and mortality caused by air, water, and food contamination, accidents, radiation exposure, excessive noise, occupational hazard, dangerous consumer products, and unsafe highway design.

Subsequently the Secretary of DHHS in 1980 presented a report, *Promoting Health/Preventing Disease—Objectives for the Nation,* outlining the national health status and objectives to be attained by the health care system by 1990. The following target areas were identified in the report: control of high blood pressure; pregnancy and infant health; immunization; sexually transmitted diseases; toxic agents; occupational health; fluoridation and dental health; surveillance of infectious disease; smoking; misuse of alcohol and drugs; nutrition; physical fitness and exercise; and stress. The objectives of the report are aimed at reducing death rates and related measures of poor health, reducing measurable risks, increasing public and professional awareness of risk and reduction possibilities, and improving services (*Health: United States,* 1980). Preliminary data indicate progress toward achieving the goal of the nation to reduce mortality at every life stage (Prevention 84/85).

Reducing the burden of avoidable illness and disability will reduce the human and economic costs imposed on the U.S. population. To accomplish the goals of prevention, changes will have to occur in environmental protection, life-styles, and orientation of health providers and institutions toward health promotion. Support will have to be gained from employers, schools, product designers and manufacturers, food distributors, and the insurance industry for preventing injury and promoting healthier life-styles.

THE VALUE OF HUMAN LIFE

The concept of human capital has evolved in economics as a way of measuring the value society places on the worth of the individual. The value is quantified and expressed in dollar amounts, and it constitutes a real limit on how much money either people or society will pay for personal health care.

The human body has often been compared to a machine,

with proper functioning dependent on its various physical and biochemical components. To maintain proper functioning and productivity, the machine must be nurtured, protected, housed, educated, and trained. These goals can only be accomplished by investing time and money in the potential capital (Hanlon and Pickett, 1984).

Since the dollar value of individual productivity is also a function of time, the potential capital worth of an individual is a function of longevity and functional capacity during a lifetime. The values the market places on different levels and types of education and work capability are basic determinants of the capital value of a human being. It has been shown that an individual's current market value increases to approximately age 25 and steadily declines thereafter and that the value of the male in society is greater than the value of the female (Landfeld and Seskin, 1982).

A major goal of the health care delivery system today is to preserve and maximize human capital by offering health-preserving and social practices that result in avoidance of disease, that is, primary prevention, and by offering diagnosis, treatment, and rehabilitative services for existing diseases, that is, secondary and tertiary prevention. The past goal of the health care delivery system has been to emphasize the "sickness system." DHHS health goals suggest a higher value should be placed on primary prevention. Table 3-10 shows the direct dollar costs and the indirect human capital costs in 1982 from diseases or deaths that might have been preventable. The direct costs are actual amounts paid for health care; the indirect costs represent loss of money from working. For example, cardiovascular diseases alone cost the consumer and society $41.2 billion for health care and $11.8 billion from lost workdays, plus $40.8 billion from potential workdays of those who died prematurely.

The outcome of health care goals should be the provision of a quality of life that will promote happiness, productivity, efficiency, and the capacity to engage in and enjoy life activities. Quantifying life is meaningless to the person unless the quality of life can be maximized and unless functional days become more valuable than dollars spent. An emphasis on primary prevention may hold the key to reducing dollars spent while increasing the quality of life.

TABLE 3-10

Direct and indirect economic costs of illness by disease category of diagnosis in United States for 1982

| Diagnosis | Amount (in billions of dollars) | | | | Percentage distribution* | | | |
| | Total | Direct costs† | Indirect costs | | Total | Direct costs† | Indirect costs | |
			Morbidity	Mortality‡			Morbidity	Mortality‡
Cardiovascular diseases	93.8	41.2	11.8	40.8	18.8	15.5	15.8	26.0
(involving blood clotting)	(27.7)	(8.9)	(3.2)	(15.6)	(5.6)	(3.3)	(4.3)	(10.0)
Lung diseases§	26.4	7.6	12.6	6.2	5.3	2.8	16.9	4.0
Blood diseases§	2.2	1.5	0.3	0.4	0.4	0.6	0.4	0.2
SUBTOTAL	$122.4	$ 50.3	$24.7	$ 47.4	24.5%	18.9%	33.1%	30.2%
Diseases of the digestive system	53.4	38.7	6.4	8.3	10.7	14.5	8.6	5.3
Neoplasms	53.7	16.5	3.0	34.2	10.8	6.2	4.0	21.8
Mental disorders	30.4	24.7	4.2	1.5	6.1	9.3	5.6	1.0
Diseases of the nervous system	26.8	21.3	2.8	2.7	5.4	8.0	3.7	1.7
Diseases of the musculoskeletal system	26.1	16.5	9.0	0.6	5.2	6.2	12.0	0.4
Diseases of the genitourinary system	20.3	15.7	3.1	1.5	4.1	5.9	4.2	1.0
Endocrine, nutritional, and metabolic diseases	14.9	9.2	2.4	3.3	3.0	3.5	3.2	2.1
Infective and parasitic diseases	10.1	5.4	2.8	1.9	2.0	2.0	3.7	1.2
Diseases of the skin	8.6	7.5	1.0	0.1	1.7	2.8	1.3	0.1
Congenital anomalies	4.5	1.7	—	2.8	0.9	0.6	—	1.8
Other	126.7	59.0	1.53	52.4	25.4	22.1	20.5	33.4
TOTAL	497.9	266.5	74.7	156.7	100.0	100.0	100.0	100.0

From 1984 fact book, 1984, National Heart Lung & Blood Institute. Data from NCHS, estimates by NHLBI.
*Numbers may not add to 100% due to rounding.
†Includes only personal health care expenditures allocated to diagnoses (83% of total direct health care expenditures).
‡Based on a 6% discount rate of loss of future earnings because of premature death.
§Does not include cancers, leukemias, and other neoplasms, or pulmonary embolism.
—Numbers too small to estimate

FACTORS AFFECTING HEALTH LEVELS

The goal of health economics is quality care leading to health and wellness of the population. Four major factors are known to affect health levels: personal behavior, environmental factors, human biology, and the health care system.

Society's investment in the *health care system* has been based on this premise: more health services equal better health. The increasing investment society has made in health care delivery is shown in Table 3-11. Although the investment has been a major one, medical services are said to have the least effect on health (Hanlon and Pickett, 1984; McKeown, 1981; McKinlay and McKinlay, 1977).

As first documented in England and Wales in the nineteenth century, health has improved throughout history, resulting in an increased life expectancy for infants and children. The reductions in deaths from the early nineteenth century causes of death—infectious diseases—were attributed to improved nutrition from increased food supplies. Major advances in hygiene and safe food and water contributed to continuing declining death rates after the 1850s.

The World Health Organization contends that experience in Third World countries today supports the premise that adequate diet reduces risk of infection, thereby leading to decreased morbidity.

Health problems of the twentieth century are being attributed primarily to *personal behavior* and *environmental* factors. Although these two factors are coming to the forefront as major influences on health, answers to the question of genetic, or human biological, influence on health are still being explored. For instance, risk factors for heart disease and stroke are being related to life-style influences such as smoking, diet, and exercise and to genetic influences such as family history of heart disease, stroke, and hypertension. The federal health goals of the 1980s focus on control of *behavioral influences* thought to be the major determinants of health, such as alcohol and drug abuse, smoking, nutrition, exercise, and stress, and *environmental influences* thought to be the major determinants of illness, such as pollution of air, water, noise, and foods. The goals also address control of and risk reduction from human *biological*

TABLE 3-11

Gross national product and national health expenditures in United States for selected years from 1929 to 1984*

| Year | Gross national product in billions | National health expenditures | | |
		Amount in billions	Percent of gross national product	Amount per capita
1929	$ 103.4	$ 3.6	3.5	$ 29
1935	72.5	2.9	4.0	23
1940	100.0	4.0	4.0	30
1950	286.5	12.7	4.4	82
1955	400.0	17.7	4.4	105
1960	506.5	26.9	5.3	146
1965	691.0	41.9	6.1	207
1970	992.7	75.0	7.6	350
1971	1,077.6	83.5	7.7	386
1972	1,185.9	94.0	7.9	430
1973	1,326.4	103.4	7.8	469
1974	1,434.2	116.1	8.1	522
1975	1,549.2	132.7	8.6	591
1976	1,718.0	150.8	8.8	666
1977	1,918.3	169.9	8.9	743
1978	2,163.9	189.7	8.8	822
1979	2,417.8	214.7	8.9	920
1980	2,631.7	247.5	9.4	1,049
1981	2,957.8	285.2	9.6	1,197
1982	3,069.2	321.2	10.5	1,334
1983	3,304.8	355.1	10.7	1,461
1984	3,662.8	387.4	10.6	1,580

From Levit, K.R., Lazanby, H., Waldo, D.R., and Davidoff, L.M.: National health expenditures, 1984, Health Care Financing Review, HCFA Pub. No. 03200, Washington, D.C., Fall 1985, U.S. Government Printing Office.
*The Health Care Financing Administration has made revisions in their health expenditure estimates. Data in this table may differ from those appearing in earlier volumes of *Health, United States*.

influences and the improvement of *health care services.* Parts Three and Four of the text will focus on the personal, environmental, and biological influences affecting the nation's health.

CLINICAL APPLICATION

The goal of health economics is to provide maximum benefit to the clients of health care services. Thus the goal of a community health nursing service should be to provide a program that will provide quality of care and meet the needs of the clients served. The amount of money the client, the community, and the agency spend in offering a service is beneficial if the client is satisfied and if there are enough clients in the community to justify the employment of nurses to provide the service.

As a student or a community health nurse, identify a specific service offered by your agency. The service may be a home health nursing program, a prenatal clinic, or a wellness clinic.

For this example, consider a home health nursing service. Ask the appropriate administrator or director of nurses if you may have the total cost of operating the nursing service for a year. Also inquire about the stated goals for offering a service. The goal is likely to be to provide nursing care in the home to reduce the need for clients to be hospitalized.

Request permission to perform a client or family satisfaction survey on a small sample of the clients of the service. An example of a satisfaction survey appears in Appendix A. To choose your sample you will need to know the number of clients served by the service for the year.

Inquire at the local hospital about the room cost per client day. Divide the number of nursing visits by the home health program into the total costs of the program for the year. This will give you some data to compare cost of care per day in the hospital to the cost of care per visit in the home.

Perform the client satisfaction survey and tally your results. If the clients are satisfied with the home health service and if the cost of visits to clients is lower than a hospital day, then the service may be considered cost effective. If clients are not satisfied, that may mean that their needs are not being met, and the more costly hospital care may be chosen by clients.

Although clients may be satisfied with the service, if the costs of visits are higher than a hospital day, the hospital service may be found to be more cost effective if clients are equally satisfied with hospital care.

The cost of home health visits may be higher if there are not enough visits or clients to support the numbers of staff employed to operate the service.

This example provides you with a very simple way of applying some of the content of this chapter. Cost studies are generally much more complex. In this example it is assumed that one home visit will equal one hospital day, that hospital nursing care costs are included in the room charge, and that the home nursing visit cost includes other agency charges such as administrative overhead.

SUMMARY

Economics is concerned with the most efficient use of resources to fulfill society's unlimited wants. Economics operates under the law of supply and demand; since our society is primarily composed of competitive organizations, when demand goes up, supply goes down and cost goes up, or vice versa.

Health economics is concerned with the distribution of health care resources to provide maximum benefit to the most people. Since the health care delivery system has been largely monopolistic, the laws of supply and demand do not hold true. As demand goes up for health care services, the supply of services also increases and costs go up. As long as the health care system remains in the control of the health provider, the usual economic principles will not hold true.

As the cost of health care services increases, the consumer has less money to spend for other needs and wants. Economic indicators show that the health care costs continue to increase per year and have risen to a cost of $387 billion, or over $1,580 per person per year.

The major factors influencing the costs of health care delivery are inflation, technology, and population changes. The availability of insurance and government funds to cover health care costs, the method of reimbursement, and the development of new and costlier methods of health care technology appear to be the major contributors to rising health care costs. The rising numbers of elderly in the population, the increasing proportion of women, and the decline in family support systems are viewed as the major population changes contributing to increased demand for services and increased costs of services.

The new financing mechanisms, competition, and alternative health care delivery methods may ultimately contribute to a three-tiered health care system providing care for all people.

One of the major problems in health care delivery is determining the efficacy of health care services and health care providers. To say whether health care costs are unreasonable, one must be able to compare the costs of those services to client benefit and to the efficiency and effectiveness of services delivered. Four methods are employed for performing cost studies in the health care system: cost accounting, cost benefit, cost efficiency, and cost effectiveness. Nursing has given minimal time to demonstrating its worth in health care delivery. Since nursing has not shown its contribution to the client in health care, the discipline has had difficulty proving that nursing services should be reimbursable and autonomous, whereas other disciplines, such as physical therapists, occupational therapists, and psychiatric social workers, have moved ahead in establishing themselves in both areas.

Another identifiable problem in health care delivery is establishing the value of primary preventive care. Today 97% of health care dollars are spent on illness care. Although history and recent studies indicate that changes in nutrition, the environment, and life-styles would provide a healthier future society, the cost studies are not readily available to show the savings society could have with a preventive emphasis in its health care delivery system. The large amount of money society annually spends on health care indicates that society values human life. However, the focus of this society's future investment should be to provide more than longevity. The goal of health economics should be to provide a quality of life that offers happiness, productivity, and the capacity to engage in life activities, through the provision of reasonably priced quality services focused on illness prevention, health promotion, and health protection.

KEY CONCEPTS

From 1800 to the 1980s the U.S. health care delivery system experienced three developmental stages, with different emphasis on health care economics. Since 1985, the health care delivery system appears to be entering a fourth developmental stage.

Three basic components provide the framework for health care delivery: labor (work force), facilities, and technology.

Three major factors have been instrumental in influencing the growth of the health care delivery system: price inflation, technology, and changes in population demographics.

Health care financing has evolved through the twentieth century from a system primarily financed by the consumer to a system primarily financed by third-party payers.

To solve the problems of rising health care costs, a number of plans for future payments of health care are being considered.

Excessive and inefficient use of goods and services in health care delivery have been viewed as the major cause of rising health care costs.

The concept of human capital has evolved in economics as a way of measuring the value society places on the worth of an individual.

The goal of health economics is maximum benefits from services of health providers leading to health and wellness of the population.

Four major factors are known to affect health levels: personal behavior, environmental factors, human biology, and the health care system.

LEARNING ACTIVITIES

1. Define in your own words the following terms: economics, health economics, gross national product, consumer price index, human capital.

2. State the goal of health economics.

3. Review Chapter 4, Ethics in Community Health Practice. Debate in class the ethical implications of the goal of health economics. Focus your debate on the implications for community health nursing practice.

4. Invite a community health nurse administrator to meet with your class or clinical conference group. Ask how inflation, changes in population, and technology have changed the community health care delivery system and community health nursing.

BIBLIOGRAPHY

Aiken. L.H.: The practice setting: an overview of health policy issues. In Aiken L.H., editor: Health policy and nursing practice, New York, 1981, McGraw-Hill Book Co.

Aiken, L., and Mechanic, D.: Applications of social science to clinical medicine and health policy, N.J. 1986, Rutgers University Press.

Ancona-Berk, V., and Chalmers, T.: An analysis of ambulatory and inpatient care, Am. J. Pub. Health 76:1102, Sept. 1986.

Beyers, M. Perspectives on prospective payment: challenges and opportunities for nurses. Rockville, Md., 1985, Aspen Systems Corp.

Bloch, H., and Pupp, R.: Supply, demand and rising health care costs, Nurs. Econ. 3(2):119, March-April, 1985.

Booth, R.: Financing mechanisms for health care: impact on nursing services, J. Prof. Nurs. Jan.-Feb. 1985.

Dornbusch, R., and Fischer, S.: Macroeconomics, ed 2, New York, 1981, McGraw-Hill Book Co.

Enthoven, A.: Health plan: the only practical solution to the soaring cost of medical care, Reading, Mass., 1981, Addison-Wesley Publishing Co., Inc.

Feldstein, R.: Health care economics, New York, 1983, John Wiley & Sons, Inc.

Freeland, M., and Schendler, C.: Health spending in the 1980's: integration of clinical practice patterns with management, Health Care Fin. Rev. 8(3):1, Spring 1984.

Fuchs, V.: The economics of health in a post-industrial society, Pub. Interest 56:3-20, Summer 1979.

Gabel, J., and Ermann, D.: Preferred provider organizations: performance, problems, and promise, Health Affairs 4(1):25, Spring 1985.

Ginzberg, E.: The economics of health care and the future of nursing, p. 28, March 1981.

Ginzberg, E.: The monetorization of medical care, N. Engl. J. Med. 310(18):1162, May 3, 1984.

Grimaldi, P., et al.: RIM's and the cost of nursing care, Nurs. Manage. 13, Dec. 1982.

Hanlon J., and Pickett, G.: Public health administration and practice, St. Louis, 1984, The C.V. Mosby Co.

Health: United States, 1985, DHEW Pub. No. (PHS) 86-1232, Washington, D.C., Dec. 1985, Department of Health, and Human Services.

Health: United States, 1980, DHHS Pub. No. (PHS) 81-1232, Washington, D.C., Dec. 1980, Department of Health and Human Services.

Health: United States and Prevention Profile, 1983, USDHHS Pub. No. (PHS) 84-1232, Washington, D.C., Dec. 1983, Department of Health and Human Services.

Healthy People: the Surgeon General's report on health promotion and disease prevention, DHEW Pub. No. (PHS) 79-55071, Washington, D.C., 1979, Department of Health, Education and Welfare.

Heider-Dorneich, P.: Social control in health economics, Rev. Soc. Economy, 36(1):1-18, April 1978.

Hicks, L.: Using benefit-cost and cost-effectiveness analysis in health-care resource allocation, Nurs. Econ. 3(2):78, March/April 1985.

Hicks, L., and Boles, K.: Why health economics? Nurs. Econ. 2(3):175, May/June 1984.

Hill, D.: Economic constraints in the health care delivery system. In Lancaster, J., and Lancaster, W., editors: Concepts for advanced nursing practice: the nurse as change agent, St. Louis, 1982, The C.V. Mosby Co.

Joel, L.: DRG's and RIM's: implications for nursing. In Beyes, M., editor: Perspectives on prospective payment: challenges and opportunities for nurses, Rockwell, Md., 1985, Aspen Publishers, Inc.

Lamm, R.: Rationing of health care: the inevitable meets the unthinkable, Nurse Practitioner 11(5):57, May 1986.

Landfeld, J., and Seskin, E.: The economic value of life: linking theory to practice, Am. J. Pub. Health 72(6): 555, June 1982.

Lauver, E.: Where will the money go? Economic forcasting and nursing's future, Nurs. Health Care p. 133, March 1985.

Lawrence, L., and McLemore T.: 1981 Summary: National Ambulatory Medical Care Survey, NCHS advance data, USDHHS, 88, March 16, 1983.

Lee, P.R.: Technology and the cost of medical care. In Lee, P., Brown, N., and I., Red, editors: The nation's health, San Francisco, 1981, Boyd & Fraser Publishing Co.

Lee, P., Brown, N., and Red, I.: Health costs: what limit? The nation's health, San Francisco, 1981, Boyd & Fraser Publishing Co.

LeRoy, L., and Solkowitz, S.: The implications of cost-effectiveness analysis of medical technology, Congress of the United States, Office of Technology Assessment, case study no. 16, Washington, D.C., 1981, U.S. Government Printing Office.

LoGerfo, J., and Brook, R.: Evaluation of health services and quality of care. In Williams, S., and P., Torrens, editors: Introduction to health services, New York, 1980, John Wiley & Sons Inc.

McKeown, T.: Determinants of health. In Lee, P., Brown, N., and Red, I., editors: The nation's health, San Francisco, 1981, Boyd & Fraser Publishing Co.

McKibbin, R., et al.: DRG's and nursing care, HCFA Grant #15-C-98421/7-02 Kansas City, Mo., June 1985. Center for Research, American Nurses' Association.

McKinlay, J.B., and McKinlay, S.M.: The questionable contribution of medical measures to the decline of mortality in the United States in the twentieth century, Milbank Mem. Fund Q. 55(3):405-H428, 1977.

Medical technology and costs of the medicare program, Congress of the United States, Office of Technology Assessment, OTA-H-228, Washington, D.C., July, 1984, U.S. Government Printing Office.

Medicare's prospective payment system: strategies for evaluating cost, quality, and medical technology, Congress of the United States, Office of Technology Assessment, OTA-H-263, Washington, D.C., Oct. 1985, U.S. Government Printing Office.

Mitchell, K.: Lean, mean and fiscally fit, Nurs. Econ. 3(3):134, May/June 1985.

National Center for Health Services Research: National health care expenditures study: changes in health insurance status full-year and part-year coverage. Data preview 21, USDHHS Pub. No. (PHS) 85-3377, Washington, D.C., July 1985, Department of Health and Human Services.

National Center for Health Services Research: National health care expenditures study, private insurance and public programs: coverage of health services, Data Preview 20, USDHHS Pub. No. (PHS) 85-3374, Washington, D.C., March 1985, Department of Health and Human Services.

National Center for Health Services Research: Research summary series. Morbidity costs: national estimates and economic determinants, USDHHS Pub. No. (PHS) 86-3393, Washington, D.C., Oct. 1985, Department of Health and Human Services.

National Center for Health Statistics: Provisional data from the health promotion and disease prevention supplement to the national health interview survey: United States, Jan.-March, 1985, USDHHS, vol. 113, Nov. 15, 1985, Department of Health and Human Services.

National Center for Health Statistics: Advance data: provisional data from the health promotion and disease prevention supplement to the national health interview survey: United States, Jan.-March 1985, USDHHS Pub. No. (PHS) 86-1250, vol. 113, Nov. 15, 1985, Department of Health and Human Services.

Nurse practitioners, physicians assistants and certified nurse midwives: quality, access, cost and payment issues, Congress of the United States, Office of Technology Assessment, Health Program, Unpublished report, May 1986.

Ostrander, V.: Consumers look to nurses, Nursing and Health Care. 7(7):368, Sept. 1986.

Prescott, P.A.: Cost-effectiveness: tool or trap? Nurs. Outlook, 27(11):722-H728, Nov. 1979.

Prest, A., and Turvey, R.: Cost-benefit analysis: a survey, The Economic J. 75(300):683-735, Dec. 1965.

Prevention 84/85, Office of Disease Prevention and Health USDHHS Pub. No. 474-512, Washington, D.C., 1985, U.S. Government Printing Office.

Prospects for a healthier America: achieving the nation's health promotion objectives, Nov. 1984, Washington, D.C., U.S. Department of Health and Human Services.

Reinhardt, U.: Rationing the health care surplus: an American tragedy, Nurs. Econ. 4(3):101, May/June, 1986.

Reitz, J.: Development of a nursing intensity index: a technical report, Baltimore, March 1985, The Johns Hopkins Medical Institutions.

Rice, D., and Hodgson, T.: The value of human life revisited, Am. J. Pub. Health 72(6):536, June 1982.

Richardson, W.: Financing health services. In Williams, S., and Torrens, P., editors: Introduction to health services, New York, 1984, John Wiley & Sons, Inc.

Rossi, P., and Freeman H.: Evaluation: a systematic approach, Beverly Hills, Calif., 1985, Sage Publications.

Rushmer, R.: Technological resources for health. In Williams, S., and Torrens, P., editors: Introduction to health services, New York, 1984, John Wiley & Sons Inc.

Schwartz, W.B., and Joskow. P.L.: Sounding board—medical efficacy versus economic efficacy: a conflict of values, N. Engl. J. Med. 299(26):1462-1464, Dec. 1978.

Sindelar, J.: Differential use of medical care by sex, J. Pol. Economy, 90(5):1003, 1982.

Tagg, P.: Feeling the effects of federal budget cuts, Nurse Practitioner, p. 36, April 1984.

Thompson, J.: The measurement of nursing intensity. In USDHHS health care financing review: 1984 annual supplement, Baltimore, November 1984, Health Care Financing Administration.

Thurow, L.: Medicine vs. economics, N. Engl. J. Med. 313(10):611, Sept. 5, 1985.

Torrens, P.: Overview of health services in the United States. In Lee, P., Brown, N., and Red, I., editors: The nation's health. San Francisco, 1984, Boyd & Fraser Publishing Co Inc.

Wilensky, G., and Rossiter, L.: The relative importance of physician induced demand in the demand for medical care, Milbank Mem. Fund Q. 61(2):252, 1983.

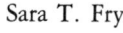

Sara T. Fry

4

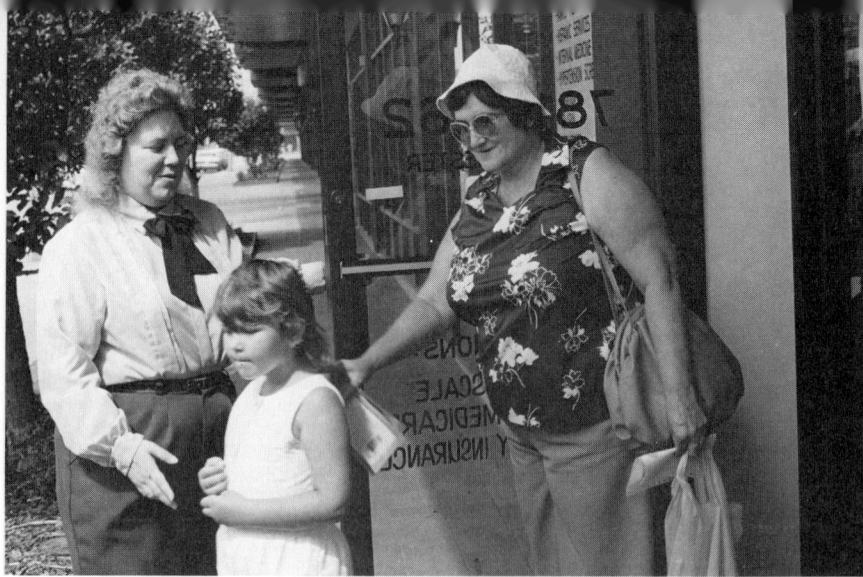

ETHICS IN COMMUNITY HEALTH NURSING PRACTICE

OBJECTIVES

After reading this chapter, the student should be able to:

Describe the meaning of accountability in community health nursing.

Identify the relationship of ethical rules, principles, and theories in community health nursing decisions.

Discuss the application of ethical principles, including their potential conflicts, in community health nursing practice.

Given an appropriate case example of community health nursing practice, identify the following:

1. The basis for clients' rights claims
2. Specific professional responsibilities in response to clients' rights
3. Limitations of clients' rights in today's health care delivery system

Given a hypothetical community health need requiring the fair and just distribution of community health nursing resources to a specific aggregate group, formulate a plan of nursing care delivery using the following:

1. A theory of distributive justice
2. Ethical principles and their priority or influence
3. Evaluation of the potential benefits and harms of the plan
4. Evaluation of the extent to which moral requirements of community health nursing practice are met by the plan

KEY TERMS

advocacy

autonomy

beneficence

Code for Nurses

codes of ethics

coercive health measures

confidentiality

client's rights

egalitarian theory

entitlement theory

informed consent

justice

maximin theory

moral accountability

Patient's Bill of Rights

principles

public health ethic

right to health

right to health care

rules

rule of utility

theories

utilitarian theory

veracity

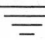

Community health nurses experience many ethical conflicts in today's health care delivery system. The nursing profession has traditionally upheld the rights and human needs of the individual client. Yet today this focus is difficult to maintain when nursing services have the additional goal of maximizing the health of populations at risk. The traditional focus is also difficult to maintain in systems where nursing resources are influenced by legislation and funding for specific population groups. One result of this latter difficulty is that other populations identified as being at risk are not adequately served by community health nursing efforts because of the lack of funds. Nurses who experience this conflict between the individualistic focus of the professional ethic and the aggregate focus of community health recognize the dilemma of professional nursing in community health settings.

The purpose of this chapter is to analyze traditional ethics of professional nursing and apply these principles to the practice of community health nursing. Since the client is the focus of all nursing actions, clients' rights are discussed first. Clients' rights to health and health care and other rights are examined from the viewpoint of traditional ethics and the expression of individual client needs, interests, and rights in community health situations.

Since clients have rights that are recognized by professional statements of ethics as well as by public documents, professionals have responsibilities or duties. These duties—telling the truth, respecting confidentiality, client advocacy, and accountability—are discussed in depth. The conflicts between these professional duties are also explored and possible solutions are suggested.

Not all nursing actions, however, are simply correlative to clients' rights. There is a relationship between general ethical principles and moral rules and the various theories of social justice that influence health care delivery and nursing services. These principles, their definitions, and applications in community health nursing are presented in terms of the moral requirements of the principles and their potential conflicts in the planning, implementation, and evaluation of nursing services.

Finally, the priority of the ethical principles in community health nursing, including the meaning of accountability, is discussed. Accountability—being answerable to someone for what has been done in the nursing role—is a strong value in nursing, directing the nurse to practice professional skills and expertise in a certain way. Thus the development of methods to measure accountability is a high priority in community health nursing. It is a priority in that community health nursing must not only demonstrate the cost-effectiveness of its services in promoting health and preventing illness but also show how it meets normal requirements for professional practice. If community health nursing can demonstrate its ability to increase the community's health while meeting requirements for accountability to clients, then great gains will be made in the name of community health nursing services.

CLIENTS' RIGHTS AND PROFESSIONAL RESPONSIBILITIES IN COMMUNITY HEALTH CARE
Clients' Rights

One of the earliest recognitions of *clients' rights* concerning health was made by the National Convention of the French Revolution in 1793. Underscoring the theme of basic human rights, the leaders of the revolution declared that there should only be one patient to a bed in hospitals (the usual practice at that time was to assign two to eight patients per bed), and hospital beds were to be placed at least 3 feet apart (Annas, 1978). This kind of direction by a government or legislating body in the recognition and assertion of clients' rights has continued to be prominent in considerations of the right to health and the right to health care as extensions of basic human rights. However, the recognition of other clients' rights—such as rights to informed consent, to refuse treatment, or to privacy—have apparently been aided by consumer groups and health care providers such as the American Hospital Association (Annas, 1978).

Right to Health

A *right to health* has been historically recognized as one of the basic human rights of all persons. When introducing the Public Health Act of 1875 to the British Parliament, Prime Minister Disraeli noted that "the health of the people is really the foundation upon which all their happiness and all their powers of state depend" (Brockington, 1956, p. 47). In modern times, the right to health has been considered comparable to the rights to life and to liberty, which obligates "the State to prevent individuals from depriving each other of their health" (Szasz, 1976, p. 478). As a natural human good, health is a fundamental right and the state is obligated to protect it, although it is the responsibility of all persons to monitor their own health state.

In the United States the recognition of a right to health is indicated in eighteenth-century quarantine laws and early nineteenth-century laws granting citizens the right to obtain, free of charge, effective cowpox vaccine (Beauchamp and Faden, 1979). These laws and early nineteenth-century public health measures such as sanitation and water supply regulations to control the spread of disease demonstrate early protective laws in matters of human health and hygiene. However, most of these measures protected a negative right to health—the right to not have one's health endangered by the actions of others. The state or government recognized its obligation to enact those measures that prevent the actions of others from adversely affecting the health of an individual.

It is important to note that positive obligations to provide services may seemingly "flow from negative rights" (Beauchamp and Faden, 1979, p. 124). In other words, the negative right to be free to enjoy good health may lead to the positive right to obtain certain services or community health safeguards. For example, the negative right to not have one's health endangered by others led to the provision of public health measures concerning sewage disposal, water supplies, and the regulation of prostitution in the past (Brockington, 1956).

The negative right to not have one's health affected by social conditions has even led to regulations concerning housing and measures to protect the health of children. In modern times, this latter view of the negative right to health has encouraged some community health advocates to propose broad, federally supported programs and services to protect citizens against preventable diseases and disability (in particular, alcoholism and smoking-related illnesses) caused, in part, by social conditions (Beauchamp, D.E., 1976, 1980, 1985).

Thus advocacy—in the guise of protecting a negative right to health—has helped open the door to consideration of the right to health as a positive right: a claim against the state and its agencies to provide actions in the form of services and programs to improve health. It has been aided by documents such as the Universal Declaration of Human Rights of the United Nations Assembly. Noting the right of all persons to a standard of living adequate to provide for health and well-being and the right "to food, clothing, housing, and medical care" (UNESCO, 1949), this document suggests that persons not only have a strong negative right to health but a strong positive right to health (or medical) care as well. It suggests that persons are entitled to certain services, programs, and goods in order to maintain or achieve health as a basic human right.

Right to Health Care

Even though it is sometimes claimed that the "right to health" is an elliptical term for the expression "the right to health care" (Daniels, 1979), the two terms denote different kinds of rights and should be kept separate. The right to health is a negative right to a natural human good, which can be of various degrees. It is a right to not have one's health interfered with by others. However, the *right to health care* is a positive right to goods and services in order to maintain and improve whatever state of health exists. It is a rights claim against the state or its agencies to provide specific health care services that one requests or is entitled to receive. For example, immunizations, kidney dialysis services, home health services for Medicare and Medicaid recipients, and federally funded prenatal and family planning services all recognize the positive right to specific health care services.

The distinction between the two terms is often blurred for two reasons. First, the World Health Organization defines *health* as "a state of complete physical, mental, and social well-being and not merely the absence of disease or infirmity" (World Health Organization, 1958). The emphasis on complete physical, mental, and social well-being in this definition tends to suggest that one is unhealthy without complete well-being. Since persons experience, as a result of the natural lottery, various degrees of health (but are not necessarily "unhealthy"), this would mean that services must be provided to bring about physical, mental, and social well-being for one to possess complete health. Thus, in recognizing a right to health, the right to health care services to achieve complete health would also have to be recognized.

This is obviously a mistake. The World Health Organization's definition of health should merely be considered as an ideal state of health—one which very few persons actually possess or maintain over a long period of time. As a definition of an ideal state of health, it has no bearing on the provision of health care services as a right of all persons and should not be construed as a state that must, in fact, exist.

A second reason why the distinction between the two terms has become blurred stems from the recent advancements of modern medicine and the willingness of government to subsidize medical treatment for specific disorders such as renal disease (Public Law 92-603, 1972) and some genetic disorders (Public Law 92-278, 1976). This tendency has created a rising escalation of expectations in terms of services to achieve optimal health. It seems as if government, in recognizing a right of citizens to be as healthy as possible, must necessarily recognize a right of citizens to those services to achieve optimal health. Therefore by subsidizing treatment of some diseases and genetic disorders, government has created the idea that the right to health means a right to good health, a state that can only be achieved through the provision of specific health care services.

Yet this is clearly wrong. In an analysis of Szasz's position (1976), Bell points out that "the right to health does not entail a right to health care because it does not entail a right to good health (only a right to good health if I already have it)" (1979, p. 162). Recognition of the right to health simply does not mean that the state is obligated to initiate health services to maintain health or improve it. Although there may be other reasons why the difference between the right to health and the right to health care are not very clear, these two reasons are certainly pertinent.

Other Rights

The right to health and the right to health care are not the only rights of clients recognized by the health care delivery system. Other basic human rights are recognized as well.

In the United States the general issue of client rights in health care did not receive widespread recognition until the early 1970s. At that time, a commission of the Department of Health, Education, and Welfare was studying medical malpractice. In its final report the commission recommended that "hospitals and other health care facilities adopt and distribute statements of patient's rights in a manner which most effectively communicates these rights to all incoming patients" (DHEW, 1973, p. 71). It is important to realize that this recommendation was intended for community health agencies as well as for acute care centers.

At the same time the American Hospital Association was also studying the issue of patients' rights. In 1972 this organization issued the results of its study, entitled *"The Patient's Bill of Rights."* The use of this document in health care facilities soon became the means by which many health care providers communicated rights to their clients. Recognizing that "the traditional physician-patient relationship takes on a new dimension when care is rendered within an organizational structure," this document affirmed the basic human rights of all clients who seek health care services (American Hospital Association, 1973). It included the rights to (1) considerate and respectful care, (2) obtain complete medical information, (3) receive information necessary for giving informed consent, (4) refuse treatment, (5) considerations of privacy, (6) confidential treatment of personal information and medical records, (7) request services, (8) information on other institutions and individuals related to care and treatment, (9) refuse participation in research projects, (10) expect reasonable continuity of care, (11) examination and explanation of financial charges, and (12) know institutional regulations.

The Patient's Bill of Rights has been criticized for several reasons. First, it seemingly grants rights to clients that have always belonged to clients (Gaylin, 1973). Second, the bill asserts a number of rights that clients have legal claims against whether or not an institution supports the document. Third, the statement "takes the circuitous route of speaking to the patient of his rights, rather than to the hospital of its duties . . ." (Gaylin, 1973, p. 142). These criticisms indicate that the problem of client rights in health care is not actually with the client. As Gaylin points out, health clients do not need to be reminded of their basic rights. Instead, society and health care providers ought to consider what their responsibilities are to clients regarding health matters. The issue of client rights is a problem in health care delivery because society does not articulate its obligations to citizens regarding health. As a result, health care providers fail to recognize and protect basic rights of clients. To correct this problem, health professionals need

to ask: What are societal obligations to citizens regarding health? What kind of responsibilities do health care providers have in response to client rights?

Societal Obligations

In a lengthy document entitled *Securing Access to Health Care* (1983), the President's Commission for the Study of Ethical Problems in Medicine and Biomedical and Behavioral Research reports the result of its study of the differences in the availability of health services as influenced by an individual's income or residence. The commission reached several conclusions concerning current patterns of access to health care and made significant recommendations for changes. The box below lists these conclusions and recommendations as contained in the commission's report to the President and to Congress.

The cornerstone of their conclusions is the assertion that "society has an ethical obligation to ensure equitable access to health care for all" (President's Commission, 1983, p. 4). It noted that this obligation "rests on the special importance of health care and is derived from its role in relieving suffering, preventing premature death, (and) restoring functioning, . . ." (p. 29). Considering these obligations, the commission recommended that costs for health care for those unable to pay ought to be spread equitably at the national level and that costs should not be "allowed to fall more heavily on the shoulders of residents of different localities" (p. 30). The commission further recommended that the federal government assume ultimate responsibility for ensuring that equitable access to health care for all is achieved "through a combination of public and private sector arrangements" (p. 29).

ETHICAL FRAMEWORK OF THE PRESIDENT'S COMMISSION

The Commission concludes that:

Society has an ethical obligation to ensure equitable access to health care for all.

The societal obligation is balanced by individual obligations.

Equitable access to health care requires that all citizens be able to secure an adequate level of care without excessive burdens.

When equity occurs through the operation of private forces, there is no need for government involvement, but the ultimate responsibility for ensuring that society's obligation is met, through a combination of public and private sector arrangements, rests with the federal government.

The cost of achieving equitable access to health care ought to be shared fairly.

Efforts to contain rising health care costs are important but should not focus on limiting the attainment of equitable access for the least well served portion of the public.

From President's Commission for the Study of Ethical Problems in Medicine and Biomedical and Behavioral Research: Securing access to health care. Vol. 1, Washington, D.C., 1983, U.S. Government Printing Office.

Professional Responsibilities

In response to clients' rights, health care professionals incur particular duties or responsibilities as illustrated in Figure 4-1. Some of these duties are supported by professional codes of ethics and are correlative to basic liberty rights of the client.

Codes of Ethics

Professional *codes of ethics* are statements encompassing rules that apply to persons in professional roles. Two questions generally arise concerning the importance of these codes in health care delivery. (1) What is their relation to universal moral principles? and (2) What is their relation to legal requirements for professional practice? (Beauchamp and Walters, 1978).

In answering the first question, we should consider the rules contained in professional codes of ethics for nurses to be specific applications of more universal moral principles. While some professional codes of ethics are merely statements about professional etiquette or conduct between professional groups and have no relation to external principles, this is not the case in nursing. The professional code of ethics for nurses prescribes moral behavior and actions based on moral principles (Fry, 1982). Thus the professional nurse has a moral obligation to follow the rules in a code of ethics such as the *Code for Nurses with Interpretive Statements* of the American Nurses' Association (1976, 1985).*

In answering the second question, we should consider many of the rules in the *Code for Nurses* to be morally obligatory and legally required. Some of the rules may even have legal ties to licensure requirements concerning professional acts. For example, the rules of respecting client confidentially and accountability are mentioned as both morally obligatory and legally required by the *Code for Nurses*.

---

*Hereafter referred to as *Code for Nurses*.

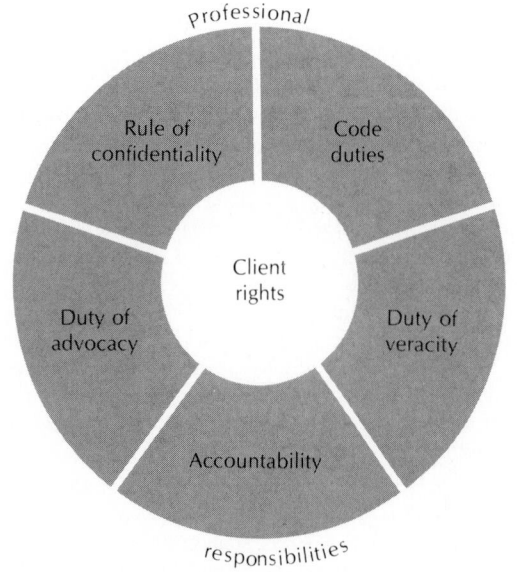

FIGURE 4-1

Client rights and professional responsibilities.

Codes of ethics also prescribe duties that are required of the professional in response to rights of the client. The duties of veracity and advocacy are specifically mentioned in the *Code for Nurses* as being correlative to clients' rights.

Duty of Veracity

Truthfulness has long been regarded as fundamental to the existence of trust among human beings. Persons have a duty of *veracity*—a duty to tell the truth and not lie or deceive people. In health care relationships several arguments are usually given for a duty to tell the truth (Beauchamp and Childress, 1983).

One argument claims that we tell the truth and forbear from lying or deceiving because this is part of the respect we owe persons. We respect persons because they are self-determining, or autonomous, individuals with all the rights and privileges of autonomous persons, including the right to be told the truth and not be lied to or deceived. Because we respect persons and their autonomy, we have a duty of veracity. For example, in community health nursing we respect persons and uphold a duty of veracity by not deceiving clients as to the nature of the care they are receiving.

A second argument claims that the duty of veracity is derived from or is a way of expressing the duty of promise keeping (Ross, 1930). Health care professionals have a duty of veracity because communicating with the client creates an implicit contract to tell the truth and not lie or deceive. The contract between client and community health nurse creates the expectation that nurses will, in interacting with the client, speak truthfully.

A third argument claims that relationships of trust are necessary for cooperation between clients and health care professionals. After all, to not tell the truth or to deceive clients will, in the long run, undermine relationships and bring about undesirable consequences for future relationships with clients. Thus the community health nurse has a responsibility to maintain truthful relationships with clients to protect and to strengthen other health care relationships in general.

Yet community health nurses often have difficulty heeding or observing a duty of veracity. Information is sometimes withheld from the client or he is deceived because the nurse may think certain information will cause the client anxiety. This tendency is illustrated by responses to a 1975 survey in which over 15,000 nurses responded to questions relating to how knowledge of the client's condition should be handled by the nurse. In response to the question, "When a patient who has a terminal illness bluntly asks you if he is dying and his physician does not want him to know, what do you usually do?"; 1% would tell him; 1% would avoid the question or try to distract him; 1% would reassure him that he is not dying, just ill; 2% would lie, saying they did not know; 14% would tell him that only the physician can answer the question; and the majority (81%) would ask why he brought up the question or try to get him to talk about his feelings (Popoff, 1975, p. 24).

Nurses also withhold information because they think that clients, particularly if very sick or dying, do not really want to know the truth about their condition. But this belief is not substantiated by surveys of the sick and dying. In a survey of 100 cancer patients, 89% preferred knowing their condition; in a survey of 100 noncancer patients, 82% said they preferred knowing, in a survey of 740 patients being diagnosed in a cancer detection center, 98.5% said they wanted to know their condition (Veatch, 1978).

Regardless of the various reasons for not telling the truth to clients or withholding information, it is clear that community health professionals have a duty of veracity. As the *Code for Nurses*** notes, "clients have the moral right . . . to be given accurate information, and all the information necessary for making informed judgments; . . ." (American Nurses' Association, 1976, 1985, p. 2). In fact, the duty to not lie or deceive is a stronger moral duty than the duty to disclose information.† The duty of veracity is a duty correlative to the patient's right to know and includes a strong moral obligation not to lie or deceive.

Rule of Confidentiality

In general social interaction certain information is regarded as confidential. Regarding information as confidential enables us to control the disclosure of personal information and to limit the access of others to sensitive information (Fry, 1984).

In community health care relationships, *confidentiality* of information is maintained for several reasons. First, if health care professionals did not follow a rule of confidentiality, clients might not seek help when they needed it. They would not reveal necessary information relating to their illnesses that would facilitate treatment for illnesses or disease processes. For example, if community health nurses could not be trusted to hold personal information in confidence, family planning clients might not reveal information relating to their reproductive history that would facilitate appropriate and safe nursing care and follow-up treatment. In short, maintaining confidentiality helps protect the functioning of professional and client relationships.

A second reason for maintaining confidentiality is derived from the sphere of privacy we recognize as a basic human right of all persons. Because persons are self-determining moral agents, they have a right to determine how personal information, especially health information, is communicated. As the *Code for Nurses* points out, "The nurse safeguards the client's right to privacy by judiciously protecting information of a confidential nature" (American Nurses' Association, 1985, p. 4). Because of respect for persons, nurses respect clients' rights to privacy by maintaining the moral rule of confidentiality.

In health care relationships, however, the duty to observe the rule of confidentiality is not always an absolute duty;

it is merely a *prima facie* duty, meaning that it may be overridden when in conflict with other duties that are morally stronger. The duty to observe confidentiality may be overridden for several reasons:

1. When in conflict with other duties toward the client. For example, the duty to preserve life may outweigh the duty to respect confidential information concerning self-destructive wishes of the client.

2. When in conflict with duties toward identified others. For example, if a mental health client tells the nurse of intent to harm or even kill another member of the community, regardless of the confidential nature of the mental health nurse/relationship, the nurse's duty to protect others from harm by warning the intended victim of the client will override the duty to keep confidentiality. This action may even be required by law (Tarasoff, 1976).

3. When in conflict with duties toward nonidentified others or the rights and interests of society in general. For example, communicable diseases such as tuberculosis or venereal disease are required to be reported by law regardless of the confidential nature of that information; this is done to protect the health of others. Another example concerns the right to keep information in one's health record private that may be overridden by duties to others in society. This occurs when health records are used for epidemiological research without the client's knowledge. There are, of course, stringent constraints placed on the use of this information by epidemiologists in health research (Gordis and Gold, 1980; Kelsey, 1981). But in general, the duty to increase or protect the health of the community through research outweighs the duty to respect the confidentiality of health records.

Duty of Advocacy

The nursing profession recognizes a strong duty of *advocacy* where the care or safety of clients is concerned. As the *Code of Nurses* states, " . . . the nurse must be alert to and take appropriate action regarding any instances of incompetent, unethical, or illegal practice by any member of the health care team or the health care system, or any action on the part of others that places the rights or best interests of the client in jeopardy" (American Nurses' Association, 1976, 1985, p. 6). In the role of advocate, the nurse speaks for or in support of the best interests of the individual client or vulnerable client populations.

This is a strong protect-the-client-from-harm duty which is derived from a general ethical principle of beneficence or the "duty to help others further their important . . . interests" (Beauchamp and Childress, 1983, p. 148). Yet the role of advocate can be difficult for the community health nurse. First, it must be recognized that clients should always determine what is in their best interests. Acting on the basis of what the nurse thinks is in the best interests of clients can lead to paternalism when the wishes of clients are never ascertained.

Second, the duty of advocacy extends to populations at risk, which may bring the community health nurse into conflict with health policy or established professional practices within a community or institution. Nurse advocates

---

*Quotations from *Code for Nurses* reprinted with permission of ANA.
†The duty to disclose information evolves from special relationships between agents. In such relationships, one agent can claim a right to information that the other agent would not be obligated to provide to a stranger. The duty to not lie, however, does not depend on special relationships. Lying threatens any relationship because, as Beauchamp and Childress point out, ". . .lying means that an agent asserts what he believes to be false in order to deceive another (1983, p. 210).

who have experienced this kind of conflict have sometimes found their jobs and other professional relationships in jeopardy (Smith, 1980). Needless to say, positions of advocacy can be difficult to maintain when they conflict with accepted professional practices.

Third, it has been questioned whether the duty of advocacy requires the community health nurse to put one's own job, health, or professional standing at risk on behalf of advocacy for the client. According to Beauchamp and Childress, this is not a moral requirement of the principle of beneficence (1983). What is required is that the nurse fulfill the primary commitment to client care and safety by protecting the client from harm. While the implicit contract of the nurse/client relationship does, in general, require positive acts of benefiting in terms of care rendered, this does not extend to the role of advocate. Thus the community health nurse is only required, in the role of advocate, to protect, speak for, and support the interests of the client to *not* be harmed in the provision of health care services.

Accountability: Moral Obligation or Moral Virtue?

The need for *moral accountability* within nursing practice in response to basic human rights has long been recognized. Even Florence Nightingale reputedly made strong objections to the overriding of a person's will for the benefit of others in the performance of nursing care (Palmer, 1977). Believing in the creativity and self-determining rights of man, Nightingale apparently included humanistic orientations in her early training programs for nurses. These orientations became the foundations on which accountability requirements in nursing were eventually constructed.

Modern leaders in nursing have also noted that means must be sought to promote progress in health care delivery while simultaneously protecting the rights of the individual. Noting the need for scientific accountability within the performance of nursing functions, Gortner called for a standard of accountability in nursing as the means by which the quality of nursing services will be provided (1974).

Yet it is uncertain what is meant by a "standard of accountability" in nursing. Further more, what does the standard of accountability require of the nurse? In the *Code for Nurses*, accountability is defined as "being answerable to someone for something one has done" (American Nurses' Association, 1985, p. 8). It includes providing an explanation to one's self, to the client, to the employing agency, and to the nursing profession for what one has done in the role of nurse. It is an obligation that has both moral and legal components and implies a contractual agreement between two parties. This means that when a community health nurse enters into a contractual agreement to perform a service for a client, the nurse will be held answerable for performing this service according to agreed terms, within an established time period, and with stipulated use of resources and performance standards. The nurse as contractor is responsible for the quality of the services rendered and is accountable to the individual client, the health service agency, the nursing profession, and even one's own conscience for what has been done (Fry, 1983a).

Referring to accountability in nursing as a moral obligation means that being answerable for what one has done is correlative to clients' rights to a certain level of competent nursing care and their rights to self-determination in health care. As a moral obligation, accountability directs the professional to act in a particular way according to moral norms (Fry, 1981, 1986b). But is accountability merely a moral obligation? Because of the central role of accountability in nursing care and its grounding in the trust relationship shared by client and nurse, accountability may also be a moral virtue, one that is peculiar to the practice of nursing.

Moral virtue may be characterized in different ways. According to Carney, moral virtue is "an ideal of human personhood at which to aim" (1978, p. 435). This statement indicates that moral virtue is apparently an ideal standard of human behavior and may help one to discern the morality of human acts.

It is generally believed that people develop virtues that support the types of moral obligations already acknowledged in daily actions. These virtues then enable people to carefully perform their duties, thus increasing the probability that performance in practice settings will closely approximate professional standards (Carney, 1978). According to this view, there is a close relationship between moral obligations already operating in a practice and moral virtues. Hence, it might be quite natural to view accountability as moral virtue.

MacIntyre had called virtue an "acquired human quality the possession and exercise of which tends to enable us to achieve those goods which are internal to practices" (1981, p. 178). MacIntyre further points out that since every practice requires a certain kind of relationship between those who participate in it, virtues are how we define our relationships to those with whom we share practices. Thus he concludes that virtues (such as justice, courage, and honesty) are essential to practices like medicine and nursing. They help define the kind of relationships we have with persons in practices and sustain the traditions that provide historical context to both practices and individual lives (MacIntyre, 1981).

In nursing, and especially in community health nursing, accountability appears to be the quality that defines the kind of relationships between client, nurse, other professionals, and the public at large that form the moral foundations of the professional ethic in nursing. Furthermore, since accountability is correlative to client's rights to competent levels of nursing care, it is responsive to the humanistic traditions that permeate nursing's history. Viewed in this manner, accountability, as a moral virtue (being derived from moral obligation), enables the nurse to achieve what is internal to the practice of community health nursing: the protection of the client's human dignity and right to self-determination in matters of health.

ETHICAL PRINCIPLES IN COMMUNITY HEALTH
Relationship of Ethical Rules, Principles, and Theories

In making moral decisions we usually appeal to various rules, principles, or theories (see Figure 4-2). *Rules* state that certain actions should (or should not) be performed

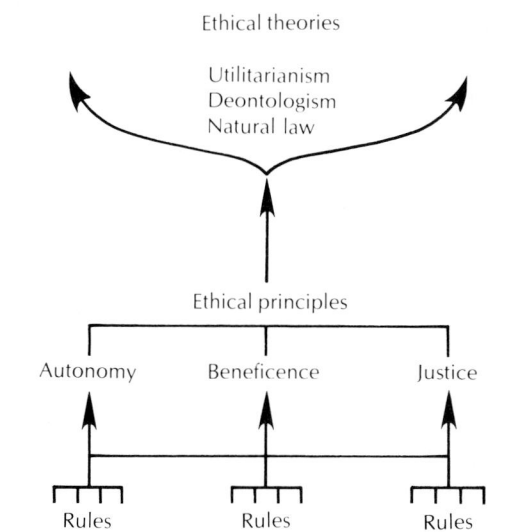

FIGURE 4-2

The relationship of ethical theories, principles, and rules.

because they are right (or wrong). An example would be that "nurses ought to always tell the truth to clients." *Principles* are more abstract than rules and serve as the foundation of rules. For example, the ethical principle of autonomy is the foundation for such rules as "always informed consent," "tell the truth," and "protect the privacy of the client." Likewise, the principle of justice serves as the foundation of rules such as "treat equals equally" and "divide your time on the basis of needs." *Theories,* however, are collections of principles and rules. They provide theoretical foundations for deciding what to do when principles or rules conflict. Examples of a few major theories are *utilitarianism, deontologism,* and *natural law* (see Glossary for exact definitions).

Within theories, the various moral rules and principles are arranged according to their importance or justifiability. For example, in utilitarianism, the principle of beneficence often carries more weight than the ethical principles of autonomy or justice. This does not mean that beneficence cannot be overridden by either principle in many circumstances.

Thus ethical principles are not absolute. Each ethical principle is always morally significant but may not always prevail when in conflict with other principles. Ethical theories simply suggest which ethical principles will more likely prevail when moral decisions have to be made.

But what makes some judgments moral and others nonmoral? Moral judgments are evaluations of what is good or bad, right or wrong, having certain characteristics that separate them from other evaluations such as personal preferences, beliefs, or matters of taste. The difference between the evaluations lies in the reasons for or the grounds on which the judgments are being made and according to the characteristics of the judgments themselves (Frankena, 1973).

Moral judgments are generally made of human actions, institutions, or character traits. What makes them moral (instead of nonmoral) is that they have the characteristics

of (1) being ultimate or preemptive, meaning that other values or human ends cannot, as a rule, override them (Fried, 1978); (2) having universality, meaning that they apply to everyone under relevantly similar circumstances (Baier, 1958); and (3) having an other-regarding focus, meaning that they treat the good of everyone alike and do not give a special place to one's own welfare (Beauchamp and Childress, 1983).

Community health nurses frequently make moral judgments. When the nurse decides to arrange a home visiting schedule on the basis of need or seriousness of illness, a moral judgment is made. When the nurse decides to refer a client to a physician for further evaluation based on the expressed wishes of the client and his condition, a moral judgment is made. When a nurse decides, regardless of personal beliefs about abortion, to inform a client of all the options available concerning a request for abortion, a moral judgment is made. When a nurse decides not to participate in political activities urged by others that might lessen health care coverage for vulnerable populations, a moral judgment is made. What makes these decisions moral rather than nonmoral are the reasons for which the judgments were made and their stated characteristics.

Principle of Beneficence
Definition

The principle of *beneficence* states that "we ought to do good and prevent or avoid doing harm" (Frankena, 1973, p. 45). It includes the idea that beneficence is a duty to help others gain what is of benefit to them but does not carry the obligation to risk one's own welfare or interests in helping others. In fact, some theorists maintain that beneficence does not morally require us to always benefit others even when we can do so. Rather we are only morally required to prevent harm to people. This may be true in general social interactions among persons. But in special relationships, the implicit contract underlying the nature of the relationship seems to indicate that positive benefiting or acts of beneficence should take place. This seems to be the case in nursing.

The need for health care forms the basis of the relationship between community health nurse and client and imposes a moral duty on the nurse to benefit the client through nursing actions. However, there may be limits on the amount of beneficial nursing care a client should expect. Certainly no nurse should be expected to provide nursing care to individual clients or client populations at physical risk to oneself or when clients' needs infringe on one's personal life or responsibilities to other clients, to oneself, or to one's own family. While the duty to prevent harm occurring to clients is a stringent one in nursing, the claim to positive benefiting is limited.

Applications in Community Health

In community health nursing, the principle of beneficence can be applied in (1) balancing harms and benefits to client populations and (2) in the use of cost benefit analyses in decisions affecting client populations.

BALANCING HARMS AND BENEFITS. Acting so as to bring about the greatest balance of good over evil, or value (benefit) over disvalue (harms), is acting in accordance with a *rule of utility.* This rule is derived from the principle of beneficence and includes the moral duty to weigh and balance benefits against harms to increase benefits and reduce the occurrence of harms (Beauchamp and Childress, 1983).

In community health a rule of utility may be appealed to in deciding whether to fund certain health programs more than others, whether to conduct screening programs for communicable disease after several cases have been found in vulnerable populations, and whether to conduct research projects where individual rights to privacy may be concerned. In each example, the decision is made by balancing the possible harms and benefits of several alternative courses of action. The community health nurse facilitates this process by accurately assessing the known benefits and harms to clients from a nursing care point of view and presenting them along with other relevant facts that might enter into the decision-making process.

COST BENEFIT ANALYSIS. Cost benefit analysis is a specific application of the principle of beneficence. It is a device for measuring the harms and benefits of providing various methods of care or health programs while also figuring the cost of the relative trade-offs that might have to be made in selecting certain courses of actions. All of the units taken into consideration, such as lives saved, costs averted, taxes saved, and illness prevented, are eventually converted into one common unit—usually money—to measure the benefits and costs of alternative approaches to a problem or to decide how to distribute health program funds.

Problems and Conflicts

Decision making in community health settings on the basis of a principle of beneficence and the weighing of harms and benefits raises moral questions concerning (1) paternalism in health care decisions and (2) the extent of the rule of utility in decision making.

PATERNALISM. Paternalism is a liberty-limiting principle that is frequently invoked to override people's actions or expressed wishes for their own good or best interests. Parents may override a child's desire to play with the interesting knobs on a stove because they do not want the child to get burned. Community health nurses may override clients' expressed wishes "not to hear any bad news" by telling them the results of laboratory testing so that their health status can be treated and improved. Nurses do this because they feel it is in client's best interests in the long run to know the status of their health.

In general, it is morally justified to restrict a person's liberty when the harm to be caused is a physical harm, possibly life-threatening, and is caused by those whose liberty is restricted. However, it is more difficult to justify paternalistic actions for perceived psychological harms. For example, it might seem morally justified to override a teenager's desire to participate in a potentially risky (to health) research project but not seem morally justified to withhold information of a defective fetus from a woman who is 6 months pregnant because it might cause her psychological harm and grief during the remaining months of pregnancy.

It is also difficult to justify paternalistic actions for the purpose of benefiting the person whose liberty is restricted. For example, it is hard to morally justify restraining and forcibly giving medication to a mental health client who has refused chemotherapy because the medication will benefit him by reducing his paranoia or irrational fears. Yet we recognize that health care practitioners often carry out paternalistic actions. If this is the case, are there some acts of paternalism which are morally justified and if so, what are the criteria for justified paternalism in community health decisions?

Since paternalism always violates the moral principle of autonomy and the moral rule to treat persons as self-determining moral agents, justified paternalism is a very limited area. According to Gert and Culver (1979), paternalism is justified only if (1) the evils that would be prevented are much greater than the evils, if any, that would be caused by the violation of the moral rule and (2) we would be willing to universally allow the violation of the moral rule in these same circumstances and be able to publicly advocate this kind of violation. Thus acts involving justified paternalism seem to be limited to those acts that prevent a person from commiting some grave bodily harm to himself—self-mutilating or self-destructing behaviors and acts committed out of ignorance such as the ingestion of harmful substances unknowingly. Beyond these and similar acts, it is hard to justify paternalism in community health. Few situations meet the previously stated criteria for justified paternalism.

EXTENT OF THE RULE OF UTILITY. Attempting to bring about the greatest possible balance of benefit over harm in community health may lead to two problems. The first is the potential overriding of individual liberties and values for the common good (Fry, 1985). For example, in calculating the benefits of a health policy to citizens in terms of tax savings and other economic benefits, the health needs of individual citizens may be overlooked or simply not deemed as important when entered into the calculations for aggregate utility. Human needs and wants that cannot be easily or accurately converted into monetary units may simply be left out in deciding for the greatest amount of overall benefit. As pointed out by MacIntyre, the methodology of cost benefit analysis in particular cannot truly represent the value choices of individuals (1979). Incommensurable value choices pertaining to health and life are distorted or ignored in figuring perceived harms and benefits into the calculations of the analysis. Thus policy decisions on the basis of the rule of utility as expressed in cost benefit analysis may be inaccurate as well as irrelevant to the health needs of individuals.

A second problem arises when the rule of utility is applied in health policy decisions having long-term effects. For example, it is often unclear how short-term harms and benefits ought to be weighed against long-term consequences in cost benefit analysis. If the benefits and harms to individual health or economic savings in the future are judged more important than present savings or health conditions, then individual and collective interests in health may be sacrificed for future benefits.

Principle of Autonomy
Definition

Autonomy refers to freedom of action as chosen by an individual. Persons who are autonomous are capable of choosing and acting on plans they themselves have decided on.

To respect persons as autonomous individuals is to acknowledge their personal rights to make choices and act according to individual determinations; they are respected as self-determining moral agents or persons. Thus when nurses respect persons as moral agents, they are acting in accordance with the requirements of the moral principle of autonomy.

Applications in Community Health

The principle of autonomy is applied in community health through considerations of (1) respect for persons, (2) the protection of privacy, (3) the provision of informed consent, (4) freedom of choice including treatment refusal, and (5) the protection of diminished autonomy.

RESPECT FOR PERSONS. In community health, clients are respected for no other reason than because they are persons and have the right to determine their own plan of life. Community health nurses acknowledge respect by seriously considering the opinions and choices of clients while not, at the same time, obstructing their actions unless they are harmful to themselves or others. Denying clients freedom

to act on their own judgments or withholding information necessary to make judgments demonstrates a lack of respect for clients.

For example, consider the elderly client who may not be treated with the respect accorded younger clients. Community health nurses often find it easier and quicker to communicate with family members or simply "tell" the client what treatment has to be performed. The elderly client may not be given a choice or even considered in the treatment plan. Age, however, does not render a client less worthy of our respect (Figure 4-3). The elderly have the right to determine their life and health plans insofar as they have the capacity to do so. To deny them the opportunity to choose according to their capacities demonstrates a lack of respect for persons and is an infringement of the principle of autonomy.

PROTECTION OF PRIVACY. The nature of community health nursing care involves close observation of clients, physical touching, and access to personal health and economic information about clients and their families. All of these aspects of nursing care may invade the privacy of clients or threaten their right to control personal information.

Since the relationship between nurse and client is built on trust, the nurse has a responsibility to protect the privacy of clients and their families insofar as clients' health is concerned. This means that personal information gathered

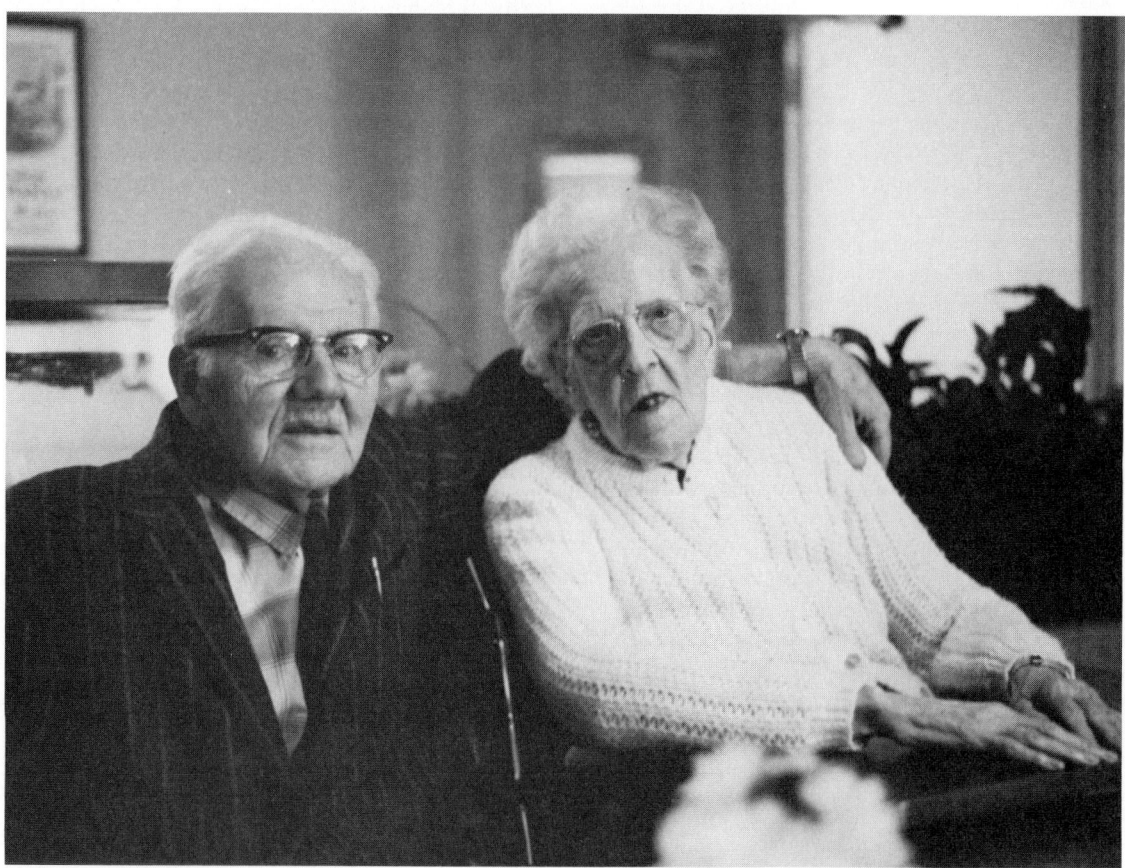

FIGURE 4-3

Age does not render clients less worthy of our respect.

in the initial home assessment of clients must be recorded in a manner that acknowledges respect for clients' privacy and is communicated only to those directly concerned with client care.

When personal economic information must be shared with third parties for payment of nursing care, clients have the right to authorize or withhold disclosure of information. Even though the information may be essential for continuity of nursing care services, the client retains control of all information generated by the nurse/client relationship.

When clients' records are examined for quality assurance purposes or notes about home or clinic visits are included in research studies to assess the effectiveness of community health nursing services, the protection of privacy may be a genuine problem. Utilization of health records in determining funding levels for community health nursing services does not justify the use of nurse-generated information about the client without the client's knowledge and permission. Health record information can only be used for quality assurance purposes or research studies and shared with others under clearly defined policies and written guidelines that protect client privacy. In addition, community health nursing services are responsible for making sure that policies and guidelines appropriately protect client privacy and that clients are informed of this protection *before* information about them is released to any source. Only when measures to protect the privacy of clients are fully carried out can it be said that community health nursing meets the requirements of the ethical principle of autonomy.

PROVISION OF INFORMED CONSENT. The principle of autonomy requires that clients be given "the opportunity to choose what shall or shall not happen to them" (National Commission, 1978, p. 10). Clients are provided this opportunity when consent is voluntarily made and when adequate disclosure standards for *informed consent* are included in the contract for community health nursing services. Three elements are essential for adequate informed consent information, comprehension, and voluntariness.

1. *Information.* For clients to have adequate information, the nurse must disclose information pertaining to treatment procedures, their purposes, any discomforts and anticipated benefits, alternative procedures for therapy, and the opportunity to question procedures or end the contract at any time. Clients should also be adequately informed as to how confidentiality of their health records will be maintained.

2. *Comprehension.* The manner and context in which information is conveyed to clients is also important for informed consent requirements. Clients must be allowed time to consider information provided by the community health nurse as well as time to ask questions. If the client is unable to comprehend because of a language barrier, such as between an English-speaking nurse and Spanish-speaking client, the nurse must provide an interpreter to remove such barriers. This, of course, implies that the client is competent to understand and can make decisions based on rational reasons. Competent clients are those able to understand a treatment procedure or proposed care plan, weigh its discomforts and benefits, and then make decisions about undertaking the procedure or plan.

3. *Voluntariness.* This element of informed consent is so important that any contract or agreement with the client constitutes valid consent only if voluntarily given, free of coercion and undue influences by other persons or the health agency. The notion of voluntariness includes the ability to choose one's own health goals and the ability to choose among several goals when offered a choice of options (Beauchamp and Childress, 1983). Again, the principle of autonomy is the main ethical principle guiding this provision.

These three elements—information, comprehension, and voluntariness—constitute informed consent in community health nursing practice. Informed consent is not valid without all elements and no contract between client and nurse is ethically acceptable without valid, informed consent.

INDIVIDUAL FREEDOM OF CHOICE. Respecting the client's right to self-determination includes respecting potential treatment refusal. The client's interest in personal freedom to follow one's own will, the potential harm to the client or other citizens, the cost of treatment refusal, and the values of society are all factors that usually enter into the nurse's acknowledgement or acceptance of treatment refusal (Capron, 1978). But as long as a client is judged competent to make this kind of decision, it is difficult to infringe on autonomy by not allowing treatment refusal.

Some of the most interesting and difficult legal cases involving treatment refusal have involved the exercise of religious beliefs *(In re estate of Brooks,* 1965). Others have involved the autonomy of the teenage minor to refuse lifesaving treatment such as kidney dialysis (Veatch, 1976). More recent cases affecting the values of entire communities have involved the right of parents to refuse lifesaving treatment for their defective newborns (Lyons, 1985, Will, 1982) and the right of the terminally ill to refuse lifesustaining food and water (Annas, 1985; Fry, 1986b; Lynn and Childress, 1983).

In community health nursing, respect for the client's or guardian's right to refuse treatment may hinge on nurse judgment of the competency of the client to make such choices. The physical competency of the elderly or severely ill client, the psychological competency of former mental patients, and the maturity or legal competency of minors may, in part, rely on the assessment of client abilities as made in the home environment by the community health nurse.

In situations of questionable competency, decisions have generally opted for the preservation of life (Beauchamp and Childress, 1983). In situations where competency to make decisions has been established, other factors such as obligations to others (such as dependent children) may determine whether or not autonomy of choice will be respected. No hard and fast rule on treatment refusal can be made. Yet community health nurses should recognize that respect for persons may involve allowing clients and their legal guardians to make decisions concerning their life and health that may be very difficult for the nurse to accept.

PROTECTING DIMINISHED AUTONOMY. The principle of autonomy is generally applied only to persons capable of autonomous choice. Persons who have diminished autonomy, whether from physical or psychological incapacities or immaturity, are not considered fully autonomous persons. Thus it is thought justifiable to interfere with the actions of those not fully autonomous to protect them from harmful results of their choices and actions without infringing on the principle of autonomy. This interference, however, requires appeals to other principles, such as beneficence, as the source of special duties toward those not fully autonomous.

The community health nurse may have difficulty recognizing when clients are not capable of self-determination because of diminished capacities. The capacity for self-determination is relative to maturity, chronological age, the presence or absence of illness, mental disability, or other social situations that restrict a person's liberty to be self-determining. Yet respect for the principle of autonomy requires that practitioners recognize when persons lack the capacity to act autonomously and therefore are entitled to protection in health care delivery (Figure 4-4).

Problems and Conflicts

Respecting the ethical principle of autonomy can be difficult in community health nursing practice. Those areas creating the most conflict for nurses have included (1) the carrying out of *coercive health measures* and (2) invasions of privacy for health reasons.

COERCIVE HEALTH MEASURES. Clients consulting a community health agency for nursing services may have a communicable disease that not only is harmful to themselves if untreated but also may affect the health of family members, neighbors, or coworkers. The client may not want to receive treatment and may even refuse to take medications or attend follow-up care recommended for the illness. For example, many areas of the United States still require clients diagnosed with active tuberculosis to be confined to a state institution until their disease process is no longer considered active or communicable to others. When diagnosed, clients must leave their jobs and families and incur the results of social stigmatization that still accompanies the diagnosis of tuberculosis. Clients have no choice in the matter. They must be admitted to the state institution and must take treatment, regardless of their own wishes, choices, or life plans.

The community health nurse may be the one to enforce these regulations or be the agent to override a client's expressed wishes in this matter. Thus nurses may find the conflict between individual rights to self-determinations in health matters and the protection of the community's health to be especially difficult when they are the agents carrying out this kind of coercive health measure.

INVASIONS OF PRIVACY. In protecting the health of vulnerable populations the community health nurse may in-

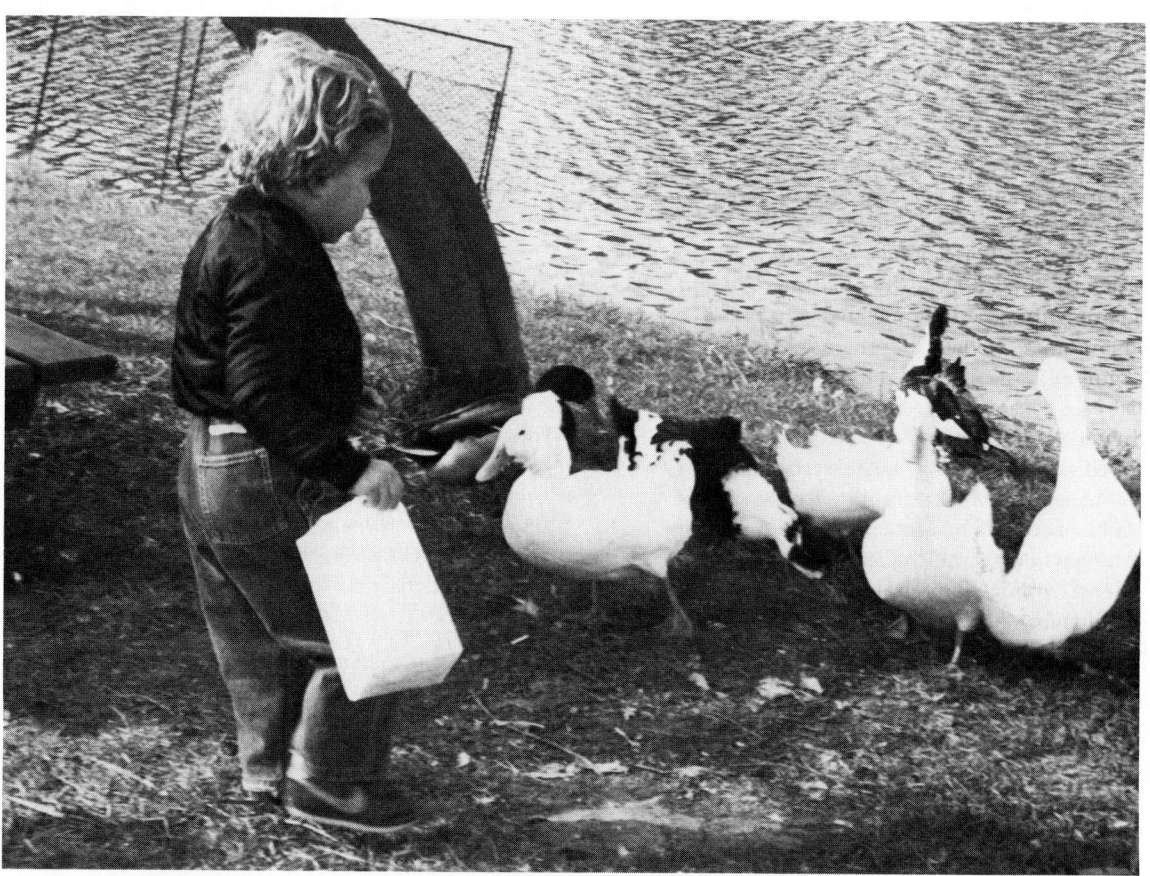

FIGURE 4-4

Children have diminished autonomy and are entitled to protection in health care delivery.

fringe on rights to privacy by actively gathering information of a private nature from those unwilling to give this information. For example, a sharp rise in the incidence of venereal disease among a high school population may require interviewing of teenagers diagnosed with disease and the accurate follow-up of all named contacts. This action may lead to invasions of individual privacy through discussion of sexual habits and preferences and potential disclosures to adults, including parents.

All of these actions are infringements of self-determining behavior but are considered justifiable on the basis of potential harms to others. Regardless, it is the nurse's responsibility to inform those whose privacy is invaded that information will be recorded and communicated in a way that does not infringe on their future privacy.

Privacy may also be invaded by the assessment and recording of personal client information. For example, the community health nurse may record information about the social habits and life-styles of pregnant women, which may subsequently be used in retrospective research studies correlating neonatal mortality and morbidity with social habits (particularly drug and alcohol use during pregnancy). This type of personal information is often freely communicated on the basis of the trust relationship between nurse and client. It may also be recorded in the client's record without full understanding of the potential impact of this information if, in fact, a child is born with anomalies related to social habits or life-styles during pregnancy. The presence of this informaton in prenatal records may mean that it might eventually be shared with other health professionals and members of the client's family, constituting further invasions of the client's right to privacy of personal information.

In community health these invasions may be justified on the basis of preventing harm to innocent third parties (the defective child), but the actual communication of this information in a way sensitive to the client's right to privacy may create many conflicts of interest for the nurse.

Principle of Justice
Definition

The formal principle of *justice* claims that equals should be treated equally and that those who are unequal should be treated differently according to their differences (Beauchamp and Childress, 1983). In considerations of community health we appeal to a principle of justice in determining the manner in which social burdens and benefits, including health goods, ought to be distributed among all individuals in the community.

Applications in Community Health

Different theories of justice may be appealed to in deciding how to distribute health care resources. These theories include (1) the entitlement theory, (2) the utilitarian theory, (3) the maximin theory, and (4) the egalitarian theory. Each theory has its advantages and disadvantages in terms of the distribution of health goods in the community.

ENTITLEMENT THEORY. The *entitlement theory* claims that everyone is entitled to whatever they get in the natural lottery at birth and there is no responsibility for government or its agencies to improve the lot of those less fortunate than others. If people have good health, are rich, and have been able to acquire possessions by purchase, gift, or legitimate exchange, they are entitled to what they have. They may also increase their possessions in any way possible as long as they do not cheat others or acquire possessions unjustly (Nozick, 1974).

It is, of course, considered unfortunate that some people are mentally or physically handicapped in society, yet others have no obligation to give some of their money to the handicapped to make their lives more comfortable. Aiding the unfortunate is simply an act of charity on the part of members in the community.

In this theory, inequalities between individuals in matters of health, position, and wealth are tolerated. Only aggressions or harms against others and the unjust acquisitions of goods are prohibited. Thus the actual distribution of goods seems more in line with a principle of autonomy or the exercise of the right to liberty than a principle of justice (Veatch, 1981).

UTILITARIAN THEORY. The *utilitarian theory* of justice claims that the best way to distribute resources among the citizenry is to decide how expenditures or the use of resources will achieve the greatest net total of good and serve the largest number of people (Mill, 1957). In times of limited resources, when all that is needed or wanted cannot be provided in the community, this method of distribution is appealing. While it does tend to overlook the needs and wants of individuals, it manages to maximize net benefits over costs and serves the greatest number of people.

In this theory the needs and wants of some individuals will not be satisfied, and they may, indeed, be harmed in the process. This would be considered unfortunate, but in distributing limited resources so that "the greatest good for the greatest number" is achieved, government and its agencies would have fulfilled their obligations to citizenry. It is easy to see that the principle of beneficence dominates other considerations in utilitarianism. Justice is served by benefiting the greatest number at the least cost.

MAXIMIN THEORY. The *maximin** theory* of justice first identifies the least advantaged members of the community (for example, the economically poor, the elderly, the mentally retarded, and children below one year of age) and decides how they might be benefited rather than deciding on greatest net aggregate benefit. It then permits free exercise of liberty on the part of all citizens and allows social and economic inequalities to evolve in such a manner that these inequalities are of benefit to the least advantaged or least well-off members in society (Rawls, 1971). Many kinds of inequalities in terms of health, health care resources, and possession of economic benefits will be tolerated and considered just as long as the position of the least advantaged is improved or benefited. For example, health professionals can charge high fees or receive substantial salaries just as

---

Maximin is a short term for maximizing the minimum position in society.

long as they also serve the interests of the disadvantaged. In a similar manner costly health care resources, such as kidney dialysis, CT scans, and artificial hearts, can be developed and purchased by those who can afford them as long as the lot of the least advantaged is also improved in the process.

Obviously, distributing health goods according to this theory will create problems in times of limited resources. Even though the maximin theory advocates distribution in accordance with a principle of justice, providing benefit to the least advantaged first is a constraint on the expansion of health care resources and technological advancement unless some way can be figured out to benefit the least advantaged in the process. Thus it is possible that technological advancement and the development of more sophisticated health care goods cannot be made widely available to the public in times of limited economic resources. The result is that interests and needs in matters of health may not be satisfied within this system of justice.

EGALITARIAN THEORY. The *egalitarian theory* of justice claims that justice requires the "equality of net welfare for individuals" (Veatch, 1981, p. 265). In this theory the distribution of good in the community takes the needs of all citizens into account equally. Thus everyone would have a claim to an equal amount of all goods and resources, including health care.

Clearly, this is a goal that cannot be achieved. It would be virtually impossible for any system of justice to guarantee equality of goods and resources for everyone, let alone equal health care. The egalitarian theory must necessarily be emended. Instead of health care being a good that everyone should have an equal amount of, basic health care should be viewed as a good that all should have equal access to. In short, everyone should have equal access to those basic health goods and resources to improve their health according to need (Green, 1976; Veatch, 1981).

This is a system that respects the autonomy of individuals to seek the health services they need or want and gives equal consideration to the positive benefiting of individuals in terms of improved health. Most important, it is just in that it follows the dictates of a principle of justice while not, at the same time, limiting the liberty of anyone in terms of basic health needs. It treats equals equally and unequals unequally and provides a just manner for the distribution of health resources in the community.

Problems and Conflicts

The application of a principle of justice in community health nursing creates conflicts in two areas: (1) establishing priorities for the distribution of basic goods and health services in the community and (2) determining which population or individuals shall obtain available health goods and nursing services.

DISTRIBUTING BASIC GOODS AND SERVICES. In deciding how to distribute basic health care assets or resources within a community, the first decision is to set the priorities for distribution. Should the protection and promotion of health be the main consideration? Or should a major portion of resources be set aside for other social goods, such as housing

or education? If community leaders agree than everyone has a right to equal access to basic health care according to need and this right must be satisfied for justice to be served, then enough community assets and financial resources will be allotted to meet the requirements of this basic right (Milio, 1975).

A second decision concerns the most effective and efficient methods of meeting this basic right while preventing death and disability among citizenry. Should the emphasis be placed on direct health care services (such as clinics and programs) or should indirect services (such as health education and transportation services) receive equal emphasis?

Third, decisions will have to be made for the appropriate relationship between rescue services and preventive services (Beauchamp and Childress, 1983). In other words, is it more effective to concentrate on kidney dialysis and terminal cancer services or should concentrated effort and economic resources be devoted to prevention of disease and disability through, for example, hypertension and diabetic screening?

Fourth, decisions will need to be made as to whether certain diseases or categories of illness receive more emphasis than others. For example, should the prevention and treatment of coronary heart disease take precedence over the prevention and treatment of venereal disease? Decisions in this area may well allocate money and services to certain socioeconomic groups or racial groups and will have to be given careful consideration to avoid conflicts of interest in matters of health.

Fifth, in establishing certain priorities, it is necessary to ascertain whether these priorities will compromise important values of principles. For example, preventive strategies aimed at discouraging alcohol consumption or smoking may well involve emphasis on behavioral change or the altering of life-styles by members of the community. The nurse might question whether priority setting in terms of these preventive strategies would have a substantial impact on the autonomy of community members, particularly their choice to engage in health risky behaviors.

Clearly, the prioritizing of health interests and the various ways to carry out these priorities may create conflicts of interests among health care providers with subsequent influence on the actual delivery of needed nursing care. These conflicts of interests continue in the next area of decision making.

DISTRIBUTING NURSING RESOURCES. Once the priorities for health within a community are designated along with the multiple ways these priorities will be carried out, community health nursing services need to decide who will receive services and what criteria can be used to distribute services equally in accordance with client needs.

One strategy may be to focus services on those who have the most reasonable chance of benefiting from services; for example, children and childbearing families (Beauchamp and Childress, 1983). Clearly, this is a utilitarian approach to distributing services aimed at providing the greatest net benefit overall. Even though it is also an approach that accommodates an interest in disease prevention, we might question whether this strategy meets the moral requirements of a principle of justice, which holds that everyone has a claim of equal access to basic health care services according to health care need. Certainly a strategy that focuses on one age group in the community wil overlook many individual wants and needs in terms of health care services and cannot be considered just.

A second strategy is to provide basic services in all categories in limited amounts and accommodate requests for nursing care services in a first come, first served basis. This approach may certainly cost more in terms of services provided and may even overlap with similar services provided in the community through health maintenance organizations or group practices of private family physicians. It does meet the basic requirement of providing the opportunity for everyone to have equal access to services even though they may have to wait a long time to be served. Yet it may not be the most efficient means of disbursing nursing resources according to the needs of clients.

A third strategy is to focus nursing services on those who are most able to pay for services, an approach that is all too frequently used in today's health care delivery system. This approach has been fostered by legislation and funding by government and its agencies. Unfortunately, this approach may have limited relevance to the needs of a particular community. For example, focusing the majority of nursing resources in a home health care program because of Medicare reimbursements in a community that has a small elderly population seems unjust when considering the health needs of other populations.

A fourth approach is to categorize those in the community according to health needs and decide who should receive first priority. Those who cannot survive without nursing resources (those receiving kidney dialysis or respiratory therapy at home) would have first priority. Those who can be assisted so as to prevent long-term disability (populations at high risk; the preeclamptic client; children with minor cardiac anomalies; close contacts of tuberculosis clients, and so on) would come next. Those who do not have an acute disabling illness or are not at risk of long-term disability (school-aged children, the elderly, and some persons with chronic diseases) would come last. Other groups whose health needs can be easily met and who can benefit the health of others (women with uncomplicated pregnancy, mothers with children under 2 years of age) may also be accorded a high priority in this system.

This approach has a decided utilitarian twist to it and limits the access of some groups to nursing services according to their priority in the schema (Figure 4-5). While it does distribute nursing resources according to who can benefit the most, some clients (such as dying cancer clients) wind up with no access to the system at all. This can hardly be considered just if we adopt the principle of justice (rather than a utilitarian principle of beneficence) as the guiding principle for distributing health goods.

As can be demonstrated by all of these various approaches to distributing nursing care resources, the moral requirements of justice create numerous conflicts of interest for health practitioners when it comes to specific choices.

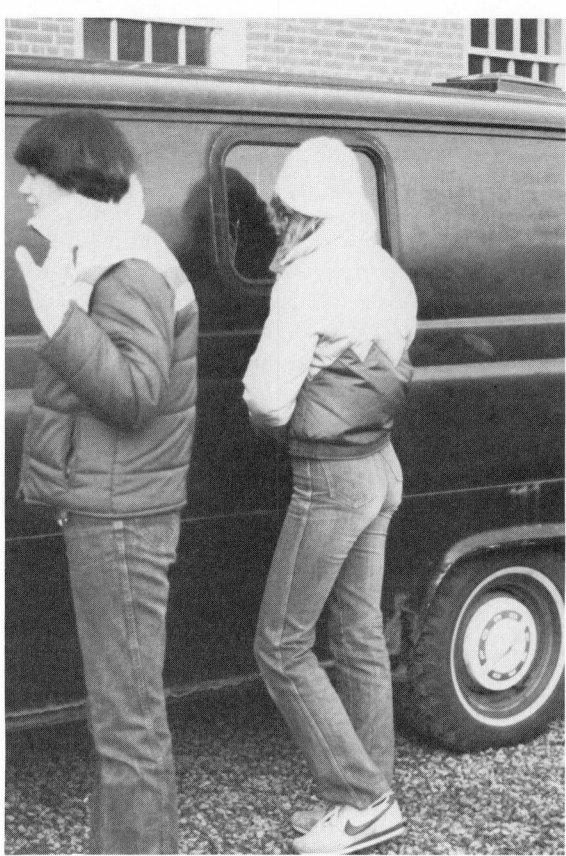

FIGURE 4-5

Teenage populations have a low priority in the allocation of health and nursing resources.

APPLICATION OF ETHICS TO COMMUNITY HEALTH NURSING PRACTICE
The Priority of Ethical Principles

In community health nursing, ethical principles direct and guide nursing actions with individuals and aggregate groups. The professional ethic, in general, places a greater emphasis on the observance of the principles of autonomy and beneficence than the principle of justice in most nursing actions (Fry, 1982). For example, in the *Code for Nurses,* respect for the principle of autonomy is emphasized by such statements as "the nurse provides services with respect for human dignity and the uniqueness of the client," that "clients have the moral right to determine what will be done with their own person," and that "the nurse's respect for the worth and dignity of the individual human being applies irrespective of the nature of the health problem" (American Nurses' Association, 1976, 1985, pp. 2, 3).

All of these statements indicate a high respect for client autonomy or claim that the nurse has a strong, primary duty to respect the client's right to self-determination.

The ethical principle of beneficence is given slightly less emphasis in the *Code for Nurses.* For example, the code claims that "the nurse's primary commitment is to the health, welfare, and safety of the client," "the nurse safeguards the client's right to privacy by judiciously protecting information of a confidential nature," and "nurses are responsible for advising clients against the use of products that endanger the client's safety and welfare. . . . The nurse may use knowledge of specific services or products in advising an individual client, since this may contribute to the client's health and well-being" (American Nurses' Association, 1976, 1985, pp. 4, 6, 15). Acts of beneficence may even include overriding the autonomy of individuals in the interests of other clients. The *Code for Nurses* describes the occurrence of this nursing action when "the nurse recognizes those situations in which individual rights to autonomy in health care may temporarily be overridden to preserve the life of the human community . . ." (American Nurses' Association, 1976, 1985, pp. 2, 3).

However, the principle of justice is not strongly emphasized in the professional code of ethics. It is noted in passing that nursing practice is not influenced by age, sex, race, color, personality, or other personal attributes or individual differences in customs, beliefs, or attitudes. The code states that "nursing care is delivered without prejudicial behavior," "the nurse adheres to the principle of non-discriminatory, nonprejudicial care in every situation and endeavors to promote its acceptance by others," and "the setting shall not determine the nurse's readiness to respect clients and to render or obtain needed services" (American Nurses' Association, 1976, 1985, pp. 3, 4). Clearly these statements related to the moral requirements of the principle of justice are not as strong as those related to the moral requirements of the principles of autonomy and beneficence.

In community health nursing, nursing actions are guided not only by the professional ethic and its priority of ethical principles; but also by the **public health ethic,** which has a different priority of principles. This ethic is strongly modeled on the priority of the principle of beneficence and follows the rule of utility in disease detection and prevention and in health maintenance (Beauchamp, 1976; Shindell, 1980). This emphasis certainly influences the practice of community health nursing, as is evidenced by the statement of the definition and role of public health nursing from the Public Health Nursing Section, American Public Health Association (1980). It describes public health nursing accomplishing its goal of improving the health of the community by identifying aggregates and by moving "away from solely meeting the needs of consumers as individually presented and toward practicing public health nursing for the 'sum' of individuals or families within the program" (American Public Health Association, 1980, p. 9).

This statement indicates an orientation in community health nursing toward following a rule of utility in matters of health pertaining to clients. The needs of aggregates as groups of individuals is determined for the purpose of providing net benefit to population groups over possible health harms (Fry, 1985). This emphasis on the moral requirements of the principle of beneficence does not align with the highly individualistic respect-for-client-autonomy emphasis of the *Code for Nurses*.

Accountability in Community Health Nursing

Moral accountability in nursing practice means that nurses are answerable for how they promote, protect, and meet the health needs of clients while respecting individual rights to self-determination in health care. In community health nursing, where the greater emphasis is on aggregates rather than individual clients, moral accountability means being answerable for how the health of aggregate groups has been promoted, protected, and met (Figure 4-6). Thus meeting accountability requirements in community health nursing will be different than meeting accountability requirements in other spheres of nursing practice.

For example, whereas the professional ethic clearly indicates that nurses are morally accountable for how they respect the client's right to self-determination and provide health services with respect for "the uniqueness of the client," the application of this ethic in community health nursing indicates that community nurses are morally accountable for how they provide health services so as to maximize total net health in population groups. It further indicates that they are accountable for demonstrating the increased health of aggregate groups through various research methods and studies while containing costs (Schlotfeldt, 1976). This is the meaning of accountability in community health nursing. Rather than being primarily accountable for how the moral requirements of the principle of autonomy are met, the community health nurse is primarily accountable for how the moral requirements of the principle of beneficence are met by nursing services.

The moral requirements of the principles of autonomy and justice are still important in community health nursing. Yet they are less important than the requirements of the principle of beneficence. In community health nursing, the emphasis of the professional ethic is slanted toward benefit to aggregates, which implies following a rule of utility in planning, implementing, and evaluating community health nursing services.

Future Directions

The emphasis on the moral requirements of a principle of beneficence in community health nursing has two implications. The first implication is heralded by the position paper *The Definition and Role of Public Health Nursing in the Delivery of Health Care,* which defines public health nursing as deriving its theoretical direction from both the public health sciences and professional nursing theories and has as its goal "improving the health of the entire community" (American Public Health Association, 1980, p. 4). If this is how community health nursing is to be defined, then it is important that the planning, implementation, and evaluation of nursing services in the community be clearly differentiated from the provision of nursing services in other spheres of health care delivery. While community health nursing is a synthesis of both the sciences of public health and nursing (Archer, 1982), there needs to be a clear understanding of how the ethical components of professional practice, including the observance of clients' rights and professional responsibilities, are considered in the provision

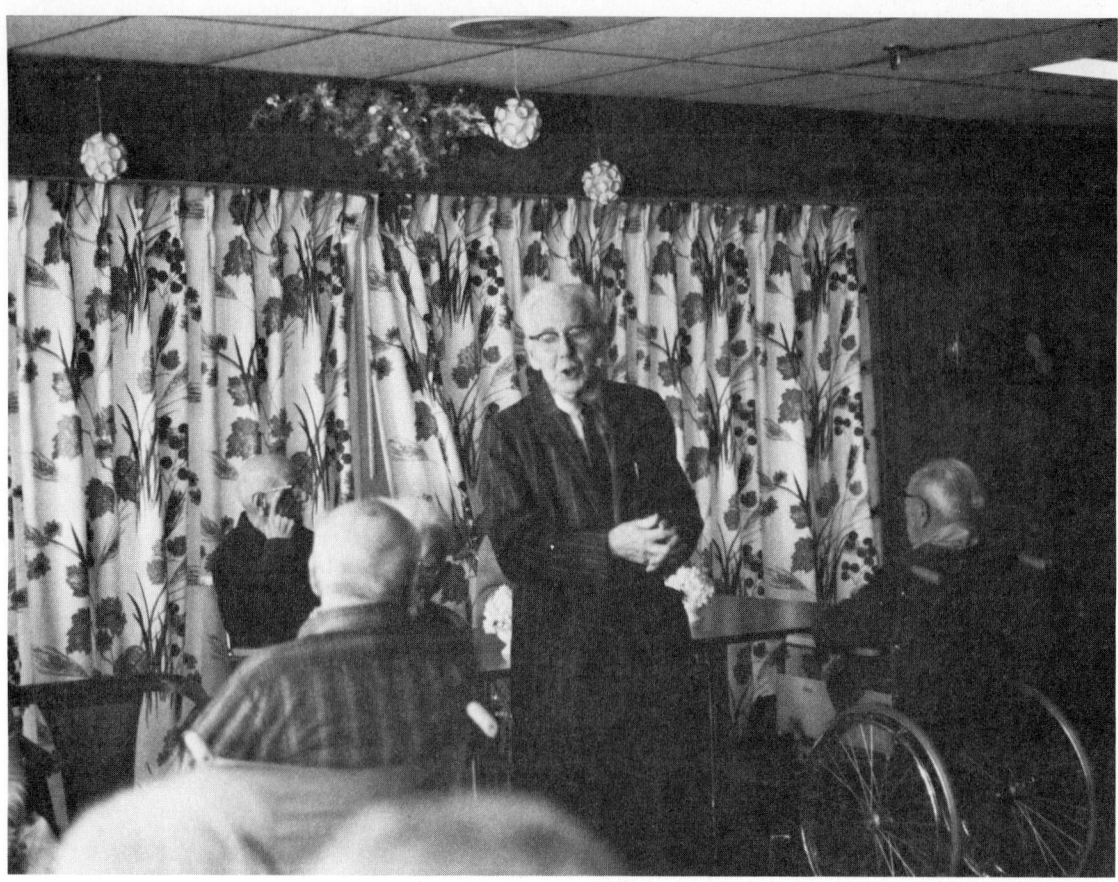

FIGURE 4-6

Community health nurses are accountable for the health of aggregate groups such as the elderly in a nursing home.

of nursing services. There is also a need for clarity and agreement on the priority of ethical principles in community health nursing. The goal of improving the health of the entire community by identifying aggregates and directing resources to them indicates an orientation toward meeting health needs according to the rule of utility. Is the ethical principle of beneficence the principle that should primarily guide community health nursing practice? Clearly, the moral underpinnings of community health nursing need to be given careful consideration in any statement defining the role of the discipline.

The second implication concerns the evaluation of accountability in community health nursing practice. Just as community health nursing has been affected by changes in both the health care delivery system and nursing practice in recent years, accountability requirements have likewise been affected by changes in public and professional expectations and the scope of nursing practice (Cushing, 1983; Warren, 1983). For example, the expanded role of the nurse has increased the legal accountability of the nurse practitioner who is certified to function as an independent care giver. Thus there is a current and future need for periodic assessment of the moral and legal requirements of accountability in community nursing services.

There is also the need to determine how accountability will be measured in community health nursing and how existing programs and services will be evaluated to determine the effectiveness of various nursing services in meeting accountability requirements. This is a task that has yet to be accomplished by today's community health nursing leaders.

CLINICAL APPLICATIONS

The following case situations are typical situations encountered in community health nursing practice. The questions after each case will help you to apply the moral concepts and ethical principles in this chapter to the nurse client relationship in community health nursing practice.

Case 1: What Are Society's Obligations to the Client?

Mr. H is a 48-year-old man referred to the visiting nurse association for evaluation and treatment of stasis ulcers on his legs and for maintenance of a weight-reduction program for both Mr. H and his wife. Mr. H is 6 feet tall and weighs over 380 pounds. The Hs have a 27-year-old mentally retarded son.

When she visited the home, Karla Lowe, the VNA nurse,

found large, oozing, sticky areas of raw tissue on Mr. H's legs. Ms. Lowe cleaned and dressed the ulcers and continued visiting the Hs every other day for the next 3 months. As the ulcers began to heal, Ms. Lowe attempted to engage the Hs in discussion about nutrition and hygiene and to encourage them to start a weight-reduction program. Mr. and Mrs. H were not interested and chose not to participate in any type of weight-reduction program.

Several months went by and Mr. H's ulcers stopped healing. When they began to deteriorate, he was hospitalized. Within a few weeks, they had healed enough that he could return home. Ms. Lowe visited his home to change dressings as before, but despite her efforts, the ulcers deteriorated once again. It was too soon for him to return to the local hospital under his SSI benefits, so it was arranged to have him admitted to the state hospital. Two days later he signed himself out of this hospital. "It was too far away and I didn't know anybody. Besides, they were too rough on me," were the reasons he gave for his action.

Angered by Mr. H's decision, his physician refused to continue treating him, and Ms. Lowe was left without any current physician orders. This meant that she could no longer give Mr. H physical care or receive reimbursement for her visits. Mr. H's unwillingness to cooperate in the development of "healthy behaviors" made him ineligible for the agency's health maintenance program. When Ms. Lowe explained the situation to her patient, Mr. H said that Mrs. H could wash his legs and apply the medicine that Ms. Lowe had been applying. Besides, he did not think that his physicians had really helped him and he had no intention of ever going to one again. He would miss Ms. Lowe's visits but he thought he would get along just fine. Ms. Lowe left the VNA number to call if they ran into any unforseen problems.

Nearly a year passed. One summer day Mrs. H called Ms. Lowe. She said that Mr. H was "awful sick" and had been in bed for nearly a month. VNA policy allowed a one-time evaluation visit, so Ms. Lowe visited the home. She found Mr. H's legs alive with the larvae of the summer flies attracted to the steamy bedroom. She urged Mr. H to seek hospitalization. He would not be turned away, even if he no longer had a physician. Mr. H agreed, an ambulance was called, and Mr. H was transported to the local hospital. Due to the condition of his legs, a bilateral leg amputation was performed.

When news of Mr. H's general condition got out (he had created quite a sensation in the emergency room of the local hospital) the people of the small town were aghast. How could a man be allowed to rot away? Where were all the services? Who was responsible? The mayor appointed a special task force to investigate the matter. Months (and endless newspapers columns) later, "no fault" was found and it was announced that the town's health services "had sufficient mechanisms to prevent such a thing from ever happening again." Mr. H recovered, obtained protheses, and moved to another state where he had family to help him.

Yet Ms. Lowe was not satisfied. Didn't the system fail patients like Mr. H? Did patients have an obligation to accept the services offered to them and the recommendations of health workers who took care of them? If they refused to follow recommendations, does this mean that health care services are totally withdrawn? Couldn't the amputations have been prevented if Ms. Lowe had, at least, continued her visits and prevented the extreme condition of Mr. H's legs prior to his last hospitalization?

Discussion Questions

1. What are society's obligations regarding health care to Mr. H?
2. How are professional obligations constrained by society's obligations?
3. Can the conclusions in the report of the President's Commission, *Securing Access to Health Care,* help Ms. Lowe?

Case 2: The Visiting Nurse and the Obstinate Patient: Are Professional Responsibilities Ever Limited?*

Mr. Jeff Williams, team leader in Home Health Care Services at the county health department, was preparing to visit Mr. Rufus Chisholm, a 59-year-old client recently diagnosed as having emphysema. Well known to the health department, Mr. Chisholm was unemployed as a result of a farming accident several years ago. Hypertensive as well as overweight, he was also a heavy cigarette smoker of long duration despite his decreased lung function. Mr. Williams's reason for visiting him today was to find out why Mr. Chisholm had missed his latest chest clinic appointment. He also wanted to find out if the patient was continuing his medications as ordered.

As Mr. Williams parked his car in front of his patient's house, he could see Mr. Chisholm sitting on the front porch smoking a cigarette. A flash of anger made him wonder why he continually tried to teach Mr. Chisholm reasons for not smoking and why he took the time out from his busy home-care schedule to follow up on Mr. Chisholm's missed clinical appointments. This client certainly did not seem to care about his own health, at least to the extent that he would give up smoking.

During the home visit, Mr. Williams determined that Mr. Chisholm had discontinued the use of his prophylactic antibiotic and was not taking his expectorant and bronchodilator medication on a regular basis. Mr. Chisholm's blood pressure was 210/114, and he coughed almost continuously. Although he listened politely to Mr. Williams's concerns about his respiratory function and the continued use of his medications, Mr. Chisholm simply made no effort to take responsibility for his health care. Even so, another clinic appointment was made and Mr. Williams encouraged the client to attend.

As he drove to his next home visit, Mr. Williams won-

---

*Cases 2 through 7 modified from Veatch, R.M., and Fry, S.T.: Case studies in nursing ethics, Philadelphia, 1987, J.B. Lippincott Co. Used with permission.

dered to what extent he was obligated as a nurse to spend time on patients who took no personal responsibility for their health. He also wondered if there was a limit to the amount of nursing care a noncooperative client could expect from a community health service.

Discussion Questions

1. What are Mr. Williams's professional responsibilities in response to Mr. Chisholm's rights to health care?
2. *Is* there a limit to the amount of nursing care nurses should be expected to give to clients?
3. What authority defines the moral requirements and moral limits of nursing care to clients in the community?

Case 3: When the Family Asks the Nurse to Tell the Truth*

Ralph Bradley, a recently widowed man in his mid-sixties, was discharged from the hospital following exploratory surgery that disclosed cancer of the colon with metastasis to the lymph nodes. His physician referred him to a community health agency for nursing care follow up. In reading the referral, the nurse learned that Mr. Bradley had been living with a married daughter and her family since his wife's death. An unmarried daughter apparently lived nearby, visiting him regularly and helping with his daily care. The referral did not explain what, if anything, the patient had been told by his physician concerning his condition.

During the first home visit it became apparent that Mr. Bradley did not know that the tumor removed from his body had been diagnosed as cancer and that it had metastasized to nearby organs. He did not realize the seriousness of his condition. But Mr. Bradley did express concern about his health. He complained of vague pain in the abdomen, asked for information about the results of tests performed before discharge from the hospital, and wanted to know how soon he would be able to return to his work as a cabinet maker. When the nurse avoided a direct answer to these questions, Mr. Bradley asked directly, "Is everything all right?" The married daughter, who was present when her father was asking these questions, assured him that, of course, everything was all right and he would be up and around the house in no time at all.

Walking the nurse to her car when the visit was over, the married daughter confided that it was the family's wish that their father not be told how serious his condition was. She said that their mother's recent death had been very difficult for him to accept. They did not want him to be further burdened with the knowledge of his condition. The nurse listened, acknowledging the difficulties posed by the wife's recent death and the father's serious condition. She told the daughter, however, that it would be very difficult, if not impossible, for anyone from her agency to continue to provide nursing care to Mr. Bradley without his knowledge of his condition.

When she returned to her office, the nurse discussed Mr. Bradley's situation with her supervisor. The nurse did not want to continue visiting the patient knowing he was being

deceived by physician and family. The supervisor suggested that she consult with the attending physician as soon as possible, explaining that Mr. Bradley was asking questions about his condition. Luckily, the nurse was able to reach the physician before it was time to make the next home visit. She asked the physician what the patient had been told about his condition. The physician said that Mr. Bradley had not been told that he had cancer at the family's request. He said that he agreed with the family that Mr. Bradley could probably not withstand the anxiety of knowing he had a terminal illness so soon after his wife's death. The physician also expressed concern about Mr. Bradley's daughters who, as he put it, "need a little time to accept the mother's death as well as accept the impending death of the old man." The physician went on to state that he would consider any act of disclosure on the nurse's part, at this time, to be inappropriate to her role as a visiting nurse and inconsistent with the well-being of the patient and his family.

Discussion Questions

1. What is the professional duty of veracity?
2. What reasons might the community health nurse give for telling the truth to Mr. Bradley?
3. What reasons might the community health nurse give for *not* telling Mr. Bradley the truth?
4. How does not telling the truth constrain nursing care in the community?

Case 4: The Nurse Who Could Not Protect the Patient's Right to Confidentiality*

Jane Sanborn was the occupational health nurse in a federal health agency. Among her responsibilities was the completion of the health status section of a form that included both personal and health history for periodic health examinations of the facility's employees. The physician completed the medical portion of the health report, recorded a decision about the employee's fitness for work, and returned the report to Ms. Sanborn, who maintained a confidential file for employees' health reports and records. Employees were asked to sign a statement on the health report to the effect that information in the report relating to employee fitness for the job could be shared with the employer as necessary.

One day, Ms. Sanborn received a memo directing her to send a copy of an employee's health report to Washington, D.C., for filing in a centralized data bank. Ms. Sanborn questioned the request and asked for an explanation of the purpose of the centralized file. No explanation was provided and the original request was repeated. Ms. Sanborn responded to the request by saying that she would send the health record as soon as she obtained the consent of the employee. The employee's original consent to share information only related to his immediate employer, not to the centralized data bank. Before she could contact the employee, however, Ms. Sanborn was again asked to send the health record immediately; additional consent from the employee was not required. When she discussed the matter with the physician and the administrator of the health facility, Ms. Sanborn was told that she should comply with the request—it was the accepted practice to send any requested employee health records to the centralized file without obtaining consent from employees. Under pressure from both the physician and the administrator, she sent the health record to the centralized data bank.

Discussion Questions

1. Why did Jane Sanborn break confidentiality in this situation?
2. Is there a morally justifiable reason to override the employee's right to confidentiality in this case situation?
3. Why is following the rule of confidentiality important in community health nursing?

Case 5: The Nurse Epidemiologist and Newborn Morbidity Statistics

Ms. Sharon Smith was the community health nurse responsible for interpreting mortality and morbidity statistics for her county health department. Based on a preliminary listing of figures, she initiated a comparative study of newborn morbidity from the death certificates of infants delivered at five county hospitals. The study revealed that one hospital had a high rate of newborn deaths. On closer look, the nurse found that the interns and residents of this hospital were using a particular kind of instrument-assisted delivery. When she presented her findings to the county health officer, he shelved the report. She persisted and eventually went public with her findings. Despite eventual investigation into the matter and a change of the procedures at the hospital in question, Ms. Smith was labeled "a traitor" by officials at her health department, and she lost the support of nurse colleagues employed by the county health agency. After several months of this treatment, she resigned her position.

Discussion Questions

1. What does the duty of advocacy mean in this case situation?
2. What is the appropriate action for the nurse to take in protecting the health, welfare, and safety of the client?
3. Does the duty of advocacy override personal concerns of the nurse? Why or why not?

Case 6: The Patient Who Did Not Want To Be Clean*

Marion Downs, a community health nurse, must decide whether or not to refer her patient, 72-year-old Sadie Jenkins, to the community fiduciary for consideration of conservatorship and guardianship. Miss Jenkins has no living relatives and lives alone in a one-room apartment furnished with a bed, refrigerator, table, chair, lamp, and small sink. Since she does not have a stove, two meals per day are supplied by her landlord. With the support of her Social Security check and food stamps, she has adequate money for her needs and has lived for over 10 years in these arrangements. She is also in good physical health.

Marion has made four home visits to Miss Jenkins to check her vital signs and medication routine following recent treatment in the Health Center's Hypertension Clinic. Although Miss Jenkins has made excellent progress and no longer requires visits from the community health nurse, her landlord, the other residents of her small apartment building, and her immediate neighbors are urging the nurse to "do something" about Miss Jenkins. Admittedly, Miss Jenkins' apartment has a strong odor from the long-term accumulation of dust, dirt, and mold. There are visible cockroaches in the apartment, and an unemptied bedpan is often sitting next to Miss Jenkins' bed (it is "too much trouble" to walk down the hallway to the hall bathroom shared by Miss Jenkins and two other tenants). Marion has noticed that Miss Jenkins has worn the same soiled clothes every time she has been to her apartment. It is also obvious that Miss Jenkins has not bathed for a long time, her hair is unwashed, and she apparently does not clean her nails and dentures. In addition, her toenails are so long that they have perforated the canvas of her tennis shoes, apparently the only shoes that she likes to wear.

Yet, Miss Jenkins is comfortable with her life-style and does not want to change her living arrangements. Although Marion has offered to contact agencies to help Miss Jenkins—homemaker service, counseling, and Senior Citizens—Miss Jenkins says that she is comfortable and does not want (or need) help from anyone.

Discussion Questions

1. Should Marion use her role of community health nurse to create an arrangement by which Miss Jenkins would lose the right to control her person, her financial resources, and her environment?
2. Can an individual in the community be forced to be clean and to live in a clean environment?
3. How far should a nurse go in providing "good" for a patient, and who determines what is "good" for Miss Jenkins?

Case 7: When Aging Parents Can No Longer Live Independently*

Joyce Fisher, a home health agency nurse, has just received a telephone call from the daughter of a patient, 82-year-old Mr. Sims, that she had visited some months before. The daughter was very distraught, telling Joyce that her father had fallen at home but refused to be seen by a physician. Mrs. Sims, her mother, had called the daughter at her place of business and pleaded with her to come to the home and stay with them. The daughter was exasperated by the frequency of these type of phone calls from her parents in recent weeks and was appealing to Joyce for help in making some long-term decisions for the care and safety of her parents.

Joyce well remembers the conversations that she had with Mr. and Mrs. Sims and their daughter several months ago following Mr. Sims's last hospitalization. Mr. and Mrs. Sims live alone in a small home and are frequently visited by their married daughter, who buys their groceries and takes them to their various health appointments. Mr. Sims has always been the decision maker of the family but allows this amount of assistance from the daughter "for Mama's sake." Another daughter lives in a nearby city but has chronic health problems that prohibit her active involvement in the affairs of her parents. A son lives on the West Coast and travels constantly in his line of business. He supports his parents by sending money for their expenses to his sister (Mr. Sims has refused direct financial aid from any of the children). All three children are concerned about the future welfare of their parents but have been unsuccessful in persuading them to change their mode of living.

The present problem is created by the fact that Mr. and Mrs. Sims are losing their ability to live independently and make their own decisions. Mr. Sims's unexplained falls are also increasing, a continued source of worry for Mrs. Sims and a genuine concern for their married daughter. They all look toward Joyce Fisher as the person who can help them make and support a decision that will preserve some autonomy for the aging parents and respect their choices and life-style. Yet Joyce doubts that what is best for all concerned (parents as well as children) can avoid infringing the choices and self-respect of the parents. Is there no happy medium for aging parents when they can no longer live independently?

Discussion Questions

1. What is the role of the home health nurse in assisting individuals to reach a decision they can live with?
2. What does it mean to respect Mr. and Mrs. Sims as autonomous individuals?

3. Do clients really have the right to refuse services or treatment from the community health nurse? Does such refusal limit future treatment? Why or why not?

SUMMARY

The practice of community health nursing is influenced by both traditional ethics of professional nursing and the aggregate focus of community health. In providing nursing care services to individuals as well as aggregate groups within the community, the nurse must necessarily balance both of these influences. Clients' rights to equal access to health care services as well as aggregate groups' needs and interests in matters of health will often compete for the attention and services of the practicing community health nurse. Thus the nurse must become familiar with the moral requirements of the practice of nursing in general and the practice of community health nursing in particular.

Community health nursing practice, as a synthesis of both public health science and nursing science, is theoretically responsive to our prevailing ideas of social justice and the methods of distributing health care resources as chosen by the community. Yet community health nursing practice, as a composite of the individualistic ethic of nursing and the aggregate ethic of public health, is also responsive to the moral requirements of ethical principles as prioritized within these ethics. How the individual community health nurse and community health nursing services view these moral requirements may well determine the future direction and influence of the discipline in meeting the health needs of communities.

☰ KEY CONCEPTS

Because clients have rights, health care professionals have responsibilities to tell the truth (veracity), respect confidentiality, function as a client advocate, and accept accountability for providing proper health care.

The development of methods to measure accountability is a high priority in community health nursing.

A right to health has been historically recognized as a basic human right.

The negative right to be free to enjoy good health may lead to the positive right to obtain certain services or community health safeguards.

"Right to health" and "right to health care" are different kinds of rights and should be kept separate.

Use of the Patient's Bill of Rights has been the means by which many health care providers communicate rights to their patients. However, the patient's Bill of Rights has been criticized for several reasons.

According to a recent presidential commission, "society has an ethical obligation to ensure equitable access to health care for all."

The professional code of ethics for nurses prescribes moral behavior and actions based on moral principles.

The need for moral accountability within nursing practice has been recognized since Florence Nightingale began her nurse training program.

The ethical principles operable in community health nursing are beneficence, autonomy, and justice.

The four major theories of justice used to decide the allocation of health care resources are the entitlement theory, the utilitarian theory, the maximin theory, and the egalitarian theory. The moral requirements of justice create numerous conflicts of interest for health practitioners when it comes to specific choices.

The professional ethic generally places a greater emphasis on observance of the principles of autonomy and beneficence than the principle of justice in most nursing actions.

In community health nursing, moral accountability means being answerable for how the health of aggregate groups has been promoted, protected, and met.

Clients' rights to equal access to health care and the aggregate's needs and interests in health matters will often compete for the attention and services of the nurse.

LEARNING ACTIVITIES

1. Hold a conference among two or three nurse students and two or three practicing community health nurses. Discuss how community health nurses assume responsibility and accountability for individual nursing judgments and actions in their areas of practice. Be sure to distinguish moral accountability from legal accountability.

2. Suggest three ways by which community health nursing might extend the scope of accountability for nurses in delivering nursing care services to aggregate groups in the community.

3. Select an aggregate group at risk in your community. Formulate a plan of nursing care delivery in response to health care need using a specific theory of distributive justice.

4. Determine how clients' rights to privacy are respected and protected in a community health care agency. To what extent do community health nurses contribute to the protection of client privacy? Are client records used in research studies? If so, how is personal information about the client protected? Suggest two methods by which client privacy could be more adequately protected. What would be the relative costs and benefits of your proposed methods?

BIBLIOGRAPHY

American Hospital Association: Statement on a patient's bill of rights, Hospitals 47:41, Feb. 16, 1973.

American Nurses' Association: Code for nurses with interpretive statements, Kansas City, Mo., 1976, 1985, The Association.

American Public Health Association, Public Health Nursing Section: The definition and role of public health nursing practice in the delivery of health care: a statement of the public health nursing section, Washington, D.C., Nov. 1980, The Association.

Annas, G.J.: Patients' rights movement. In Reich, W.T., editor: Encyclopedia of bioethics, vol. 3, New York, 1978, The Free Press, pp. 1201-1205.

Annas, G.J.: Fashion and freedom: When artificial feedings should be withdrawn, Am. J. Pub. Health 75:685-688, 1985.

Archer, S.E.: Synthesis of public health science and nursing science, Nurs. Outlook 30:442-46, Sept.-Oct. 1982.

Baier, K.: The moral point of view, Ithaca, N.Y., 1958, Cornell University Press.

Beauchamp, D.E.: Public health and social justice, Inquiry 13:3-14, March 1976.

Beauchamp, D.E.: Public health and individual liberty, Ann. Rev. Pub. Health 1:121-36, 1980.

Beauchamp, D.E.: Community: the neglected tradition of public health, Hastings Center Rep. 15:28-36, Dec. 1985.

Beauchamp, T.L., and Childress, J.F.: Principles of biomedical ethics, New York, 1983, Oxford Press.

Beauchamp, T.L., and Faden, R.R.: The right to health and the right to health care, J. Med. Philos. 4:118-31, June, 1979.

Beauchamp, T.L., and Walters, L.: Patients' rights and professional responsibilities. In Beauchamp, T.L., and Walters, L., editors: Contemporary issues in bioethics, Belmont, Calif. 1978, Wadsworth Publishing Co.

Bell, N.K.: The scarcity of medical resources: are there rights to health care? J. Med. Philos. 4:158-69, June 1979.

Brockington, C.: A short history of public health, London, 1956, Churchill.

Capron, A.M.: Right to refuse medical treatment. In Reich, W.T., editor: Encyclopedia of bioethics, vol. 4, New York, 1978, The Free Press, pp. 1498-1507.

Carney, R.S.: Theological ethics. In Reich, W.T., editor: Encyclopedia of bioethics, vol. 1, New York, 1978, The Free Press, pp. 429-437.

Cushing, M.: Expanding the meaning of accountability, Am. J. Nurs. 83:1202-1203, Aug. 1983.

Daniels, N.: Rights to health care and distributive justice: programmatic worries, J. Med. Philos. 4:174-91, June 1979.

Department of Health, Education, and Welfare, Commission on Medical Malpractice: Report of the secretary's commission on medical malpractice, vols. 2, DHEW Pub. Nos. (OS) 73-88, (OS) 73-89, Washington, D.C, 1973, U.S. Government Printing Office.

Feinberg, J.: Social philosophy, Englewood Cliffs, N.J., 1973, Prentice-Hall, Inc.

Frankena, W.K.: Ethics, Englewood Cliffs, N.J., 1973, Prentice-Hall, Inc.

Fried, C.: Right and wrong, Cambridge, Mass., 1978, Harvard University Press.

Fry, S.T.: Accountability in research: the relationship of scientific and humanistic values, Adv. Nurs. Sci. 4:1-13, 1981.

Fry, S.T.: Ethical principles in nursing education and practice: a missing link in the unification issue, Nurs. Health Care 3:363-68, Sept. 1982.

Fry, S.T.: Dilemma in community health ethics, Nurs. Outlook, 31:176-179, May/June 1983a.

Fry, S.T.: Rationing health care: the ethics of cost containment, Nurs. Economics 1:165-169, Nov./Dec. 1983b.

Fry, S.T.: Confidentiality in health care: a decrepit concept? Nurs. Economics 2:413-418, Nov./Dec. 1984.

Fry, S.T.: Individual vs. aggregate good: ethical tension in nursing practice, Int. J. Nurs. Studies 22:303-310, Dec. 1985.

Fry, S.T.: Ethical aspects of decision-making in the feeding of cancer patients, Semin. Oncol. Nurs. 2:59-62, Feb. 1986a.

Fry, S.T.: Ethical inquiry in nursing: the definition and method of biomedical ethics, Periop. Nurs. Q. 2:1-8, June 1986b.

Gaylin, W.: The patient's bill of rights, Sat. Rev. Sci. 1:22, Feb. 24, 1973.

Gert, B., and Culver, C.M.: The justification of paternalism. In Robinson, W.L., and Pritchard, M.S., editors: Medical responsibility: paternalism, informed consent, and euthanasia, Clifton, N.J., 1979, Humana Press, pp. 1-14.

Gordis, L., and Gold, E.: Privacy, confidentiality, and the use of medical records in research, Science 207:153-56, Jan. 11, 1980.

Gortner, S.R.: Scientific accountability in nursing, Nurs. Outlook 22:764-68, Nov. 1974.

Green, R.: Health care and justice in contract theory perspective. In Veatch, R.M., and Branson, R., editors: Ethics and health policy, Cambridge, Ma. 1976, Ballinger Publishing Co.

In re estate of Brooks, 32 Ill. 2d 361, 205 N.E. 2d 435, 1965.

Kant, L.: Groundwork of the metaphysic of morals, New York, 1964, Harper & Row Publishers, Inc. (Translated by H.J. Paton: originally published in 1785.)

Kelsey, J.L.: Privacy and confidentiality in epidemiological research involving patients, IRB 3:1-4, Feb. 1981.

Lynn, J., and Childress, J.: Must patients always be given food and water? Hastings Center Rep. 13:17-21, Oct. 1983.

Lyons, J.: Playing god in the nursery, New York, 1985, W.W. Norton Co.

MacIntyre, A.: Utilitarianism and cost-benefit analysis. In Beauchamp, T.L., and Bowie, N.E., editors: Ethical theory and business, Englewood Cliffs, N.J., 1979, Prentice-Hall, Inc.

MacIntyre, A.: After virtue, Notre Dame, Ind., 1981, University of Notre Dame Press.

Milio, N.: The care of health in communities: access for outcasts, New York, 1975, Macmillan Publishing Co., Inc.

Mill, J.S.: Utilitarianism, New York, 1957, The Bobbs-Merrill Co., Inc. (Edited by O. Priest; originally published in 1863.)

National Commission for the Protection of Human Subjects of Biomedical and Behavioral Research: The Belmont report ethical principles and guidelines for the protection of human subjects of research, DHEW Pub. No. (OS) 78-0012, Washington, D.C., 1978.

Nozick, R.: Anarchy, state, and utopia, New York, 1974, Basic Books Inc. Publishers.

Palmer, L.S.: Florence Nightingale: reformer, reactionary, researcher, Nurs. Res. 26:84-89, March-April 1977.

Popoff, D.: What are your feelings about death and dying? Part 1, Nursing 5:15-24, 1975.

President's Commission for the Study of Ethical Problems in Medicine and Biomedical and Behavioral Research: Securing access to health care. Vol. 1, Report on the ethical implications of differences in the availability in health services, Washington, D.C., March 1983, U.S. Government Printing Office.

Public Law 92-603, Social Security amendments of 1972, 92nd Congress, Oct. 30, 1972.

Public Law 92-278, The national sickle cell anemia, Cooley's anemia, Tay-Sachs and genetic disease act, Title IV, 90 stat., Section 410, 1976.

Rawls, J.: A theory of justice, Cambridge, Mass, 1971, Harvard University Press.

Rosen, G.: Preventive medicine in the United States: 1900-1975, New York, 1975, Science History Publishers.

Ross, W.D.: The right and the good, Oxford, 1930, Oxford University Press.

Schlotfeldt, R.M.: Accountability: a critical dimension of health care, Health Care Dimen. 3:137-48, 1976.

Shindell, S.: Legal and ethical aspects of public health. In Last, J.M., editor: Maxcy-Rosenau public health and preventive medicine, ed. 11, New York, 1980, Appleton-Century-Crofts, pp. 1834-1845.

Smith, C.S.: Outrageous or outraged: a nurse advocate story, Nurs. Outlook 28:624-25, Oct. 1980.

Szasz, T.: The right to health. In Gorovitz, S., et al., editors: Moral problems in medicine, Englewood Cliffs, N.J., 1976, Prentice-Hall Inc.

Tarasoff v. Regents of The University of California, 131 Cal. Rptr. 14, 551 P.2d 334, 1976.

UNESCO: Human rights, a symposium, New York, 1949, Allan Wingate.

Veatch, R.M.: Death, dying, and the biological revolution, New Haven, Conn. 1976, Yale University Press.

Veatch, R.M.: Truth-telling: attitudes. In Reich, W.T., editor: Encyclopedia of bioethics, vol. 4, New York, 1978, The Free Press, pp. 1677-1682.

Veatch, R.M.: A theory of medical ethics, New York, 1981, Basic Books, Inc. Publishers.

Warren, J.J.: Accountability and nursing diagnosis, Am. J. Nurs. Admin. 13:34-37, Oct. 1983.

Will, G.F.: The killing will not stop, The Washington Post, April 22, 1982, p. A-29.

Williams, C.: Community health nursing: what is it? Nurs. Outlook 25:250-52, 1977.

World Health Organization: The first ten years of the World Health Organization, New York, 1958, WHO.

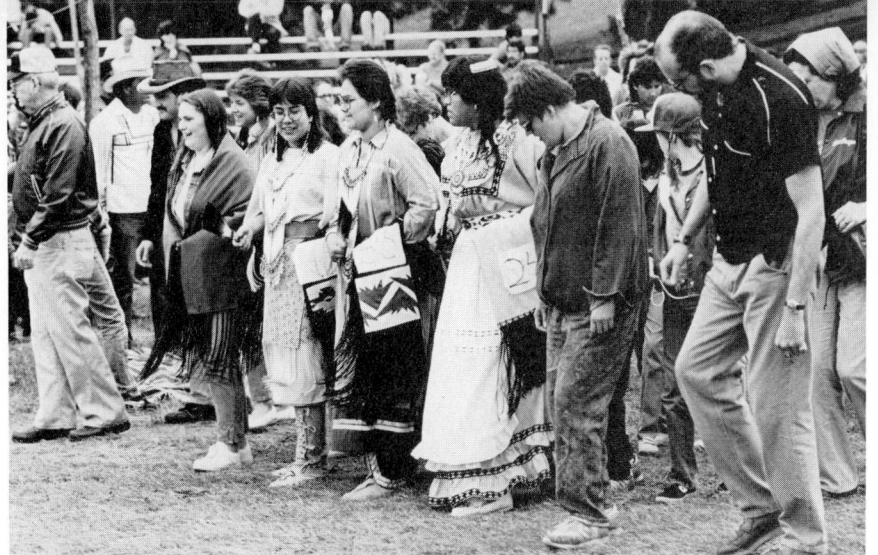

Eleanor Bauwens
Sandra Anderson

5

SOCIAL AND CULTURAL INFLUENCES ON HEALTH CARE

⩦ OBJECTIVES

After reading this chapter, the student should be able to:

Define culture and how it relates to health and illness behavior.

Identify concepts relevant to culture and health care.

Recognize the variety of influences that cultural differences have on the interpretations of health and illness.

Evaluate the effects of variation between one's own value and belief systems and those of clients from different cultures, particularly as they have implications for nursing care.

List factors that produce diversity in health-seeking behavior between and within ethnic groups.

Describe the nature of poverty and its effect on health status and health behavior.

Assess sociocultural factors and their impact on health care for the individual, family, and community.

Provide culturally appropriate nursing care based on assessment, planning, and evaluation.

⩦ KEY TERMS

beliefs	cultural shock	holism
bicultural	cultural values	iatrogenic
culture	enculturation	minority
culture-bound	ethnic collectivity	poverty
culture change	ethnicity	race
culture of poverty	ethnocentrism	stereotype
cultural relativism		

The premise of this chapter is that health care is based not only on knowledge of the physical causes of disease but also on sociocultural influences. Often nurses must plan and give care to individuals and families whose health beliefs and practices differ from their own. If the care is to be effective and appropriate, the nurse must have knowledge of the importance of cultural influences and of specific cultural values.

This chapter will help nurses deliver more personalized, culturally appropriate care to all clients. Ideally it will increase nurses' sensitivity to sociocultural influences on health care and thereby improve their ability in the assessment, intervention, and evaluation of health problems. We explore the meaning of culture, cultural differences, specific cultural groups in the United States, and poverty, and we provide guidelines for cultural assessment and culture-relevant health care.

MEANING OF CULTURE

Culture enables us to interpret our surroundings and the actions of people around us and to behave in ways that make sense. "Culture consists of standards for deciding what is, what can be, how one feels about it, and how to go about doing it" (Goodenough, 1966, pp. 257-258). Some anthropologists conceive of culture as a set of rules that provide the individual with a means for behaving and interpreting the behavior of others. This set of rules can be compared to a cultural grammar. Harrison and Ritenbaugh (1981) elaborate on the idea that "culture is to behavior" as "language is to speech." This definition implies that people are not always consciously aware of the rules, but if they are broken, people become uncomfortable. For example, if greetings and farewells are not exchanged in an appropriate manner, either party may feel uncomfortable and the relationship may be awkward.

Viewing culture as a set of rules also implies that there are methods by which to learn explicit and implicit cultural rules. Explicit cultural rules are those in people's conscious awareness; implicit rules are those that people do not consciously recognize. Explicit cultural rules are more easily learned than implicit rules; however, there are ways to learn about the implicit rules through talking with people and observing their behavior. The rules can then be inferred from what people say they should do and from observations and descriptions of what people actually do.

One individual does not need to know all the rules of grammar to communicate by speech; neither does a person need to know all the cultural rules to act appropriately and understand the behavior of others. In other words, individuality in behavior, perception, and feelings is taken into account. When enough grammar is known, individuals can create new sentences and make themselves understood in a variety of situations. Understanding cultural rules allows for the interpretation of behavior and helps a person act appropriately.

CONCEPTS RELEVANT TO CULTURE
Holism

Anthropologists believe that culture is a functional, integrated whole with interrelated and interdependent parts. The concept of *holism* requires that human behavior not be isolated from the context in which it occurs and that the culture is best viewed and analyzed as a whole. The various components of a culture, such as the political, economic, religious, kinship, and health systems, perform separate functions and mesh to form an operating whole; thus to understand any one system, one must view each in relation to the others and to the entire culture. A culture is often said to be more than the sum of its parts (Benedict, 1934).

Culture Change

Any change in one or more systems affects the whole. Culture is never static but is in a constant process of adding or deleting elements. This process of *culture change* is a result of contact between groups and of forces within a group. Culture change usually creates new challenges and problems; it involves creative adaptation and retention of behavioral precedents that are passed on through language, customs, beliefs, attitudes, values, goals, laws, traditions, and moral codes. At times precedents become outmoded or maladaptive and thus provide a potential source of conflict (Elling, 1977). The health status of a society is related to its ability to adapt to change.

In a society such as the United States, which has become increasingly technological as scientific medicine has steadily advanced, some individuals have become alienated from orthodox medicine. The search for treatment goes beyond allopathic methods of healing. For example, chiropractic medicine contradicts the monolithic concept of scientific medicine, but it has gained status because of political, social, and legal changes.

Enculturation

Cultural behavior, or how to act appropriately, is socially acquired, not inherited. Patterns of cultural behavior are learned through the process of *enculturation,* sometimes called socialization. Enculturation is the process of acquiring knowledge and internalizing values; through this process persons achieve competence in their own culture. Children acquire their culture by watching adults and making inferences about the rules for behavior. Cultural behavior patterns provide explanations for life events, which are important for nurses to understand. These events include such things as birth, death, puberty, childbearing, rearing of children, illness, and disease. As children grow in society, they learn certain beliefs, attitudes, and values about these life events, and this knowledge is carried throughout the life span, unless necessity or force compels them to learn different ways.

Culture-Bound

Whenever people learn a culture, they are to some extent imprisoned without knowing it. Anthropologists refer to this existence as being *culture-bound;* that is, living within a particular reality that is considered as *the* reality. All of us have learned ways to interpret our world based on our enculturation. Our interpretations are understandable and persuasive to those brought up to share the same frame of reference, but our interpretations may sometimes make little sense out of context. We are culture-bound within our own culture and profession, nursing. Being culture-bound within nursing means that we are likely to view our modern scientific approach to health and illness as the only way. Clients may view this modern scientific approach differently, judging that in some ways it meets their needs, and in other ways it does not. Dissatisfaction with medical treatment and practitioners, the movement toward self-care, and the striving for freedom of choice and individual responsibility have led to an increased interest in alternative health services. Western medicine is often practiced in unscientific ways. Desirable outcomes may occur independently of the physician's intervention, or the intervention may lead to *iatrogenic* consequences (Young, 1978).

Ethnocentrism

Because we look at the world from our own particular cultural viewpoint, we often believe our way is best; called *ethnocentrism.* It is important for nurses not to consider their own way the best and other people's ideas as ignorant or inferior. The ideas of lay individuals may be valid and certainly influence their health care behavior. The beginning of culturally appropriate health care lies in the awareness of the community health nurse that people may live by different rules and priorities from those of the health care provider, and these rules and priorities decisively influence health-related behavior. Health care providers tend to act on the assumption that their world view conforms to the way the world really is or ought to be. When people are judgmental of other cultures, they go beyond healthy cultural identification. Anthropologists use the term *cultural relativism* to denote that cultures are neither inferior nor superior to one another. Cultural relativists believe that there is no single scale for measuring the value of a culture; rather the value of a culture can only be defined by its meaning to its members. The following comment by Jelliffe (1969, p. 61) refers to nutrition specifically, but it can be applied to any aspect of culture:

> . . . all different cultures, whether in a tropical village or in a highly urbanized and technologically sophisticated community, contain some practices and customs which are beneficial to the health and nutrition of the group, and some which are harmful. No culture has a monopoly on wisdom or absurdity.

Health professionals must recognize the existence of cultural relativism in regard to modern scientific medicine. Nurses must realize that not even their own beliefs and professional practice are immune to scientifically unsound behavior. Tripp-Reimer (1982) studied the concepts of ethnocentrism and cultural relativity in an Appalachian population served by Appalachian and non-Appalachian health professionals. She observed that both the client and the health care provider enter the clinical situation with predetermined values, beliefs, and perceptions. She noted that "the provider's culture biases the interpretation and understanding of client behavior. . . (and) it will diminish the quality of care available for minority clients" (Tripp-Reimer, 1982, p. 188).

Stereotypes

Stereotypes are exaggerated beliefs and images that are popularly depicted in the mass communication media and folklore. Usually these images are false; they obscure important differences among members of a group and exaggerate those between groups. The perceived, exaggerated differences between two groups help to justify negative behavior of people in one group toward others. Individuals can be found to fit the stereotypes, but there are many more who do not. Stereotypes are commonly reflected by false and insensitive expressions such as "Indians are drunks," "blacks are lazy," "poor whites are trash," or "nurses are passive." Stereotyping can lead to inaccurate assessments and interventions based on preconceived notions rather than on unbiased, nonprejudicial observation and questioning. Health professionals must remain sensitive to individual variation within groups.

Cultural Values

The cultural system is composed of value orientations. A *value* is a type of belief about how one should or should not behave. *Beliefs* are "statements which the subject holds as true, but which may or may not be based on empirical evidence: thus, the strength of a belief does not depend on its degree of correspondence with objective fact. . ." (Horn, 1979, p. 63). All belief systems are culture-bound because they are based on cultural factors and the meaning that individuals ascribe to these factors. Individuals assign meaning to health and illness based on their values and beliefs. Thus the behavior of clients in regard to health and illness can be more accurately understood by knowing something about their beliefs and values.

Cultural values are the prevailing and persistent guides influencing thinking and actions of people. Individuals' beliefs and values influence the kind of health care considered acceptable or desirable. Values provide powerful motivation and standards for behavior. For instance, if people value prevention, they will generally have their children immunized against disease. If prevention of illness is not valued, immunizations are likely to be ignored, even if provided free of charge.

There are two types of values: public and personal (Goodenough, 1966). Public values tend to be objectified by policies and laws; personal values are usually unverbalized and individualized. People may agree on public values but may vary greatly on personal values. Acceptance of rules requires that public values be reasonably compatible with personal values. When incompatibility exists, the society strives for agreement between public and personal values. An example of this is the conflict over abortion in the United States.

One of the most important elements shared by a culture is its values. Shared values give a culture stability and security; they provide a standard for behavior. If two people share a similar culture and their experiences tend to be similar, their values tend to be similar. Although no two people have exactly the same value pattern, they are enough alike to recognize similarities and to identify the other as "one of my kind" (Goodenough, 1966).

The nurse should not expect to understand the value system of a family or cultural group after the first contact. The nurse should realize the importance of gathering data to help understand the values people have regarding health care because cultural values determine what people believe to be good or bad, adequate or inadequate health care (Leininger, 1976). Even in situations when the cultural backgrounds of the client and nurse are assumed to be similar, problems can arise if the nurse concentrates only on the disease and fails to recognize the sociocultural aspects influencing health and illness.

Although it is important to understand the client's ideas about disease, it is equally important to understand what the client views as appropriate treatment and acceptable behavior on the part of the health care provider. The degree to which the client's actions taken to resolve a health problem fall into the professional health care arena is influenced by the similarity between the client's and the health care provider's cultural, economic, and social conditioning (Chrisman and Kleinman, 1983). If health care providers have a working knowledge of the culture, they can more accurately interpret and influence the client's behavior.

CULTURAL DIFFERENCES

All segments of the population in the United States share certain common elements in life patterns and basic beliefs. However, because of different cultural traditions and increasing mobility, a homogeneous culture is seldom found. In a homogeneous culture individuals tend to share the same attitudes, interests, and goals. Generally people are likely to do what is expected or to follow the norms, but discrepancies occur in all cultures. Society presents to individuals what they should do (ideal), but their actual behavior (real) only approximates the norm, especially if the norm is not highly valued. The actual behaviors tend to cluster toward a trend or mode. Individuals who grow up in the same society acquire certain standardized ways of dealing with objects and people. This means that even among total strangers in a completely unique situation there is some level of subjective understanding of what is normal and abnormal in overt behavior, that is, what people actually do.

Ethnic Collectivity

People who have been reared in an *ethnic collectivity* (a group with common origins, a sense of identity, and shared standards for behavior) often acquire from that experience cultural norms that determine the thought and behavior of individual members (Harwood, 1981). The effects of this enculturation carry over to health care and become an important influence for activities relative to health and illness behavior.

Social scientists speak about American culture as if it included a set of values shared by everyone. However, even within an ethnic collectivity intraethnic variations can be expected and are apparent in health behaviors. For example, variations are seen in conceptions of mental illness (Guttmacher and Elinson, 1971), in definitions of health and illness, in skepticism about medical care, in use of health care services (Berkanovic and Reeder, 1973), and in willingness to assume a dependent role when ill (Greenblum, 1974; Suchman, 1964).

The term *bicultural* implies that a person straddles two cultures, life-styles, and sets of values. To understand biculturalism it is necessary to discuss differences in the terms ethnicity, race, and minority. Ethnicity is frequently used to mean race, but it includes more than a biological identification. *Ethnicity* refers to groups whose members share a common social and cultural heritage passed on to each successive generation. Members of an ethnic group feel a sense of identity. *Race* is a biological term. Racial group members share distinguishing physical features like skin color, bone structure, and genetic traits such as blood grouping. Ethnic and racial groups may overlap. In such cases the biological and cultural similarities can reinforce one another. A *minority* may consist of a particular racial, religious, or occupational group that constitutes less than a numerical majority of the population. In this sense all of us belong to various kinds of minorities (Bullough and Bullough, 1982). Sometimes a minority group is designated because of its limited access to power or assumed inferior traits and undesirable characteristics. A numerical majority may be considered a minority because they lack the kind of power that usually accompanies majority status. Bicultural group members may share ethnic and racial characteristics of the larger group of which they are a part, but they also share a common culture different from that of the larger group.

Cultural Shock

"Cultural shock" is one of the effects of working with individuals from different cultural backgrounds. Leininger (1976, p. 7) describes *cultural shock* as "the feelings of helplessness and discomfort and the state of disorientation experienced by an outsider attempting to comprehend or effectively adapt to a different cultural group because of differences in cultural practices, values, and beliefs." Cultural shock sometimes makes health care providers feel uncomfortable or even angry. Kubricht and Clark (1982) surveyed nurses and foreign clients to identify areas in which needs were unmet and problems were encountered by nurses who were caring for these people. The survey revealed that foreign clients experienced feelings of boredom, anxiety, and fear; nurses experienced feelings of frustration and inadequacy; communication was either inadequate or nonexistent; the lack of culture-specific information was a significant problem; and resources to meet these needs were not consistently available.

Nurses can help reduce cultural shock by knowing about the different cultural groups with whom they are working. Ways of learning about culturally different clients include transcultural course work and experiences. Even with some knowledge of a variety of cultures, the nurse may regard clients as strange and have difficulty communicating; likewise, the client may perceive the health system and health care providers as unusual and incomprehensible. During a period of adaptation it is important for nurses to develop respect for others who are culturally different but at the same time maintain their own sense of worth. Community health nursing practice requires tolerance of beliefs that may be counter to those of the nurse.

Communication Patterns

Obvious barriers are present when two people speak different languages. Familiarity with the language of the client is one of the best ways to gain insight into a culture. Kluckhohn (1972) wrote that every language is also a special way of looking at the world and interpreting experiences. Each different language has a whole set of unconscious assumptions about the world and life. Kluckhohn believed that people see and hear what the grammatical system of their language makes them sensitive to. It is a high priority of the community health nurse working with clients who speak another language to comprehend at as many levels and with as many senses as possible.

However, barriers to communications also may exist when individuals speak the same language. Nurses may have difficulty explaining things in simple jargon-free language that clients can understand. It is important to ascertain that the message is received and understood as the sender intended it. The nurse and client can employ a feedback mechanism to facilitate communication. Much of the information we transmit to each other is conveyed by facial expression, posture, body movement, and voice tone. For example, an Anglo may value straightforward criticism to the person's face, but a Papago Indian finds that action impolite. Thus, Papago clients may be unwilling to criticize health personnel directly even if they are dissatisfied with their care.

Cultural differences are reflected in communication patterns. For instance, the actual terms used may vary according to whom you speak, when you speak, acceptable and taboo topics, and the social situation. For example, Saunders (1954, p. 116) describes the effect that the inability to understand Spanish-speaking people's ways of looking at things may have on the English speaker's assessment of their worth: ". . . in English a clock runs, while in Spanish, it walks *(el reloj anda)*. Such a simple difference as this has enormous implications for appreciating differences in the behavior of English- and Spanish-speaking persons. If time is moving rapidly, as Anglo usage declares, we must hurry. . . . If time walks, as the Spanish-speaking say, one can take a more leisurely attitude toward it. . . ." An attempt to understand a people's world view through their language can avert some major misunderstandings.

Personal Space and Contact

Personal space is an invisible, flexible boundary. Insel (1978) describes personal space as a "portable bubble" that continuously surrounds the individual. This invisible cushion of air provides a margin of safety and security. The bubble expands, shrinks, and changes in permeability according to the social situation, the physical area, the culture of the individual, and the relation to others present (Meisenhelder, 1982). Body or eye contact accepted or even expected in one culture may be taboo in another. Touching may be considered an intrusion of personal space in some cultures, but in others many forms of traditional healing require touching as part of the healing process or as a comfort measure.

Hall (1966) observed and interviewed northeastern Americans to learn about their use of personal space. He identified four zones: (1) intimate distance that extends up to 18 inches from the body, (2) personal distance as an area of 18 inches to 4 feet from the individual, (3) social distance of 4 to 12 feet, and (4) public distance of 12 feet or more. People are usually not aware of the use of personal space according to zones; nevertheless, the use of personal space is certainly influenced by culture.

Watson (1970) studied cultural differences in the use of personal space. He compiled a range of space by nationality and found that Americans, Canadians, and British require the most personal space, whereas Latin Americans and Arabs need the least. He noted that within the same cultural group individuals interacted at a uniform distance according to the situation. Because people do not consciously recognize their use of personal space, they have difficulty understanding a different cultural pattern. As a result, acts of friendliness may be misinterpreted as threatening behavior if personal space has been invaded.

An understanding of personal space by the community health nurse can facilitate the nursing assessment process and has significance for nurse-client interaction. Health professionals often feel that they have access to any area of the client's body. The client may develop patterns of avoidance and withdrawal to protect personal space. Nevertheless, close contact is necessary when performing a physical assessment, for example. The nurse should attempt to reduce anxiety by recognizing the individual's need for personal space and taking the appropriate action to provide privacy. Clients should be allowed to direct the use of their personal space whether they are in their homes or in the hospital so that individual identity and integrity are preserved.

Sociocultural Views of Disease and Illness

In countries such as the United States there is an extremely complex system of health beliefs and practices. Variation in these beliefs and practices may be found across ethnic and social class boundaries and even within families. Currently the generally accepted approach is the biomedical model, which emphasizes biological concerns. These concerns are often considered more "real," significant, and interesting than psychological and sociocultural issues (Kleinman et al., 1978). Most health professionals in modern Western settings are primarily interested in the treatment of diseases and abnormalities in the structure and function of body systems. Kleinman et al. view the biomedical approach as culture-specific (culture-bound) and value-laden. The biomedical model represents one end of a continuum. At the other end is traditional content, the popular beliefs and practices that usually diverge from medical science (Chrisman, 1977). Health beliefs and practices of individuals vary along this continuum.

In the last decade anthropologists and sociologists have made a distinction between illness and disease. The human experience of illness is not necessarily identical to the biomedical interpretation of disease. Illness is the individual's perception of being sick. Disease is only diagnosed when the condition is a deviation from norms as established by Western biomedical science (Fabrega, 1971). Illness may occur in the absence of disease; for instance, 50% of the visits to a physician are for complaints without a definite biological basis. "Illness is culturally shaped in the sense that how we perceive, experience and cope with disease is based on our explanations of sickness" (Kleinman et al., 1978, p. 252). Disease is described in medical-surgical nursing textbooks; however, nurses must also be familiar with the personal and cultural reactions to disease or discomfort.

Culture influences our expectations and perceptions of symptoms; the way we label sickness; when, how, and to whom we communicate our health problem; and how long we remain under care. Because health and illness are shaped by cultural factors, there is variation in health care behavior, health status, and patterns of sickness and care within and between different cultures. Health care behavior refers to social and biological activities of the individual based on maintaining an acceptable health status or on altering an unacceptable condition. Health status refers to the success with which a person has adapted to the total environment. Health care behavior influences health status, which influences health care behavior, and both are affected by sociocultural forces such as economics, politics, environmental influences, and the health system (Elling, 1977).

The model in Figure 5-1 shows the relation of sociocultural patterns to the health care system and many other factors that have a bearing on health. As the model illustrates, sociocultural influences affect not only the individual's health status but also the entire health system. Other factors depicted in the model also produce changes in the health status of a population. For example, demographic structure traditionally has been linked to the health status of a population. Among demographic factors, characteristics such as age, gender, marital status, and migration have a strong influence on health status. The arrows indicate a causal direction of influence where the effects are clear and/ or important. Biomedical factors, including race, weight, height, and genetic inheritance are linked to various deviations from the normal functioning of the body, influencing the health status of an individual. Most of the relationships depicted in the model are reciprocal. The many interrelations also indicate that a change in any one factor affects the others.

Health care providers and clients may define disease and illness differently. If so, they may disagree about the best method of care for the client. Such a disagreement may cause the client to be uncooperative. If the provider and the client share the same beliefs and values, agree on a plan of care, and desire the same outcome from the care, the client is more likely to accept the care. The community health nurse should not attempt to compete with or change clients' values but instead should involve the client in making decisions about the plan of care. If the client is involved, cooperation is more likely to occur, and the client's health status will be improved.

People who have been reared in a group with common origins and a sense of identity often share basic concepts and attitudes toward health and illness as well as styles of behavior and concerns about the world. Their knowledge about health and their behaviors relative to preventing illness and treating disease are learned within the group. Although a group within a culture may practice certain health behaviors, individuals within the group may stray from the group values and may be willing to accept care not normally acceptable to the total group. An appreciation of individual differences within a cultural group will help providers avoid the common tendency to stereotype ethnic group members. An accurate description of the culture and the health behaviors of ethnic group members ideally provides an assessment of the values the group places on health care and treatment. However, only an assessment of the individual will indicate to the provider what is acceptable to the client.

DIVERSE CULTURES OF THE UNITED STATES

The United States has many diverse cultures as a result of the history of immigration by a variety of ethnic groups to this country. Although broad cultural values are shared by most people, a rich diversity of values and beliefs exists, including variation in health and illness beliefs. Nevertheless, nursing tends to be practiced in an ethnocentric manner. Generally, nursing has been taught and practiced as if all clients were members of the dominant American group, white, Christian, and of European ancestry (Ruiz, 1981). Because familiarity with this American group is widespread, it is not discussed in this chapter. (For information on low-

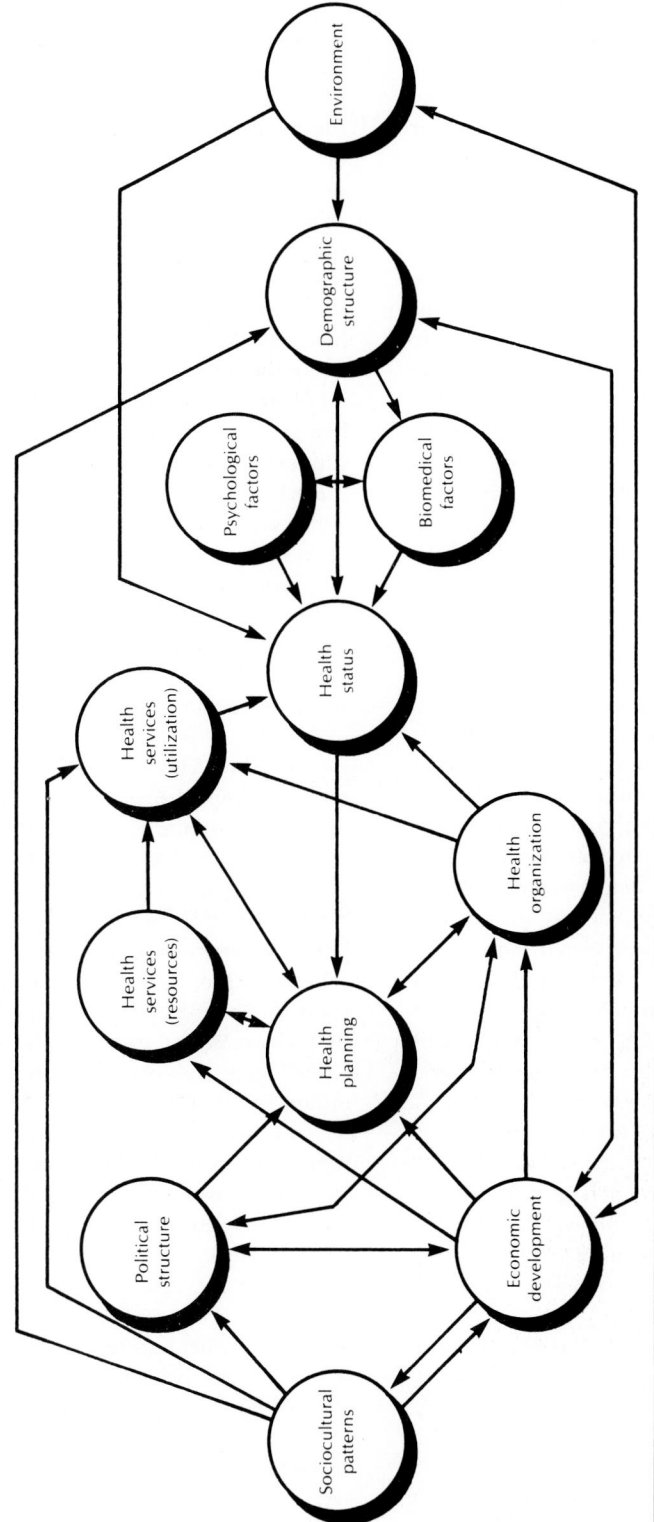

FIGURE 5-1

Sociocultural patterns and the health system. (From De Miguel, J.M.: A framework for the study of national health systems, Inquiry 12(2):10-24, 1975. Reprinted with permission of the Blue Cross Association.)

income Anglos see Bauwens [1977], and for middle-income Anglos see Hautman and Harrison [1982].)

Information about the cultural backgrounds of Asian Americans, black Americans, Mexican Americans, Middle Eastern-Arab Americans, and Native Americans is presented to help understand how cultural factors can and do influence client behavior and to highlight the importance of using cultural background data in providing nursing care. Factors that produce diversity between and within ethnic groups include historical factors, education, sex, place of birth, geographical location, socioeconomic status, and religious affiliation. The purpose of these examples of specific ethnic groups is not to present a detailed description of their culture and health behavior but to introduce to nurses and other health workers an appreciation of the multiple factors that influence health and illness beliefs.

Asian Americans

The likelihood of nurses having contact with Asians in the United States is greater than ever before. Historically the largest groups have been the Japanese, Chinese, Filipino, and Korean. A more recent influx of refugees from Viet Nam, Cambodia, and Laos has increased the Asian population, especially on the West Coast. A wide range of health beliefs and behaviors exists not only between the various groups but also within each group.

Early Chinese settlers in the United States were predominantly men who arrived in large numbers around 1850 to further their economic situation. They came with the idea of temporarily leaving their families to earn money and then returning to their homeland or eventually reuniting the family in the United States. Immigration laws intervened, and for those Chinese men who chose to stay, it meant that their families were restricted from joining them (Spector, 1979).

The form of extended household associated with traditional China in which grandparents, parents, siblings, and even aunts, uncles, and cousins lived under one roof is rare in the United States today. However, often members of Chinese families still maintain strong emotional bonds and a sense of responsibility for mutual assistance as needed. Traditional customs and preferences that may or may not be present in Chinese American families include a male-dominated household, women viewed as liabilities because of the transfer of their loyalties to the husband's family at the time of marriage, preference and indulgence of boys, and respect for and deference to the elderly (Henderson and Primeaux, 1981).

If nurses are knowledgeable about the prescribed roles in the particular Chinese American families, they will be able to assess and intervene more appropriately. Special care is needed when dealing with individual's and family's expressions of feelings even though they may be nonverbal (Henderson and Primeaux, 1981). Most Asians strongly emphasize harmony and avoidance of conflict in groups. Direct confrontations are usually avoided even if one must accept the blame. It is important for all to maintain self-esteem and not lose face, and this is achieved at times by nonresponsiveness.

Recent examination by Yu (1982) of available vital statistics showed that Chinese Americans have a lower infant mortality than white Americans. What are some plausible explanations for this low infant mortality among Chinese Americans? One explanation may be the reporting errors of births and deaths. Misreporting of race, especially when interracial marriages are involved, may be a source of error. Some researchers suggest that the low death rates, if not the result of errors in reporting, might be accounted for by rarity of teenage pregnancies in Chinese Americans. However, it seems the Chinese advantage is evident in every age group. The larger proportion of educated women among Chinese Americans has been considered. Again, Chinese American women have the lowest death rate at every level of education. Cultural influence on the health habits and life-style of Chinese Americans may be part of the explanation for differential statistics in infant mortality. Cultural influence on behaviors of women during pregnancy might include the following: (1) eating one or more types of Chinese herbs during pregnancy and just before delivery of the baby, (2) eating traditional foods, and (3) giving special herbs to the infants. At the present time all of these practices have been minimally studied to understand any possible association with infant mortality (Yu, 1982). Additional factors influencing the apparent differential in infant mortality among whites and Chinese might be found in other culturally determined health practices and life-styles, such as higher prevalence of smoking and substance abuse among white women as compared with Chinese American women. Precisely how the maternal intrauterine environment may be shaped by cultural health habits and practices is becoming more clear and is currently receiving attention through research.

Black Americans

In the past various terms have been used to describe blacks: colored, negro, Afro-American, and black. Caution is advised in labeling clients because, depending on their age, they may prefer a term to which they attach dignity. Jackson (1981) notes that blacks constitute a highly heterogeneous group; in other words, no typical black individual exists. Because blacks have highly visible physical traits such as skin color, many health professionals have a tendency to treat blacks as if they were all alike. However, black Americans display considerable variation in their health attitudes and behaviors.

Most of the black Africans who came to this country during the seventeenth and eighteenth centuries were different from other immigrants because they came unwillingly on slave ships, primarily from West Africa. Emancipation did not end the problem of being black in this country.

Some of the differences in health problems are the result of varying genetic pools and hereditary immunity. However, many of these differences are more closely associated with economic status than with race. Poverty, discrimination, and social and psychological barriers tend to keep people from using services that are available. These three factors interact and reinforce each other, which partially explains the fact that mortality and morbidity are higher for blacks (Bullough and Bullough, 1982). Black Americans have a higher infant mortality (18.4 per 1000 live births in 1984) than white Americans (9.4 per 1000 live births in 1984). The infant mortality rate for black infants was almost twice that for white infants in 1984, as it was 20 years earlier (Figure 5-2). However, the infant mortality rate for both the white and black populations has been decreasing by the same average annual percent (3.6% per year) between 1960 and 1984.

The black family is often oriented around women (matrifocal). Within the family the wife and/or mother is often charged with the responsibility for protecting the health of family members. She is expected to assist them in maintaining good health and in determining treatment if a family member is ill.

In general, black Americans have a strong religious orientation. Most belong to protestant faiths. The most common and frequently cited method of treating illness is prayer (Spector, 1979). Snow (1977) stated that many of her informants found it impossible to separate religious beliefs from medical ones. In some instances illnesses may be viewed as punishment for failure to abide by God's rules. Thus spiritual healers may be sought for curing illnesses; they generally have their own special curing techniques. Snow found that whether an individual comes from a rural or urban background is important in the selection of a health care provider. In general, those individuals who were reared in the rural South grew up being treated by folk practitioners. In many cases they did not encounter a physician until adulthood; thus they are most likely to turn to a neighborhood folk practitioner when ill. White (1977) claimed that folk medicine is still used within the black community because of humiliation in the mainstream health care system, lack of money, and lack of trust in health workers. Many go to physicians mainly because of the control of medicines and not because they feel the physician is superior in knowledge or training.

It is important for the community health nurse to recognize that black Americans are a heterogeneous group. Nevertheless, many are still influenced by ethnic group customs and traditions. Nurses have a responsibility to improve accessibility to health care, to provide culturally relevant health care, and to assist blacks to improve their own health status.

Mexican Americans

In this chapter the term *Mexican American* is used as a general designation for individuals of Mexican ancestry who live in only the southwestern states where studies were conducted. Given the regional enculturation and socioeconomic variation existing within the Mexican American populations, it is difficult to formulate conclusions about an entire ethnic

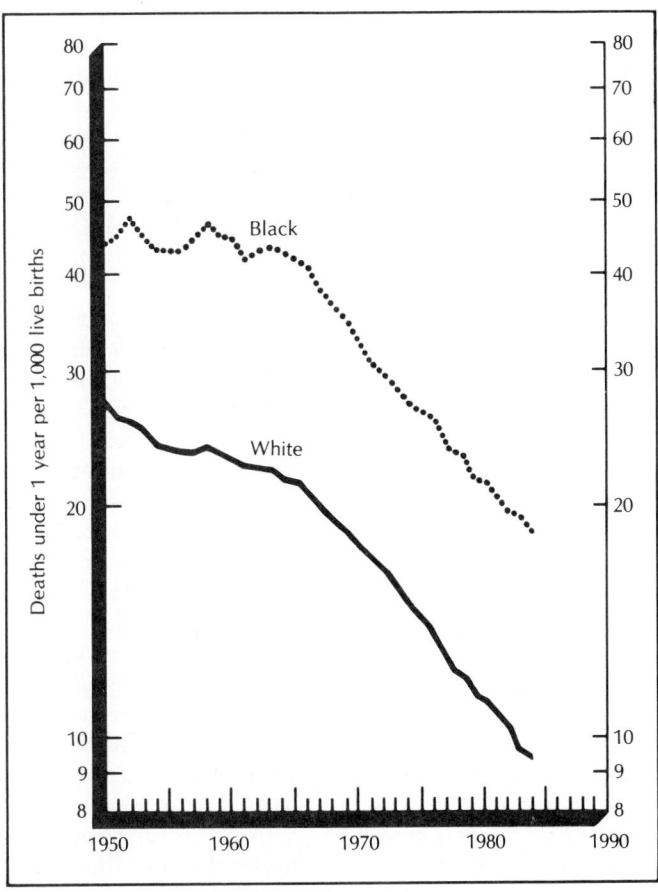

FIGURE 5-2

Infant mortality rates by race: United States, 1950-84. (From National Center for Health Statistics.)

group with such diversity as rural villagers in New Mexico and Colorado (Saunders, 1954; Weaver, 1970), agricultural laborers in Texas (Rubel, 1966), low-income residents in Arizona (Kay, 1977), or urban lower-class individuals in California (Clark, 1970). Not only do studies represent different populations but also differing definitions of Mexican American are used (Quesada, 1973). Thus any discussion of Mexican Americans is complicated by the problem of defining this population.

Mexican Americans moved northward from Mexico into the southwestern section of the United States. Therefore unlike most other immigrants, they are close to their homeland. There is also geographical similarity between the southwestern United States and northern Mexico, so that the Mexicans who moved north were more or less at home. Because of the geographical closeness, there is considerable movement of Mexican Americans back and forth between the two countries, since many still have relatives in Mexico.

Traditionally the family is important in Mexican-American culture and is characterized by a close-knit kin group. Ties beyond the nuclear family link grandparents, uncles, aunts, and cousins. A Mexican American is expected to turn to the family first to fulfill needs; seeking outside help often is done at the expense of pride and dignity of both the individual and the family. Practices are passed from generation to generation. If strong ties exist between the client and the family, the advice of the family may be followed rather than that of the community health nurse. The nurse may suggest that the client solicit the opinions of other family members regarding proposed actions. This demonstrates that the nurse understands the family's importance in health matters.

Language is also a cultural factor that influences health care practices. If a language barrier exists, it can be overcome by providing translators or Spanish-speaking health care providers. Mexican-American clients may be fairly fluent in English, yet when exposed to treatment plans in technical language, they may not comply with the regimen because of its unfamiliarity or miscommunication.

Religion is often an important cultural factor affecting health beliefs and practices. Many Mexican Americans are members of Catholic churches and turn to religious practices to overcome illness. Folk cures today often include prayers before the treatment begins (Kay, 1977).

Health is viewed as harmonious relations within the social and spiritual realms. Disruptions in social relations or breaking cultural rules are believed to have a bad effect on an individual's mental and physical well-being (Madsen, 1964). Rubel (1966) noted that Mexican Americans structure folk illness concepts into two major categories: (1) *males naturales* (natural illnesses) and (2) *mal puesto* (bewitchment). The first category includes four prominent folk syndromes: *molera caida* (fallen fontanel), *empacho* (indigestion infection), *mal ojo* (evil eye), and *susto* (fright); the second category includes such disorders as *brujeria* (witchcraft). Mal puesto is a declining belief and is generally used after several other diagnoses have been tried and treatment has been unsuccessful (Madsen, 1964; Rubel, 1966).

A wide variety of folk practitioners is used, including *curanderos* (folk healers), *sobadoras* (masseuses), and *parteras* (lay midwives). Generally an individual is referred to these folk practitioners by a family member, relative, or friend who has previously used their services or is aware of their reputations (Madsen, 1964).

Mexican Americans recognize a number of scientific disease categories and folk concepts of illness. However, recognition does not necessarily imply acceptance of scientific causes of disease. Causation may still be attributed to a lack of harmonious relations (Kay, 1977). Folk or scientific beliefs may be selectively chosen depending on such factors as the nature of the illness or the ability of folk or scientific treatment to produce a satisfactory outcome. Kay indicated that curanderos refer individuals to biomedical practitioners for serious illness and sometimes encourage treatment for folk illnesses by traditional and scientific means.

Nurses should elicit the client's view of the illness and recognize that Mexican Americans come with a culturally determined set of norms, and many have their own culturally derived concepts and interpretations about specific health problems. Denial of folk disorders by health professionals only reinforces the belief that these disorders lie outside scientific medicine's competence. Thus the client is encouraged to continue other forms of treatment. "The pervasiveness of folk medicine, its vitality, and self-sufficiency are noteworthy. It is not a question of a random collection of beliefs and superstitions. Folk medicine flourishes today because it is a functional part of the people's way of life" (Foster, 1952, p. 5).

Identifying cultural patterns is important in collecting data for planning nursing care. It is essential that the community health nurse be familiar with and understand the various cultural factors that may influence the health beliefs and practices of Mexican Americans and may determine their acceptance of health care services.

Middle Eastern—Arab Americans

Little attention has been given in the literature to the health care needs of Middle Eastern—Arab Americans. Only recently have Arabs immigrated to the United States in significant numbers. There are now between 2 and 3 million permanent and temporary residents in the United States, originally from the Middle East (Meleis and Sorrell, 1981). In addition to geographical origination, Arabs are frequently characterized by use of the Arabic language and practice of the Islam religion. They share the values, customs, and beliefs of the Arab culture.

Social properties of the Arab culture that are of interest to health care providers have been described by Meleis (1981) and Meleis and Sorrell (1981) and are listed as follows: (1) Affiliation with family is needed if an Arab American is to cope satisfactorily with daily events and/or life crisis. Arab Americans usually do not actively seek advice but feel help should be offered without a specific request. Visiting between family members is viewed as a social obligation during illness and other significant life events, which should be remembered in regard to hospital visitation. (2) Western medicine is usually highly valued even though the will of God, the "evil eye," and hot and cold shifts may be used to explain certain diseases. An effective cure and not personal care is expected of the health care system. They prefer to receive personal care from their families. Many Arab Americans believe that the more intrusive the procedure, the better the chance for recovery. (3) Arab Americans tend to give as little information as possible about themselves and their families to strangers. They may wonder about the personal nature of questions that may appear to others as routine. Arab American clients frequently present a general description of their health status as any illness that is thought to affect the whole individual and the well-being of the entire family. Pain is also experienced in a generalized way. (4) Arab society is oriented to the present, and many believe that planning ahead has the potential of defying God's will. Arab American women tend not to plan ahead for labor, delivery, and a new baby. Lack of planning should not be interpreted as maternal disinterest in the infant. Their values concerning planning and prevention make it difficult for some Arab Americans to use contraceptives. When birth control is practiced, Arab American women are more likely to prefer intrauterine devices because of the value placed on intrusive treatment. (5) Arab American women usually dress conservatively. Since they value modesty, it is important to protect patients from unnecessary exposure. Topics related to sex and reproduction are discussed with female relatives and friends but not with men or strangers. "Extreme tact needs to be exercised when involving the wife in any discussion without the husband . . . he can be employed to enhance the compliance of the family in all areas of health care including contraception" (Meleis and Sorrell, 1981, p. 176).

This general profile of Arab Americans does not fit any individual exactly but fits most of them in some way. Meleis (1981, p. 1183) offers an important caveat: "The line between individualizing care based on cultural diversity and stereotyping is a very fine one."

Native Americans (American Indians)

Confusion over who is a Native American is compounded by the lack of an adequate definition. In 1954 the United States Bureau of Indian Affairs admitted that it could not determine an adequate definition of who an Indian is or was (Josephy, 1969). Thus the term *Indian* in government reports can refer to a cultural group, a racial group, or a legal concept. As defined by the 1979 census, the largest concentrations of Native American populations in the United States were in Arizona and Oklahoma with 95,000 Native Americans each and New Mexico with approximately 72,000. Alaska, California, North Carolina, South Dakota, New York, Montana, Washington, and Minnesota are other states with large numbers of persons classified as Native Americans.

Among the Navajo, a southwestern Native American tribe, infant mortality has been reduced dramatically in recent years. In 1955 there were approximately 139 Navajo infant deaths per 1000 live births (Kunitz and Levy, 1981); in 1980 the Navajo death rate was 10.4 per 1000 population (Indian Health Service, 1981). The infant mortality for Native Americans fell from 62.5 per 1000 in 1955, to 16.4

per 1000 live births in 1976 to 1978, to 10.6 per 1000 live births in 1982. The rate is recently 4% lower than the United States and the all races rate for 1982, which is 11.5 per 1000 live births (Indian Health Service, 1986).

Infant mortality is influenced by the use of prenatal care, birth weight of the infant, feeding patterns, nutritional status of the infant and mother, and complicated pregnancies. Improvements in the future will probably be associated with improved living conditions and increased socioeconomic status rather than improved medical care (Oakland and Kane, 1973).

Providing effective health care to Native Americans is complicated by the fact that each nation or tribe has its own language, religion, and belief system regarding health and illness and its treatment. There are also variations in geography, distribution of wealth, and social organization. What is effective among one group may not be among another group (Vogel, 1970). The problem for the community health nurse is to fit traditional customs into effective preventive health care. The nurse must be aware that all Native Americans are not the same; they are not even members of the same tribe. Individuals range from those uneducated in Anglo ways to those well educated in their own and Anglo cultures. The nurse has to determine the client's level of knowledge.

The Native American family is frequently an extended family that includes several households. In addition, other individuals, formalized through a religious ceremony, can become the same as parents in the family network. Grandparents are family leaders, and respect for individuals increases with age. The family is important during periods of crises when family members serve as sources of support and security. The family structure has implications for the community health nurse, since family members need to be included in actively caring for the client (Primeaux and Henderson, 1981).

Religion is integrated into a distinct way of living and interpretation of life and is constantly present, whereas in the Western world religion generally is viewed as a discrete body of knowledge practiced in a specific place. Traditional healing ceremonies are ritualistic ways to handle illnesses and deaths. Some rituals may be performed by the family, or a traditional specialist may be sought to perform the ceremonies (Primeaux and Henderson, 1981). It is important for the community health nurse to recognize that Native Americans' health beliefs and practices today are a combination of Western medicine and traditional religious practices. Even though Anglo physicians and hospitals have been made available to Native Americans on reservations, old ways to treat illnesses continue to exist and are incorporated into the modern referral system in some places. As Ackerknecht (1942, p. 508) noted, " . . . the strong connection between these (healing) rites and the whole religion and tradition of the tribe produce certain psychotherapeutic advantages for the medicine man which the modern physician lacks." For example, a Navajo nursing student related an incident about her mother-in-law who lives on the Navajo reservation. A physician diagnosed the woman as having breast cancer, based on positive mammography and a biopsy. Surgery was recommended (radical mastectomy), but her mother-in-law refused. Instead she went to a medicine man who sucked out the inflicting cause. The mother-in-law still returns to the physician for periodic checks that include mammography. The student stated that she is thankful that her mother-in-law is well, but the physician remains appalled by this outcome, which included no further problems.

The knowledge of health beliefs and practices can assist the community health nurse in the management of the individual client and in the planning of health care delivery to specific cultural groups. Knowledge of the culture enhances the ability of the nurse to understand clients' problems, since cultural beliefs and values affect the way in which individuals recognize illness, select a health care provider, and determine their expectations of the provider. There may be the simultaneous use of various health services by clients and the switching serially from traditional to Western scientific medicine or other forms of practice. As illustrated in the example about the nursing student's mother-in-law, there is a strong ideological tendency to accept orthodox medicine, but at the same time there are pragmatic reasons to use unorthodox practitioners.

Refugee and Immigrant Populations

Immigrants are a growing segment of the American population. These individuals are first-generation immigrants and, therefore, are unacculturated to prevailing American norms of health belief or behavior. Changes in health status and health practices doubtless occur. To assess the appropriateness of a given health behavior would require broad research into the client's life and social context.

Social factors such as settlement patterns, communication networks, social class, and education also help immigrants and refugees to maintain their cultural traditions. In addition, most have their own community churches, stores, newspapers, physicians, and folk healers. Pattern of settlement by area of origin assists immigrants to adapt to new demands and assures that they have someone to call on for illness or other crises. The social class to which an individual belongs, education, and residential background also help to predict health practices. Fear of disease and past illness experience may also inhibit seeking treatment.

Immigrants often first experience medical culture conflict when their expression and interpretation of discomfort conflicts with that of current Western medical practice. Most health care professionals cannot learn all the folk health care of their client groups. Without a holistic view of the immigrant or refugee culture, health professionals find themselves confronted with what appears to them as the strange and curious notions of the individuals concerned. They begin to overgeneralize and say all individuals in this group are alike; for example, "Vietnamese have a present time orientation." This leads to stereotyping, which can lower the quality of care Vietnamese immigrants or refugees receive because the provider will give the Vietnamese immediate care to treat the illness but may not be inclined to plan for prevention of future problems.

The community health nurse should evaluate each person individually to determine the needs of that particular client and the degree to which the client adheres to cultural standards of health behavior. The nurse must recognize that the behavior of all members of a specific ethnic group is not necessarily uniform and may vary according to factors such as income, occupation, education, length of time since immigration, and experiences with health care services.

Southeast Asian Refugees

Since 1975, over 0.5 million persons from Vietnam, Cambodia, and Laos have entered the United States under federal and private assistance. Many have been forced into involuntary migration from their homelands. There is much variation among these individuals based on sociocultural factors such as ethnic group membership, socioeconomic status, geographical residence, gender, and degree of urbanization (Montero, 1978).

One ethnic group, the Hmong, are sufficiently similar to the other refugee groups from Southeast Asia to serve as a model for discussion. The Hmong in Southeast Asia are members of a large group found in China, Northern Vietnam, Thailand, and Laos. The Hmong were probably originally from the far north in China and spread southward in search of new lands for cultivation (see Geddes, 1976, for a review of Hmong history).

Nonrefugee Hmong in Southeast Asia have very high birth rates, large extended family households, and relatively low infant and crude mortality rates. The Hmong in the United States have posed special problems because of low use of health care services and psychiatric problems associated with refugee migration (Westermeyer et al., 1983). The cause of low utilization of services may be due to experienced difficulties in communicating with American providers. Migration may change family and network structures, and this disruption or loss of social support systems may have adverse effects on health. The Hmong in the United States can be expected to face challenges to their belief that spirits cause illness, since this belief conflicts with modern medical understanding of illness (Kunstadter, 1985). This affects their use of health services and their health.

The community health nurse must communicate a genuine respect for the Hmong cultural heritage and recognize this group's dependence on folk medicine. Often they do not distinguish religion and medicine and, although they are not opposed to Western medicine, traditional folk medicines are given first choice. Awareness of the influence of culture on behavior should assist the nurse to suspend judgment and to seek help from someone who knows the cultural pattern in question. The nurse will need to recognize her own folk beliefs, ethnocentrism, and assumptions about refugees and to be alert to culturally diverse expectations and other significant clues as to how health care might be better directed.

POVERTY

There is no agreement about how *poverty* should be defined or measured; in fact, no one really knows the extent of poverty in the United States. Any attempt at defining and measuring poverty must consider numerous variables. The federal government's poverty standards are defined and measured strictly in terms of income; that is, an absolute standard is used. Some have agreed that poverty should be defined by relative standards, accepted standards of what human life requires.

Absolute and Relative Standards

Poverty may be defined in absolute or relative terms. An *absolute standard* attempts to define some basic set of resources necessary for adequate existence. The federal government defines poverty in absolute terms using the Social Security Administration (SSA) standard as the official measure. This standard varies by place of residence, family size, and sex of the family head. The basis for the standard is the cost of food. Farm families are presumed to need 85% of the cash income required by nonfarm families because they can grow crops and thus not spend as much money for food. In 1985 the poverty income for a nonfarm family of four was $10,989 and for a farm family of four, $9,341. Increases in the SSA poverty standard are based on the consumer price index. The consumer price index reflects, among other factors, current market prices for food as determined by the United States Department of Agriculture. (See Chapter 3 for a discussion of the Consumer Price Index.)

A *relative standard* attempts to define poverty in terms of the median standard of living in a society. Townsend (1974, p. 15) stated the "Individuals, families and groups . . . can be said to be in poverty when they lack the resources to obtain the type of diets, participate in activities, and have the living conditions and amenities which are customary, or are at least widely encouraged or approved, in the societies to which they belong." If a relative standard were to be used, the poor might be defined as those who earn 50% of the median income for their family size. For example, in 1985 the median income for four-person families was $27,740. Any four-person family with an income of less than $13,870 would be considered poor. This would raise the poverty level for a four-person family in 1985 by $2,881 over the estimated 1985 SSA standard of $10,989, which would increase the poverty count significantly. A major attraction of the relative standard is that it more clearly delineates the overall distribution of wealth in the United States.

Health and welfare programs for the poor are based on absolute standards, which are misleading because they do not consider all of the dimensions, such as access to basic services, regional variations, and assets. As a result, many of the deserving poor do not receive assistance. The working poor have incomes too high to be considered eligible for public assistance programs, yet because of inflation, common needs such as food and health care are inaccessible.

Culture of Poverty

Oscar Lewis was an early formulator of the concept, *"culture of poverty"* in his works, *The Children of Sanchez* (1961) and *La Vida* (1966). The main idea of this concept is that poverty is not merely economic deprivation but also entails personality traits, some of which are psychologically compensatory

and rewarding. Like other aspects of culture, such elements are passed from generation to generation through enculturation. Many of the poor have beliefs, values, and lifestyles that are not an adjustment to low income but an ingrained way of life that is self-perpetuating and reinforced by each new generation. Lewis (1966) noted that the socioeconomic interests and values of the larger society are causal factors in the development and perpetuation of poverty. He contended that to eliminate poverty, these lifestyles and ways of perceiving the world and one's place in it must be abolished if poverty is to be eradicated.

Numerous critics have disagreed with Lewis' rationale. Valentine (1968) disagrees with the causes of behavior, the reasons for the deprivation of the poor, and the directions that social policies should take. He and other critics (Kahn, 1969; Leacock, 1971) of the concept fear that those unsympathetic to the poor will use the concept to withdraw aid or institute programs that will require some type of menial work to receive aid.

There are dangers associated with the use of the culture of poverty concept. For example, if the existence of a distinct and self-perpetuating culture of poverty were widely accepted, public funds might be diverted from programs to create more jobs, more housing, and better schools to those for more social work and reeducation of a psychiatric nature. Moreover, the culture of poverty concept serves to sustain the complacency of the more affluent by shifting the onus away from themselves and onto the shoulders of the poor, referred to by Ryan (1971) as "blaming the victim." Another danger that may be associated with the concept is that if the poor can be characterized as disorganized, deviant, or even sick, it would be foolhardy to permit them to share in decisions about the allocation of funds or to give them any control over their lives.

However, the culture of poverty concept may be handy if carefully used. For example, the controversy and research about the concept may help us understand the range of values of the poor, the function of their specific values, and in what situations they emerge. Attention to life-styles can tell us how and why certain groups are excluded from the mainstream and are unable to obtain adequate services. The insight gained can guide health care planners and others to restructure health care so that it is equally available to the poor.

Poverty and Health

There is a reciprocal relation between poverty and health. It has long been recognized that economic deprivation and health status are intertwined. For example, in 1828 Villerme showed that mortality in France was closely linked to the living conditions of different social classes (Rosen, 1963).

In the early twentieth century the health of the poor was deplorable. In the United States industrial expansion, urban growth, and immigration coincided to produce congested areas with inadequate housing. Poverty, malnutrition, and disease were widespread. Campaigns demanded governmental action to eliminate or ameliorate the consequences of poverty with respect to health. Between 1910 and 1920

American social policy was formulated, and legislation in relation to health was passed. The depression of the 1930s forced on the United States an urgent need to reconsider and to change established patterns of federal and state aid. Through these measures there was a recognition of the health hazards and poor health to which people were subjected because of economic instability.

By the 1960s it was evident that poverty and its attendant ills had not disappeared. With the passage of the Economic Opportunity Act in 1964, the United States declared war on poverty and rediscovered the poor. Congress passed antipoverty legislation to coordinate federal agencies with services and resources related to poverty and to enable the poor to become the recipients. In 1965 Congress enacted the Medicare and Medicaid programs.

From the standpoint of most indicators, the health status of rural people is poor, particularly when contrasted with the health of the total population. The death rates of infants and mothers are significantly higher in rural areas than in urban areas. Additionally, work-related disability rates are high because of accidents resulting from hazardous work environments (Health Status in Rural America, 1977). Most sparsely settled rural areas lack medical personnel and resources as well as strong lobbies in special interest areas. The poor are unlikely to use preventive health care because of more pressing priorities (Bauwens, 1977; Koos, 1954).

Although the health problems of the general rural populations are severe, they are even more critical for migrant farm workers. Migrants generally are more frequently ill, acutely and chronically, than the majority of Americans (Shenkin, 1974). Bissell (1976) noted that "the infant mortality rate is 125 percent above the national average." The accident rate among children of migrants is high because there is little supervision while the mother is working in the fields. Lack of sanitary facilities and overcrowding contribute to the spread of infectious diseases. Housing is frequently improvised and inadequate. The migratory conditions and poverty render the migrants less able to seek health care and these conditions account for the greater probability of their acquiring diseases. In general, poor people get sick more and stay sick longer because of inadequate health maintenance, lack of prevention, poor nutrition, and limited access to adequate personal health services.

The poor are more vulnerable to disease and less able to cope with it than the nonpoverty population. Because of this vulnerability, community health programs should ideally focus attention on populations in which there are high incidences of chronic and communicable diseases, high infant death rates, high birth rates, environmental hazards, and multiple social problems. The community health nurse needs to be involved in the planning and implementing of such programs. The programs ideally take into account social and cultural factors, respect values, mobilize local resources, and concentrate on meeting the needs of the poor. To meet these needs, health programs may encounter difficulties for at least four reasons:

1. The methods used may have to be adapted or especially designed to reach the individuals.

2. Geographically the individuals may be remote from the health centers, adding to problems of transport.
3. Politically the individuals may have little access to power and therefore little influence on the allocation of resources.
4. The values held by the individuals may be different from those of the program planners and administrators, and the setting of objectives and appraising of results of the programs may have to follow criteria that differ from those adopted by the rest of the population.

When working with the poor, nurses need to be able to identify the strengths and weaknesses of poor clients without imposing their own values. Facts regarding poverty lifestyles need to be distinguished from myth and prejudice. The following questions should be considered by the nurse: Do I perceive the values of the poor client as different from my own? If yes, how do the values differ? Do I expect the poor client to conform to my values? What does the client expect of me as a health professional? This value clarification is necessary for nurses to examine their own attitudes with respect to poor clients.

SOCIOCULTURAL ASSESSMENT

The material in this section is meant to assist nurses to be aware of and sensitive to sociocultural factors that affect health and the health care system. Awareness of sociocultural factors is necessary when assessing a community, family, and individual. Sociocultural assessment provides a data base from which the nurse can obtain an idea of the client's attitudes, values, and beliefs about the world in which the client lives. If culture consists of standards for what is correct and the background for behavior, then the nurse should assess his or her own culture of health care, both from the viewpoint of the culture of origin (what the nurse was taught to believe when growing up) as well as from the system into which the nurse has been socialized. The nurse needs to explore values, since values form one basis for behavior. What were the nurse's earliest experiences with deviations from health? Which symptoms was the nurse taught to notice and attend to?

Assessment tools or guides may be specific to a particular area (e.g., mental health) or have a narrow focus specific to nutrition practices, for example. A number of sociocultural assessment guides for nurses are available (Branch and Paxton, 1976; Leininger, 1976; Kay, 1977; Block, 1983; Orque, 1983; Tripp-Reimer, et al., 1984; Steiger and Lipson, 1985). Brownlee (1978) has identified several relevant factors to guide the nurse on the assessment of community, family and/or individual sociocultural factors.

Community Sociocultural Factors

The following is a list of pertinent sociocultural factors to be assessed in the community:

1. Existing influences that divide people into groups within the community, such as ethnicity, religion, social class, occupation, place of residence, language, education, sex, race, and age
2. Conditions that lead to social conflict and/or social cohesion

3. Attitudes toward minority groups, youth and the elderly, and males and females
4. Division of the community into neighborhoods or districts and the characteristics of these
5. Formal and informal channels of communication between health programs and the community
6. Barriers that may be the result of differences in cultural beliefs and practices
7. Political orientation in the community (attitudes toward authority and its use in health problems)
8. Patterns of migration either in or out of a community and their effect on health care services
9. Relation of religion and medicine within the community (who and what causes various illnesses and how they can be prevented)
10. Types of diseases or illnesses thought by various members of the community to exist (culture-specific conditions, such as illnesses caused by hot and cold imbalances and diseases of magical origin)

Family and/or Individual Sociocultural Factors

When assessing families or individuals, the community health nurse needs to be aware of the following:
1. Typical family households, roles played by family members and kinship groups, and patterns of residence
2. Events, rituals, and ceremonies considered important within the life cycle, such as birth, baptism, puberty, marriage, and death
3. The health beliefs and values of the family members and the social meaning attached to wellness and illness
   a. Beliefs concerning body organs and/or systems and how they function
   b. Particular methods used to help maintain health, such as hygienic and self-care practices
   c. Attitudes toward immunizations, screening tests, and other preventive health measures
   d. Beliefs and practices surrounding conception, pregnancy, childbirth, lactation, and rearing of children
   e. Attitudes toward mental illness, deformities, and death and dying
4. The person(s) in a family responsible for various health-related decisions, such as what to do when ill, where to go, who to see, and what advice to follow
5. Health topics that may be sensitive or taboo to the client
6. Possible conflicts between family health beliefs and practices and the teachings and practices of an established health program
7. Beliefs, rules, and preferences or prejudices concerning food, such as those believed to cause or cure illness
8. Culturally appropriate ways to enter and leave situations, including greetings, farewells, and convenient hours to make a home visit

Sociocultural assessment of the community, family, or individual includes all the preceding factors. The community health nurse needs to spend time to learn the culture before beginning any efforts at intervention or change. Specific families and individuals do not always reflect the "typical" cultural pattern. The nurse must remain sensitive to individual variations.

The nurse should also assess cultural standards about appropriate roles for participants in a health care system. How does the nurse feel about the use of medical doctors, osteopaths, chiropractors, Christian Science practitioners, psychologists? What about faith healers and folk curers? The client is also expected to cooperate with treatment recommendations. What constitutes "cooperation" is, however, culturally determined. Which aspects of care and treatment are the responsibility of the client? Should the client question health care management or is that disrespectful?

Assessment in the nursing process is done to meet certain of the client's needs. Culture affects the way these needs are perceived, understood and attended to. Social factors, such as age, education, income, religion, generation removed from mother country, and opportunities for obtaining health care, all influence health beliefs and practices. Sociocultural assessment leads to relevant nursing diagnoses, planning, and interventions. Interventions may be adapted toward those the client expects or an acceptable compromise for treatment may be necessary. Not every element of culture needs to be included in any one assessment; sociocultural factors will vary in importance based on the particular situation.

GUIDELINES FOR CULTURALLY APPROPRIATE HEALTH CARE

Modern Western medicine considers the biomedical model to be the best if not the only view of disease. This cultural conditioning of health professionals leads to depreciation or even denial of the client's view. To compensate for this inherent bias it is suggested that nurses elicit clients' interpretations of their health problems.

Client's Explanatory Model

Kleinman (1980) developed the concept of a client explanatory model by which an individual pulls together various beliefs and applies them to an illness to provide a meaningful explanation of the events surrounding the illness and to choose an appropriate course of action. The client's model deals with one or more of the same five questions for illness as used in the medical model: (1) etiology, (2) onset of symptoms, (3) pathophysiology, (4) course of illness, and (5) treatment. Usually the client's model is more concrete, is not completely articulated, and may be inconsistent and based on erroneous evaluation of evidence. "Nonetheless, they (clients' models) are comparable to clinical models . . . as attempts to explain clinical phenomena" (Kleinman et al., 1978, p. 256). The client's model reflects cultural beliefs, social class, education, occupation, religious affiliation, and past experience with illness and health care.

Clients often hesitate to disclose their models to health professionals. Once the client is assured that the health care provider is genuinely interested, his model can usually be elicited by the nurse with a few simple, direct questions. The following set of questions will help to elicit the client's explanation of the illness (Kleinman et al., 1978, p. 256):
1. What do you think caused your problem?
2. Why do you think it started when it did?
3. What do you think your sickness does to you? How does it work?

4. How severe is your sickness? Will it have a short or
   long course?
5. What kind of treatment do you think you should
   receive?

Client's Perception of Symptoms

A model developed by Jackson (1981) illustrates the process
that a client might use from the initial self-perception of
illness symptoms to treatment, whether that treatment is
self-care, medical, or nonmedical (Figure 5-3). The model
begins with the perception of a symptom, which implies
that the individual has identified that something is wrong.
The individual then evaluates the significance of the symptom. Many factors influence the interpretative process, such
as cultural beliefs and values, extent of discomfort, and
previous experience with illness. Jackson (1981) believes
that the level of income, social class, education, and disruption of activity are major variables that determine the
client's process of symptom management. Based on the
interpretation, the client may or may not initiate further
action. If further action is considered necessary, the person
can choose self-treatment or treatment by others, medical
or nonmedical. The client then makes a decision about the
success or failure of the selected treatment. If the treatment
is deemed a failure, vacillation among alternative sources
of health care or simultaneous use of two or more alternatives
is likely to occur.

Cultural Health Practices

Cultural health practices can be considered as efficacious,
neutral, or dysfunctional (Pillsbury, 1982). Efficacious practices are recognized by Western medicine as being beneficial
to health even though they may be very different from
scientific practices. Beneficial practices should be actively
encouraged by community health nurses, although they may
seem foreign to other health professionals. A treatment
strategy congruent with the client's own beliefs has a better
chance of being successful. For example, cultural beliefs

about the efficacy of herbal teas must be considered by the
community health nurse, since some are therapeutic (dehydration can be treated with tea). Treatment with tea may
be as efficacious as water. Another example is the use of the
traditional birthing position of kneeling, which seems to
be more beneficial for women than the horizontal position
advocated by Western medical practice (Cominsky, 1977).

Neutral (harmless) practices are of no significance one
way or another to the health of the individual. They may
be considered unimportant by the health professional, but
for the individual the health practices may be linked with
beliefs that are closely integrated into everday behaviors.
Examples of practices that are neutral include "the ritual
disposal of the placenta and cord, interpretation of signs in
the cord, avoidance of sexual activity during various stages
of pregnancy, culturally prescribed hygiene practices and
avoidance of exposure during a lunar eclipse" (Johnston,
1980, p. 13). Even though these practices do not require
intervention by the practitioner, the nurse should respect
their significance and meaning to the individual.

In all cultures there are practices that are dysfunctional
or harmful from a health point of view. In Western countries
the excessive use of sugar and overrefined flour is partially
responsible for the high incidence of dental caries and obesity. Health education should be focused on dysfunctional
or harmful health practices. Efforts should be made to assist
clients to modify harmful practices.

Williams and Jelliffe (1972) included a category of uncertain practices in their cultural assessment system. This
category includes practices with unknown effects, such as
swaddling newborns and the use of abdominal binders for
mothers and infants. In most instances practices do not
perfectly fit into one category or another. "Health practices
are relatively more or less beneficial or harmful when compared to alternative practices" (Greene and Johnston, 1980,
p. 13).

In addition to culturally specific health care practices,
individuals may turn to alternative health practitioners for

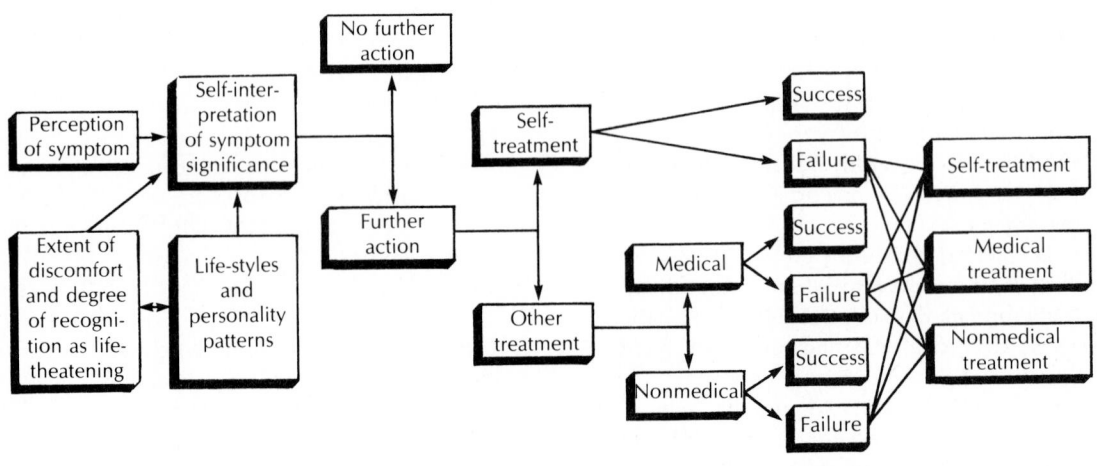

FIGURE 5-3

Process of symptom management. (From Jackson, J.J.: Urban black Americans. In Harwood,
A.I., editor: Ethnicity and medical care, Cambridge, Mass., 1981, Harvard University Press.
Reprinted by permission.)

a variety of reasons. Harwood (1981) listed the following general reasons why individuals might use alternative healers: (1) lack of availability and accessibility of mainstream health services, (2) lack of satisfaction with treatment, (3) lack of trust in the ability of Western medical practitioners to effectively treat psychosocial problems, and (4) lack of knowledge of Western medical practitioners in the treatment of culture-bound syndromes.

In many cases alternative healers complement the delivery of mainstream health care services. Often they are more available and accessible than Western health care providers. They are familiar with culture-bound syndromes and cultural traditions. In addition, they often establish warm relations with clients and their families.

CLINICAL APPLICATION

Based on the discussion of culture and cultural differences, principles for nursing practice can be identified for application in clinical practice:

The nurse should be aware of the client's cultural interpretation of health, illness, and health care. A client's perception and definition of an experience as an illness is partially the result of culturally learned beliefs and the amount and kind of exposure to mainstream health culture. Clarification of the variety of client interpretations by different cultural groups is important. The objective is to be aware of and sensitive to the fact that there are multiple factors underlying client behaviors. The nurse should question clients concerning their ideas about health and illness in a nonjudgmental way that elicits the client's concepts and communicates genuine interest.

The nurse should identify sources of discrepancy between clients' and health providers' concepts of health or illness. A frequent source of poor communication between clients and nurses is when one party uses a term to label an illness or a symptom and that term is unfamiliar to the other person. Another source of miscommunication occurs when the client and the nurse use the same term but mean different things. For example, the term *family* has a variety of meanings for different segments of the community. Lack of communication may go undetected because the client and the nurse are using the same term. The nurse should check with the client as to the meaning for the unknown term, and the client should be encouraged to request clarification from the nurse. Discrepancies will then become apparent and should be discussed. Methods of handling discrepancies include educating the client; adapting the nursing care plan to the client's system (i.e., agreeing to a therapeutic plan that accommodates the client and the nurse to some degree); or working within the client's system by using a therapeutic care plan that is considered effective by the nurse and appropriate for the client's culture.

The nurse should be aware of the cultural values that affect client's use of the health care system. Cultural values shape human health behaviors and determine what individuals will do to maintain their health status, how they will care for themselves and others who become ill, and where and from whom they will seek health care. Cultural preferences for certain modes of treatment suggest that nursing inter-

ventions may be more effective if they include culturally preferred treatment modes. For example, the nurse might mention the use of herbal teas in addition to the usual use of water or juice when caring for Mexican American clients.

The nurse should evaluate the effectiveness of nursing actions with clients from diverse cultural groups. One way to evaluate the effectiveness of nursing actions is by monitoring the client's adherence to treatment regimens. Clients judge regimens not only on a medical basis but also on a social and cultural basis. Whether the regimen is adhered to or not may depend on such conditions as explaining the regimen using terms that the client can understand; accommodating the client's life-style, dietary patterns, and health beliefs; and enlisting the client's family in reinforcing treatment regimens. The specific family members enlisted for support may differ according to the client's ethnic affiliation.

Knowledge of cultural patterns enhances the ability of the nurse to assess and understand the client's health beliefs and practices. Assessment of sociocultural factors enables the nurse to identify ways in which individuals and families may differ from the typical cultural pattern. Sensitivity to individual variations makes it possible to plan culturally appropriate interpretation of health problems. It is important to be aware of the process that clients use from the initial self-perception of their illness symptoms to treatment. The nurse must be aware of how clients evaluate the success or failure of the treatment. Cultural health practices are described as being beneficial, neutral, or harmful.

The overall purpose of this chapter has been to help nurses deliver more personalized, culturally appropriate care to all clients. If clients are to be treated in a holistic manner, the nurse must constantly be aware of their attributes and health beliefs and practices.

SUMMARY

Sociocultural variables related to health care have been discussed. The premise that health care is based not only on knowledge of the physical causes of a disease but also on sociocultural influences has been introduced. Culture has been defined as a set of rules that help people act appropriately. The following cultural concepts that have relevance for nurses have been discussed: holism, culture change, enculturation, culture-bound, ethnocentrism, stereotypes, and cultural values.

The mobility of people and their cultural diversity increase the likelihood that nurses will come in contact with a variety of cultural life-styles and traditions. Often nurses must provide care for individuals from different cultural groups. This chapter has explored cultural trend items in the following areas: ethnic collectivity, cultural shock, communication patterns, personal space and contact, and cultural views of disease and illness. Diverse cultures of the United States, namely, Asian, black, Mexican, Arab, and Native American, have been presented as examples to provide cultural background data to assist nurses in providing culturally relevant nursing care. Poverty has been addressed from the economic, psychological, and cultural perspective, and the reciprocal relation between poverty and health has been discussed.

≡ KEY CONCEPTS

Culture enables us to interpret our surroundings and the actions of people around us and to behave in ways that make sense.

Some anthropologists conceive of culture as a set of rules that provide the individual with a means for behaving and interpreting the behavior of others.

The concept of holism requires that human behavior not be isolated from the context in which it occurs and that the culture is best viewed and analyzed as a whole.

Culture is never static but is in a constant process of adding or deleting elements.

Enculturation is the process of acquiring and knowledge and internalizing values; through this process persons achieve competence in their own culture.

Because we look at the world from our own particular cultural viewpoint, we often believe our way is best; such a viewpoint is called "ethnocentrism." It is important for nurses not to consider their own way as best and other people's ideas as ignorant or inferior.

Stereotypes are exaggerated beliefs and images that are popularly depicted in the mass communication media and folklore. Usually these images are false; they obscure important differences among members of a group and exaggerage those between groups.

Cultural values are the prevailing and persistant guides influencing thinking and actions of people.

People who have been reared in an "ethnic collectivity" (a shared group with common origins, a sense of identity, and shared standards for behavior) often acquire from that experience cultural norms that determine the thought and behavior of individual members.

"Cultural shock" is one of the effects of working with individuals from different cultural backrounds. Nurses can reduce cultural shock by knowing about the different cultural groups with whom they are working.

Poverty may be defined in absolute or relative terms. An absolute standard attempts to define some basic set of resources necessary for adequate existence. A relative standard attempts to define poverty in terms of the median standard of living in a society.

There is a reciprocal relationship between poverty and health. It has long been recognized that economic deprivation and health status are intertwined.

The mobility of the population and its cultural diversity increase the likelihood that nurses will come in contact with a variety of cultural life-styles and traditions.

LEARNING ACTIVITIES

1. Define culture and how it relates to health and illness behavior.

2. Identify concepts relevant to culture and health care.

3. Before asking clients questions that have cultural relevance, ask yourself the same question about your own culture.

4. Recognize the variety of influences that cultural differences have on the interpretation of health and illness.

5. Identify factors that produce diversity in health-seeking behavior between and within ethnic groups.

6. Describe the nature of poverty and its effect on health status and health behavior.

7. Assess sociocultural factors and their impact on health care for the individual, family, and community.

BIBLIOGRAPHY

Ackerknecht, E.H.: Problems of primitive medicine, Bull. Hist. Med. 11:508-509, 1942.

Arizona Department of Health Services: AHCCCS (Arizona Health Care Cost Containment System) Bulletin, Phoenix, Dec. 14, 1982, AHCCCS Public Information Office.

Bauwens, E.E.: Medical beliefs and practices among lower-income Anglos. In Spicer, E.H., editor: Ethnic medicine in the Southwest, Tucson, 1977, University of Arizona Press.

Benedict, R.: Patterns of culture, Boston, 1934, Houghton Mifflin Co.

Berkanovic, E., and Reeder, L.G.: Ethnic, economic and social psychological factors in the source of medical care, Soc. Prob. 21:246-259, 1973.

Bissell, K.A.: The migrant farmworker, Washington, D.C., 1976, The Catholic University of America.

Bloch, B.: Bloch's assessment guide for ethnic/cultural variations. In Orque, M.S., Bloch, B., and Monrroy, L.S., editors: Ethnic nursing care, St. Louis, 1983, The C.V. Mosby Co.

Brownlee, A.T.: Community, culture and care, St. Louis, 1978, The C.V. Mosby Co.

Bullough, V.L., and Bullough, B.: Health care for the other Americans, New York, 1982, Appleton-Century-Crofts.

Calhoun, M.A.: Providing health care to Vietnamese in America: what practitioners need to know, Home Healthcare Nurse 4(5):14-22, May 1986.

Chrisman, N.J.: The health seeking process, Cult. Med. Psychiatry 1:351-377, 1977.

Chrisman, N.J., and Kleinman, A.: Popular health care, social networks and cultural meanings: the orientation of Medical Anthropology. In handbook of Health, Health Care, and the Health Professions, New York, 1983, The Free Press.

Clark, M.: Health in the Mexican-American culture, Berkeley, 1970, University of California Press.

Cominsky, S.: Childbirth and midwifery on a Guatemalan finca, Med. Anthropol. 1:94, 1977.

De Migul, J.M.: A framework for the study of national health systems, Inquiry 12(2):10-24, June 1975.

Dohrenwend, B.P.: Sociocultural and social-psychologist factors in the genesis of mental disorders, J. Health Soc. Behav. 16:365-392, 1975.

Dohrenwend, B.P., and Dohrenwend, B.S.: Social status and psychological disorder: a causal inquiry, New York, 1969, John Wiley & Sons, Inc.

Dohrenwend, B.S., and Dohrenwend, B.P.: Stressful life events: their nature and effects, New York, 1974, John Wiley & Sons, Inc.

Dunham, H.W.: Community and schizophrenia: an epidemiological analysis, Detroit, 1965, Wayne State University.

Elling, R.H.: Socio-cultural influences on health and health care, New York, 1977, Springer Publishing Co., Inc.

Fabrega, H.: Medical anthropology. In Siegel, B.J., editor: Biennial review of anthropology, Standard, Calif., 1971, Stanford University Press.

Foster, G.M.: Relationships between theoretical and applied anthropology: a public health analysis, Hum. Organization 11:5-16, 1952.

Geddes, W.: Migrants of the mountains: the cultural ecology of the Blue Miao (Hmong Njcca) of Thailand, Oxford, 1976, Clarendon Press.

Goodenough, W.H.: Cooperation in change, New York, 1966, Russell Sage Foundation.

Greenblum, J.: Medical and health orientations of American Jews: a case of diminishing distinctiveness, Soc. Sci. Med. 8:127-134, 1974.

Greene, L., and Johnston, F.: Social and biological predictors of nutritional status, growth, and development, New York, 1980, Academic Press, Inc.

Guttmacher, S., and Elinson, J.: Ethno-religious variation in perceptions of illness: the use of illness as an explanation for deviant behavior, Soc. Sci. Med. 5:117-125, 1971.

Hall, E.T.: The silent language, New York, 1959, Doubleday & Co., Inc.

Harrison, G., and Ritenbaugh, C.: Anthropology and nutrition: a perspective on two scientific subcultures, Fed. Proc. 4(11):2595-2600, Sept. 1981.

Harwood, A., editor: Ethnicity and medical care, Cambridge, Mass., 1981, Harvard University Press.

Hautman, M.A., and Harrison, J.K.: Health beliefs and practices in a middle-income Anglo-American neighborhood, Adv. Nurs. Sci. 4(3):49-64, 1982.

Health status in rural America, Rural Health Report no. 1, Washington, D.C., 1977, Rural America.

Henderson, G., and Primeaux, M.: Transcultural health care, Reading, Mass., 1981, Addison-Wesley Publishing Co., Inc.

Hollander, J.: The abolition of poverty, Boston, 1914, Houghton Mifflin Co.

Hollingshead, A.B., and Redlich, F.C.: Social class and medical illness, New York, 1958, John Wiley & Sons, Inc.

Horn, B.M.: Transcultural nursing and child-rearing of the Muckleshoot people. In Leininger, M., editor: Transcultural nursing, New York, 1979, Masson International Nursing Publications.

Indian Health Service: Indian Health Service "Chart Series" tables, Office of Program Statistics, Rockville, MD., 1981.

Indian Health Service: Indian Health Service "Chart Series" tables, Office of Program Statistics, Rockville, MD., 1986.

Insel, P.M.: Too close for comfort, Englewood Cliffs, N.J., 1978, Prentice-Hall, Inc.

Jackson, J.J.: Urban black Americans. In Harwood, A., editor: Ethnicity and medical care, Cambridge, Mass., 1981, Harvard University Press.

Jelliffe, D.B.: Child nutrition in developing countries, Washington, D.C., 1969, U.S. Department of Health, Education, and Welfare.

Josephy, A.M., Jr.: The Indian heritage of America, New York, 1969, Alfred A. Knopf, Inc.

Kahn, A.O.: Studies in social policy and planning, New York, 1969, Russell Sage Foundation.

Kay, M.A.: Health in the Mexican-American barrio. In Spicer, E.H., editor: Ethnic medicine in the southwest, Tucson, 1977, University of Arizona Press.

Kleinman, A.: Patients and healers in the context of culture, Berkeley, 1980, University of California Press.

Kleinman, A., Eisenberg, L., and Good, B.: Culture, illness and care, Ann. Intern. Med. 88:251-258, 1978.

Kluckhohn, C.: The gifts of tongues. In Samover, L.A., and Porter, R.E., editors: Intercultural communication: a reader, Belmont, Calif., 1972, Wadsworth, Inc.

Kniep-Hardy, M., and Burkhardt, M.: Nursing the Navajo, Am. J. Nurs. 77:95-96, 1977.

Koos, E.: Health in Regionville, New York, 1954, Columbia University Press.

Kubricht, D.W., and Clark, J.A.: Foreign patients: a system for providing care, Nurs. Outlook 30(1):55-57, Jan. 1982.

Kunitz, I.J., and Levy, J.E.: Navajos. In Harwood, A., editor: Ethnicity and medical care, Cambridge, Mass., 1981, Harvard University Press.

Kunstadter, P.: Health of Hmong in Thailand: risk factors, morbidity and mortality in comparison with other ethnic groups, Cult. Med. Psychiatry 9(4):329-351, Dec. 1985.

Leacock, E.: The culture of poverty: a critique, New York, 1971, Simon & Schuster.

Leininger, M.: Transcultural health care issues and conditions, Philadelphia, 1976, F.A. Davis Co.

Lewis: O.: The children of Sanchez, New York, 1961, Random House, Inc.

Lewis, O.: La Vida, New York, 1966, Random House, Inc.

Madsen, M.: The Mexican-Americans of south Texas, New York, 1964, Holt, Rinehart & Winston General Book.

Mechanic, D.: Illness and cure. In Kosa, J., Antonovsky, A., and Zola, I., editors: Poverty and health: a sociological analysis, Cambridge, Mass., 1969, Harvard University Press.

Meisenhelder, J.B.: Boundaries of personal space, Image 14(1):16-19, Feb.-March 1982.

Meleis, A.I.: The Arab American in the health care system, Am. J. Nurs. 81:1180-1183, 1981.

Meleis, A.I., and Sorrell, L.: Arab American women and their birth experiences, Am. J. Matern. Child Nurs. 6:171-176, 1981.

Moccia, P., and Mason, D.J.: Poverty trends: implications for nursing, Nurs. Outlook 34(1): 20-24, Jan./Feb. 1986.

Montero, D.: The Vietnamese refugees in America: patterns of socioeconomic adaptation and assimilation, College Park, M.D., 1978, Institute of Urban Studies, University of Maryland.

National Center for Health Statistics: Vital statistics of the United States, 1977, vol. II, Mortality, Part A, Hyattsville, M.D., 1981, U.S. Government Printing Office.

National Center for Health Statistics: Monthly vital statistics: 34(6), Supplement No. 2, Sept. 1985.

Oakland, L., and Kane, R.L.: The working mother and child neglect on the Navajo reservation, Pediatrics 51:849-853, 1973.

Orque, M.S.: Orque's ethnic/cultural system: a framework for ethnic nursing care. In Orque, M.S., Bloch, B., and Monrroy, L.S., editors: Ethnic nursing care, St. Louis, 1983, The C.V. Mosby Co.

Pillsbury, B.: Doing the month: confinement and convalescence of Chinese women after childbirth. In Kay, M., editor: Anthropology of human birth, Philadelphia, 1982, F.A. Davis Co.

Primeaux, M., and Henderson, G.: American Indian patient care. In Henderson, S., and Primeaux, M., editors: Transcultural health care, Philadelphia, 1981, F.A. Davis Co.

Quesada, G.M.: Mexican Americans: Mexicans or Americans? Lubbock, Tex., 1973, Southwestern Council of Latin-American Studies.

Reinert, B.R.: The health care beliefs and values of Mexican-Americans, Home Healthcare Nurse 4(5):23-31, May 1986.

Rosen, G.: The evalution of social medicine. In Freeman, H.E., Levin, S., and Reeder, L.B., editors: Handbook of medical sociology, Englewood Cliffs, N.J., 1963, Prentice-Hall, Inc.

Rubel, A.: Across the tracks: Mexican Americans in a Texas city, Austin, 1966, University of Texas Press.

Ruiz, M.C.J.: Open-closed mindedness, intolerance of ambiguity and nursing faculty attitudes toward culturally different patients, Nurs. Res. 30(3):177-181, 1981.

Ryan, W.: Blaming the victim, New York, 1971, Pantheon Books. Samora, J.: Conceptions of health and disease among Spanish-Americans, Am. Cath. Sociol. Rev. 22:314-323, 1961.

Saunders, L.: Cultural difference and medical care, New York, 1954, Russell Sage Foundation.

Shenkin, B.N.: Health care for migrant workers, Cambridge, Mass., 1974, Ballinger Publishing Co.

Snow, L.F.: Popular medicine in a black neighborhood. In Spicer, E.H., editor: Ethnic medicine in the southwest, Tucson, 1977, University of Arizona Press.

Spector, R.E.: Cultural diversity in health and illness, New York, 1979, Appleton-Century-Crofts.

Suchman, E.A.: Sociomedical variations among ethnic groups, Am. J. Sociol. 70:319-331, 1964.

Townsend, P.: Poverty as relative deprivation: resources and style of living. In Weaderburn, D., editor: Poverty inequality and class structure, London, 1974, Cambridge University Press.

Tripp-Reimer, T.: Barriers to health care: variations in interpretation of Appalachian client behavior by Appalachian and non-Appalachian health professionals, West. J. Nurs. Res. 4(2):179-191, 1982.

Tripp-Reimer, T., Brink, P., and Saunders, J.: Cultural assessment: content and process, Nurs. Outlook 32(2):78-82, March/April 1984.

U.S. Bureau of the Census: Statistical abstracts of the United States, 1979, Washington, D.C., 1979, U.S. Government Printing Office.

Valentine, C.A.: Culture and poverty, Chicago, 1968, University of Chicago Press.

Vogel, V.J.: American Indian medicine, Norman, Okla., 1970, University of Oklahoma Press.

Watson, O.M.: Proxemic behavior: a cross-cultural study, The Hague, Netherlands, 1970, Monitor & Co.

Weaver, T.: Use of hypothetical situations in a study of Spanish-American illness referral systems, Hum. Org. 29:140, 1970.

Westermeyer, J., Vang, T.F., and Neider, J.: Migration and mental health among Hmong refugees, J. Nerv. Ment. Disorders 171(2):92-96, 1983.

White, E.H.: Giving health care to minority patients, Nurs. Clin. North Am. 12:27-40, 1977.

Williams, C., and Jelliffe, D.: Mother and child health: delivering the services, London, 1972, Oxford University Press.

Young, A.A.: Rethinking the Western health enterprise, Med. Anthropol. 2(2):1-9, 1978.

Yu, E.: The low mortality rates of Chinese infants: some plausible explanatory factors, Soc. Sci. Med. 16(3):253-265, 1982.

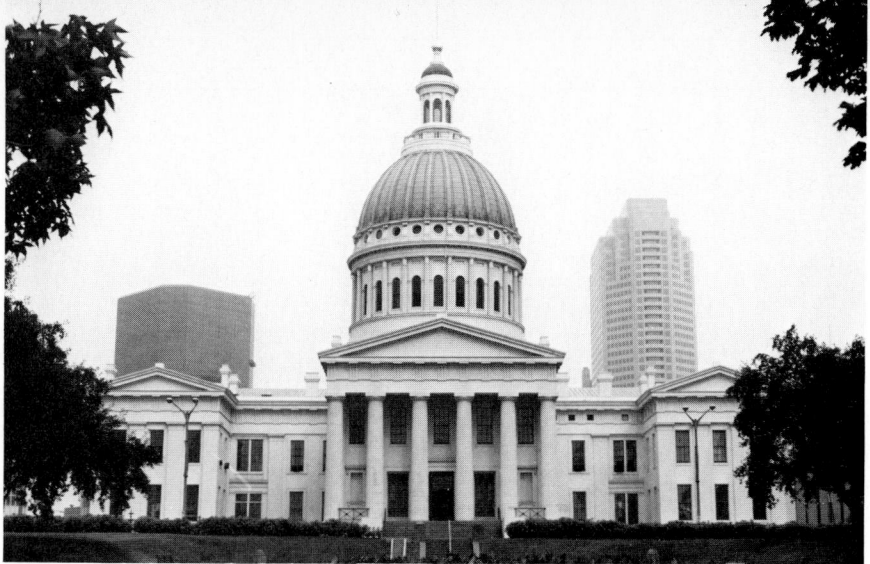

Cynthia E. Northrop

6

GOVERNMENTAL, POLITICAL, AND LEGAL INFLUENCES ON THE PRACTICE OF COMMUNITY HEALTH NURSING

≡ OBJECTIVES

After reading this chapter, the student should be able to:

Describe the trends and roles of several levels of government.

Identify the impact of changing governmental roles and structures on health care.

Describe the major governmental functions in health care.

Discuss community health nursing roles in selected governmental agencies.

Shape health policy by participating in the regulation-making process and the political arena.

Identify self-regulatory activities as a professional nurse.

Describe selected laws that affect community health nursing practice, both generally and in special areas of practice.

Conduct a brief exercise in legal research as one means of staying current with the law.

≡ KEY TERMS

Department of Health and Human Services (DHHS)

Federal Register

Codes of Regulation

judicial and common law

legislation

Lexis

legislative process

National Center for Nursing Research

Occupational Safety and Health Act (OSHA)

police power

Practice Acts

private sector

professional negligence

Public Health Service (PHS)

regulation

scope of practice

Scorpio

self-regulation

World Health Organization (WHO)

Community health nurses are an integral part of the health care system and are significantly affected by the government and the legal system. This chapter will provide descriptions of these institutions, including organization and primary functions of governments, governmental regulation, and professional self-regulation. The chapter concludes with an overview of laws affecting community health nursing practice.

GOVERNMENTAL ROLE IN HEALTH CARE

Many nurses who select community health nursing as an area of practice are intrigued by the interdependence of law, health, nursing practice, and government. They often seek additional coursework beyond their initial degree and unique work experiences to further their understanding of how law and government relate to health care.

Legal Basis for Governmental Role in Health Care

One of the first constitutional challenges to congressional legislation in the area of health and welfare came in 1937, when Congress established unemployment compensation and old-age benefits. Although Congress had created other health programs, its legal basis for doing so had never before been challenged. The Supreme Court decided that such federal government action was within congressional powers to promote the general welfare found in Article I, Section 8, of the U.S. Constitution. Most legal bases for congressional action in health care are found in Section 8. They include the following:

1. Provide for the general welfare
2. Regulate commerce among the several states
3. Raise funds to support the military
4. Provide spending power

These statements within Section 8 of Article I have been interpreted by the Court to include a wide variety of federal powers and activities.

The legal basis for state and local activities in the area of health does not require the identification of an explicit power within a state constitution. Most state power that concerns health care is known as the state's *police power*. This means that states may act to protect the health, safety, and welfare of their citizens. Such police power must be reasonably exercised, and the state must demonstrate that it has a compelling interest in taking actions, especially actions that might infringe on individual rights.

An example of a state exercising its police powers is that of a state legislature requiring immunization of children before school admission. The state's reasonable actions must be to protect the health, safety, and welfare of its citizens. In the immunization of preschool children the state is attempting to eliminate communicable diseases and to prevent death and disability. These goals involve activities that protect the health, safety, and welfare of state citizens.

Trends and Shifts in Government Roles

Governmental involvement in health care at both the state and federal level began gradually. Many historical events align closely with the role that has developed. Wars, economic instability, depression, plurality of viewpoints, and political parties all have shaped the governmental role. Post-depression plans to revive the country, Roosevelt's New Deal, established major precedents for government spending on health care for Americans. In 1930 federal laws were passed to promote the public health of merchant seamen and the American Indians. The Social Security Act of 1935 was a substantial piece of legislation, which has grown since then to include not only the aged and unemployed but survivors' insurance for widows and children, child welfare, health department grants, and maternal and child health projects. In 1934 Senator Wagner of New York initiated the first national health insurance bill. Debate still continues on the extent of governmental responsibilities in health care.

Before the 1930s the only major governmental action relating to health was the creation of the Public Health Service in 1798. The *Department of Health and Human Services (DHHS),* known until 1980 as the Department of Health, Education, and Welfare (DHEW), was not created until 1953. It had a small predecessor that was established in 1939, the Office of Defense, Health, and Welfare Services. In 1946 Congress enacted a mental health bill and the Hospital Survey and Construction Act and created the National Institutes of Health in 1948. These legislative acts created entities that became part of the executive branch, now within the DHHS.

In a democracy, what governments should and can do for the citizens in the area of health care depends on the beliefs of those citizens. Strong beliefs of self-determination and self-sufficiency mixed with beliefs about social responsibilities are hallmarks of a pluralistic approach to solving societal problems. Political party platforms provide the best example for demonstrating how different beliefs yield different approaches to problems.

Goldsmith (1973) studied 12 health platforms written by the two major parties between 1948 and 1968 and found them to be predictable of future governmental direction in health care. In particular, Goldsmith stated that the platform pointed to areas of future health legislation. He recommended that influential health policy leaders in each party be identified and that health care providers and others examine the party platforms.

A major effort of the Reagan administration from 1980 to 1988 was to shift federal government activities to the states. In addition, passage in 1986 of the Gramm-Rudman Act, which was designed to decrease the federal budget deficit, not only will continue the shift of federal programs to states but also may mean significant cutbacks in health and social programs.

This discussion has focused primarily on trends and shifts among and within government levels. An additional aspect of governmental responsibilities is the relationship between government and individuals. Freedom of individuals must be balanced with government powers. Citizens also express their views of what amount of governmental interference will be tolerated. For example, the issue of sex education in public schools delineates at least two viewpoints on the governmental and individual relationship:

1. Since the government through the legislative branch established a system of education, some citizens believe that education should include content on sex.
2. Some citizens believe sex education belongs in the family and should not be interfered with by a governmental body (public schools).

These are only two of the views expressed in the public literature. Although many have strong feelings about this issue, the purpose of the example is to stress how responsibilities of governments and individuals can shift back and forth between them as well as between levels of government.

Major Governmental Health Care Functions

Although the amount and degree of health care functions that governments carry out may shift and vary, there are four general categories of functions: (1) Direct services, (2) Financing, (3) Information, and (4) Policy setting. These four functions are found at all levels of government—federal, state, and local.

Direct Services

Federal, state, and local governments provide direct health services to individuals and groups based on certain criteria, although provision of direct services is not the major function of government in health care. Examples of this governmental function are provision of health care for American Indians, members and dependents of the military, veterans, and federal prisoners. State and local governments employ community health nurses to deliver services to individuals and families, usually based on financial need. However, state and local governments also may provide direct services to all individuals for particular purposes, such as hypertension screening, tuberculosis screening, and well-child immunizations. Health services are also provided for prisoners in local jails or state prisons by state and local governments.

Financing

Governments pay for some health care services, training of personnel, and research. Financial support in all three areas has made a significant contribution and major impact on consumers and health care providers. State and federal governments finance the direct care of clients through Medicare, Medicaid, and Social Security programs. Many nurses have been educated with government funds; schools of nursing have been built and equipped through federal capitation funds. Other health care providers have also been supported financially by governments. Finally, monies in the form of grants have been given by governments for specific research and demonstration projects. Probably one of the best known centers of medical research is the federally funded National Institutes of Health.

Information

All branches and levels of government at one time or the other have collected, analyzed, and made available data about health care and health status in this country. An example is the annual report, *Health: United States,* compiled by the DHHS (1986). Collection of vital statistics, including mortality and morbidity data, gathering of census data, and health care status surveys are all governmental activities. Table 6-1 lists available international and federal govern-

 TABLE 6-1

International and National Sources of Data on the Health Status of the U.S. Population

Organization	Data source
INTERNATIONAL	
United Nations	Demographic Yearbook
World Health Organization	World Health Statistics Annual
FEDERAL	
Public Health Service	National Vital Registration System
	National Survey of Family Growth
	National Health Interview Survey
	National Health Examination Survey
	National Health and Nutrition Examination Survey
	National Master Facility Inventory
	National Hospital Discharge Survey
	National Nursing Home Survey
	National Ambulatory Medical Care Survey
	Medical Specialist Supply Projections
	National Morbidity Reporting System
	U.S. Immunization Survey
	Surveys of Mental Health Facilities
	Estimates of National Health Expenditures
Department of Commerce	U.S. Census of Population
	Current Population Survey
	Population Estimates and Projections
Department of Labor	Consumer Price Index
	Employment and Earnings

ment data sources on the health status of the total U.S. population. These sources are available in the government documents section in most large libraries.

Policy Setting

Policy setting, the last major category of government functions to be discussed, relates to all the functions. Decisions about health care are made by the government at all levels and within all branches of government. Decisions that shape health care are policy-making and policy-setting activities. As mentioned earlier, governments often give financial support to one group of individuals rather than to another group. Such a decision influences health care resources for both groups and is a policy-setting function of government as well. Health policy decisions usually have broad implications for economic growth, resource allocation, and development in the health care field. Examples of policy setting include the Health Planning, Resources and Development Act and the Professional Standards Review Organization.

ORGANIZATION OF GOVERNMENTAL AGENCIES

Community health nurses (CHNs) are actively involved with many levels of international and national government. This section provides information about international organizations and their activities in the health care field and the roles of community health nurses in different national governmental agencies.

International Organizations

In June of 1945 many national governments joined together to create an international organization, the United Nations. Its charter describes its aims and goals. Several goals deal with human rights, world peace, and security, and promotion of economic and social advancement of all people. The United Nations (Figure 6-1) is headquartered in New York City and is made up of six principal organs. Several other organs and many specialized agencies and autonomous organizations are also within the system. One of these special, autonomous organizations is the *World Health Organization (WHO).*

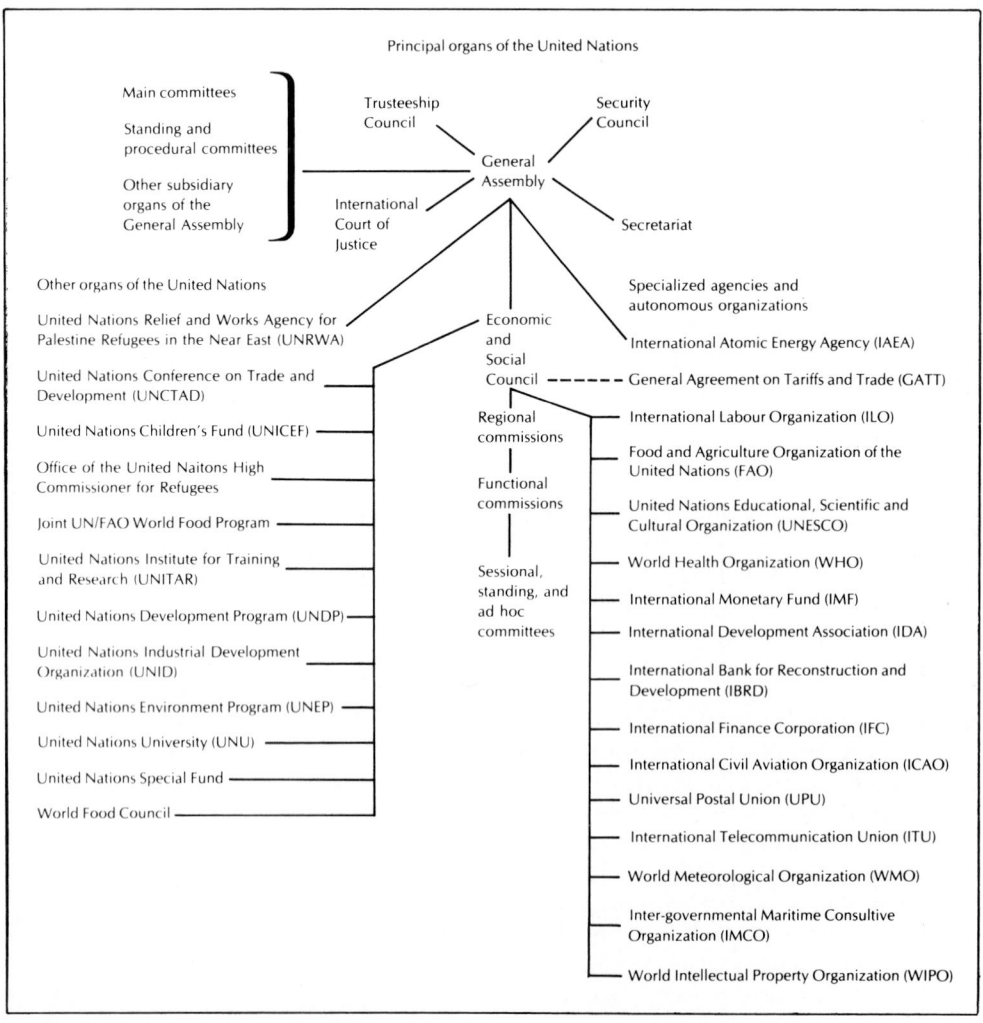

FIGURE 6-1

The United Nations system. (From United Nations: Basic facts about the U.N., New York, 1984, United Nations.)

Established in 1948, WHO relates to the United Nations through the Economic and Social Council. Its goal is the attainment by all people of the highest possible level of health. Headquartered at 20 Avenue Appia, 1211 Geneva, Switzerland, WHO is composed of three main organs: the Assembly, Executive Board, and Secretariat. The Secretariat is described in detail in Figure 6-2. The organization has six regional offices. The office for the Americas is located in Washington, D.C. and is known as the Pan American Health Organization (PAHO). Glancing over Figure 6-2 one can get an idea of the variety of activities in this organization.

The World Health Assembly, to which all United Nation members belong, meets annually. It is the policy-making body of WHO. The executive board, which consists of 30 members elected by the assembly, meets at least twice a year. WHO provides worldwide services to promote health, cooperates with member countries in their health efforts, and coordinates biomedical research. Its services, which benefit all countries, include a day-to-day information service on the occurrence of internationally important diseases; publication of the international list of causes of disease, injury, and death; monitoring of adverse reactions to drugs; and establishment of world standards for anti-

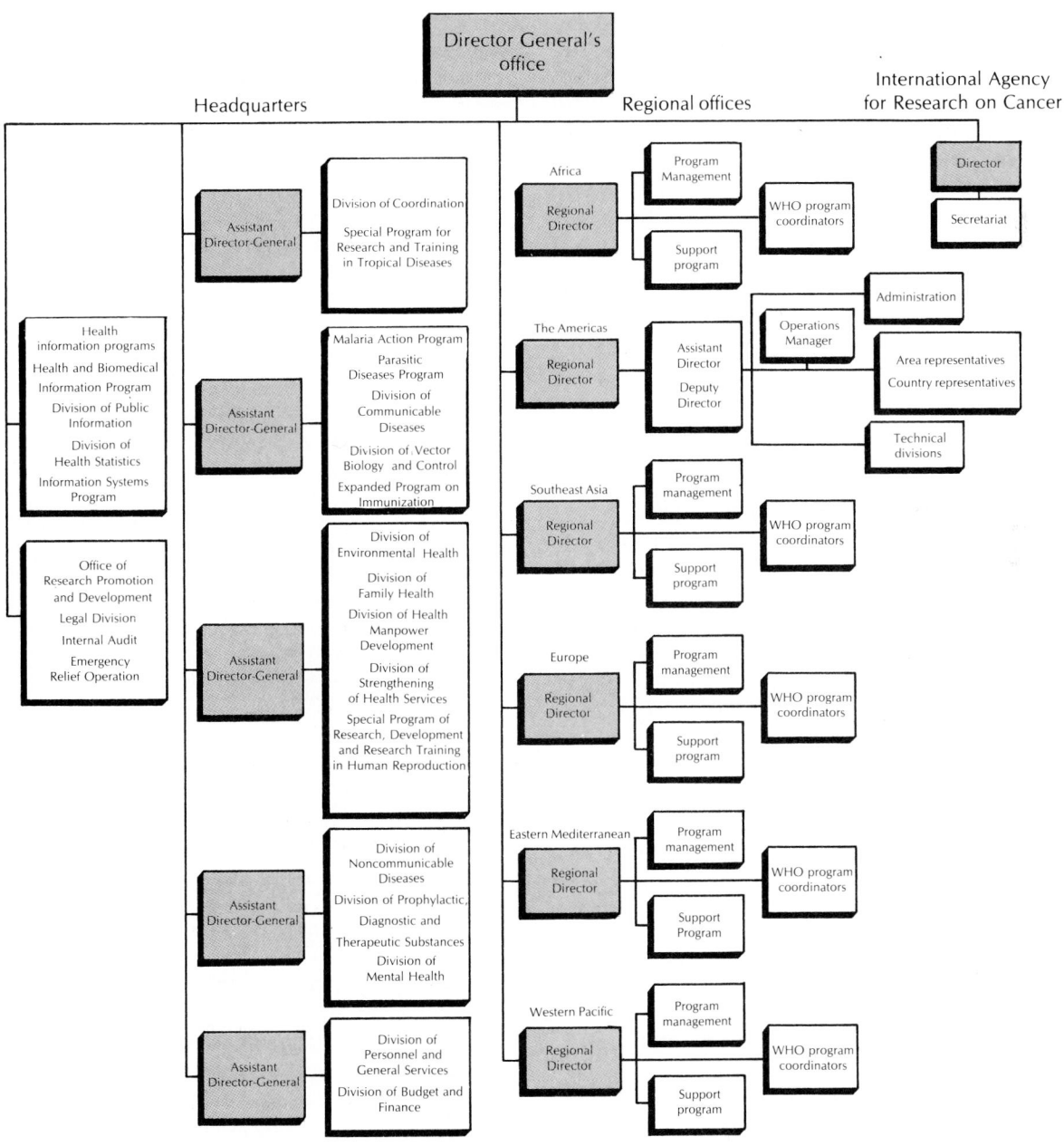

FIGURE 6-2

Structure of the World Health Organization. (Used with permission of the Office of Publication, WHO, Geneva, 1982.)

biotics and vaccines. Assistance rendered to individual countries at their request includes support to national programs to fight disease, train health workers, and strengthen health services. An example of biomedical research collaboration is a special program for research in six widespread tropical diseases—malaria, leprosy, "snail-fever," filariasis, leishmaniasis, and "sleeping sickness."

The number of community health nursing roles in international health is increasing. Besides offering direct health services, nurses serve as consultants, educators, and program planners and evaluators. They focus their work on a variety of community health concepts, including environment, sanitation, communicable disease, wellness, and primary care.

Federal Agencies

Many federal agencies are involved in governmental health care functions. Legislation passed by Congress may be delegated to any agency within the executive branch for implementation, surveillance, regulation, and enforcement. Congress decides which agency will monitor specific laws. For example, most health care legislation is delegated to the DHHS. However, legislation on the environment or on occupational health may be within another agency's realm, for example, the Environmental Protection Agency or Labor Department. Examples of those most involved with health care will be included in the following discussion.

Department of Health and Human Services

DHHS is the agency most involved with the health and welfare concerns of Americans. It touches more American lives than any other federal agency. As mentioned earlier, it was created in 1953 as the Department of Health, Education, and Welfare and renamed DHHS in 1980 when a separate cabinet department, the Department of Education, was established. The organizational chart of DHHS (Figure 6-3) depicts an office of the Secretary and four principal operating components: Social Security Administration, Health Care Financing Administration, Office of Human Development Services, and the Public Health Service. The last component is highly involved with health care and health status of Americans.

Public Health Service

The major components of the *Public Health Service (PHS)* include the following (Office of Federal Register, 1985):
1. Office of the Assistant Secretary for Health and Surgeon General
2. Alcohol, Drug Abuse, and Mental Health Administration
3. Centers for Disease Control
4. Agency for Toxic Substances and Disease Registry
5. Food and Drug Administration
6. Health Resources and Services Administration
7. National Institutes of Health

The PHS has been a long-standing, significant contributor to the improved health status of Americans. The Health Resources and Services Administration, the sixth component listed above, contains the Bureau of Health Professions,

which includes a Division of Nursing. Medicine and dentistry have divisions of their own, and a division exists for allied health professionals.

The Division of Nursing has the following specific goals: (1) provides the professional nursing expertise and leadership required by the Bureau of Health Professions in planning, coordinating, evaluating, and supporting development and utilization of the nation's health work force resources; (2) supports and conducts programs on the development, use, quality, and awarding of credentials of nursing personnel, including registered nurses, practical or vocational nurses, and nursing aides; (3) in cooperation with others, assists state and local areas in planning, developing, and improving nursing services and educational programs; (4) conducts and supports programs related to the provision of nursing care to advance the health status of individuals, families, and communities; (5) engages with other bureau programs in cooperative efforts of research, development, and demonstration on the interrelationships between individual members of the health care team, their tasks, education requirements, and related training modalities; (6) maintains liaison with health professional groups and others, including consumers, having common interest in the nation's capacity to deliver nursing services; (7) fosters, supports, and conducts projects to expand the scientific base of nursing practice and role reformulation and to develop and incorporate new knowledge into practice and education; and (8) provides consultation and technical assistance to public and private organizations, agencies, and institutions, including the PHS regional offices and other agencies of the federal government, on all aspects of nursing relevant to the division's functions (Division of Nursing, PHS, 1985).

In late 1985 Congress overrode a Presidential veto, creating the *National Center for Nursing Research.* The research and research-related training activities previously supported by the Division of Nursing have been transferred to the National Center for Nursing Research within the National Institutes of Health. This center will be the focal point of the nation's nursing research activities. It will promote the growth and quality of research in nursing and patient care, provide important leadership, expand the pool of experienced nurse researchers, and be a point of interaction with other bases of health care research.

Other Federal Government Agencies

DHHS has primary responsibility for federal health functions. However, the cabinet departments of the federal government have been delegated by Congress to carry out certain other health functions. Those departments that will be described in this chapter are Commerce, Defense, Labor, Agriculture, and Justice.

DEPARTMENT OF COMMERCE. Within the Department of Commerce (DOC) is the Bureau of the Census, which carries out an information function in health care. Established in 1902, this bureau conducts a census of the population every 10 years. Information collected from individual persons and households is confidential and used only for statistical purposes. Also a part of the DOC is the National Oceanic and Atmospheric Administration, which provides special ser-

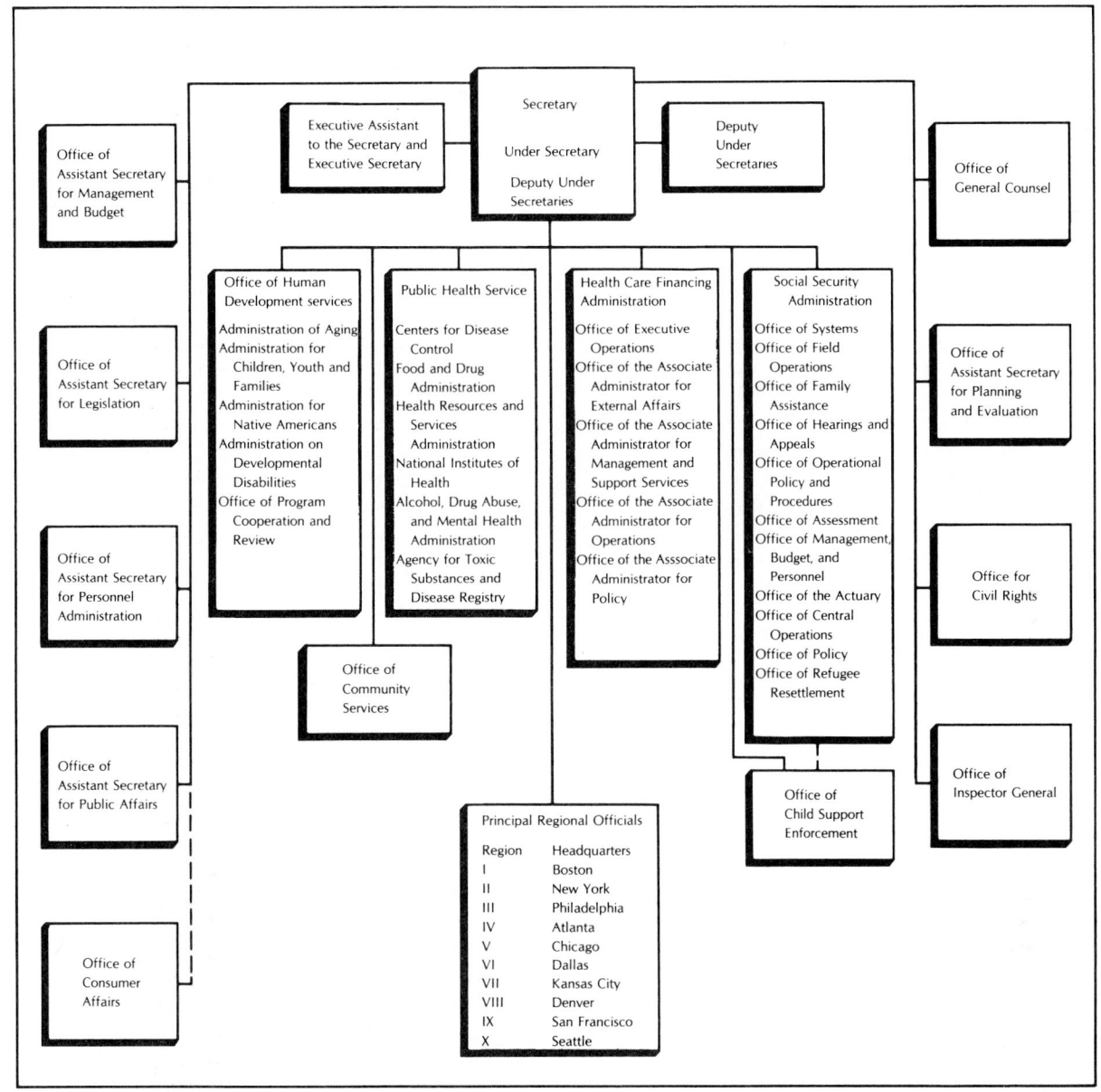

FIGURE 6-3

Organizational chart of the Department of Health and Human Services. (From Office of Federal Register: United States Government Manual, Washington, D.C., 1985, U.S. Government Printing Office, p. 842.)

vices in support of urban air quality control.

DEPARTMENT OF DEFENSE. The Department of Defense (DOD) delivers health care to members of the military and their dependents. The Assistant Secretary of Defense for Health Affairs administers the Civilian Health and Medical Program of the Uniformed Services (CHAMPUS). Established in 1956, CHAMPUS has the mission of delivering civilian health care services primarily for spouses and dependents of active, retired, or deceased service members. The departments within Defense (Army, Navy, Air Force & Marines) each have a surgeon general. Health services, including community health services for members of the military, are delivered by a Health Services Command in each department. In each command nurses of high military rank, including brigadier general, are part of the administration of health services.

DEPARTMENT OF LABOR. The Department of Labor has two administrations with health functions: Occupational Safety and Health Administration and the Mine Safety and Health Administration. Both are charged with writing safety and health standards and ensuring compliance in the workplace, including inspections, investigation of complaints, and citations if necessary. Each coordinates its activities with state departments of labor and of health.

DEPARTMENT OF AGRICULTURE. The Department of Agriculture is involved in health care primarily through administering the Food and Nutrition Service. Although plant, product, and animal inspection by the Department of Agriculture is also related to the health of Americans, the Food and Nutrition Service established in 1969 oversees a variety of food assistance activities. In collaboration with state and local government welfare agencies, food stamps are provided to needy persons to increase their food purchasing power. Other programs include school lunch and breakfast programs; Supplemental Food Program for Women, Infants, and Children (WIC); and grants to states for nutrition education and training.

DEPARTMENT OF JUSTICE. Health services to federal prisoners are administered within the Department of Justice. The Bureau of Prisons, Medical and Services Division includes medical, psychiatric, dental, and health support services along with environmental health and safety, farm operations, food service, commissary, laundry, and other personal services for inmates.

The fact that many federal executive branch agencies are involved in direct service, funding, collecting and disseminating information, and setting policy reinforces the pluralistic approach of American government to health care.

State and Local Government Departments

Most state and local (county and city) jurisdictions have governmental activities that affect the health care field. At the state level three executive branch departments will be described: health, education, and corrections. The organization of a local health department will also be described and community health roles will be included.

State Health Departments

Selected programs within a typical state health department are as follows:

    Legal services
    Services to the chronically ill and aging
    Juvenile services
    Medical assistance: policy, compliance, operations
    Mental health and addictions
    Mental retardation and developmental disabilities
    Environmental programs
    Departmental licensing boards
    Division of vital records
    Health services cost review
    Health planning and development
    Preventive medicine and medical affairs

CHNs serve in many capacities throughout most state health departments. These capacities are similar to those in international and federal agencies: consultation, direct services, research, teaching, supervision, planning, and evaluation of health programs. Most health departments have a division or department of community health nursing. Most also have a board of examiners of nurses, which usually is found in the department of licensing boards. Created by state legislation known as a state nurse practice act, the examiner's board is made up of nurses and consumers. A few states have other providers or administrators as members. The functions of this board are described in the practice act of each state and generally include licensing and ex-

amination of RNs and LPNs; approval of schools of nursing in the state; revocation, suspension, or denial of licenses; and promulgation of regulations about nursing practice and education. Nurse practice acts will be discussed later under a section on scope of nursing practice.

State Education Departments

Some state departments of education coordinate health curricula and services provided within local school systems. Other state legislatures mandate coordination of services solely within the health department or jointly between health and education departments. Often liaison groups or councils are formed to facilitate joint coordination. Consisting of members from state health departments and state departments of education, these councils develop policy and guidelines for school health services and health education. Community health nurses often represent health and education departments at these councils and help shape health policy. Community health nurses also serve in departments of education in similar capacities as in health departments.

State Departments of Corrections

Community health nurses also work in state departments of corrections as planners, implementors, coordinators, and in some cases, supervisors of health and nursing services for inmates in state prisons. Community health nurses in such state positions may also coordinate the health service efforts of local jails. Some local jails hire a nurse directly whereas others use the services of community health nurses in local health departments.

Local Health Departments

Depending on funding and other resources, programs offered by local health departments along with state departments vary greatly. A fairly comprehensive list of such programs, taken from an urban-suburban county health department in a mid-Atlantic state, is shown in the box at right. At the local level, as at the state level, coordination of health efforts is essential between health departments and other county or city departments. For example, local boards of education and departments of social services are an integral part of activities of local governments. More often than at the other levels of government, community health nurses at the local level provide direct services. Some community health nurses deliver special or selected services, such as tuberculosis or venereal disease contact studies or child immunization clinics. Other community health nurses have a more generalized practice, delivering services to families in certain geographic areas called census tracts; this method of delivery of community health nursing services involves broader needs and a wider variety of nursing interventions.

Social Welfare Programs

The focus thus far in this discussion of governmental programs has been on health programs. Federal, state, and local governments also provide social welfare programs. Generally, these programs provide monetary benefits to the poor, elderly, disabled, and unemployed.

The federal Social Security Act establishes a number of programs, principally, the social insurance programs, Social Security, unemployment insurance, and welfare programs.

The Social Security Administration within the Department of Health and Human Services administers the following programs:

1. Old Age Survivors and Disability Insurance (OASDI)
2. Aid to Families with Dependent Children (AFDC);
3. Supplemental Security Income (SSI).

OASDI provides monthly benefits to retired and disabled workers, their spouses and children, and to survivors of insured workers. AFDC, which is a federal and state program, helps needy families in which there are children. AFDC subsidizes children deprived of financial support of one of their parents as a result of death, disability, absence from the home, or, in some states, unemployment.

SSI is a program for the aged, blind, and disabled. Some states have chosen to supplement the federal SSI program.

The funds for these programs are provided by contributions from employees, employers, and self-employed individuals. These contributions are pooled into a special trust fund that is paid to a worker on retirement, death, or disability as partial replacement of the earnings the family has lost.

In 1965 amendments to the Social Security Act created Medicare and Medicaid. These two distinct programs serve different purposes. Medicare is a federal health insurance program for persons over 65 years of age and certain disabled individuals. It is funded through social security contributions, premiums, and general revenue. The Medicaid program, through federal grants to states and through funding from states themselves, provides medical services to the needy. These programs are administered by the Health Care Financing Administration (HCFA) within the Department of Health and Human Services and for Medicaid in conjunction with state governments.

HCFA develops and implements policies, procedures, and guidance related to program recipients, the providers of services such as hospitals, nursing homes, physicians, and the contractors that process claims. Most notably among HCFA's policies is the prospective payment system known as diagnostic related groups (DRGs).

HCFA also oversees the portions of Medicare/Medicaid programs that deal with quality assurance, health and safety standards for providers of care in federal health programs, end-stage renal disease program (ESRD), and the professional standards review organization (PSRO) provisions of the law. (See Chapter 3 for additional discussion of Medicare and Medicaid programs.)

In addition, there are human development services coordinated by the Office of Human Development Services within DHHS. Specifically, programs are focused on the aging, children, youth and families, Native Americans, and the developmentally disabled.

The Older Americans Act is designed to promote the welfare and needs of older people. Through this act the federal government promotes the development of state-administered community-based systems of comprehensive social services for the elderly.

Social programs focused on children and families include programs on adoption opportunities, Head Start services, runaway youth facilities, child abuse prevention and treatment, juvenile justice, and deliquency prevention.

There are also programs to promote the social and economic development of Native Americans. The Administration on Developmental Disabilities assists states in increasing the provision of quality services to persons with developmental disabilities. Grants are administered that support projects aimed at removing physical, mental, social, and environmental barriers for these disabled individuals.

Impact of Governmental Health Functions and Structures on Community Health Nursing

The variety and range of functions of governmental agencies has had a major impact on community health nursing. Funding, in particular, has shaped roles and tasks of community health nurses. The categorization of money by governments to special needs has led to special, more narrowly focused community health nursing roles. Generalized community health nursing practice usually declines with more specifically identified funding. For example, funds earmarked for communicable disease programs usually will not pay for and support home care services.

Many community health nursing roles have been influenced by federal, state, or local government. Training grants

EXAMPLES OF PROGRAMS PROVIDED BY LOCAL HEALTH DEPARTMENTS

Addictions and alcoholism clinics
Adult health
Birth and death records
Child day care and development
Child health clinics
Crippled children's services
Dental health clinic
Environmental health
Epidemiology and disease control
Family planning
Geriatric evaluation
Health education
Home health agency
Hospital discharge planning
Hypertension clinics
Immunization clinics
Information services
Maternal health
Medical social work
Mental health
Mental retardation and developmental disabilities
Nursing
Nursing home licensure
Nutrition division
Occupational therapy
Physical therapy
School health
Speech and audiology
Vision and hearing screening

for nurse practitioners in primary care have provided incentives to individual nurses to attend programs and develop new community health nursing roles within the health care system. Family, school, adult, or pediatric nurse practitioners emerged primarily because of the funding provided by governmental agencies. Education in public health has also been changed by governmental policies and funding.

Other health policy information, funding, and direct service functions of government have influenced community health nursing. Health care to special populations such as migrant workers, pregnant women, or at-risk children has taken the form of law. Legislatures have identified special needs and programs to meet those needs. Often community health nurses are called on to implement these programs. Vital statistics and other epidemiological data collected by governmental agencies have influenced the location, work force, planning, and evaluation of community health nursing services.

According to the evolving economic policies of the Reagan administration, whatever federal money is given to the states will be in the form of block grants. A sum of money with no specific program tags, the block grant may have a great impact on community health nursing. Having less money in special programs will mean a shift of community health nursing roles toward more generalized practice. Whether community health nursing should be a specialty or a generalized practice is an age-old debate. The purpose of mentioning the debate here is to show how government funding has clearly shaped the functions of community health nurses within all levels of government.

PRIVATE SECTOR INFLUENCE ON REGULATION AND HEALTH POLICY

Most of the roles of government in health care previously discussed were related to legislation passed by the legislative branch and administration of the laws by the executive branch. One power that the legislature grants to the executive branch agencies when it passes a law and delegates the law's administration to an agency is the power to make regulations. Laws precede and dictate who writes what kind of regulation. Because regulations flow from legislation, they have the force of law.

The *private sector,* which includes anyone who is not part of the government or public sector, can influence and shape legislation through many means. These same means can be used by the private sector to influence the writing of regulations. This part of the chapter will describe the process of regulation writing and ways to influence it. This section concludes with a discussion of self-regulation activities in the private sector.

Process of Regulation

In each level of government the executive branch can and in most cases must prepare regulations. These rules are more detailed than the law they are based on and relate to the subject of the executive department. These rules establish, fix, and control standards and criteria for carrying out a certain law. Figure 6-4 gives the steps in the usual regulation-writing process.

After receiving a legislative directive, the department in the executive branch begins the process of regulation by studying the topic or issue. Advisory groups or special task forces including nondepartment members sometimes are formed to provide early input on the content of the regulations. As the work of the groups or individual department members progresses, initial drafts of the proposed regulations are written.

After refinement, the proposed regulations are placed in final draft form and published in the legally required document. At the federal level that document is called the

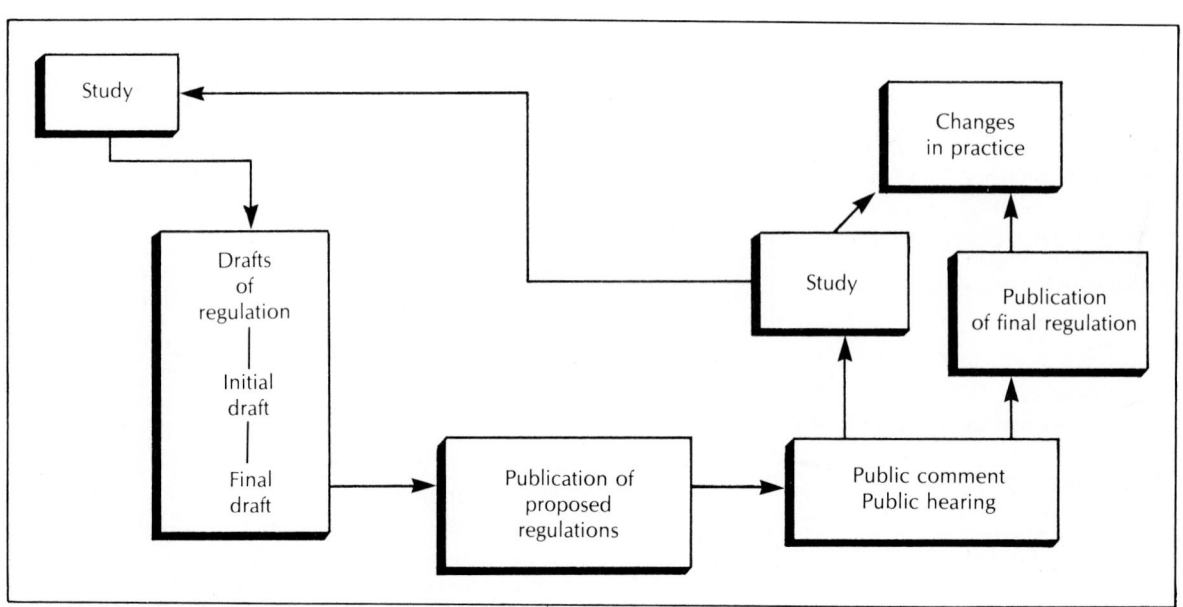

FIGURE 6-4

Process of regulation writing.

Federal Register. Similar state registers exist in most states where regulations from state departments are published. The publication of proposed regulations includes notice about a time period within which public comment will be accepted. Public comment in this situation usually is written. The notice may also give a date, time, and place for a hearing that is open to the public. Anyone may attend; if one wishes to speak at the hearing, published rules for that procedure must be followed. Usually, speaking involves some type of notification and the limiting of testimony to a certain amount of time of which the speaker is informed beforehand.

Revisions to the proposed regulations are made based on public comment and public hearing. Depending on the amount and content of the public reaction, final regulations are prepared or more study is done of the area and issues involved. Final published regulations carry the force of law. The date when regulations become effective is also published.

Close monitoring by and participation of the private sector in regulation writing can begin as soon as a law is passed and delegated to an executive branch agency. Government manuals, updated at least yearly, list names and phone numbers of individuals within the executive branch. Early contact and expression of interest on how a particular law gets administered may result in membership on a task force or advisory board. If not, the membership of such groups is public information, and one could contact these members to determine their thoughts on what shape the regulations will take.

Surveillance of the *Federal Register* or state registers on a regular basis is essential. Once proposed regulations are published, members of the private sector may influence regulations by attending the hearings, providing comments, testifying, and engaging in lobbying aimed at individuals involved in the writing. Concrete, written suggestions for revision submitted to these individuals is usually a persuasive manner in which to proceed.

Final regulations, published in a *Code of Regulations* (both federal and state), usually mean changes in practice. Regulations need to be disseminated to all individuals whose practice is affected by them. This dissemination can be effectively helped along with private sector involvement. Regulations need to become part of policy and procedure manuals of agencies affected by them.

Community Health Nurse's Role in the Political Process

The number and type of laws influencing health care are increasing. Because of this, involvement in the political process at all possible points is most important to community health nursing. The community health nurse's basic understanding of this political process should include knowing who the lawmakers are, how bills become law, and methods of influencing the process and shaping health policy.

The legislatures, federal and state, are composed of two houses: an assembly or house, and a senate. Representatives and senators are elected by the people within a particular geographic jurisdiction. Each state has two federal senators and one or more representatives, depending on the state's population. States have their own rules for apportioning representation across their state for the state legislature.

Although the Congress meets throughout the year, state legislatures have sessions of varying lengths. Each legislature has its own leadership, usually dominated by either the Democrat or Republican party. Roles include the presiding officers, party floor leaders, and committee chairpersons.

An important part of this *legislative process* is the work of the staffs of the legislatures. These individuals do the legwork, research, paperwork, and other activities that move ideas into bills and then into law. In addition to the individual legislator's staff, committee staffs are also important. Both of these can provide valuable information for constituents as well as for their legislators.

The legislative process begins with ideas that are developed into bills written by the sponsor of the ideas. After the bill is drafted, it is introduced to the legislature, given a number, read, and assigned to a committee. Hearings, testifying, lobbying, education, research, and informal discussion follow. If the bill is passed from the committee, the entire house hears the bill, perhaps amending it, but making a decision on the bill. The decision takes the form of a vote. A majority vote moves the bill to the other house where it is read, amended, and voted on.

Community health nurses can be involved in the process at any point. Many professional nursing associations have professional lobbyists, legislative committees, and political action committees (PACs) devoting full time to shaping health policy.

Common methods of lobbying include face-to-face encounters, personal letters, mailgrams, telegrams, telephone calls, testimony, petitions, reports, position papers, fact sheets, letters to the editor, news releases, speeches, coalition-building with others, demonstrations, and litigation. Depending on the issue, each of these can be equally effective.

Behind the scenes of this process lies the political party activity that community health nurses should consider becoming involved in. A wide variety of activities are available to the citizen, including voting, participating in the party organization, registering voters, getting out the vote, fundraising, building networks or communication links, and political action committees.

Self-Regulatory Activities

Self-regulation is an essential characteristic of a profession (American Nurses Association, 1985). It can involve many activities that have as their goals overseeing the rights, obligations, responsibilities, and relationships of a nurse to society, to nursing as a profession, and to clients. On entering the nursing profession, an individual assumes a position of responsibility and trust. That position involves accountability for all outcomes of nursing practice. The importance of professional responsibility cannot be underrated. It has been said that as a last resort a profession should regulate itself before others (the government, for

---

SELECTED SELF-REGULATORY ACTIVITIES

INDIVIDUAL NURSES

Being knowledgeable about the Nurse Practice Act

Initiating reports of nursing misconduct according to the Nurse Practice Act to state boards

Being knowledgeable about the *Code for Nurses*

Initiating reports of nursing misconduct according to the *Code for Nurses* to state nursing associations

Supporting organizational activities of self-regulation

Encouraging consumers to register legitimate complaints

Participating in institutional ethics committees, infant bioethics committees, and institutional review boards

Seeking continuing education opportunities

PRIVATE NURSING ORGANIZATIONS

Accreditation of nursing education

Certification of excellence in nursing

Ethics committees

Continued development of ethical guidelines

Research committees on human rights

Peer review systems, audits, and quality assurance activities

---

example) impose regulation. It is with this idea that suggested self-regulatory activities are made in this chapter.

Not only should community health nurses devote energies to monitoring and participating in regulation writing and other political processes (lobbying, voting, working for candidates, running for offices), but they should develop and participate in self-regulatory activities. These activities emanate from the private sector (nongovernmental groups and individuals) and, as mentioned above, are devoted to governing one's own actions. However, self-regulation is never the only activity that governs one's own actions. Other activities discussed in this chapter, law and government, are also governing or controlling practices of the professions.

Examples of self-regulation are listed in the box above. Belonging to an organization is not enough; contributing to the policy statements, attending meetings, and so on give essential support to organizations providing self-regulation. Activities listed in the box are divided into those that individual nurses are accomplishing and those that, with support of individuals, organizations are accomplishing. This is a selected list, and additional areas of self-regulation can be identified.

LAWS AFFECTING COMMUNITY HEALTH NURSING PRACTICE

The practice of community health nursing is the synthesis of nursing practice and public health practice applied to promoting and preserving the health of populations. (American Nurses Association, 1986). This abbreviated definition recognizes the diversity of community health nursing and the inherent relationship of law to that practice. Not only are there legal aspects that relate to nursing practice, but nurses are also subject to legal aspects of public health practice.

Getting advice and review by legal counsel of the community health agencies where nurses are employed should

be an integral part of the decision-making process. If a nurse is in private practice or self-employed, a lawyer in the community should be sought for assistance. The American Association of Nurse Attorneys* can provide the names of nurse attorney members who are available for consultation, speaking, writing, and legal advice.

Types of Laws

Several definitions of law are available. However, many of these tend to describe what law is *not* rather than what it is. Definitions of law include the following:

1. A rule established by authority, society, or custom
2. The body of rules governing the affairs of people within a community or among states; social order; the common law
3. A set of rules or customs governing a discrete field or activity, for example, criminal law, law of contracts
4. The system of courts, judicial process, and legal officers giving effect to the laws of a society; profession of a lawyer

These definitions reflect the close relationship of law to community and to society's customs and beliefs. Since community health nursing practice in the community reflects society's beliefs and customs, law has had a major impact on it. While, historically, community health nursing practice emerged out of individual voluntary activities, soon society recognized the need for it and, through legal mandates, created positions and functions for nurses in community settings. These functions in many instances carry with them the "force of law." For example, if the community health nurse discovers a person with smallpox, the law directs that the nurse, along with others legally designated in the community, take specific direct action. The law provides mechanisms whereby if the person with smallpox does not comply, other, more invasive interventions can be carried out. This is just one example of how the law has shaped community health nursing practice.

There are three types of laws that are part of our society. Each type has a different source or legal base that will be described in the following discussion:

1. Constitutional law
2. Legislation and regulation
3. Judicial and common law

Constitutional Law

Constitutional law emanates from federal and state constitutions. As discussed earlier in this chapter, both documents describe, among other things, the powers and duties of officials; the responsibilities and division of government into three branches (executive, legislative, and judicial), and the rights of individuals. From this type of law community health nurses can get answers to questions in selected practice situations. For example, on what basis can the state require quarantine or isolation of individuals with tuberculosis? The answer to this question can be found in constitutional law.

The U.S. Constitution contains explicit and limited

---

*113 West Franklin Street, Baltimore, MD 21201.

functions of the federal government. All other powers and functions are those that the individual states hold. The major power of the states that relates to community health nursing practice is that a state may intervene in a reasonable manner to protect the health, safety, and welfare of the citizenry. As described earlier in this chapter, the state's "police power" is not without limitation. First, it must be a "reasonable" exercise of power. Second, if the power interferes or infringes on individual rights, the state must demonstrate that there is a "compelling state interest" in exercising its power. Hence, isolating an individual or separating one from a community because he has a communicable disease has been deemed an appropriate exercise of state powers. The state can isolate even though it is an infringement on individual rights (freedom, autonomy) under the following conditions:

1. If the isolation is done in a reasonable manner
2. If a compelling state interest exists in the prevention of an epidemic
3. If the isolation is necessary to protect the health, safety, and welfare of individuals in the community or the public as a whole

Legislation and Regulation

Legislation is the type of law that comes from the legislative branches of government at different levels; state, local, or federal. Much legislation has an impact on community health nursing. In the previous situation dealing with the person with a communicable disease, the state exercised its power through legislation. As mentioned above, *regulations* are very specific statements of law that relate to individual pieces of legislation.

Community health nurses are often employed within the executive branch. The state or local health department is part of this branch. Hence, nurses become an instrument of the state's police power, in that nursing interventions often are done to implement legislation and regulations. Nurses employed in other community settings, those with no governmental responsibilities or legal mandates, are still often subject to legislation and regulations. For example, community health nurses rendering home health care in a private agency must deliver care according to Medicare (federal law) legislation and regulations or Medicaid (state law) legislation and regulations for the agency to be reimbursed for those services. Private and public health care services rendered by community health nurses are subject to many government regulations.

Judicial and Common Law

Judicial and *common law* is the last group of laws having an impact on community health nursing. Judicial law is that law based on court or jury decisions. Federal or state legal procedure, depending on the jurisdiction, outlines the details of how disputes are to be settled. Representatives from both sides of an issue present evidence, written or oral, before a court and/or jury who decide the outcome. Either party may have a basis on which to appeal the first decision; a higher court reviews that decision and renders a second one. Other appeal routes may be sought, depending on the outcome and issue. Special legislatively designed

processes of settling claims may exist, depending on the jurisdiction. For example, medical malpractice panels exist in many states and may be the body that reviews a claim first.

The opinions of the courts are judicial opinion and also referred to as "case law." The court uses other types of laws to make its decision, including previous court decisions or cases. Precedent is one principle of common law. Judges are bound by previous decisions unless they are convinced that the "old law" is no longer relevant or valid. This process is called "distinguishing" and usually involves a demonstration of how the currently disputed situation differs from the previously decided situation. Other principles of common law are part of a court's rationale and the basis of making a particular decision. Such principles include justice, fairness, respect for individuals, autonomy, and self-determination. These common law principles are part of our traditions and heritage as a society and play an important role in decisions made by courts.

General Community Health Nursing Practice and the Law

Despite the broad nature and the varied roles of community health nursing practice, there are two legal aspects that apply to most of these practice situations. The first aspect is *professional negligence* or malpractice; the second is the *scope of practice* defined by custom and state practice acts. Each of these aspects is discussed in some detail.

Professional Negligence

Professional negligence or malpractice is defined as an act or failure to act when a duty is owed to another that was not reasonable and that leads to injuries compensable by law. For a client to succeed in persuading the judge or jury that a nurse was negligent, one has to prove *all* of the following:

1. The nurse owed a duty to the client.
2. The duty to act as a reasonable, prudent nurse under the circumstances was breached or not fulfilled.
3. The failure to be reasonable under the circumstances led to or was the proximate cause of the alleged injuries.
4. The injuries claimed are compensable through usual legal remedies.

Reported cases, those cases appealed to higher courts, involving negligence and community health nurses are almost nonexistent. As one example, a case involving an occupational health nurse is discussed.

The California case of *Cooper vs National Motor Bearing Co.* 288P 2d 581, 1955, involved an occupational health nurse who negligently implemented standing orders on an injury involving a puncture wound. The nurse, by her own testimony, admitted that she did not examine or probe the wound or refer the injured worker to the physician but just swabbed and bandaged it. Only after 10 months, documented by many visits to the dispensary and the worker's complaints of the wound not healing, did the nurse refer the worker to the company doctor. On referral basal cell carcinoma was found and surgery followed.

The fact that the nurse was employed by the industry

to render first aid established the first element of negligence: a duty was owed the worker. By her own testimony the nurse stated that it was her duty to refer any condition or injury she was not familiar with, or not sure about, to the doctor for diagnosis. The standard of good nursing care in the community was to examine the wound for foreign bodies. The nurse knew the normal healing time was 1 to 2 weeks. If a wound persisted and did not heal, proper nursing care would indicate referral to a physician. Testimony was given that the practice of an occupational health nurse in this particular type of industry is to probe wounds for foreign bodies. According to the nurse's education and experience, she should have been aware of the possibility of foreign objects in such a wound.

In this case the nurse's failure to detect the foreign body was the proximate cause of the basal cell carcinoma. The injuries were compensable through existing legal remedies. The pain, suffering, loss of wages or time from work, and bodily disfigurement were all injuries that could be calculated and totaled as a monetary amount. The nurse and the company were found negligent by the California Court.

An integral part of negligence suits is the question of who should be sued. Obviously, those who made the mistakes should be sued, but part of the consideration of who to sue relates to who can best compensate for the injuries. When a nurse is employed and functioning within the scope of that employment, the employer is responsible for the nurse's negligent actions. This is referred to as the doctrine of *respondeat superior.* By directing a nurse to carry out a particular function, the employer becomes responsible along with the individual nurse for the negligence. The scope of employment is usually more inclusive than a job description and does not include criminal activities. Because employers are usually better able to compensate for the injuries suffered, they are most often sued and not nurses.

Community health nurses employed by governmental agencies need to ascertain whether that agency has *sovereign immunity.* Under this doctrine, the agency may be exempt from suit for particular kinds of actions, such as negligence. However, sovereign immunity will not shield from suit certain individuals within an agency, including nurses, who are acting under the auspices of the government when the negligence occurs. Individual public health nurses may have personal immunity for particular practice areas, such as giving immunizations, or in some states the legislature has granted personal immunity to community health nurses to cover all aspects of their practice.

Scope of Practice

The scope of practice issue involves differentiating between the practices of physicians, nurses, and other health care providers. *Scope of practice* is assessed (1) by examining the usual and customary practice of a profession and (2) by taking into account how legislation defines the practice of a particular profession in a jurisdiction. The issue is particularly important to community health nurses who have traditionally practiced in a wide scope.

The usual and customary practice of community health nursing can be determined through a variety of sources, including the following:

1. Content of community health nursing educational programs, general and special
2. Experience of other practicing nurses (peers)
3. Activities and statements, including standards, of community health nursing professional organizations
4. Policies and procedures of agencies employing nurses
5. Needs and interests of the community
6. Literature, including books, texts, and journals

All these sources can describe the usual practice of a community health nurse and the scope of that practice.

Every community health nurse should know and follow closely the proposed changes in nursing, medicine, and other related practice acts. As mentioned earlier, these pieces of state legislation define a scope of practice for these professionals. The nurse should always examine *all* related definitions to nursing practice. For example, the definitions of practice of registered nursing, medicine, and pharmacy in Maryland are given in the box at right.

These three definitions along with customary practice are pertinent, for example, to the question of whether a community health nurse is "dispensing" medications in a methadone clinic in a local health department when following physician prescription and preparing several identical doses for the client to take between clinic visits. The question of scope forces one to clarify both independent and dependent community health nursing functions. The failure to know one's limitations may lead to charges of practicing another profession without a license, fines, and possible suspension or revocation of the license. Because practice acts vary, so does the scope of practice issue. It is best to refer directly to practice acts for a particular state code.

This section has examined two legal aspects that generally have an impact on community health nursing practice. Because of the variety of work experiences of community health nurses and hence the variety of legal aspects, the following section will deal with areas of practice with a special focus.

Special Community Health Nursing Practice and the Law

The field of community health nursing includes nurses prepared as generalists who practice in community health settings and nurses prepared as community health nursing specialists. An essential component of community health nursing practice is knowledge of community resources and other health professionals. The community health nurse typically delivers care to clients or groups where they live, work, play, or go to school. In addition, the nurse encompasses further specialization in clinical areas such as family health, school and college health, occupational health, and community mental health and fulfills functional roles in administration, education, research, and consultation (American Nurses Association, 1980). Legal aspects of community health nursing vary, depending on (1) the setting where care is delivered, (2) the clinical specialty, and (3) the functional role.

For the purposes of this chapter, four special areas of community health nursing practice and their respective legal aspects will be highlighted. Those four areas are school

PRACTICE OF REGISTERED NURSING, MEDICINE, AND PHARMACY IN MARYLAND, 1986

REGISTERED NURSING—HEALTH OCCUPATIONS 7-101(f)

Practice registered nursing means the performance of acts requiring substantial specialized knowledge, judgment, and skill based on the biological, physiological, behavioral, or sociological sciences as the basis for assessment, nursing diagnosis, planning, implementation, and evaluation of the practice of nursing to maintain health, prevent illness, or care for or rehabilitate the ill, injured, or infirm.

For these purposes, practice registered nursing includes administration, teaching, counseling, supervision, delegation, and evaluation of nursing practice; execution of therapeutic regimen, including the administration of medication and treatment; independent nursing functions and delegated medical functions; and performance of additional acts authorized by the Board under section 7-205.

MEDICINE—HEALTH OCCUPATIONS 14-101(k)

Practice medicine means to engage, with or without compensation, in medical diagnosis, healing, treatment, or surgery. Practice medicine includes doing, undertaking, professing to do, and attempting any of the following: diagnosing, healing, treating, preventing, prescribing for, or removing any physical, mental, or emotional ailment or supposed ailment of an individual by physical, mental, emotional, or other process that is exercised or invoked by the practitioner, the patient, or both; or by appliance, test, drug, operation, or treatment; ending of a human pregnancy; and performing acupuncture.

Practice medicine does not include selling any nonprescription drug or medicine, practicing as an optician, or performing a massage or other manipulation by hand, but by no other means.

PHARMACY—HEALTH OCCUPATIONS 12-101(j)

Practice pharmacy means to engage in any of the following activities: selecting, preparing, and dispensing drugs, medicines, or devices; providing information and explanation to patients and health care practitioners about the safe and effective use of drugs, medicines, or devices; or identifying and appraising problems concerning the use or monitoring of drug therapy.

and family health, occupational health, home care and hospice services, and correctional health. Examples of legislation and judicial opinions affecting community health nurses within these selected areas will be included.

School and family health nursing may be delivered by community health nurses employed by health departments or boards of education. School health legislation provides a framework for nursing functions. The legislation establishes a minimum of services that must be provided to children in school systems including public and private schools. For example, most states require that children be immunized against certain communicable diseases before entering school. Children must have had a physical examination at that time, and most states require at least one physical at a later time in the course of their schooling. Legislation also specifies when and what type of health screening will be conducted in schools, such as vision and hearing testing. Many jurisdictions carry out these activities specified by the legislature plus many other activities. In financially "good times" there is usually an increase in the services community health nurses render in school and family health nursing. When the economic situation deteriorates, usually the services delivered are only those specified by the legislature.

A major area of legislation that makes an impact on community health nursing practice with schools and families is child abuse and neglect. Most states require nurses to report to police or a social service agency any situation in which they suspect a child is being abused or neglected. This is one instance in which society has said a professional may breach confidentiality to protect someone who may be in a helpless and harmful position. There is civil immunity for such reports and nurses may be called as witnesses should

a hearing follow the investigation made by a social service agency. As a matter of fact the majority of litigation in which community health nurses are involved is the area of child abuse.

Much federal legislation affects community health nursing practice with schools and families; Head Start, early diagnostic screening programs, nutrition programs, services for the handicapped, and special education are just a few examples. Most of this legislation, although written by Congress, requires cooperative federal and state funding, planning, and implementation. Each nurse working within a service based on legislation should be oriented to the legislation. It is advisable that the legislation and its regulations become part of the agency's nursing policies and procedures so that the nurse may refer to it.

Occupational health is another special area of practice that is greatly affected by state and federal laws. The *Occupational Safety and Health Act (OSHA)* places many requirements on industries. These requirements shape the types of services given to workers and functions of community health nurses. OSHA also established a reporting system for workers exposed to toxic agents in the workplace. A record-keeping system required by OSHA greatly affects health records in the workplace. Each state has an agency similar to the federal agency that also monitors and inspects industries, including the health services rendered by nurses. Most states have a "worker's right to know" law that requires employers to give information to their employees concerning the nature of toxic substances that they may encounter in the workplace during their employment. In addition, all states have worker's compensation statutes that provide the sole remedy for workers injured on the job. Access to records, confidentiality, and the use of standing orders are legal issues of great significance to nurses employed in industries.

Home care and hospice services rendered by community health nurses are greatly affected by state laws that require licensing and certification. Compliance with these laws is integrally linked to the method of payment for the services. For example, a service must be licensed and certified to obtain payment for services through Medicare, which is federal law. Federal regulations implementing Medicare have had an impact on much of community health nursing practice including how nurses record the details of their visits.

Many states have passed laws requiring nurses to report elder abuse to proper authorities. In some states there is an impact on home care and hospice services through legislation related to rights to death with dignity, rights of residents of long-term care facilities, definitions of death, and use of living wills. The legal and ethical dimensions on community health nursing practice are particularly important in this area of practice. Individual rights, such as the right to refuse treatment, and nursing responsibilities, such as the legal duty to render reasonable and prudent care, may often be in conflict in delivering home and hospice services. Much case discussion, sometimes including outside consultation, is required when rights and responsibilities are in conflict and a decision must be made to resolve that conflict.

Nursing practice in correctional health systems is controlled by state and federal law and regulation as well as by recent Supreme Court decisions. The laws and decisions relate to the type and amount of services that must be given or made available to incarcerated individuals. For example, physical examinations of each prisoner after they are sentenced are required. Prisoners must be provided minimum care, especially care when they are sick. Court decisions requiring that health services be adequate are based on constitutional law. If minimum services are not provided, it is a violation of a prisoner's right to be free of cruel and unusual punishment. Such decisions provide a framework that strongly influences the setting of nursing priorities. For example, providing sick calls would be a first priority rather than nutrition classes.

Each area of special community health nursing practice mentioned in this chapter and other areas are significantly shaped by legislation and judicial opinion. Those nurses responsible for setting and implementing program priorities need to identify and monitor laws related to each special area of practice. Suggested legal resources that might be used to stay current with laws will be described in the following section.

Legal Resources

In addition to seeking legal counsel, one can find many resources in public libraries as well as law libraries that can help community health nurses find laws pertinent to their practice. Possible legal resources include the following:

State bar associations
State code
State annotated code
Indexes to codes
Supplements to codes and indexes
Federal Register and state registers
Codes of regulations (federal and state)
Administrative agency rules and decisions
Case law
Opinions of attorney generals
Legal dictionaries
Legislative histories
Legal periodicals

In using these legal resources, begin by reviewing the topical index to each source. As the headings are reviewed, several can be identified as having something to do with the content areas of practice (such as immunizations or family planning) and the types of clients (e.g., minors, adolescents, and children) served by the community health nurse. Computer search tools are often available to one looking for laws and regulations relevant to one's practice. One legal computerized search is called *Lexis.* The Library of Congress has a service called *Scorpio.* Both services will not only search books and journals but recent case law, bills, amendments, and legislation. One of the best ways to stay informed is to monitor and read the area newspaper.

CLINICAL APPLICATION

Each community health nurse must consider legal implications of practice in each clinical encounter. Because the community health nurse may be the agent of the government when implementing a particular health program, consideration must be given to the power of the state or relationship of this power to individual rights.

Attention in daily practice to quality assurance, risk management, and documentation will help to assure that injuries to clients are minimized and that adequate community health nursing services are delivered.

In each clinical encounter, the community health nurse should know, before the activity, what standard of care applies to the situation. Standards of care can be found in agency policies, procedures, nursing and health care literature, ANA and other professional association's standards, expert nurse witnesses, community health nursing curriculum, legislation such as the state nurse practice act, and accreditation and certification criteria. Lastly, a community health nurse can review nursing documentation to see if agency policy requirements were met. Conducting a self-audit assures that standards of care are met.

SUMMARY

This chapter has presented information about the governmental and legal influences on the practice of community health nursing. The influence of government and law on community health nursing is significant. However, community health nurses can be part of the influence on government through regulation writing and lobbying. Organization, functions, and structures of government and the process of regulation writing are all important areas for community health nurses to know. Legal aspects of the roles and functions of general and specific areas of community health nursing, especially scope of practice and negligence, will prove to be useful information for nurses in community health.

⬒ KEY CONCEPTS

Many historical events have played a significant part in developing the role of government in health care.

The legal basis for most congressional action in health care can be found in Article I, Section 8 of the U.S. Constitution.

The four major health care functions of the federal government are direct services, financing, information, and policy setting.

The goal of the World Health Organization is the attainment by all people of the highest possible level of health.

Many federal agencies are involved in government health care functions. The agency most directly involved with the health and welfare of Americans is the Department of Health and Human Services (DHHS).

Most state and local jurisdictions have government activities that affect the health care field.

The variety and range of functions of government agencies have had a major impact on community health nursing. Funding in particular has shaped the role and tasks of community health nurses.

The private sector can influence legislation in many ways, especially through influencing the process of writing regulations.

The number and types of laws influencing health care are increasing. Because of this, involvement in the political process is most important to community health nurses.

Self-regulation is an essential characteristic in many professions, including the nursing profession.

Professional negligence and the scope of practice are two legal aspects particularly relevant to nursing practice.

Community health nurses must consider the legal implications of their own practice in each clinical encounter.

LEARNING ACTIVITIES

1. Conduct an interview with the local health officer. Ask for information from a 10-year period. See if you can see trends in population size and needs and roles/activities of government that were implemented to meet these changes.

2. Examine a current health department budget. Compare that with a budget from previous years. Has there been any impact on health care because of changes in government spending?

3. Select a community health nursing role you would like to examine closer. Interview that person, asking questions about job functions, organizational structure, agency goals, salary, mobility within the agency, and potential contributions of this role to the health of the community.

4. Locate your *State Register* or other document such as newspapers that publish proposed regulations. Select one set of proposed regulations and critique them. Submit your opinion in writing as public comment or attend the public hearing and testify on the regulations. Be sure to submit something in writing. Evaluate your participation by stating what you learned and whether the proposed regulations were changed in your favor.

5. Find and review your state nurse practice act.

BIBLIOGRAPHY

Altman, S., and Sapolsky, H.: Federal health programs, Lexington, Mass., 1981, D.C. Health & Co.

American Nurses' Association: Guidelines for implementing the code for nurses, Kansas City, Mo., 1980, The Association.

American Nurses' Association: A conceptual model of community health nursing, Kansas City, Mo., 1982, The Association.

American Nurses' Association: Code for nurses, Kansas City, Mo., 1985, The Association.

American Nurses' Association: Standards of community health nursing practice, Kansas City, Mo., 1986, The Association.

American Public Health Association: The definition and role of public health nursing in the delivery of health care, Washington, D.C., 1981, The Association.

Aroskar, M.A.: Ethical issues in community health nursing, Nurs. Clin. North Am. 14(1):35-44, March 1979.

Bagwell, M., and Clemens, S.: A political handbook for health professionals, Boston, 1985, Little, Brown & Co.

Beauchamp, T., and Childress, J.: Principles of biomedical ethics, ed. 2, New York, 1983, Oxford University Press.

Blum, H.: Planning for health, New York, 1981, Health Sciences Press.

Bullough, B.: The law and the expanding nursing role, ed. 2, New York, 1980, Appleton-Century-Crofts.

Campazzi, B.: Nurses, nursing and malpractice litigation, Nurs. Adm. Q. 5(1):1-18, 1981.

Christofel, T.: Health and the law: a handbook for health professionals, New York, 1982, MacMillan, Free Press.

Curtin, L., and Flaherty, M.: Nursing ethics theories and pragmatics, Bowie, Md., 1982, Robert J. Brady Co.

Dahl, R.: Democracy in the United States: promise and performance, ed. 2, Chicago, 1972, Rand McNally & Co.

Davis, A., and Aroskar, M.: Ethical dilemmas and nursing practice, ed.2, New York, 1983, Appleton-Century-Crofts.

Division of Nursing, Bureau of Health Professionals, Health Services and Resources Administration, Public Health Service: The division of nursing, Hyattsville, Md., 1985, The Division.

Fox, J.: Controversial and legal issues, Family Comm. Health 2(3):62-68, Nov. 1979.

Fromer, M.: Ethical issues in health care, St. Louis, 1981, The C.V. Mosby Co.

Goldsmith, S.: Political party platform health planks: a mechanism for participation and prediction? Am. J. Public Health 63(7):594-601, 1973.

Health: United States, 1984, DHHS Pub. No. (PHS) 85-1232, Washington, D.C., 1984, Department of Health and Human Services.

Healthy People: the Surgeon General's report on health promotion and disease prevention, DHEW Pub. No. (PHS) 79-55071, Washington, D.C., 1979, Department of Health, Education and Welfare.

Hemelt, M., and Mackert, M.: Dynamics of law in nursing and health care, ed. 2, Reston, Va., 1982, Reston Publishing Co., Inc.

Miles, R.: The Department of Health, Education and Welfare, New York, 1974, Praeger Publishers, Inc.

Northrop, C., and Kelly, M.: Legal issues in nursing, St. Louis, 1987, The C.V. Mosby Co.

Northrop, C.: Current status of nursing litigation, Nursing Economics 2(6):423-427, 1984.

Northrop, C., and Mech, A.: The nurse as expert witness, Nurs. Law Ethics 2(2):1,2,6,8, March-April 1981.

Office of Federal Register: United States government manual, 1985-86, Washington, D.C., 1985, U.S. Government Printing Office.

Solomon, S., and Roe, S.: Integrating public policy into the curriculum, 1986, National League for Nursing.

Solomon, S., and Roe, S.: Key concepts in public policy, student workbook, 1986, National League for Nursing.

United Nations: Basic facts about the UN, New York, 1984, The UN.

Weaver, J.: National health policy and the underserved, St. Louis, 1976, The C.V. Mosby Co.

Wiley, L.: Liability for death: nine nurse's legal ordeals, Nursing '81 2(9):34-43, 1981.

Wing, K.: The law and the public's health, ed. 2, Ann Arbor, Mich. 1985, Health Administration Press.

World Health Organization: The work of WHO, 1978-79: biennial report of the Director-General, Geneva, 1980, WHO.

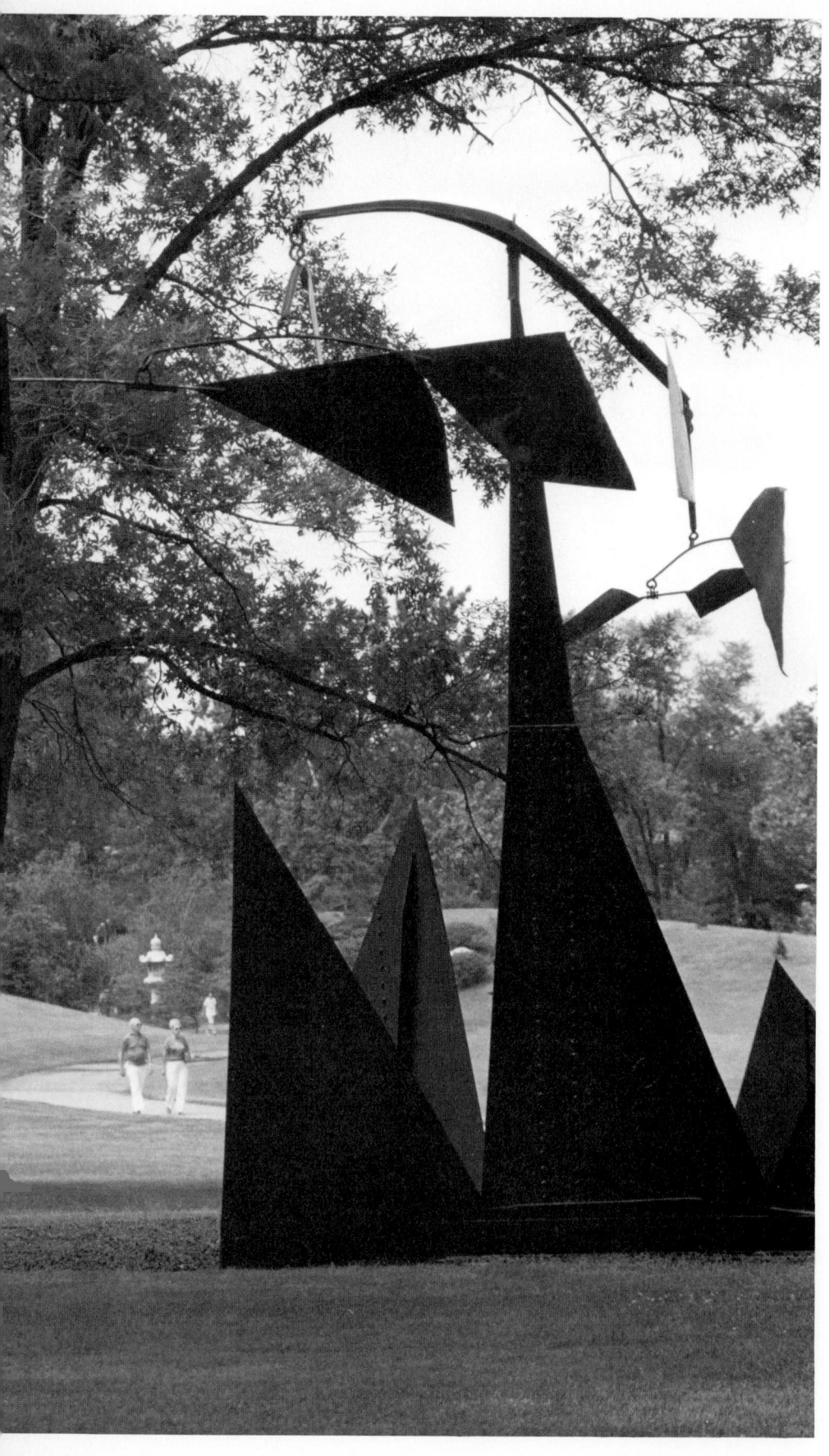

CONCEPTUAL FOUNDATIONS FOR COMMUNITY HEALTH NURSING PRACTICE

There is no question that nursing is struggling in its quest for a scientific base for practice. Great strides have been made in this effort in recent years. Community health nurses must continue to develop and evaluate conceptual models and move forward in theory development. No one conceptual model meets the needs and demands in community health nursing practice. Chapter 7 is a review of a variety of conceptual models from nursing and the social sciences, which offer promise of usefulness for practice. In addition, because of its integral role in community health nursing, the epidemiological model for practice is detailed in Chapter 8.

Chapters 9 through 12 describe components of community health nursing that are the foundation of role implementation. To effectively provide health promotion, community health nursing largely relies on educational strategies. Clients, whether individuals, families, or groups within the community, benefit from the educational aspect of community health nursing. Research documents the effectiveness of practices, and the models described in Chapters 7, 8, 10, and 11 provide frameworks for organizing practice.

Likewise, as programs are developed in all aspects of community health nursing, effective methods of evaluation are essential. As funds decrease in the health sector, the need for programs to be cost effective will increase. Planning, evaluation, record keeping, and quality assurance are integral tools for effective community health nursing practice.

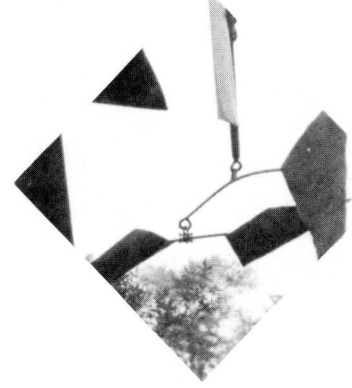

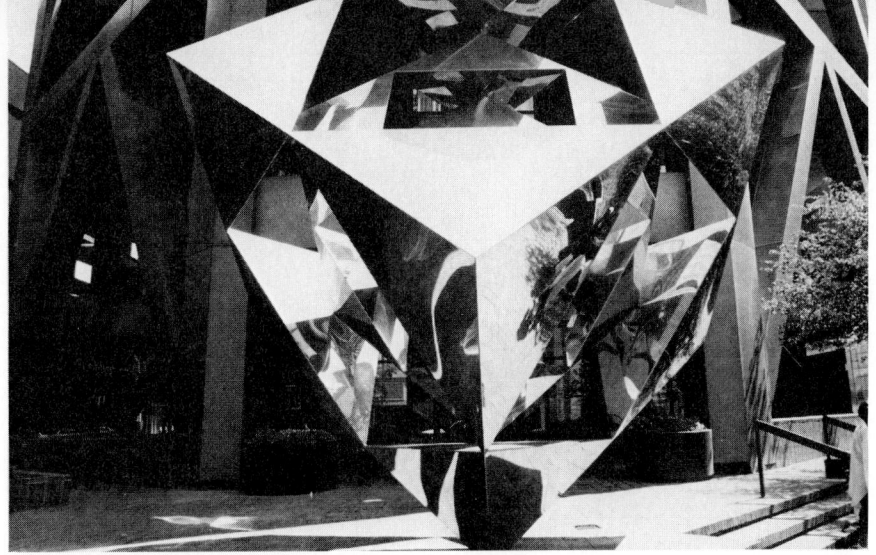

Gwendolen Lee
Jeanette Lancaster

7

CONCEPTUAL MODELS FOR COMMUNITY HEALTH NURSING

OBJECTIVES

After reading this chapter, the student should be able to:

Name three general themes of inquiry in nursing.

Define the terms *theory, model, concept,* and *conceptual framework.*

Differentiate between conceptual model and theory.

Describe key components of contemporary conceptual models in nursing.

Identify at least three uses of conceptual models in nursing.

Describe the conceptual models of community health nursing as delineated by the ANA and the APHA.

List the chief characteristics of the following interdisciplinary theories: systems, developmental, interaction.

Give an example that illustrates the applicability of the following interdisciplinary theories to nursing: systems, developmental, interaction.

List the chief characteristics of the following conceptual frameworks for nursing practice: Roy, Rogers, Johnson, Orem, Neuman, King.

KEY TERMS

boundary

concept

conceptual model

construct

Denver Developmental Screening Test (DDST)

developmental theory

energy fields

entropy

equifinality

feedback

four-dimensionality

General Systems Theory (GST)

hypothesis

Interaction models

Johnson's behavioral systems

King's theory

Maslow's hierarchy of needs

model

negentropy

Neuman's health care systems model

openness

Orem self-care nursing model

pattern and organization

proposition

Rogers' science of unitary man

Roy adaptation model of nursing

theory

Tridimensional leader effectiveness model

As described in Chapter 1, community health nursing has historically reflected the qualities of both art and science in the early accounts of home visiting, health teaching, and drawing on epidemiological concepts to determine the focus of actions. In recent years there has been considerable argument about the extent of a scientific basis for nursing. According to Walker and Avant (1983, p. vii), "As nursing has come of age, not only as a practice but also as a scholarly discipline, there has been increasing concern with delineating the theory base for nursing."

Since the time of Florence Nightingale, three general themes of inquiry have been explored:
1. Concern with principles and laws that govern the life processes, well-being, and optimal functioning of human beings, sick or well.
2. Concern with the patterning of human behavior in interaction with the environment in critical life situations.
3. Concern with the processes by which positive changes in health status are affected.

To develop and refine these concerns, nursing must advance as a theory-based profession. A study of theory calls attention to relationships that influence the practice of nursing. The development of conceptual models has stimulated the development and refinement of theory and research. Throughout this chapter some theories based on classic writings will be discussed. These theories reflect current thinking in theory development in nursing.

This chapter contains a discussion of selected conceptual models for guiding community health nursing practice. Several terms are defined, and the usefulness of conceptual models for guiding practice is explained. Additionally, the Division of Community Health Nursing of the American Nurses' Association (ANA) has developed a "Conceptual Model of Community Health Nursing," and the American Public Health Association (APHA) has written a position paper entitled "The role and definition of public health nursing in the delivery of health care." These models are summarized and compared regarding major themes and inherent differences.

DEFINITION OF KEY TERMS

To fully appreciate the usefulness of models, it is necessary to sort through the semantic jungle surrounding this topic. Frequently the terms *model* and *theory* are used inter-

changeably. All theories are models, but the converse is not true; all models are not theories because not all models have the requisites of theoretical construction. A model expresses structure, whereas a theory adds substance to that structure. A *theory* is an internally consistent group of relational statements that presents a systematic view about the subject being studied and is useful in describing, explaining, or predicting (Walker and Avant, 1983). Theory sets limits on what questions to ask and what methods to use in seeking answers (Meleis, 1985).

Concepts are the building blocks of theory. A concept is not a thing or an action, but the image of the phenomenon. Concepts can be primitive, concrete, or abstract. A primitive concept, such as the color red, has a common meaning to all people. A concrete concept is defined by primitive concepts, is limited by time and space, and is observable. A chair is an example of a concrete concept. In contrast, an abstract concept, although definable by primitive concepts, is independent of time and space; an example is an idea (Walker and Avant, 1983).

Concepts that refer to phenomena not directly observable are usually considered *constructs*. In contrast, *hypotheses* or *propositions* specify the relationship between two or more concepts (Williams, 1979). Examples of concepts include nurse, chair, and house; less observable constructs might be society, intelligence, and age. A hypothesis might be "the more information hypertensive clients have about their disease, the more they will adhere to the therapeutic regimen." The last term to be defined to describe theory is *variable*, which is a concept that takes on more than one value. A theory then has certain attributes: clearly defined concepts, and hypotheses that are interrelated and testable and tie the concepts together.

An additional term that needs to be defined is *conceptual framework*, "a group of concepts plus a set of propositions which spell out the relationships between those concepts . . ." (Williams, 1979, p. 93). According to this description, all theories are conceptual frameworks.

A *conceptual model* can be defined as "a set of concepts and those assumptions that integrate them into a meaningful configuration" (Fawcett, 1980, p. 10). Conceptual models provide a certain frame of reference for members of a discipline, telling them what to look at; their utility comes from the organization they provide for thinking, for observations, and for interpreting what is seen (Fawcett, 1984). As can be seen, the terms *conceptual model* and *conceptual framework* are essentially the same. For the purposes of this discussion, conceptual model will be the term of choice.

At present most of what are referred to in nursing as theories actually fall within the realm of conceptual models or sets of concepts and a group of statements that explain how these concepts are interrelated. The aim of nursing research is to clarify, test, and refine the current models so that they reach the specificity of theory. Conceptual models constitute a key stage in theory development by providing focus, ruling some variables in as relevant and others out as unrelated.

Contemporary conceptual models of nursing specify varying relationships and interactions among four essential components: person, environment, health, and nursing. Each of the nursing models discussed in this chapter has a unique view of the four primary concepts, and each conceives of the interactional pattern in a different fashion; however, several commonalities do exist. Most nursing models view people as holistic beings who have biophychosocial qualities. People are viewed also as being interactive and part of a family, community, and society. Each model views health and nursing in a different way and delineates the nursing process in accordance with its unique tenets. Conceptual models having the greatest application to community health nursing view people as being in continuous interaction with their environment. The environment affects its inhabitants and vice versa. Additionally, environment refers to that which is internal as well as the more easily observable external environment. The environment in community health is dynamic and ever-changing and can be either a positive or negative force in health.

In community health nursing, the major focus of attention is on health. The unique feature of this area of nursing is its emphasis on assisting individuals, families, groups, and communities to maintain health. To do this, the community is viewed from a holistic perspective as a motivator or disruptor of health care. The nursing goal is to assess, plan, implement, and evaluate ways to make the designated community a healthy place to live. The aim of community health nursing is also directed toward assisting recipients of care to assume personal responsibility for their health; teaching, counseling, and advocacy are essential features of the nursing role.

USING CONCEPTUAL MODELS

To some extent everyone has a conceptual model because all people have assumptions and beliefs about how the world operates. Everyone has a unique set of concepts guiding the categorization of ideas and information within their belief system. In nursing practice, people view situations differently and have personalized ways of responding to others. Whether implicit or explicit, a person's conceptual models play a major role in determining behavior. Conceptual models guide actions and are either consciously or unconsciously recognized. As will be seen in the latter part of this chapter, a variety of conceptual models have potential usefulness in

community health nursing, and many nurses already practice in accordance with a model such as systems theory or a developmental framework.

Conceptual Models in Nursing Education

Conceptual models often provide the general outline for organizing curricular content and for selecting teaching-learning approaches. To guide curriculum, conceptual models must be linked with theories about education and the teaching-learning process and must draw upon substantive theoretical content from nursing and other relevant disciplines (Fawcett, 1984).

Conceptual Models in Research

Nursing research has received a major impetus to include a conceptual basis for study. Just as in education, conceptual models focus the study and also guide the delineation of variables to be included and those to be logically omitted. However, some differences exist in the ways conceptual models are used in research and in curriculum design. In research the use of models must be more explicit and precise, whereas in curriculum design it can be broader to allow flexibility and creativity in the delineation of content. To verify the effectiveness of the research process, concepts must be clearly defined and carefully developed to allow for accurate measurement.

In nursing research, conceptual models provide the essential conceptual, instrumental, and methodological rules for guiding the work. The model helps define the concepts from which specific variables are derived; it defines research questions and thereby serves as an overall map for the study. Specific research endeavors may focus on one or a few aspects of a conceptual model (Fawcett, 1984). Currently, many models convey more of a philosophy of care than a model of care because the relational statements have not clearly been delineated. Most models do have carefully articulated concepts, and once they have been tested and relationships have been documented, the models will offer greater usefulness for education, research, and practice.

Conceptual Models in Nursing Practice

In practice, just as in education and research, conceptual models give direction, simplify, and help organize information. Models can be used in clinical practice to order existing knowledge or concepts and to examine the relationships among objects or events. The use of a specific model determines the kind of information that will be gathered and the way the information will be organized and interpreted. Currently, most nursing models are useful for testing specific theories. Models such as those described in the next section do guide nursing practice through the structure for assessing and diagnosing health deficits in individuals, families, and communities.

Nurses have historically used models in their actions; the work of Florence Nightingale and Lillian Wald provide clear evidence of an epidemiological model for practice. Nightingale, in early work in the Crimean War, recognized both the role of the environment on health and the destructiveness of disease patterns. Similarly, Wald devoted much of her life to campaigning for better living conditions in New York City so that disease would not run rampant among the people she served.

Historically, community health nurses have relied heavily on an epidemiological model to guide practice. Because of its key role in community health, the epidemiological model is discussed in depth in Chapter 8. The next two sections focus on two recently developed and, in many ways, similar models for practice: the model of the ANA Division on Community Health Nursing Practice and the model of the APHA Public Health Nursing Section. When using models for practice, be aware that some are not carefully developed and can confuse rather than guide practice.

THE ANA CONCEPTUAL MODEL OF COMMUNITY HEALTH NURSING PRACTICE

The definition of community health nursing set forth in the ANA *Conceptual Model of Community Health Nursing* is futuristic with its emphasis on health promotion and consumer involvement and its consideration of health as being influenced by multiple factors within people and by the environments in which they seek to live. The definition reads as follows (American Nurses' Association, 1980, p.2):

> Community health nursing is a synthesis of nursing and public health practice applied to promoting and preserving the health of populations. The practice is general and comprehensive. It is not limited to a particular age group or diagnosis, and is continuing, not episodic. The dominant responsibility is to the population as a whole; nursing directed to individuals, families, or groups contributes to the health of the total population. Health promotion, health maintenance, health education, and management, coordination, and continuity of care are utilized in a holistic approach to the management of the health care of individuals, families and groups in a community.

This definition encompasses both direct and indirect services to individuals, families, groups, and communities. Its scope is concerned with both wellness and illness in providing, as well as facilitating, the delivery of services. A set of assumptions and beliefs further elaborate on the goal of community health nursing and describe the scope of practice.

Assumptions and Beliefs

The following assumptions and beliefs about community health nursing are set forth* (American Nurses' Association, 1980):

Assumption 1: The health care system is complex.
Assumption 2: Primary, secondary, and tertiary health care are components of the health care system.
Assumption 3: Nursing, as a subsystem of the health care system, is the product of education and practice based upon research.
Assumption 4: The provision of primary care predominates in community health nursing practice, with lesser involvement in secondary and tertiary health care.
Assumption 5: Community health nursing occurs principally in primary health care settings.

---

*Reprinted with the permission of ANA.

Belief 1: Health care should be available, accessible, and acceptable to all persons.
Belief 2: The making of health policy should include participation by recipients of health care services.
Belief 3: The nurse as a provider and the client as a consumer of health care services can form a conjoint relationship to advocate and effect change in health policies and services.
Belief 4: The environment affects the health of populations, groups, families, and individuals.
Belief 5: Prevention of illness is essential to promote health.
Belief 6: A health axis intersects with the life span axis.
Belief 7: The client is the only constant member of the health care team.
Belief 8: Individuals within a community are ultimately responsible for their own health and must be encouraged and taught to be active participants in their own health care.

Scope of Practice

According to the ANA conceptual model, the focus of community health nursing is on the prevention of illness and promotion and maintenance of health. Nursing activities to achieve these goals include client education, counseling, advocacy, and management of care. The major emphasis in community health nursing is on primary care, which begins when clients enter the health care system and continues throughout the duration of the client's care. Secondary and tertiary care are afforded less emphasis. Clients are considered to be active members of the health care team, and the goal of care is to help clients assume self-responsibility for health care.

The specific functions viewed as priorities in the role of the community health nurse are seen in the nine standards identified by the Division on Community Health Nursing Practice and given in Appendix F (American Nurses' Association, 1980).

The major goal of the community health nurse, as pointed out in Chapter 1, is the preservation and improvement of the health of the community. This overall objective is accomplished through two major modes or routes. The first community health nursing mode is direct care to individuals, families, and groups within a designated community. The second mode directs attention to the health of the total population and considers how community health problems and issues affect individuals, families, and groups. For example, the problem of improper waste disposal or stagnant water near a residential area would be considered a community health nursing problem in terms of how the residents of that area were affected.

Practicing in the first mode, community health nurses work directly with clients to promote optimal health, and where health has been disrupted, to assist in restoration and stabilization of chronic conditions. The pattern of practice takes place through clinics, home health care, and group work with clients having common health needs. Practice is collaborative with other members of the health care team, is holistic in orientation, and emphasizes the evaluation of nursing care to individuals, families, and the community.

In the second mode the focus is on the community as client, and the aim is to assist communities to identify health needs, establish priorities, plan and implement actions, and identify and intervene in factors affecting the health of the community. This mode emphasizes the on-going interaction between people and their environment in which each is affected by the other. The role of the community health nurse embraces all three levels of prevention—primary, secondary, and tertiary, with emphasis on primary. As will be noted in the following discussion, many similarities exist between the ANA *Conceptual Model of Community Health Nursing* and the definition and role delineation established by the APHA Public Health Nursing Section.

THE APHA DEFINITION OF PUBLIC HEALTH NURSING AND ITS ROLE IN THE DELIVERY OF HEALTH CARE

Like the ANA, a work group of the APHA Public Health Nursing Section was established as an ad hoc committee to define public health nursing* and delineate its scope of practice. To state a clear and concise position, the following definition of public health nursing was recommended (American Public Health Association, 1981, p.4):

> Public health nursing synthesizes the body of knowledge from the public health sciences and professional nursing theories for the purpose of improving the health of the entire community. This goal lies at the heart of primary prevention and health promotion and is the foundation for public health nursing practice. To accomplish this goal, public health nurses work with groups, families, and individuals as well as in multidisciplinary teams and programs. Identifying the subgroups (aggregates) within the population which are at high risk of illness, disability, or premature death and directing resources toward these groups is the most effective approach for accomplishing the goal of public health nursing. Success in reducing the risks and in improving the health of the community depends on the involvement of consumers, especially groups experiencing health risks, and others in the community, in health planning, and in self-help activities.

The position paper of the APHA committee further noted that public health nursing practice is a systematic process in which the following occur (American Public Health Association, 1980, pp. 4-5):

1. The health and health care needs of a population are assessed by nurses or in collaboration with other disciplines in order to identify subpopulations (aggregates), families, and individuals at increased risk of illness, disability, or premature death.
2. A plan for intervention is developed to meet these needs that includes available resources and those activities that contribute to health and its recovery and to the prevention of illness, disability, and premature death.
3. A health care plan is implemented effectively, efficiently, and equitably.
4. An evaluation is made to determine the extent to which these activities have an impact on the health status of the population.

Both the ANA and APHA definitions emphasize the blending of nursing and public health knowledge as a foundation for determining the scope of practice. They both

acknowledge that community health nursing efforts are directed toward all people whether they are cared for as individuals, as part of a family, in a community, or as a community at large. Each definition emphasizes a multidisciplinary role for the successful implementation of public health practice, and they both focus on the increasing priority of health promotion. The APHA definition emphasizes primary care more than the ANA definition does, and it also clearly points out the need to determine within a community those groups at greatest risk for health disruption so that nursing interventions can be targeted toward them to prevent the onset of disease.

INTERDISCIPLINARY MODELS APPLICABLE TO COMMUNITY HEALTH NURSING

Several models retain their basic structure and order even though they cross interdisciplinary lines; that is, they can be used or adapted appropriately by more than one of the physical, biological, and social sciences, as well as by the professions. These are generally referred to as "types" or "categories" of models. Those to be considered here are systems theory, developmental theory, and interaction models.

Systems Theory

Systems theory, also referred to as *general systems theory* (GST), was described as a conceptual model to illustrate the unity in the sciences. Advocating an organismic (as opposed to the mechanistic) view, Bertalanffy (1952, p. 11) wrote that "every organism represents a *system,* by which term we mean a complex of elements in mutual interaction." The elements in interaction to which he referred were wholeness, organization, and dynamic order (pp. 9-13), and he delineates how these concepts are important phenomena in the realms of physics, biology, psychology, and philosophy (1952, pp. 176-204). The rationale for such a model was its allowance for the transfer of laws from one realm (or science) to another. Just as Bertalanffy thought, the model has proved useful because it permeates the literature of many disciplines and professions.

Characteristics of Systems Theory

Several concepts generally discussed in relation to general systems theory are wholeness, organization, openness, boundary, entropy, negentropy, and equifinality. *Wholeness* refers to that property of a system in which a collection of parts responds as an integrated single part. The arrangement of the elements and the order of their relationship to each other refers to their *organization*.

Openness of a system refers to the extent to which it exchanges energy in any form with the environment. An open system is affected by the environment (receives input) and in turn affects the environment by its output. In a closed system, no energy is exchanged.

Boundary refers to a line or border showing what elements constitute the system, that is, what elements are inside the system. In biological terms the cell membrane is a boundary regulating what goes in and comes out of the cell. In social systems the boundary is more like an imaginary line used referring to given individuals as a group.

---

*The term *public health nursing* will be used in this section of the discussion instead of *community health nursing* because APHA uses this term to refer to their nursing clinical section.

Entropy is a concept based on a major implication of the second law of thermodynamics, which states that elements in a closed environment will proceed toward greater randomness or less order. Entropy is also described as disordered energy, or energy that is bound and cannot be converted to work. *Negentropy* is the energy that is "free," can be used for work, and tends toward order. Because living systems are open systems, they do not adhere to the implications of the second law of thermodynamics. The final term is *equifinality,* which means that the end state of the open system is independent of the beginning state or starting point.

Feedback is the process whereby the output of the system is redirected as part of the input of the same system. The regulation of the body as a physiological system uses feedback to regulate temperature, heart rate, and respiration, to mention only a few functions. However, the discussion of input, thruput, output, and feedback characterizes all explanation of systems.

Advantages and Disadvantages

Systems theory can be applied (1) across disciplines so that universal laws are identified and useful and (2) to individuals, groups, and communities. Further, it emphasizes how each isolated variable affects the whole and how the whole affects each part. A disadvantage is that it does not explicitly emphasize growth and change toward a higher level of organization.

Application to Community Health Nursing

WHOLENESS. The community as a whole is a social system made up of interrelated and interdependent subsystems. The subsystems include the economic, educational, religious, health care, political, welfare, law enforcement, energy (health, light, and water), and recreational systems. When any one of the subsystems is affected, it affects the community as a whole. A subsystem in which changes are seen immediately and obviously in the whole is the economic system.

ORGANIZATION. All of the subsystems of the larger social system, the community, are organized and related to each other in a specific way. Specific communication channels exist for the organizations to relate to each other and to the whole.

OPENNESS. According to systems theory, the community is an open system that exchanges materials such as energy and goods and services, values, and ideals with the environment outside the community. The community as a system has boundaries, the most obvious being geographical lines. The imaginary boundary is one that encompasses all the subsystems in the community and identifies what is inside and outside the community. Entropy can be compared with the landfill garbage dumps (waste) or problems such as crime, violence, and poor health in the community, whereas negentropy can be compared with the resources, health, wealth, and altruistic values of the people. Equifinality indicates that wherever the community begins (e.g., the poor and unattractive), given the resources and energy, it may attain economic balance and beauty.

FEEDBACK. An excellent example of feedback in the community, according to systems theory, is in the economic system. If the output is good, it provides good input and further contributes to the growth of the economy in the community.

Developmental Theory

Developmental theory as a way of thinking about how changes occur is based on theories of development of the human organism. Lewis (1982) classifies theories of child development as reactive and structural. Reactive theories emphasize the influence of the environment on the development of the child. These include stimulus-response theory, learning theories, classical conditioning, and operant conditioning. Structural theories emphasize the genetically determined program for development, which is usually described in stages (Lewis, 1982, p. 10). Examples of structural theories include Freud's psychosexual stages (oral, anal, phallic, latency, and genital), Erikson's psychosocial phases (trust vs mistrust, autonomy vs shame and doubt, initiative vs guilt, industry vs inferiority, identity vs role confusion, intimacy vs isolation, generativity vs self-absorption, and integrity vs despair), and Piaget's stages of cognitive development (sensorimotor, period of preoperational thought, stage of concrete operations, and formal operations) (Lewis, 1982, pp. 12-13). Although Lewis (1982) refers to these as structural theories, they are generally referred to as developmental theories.

Characteristics of Developmental Theory

Chinn (1980, pp. 30-31), describes the major characteristics of developmental models as direction, stages or phases, progression, potentiality, and forces. These characteristics refer to the process of growth or change.

Direction refers to the fact that growth proceeds in a specific direction toward an end state or goal. In development of the individual, a direction of physical growth is toward being taller, and a direction of mental growth is toward complexity in thought and language.

Stages, phases, and levels, are synonymous terms used to describe periods when the individual or group is concentrating on a particular task or developmental milestone. Each stage has facets of growth or behavior that are unique to it. For example, the development of motor capabilities at different ages proceeds sequentially; that is, an infant crawls, pulls to a standing position, and then walks over a period of months.

Progression suggests that the way in which changes occur over time have a characteristic form. Chinn (1980, p. 31) describes four forms of progression: linear, spiral, oscillation, and differentiation. Linear refers to changes, such as aging, that proceed in a unidirectional manner. Spiral refers to the fact that some similar behaviors are performed at a more complex level; for example, thinking and problem solving are behaviors that are repeated but performed at higher levels. Oscillation is the individual going back and forth for a time between behaviors of a stage he or she is growing out of and a more complex stage he or she is growing toward. Differentiation refers to changes in which the functions of the individual become more specialized.

Forces include genetic and environmental factors. Individuals are genetically programmed for growth and development. The environmental forces can enhance or deter the development.

Potentiality refers to the capabilities offered by the genetic endowment of the individual given a supporting and nurturing environment. Although it is easier to understand these characteristics in the development of the individual organism, the reader should remember that the developmental model is also applied to change in groups or social organizations such as health care delivery systems.

Advantages and Disadvantages

Advantages of developmental models are these: (1) characteristics are easy to understand and when considered in relation to the human organism, the developmental changes can be observed, and (2) growth is emphasized and viewed as a positive event, which may be experienced psychologically even when physical growth has ceased. A disadvantage of developmental models is that major variables such as environment, sociocultural factors, or circumstances may not be taken into consideration or may be minimized.

Application to Community Health Nursing

The usefulness of developmental theory in working with infants and children is evidenced by the fact that growth and development is an inherent part of every nursing curriculum. A major part of the nurse's role in working with infants and children is assessing their developmental progress and helping parents promote that progress with a stimulating environment. One of the most widely used screening tools that assess child development is the **Denver Developmental Screening Test (DDST)**. The DDST was developed and tested to yield a developmental profile in the areas of gross motor, language, fine motor–adaptive and personal-social skills (further details of the DDST are in Chapter 21 and the appendixes). The developmental approach also has been widely discussed and written about as a way of working with families (see Chapters 18 and 19). Duvall (1977, p. 144) described the family life cycle in eight stages: beginning, early childbearing, preschool, school, teenagers, launching center, middle years, retirement, and old age. The nurse can use each of these stages of development and their respective tasks for each stage in the assessment and the promotion of family development. Peplau's developmental model (Blake, p. 54), Maslow's hierarchy of needs, and crisis intervention are examples of widely used developmental models (Thibodeau, pp. 45, 47).

Interaction Models

Interaction models are based on theories that stem from philosophical writings such as those of Cooley (1909) and Mead (1934). Mead, influential in the development of social psychology, viewed a human being as a reflection of human society, that is, primarily a social and cultural being. Further, he contended that a newborn develops a self as a consequence of relationships with others and the environment. Contemporary social psychologists such as Rose (1962) use the term *symbolic interactionism,* and Burr (1981, p. 102) uses the framework of interactionism to encompass role theory and self theory. The major concepts used in interaction models are communication, perception, role, and self-concept.

Characteristics of Interaction Theory

Communication is the act of giving and receiving information and consists of both verbal and nonverbal language.

Perception is the way a person perceives a situation or an event. It is influenced by antecedent, cognitive, and emotional factors already present in the person's background.

Role refers to the set of prescriptions defining what the behavior of a position member should be (Burr, 1981, p. 54). Variations in meanings attached to role are best illustrated by the qualifiers or descriptors attached to role. Multiple roles refer to the fact that one human being has several roles. Each role brings expectations, and sometimes role strain occurs as a result of role conflict.

Self-Concept refers to the way in which persons visualize and think about themselves. The picture that we have of ourselves influences the way we interact with others.

Advantages and Disadvantages

Interaction theory calls attention to how elements affect each other and especially the individuality of human beings. However, attention can be focused on interaction to the exclusion of other variables.

Application to Community Health Nursing

The phenomenon of family dynamics is frequently addressed in the nursing literature. The interaction model can be useful in analyzing the family dynamics.

COMMUNICATION. Community health nursing presents many occasions when, to be more helpful to a family, assessment of the communication patterns are indicated. The reason for the contact with the nurse may be health related, but the manner in which the family is coping with the health problems may be intricately related to communication patterns. That is, who talks to whom about what and in what way? Furthermore, it is important to know who listens, what is heard by the person listening, if the message sent is the message received, and finally what kind of feedback the members of the family give to each other.

ROLE. Assessment of the role structure is also important in working with families. Role refers to a set of expected behaviors by virtue of occupying or holding a given position, and every person assumes multiple roles. The person who enters the health care system inevitably has multiple roles; problems or illnesses that generally bring the person to the health care system will affect the person's ability to function in many of the roles. The person may worry about the inability to function in all the roles. An obvious, and perhaps overused, example is the person in the executive position who worries that illness such as heart attack will interfere with the role as provider for the family. In the health maintenance function, the nurse uses knowledge about role to identify such things as role conflict, a situation in which a person is confronted with incompatible expectations, or role strain, anxiety, work, and stress associated with the role. The nurse will also have contact with first-time parents who are undergoing the role transition from couple to parents and adding the roles of mother and father to that of husband and wife.

SELF-CONCEPT. Self-concept, or the way a person sees himself or herself, is an important aspect of health and well-being. It probably influences health-seeking behaviors and adaptation to problems of a health-illness nature. The change from being a well person to someone who is not in total control of his or her life and especially health may result in a lower self-concept. Thus it is important that the nurse listen for cues and help the person use self-concept positively.

PERCEPTION. Just as perception of events and situations such as auto accidents differs from one person to another, persons' perceptions of events and situations happening to them are affected by previous experiences including attitudes, beliefs, and socialization into a particular culture. It is useful to the nurse to recognize the differences in perception. The perception of the patient/client of the situation may not be the same as that of the nurse.

NURSING MODELS WITH APPLICATION TO COMMUNITY HEALTH NURSING

Several conceptual models have been developed and described by nurses for use in nursing. Among the more prominent are models developed by Roy, Rogers, Johnson, Neuman, Orem, and King. These are described briefly.

Roy

The *Roy Adaptation Model of Nursing* was first presented in the periodical literature (Roy, 1970) and has since been used as a conceptual framework for nursing curricula, nursing practice, and nursing research. This model has some of the characteristics of a systems theory and some of the characteristics of interaction theory. Roy (Riehl and Roy, 1981, p. 179) describes it a "systems theory though it also contains interactionist levels of analysis."

Characteristics and Key Assumptions

A human is viewed as an adaptive system. Changes occur in the system in response to stimuli (input). If the changes promote integrity of the individual (such as growth or self-mastery), the response is adaptive; otherwise, the response is considered maladaptive. The system has two major mechanisms for adapting or coping: the regulator and cognator. The regulator system is concerned with the neural, endocrine, and perception-psychomotor processes, and the cognator mechanism is concerned with the processes of perception, learning, judgment, and emotion (Roy and Roberts, 1981, pp. 60-63). Additionally, four modes for effecting adaptation of the system include physiological needs, self-concept, role function, and interdependence.

Application to Practice

Goal: The goal of the nurse is to "maintain and enhance adaptive behavior and to change ineffective behavior to adaptive" (Roy, 1984, p. 59). The nurse achieves the goal by manipulating or changing the stimuli causing the stress

to help the person cope more effectively. When individuals encounter more than the usual amount of stress, such as that caused by illness, their established coping mechanisms may be ineffective. Thus a nursing intervention is required.

Strengths and Limitations

Strengths of the model include the following: (1) most of the terminology is familiar or is clearly described, (2) the nursing process is similar to the standard of assess, plan, implement, and evaluation, (3) the focus is on behaviors, which offers greater individuality to the client assessment, (4) assessment of psychosocial needs is emphasized, and (5) it has been applied in practice, education, and research (Fawcett, 1984, pp. 270-285).

Limitations of the model are the following: (1) the adaptive modes overlap, especially in the modes of self-concept, role function, and interdependence, (2) the judgment of behavior as adaptive or maladaptive will be influenced by the value system of the nurse assessing the client, and (3) the term adaptation generally does not convey a meaning of growth as intended in the model.

Nursing Process

The nursing process, according to Roy, consists of a first and second level assessment, problem identification, nursing diagnosis, setting priorities, goal setting, intervention, and evaluation (Roy, 1984, p. 43). In the first level assessment, client behaviors in each of the adaptive modes (physiological, self-concept, role function, and interdependence) are observed and described. In the second level assessment, the nurse identifies the focal, contextual, and residual factors influencing client behavior. The focal stimuli is the situation, such as stress, injury, or illness, immediately confronting the individual. The contextual stimuli are the other factors present such as family milieu or environment. The residual stimuli are influencing factors from the client's background: beliefs, attitudes, experiences, and traits. Following the second level assessment, problems are identified, nursing diagnoses are made, priorities are set, and then goals are formulated. The next step, intervention, manipulates the stimuli to promote adaptation, and the evaluation is used to judge the effectiveness of the nursing approach.

Rogers

Martha Rogers' *Science of Unitary Man* first appeared in the literature in 1970. It has been used as the conceptual base for the curriculum at New York University, for several research projects, and to a lesser extent in nursing practice.

The Roger's model has strong ties to general systems theory, which are reflected in her basic assumptions (1970, pp. 49-77), and elements of the developmental model are inherent in it.

Characteristics and Key Assumptions

Energy fields, universe of open systems, pattern and organization, and four dimensionality are described by Rogers as the four building blocks for her conceptual system (Rogers, 1980, p. 330). *Energy fields* refers to the conceptualization of humans and their environment as matter or energy evidenced by wave patterns. Rogers emphasizes the energy field as part of a person's wholeness: "The human field is more than and different from the sum of its parts" (Rogers, 1980, p. 330). *Openness* refers to the view of persons as open systems who interact continuously with the environment. *Pattern and organization* refer to the way the energy fields emerge, and are characterized by wave pattern and organization. *Four dimensionality* is another characteristic of energy fields. This has been described by Johnson and Fitzpatrick 1982 (p. 10) as "transcendence of the time-space interaction." Four dimensionality is easier to understand by thinking of the phenomenon of clairvoyance; a person who is clairvoyant sees the future and transcends time for an instant.

Rogers (1980, p. 333) postulates the development of unitary persons by use of three principles of homeodynamics. *Helicy* refers to life as proceeding in one direction and rhythmically along a spiral. *Resonancy* refers to the wave pattern and organization of the energy fields. *Complementarity* refers to *integrality,* formerly called the simultaneous mutual interaction of the human and environmental fields.

Application to Practice

Goal: Rogers' background in public health obviously influenced her statement of nursing's goal: "Maintenance and promotion of health, prevention of disease, nursing diagnosis, intervention, and rehabilitation encompass the scope of nursing's goals" (Rogers, 1970, p. 86). She also emphasizes that nursing is for the well and the sick, rich and poor, in all settings—home, school, work, and play.

Rogers made the goal of nursing clear: individuals should achieve their maximum health potential (1970, p. 86). However, it was others who developed her model into a framework for the nursing process. Therapeutic touch (Krieger, 1981; Heidt, 1981) is an application of the Rogers framework to nursing process. Whelton (1979, pp. 10-14) illustrates areas of assessment and nursing process in the areas of wholeness, openness, pattern and organization, unidirectionality, and sentience and thought.

Falco and Lobo (1985) illustrated the process of assessment using the principles of homeodynamics: integrality, resonancy, helicy. Whall (1981, pp. 33-34) operationalized Roger's theory by illustrating the assessment of families under the categories of (1) individual sub-system, (2) interactional patterns, (3) unique characteristics of the whole, and (4) environmental interface synchrony.

Strengths and Limitations

Strengths of this model are (1) emphasis on the total context of the universe, (2) the goal of maximum health potential, and (3) emphasis on the effect of environment (not only air pollution, but also life-style) on a person's health. Limitations of the model follow: (1) terminology is not easily understood and (2) application to practice needs to be more clearly operationalized.

Johnson

Dorothy Johnson's Behavioral Systems Model was first presented as an unpublished paper at Vanderbilt University in 1968. It was subsequently used in the graduate program at the University of California at Los Angeles. It has also been tested to some extent by research studies (Derdiarian, 1983) and has been applied in practice (Auger, 1983). It is clearly a systems model with the behavioral system having subsystems; the system and the subsystems are linked to each other and are open.

Characteristics and Key Assumptions

Johnson assumed that the person can be viewed as a behavioral system in the same way that physicians view a human as a biological system. The *behavioral system* consists of seven subsystems: achievement, affiliative, aggressive, dependency, eliminative, ingestive, and sexual. Each subsystem has four structural elements: drive or goal, set or predisposition to act, choices of action alternatives from which he can choose, and the person's action or behavior. The behavioral system as a whole and each of the subsystems has functional requirements: protection, nurturance, and stimulation. The outcome of the behavioral system is the patterned, repetitive, and purposeful ways of behaving. If behavior is efficient and effective, it will be orderly, purposeful, and predictable.

Application to Practice

Goal: "The goal of nursing action in each case is to restore, maintain, or attain behavioral system balance and stability at the highest possible level for the individual" (Johnson, 1980, p. 214). This means the nurse is concerned with promoting efficient and effective behavior related to health.

Assessment to begin the nursing process consists of listing all significant behaviors in each of the seven subsystems. The behaviors are identified as functional or dysfunctional. The variables influencing or causing the behaviors are also identified. The nursing problem or diagnosis is made and is placed in one of four diagnostic classifications: (1) insufficiency, which indicates the subsystem is not functioning because of inadequacy of functional requirements; (2) discrepancy, which indicates the behavior is not meeting the intended goal; (3) incompatibility, which indicates that goals or behaviors of two subsystems are in conflict, and (4) dominance, which indicates that the behavior in one subsystem is used more than any other. Before the intervention, long- and short-term goals are set. There are also four modes of nursing intervention: (1) restrict or place limits on behavior, (2) defend or protect from negative stressors, (3) inhibit or suppress ineffective responses, and (4) facilitate or give nurturance and stimulation. Following intervention, evaluation is made in terms of long- and short-term goals.

Strengths and Limitations

The conceptualization of man as a behavioral system gives an alternative to the medical model as a way of viewing a human. In this way the nursing role can be differentiated from medicine's role. Johnson has demonstrated how the model can be used as a comprehensive and complex system for nursing care. The complexity of the model and the terminology requires considerable effort to understand and apply in practice.

Orem

The *Orem Self-Care Nursing Model* began when Orem (1959, p. 5) described the nurse's role as giving assistance to the person having inabilities in self-care. It was further developed by the Nursing Model Committee of the School of Nursing Faculty of the Catholic University of America, initiated in 1965 (Nursing Development Conference Group, 1973). The first full description, *Nursing: Concepts of Practice,* was published in 1971. The model is also described in later works (Nursing Development Conference Group, 1973; Orem, 1981, 1985). Orem's model was categorized by Riehl and Roy (1980) as a systems model; however, Bush (1979) characterizes it as an interaction model. She uses the concept of nursing systems (Orem, 1981, p. 92) and discusses role (Orem, 1981, pp. 8-16) and self-concept (Orem, 1980, p. 88), but the analogy between the model and systems theory or the model and interaction theory is somewhat tangential.

Orem's model evolves from the way she conceptualizes nursing and especially from the fact that nursing is concerned with self-care. Important terms in the model are self-care, self-care agency, therapeutic self-care demand, and self-care deficit.

Self-care consists of those activities that an individual does for himself to maintain life, health, and well-being. *Self-care agency* refers to the person who provides the self-care. Every individual has need of a composite of self-care actions called *therapeutic self-care demand.* If the therapeutic self-care demand is greater than the self-care agency, a *self-care deficit* exists. When this occurs nursing intervention is needed.

Application to Practice

Goal: The goal of nursing is to meet the patient's self-care demand until he or his family is capable of providing it.

Orem categorized self-care requirements into three types: (1) universal, which consists of self-care to meet physiological and psychosocial needs, (2) developmental, the self-care required when one goes through developmental stages, and (3) health deviation, the self-care required when an individual has a deviation from health. Using the Orem model, assessment is made of the therapeutic self-care demand, the self-care agency and the self-care deficits in the areas of knowledge, skills, motivation, and orientation.

Following the nursing assessment, a design is formulated for the nursing system, which is the approach the nurse uses to meet the patient's self-care deficit. These are categorized into three systems: (1) wholly compensatory in which the patient has no active role; (2) partly compensatory in which the patient and the nurse have an actual role; and (3) educative development in which the patient can meet his need for self-care with some assistance from the nurse.

To implement the nursing system the nurse uses one of the following actions: (1) acting for or doing for, (2) guiding, (3) supporting, (4) providing, and (5) teaching.

Strengths and Limitations

The model builds on self-care a function that nurses have assumed responsibility for historically. Orem emphasized the client's role in planning and implementing care ac-

cording to his or her capability. Structure in the model focuses on the client as a learner and the nurse as a teacher. Elipoulos (1984) advocates its use with older adults. However, Anna (1978) reported that the terminology for the concepts was confusing.

Newman

Betty Neuman's *Health-Care Systems Model* was first introduced as a total person approach to viewing patient problems (1972, Neuman and Young). She refers to her conceptual framework as an "open systems model of two components—stress and reaction to it" (Neuman, 1980, p. 122). Her model also draws from the Gestalt and field theories in psychology.

Characteristics and Key Assumptions

The total person model was designed to bring together simultaneously the behavioral, biological, developmental, and interacting components of the person. A human is depicted graphically as a series of concentric circles having stressors impinging on them. The basic structure (factor common to all organisms) is viewed as the center of the concentric circle. Surrounding the basic structure are the following: (1) flexible lines of resistance, or the organism's internal mechanisms for defense against stress; (2) normal line of defense, or what the individual has become over time; and (3) flexible line of defense, which is a protective buffer around the normal line of defense.

Stressors and reaction to stress can be viewed as intrapersonal, interpersonal, or extrapersonal. Intrapersonal refers to factors within the individual, interpersonal refers to factors between individuals, and extrapersonal refers to factors outside the individual.

Application to Nursing Practice

The "major goal of nursing is conceptualized as keeping stabilized both the individual and the family system, as clients, within their environment" (Neuman, 1983, p. 252).

Assessment, according to Neuman (1982, p. 27), includes the client's perception of stressors and the nurse's perception of stressors. She also included assessment of intrapersonal, interpersonal, and extrapersonal factors as perceived by client and caregiver. Neuman (1983, p. 244) proposed a new nursing process tool for determining status of family on a stability (wellness)/instability (illness) scale. This assessment is organized according to four categories: (1) psychosocial relationship characteristics, (2) physical status, (3) developmental characteristics, and (4) spiritual influence.

Nursing intervention is implemented through primary prevention such as reducing stress, secondary prevention such as early case finding, and tertiary prevention such as reeducation.

Strengths and Limitations

The model builds on the function of primary, secondary, and tertiary prevention, which is supported by the discipline of public health and has been a major contribution of the nursing profession. In addition to emphasizing the total person, Neuman (1983, p. 244) provides a format for assessing the family. However, it is so broad in scope that it may fail to delineate a distinct role or function of nursing.

King

Imogene *King's theory* (1968) was first introduced as a "conceptual frame of reference." The framework was used in the curriculum at Ohio State when King was director of that school of nursing, and King has reported its use in her own research (1978). King refers to her work as systems theory, and it does reflect some properties of the systems model. It also reflects properties of interaction theory, and it is sometimes described as an interaction model (Bush, 1979).

Characteristics and Key Assumptions

A human is a social, sentient, rational, reacting, perceiving, controlling, purposeful, action-oriented, and time-oriented being (King, 1981, p. 143). King describes her conceptual framework as a general systems theory with three subsystems: personal system, interpersonal system, and social system. The *personal* system is made up of the concepts of perception, self, growth and development, body image, space, and time. The *interpersonal* system is made up of the concepts of human interactions, communication, transactions, role, and stress. The *social system* is made up of the concepts of organization, authority, power, status, and decision making. The three systems are dynamic and interacting (King, 1981).

Application to Nursing Practice

Goal: The goal of nursing is health.

Nursing intervention is carried out through the process of action, reaction, interaction and transaction between the client and the nurse. King also described a theory of goal attainment, which is implemented through a goal-oriented nursing record. This consists of five major elements: a data base, a problem list, a goal list, a plan, and progress notes (King 1981, p. 165)

Strengths and Limitations

Two strengths of the model are its emphasis on client perception and client participation in planning his or her own care by King's emphasis on the transaction. The empirical testing of the model for application to practice and for research is limited.

Similarities and Differences of Models

One way to examine the similarities and differences in nursing models is to consider how each author defines components of the nursing paradigm: person, environment, health, and nursing (Table 7-1). Similarities in the models include their consideration of the impact of environment on humans and human interaction with the environment. Behavioral patterning, the holistic human, and maximum functioning of the organism are common themes. For the most part, the differences are more in their emphasis al-

though there are some unique views (e.g., Rogers' emphasis on energy fields and Johnson's conceptualization of a human as a behavioral system). In others particular attention is focused on themes previously introduced in nursing. Neuman emphasizes primary, secondary, and tertiary prevention; Orem's model is organized around self-care; Roy recognizes the human as a psychosocial human being. King's emphasis on transaction fits with Peplau's attention to interpersonal process and more recent literature on contracting.

PSYCHOSOCIAL THEORIES APPLICABLE TO COMMUNITY HEALTH NURSING
Motivation

The influence of motives on behavior and the influence of motivation on achievement or work productivity has long been recognized (Hersey and Blanchard, 1977, p. 5). Between 1900 and 1930 classical theory, also referred to as "scientific management," postulated that the basic motive of man was for economic gain; the emphasis in organizations was on tasks. However, following the studies at the Hawthorne Plant of the Western Electric Company, the classical theory was abandoned for the human relations theory. The human relations theory advocated the importance of job satisfaction and the feeling of belonging to a group (interpersonal relations); thus in the work setting the emphasis in organizations should be on relationships (Hersey and Blanchard, 1977, p. 91).

An early advocate of the human relations movement was Elton Mayo, who noted that the assumptions of many managers about workers was that workers wanted to make as much money as possible for as little work as possible (Hersey and Blanchard, 1977, p. 54). Douglas McGregor developed this thesis further and is now widely known for his list of assumptions about human nature and human motivation, called Theory X and Theory Y. McGregor (1960) drew heavily from Maslow's work on motivation. Although there are other motivation theories, including that of Herzberg (1976), Maslow's are described because his writings have been used most widely in nursing.

Chief Characteristics

Maslow's theory (1970) postulates that the basic driving force or basic motive of people arises from a hierarchy of needs. When needs of the lower hierarchy are met, the need at the next higher level becomes the basic motivating need. The hierarchy of human needs progresses from lower to higher needs as follows: physiological requirements, to safety and security, to social affiliation (love and belonging), to esteem and to self-actualization.

Advantages and Disadvantages

Perhaps more than any other single work, Maslow's writings have given nursing the impetus to view clients as human beings with needs beyond physiological ones. It promoted a movement to look beyond the pathophysiology of disease to the psychosocial needs of clients. However, the broad categories may obscure individuality of clients and their unique reaction to illness.

TABLE 7-1

Definitions of Person, Environment, Health, and Nursing

Nurse Author	Person or Patient/Client	Environment	Health	Nursing
Roy	An adaptive system (Roy, 1980, p. 43); "a complex and dynamic interaction of parts that make a whole . . . functions as a unity for some purposes" (Roy, 1983, p. 262).	"All conditions, circumstances, and influences surrounding and affecting the development and behavior of persons or groups" (Roy, 1983, p. 269).	"A state and a process of being and becoming an integrated and whole person. Integrity means soundness or an unimpaired condition that can lead to completeness or unity" (Roy, 1983, p. 269).	"The science that observes, classifies, and relates the processes by which persons positively affect their health status, and (2) the practice discipline that uses this particular scientific knowledge in providing a service to people" (Roy, 1983, p. 2).
Rogers	"Unitary man—a four-dimensional, negentropic energy field identified by pattern and organization and manifesting characteristics and behaviors that are different from those of the parts and which cannot be predicted from knowledge of the parts" (Rogers, 1980, p. 332).	A four dimensional, negentropic energy field identified by pattern and organization and encompassing all that outside any given human field" (Rogers, 1980, p. 332).	Health not specifically defined; however, she does state that disease and pathology are value terms (Rogers, 1980, p. 336,) and since values change, phenomena perceived as disease such as hyperactivity may change over time and not be perceived as disease.	Goal of nursing is that individuals achieve their maximum health potential through maintenance and promotion of health, prevention of disease, nursing diagnosis, intervention, and rehabilitation (Rogers, 1970, p. 86).
Johnson	Behavioral system (Johnson, 1980, p. 207).	Malfunctions in behavioral systems are frequently caused by "sudden internal or external environmental change" (Johnson, 1980, p. 212; refers to man's interaction with environment p. 209).	"It seems reasonable to assume that health would be considered behavior that is orderly, purposeful, predictable, and functionally efficient and effective" (Johnson, 1980, p. 209).	Goal of nursing is to "restore, maintain, or attain behavioral system balance and stability at the highest possible level for the individual" (Johnson, 1980, p. 214).
Orem	"A psycho-physiological organism with rational powers" (Nursing Development Conference Group 1979, p. 83); "a unity that can be viewed as functioning biologically, symbolically, and socially" (Orem, 1980, p. 120).	Although not explicitly defined, speaks to the role of the nurse in providing a developmental environment (Orem, 1980, p. 66); "environmental elements" (p. 66); "environment as physical and social" (p. 66).	"The state of wholeness or integrity of human beings" (Orem, 1980, p. 118).	"A service, a mode of helping human beings" (Orem, 1980, p. 5); special concern is "the individual's need for self-care action and the provision and management of it on a continuous basis in order to sustain life and health, recover from disease or injury, and cope with their effects" (Orem, 1980, p. 6); "creative effort of one human being to help another human being" (Orem, 1980, p. 55).

TABLE 7-1

Definitions of Person, Environment, Health, and Nursing—cont'd

Nurse Author	Person or Patient/Client	Environment	Health	Nursing
Neuman	"A composite of the inter-relationship of the four variables (physiologic, psychologic, sociocultural, and developmental) that are always present" (Neuman, 1980, p. 121).	"All that which surrounds an individual, all internal and external forces that could affect life and development" (Neuman, 1983, p. 246); "consists of the internal and external forces surrounding man at any point in time. Man is viewed as in constant change or motion—in reciprocal action with the environment" (Neuman, 1982, p. 9).	"Health or wellness is the condition in which all parts and subparts (variables) are in harmony with the whole of man." Disharmony "reduces the wellness state." (Neuman, 1983, p. 246); "consists of the internal and external forces surrounding man at any point in time. Man is viewed as in constant change or motion—in reciprocal action with the environment" (Neuman, 1982, p. 9).	"Nursing can use this model to assist individuals, families, and groups to attain and maintain a maximum of total wellness by purposeful interventions" (Neuman, 1982, p. 11).
King	A social, sentient, rational, reacting, perceiving, controlling, purposeful, action-oriented, and time-oriented being (King, 1981, p. 143).	Writes about environment, but does not define it "the internal environment of human beings transforms energy to enable them to adjust to continuous external environmental changes. . . ." (King, 1981, p. 5)	"dynamic life experiences of a human being, which implies continuous adjustment to stressors in the internal and external environment through optimum use of one's resources to achieve maximum potential for daily living" (King, 1981, p. 5).	"Nursing is perceiving, thinking, relating, judging, and acting vis-a-vis the behavior of individuals who come to a nursing situation" (King, 1981, p. 2). "Nursing is a process of human interactions between nurse and client whereby each perceives the other and the situation; and through communication, they set goals, explore means, and agree on means to achieve goals."

Application to Community Health Nursing

Many nursing programs have used Maslow's **hierarchy of needs** as a model for curriculum. An example of how it generally is applied to nursing care planning is as follows: (1) Problem: Failure to thrive, (2) Interference with basic human need: Social affiliation or love and belonging, (3) Nursing plan and implementation: Set goals for mother or mother-surrogate to meet need of social affiliation, and (4) Evaluation: Assess alleviation of problem.

As mentioned above, the categories of needs are broad, and often how the need is being interfered with has to be further delineated before action can be taken.

Change

Change is constant and inevitable; some changes are planned, others are unplanned. Since an objective of most baccalaureate programs is for their graduates to be change agents, planned change is of concern here. "Planned change is a conscious, deliberate, and collaborative effort to improve operations of human systems . . . through the utilization of valid knowledge" (Bennis, Benne, Chin, and Corey, 1976, p.4). Lewin (1951), the noted psychologist, applied concepts from field theory to the process of change.

Chief Characteristics of Change

According to field theory, change occurs in a three-step process: unfreezing, moving, and refreezing. Unfreezing begins with dissatisfaction with the present system or a feeling that things need to be different. The dissatisfaction may occur first among or within the group members. The leader must promote the unfreezing process or the willingness of the group members to give up their old or familiar ways of doing things and to be willing to consider alternatives to the present situation. A major part of unfreezing is called force field analysis, or identifying forces in support of the change (driving forces) and those forces that fail to support or are against the change (restraining forces) (Bernhard and Walsh, 1981, p. 143).

The second step in the change process, moving, involves implementing the change. Three change strategies are: empirical-rational, normative-reeducative, and power-coercion (Chin and Benne, 1976, p. 23). The empirical-rational strategy provides people with knowledge that the change will make things better; for example, chlorine added to the water supply makes it safe for drinking. The normative-reeducative strategy goes beyond an increase in knowledge to include change in values and attitudes. For example, a change in format of a nursing procedure or a nursing process would require a change in the nurse's value and attitude that the change was for the better. The power-coercive strategy implements change by the use of power. An administrator may make a change without any input from the staff members, that is, the individual uses the power base for the change.

The final stage in the change process is called refreezing. In refreezing the newly acquired behavior has been practiced and is stable.

Advantages and Disadvantages

The model of change as related to field theory enables people who want to implement change to recognize the elements in a situation that must be assessed and known and to develop a way to proceed. A change agent who has taken into consideration the elements that must be considered in the change process is much more likely to benefit from an accepted and lasting change.

Application to Community Health Nursing

Suppose a community health nurse in a middle management position has just attended a conference on problem-oriented records and thinks that system would be an improvement over the system currently being used. According to the first stage in change theory, unfreezing, the manager would need to determine if any of the staff were dissatisfied with their own method. If dissatisfactions about the current method exist, the unfreezing process has begun. The nurse then needs to ask the staff to discuss their views on the process currently used. In this way the nurse can identify the driving and restraining forces in the staff and move toward presenting the proposed change to administration to see if they support the change. If there is enough support for the next stage, then it is time for the moving stage. This stage may mean sending others to a conference on problem-oriented medical records or inviting someone to come in and present a conference. This would be the normative-reeducative strategy. Then the change would be implemented and the refreezing phase would begin.

Communication

Communication or the act of transmitting, giving, or exchanging information (Webster's New World Dictionary, 1978) can be described by use of two simple models. The first model (Figure 7-1) is linear and consists of a sender, a message, and a receiver. The second, seen in Figure 7-2,

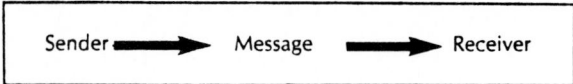

FIGURE 7-1

Linear model of communication.

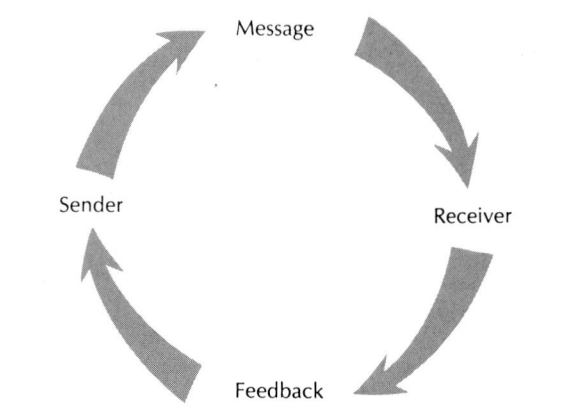

FIGURE 7-2

Circular model of communication.

is circular and includes a sender, a message receiver, and feedback.

More elaborate models exist in the literature, and Lancaster (1982, pp. 111-112), has described four models of communication theory:

1. The systems approach which consists of input—processing—output and feedback.
2. The questioning approach which consists of asking the questions of who? what? how? to whom? and to what effect? (feedback).
3. Human relations model described as generation of idea, encoding, transmission, receipt of message, decoding, and action.
4. A composite model which consists of generation of idea, encoding transmission, receipt of message, decoding, action, and feedback to encoding.

Chief Characteristics

FORM. Communication is the expression of a message in at least four forms: art, written, verbal, and non-verbal. Music, art, poetry, and literature are all forms of expression and communication. Written words in the form of books, articles, and letters are another way of communicating. Verbal communication is through language or symbols; the most obvious example is television. The nonverbal form of communication includes body movements and facial expression, voice tone and quality, allocation of personal space, touch, and personal expression such as style of dress.

PURPOSE. Human communication is generally carried out for the following purposes: (1) to give information, (2) to obtain information, (3) to release tension and, (4) to problem-solve.

SITUATIONAL VARIABLES. Variables that affect the communication and have a part in whether it is successful or unsuccessful include: (a) relationship between those communicating, (b) perception of the topic by those communicating, and (c) beliefs, values, and attitudes of those involved in the communication.

Advantages and Disadvantages

The communication model illustrates that communication is a circular process, an exchange, that requires processing and interpretation.

Application to Community Health Nursing

The community health nurse is most often a person who elicits information from a patient and consequently is the receiver of information. Some general guidelines or techniques for more effective communication are as follows:

1. Attend and receive the message as an active listener.
2. Clarify the message by asking for an illustration.
3. Reflect and paraphrase to check accuracy of message received.
4. Validate and summarize at the close of the session.

Leadership

Leadership is the "process of influencing the activities of an individual or a group in efforts toward goal achievement" (Hersey and Blanchard, p. 85). Two ways of describing leadership are generally used. One way is to describe styles of leadership. Style refers to the way in which a person practices leadership, or the way of acting. Although there are others, the three most recognized styles of leadership are autocratic, democratic, and laissez-faire. The second way of describing leadership is by theories of leadership. As defined previously in this chapter (p. 132), the purpose of a theory is to describe, predict, and explain. Thus theories on leadership attempt to describe the concepts in leadership and the relationship between them; in other words, it tries to determine what elements constitute leadership or, in some cases, what elements constitute a leader.

Chief Characteristics

STYLES. Style refers to the amount of control the leader exerts over subordinates vs the amount of freedom allowed to them. The autocratic style uses maximum control, makes decisions, and tells the subordinates what to do, when to do, how to do, and then how well they did it in either the form of praise or criticism. The democratic leader invites input from the group in decision making and allows some flexibility in how and when to implement the decision. The group receives feedback from the leader in a more factual way rather than in a judgmental way. The democratic group also receives feedback from each other. The laissez-faire leader gives the group total freedom and is sometimes seen as a person who abdicates leadership responsibility. Stogdill (1974, pp. 365-370), reported that autocratic and democratic groups show about the same productivity, whereas the laissez-faire group showed less productivity, less satisfaction, and less cohesiveness. The democratic group showed more group cohesiveness, and the autocratic group demanded more attention from the leader.

THEORIES. Earlier theories of leadership can be considered descriptive in that they describe a single factor as the key to effective leadership. The first of these was the great man theory. The great man theory postulated that some are "born leaders." This was consistent with the practice of passing the leadership role from the king, who was father and leader, to his son. A second descriptive theory of leadership is trait theory. This theory put together all the traits that make a good leader. These traits included physical stature, intelligence, education, personality, charisma, and socioeconomic status.

A third theory of leadership, called situation theory, used the idea of the right person being in the right place at the right time. The question is often asked about some leaders, for example: Did Napoleon make history or did history make Napoleon? According to situation theory, history made Napoleon. A fourth theory was called interaction theory, which postulated that it was neither the person's personality nor the situation, but a combination of the two. Thus anyone could become a leader in the right situation (Bernhard and Walsh, pp. 45-47).

More recently, especially since the early 1960s, theories of leadership have evolved that emphasize consideration of multiple factors in determining effective leadership. These reflect influence from motivation theories, but they have also considered the styles of leadership, the followers themselves, and the situation. Studies at the University of Michigan identified two important aspects of leadership, which they called employee orientation and production orientation. Leadership studies at Ohio State identified the two dimensions of leadership as initiation of structure and consideration. *Structure* was concerned with the task behavior, and *consideration* was concerned with relationship behavior. During the Ohio State studies, these dimensions were plotted on vertical and horizontal axes to form four quadrants. Blake and Mouton also used this way of showing leadership dimension, referred to it as a managerial grid, and used the terms "concern for people" and "concern for production." The outcome of these and other studies led Hersey and Blanchard (1977, p. 100) to conclude that it was unrealistic to think of a single ideal type of leadership behavior. They used the two axes to plot leadership, with task behavior on the horizontal axis and relationship behavior on the vertical axis. They added maturity of followers on the horizontal axis, projected effectiveness, and called it the *Tri-Dimensional Leader Effectiveness Model* (Hersey and Blanchard, 1977, p. 105). The effectiveness of the leadership behavior demands that the leader use the appropriate style of leadership for the appropriate situation. This meant that the leader's style varied from one situation to another. This has led to the general acceptance that effectiveness of leadership depends on the leader's ability to behave according to the situation and the followers.

Advantages and Disadvantages

The Tri-Dimensional Leader Effectiveness Model by Hersey and Blanchard supports the position that leadership skills can be taught and learned. It does not give credence to the idea that leadership is a bit of magic and that only certain individuals are born with the necessary characteristics. Every nurse is a leader in some arena and will be a more effective leader if she can take into consideration all the variables that influence leadership effectiveness.

Application to Community Health Nursing

A large number of health professionals are involved in the delivery of health care, and the nurse is often expected to offer the needed leadership. The leader must take into consideration the task or goal to be accomplished, group needs, including their relationship needs, and the situation.

The nurse brings to the situation knowledge about change theory, motivation theory, group process skills, and interactional skills. All of these are needed for effective leadership.

CLINICAL APPLICATION

To illustrate the clinical application of conceptual framework to practice, a case is presented, two nursing diagnoses are identified, and the approach to assessment is presented using the framework of seven conceptual frameworks, which would lead to identification of the problems and the formulation of nursing diagnoses.

Case Example

Timothy is a 2-week-old infant of a teenage mother. When the infant returns to the well baby clinic, at age 2 weeks, he has not regained his birth weight. Two obvious areas the nurse would want to assess would be the food intake of the infant and the interaction between mother and her infant. For purposes of this case example these will be referred to as nutrition and mother-infant interaction.

NUTRITION: ALTERATION IN

Maslow's basic human need	Physiological need for nutrition
Orem	Universal self-care requisite of food
Roy	Physiological need of nutrition
Johnson	Ingestive system
Rogers	Openness (intake and output of food)
Neuman	Intrapersonal factors
King	Personal system

PARENTING: POTENTIAL FOR ALTERATION IN

Maslow's basic human need	Need for love and belonging, or need for security
Orem	Universal need for social interaction
Roy	Adaptative mode of role
Johnson	Affiliative subsystem
Rogers	Energy fields
Neuman	Interpersonal factors
King	Interpersonal system

Comparison

In the assessment of this infant, the nurse as she uses each framework, would employ terms and phrases that match the broader frame of reference of the particular conceptual model. However, in this particular case, the nursing diagnosis would be the same.

SUMMARY

This chapter has presented selected conceptual models and their usefulness in guiding the practice of community health nurses. The importance of theory development and scientific inquiry to nursing was reviewed, key terms were defined, and the usefulness of conceptual models to nursing education, nursing research, and nursing practice was described. The ANA and the APHA conceptual models specific to community health nursing, as well as interdisciplinary, nursing, and psychosocial models, were included.

Interdisciplinary models applicable to community health nursing presented included systems, developmental, and interaction; for each of these models an evaluation was made about its main characteristics, general advantages and disadvantages, and its application of community health nursing. Descriptions of the conceptual models from the nursing literature by Roy, Rogers, Johnson, Orem, Neuman, and King included characteristics, application to practice, and strengths and limitations. Only if such models are clearly understood, including their good and bad points, can they ultimately become useful in practice, education, and research.

Finally, the psychosocial theories of motivation, communication, and change were explored. As in the discussion of both nursing and interdisciplinary models, the reader's attention was directed to the overview, chief characteristics, advantages and disadvantages, and application to community health nursing.

KEY CONCEPTS

Community health nursing has historically reflected the qualities of both art and science; however, for nursing to advance it must develop as a theory-based profession.

Most of what are referred to in nursing as theories are actually conceptual models.

A conceptual model is a "set of concepts and those assumptions that integrate them into a meaningful configuration."

Conceptual models of nursing specify varying relationships and interactions among four essential components: person, environment, health, and nursing.

Conceptual models having the greatest application to community health nursing view people as being in continuous interaction with their environment.

In nursing practice, education, and research, conceptual models give direction and simplify and help organize information.

Both the ANA and APHA definitions of community health nursing emphasize the blending of nursing and public health knowledge as a foundation for determining the scope of practice. Both models acknowledge that CHN efforts are directed toward all people, emphasize a multidisciplinary role for nurses, and focus on the increasing priority of health promotion.

Interdisciplinary conceptual models with applications to community health nursing are systems theory, developmental theory, and interaction models.

Conceptual models specific to nursing have been developed by Roy, Rogers, Johnson, Orem, and King.

Among the psychosocial theories applicable to nursing, the writings of Maslow have been most widely used. Maslow's theory states that the basic motivations of individuals arise from a hierachy of needs.

Change is an important concept in community health nursing. According to Lewin's application of field theory to the change process, change occurs in three steps: unfreezing, moving, and refreezing.

Along with change, communication and leadership are important psychosocial concepts with applications to community health nursing.

LEARNING ACTIVITIES

1. Write down what you consider to be the major themes in nursing. Compare with the general themes cited in this chapter. How are they alike? How do they differ?

2. Select one of the conceptual models used by an early nursing leader and evaluate its potential usefulness to contemporary practice.

3. Identify several concepts in nursing that you think are related. Using the concepts, try to construct a conceptual framework, a model, and a theory. Do not be discouraged that it is not an easy task. It will help you understand the terms.

4. Debate one of these issues; (1) conceptual models should (should not) guide nursing practice or (2) conceptual models help (hinder) community health nursing practice.

BIBLIOGRAPHY

American Nurses' Association: A conceptual model of community health nursing practice, Kansas City, Mo., 1980, The Association.

American Public Health Association: The definition and role of public health nursing in the delivery of health care, Washington, D.C., 1981, The Association.

Anna, D.J., et al: Implementing Orem's conceptual framework . . . core of Orem's philosophy is the belief that man has an innate ability to care for himself. J. Nursing Admin. 8:8-11, 1978.

Auger, J.A., and Dee, V.: A patient classification system based on the behavioral system model of nursing, Part 1, J. Nurs. Adm 13(4):38-43, 1983.

Bennis, W.G., et al., editors: The planning of change, New York, 1976, Holt, Rinehart and Winston.

Bertalanffy, L.V.: Problems of life: an evaluation of modern biological and scientific thought, New York, 1952, Harper Brothers.

Bernhard, L.A., and Walsh, M.: Leadership—

the key to the professionalization of nursing, New York, 1981, McGraw-Hill Book Co.

Burr, W.R., et al., editors: Contemporary theories about the family, New York, 1979, Free Press.

Bush, H.A.: Models for nursing, Adv. Nurs. Science 1:13, 1979.

Chin, R.: The utility of system models and developmental models for practitioners. In Riehl, J.P., and Roy, S.C., editors: Conceptual models for nursing practice, ed. 2, New York, 1980, Appleton-Century-Crofts.

Chin, R., and Benne, K.D.: General strategies for effecting changes in human systems. In Bennis, W.G., et al., editors: The planning of change, New York, 1976, Holt, Rinehart and Winston.

Cooley, C.H.: Social organization, New York, 1909, Scribner's.

Derdiarian, A.K., and Forsythe, A.B.: An instrument for theory and research development using the behavioral systems model for nursing: the cancer patient, Nurs. Res. 32:260, 1983.

Eliopoulos, C.: A self care model for gerontological nursing, Geriatric Nurs. 5(8):366-9, 1984.

Duvall, E.M.: Marriage and family development, ed. 5, Philadelphia, 1977, J.B. Lippincott.

Fagan, J., and Shepherd. I.L.: Gestalt therapy now, Palo Alto, Calif., 1970, Science and Behavior Books.

Falco, S.M., and Lobo, M.L. In George, J.: Nursing theories: the base for professional nursing practice. Englewood Cliffs, N.J., 1980, Prentice-Hall, Inc.

Fawcett, J.: A framework for analysis and evaluation of conceptual models of nursing, Nurse Educator 5(6):10, 1980.

Fawcett, J.: Analysis and evaluation of conceptual models of nursing, Philadelphia, 1984, F.A. Davis.

Fitts, W.H.: Tennessee self-concept scale manual, Nashville, Tenn., 1965, Counselor Recording and Tests.

George, J.B.: The base for professional nursing practice, ed. 2, Englewood Cliffs, N.J., 1985, Prentice-Hall, Inc.

Heidt, P.: Effect of therapeutic touch on anxiety level of hospitalized patients, Nurs. Res. 30(1):32, 1981.

Hersey, P., and Blanchard, K.H.: Management of organizational behavior: utilizing human resources, ed. 3, Englewood Cliffs, N.J., 1977, Prentice-Hall, Inc.

Herzberg, F.: The managerial choice: to be efficient and to be human, Homewood, Ill., 1976, Dow Jones-Irwin, 1976.

Johnson, D.E.: The behavioral system model for nursing. In Riehl, J.P., and Roy, S.C.: Conceptual models for nursing practice, ed. 2, New York, 1980, Appleton-Century-Crofts.

Johnston, R.L., and Fitzpatrick, J.J.: Relevance of psychiatric mental health nursing theories to nursing models. In Fitzpatrick, J.J., et al.: Nursing models and their psychiatric mental health applications, Bowie, Md., 1982, Robert J. Brad Co.

King, I.: A conceptual frame of reference for nursing, Nurs. Res. 17(1):27, 1968.

King, I.: A theory for nursing: systems, concepts, process, New York, 1981, John Wiley & Sons.

King, I.: The "why" of theory development. In National League for Nursing: Theory development, what, why, how? New York, 1978.

Krieger, D.: Foundations for holistic health nursing practices: the renaissance nurse. Philadelphia: 1981, J.B. Lippincott.

Lancaster, J., and Lancaster W., editors: Concepts for advanced nursing practice: the nurse as change agent. St. Louis, 1982, The C.V. Mosby Co.

Lewin, K.: Field theory in social science, New York, 1951, Harper.

Lewis, M.: Clinical aspects of child development, ed. 2, Philadelphia, 1982, Lea & Febiger.

Mead, G.H.: Mind, self and society, Chicago, 1934, University of Chicago Press.

Maslow, A.H.: Motivation and personality, ed. 2, New York, 1970, Harper & Row.

McGregor, D.: The human side of enterprise, New York, 1960, McGraw-Hill Book Co.

Melis, A.: Theoretical nursing: Development and progress, Philadelphia, 1985, F.A. Davis.

Neuman, B.: Family intervention using the Betty Neuman Health care. In Clements, I.W., and Roberts, F.B.: Family health: a theoretical approach to nursing care, New York, 1983. John Wiley & Sons.

Neuman, B., and Young, R.J.: A model for teaching total person approach to patient problems, Nurs. Res. 21:264, 1972.

Neuman, B.: The Betty Neuman health care systems model: a total person approach to patient problems. In Riehl, J.P., and Roy, S.C., editors: Conceptual models for nursing practice, ed. 2, New York, 1980. Appleton-Century-Crofts.

Neuman, B.: The Neuman systems model: application to nursing education and practice, Norwalk, Conn., 1982, Appleton-Century-Crofts.

Orem, D.: Nursing: concepts of practice, ed. 2, New York, 1980, McGraw-Hill Book Co.

Orem, D.: Nursing: concepts of practice, ed. 3, New York, 1985, McGraw-Hill Book Co.

Riehl, J.P., and Roy, C.: Conceptual models for nursing practice, 2nd ed., New York, 1980, Appleton-Century-Crofts.

Rogers, M.E.: Nursing: a science of unitary man. In Riehl, J.P., and Roy, C.S., editors: Conceptual models for nursing practice, New York, 1980, Appleton-Century-Crofts.

Rogers, M.E.: An introduction to the theoretical basis of nursing, Philadelphia, 1970, F.A. Davis.

Rose, A., editor: Human behavior and social processes: an interactionist approach, Boston, 1962, Houghton Mifflin.

Roy, C.: Introduction to nursing: an adaptation model. Englewood Cliffs, N.J., 1976, Prentice-Hall, Inc.

Roy, C.: Introduction to nursing: an adaptation model, ed. 2, Englewood Cliffs, N.J., 1984, Prentice-Hall, Inc.

Roy, S.C., and Roberts, S.L.: Theory construction in nursing: an adaptation model. Englewood Cliffs, N.J., 1981, Prentice-Hall, Inc.

Stogdill, R.N.: Handbook of leadership: a survey of theory and research, New York, 1974, Free Press.

Thibodeau, J.A.: Nursing models: analysis and evaluation, Monterey, Calif., 1983, Wadsworth Health Sciences Division.

Walker, L.O., and Avant, K.C.: Strategies for theory construction in nursing, Norwalk, Conn., 1983, Appleton-Century-Crofts.

Williams, C.A.: The nature and development of conceptual frameworks. In Downs, F.S., and Fleming, J.W.: Issues in nursing research, New York, 1979, Appleton-Century-Crofts.

Yura, H., and Torres, G.: Todays' conceptual framework within baccalaureate nursing programs. In Faculty-Curriculum Development. Part III. Conceptual Framework—Its Meaning and Function, New York, 1975, National League for Nursing.

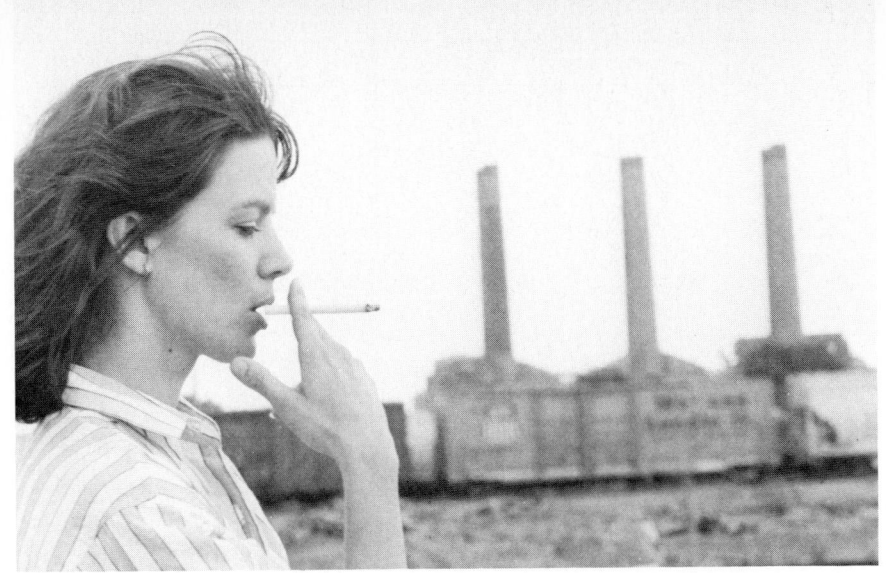

Barbara Valanis

8

THE EPIDEMIOLOGICAL MODEL IN COMMUNITY HEALTH NURSING

OBJECTIVES

After reading this chapter the student should be able to:

Describe the science of epidemiology, its concepts, principles, and methods.

Illustrate general uses of epidemiology.

Interpret the relevance of epidemiological research findings to community health nursing practice.

KEY TERMS

advanced disease

agent

attack rates

causality

confounding variable

descriptive epidemiology

ecological fallacy

ecological studies

endemic

environment

epidemic

epidemiology

immunity

incidence

incubation period

inherent resistance

levels of prevention

morbidity

mortality

natural history

pandemic

pathogenesis

person-year

prepathogenesis

prevalence

rate

relational studies

risk

specific protection

substantive epidemiology

surveillance

susceptibility

transmission cycle

web of causation

Epidemiology is a community health science and is essential to nursing practice. In the same way that knowledge of human physiology provides a basis for diagnostic and treatment decisions in medical practice, epidemiology provides a basis for diagnosis and treatment in community health practice. Whereas a physician uses the basic medical science of physiology in diagnosing and treating an individual patient, the community health practitioner uses epidemiology in diagnosing and treating a community.

HISTORY AND DEFINITION

The term *epidemiology* is derived from three Greek words: (1) *epi,* upon; (2) *demos,* the people; and (3) *logos,* science. Thus it is the science of events that occur in a community of people. The following definition reflects the major components of the modern discipline: "Epidemiology is the study of the distribution of states of health and of the determinants of deviations from health in populations." The purpose of epidemiology is to identify the etiology of deviations from health and to provide the data necessary to prevent and control disease through community health intervention.

Epidemiologists study a variety of factors related to the environment and the people in that environment in an attempt to identify the determinants of observed patterns of health. Epidemiologists function as detectives concerned with the entire spectrum of health status from health to serious illness. They seek to identify the who, what, where, when, and how of disease causation. By comparing the characteristics of persons, places, and time associated with a particular illness with these same characteristics for those who do not have the illness, epidemiologists narrow down the suspected causal agents of that illness. Once an agent is identified and the susceptible population recognized, epidemiologists attempt to identify the means by which the agent is transmitted to the susceptible human population. This information provides a basis for intervention by community health officials who can act to prevent or control occurrence of the disease by removing the agent, by reducing the susceptibility of the population, or by interfering with the transmission of the agent to the human population.

Epidemiology is an ancient and for the most part observational science. People have been trying for thousands of years to determine what causes disease. Supernatural events were one of the first factors used to explain the occurrence of illness. As long ago as 460-377 BC, Hippocrates, considered by some to be the first epidemiologist, tried to explain disease occurrence on a rational rather than a supernatural basis, pointing out that environment and lifestyle are related to the occurrence of disease.

During Biblical times, public health measures were instituted on the basis of observations about occurrence of disease, even when the actual disease agent was unknown. For example, the ancient practice of isolating lepers arose from the observation that the disease often developed in those persons who came in close physical contact with a leper.

In more recent years the investigative observations of John Snow in England resulted in the initiation of intervention measures to prevent the use of certain water supplies. His work in the 1850s led him to suspect contaminated water as the source of cholera outbreaks. By measuring the frequency of cholera deaths in relation to the number of people living in a geographical area, he determined that rates of cholera mortality were much higher among certain parts of the city with a common water supply than among other sections with a different water supply. Thus measures could be taken by public health officials to limit the occurrence of cholera by control of contaminated water even though the actual agent, the cholera vibrio, was as yet unknown (Snow, 1936). Koch finally isolated the cholera vibrio in 1883.

Most early epidemiological observations and investigations were related to occurrences of infectious disease and lacked a systematic approach to investigation. The development of rates such as Snow's mortality observations provided a scientific basis for systematic study of health and illness distributions. As data on infectious diseases accumulated and led to public health intervention, infectious diseases were largely controlled. After that, disease of a chronic nature with noninfectious origins became more common, taking over as major causes of morbidity (illness) and mortality (death), particularly in industrialized nations (Figure 8-1). In 1900, infectious diseases accounted for over 40% of deaths and heart disease, cancer, and stroke for less than half of deaths from noninfectious diseases. By 1982, death from infectious disease was uncommon. Heart disease, cancer, and stroke respectively accounted for 49%, 22%, and 8% of all deaths (NCHS, 1985).

However, infectious diseases are again becoming a focus

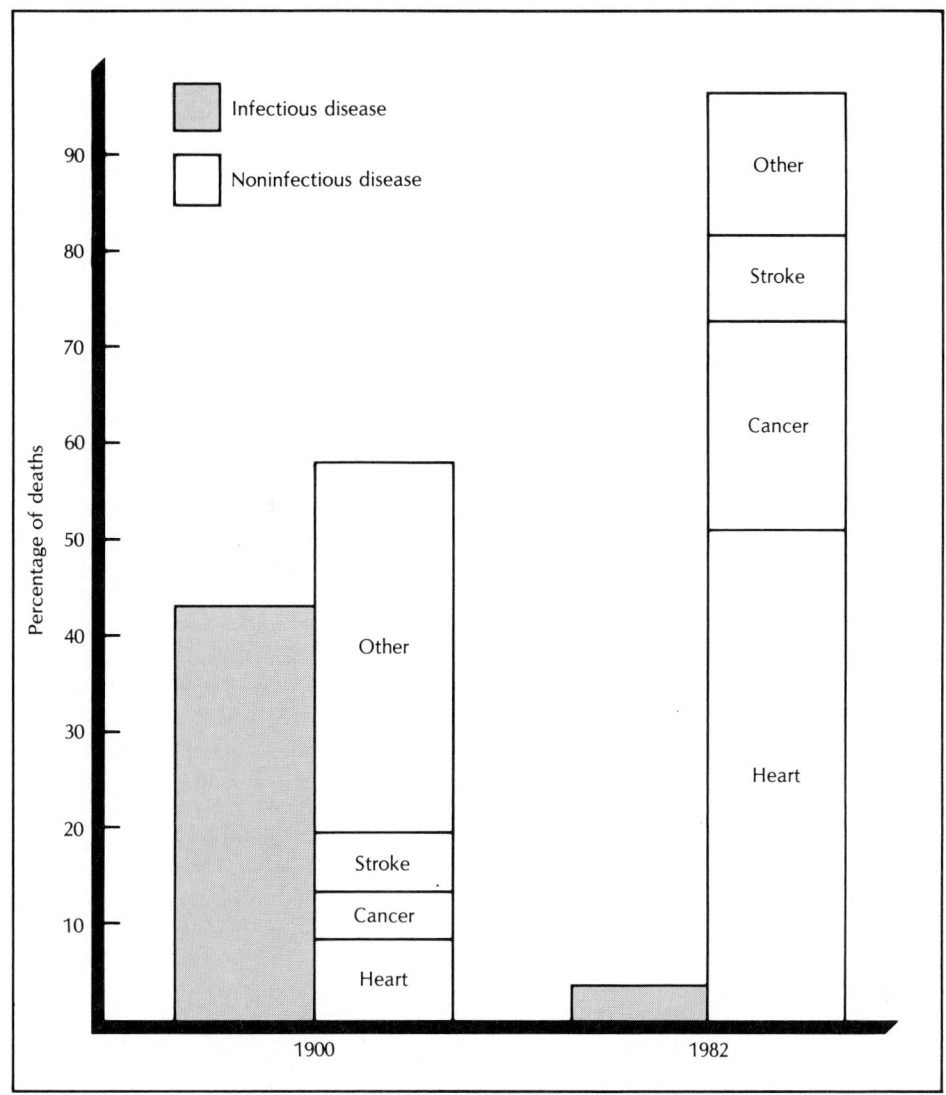

FIGURE 8-1

Proportional distribution of deaths from infectious and major noninfectious diseases, United States, 1900 and 1982.

of attention. The advent of procedures such as organ transplants requiring concurrent use of immunosuppressive drugs and widespread use of chemotherapy for cancer have contributed to the presence in hospitals of immune-suppressed or immune-impaired patients, who are highly susceptible to infection. For these patients, common organisms in the hospital environment, including staphylococci, gram-negative bacteria, and fungal organisms can be lethal. Elderly persons and others whose resistance is lowered by their disease process are also at risk. As a result, infection control has become a major program in most hospitals. Similarly, infectious disease has emerged as a community problem. For example, gonorrhea incidence has risen dramatically in response to a variety of factors, including funding cutbacks in venereal disease programs during the 1960s and 1970s, virulence of new strains introduced by veterans returning from Vietnam, and changing sexual mores subsequent to widespread introduction of the contraceptive pill in the 1960s. Genital herpes is on the rise. In 1983 and

1984, outbreaks of measles were observed among students at several universities. Other infectious diseases in the news in the past 10 years include Legionnaire's disease, toxic shock syndrome, listeriosis, and most recently acquired immune deficiency syndrome (AIDS). Except for AIDS, however, these are primarily associated with morbidity; relatively few deaths are involved.

Epidemiological investigations today focus on infectious disease; noninfectious, chronic conditions such as heart disease, cancer, and stroke; acute events such as spontaneous abortion or accidents; and a wide spectrum of emotional and mental health conditions such as depression or alcoholism. In addition, epidemiology is no longer limited to the study of diseases or patterns of ill health; it also focuses on description of normal characteristics of populations. Instances of such focus include studies of body weight in relation to height and of blood group subtypes in different population groups. By extending its scope to include mental and social conditions in addition to disease, epidemiology has helped behavioral scientists, social workers, community health planners, and all those concerned with the health and well-being of human populations. It is truly multidisciplinary, both providing information to the medical, social, and behavioral sciences and drawing on these sciences in its research.

COMPONENTS OF EPIDEMIOLOGY

The term *epidemiology* has come to refer both to the particular methods applied in studies of disease causation and to the body of knowledge that arises from such investigations. The collection of epidemiological knowledge is usually termed substantive epidemiology, although some authors may refer to it as descriptive epidemiology. In this chapter, the term *descriptive epidemiology* refers to the first phase of epidemiological research, which includes observations and recordings of the existing patterns of a disease occurrence. The term *substantive epidemiology* refers to the body of knowledge, the known epidemiological characteristics of a particular disease or illness. This epidemiological description of a particular disease, which constitutes the substantive epidemiology for that condition, includes the natural history of the disease, patterns of occurrence; and factors associated with high risk for developing the disease (risk factors).

There are two ways to describe a disease—the clinical description and the epidemiological description (see Table 8-1). The clinical description relates to the onset and progression of symptoms in individuals similarly affected. The

epidemiologist has to single out in terms of probabilities, averages, and means those demographic and physiological characteristics that are most common in the diseased population. Hence statistics are a crucial tool for the epidemiologist.

An episode of food poisoning illustrates the distinction between a clinical and epidemiological approach to illness. Clinicians (nurse practitioners, physicians) record the signs and symptoms such as elevated temperature, presence of nausea and vomiting, or diarrhea that are experienced by the patient. After taking a careful history and performing a thorough physical examination, supplemented if necessary by laboratory tests, clinicians consider the differential diagnoses and come to the conclusion that the most likely diagnosis is gastroenteritis attributable to food poisoning. They then institute treatment and record the patient's progress in terms of when symptoms were relieved.

Epidemiologists describe this event in terms of how it affects the group. They note the time and place of onset of symptoms in all the sick individuals who can be identified, preferably including those with symptoms too mild to require medical treatment. They also assemble data on the circumstances related to the illness for all individuals in the group to determine if they share a common circumstance. This may lead to a suspected common source of infection, such as food at a church supper. To identify the likely food item responsible for the poisoning, precise information is gathered on all the various foods eaten by those present. A comparison is made of illness rates among all those present

---

=== **TABLE 8-1**

Comparison of epidemiology and physiology

	Epidemiology	Physiology
	Scientific method	
Tools	Epidemiological methodology	Physiological methodology
Knowledge Outcome	Trends in disease occurrence	Physiology of human body
	Distribution of populations at high risk of disease	
	Social, economic, biological, and genetic determinants of disease	
	Natural history of disease	
Purpose	Diagnosis and treatment in community health practice	Diagnosis and treatment decisions in medical practice
Focus	Group	Individual

=== **TABLE 8-2**

Distribution of blood pressure and weight as independent and nonindependent factors

Weight	Independent factors			Nonindependent factors		
	High blood pressure (%)	Low blood pressure (%)	Total (%)	High blood pressure (%)	Low blood pressure (%)	Total (%)
Overweight	2	18	20	7	13	20
Not overweight	8	72	80	3	77	80
TOTAL	10	90	100	10	90	100

at the supper who ate each food and those who did not. Once the contaminated food is identified, attempts are made to determine the source of the contamination. Often the source is someone involved in the food preparation. Once the source is identified, community health measures such as treatment of the person carrying the organism and instruction in hygienic food practices must be instituted to assure that the event does not recur.

BASIC EPIDEMIOLOGICAL CONCEPTS
Causality

In common usage the term *cause* is generally understood to mean a stimulus that produces an effect or outcome. Cause in epidemiology also deals with something that produces an effect or outcome. However, since an epidemiologist must investigate causal relationships between a stimulus and an outcome by use of statistical measures of association, it is important to understand ways in which events or circumstances may be related in statistical terms. The first level of relationship to be ascertained is that of statistical association or independency. In statistical terms, two events are said to be independent if the probability that the two events occur together is equal to the probability that one occurs times the probability that the other occurs. For example, in Table 8-2 under Independent Factors, we find that in a given community 20% of the adult population is overweight and 10% of this population has high blood pressure. If the proportion of individuals exhibiting both characteristics (overweight and high blood pressure) is exactly 2% (the product of 20% × 10% = 2%), these two events are considered statistically independent of each other. The grouping for high blood pressure and overweight does, in fact, contain 2% of the population. By contrast, in Table 8-2 under Nonindependent Factors, although the percent who are overweight remains at 20% and the percent who have high blood pressure remains at 10% of the population, the proportion of individuals who are overweight and also have high blood pressure is 7%. This is more than three times the 2% that we calculated would be expected by chance alone. In this case these two factors are not independent. A variety of statistical tests for independence of factors is used in analysis of epidemiological data. The type of test depends on the structure of the data. Thus in sta-

tistical terms, before a relationship between two factors is considered for further investigation of *causality,* the distribution of the two factors must be one that cannot be accounted for by chance alone; that is, they have a statistically significant association.

It is important to stress that statistical associations are determined for *categories or groups* and not for individual instances. In the example given in Table 8-2, under Independent Factors it is not possible to say that high blood pressure and overweight caused any individual to have heart disease. However, the information under Nonindependent Factors may suggest the possibility of causal association in an individual instance. This is particularly true if the association between two categories of events is strong.

Once it has been determined that two factors are not independent but that they have a significant association, the next step is to determine whether the relationship is causal. As illustrated in Figure 8-2, nonindependent associations may be causally or noncausally related. *Direct causal associations* are those in which a factor causes a disease with no other variables intervening.

$$A \longrightarrow B$$

Apparent directness depends on the limitations of current knowledge, and what is considered a direct association may become indirect, since further studies of causal mechanisms may reveal a new, more direct cause for the association. For example, the early studies of toxic shock syndrome implicated tampons as the probable cause. More recent research has indicated that the presence of staphylococcal organisms in the vagina is the actual direct cause. The tampons are a contributing cause in that they create an ideal environment for proliferation of the organism (Centers for Disease Control, 1980).

In *indirect causal associations* a third variable called *intervening variable* occupies an intermediate stage between the cause and effect.

$$A \longrightarrow B \longrightarrow C \longrightarrow D$$

For example, breathing air polluted by cigarette or other smoke (A) causes damage to the respiratory epithelium (intervening variable B); this damage increases the suscepti-

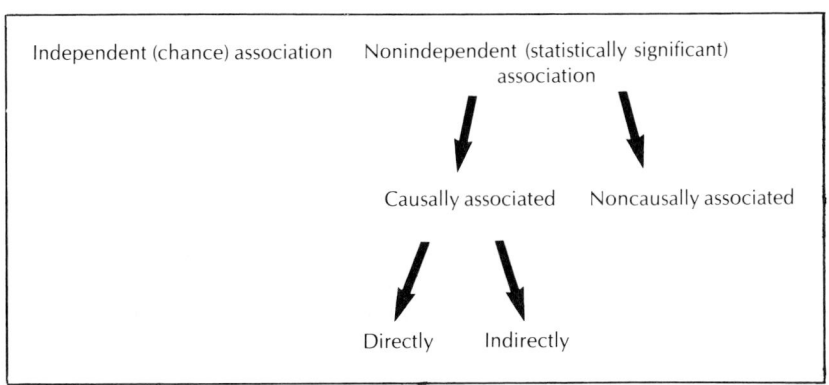

FIGURE 8-2

Types of statistical associations.

bility of the epithelium to infection (intervening variable C); this results in chronic bronchitis (D).

Finally, as illustrated in Figure 8-2, although an association may be nonindependent, it may also be *noncausally associated*. This type of variable rides with the causal variable and varies systematically with it. It is called a **confounding variable**. When uncontrolled, its effect cannot be distinguished from the effects of a hypothetical causal variable under study with which it is highly correlated. Age, if uncontrolled, is a confounding variable for an association between duration of exposure to a toxic chemical and its associated health outcome. If the health outcome increases in frequency with age, an analysis looking at duration might show an increase in duration. However, since age and duration increase together, removing the aging effect may also remove the association with duration.

The ultimate determination of whether an association is causal is through an epidemiological experiment. Thus for practical purposes a factor is considered causal if reducing the amount or frequency of occurrence of the suspected cause reduces the frequency of the effect, in this case the frequency of the illness of interest. For example, if treating hypertensive individuals to keep their blood pressure low reduces the frequency of stroke compared with the frequency of stroke in an equivalent, untreated group of hypertensive individuals, hypertension would be considered a cause of stroke.

There are instances when an epidemiological experiment is not feasible or desirable. In these instances, criteria are needed for making decisions regarding intervention based on available epidemiological data. The five criteria generally used for assessing causality in such instances were presented in the 1964 Surgeon General's report, in which they were used for assessing the causal relationship between smoking and a variety of health outcomes. They are (1) evidence that exposure to the causal factor occurred before the disease process began, (2) strength of the association, (3) specificity of the association, (4) consistency of the association among various epidemiological studies, and (5) the existence of a biological mechanism to explain how an agent could produce the disease.

A cause can be any of a large number of characteristics relating to time, place, person, or events. Modern epidemiology has moved ahead from the "single-cause idea" and recognizes the presence of multiple causes in any biological phenomenon. However, the single-cause model of the past has its usefulness, particularly in the control of infectious diseases in which the identification of the source of infection leads the way to the isolation of the causal organism and provides a means for eliminating or controlling the frequency of disease occurrence by restricting exposure of noninfected, susceptible individuals to the bacillus. The tubercle bacillus, for instance, was identified as *the* cause of tuberculosis because this organism must be present for tuberculosis to occur. This does not necessarily mean that it will always cause clinically recognizable disease. There are circumstances when the bacillus is present and no disease occurs. The host has to be susceptible to the organism; susceptibility reflects previous exposure to the organism,

immune response, and so on. If the host is not susceptible, no disease occurs. The environment is also important, since the likelihood of exposure to the organism may vary greatly in different geographical areas.

In the case of noninfectious disease agents, the single-cause model is of limited usefulness, since there is no single factor or agent that must be present to cause the disease. For example, even though smoking is recognized as a major cause of lung cancer, nonsmokers and individuals who have never been exposed to the cigarette smoke of others do get lung cancer. Clearly, there must be other substances that cause the disease. Nonsmokers exposed to asbestos may develop lung cancer. Also, smokers who are exposed to other substances, such as asbestos, are much more likely to develop lung cancer than are smokers not exposed to these substances. Exposure to multiple causal factors may have an additional or multiplicative effect.

In a different example, home accidents may result from numerous factors such as clutter in the environment, loose throw rugs, curled edges of linoleum, electrical wires running across the room, wet floors, poor lighting, or physical impairments of residents such as problems with balance, musculoskeletal function, or eyesight. Any of these factors could cause a home accident. All are amenable to intervention through public education, better engineering design or maintenance, or devices such as corrective lenses or walkers, which supplement physical functioning. Presence of several of these factors increases the probability of an accident occurring. Such interrelationships between a multitude of factors, some known and some unknown but all bearing ultimately on the cause of the disease, constitute the **web of causation.** It is, fortunately, not necessary to understand completely the intricacy of relationships between factors to institute adequate preventive measures.

Numerous factors such as smoking, obesity, blood cholesterol level, and stress are causes of heart attack by our earlier definition. The more of these factors present in an individual, the greater the risk of heart attack. Since presence of these factors increase the risk for contracting a disease, we call them *risk factors*. While we do not understand how these factors work or how they interact, we can intervene and reduce the risk of heart attack by persuading individuals to give up smoking, to lose weight, or to change their diet to reduce cholesterol. Planning of such interventions is based on understanding the natural history of disease.

Natural History

Natural history of the disease, the process by which diseases occur and progress in humans, involves the interaction of three different kinds of factors: the causative agent(s), a susceptible host (man), and the environment. The web of causation is one model of the interrelationship among these factors. Another model illustrating the relationship among these factors, the ecological model, is shown in Figure 8-3. Humans are seen as surrounded by their social, biological, and physical environments. Change in any of these environments may initiate change in the others, affecting the relationship between humans and agents in these en-

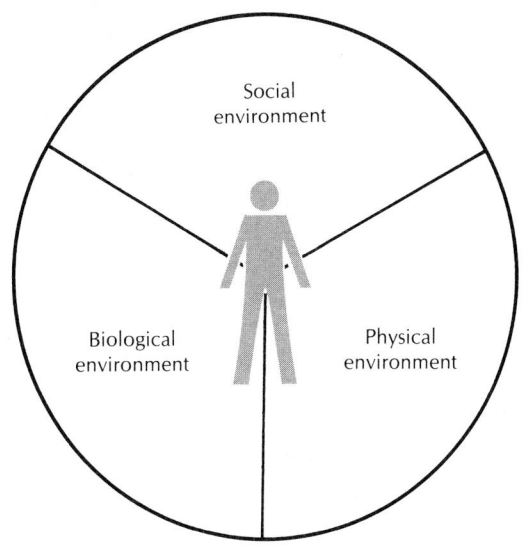

FIGURE 8-3

Ecological model of host, agent, and environment relationships.

vironments. As long as a state of equilibrium exists between host, agent, and environment, a state of health is maintained. For example, an increase in the amount of the agent resulting from a change in environmental conditions increases the likelihood that a susceptible host will be exposed. An increase in host susceptibility resulting from lack of sleep, malnutrition, excessive stress, aging, or a variety of other factors also increases the risk of disease. Changes in the environment contribute to changes in host susceptibility as well as to the conditions for viability of the agent.

The Agent

An *agent* can be either a factor whose presence causes a disease or one whose absence causes disease. An example of the former is the gonococcus that causes gonorrhea; an example of the latter is insufficient intake of vitamin C, which may lead to scurvy. Categories of causative agents include physical, chemical, nutrient, biological, genetic, and psychological agents. Physical agents include various mechanical forces or frictions that may produce injury as well as atmospheric abnormalities such as extremes of temperature or excessive radiation. Chemical agents include substances that may occur as dusts, gases, vapors, fumes, or liquids. The term *nutrient agents* refers specifically to basic dietary components. All living organisms, including insects, worms, protozoa, fungi, bacteria, rickettsia, and viruses, are biological agents; this is the class of agents that are infectious. Genetic agents are agents transmitted from parent to child through the genes. Psychological agents are stressful circumstances in the environment.

Certain characteristics of agents affect their ability to produce disease in the host. For infectious agents these characteristics are infectivity, pathogenicity, and virulence. Measures of these characteristics (i.e., the infection rate, pathogenicity rate, and case fatality) provide a means of population surveillance, allowing public health officials to assess the nature of the problem they are dealing with in

order to plan for intervention. These characteristics are discussed further in Chapter 17. Important characteristics of the noninfectious agents include toxicity for chemical agents, size and shape of physical agents, chronicity or suddenness of psychological agents, and homozygocity or heterozygocity of genetic material.

The Environment

Environment refers to all external conditions and influences affecting the life of living things. Physical, socioeconomic, and biological environments provide reservoirs and modes of transmission for agents. The physical environment includes the geological structure of an area and the availability of resources such as water and flora which influence the number and variety of animal reservoirs and arthropod (i.e., insects) vectors. Weather, climate, and season are important influences on these factors.

The socioeconomic environment contributes to the types of infectious agents in a location, since social and economic conditions relate to the extent of environmental sanitation, pasteurization of milk, disposal of garbage and excreta, and the availability of medical facilities for immunization and medical care. The socioeconomic environment may also influence the noninfectious agents; that is, more psychological stressors may be found in low-income neighborhoods than in higher income neighborhoods. Low-income neighborhoods are more likely to be located near industrial plants, which may produce dangerous chemicals or emit physical particles of agents such as asbestos or coal tar.

Finally, there is the biological environment, including other living plants and animals, which may serve as either the reservoir or as the vector for transmission of an infectious agent. Because these agents are living organisms, they require a place to live and multiply. The habitat of these agents are called reservoirs and may be any human, animal, arthropod, plant, soil, or inanimate matter that provides an environment for survival or reproduction. The reservoir is thus intimately related to the *transmission cycle* of the agent in nature. The transmission cycle, or life cycle, refers to where the agent resides and to how it is transported from here to a susceptible host.

The Host

Disease can only occur in a susceptible human host. The concept of immunity is important to the understanding of host resistance to disease caused by infectious agents. *Immunity* refers to the increased resistance on the part of a host to a specific infectious agent. Immunity can be humoral (antibodies in the blood) or cellular (specific to each type of cell). The role of each of these varies with the infectious agent and with the immune response of the host. Immunity can be passive or active. Passive immunity is attained either naturally (maternal transfer of antibodies to the fetus) or artificially (inoculation of specific protective antibodies, for example, immune serum globulin for infectious hepatitis or diphtheria antitoxin for diphtheria prevention). Passive immunity is temporary; in the newborn it usually lasts 6 months, during which time the infant is only protected against infection experienced by the mother and for which she has made antibodies. By contrast, active immunity is long lasting and may protect an individual for life. It is attained naturally by infection, with or without clinical manifestations, or artificially by the inoculation of vaccine obtained from fractions or products of the infectious agent or of the agent itself in killed, modified, or variant form. The principle of active immunity is used in many of the major vaccination programs such as for diphtheria and polio. It was also the basis for the successful program to eradicate smallpox from the world through an international vaccination and surveillance program.

In contrast to immunity, the term *inherent resistance* refers to the ability to resist disease independently of antibodies or of specifically developed tissue response. It commonly rests in anatomical or physiological characteristics of the host; it may be genetic or acquired, permanent or temporary. The concept of inherent resistance is useful in understanding host resistance to both infectious agents and other types of agents. For example, factors such as general health status or nutrition may affect resistance to disease. Someone in good health who maintains good nutrition and a regular schedule of rest and exercise may be exposed to the tubercle bacillus and resist infection even though he is not immune to the organism. Similarly, this individual, if exposed to psychological stress, may resist ulcers better than someone in poorer general health.

The Disease Process

Table 8-3 gives the stages of the natural history of any disease and lists points of intervention for each stage. Basically, there are three stages in the natural history (Leavell and Clark, 1958). The first of these is the stage of *prepathogenesis,* or *susceptibility.* In this stage, disease has not developed, although the groundwork has been laid through the presence of factors that favor its occurrence. For example, the poor eating habits and fatigue resulting from lack of sleep that are often present among college students during exam week represent risk factors that favor the occurrence of the common cold.

The second stage in the natural history is *pathogenesis.* Within this stage there are two substages: the first substage is *presymptomatic disease,* sometimes called *early pathogenesis.* At this substage, the individual has no symptoms indicating the presence of illness. However, pathogenic changes have begun. In the second substage, *discernible early lesions,* there are changes that may be detectable through sophisticated laboratory tests. These changes are called *subclinical* because they are below the level of the *clinical horizon,* which is an imaginary line dividing the point where there are detectable signs and symptoms from that where there are not. In this substage the client may develop early signs and symptoms. For example, premalignant changes or early malignant tissue changes in the cervix may be detected by a Pap smear long before a woman would experience symptoms and before signs would be visible to an obstetrician on visual examination.

Stage three in the natural history is *advanced disease.* By this stage, sufficient anatomical or functional changes have occurred to produce recognizable signs and symptoms.

This stage includes disease so advanced that death is inevitable. Once a client has entered this stage, possible outcomes may be complete recovery, residual defect that produces some degree of disability, or death. In an attempt to further understand this stage, clinicians and researchers have developed classification schemes for varying degrees of disease severity, including the staging systems used for malignancies, and the functional and therapeutic classifications used for cardiac disease.

Exposure of the host to an agent occurs during the stage of prepathogenesis. In the case of infectious agents, exposure is followed by an *incubation period,* a time when the organism multiplies to sufficient numbers to produce a host reaction and clinical symptoms. This period is relatively brief, usually hours to months. For diseases caused by noninfectious agents, however, this time from exposure to onset of symptoms, called the induction period or latency period, may be from years to decades. Accidents resulting from a severe psychological stressor may happen shortly after initial exposure to the stressor. By contrast, ulcers as a consequence of psychological stress may require years of exposure.

One of the shorter known latency periods for cancer is the 5-year latency period of leukemia in children resulting from radiation exposure. On the other hand, lung cancer resulting from asbestos exposures may have a latency period of 40 years between exposure and detection of the disease. Exceptions to the general rules governing latency periods as just described, do occur—for example, some chemical agents cause almost instantaneous, acute episodes of poisoning.

In contrast to diseases caused by infectious agents, those diseases caused by noninfectious agents or by still unidentified agents are more likely to be conditions of a chronic nature. Most, but not all, diseases with infectious causes are of relatively short duration. The patient is usually ill for a period ranging from a few days to several months and generally recovers without any residual disability or, if the illness was severe, may die from the illness. The patient who has recovered rarely requires long-term follow-up, although there are exceptions. Tuberculosis and rheumatic heart disease, which results from a staphylococcal infection, are examples of diseases caused by infectious agents that are chronic in nature. In the case of noninfectious agents, there is often residual disability requiring ongoing medical treatment and rehabilitation programs. For example, patients with cardiovascular disease are likely to require ongoing supervision of prescribed medications such as digitalis, control of diet, and modification of life-style.

Levels of Prevention

The natural history of a disease provides the basis for community health intervention. Because a disease evolves over time and pathological change becomes less reversible as the disease process continues, the ultimate aim of intervention programs is to halt or reverse the process of pathological change as early as possible, thereby preventing further damage. A three-level model for intervention, based on the stages of disease natural history, has been developed (see Table 8-3). The goal of intervention at each of the three

TABLE 8-3

Natural history of disease and application of preventive measures

Stage	Events	Level of application of preventive measures	Specific interventions
Prepathogenesis	1. Interrelations of various host, agent, and environmental factors bring host and agent(s) together	Primary prevention	Health promotion (health education, nutrition counseling, adequate housing, personal hygiene, etc.)
	2. Disease-provoking stimulus is produced in the known host		Specific protection (immunizations, sanitation, removing occupational and environmental hazards, use of specific nutrients, etc.)
Pathogenesis Early pathogenesis	1. Interaction of host and stimulus 2. Stimulus or agent becomes established (if infectious agent, increases by multiplication) 3. Beginning tissue and physiological changes	Secondary prevention	Early diagnosis and prompt treatment (screening, case-finding, selective examination)
Discernible early lesions	1. Clinical recognition of disease is possible through laboratory or other tests that detect early physiological changes 2. Patient develops early symptoms	Tertiary prevention	Disability limitation (treatment to arrest disease process)
Advanced disease	1. Disability 2. Defect 3. Chronic state 4. Death		Rehabilitation (retraining for maximum use of remaining capacities, facilitating reentry to the family unit and to the workplace)

Adapted from Leavell, H.R., and Clark, E.G., Preventive medicine for the doctor in his community, New York, 1958, McGraw-Hill Book Co.

levels is to prevent the pathogenic process from evolving further. The three *levels of prevention* are called primary, secondary, and tertiary prevention.

Primary prevention is aimed at intervention before pathological changes have begun and during the natural history stage of susceptibility. Primary prevention seeks to keep the agent away from contact with the host or to eliminate host susceptibility. Primary preventive efforts are of two types, general health promotion and specific protection.

General health promotion includes all activities that optimize the environment and favor healthy living. Thus efforts to improve the physical environment, whether that of the outdoors, the home, school, or work, would be included. Health education aimed at educating the population about good nutrition, the need for rest and recreation, preparation for retirement, hygiene, or the harmful effects of smoking or drug use is a form of general health promotion.

Efforts aimed at primary prevention of chronic, noninfectious diseases such as heart disease must focus on such things as maternal diet during pregnancy, the diet of the child during early life, regular exercise, and education programs regarding the hazards of smoking. Although success cannot be guaranteed, prospects for success are greatest if intervention occurs early in life, before physiological risk factors such as obesity and elevated cholesterol levels are permitted to develop. These physiological states involve cellular changes that are steps in the development of disease, and therefore reduction of these risk factors is already secondary prevention.

Since 1900 effects of primary prevention can be seen in the dramatic reduction in mortality from infectious disease resulting largely from environmental manipulation and immunization programs (Figure 8-1). This reduction in infectious disease mortality, particularly among infants, young children, young women, and the elderly, has led to an increased size of the total population as well as to the advent of chronic disease as a major community health concern. Because fewer people die of infectious disease, more live to older ages at which chronic diseases are common. Also, industrialization and changes in life-style have increased exposure to potential causal agents for noninfectious disease.

Secondary prevention efforts seek to detect disease early and treat promptly to cure disease at its earliest stage or to slow its progression, prevent complications, and limit disability when cure is not possible. Thus secondary prevention is focused primarily on presymptomatic disease or very early clinical disease. Screening is the most common form of secondary prevention. Many screening tests can detect early physiological indicators of disease before the people have any indication that they are ill. Examples include cervical cancer tests, hearing tests for deafness, the tuberculin test for tuberculosis, and the phenylalanine test for PKU in infants. Such screening programs have become popular in recent years as improved technology has led to a proliferation of available test procedures.

Detection and treatment of conditions at the stage allowed by screening tests provide benefits ranging from prevention of mental retardation in children with PKU by use of a special diet maintained until adulthood to preservation of life for cancer patients whose disease is detected while in the early stage where it is curable. In the case of communicable disease, not only do early detection and treatment (secondary prevention) benefit those who are affected, but the screening program provides primary prevention for those in proximity to affected individuals who will no longer be exposing these others to the infectious agent. For example, the VDRL as a screen for sexually transmitted diseases identifies clients who are then referred for further diagnostic follow-up and for treatment. Once treated, they cannot transmit the disease to others.

A word of caution: screening tests are given to individuals who assume they are well. Because the tests are not diagnostic, they merely separate persons who are more likely to have the disease from persons who probably do not. Individuals screened as positive require a diagnostic follow-up to determine if they actually have the disease. For example, in a routine physical examination a complete blood count may be performed to screen the person for potential health problems such as the presence of infection or anemia. This is called casefinding. A low hemoglobin count may require further diagnostic follow-up to ascertain the cause of anemia. A high white blood count may require further diagnostic follow-up to determine the location of the infection. Thus from an ethical point of view, certain criteria should be met before a screening test is indiscriminately administered:

1. An effective treatment that will change the course of the disease must be available.
2. There must be evidence that the test does, in fact, detect the disease at an earlier stage in the natural history than when symptoms are present.
3. The test must have the ability to screen as positive those individuals with the disease (sensitivity) and the ability to screen as negative those persons without the disease (specificity).
4. Follow-up services must be available and accompanied by an adequate notification and referral service for those positive on the screening.

These criteria are necessary because the sensitivity of screening tests is always less than 100%. Conversely, individuals without the disease are not necessarily screened as negative because the specificity of a screening test is never 100%. It is therefore useful to teach clients about early symptoms

as a part of the screening program so they will be alerted to the significance of symptoms that might appear several months later.

Tertiary prevention includes limitation of disability for persons in the earlier stages of illness and rehabilitation in those persons for whom residual damage already exists. Tertiary prevention activities are focused on the middle to later phases of the stage of clinical disease when irreversible pathological damage produces disability. For a client recovering from a stroke, exercise therapy to preserve muscle tone, restore motion, and prevent contractures is a form of tertiary prevention, since it both limits disability and begins the process of rehabilitation by maximizing the individual's residual capacities. Psychosocial and vocational services are usually part of a rehabilitation program as well.

Measures for the control of communicable disease are aimed at preventing the spread of the infectious agent from those environments harboring it to individuals who are susceptible and who may be exposed. This can be achieved by modifying or eliminating the environment in which the infectious agent lives, by interfering with the means of transmission to the human host, or by increasing host immunity—all measures aimed at primary prevention. Control is facilitated by maintaining surveillance programs that quickly identify new cases for follow-up with isolation methods to prevent exposure of those susceptible or by instituting specific treatments to limit the period of communicability and progression of pathological conditions (secondary prevention). Tertiary prevention plays a smaller role in infectious disease programs than in noninfectious programs, since infectious disease less often results in permanent disability.

Specific protection refers to measures aimed at protecting individuals against specific agents such as immunization against polio or to attempts to remove agents from the environment such as sewage treatment, pasteurization of milk, or chlorination of water.

In infectious disease, illness can be prevented if the agent is destroyed or otherwise removed from the environment or if specific protection is instituted through vaccination programs. This works because the infectious agent is necessary to produce the disease. As previously noted, for chronic conditions caused by noninfectious agents there is no single necessary agent. For example, chronic obstructive pulmonary disease, may result from smoking, from asbestos exposure, from air pollution, or from a variety of other agents. Each agent must be eliminated to assure control of disease. Specific protection measures, such as removal of hazardous substances from the workplace, will reduce occurrence of the disease but will not eliminate it.

The combined effects of two or more agents (synergism) are frequently seen in instances of causation by noninfectious agents. For example, nonsmoking workers exposed to asbestos do not have a statistically significant increase in the risk of dying from lung cancer when compared with nonsmoking, nonexposed individuals. However, workers who smoke and are exposed to asbestos are estimated to have 92 times the risk of the nonsmoking, nonexposed individuals (Kleinfeld et al. 1967). This is of concern because control efforts often must settle for minimizing rather than eliminating workplace exposures. The synergistic effect of other exposures could mean that substantial risk remains even with low-level exposures. It was hoped that if exposures to harmful environmental agents were kept low, the latency period before onset of symptoms would be so long that the average individual would not develop problems until old age. Since synergism may shorten latency periods and produce illness in the prime of life at low exposure levels, reducing behavioral risks such as smoking is crucial.

EPIDEMIOLOGICAL METHODS
Sources of Data

Epidemiological investigations use data from a variety of existing sources, such as census data collected by the government or records maintained by hospitals. In other instances the data may be generated for a specific study through surveys that include interviews and physical examination. Basically, there are three types of data required: population statistics, mortality data, and morbidity data.

A population census, carried out every 10 years in many countries, is the main source of population statistics. Census data include information about the geographical and economic characteristics of the population and the personal and demographic characteristics of individuals and households. Certain of these data provide the denominator for routine health statistics.

Mortality statistics are generally based on the numbers and causes of death listed on death certificates, since in most of the world registration of deaths is required by law. As a result, this provides a fairly complete record of the number of deaths. Accuracy of the reported cause of death varies from place to place, but the reported data are probably adequate indicators of the mortality count for major causes of death.

Morbidity data as a rule are not routinely recorded and therefore are less readily available and less accurate than are mortality statistics. Probably the two major sources of morbidity data are hospital records and notification systems, such as the reporting of some 37 infectious diseases decreed as reportable in most states in the United States (see Appendix J) or reporting required by disease registries such as cancer registries or birth defects registries. Surveys are often conducted when data are not otherwise available. Birth certificates provide information for the numerator and for the denominator of various rates measuring health aspects of childbirth and infancy.

Summary statistics for a community are frequently available from organizations that routinely use them for health planning purposes. These organizations include the health department, regional planning agencies, hospitals, and a variety of government agencies.

Rates in Epidemiology

In epidemiology a count or frequency of events is of limited interest by itself. However, when frequency is used as the numerator of a fraction that expresses a proportion and specifies time, it is of great value and is a called a *rate.* The rates most frequently used as indexes of community health are listed in Table 8-4. The reporting, for example, of three cases of infectious hepatitis in one month without indicating if they occurred among 1000 students in a school (3 ÷ 1000 = 0.3%) or among 20 in a dormitory (3 ÷ 20 = 15%) is of little practical value to the epidemiologist or to community health practitioners except for the fact that the number of cases of this disease may be useful to estimate the need for additional medical services. Rates serve as a means of summarizing large amounts of information in a way that allows comparison between populations in different places and at various points in time. This facilitates the assessment of trends, identification of excesses of disease occurrence, and evaluation of progress in control efforts. For example, public health officials have recently observed that the rates of lung cancer deaths among females have been increasing rapidly since 1965 (see Figure 8-4). It has been estimated that if these rates continue to rise at the present rate, lung cancer will overtake breast cancer as the leading cause of cancer mortality for women. In an attempt to reduce these preventable deaths, public health officials have instituted antismoking campaigns aimed heavily at young women.

In Cook County, Illinois, in 1976 high rates of measles were observed among high school students by school nurses. Measles are unusual among this age group, and highest rates usually occur among primary school children. When these cases were reported to the county health department, an investigation was begun. As a result of an investigation of the exposure and immunization histories of these cases, it was learned that these cases were among the earliest groups vaccinated after the measles vaccine first became available. They had been vaccinated before 6 months of age. Because there was residual maternal antibody still present in their blood, the vaccination did not stimulate active antibody production as intended. Thus when maternal immunity waned, these persons were susceptible to the disease. After the investigation, such susceptible individuals were actively sought by county officials so they could be revaccinated before a new epidemic occurred.

Both the increase in female lung cancer mortality and the increase in measles rates among the students in Cook County represent epidemics. *Epidemics* are defined as rates of disease significantly higher than the usual frequency. The usual frequency represents the *endemic* level. A third term, *pandemic,* is used to describe epidemics that include large areas of the world—a worldwide epidemic. Figure 8-5 illustrates the endemic fluctuation of rates. The peak in 1976 represents an epidemic as it is clearly in excess of normal rates.

Rates are expressed by a *numerator,* a *denominator,* and specification of *place* and *time.* Both the numerator and denominator have to be similarly restricted by population characteristics (age, sex, race) and by time. When the denominator refers to a population that includes the numerator, the relative frequency is expressed as a *rate,* as in the following example:

$$\frac{\text{No. of new cases of cervical cancer in Cincinnati in 1983}}{\text{No. of women in Cincinnati in 1983}} \times 100,000$$

Because cervical cancer can only occur among women, only women are included in the denominator. The women

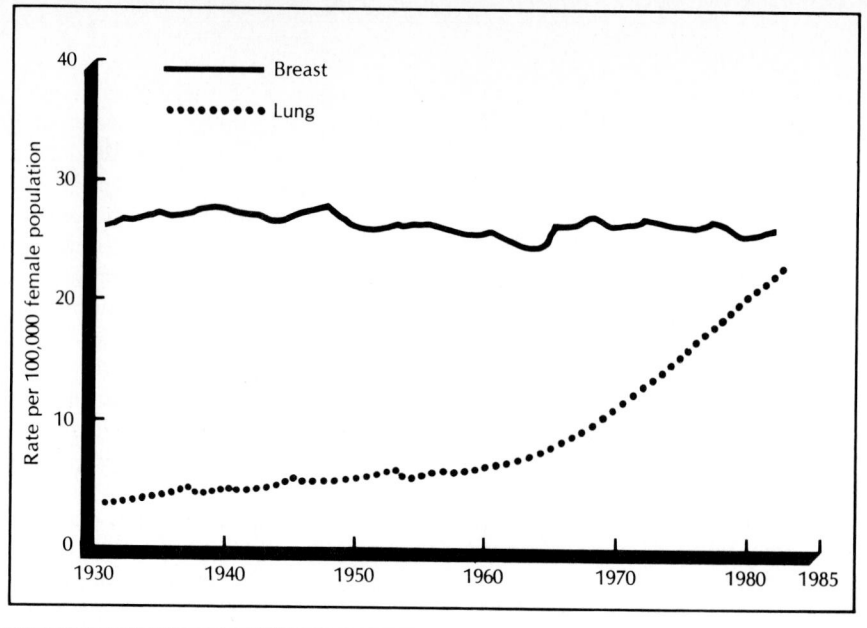

FIGURE 8-4

Age-adjusted death rates for women with breast and lung cancer in the United States from 1930 to 1985.

TABLE 8-4

Rates most frequently used as indexes of community health

Type of rate	Usual population factor
GENERAL MORTALITY	
Crude rate $= \dfrac{\text{No. of deaths during a year}}{\text{Average (midyear) population}}$	Per 100,000 population
Cause-specific rate $= \dfrac{\text{No. of deaths from a stated cause in a year}}{\text{Average (midyear) population}}$	Per 100,000 population
Age-specific rate $= \dfrac{\text{No. of deaths among persons in given age group in a year}}{\text{Average (midyear) population in same age group}}$	Per 100,000 population
Proportional rate $= \dfrac{\text{No. of deaths from a specific cause in given time period}}{\text{Total deaths in same time period}}$	Per 100 population
MORBIDITY	
Incidence $= \dfrac{\text{No. of new cases of disease in a place from time}_1 \text{ to time}_2}{\text{No. of persons in a place at midpoint of time period}}$	Per 100,000 population
Prevalence $= \dfrac{\text{No. of existing cases in a place at given time}}{\text{No. of persons in a place at same time}}$	Per 100,000 population
MATERNAL AND INFANT MORTALITY	
Maternal (puerperal) rate $= \dfrac{\text{No. of deaths from puerperal causes in a year}}{\text{No. of live births in same year}}$	Per 100,000 live births
Infant rate $= \dfrac{\text{No. deaths of children less than 1 year of age during a year}}{\text{No. of live births in same year}}$	Per 1000 live births
Neonatal rate $= \dfrac{\text{No. of deaths of children in a year}}{\text{No. of live births in same year}}$	Per 1000 live births
Fetal rate $= \dfrac{\text{No. of fetal deaths during year}}{\text{No. of live births and fetal deaths in same year}}$	Per 1000 live births and fetal deaths
Perinatal rate $= \dfrac{\text{No. of fetal deaths at 28 weeks or more and infant deaths under 7 days of age during a year}}{\text{No. of live births and fetal deaths at 28 weeks or more in same year}}$	Per 1000 live births and fetal deaths
FERTILITY	
General fertility rate $= \dfrac{\text{No. of live births during a year}}{\text{No. of females aged 15-44 at midyear}}$	Per 1000 population

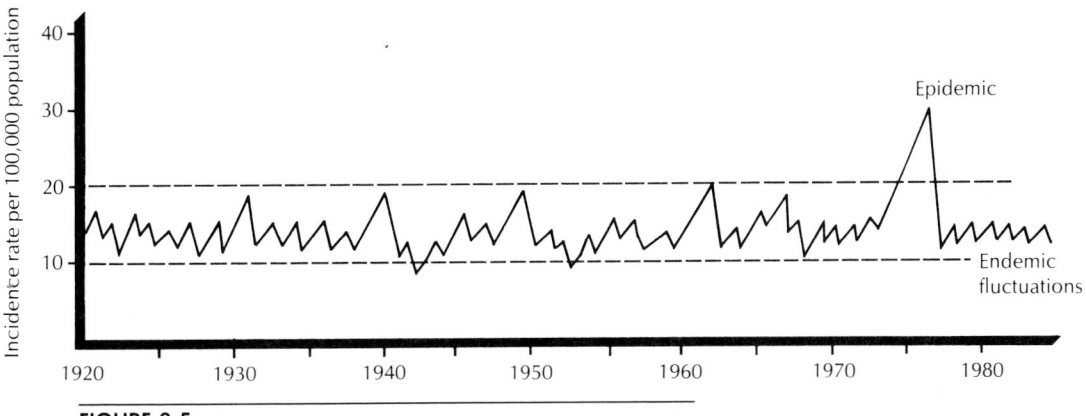

FIGURE 8-5

Schematic representation of endemic and epidemic rates.

in both the numerator and denominator are those living in Cincinnati in 1983. The resulting rate is generally multiplied times some constant value, usually 100,000, so that rates for different-sized populations can be compared.

By contrast, if the numerator is not included in the denominator, a *ratio* is obtained. The annual fetal death rate is the number of fetal deaths in a year related to the total number of annual births plus fetal deaths. The annual fetal death *ratio* is the number of fetal deaths in relation to only the total number of live births. Here the denominator does not include both the total population of affected and unaffected persons (live births and fetal deaths) but only the unaffected.

The numerator and denominator of rates may be *general* or *specific*. General rates refer to rates that include the total population whereas specific rates apply only to the population subgroup specified, for example, women, children under 17 years of age, or black males.

Death Rates (Mortality)

General **mortality** rates are called *crude rates*. The numerator of these rates includes all relevant deaths in the entire population of the geographic area of interest. The denominator is the number of persons in the population. When the numerator of these rates includes only deaths from a particular cause occurring in that total population, for example coronary heart disease (CHD), they are called disease-specific or cause-specific rates (see Table 8-4 for the calculation of these rates). Because such rates provide one measure, an average rate, for the experience of the entire population, there may be a problem in interpreting comparisons of such rates; the mortality experience of everyone, including men, women, whites and nonwhites, young and old are averaged. The resulting rate is therefore dependent on the distribution of population subgroups. If these subgroups have very different rates of mortality, for example if young persons have low rates and elderly persons have high rates, then the crude rate for a population comprised mostly of older persons would be high while the crude rate for a population comprised mostly of young persons would be low, even if the rates for each specific age group were the same in the two populations. We might observe such a situation when com-

paring crude rates for a state with a young population, such as Alaska, with a state that has a substantial elderly population, such as Florida.

If one is comparing only two or three locations, it may be feasible to compare *specific rates* for subgroups, for example, sex-specific mortality for men and women or age specific mortality rates for various age subgroups. These rates contain the number of deaths from a particular cause among the subgroup (e.g., number of CHD deaths among males) in the numerator and the number of persons in the subgroup (men) in the denominator (see calculation of age-specific rate in Table 8-4). However, if one wanted to compare mortality for a large number of geographical locations or a large number of time periods, use of specific rates becomes confusing because so many rates are involved. Imagine that you wanted to compare CHD rates for all 50 U.S. states. Even if you compared only four age groups—less than 18 years, 18 to 44, 45 to 64, and 65 and older—you would be dealing with 200 rates! Use of a *standardized*, or *adjusted*, rate allows the use of a single rate for each population being compared, reducing the number to 50. These rates adjust for differences in the distribution of age, sex, race, or other factors in the populations being compared. Use of age-adjusted rates would allow one to answer the question, "If these populations had the same age distribution, how would their overall experience with this disease compare?" Comparison of the 50 age-adjusted rates would thus allow one to determine which states had excessively high or unusually low rates of mortality relative to the others.

Another kind of mortality rate often used is the *proportional mortality rate* (see Table 8-4 for calculation). This rate reflects the relative contribution of different causes of death to total mortality. Figure 8-1, showing the proportional distribution of death from various causes is based on proportional mortality rates. The rates in the figure are general—including the total population—but these rates may also be specific to subgroups such as men or women.

Morbidity

The two most commonly used **morbidity rates** are incidence and prevalence. **Incidence** is a measure of all new cases arising during a defined period of time, usually 1 year, in a population at risk, and is calculated as follows:

$$\text{Incidence} = \frac{\substack{\text{No. of new cases of disease in a} \\ \text{place from time}_1 \text{ to time}_2}}{\substack{\text{No. of persons in a place at} \\ \text{midpoint of time period}}}$$

For this rate the denominator uses the population size at the midpoint of the time period. This rate, called a *cumulative incidence,* is the one commonly used for large general population estimates. Other measures of incidence, such as incidence density, are modifications of this rate, used in cohort studies where a defined group of persons is followed over time. To account for persons who die, who are lost to follow-up, or who have contracted the disease and are therefore not at continued risk, a measure called person-years is used as the denominator of these incidence rates. A *person-year* is one person at risk for 1 year. The numerator is the total number of cases accumulated over the study period. The rate yielded by dividing the numerator by the denominator is subsequently divided by the number of follow-up years to yield an average incidence.

Incidence represents the risk of developing a particular disease. Thus these rates are useful in studies of disease etiology where incidence for groups exposed to a putative etiological agent is compared with incidence for groups not exposed. This measure comparing the risk for two groups is the relative risk ratio discussed earlier.

Incidence is useful for monitoring occurrence of a disease in defined populations over time. Incidence is preferable to mortality for this purpose, since incidence reflects only diagnosed occurrence of the disease and unlike mortality does not reflect additional factors such as improvements in treatment leading to improved survival. Such monitoring of disease can alert community health personnel to the presence of new hazards in the environment. For example, a sudden increase in a particular congenital malformation, could indicate an environmental hazard recently introduced to that geographical area.

Special rates expressing incidence, called **attack rates,** are frequently used in surveillance and control of infectious disease. Attack rates are calculated when a clearly defined population has been exposed to an infectious agent; the rate represents the incidence of illness among that exposed population. An example is the incidence of hepatitis B among a classroom of children at a day-care center exposed to a contagious classmate. Changes in attack rates may indicate a change in the immune status of a population, as in the Cook County measles epidemic discussed earlier, or may be an indication of a more virile strain of an organism. These rates are discussed further in Chapter 17.

Prevalence is a measure of the existing number of cases present in a population at a given time:

$$\text{Prevalence} = \frac{\substack{\text{No. of existing cases in a} \\ \text{place at given time}}}{\substack{\text{No. of persons in a place at} \\ \text{midpoint of year}}}$$

This rate is a function of incidence and duration of the disease. The number of cases of chronic disease with low mortality will tend to accumulate and will result in an increasing prevalence. Death and recovery are the two most common factors that remove cases from the case load requiring care. A less common factor is substantial migration from the community. To evaluate adequacy of existing services and to plan for future needs, public health officials require a measure of the case load requiring care. Prevalence is the measure generally used. In addition, future prevalence can be projected by using incidence, recovery, and mortality to estimate changes in prevalence over time.

THE SEQUENCE OF EPIDEMIOLOGICAL INVESTIGATION

Epidemiological investigations generally proceed in an orderly fashion, beginning with observing and recording the existing patterns of occurrence for the condition under study. These observations are recorded in terms of person, place, and time. From these recorded observations, a description of which specific characteristics are associated with high versus low frequency of disease occurrence is generated. This first phase of investigation, called *descriptive epidemiology,* suggests hypotheses concerning etiology.

Consider the approach of investigators interested in trying to learn what causes breast cancer. The first step is to obtain the rates of breast cancer for groups of people with different characteristics, rates in different geographical locations, and rates at various points in time. Although epidemiologists would prefer to have the rates of newly occurring cases, *incidence,* these are not generally available without a special survey or a disease registry, so the rates of death from the disease, *mortality,* are generally used in early stages of the investigation.

In examining these rates, it is observed that breast cancer is rare among men compared with women and more frequent among whites than nonwhites, among single women than married women, and among those in higher socioeconomic groups than those in lower socioeconomic groups. Breast cancer occurs with increasing frequency in successively older age groups and shows a decreasing frequency as number of liveborn children increase and age at first full-term pregnancy decreases. By geographical area, rates of breast cancer are higher in the developed, Western countries than in less developed countries. Rates are lowest in Asian countries such as Japan. In the early 1900s breast cancer mortality was increasing steadily, but these rates have leveled off during the past 50 years or so, reflecting improvements in early detection and treatment. Incidence now shows little change for whites but continues to rise for nonwhites.

These observed patterns may suggest hypotheses to the epidemiologist, for example, that hormonal factors may be operating as a causal mechanism.

Hypotheses suggested by the descriptive epidemiology of a condition are tested in the second investigative phase, called *analytic epidemiology.* Because these analytic studies are based on observational data, the suspicion exists that the observed association of a suspected causal factor with occurrence of a particular disease may be caused by other factors, such as genetic self-selection of individuals for use of harmful substances or the presence of other confounding variables, which interact in some unknown way with the factor under study to cause the disease. Genetic self-selection in this discussion refers to hereditary chemical imbalances that are thought to predispose an individual to craving for substances like alcohol and cigarettes. Confounding variables may be identified at a later stage of investigation. Suppose that a researcher noted that rates of spontaneous abortion increased with the number of pregnancies. Having babies might not be a causative factor; the number of pregnancies may be related to age of the mother. If physiological aging leads to a decreased capacity for carrying a pregnancy to term, then age would be confounding the original association between parity and spontaneous abortion rates. Because of this problem, multiple analytic studies on the same hypotheses are usually required.

Analytic studies may be done on either an ecological level or a relational level. *Ecological studies* compare large aggregates of people, usually of a defined geographical area, with another such large population. For example, cancer rates may be compared for the populations of towns with polluted drinking water and those of towns with pure drinking water to assess whether water pollution is associated with elevated rates of cancer. Or, per capita data on fat consumption may be compared for countries with high and low rates of colon cancer to investigate a hypothesized causal role for fat consumption in development of colon cancer. Such studies, while a useful first step in the analytic phase of investigation, are subject to the *ecological fallacy.* There is a fallacy in assuming that relationships observed among groups can be assumed for individuals. Although there may be a striking relationship between high cancer rates and polluted drinking water in the populations studied, there is not necessarily the same relationship observed on individual levels. Imagine for example, that the majority of residents of the towns with polluted water who developed cancer were men who worked in other towns where they were exposed to carcinogens in the workplace. They actually drank less of the polluted water than did the individuals remaining in the town.

Relational studies, on the other hand, do relate exposure and disease in the same individuals. The presence or absence of exposure and disease is determined for each individual. Then the frequency of joint presence of disease and exposure is assessed.

Four basic types of studies are commonly used: (1) cross-sectional studies; (2) case-control studies; (3) cohort studies; and (4) historical cohort studies. Other names used synonomously with these terms are listed in Table 8-5 along with the design of each.

Cross-sectional and case-control studies are generally used as first steps in the analytic phase of investigation as they can be done quickly, require small samples, and are relatively inexpensive. These studies provide preliminary evidence of an associaton between an hypothesized causal variable and a particular health outcome. Cohort and his-

torical cohort studies generally require large samples, take longer to complete, and are expensive. On the other hand, they do yield measures of incidence or risk; no incidence can be derived from the cross-sectional or case-control studies, and any risk measures must be obtained by indirect means. They are not, however, a practical design for studies of rare disease because of the size of the populations that have to be followed to generate incidence cases.

When sufficient evidence from analytic studies has accumulated in support of a specific factor being causally related to the occurrence of a particular disease, the experimental phase of epidemiological investigation is begun. This is the third phase of the investigation, which uses an experimental design to confirm the causal nature of relationships identified through observational studies.

Because it would be unethical to expose humans to an agent thought to be harmful, in most epidemiological experiments the study sample is chosen from individuals already exposed to the causal agent under study. The suspected causal factor is then taken away from one study group, and their disease experience is compared with that of the group who remains exposed to the suspected factor. For example, if hypertension is thought to be a causal agent for stroke, patients with hypertension may be randomly assigned to a treatment group that is given medication to reduce blood pressure, while the remaining subjects receive either no treatment or diet treatment only. The two groups are then compared for the incidence of stroke. Because in the experimental phase the investigator has control over who is or is not exposed as well as over the experimental conditions, the problems of the analytic studies are not generally present. As a result, data from experimental studies are typically used to prove causal relationships.

Although ideally, experimental data demonstrating cause would be available before decisions must be made, such as whether to set up programs to reduce or eliminate a particular exposure or to answer clients' questions about a particular risk, often this is not possible. Epidemiological research is proliferating. Results of studies are discussed in the lay press, sometimes before the relevant issue of a journal has arrived in the library. Health professionals are often besieged by clients who want interpretation and guidance about what to do. Should they ask their doctor to take them off reserpine for their hypertension in view of a report showing an association of reserpine use with breast cancer? What about all the advertisements the client has been seeing for mammography? Is it important to have a mammogram? How often? Should all women have them regularly or only women in specific age and risk groups? What about school nurses teaching breast self-examination to high school girls? Is this a good idea? Why? Why not? Epidemiological research provides data for answering these questions, but study results may be conflicting. Quality of study designs vary and results may be attributable to biases in the study design. Thus to reach appropriate conclusions to guide practice, nurses need to have sufficient understanding of epidemiological methods to allow them to read the literature critically.

TABLE 8-5

A comparison of ecological and relational studies

Level of studies	Types of studies	Other common terms for study design	Basic design
Ecological	Cross-sectional	Correlational Ecological correlational	Rates of disease frequency are correlated with frequency of factor at various points in time
	Case-control	Retrospective	Places with high rates of a disease are compared with places with low rates for levels of factors thought to be related to causing that disease
	Cohort	Prospective Longitudinal	Rates of disease occurrence are compared into the future for places with current environmental exposures and places known not to have such exposures
	Historical cohort	Retrospective-prospective Nonconcurrent cohort	Rates of disease occurrence are compared for places with known past exposure to an environmental factor and places known not to have such exposures; tracking of rates begins in the past at the time of exposure and continues to the present
Relational	Cross-sectional	Correlational	Current rates of exposure among individuals are correlated with current rates of disease frequency among these same individuals
	Case-control	Retrospective Case comparison	Individuals with the study disease are compared with a group of individuals without the disease, who are similar in regard to other characteristics, for frequency of prior exposure to the study factor
	Cohort	Prospective Longitudinal Prospective population	A group of individuals known to be exposed to a factor and a group of similar individuals not exposed are followed into the future for occurrence of the study disease and comparison of its incidence
	Historical cohort	Retrospective-prospective Nonconcurrent cohort Retrospective cohort Retrospective mortality Retrospective incidence	A group of individuals known to have been exposed to a factor at a time in the past is compared with a group of individuals not exposed and their disease incidence or mortality is compared from the time of exposure to the present

It is beyond the scope of this chapter to discuss in depth the methological design considerations that need to be considered. To obtain the necessary skills, an epidemiology course is highly recommended. In the absence of a course, any of the following epidemiology texts provide some useful background: Valanis, 1986; Mausner and Kramer, 1984; Friedman, 1981.

The following discussion of a recently published study which generated national media attention illustrates the type of critical analysis required when reading the literature. The case-control study by MacMahon, et al. (1983) illustrates biases inherent in research design which may affect validity of results. These researchers reported a finding that coffee drinking was associated with occurrence of pancreatic cancer. Cases were pathologically documented incidence cases of pancreatic cancer treated at the study hospitals during a defined time period. Control subjects were other patients with gastrointestinal disease treated by the same physicians at the study hospital during the same period. Use of coffee was assessed for the period immediately before diagnosis. This time frame for assessing coffee exposure together with the use of patients with gastrointestinal disease as controls may have introduced a bias leading to the findings reported. Because of the slow onset of many gastrointestinal diseases, control patients may have experienced mild gastrointestinal discomfort for an extended period before diagnosis. Because coffee drinking tends to produce gastrointestinal discomfort for many people, it is quite likely that these control subjects had decreased or eliminated use of coffee considerably before diagnosis. If so, the finding that pancreatic cancer patients drank more coffee than control subjects is not surprising.

USES OF EPIDEMIOLOGY
Investigation of Disease Etiology and Determination of the Natural History of Disease

Because the purpose of epidemiological investigation is to determine the cause of disease, thus providing the data needed for control or eradication, etiological studies represent a major use of epidemiological methods. To prevent disease, one must identify the causes(s) of the disease and understand the means by which causal agents are transmitted to the human host. In contrast to epidemiological studies, which emphasize the prepathogenic or early pathogenesis of disease, research carried on by clinicians, whether by physicians, nurses, or other groups, is largely concerned with patient responses to treatment (physiological and psychological) during the later stages in the natural history, since the patients usually studied have sought treatment for symptoms of illness.

Although there are numerous epidemiological studies based solely on hospitalized cases, it is essential to look at studies that are concerned with all cases of a disease in a population, regardless of their location. Without this spectrum of disease severity, it is impossible to understand the natural history. Thus epidemiological research often produces a different picture of the disease than do studies derived only from hospital data. As an example, recent data show that half or more of the deaths of middle-aged men from CHD occur in the initial days of the first clinical attack of coronary thrombosis. A substantial portion of these deaths occur in the first hours before the patient reaches the hospital, so these cases are never part of clinical research. In addition, there are many cases of silent myocardial infarction (MI) that are generally unknown to the clinician. These data provide important information that can be used for planning early intervention directed toward identification and treatment of the silent MI group. In addition, the data on the high early mortality of clinical attacks suggest the need for lifesaving squads trained in cardiopulmonary resuscitation with readily available equipment.

Identification of Risks

Risk refers to the probability of an unfavorable event. In epidemiology, the term generally refers to the likelihood that people who are without a disease but who come in contact with certain risk factors thought to increase disease risk will acquire the disease. In general, the risk to an individual of developing a particular disease can be estimated only on the basis of the experience of whole populations of individuals. Once this experience is known, the relevant risks can be calculated for persons who are similar to those in that population. Further, population data on disease occurrence can provide data for estimating the effect on disease rates of a community intervention. Epidemiological methods are used to collect the appropriate data and to estimate these risks.

Risk to an individual of developing a disease caused by a particular exposure is derived by comparing the occurrence of disease in a population exposed to the causal agent to the occurrence of disease in a nonexposed population. This measure, called a *relative risk ratio,* estimates how much the risk of acquiring a disease increases with exposure to a particular causal agent or known risk factor. Thus a relative risk ratio of 5:1 implies that the risk of acquiring that disease is five time greater for someone exposed to an etiological agent than for someone not exposed.

Relative risk ratios are a useful tool for identifying factors that represent increased risk for development of a disease. Diabetes, obesity, hypertension, and smoking are considered risk factors for cardiovascular disease because populations with these characteristics show a rate of that disease several times greater than that of populations without those conditions or behaviors. Once these risk factors are identified, community health programs can be instituted to change high-risk behaviors such as smoking and to identify high-risk individuals through comprehensive screening programs that ensure medical treatment to reduce risk. In addition, nurses and other clinicians can counsel high-risk individuals regarding methods to reduce their risk by adopting healthier life-styles.

An estimate of the effect on disease occurrence of community intervention to eliminate exposure to a causal agent is provided by a measure called *attributable risk.* This measure subtracts the rate of disease occurrence (incidence) in the nonexposed population from the rate of disease occurrence (incidence) in the exposed population. If a nonsmoking population develops cardiovascular disease at a rate of 350 cases per 100,000 population and a smoking population develops cardiovascular disease at a rate of 685 cases per 100,000, then 335 cases per 100,000 population are attributable to cigarette smoking and should be preventable if cigarettes were banned.

Identification of Syndromes and Classification of Disease

Identification of syndromes and disease classification relate directly to clinical medicine. Broad descriptive clinical and pathological categories often include very different elements. Their different statistical distribution and the different ways in which the disease progresses or behaves in a population may make it possible to distinguish one element from another and thus to identify characteristic syndromes. Previously all vascular diseases were classified together. As epidemiological data accumulated, it became clear that cerebrovascular disease and cardiovascular disease were distinct conditions, although both shared the characteristic narrowing or occlusion of a blood vessel as a preceding mechanism. However, populations with high rates of cerebrovascular disease, such as the Japanese, had low rates of cardiovascular disease and the converse was true (Morris, 1975). The rubella syndrome was identified as a collection of malformations and functional problems common to offspring of mothers infected with rubella during pregnancy, particularly during the first trimester (Gregg, 1941). More recent examples include the identification of toxic shock syndrome as a definable group of symptoms characterized by fever of greater than 39° C, rash, desquamation of skin, particularly on the extremities, hypotension, and involvement of three or more of the following organ systems: gastrointestinal, muscular, mucous membrane, renal, hepatic, hematological, and central nervous (Centers for Disease Control, 1980) and the identification of AIDS among homosexual men (MMWR, 1981).

Differential Diagnoses and Planning
Clinical Treatment

Descriptive data on, for example, the age and sex incidence of disease, aid the clinician in understanding the condition and in sorting through multiple possible diagnoses with the same or similar symptoms. Recognizing the association of age with prognosis for long-term survival in breast cancer will probably influence treatment and may influence control programs. Breast cancer diagnosed premenopausally tends to be more lethal than postmenopausal breast cancer, thus requiring more aggressive treatment and closer follow-up. Mumps may be a mild, self-limiting disease in childhood, but in adult men it can lead to infertility. Thus community health intervention to reduce susceptibility or to prevent exposure of men who did not acquire infection during childhood is important.

Surveillance of the Health Status of Populations

Surveillance means keeping watch over. Epidemiological descriptions of diseases provide data regarding who is at high risk of contracting a disease, in which geographical locations it is more likely to occur, and when in time it was most frequently observed. This information alerts health workers to situations that should be monitored for early indication of a disease outbreak so that early detection programs may be set up and intervention promptly instituted. As an example, influenza rates tend to increase during late fall and early winter. Specific types of influenza are likely to recur in 2- to 3-year or 4- to 6-year cycles (Benenson, 1985). Groups at high risk of becoming seriously ill and dying of influenza are infants, young children and elderly persons. By monitoring the population for early indication of influenza through reports of deaths from influenza, of increases in cases seen at emergency rooms, or of increased rates of absence from schools or work because of respiratory illness, public health officials can identify the signs of an outbreak early and can take steps to immunize susceptible, high-risk populations to prevent occurrence of the illness.

In an additional example, the descriptive epidemiology of measles indicates that it occurs most frequently among school-age children, that rates vary by season with highest rates in the fall, and that there are long-term cycles with increased rates every other year in large communities and at less frequent intervals in smaller communities, where outbreaks tend to be more severe. Measles is transmitted from person to person by close contact; it therefore tends to occur in locations where children congregate (Benenson, 1975). Armed with this information, the school nurse can be alert to signs and symptoms of measles during the fall and can follow up on absences to determine if measles caused the absence. Numerous such absences may indicate a need to review the immunization status of the school population. Although most schools, in theory, require up-to-date immunizations for a child to enter, all too often monitoring does not occur and follow-up programs must be instituted to obtain immunizations for the susceptible children.

Monitoring of newly diagnosed cancer cases or of birth defects can alert officials to clusters of cases that may suggest clues as to their causes. The occurrence of several cases of adenocarcinoma of the vagina of young girls was noted by physicians in Boston. They realized that the occurrence of several cases in a short period of time in this age group was a highly unusually event. Their follow-up investigation led to identification of diethylstilbestrol, a drug given to the mothers of the girls during their pregnancies, as the probable causal agent (Herbst and Scully, 1972).

Community Diagnosis and Planning of Health Services

Epidemiology provides the facts about community health. It describes the nature and relative size of the health problems to be dealt with, as well as how they are distributed in terms of geographical location, age group, socioeconomic group, and so on. This kind of information forms the basis for planning the number and types of services required to meet the needs of a particular community. A neighborhood with a high proportion of elderly individuals is likely to have high rates of cardiovascular disease, cancer, and other chronic, debilitating diseases. Particularly if it is a low-income neighborhood, elderly residents may lack the financial resources to travel to a distant source of medical care. Thus health planners need to consider setting up a satellite clinic in the neighborhood or providing transportation or home services. Maternity and child health services can be planned to meet the needs of a community with a young population with a high birth rate. Family planning facilities, well-child centers that include immunization services, and health education programs aimed at prevention of disease through promotion of good health habits may be appropriate.

Evaluation of Health Services

Since many health services are initiated as an effort to treat a community problem identified by epidemiological data, these same data, used as a monitoring device, are useful in the evaluation of these services. For example, one means of evaluating the effectiveness of a maternity and child health center established to reduce the rates of morbidity and mortality among mothers and children is to follow closely the morbidity or mortality to see whether they drop and remain low after the health center is in operation.

APPLICATIONS OF EPIDEMIOLOGY IN COMMUNITY HEALTH NURSING

Most nurses working in community health are employed by agencies that interact directly with individual clients and families, such as visiting nurse associations, community-based maternity and child health or mental health centers, alcohol and drug intervention programs, health maintenance organizations, or nursing centers. Nursing in occupational health settings, although usually limited to contact with the individual client, requires consideration of the family resources and needs in planning care. Some nurses will be employed as health planners or administrators involved in planning and evaluating services of their agency, for example, the director of a visiting nurse association. Nursing administrators in a health department, in contrast, may be involved both in planning services of that agency and in coordinating the services of a variety of community agencies. Similarly, nurses serving on community boards need to be concerned with coordination of existing services and planning to meet currently unmet needs. Regardless of the agency or the nurses' position, they will be involved in some phase with the epidemiological process.

Care of patients and families is based on the following steps of the nursing process: (1) assessment, (2) planning, (3) implementation, and (4) evaluation. The same process is used in providing care for communities. In both instances, epidemiology provides the baseline information for assessment of needs, for setting priorities in developing a plan of care, and for evaluating the effectiveness of care.

Agencies providing care to communities through surveillance of health indicators for planning, provision, and evaluation of services interrelate through referrals, required reporting, and feedback mechanisms with agencies such as visiting nurse services whose primary purpose is provision of direct services to clients. Because of the interrelationships between the various levels of health agencies, observations of need based on a common baseline of information are necessary if nurses at various levels and in various settings are to provide appropriate care. If such a baseline of information is not shared, each nurse would collect only the data she considered important; interpretations of the data would vary from nurse to nurse. Epidemiological concepts, such as natural history of disease and primary, secondary, and tertiary prevention, provide a unifying approach for defining which data should be collected and how they should be interpreted.

If such common information is available at all levels and common interpretation is likely, then the referral and reporting system within a community is facilitated and effective response of the system to a need should result. To assess needs, the nurse providing direct care requires data on the presence or absence of risk characteristics, including family composition and relationships, socioeconomic and cultural factors, environmental factors, and medical and health history (incidence, prevalence, and mortality, both current and over a period of time). The nurse involved in planning services for the community requires parallel data for the community: presence and distribution of risk characteristics for the community, including composition by age, race, socioeconomic and cultural factors, environmental factors, and rates measuring the medical and health history.

CLINICAL APPLICATION

The following situation illustrates the use of epidemiological data by nurses providing direct services and by those involved in planning at the community level:

A nurse at the Visiting Nurse Service receives a referral for a home visit to a 15-year-old mother whose premature infant has just been discharged from the hospital. The mother of the infant lives with her 40-year-old mother, a heavy smoker who is 50 pounds overweight, and her 45-year-old father, who has high blood pressure and is employed by a company that manufactures pesticides. On her way from the bus stop to the house, the nurse passes overturned trash cans with garbage strewn in the street and numerous teenagers lounging on the doorstep of a neighboring house. When she arrives, she finds that the baby has a temperature of 39°C and diarrhea but no signs of an upper respiratory infection. The grandmother reports that the temperature was normal late yesterday when the infant was discharged from the hospital. The baby's mother has returned to school and the grandmother is caring for the baby. She states that she quit a part-time job so she could do this and that they can just scrape by on her husband's salary of $12,000 a year.

The apartment is hazy with cigarette smoke but appears clean and tidy. Grandmother has a hacking cough and appears slightly short of breath. Her pulse is 96. She had been preparing a dinner of baked ham, canned green beans, and boxed macaroni and cheese when the nurse arrived. An interview with the grandmother reveals a family history of CHD on both sides of the family. The nurse also learns that the baby's mother is continuing to see the baby's father and that she is irritable and impatient when the baby cries. About this time the grandfather arrives home from work, tired and hungry. His clothing and hair are sprinkled with a light but visible dusting of powder. After being introduced, he has a beer, then excuses himself to shower and change.

Table 8-6 lists the observations of the nurse, the pertinent epidemiological facts that facilitate interpretation of the observation, the implications for nursing care, and the possible courses of action based on her assessment. For example, the nurse has observed an elevated temperature in the infant accompanied by diarrhea. The infant was fed once during the night and once in the morning with bottles of milk sent home from the hospital. Only the afternoon feeding was from formula mixed in the home. The nurse's knowledge of the natural history of infectious diseases reveals these important facts: (1) an elevated temperature and diarrhea in the absence of respiratory symptoms suggest a milk-borne infection or some other infection transmitted by oral entry, and since the temperature is elevated, the symptoms are probably caused by an infection rather than by a toxin; (2) most gastrointestinal infections have incubation periods longer than 24 hours and most feedings were from hospital-supplied formula. The nurse concludes that the infection may have originated in the hospital and initiates appropriate action, both to secure treatment for the infant and to notify appropriate persons who can evaluate and control any infection problem at the hospital.

Similar assessment processes are illustrated in Table 8-6 for the other observations of the nurse. In each instance the nurse can evaluate her care by referring back to the epidemiological risk factors that suggested the approach to care and can evaluate whether her actions have been effective by determining whether the risks have been eliminated.

Her interventions with this family will bring her into contact with nurses in other community agencies—the health department nurse, the school nurse, and the occu-

TABLE 8-6

Example of use of epidemiological data in clinical practice

Observation(s)	Relevant epidemiological data	Assessment of implications	Intervention(s)
Baby			
Elevated temperature accompanied by gastrointestinal symptoms less than 24 hours after hospital discharge	Elevated temperature indicates infection, not toxin as source of gastrointestinal symptoms	Because most infectious agents have incubation periods longer than 24 hours, infection could have originated in hospital	Refer to pediatrician for culture and treatment; report possible hospital-related infection in premature nursery to health department nurses who may need to follow up on other recent discharges and to work with hospital epidemiologist to identify source of infection
Mother			
Still dating father of baby; not using birth control Irritable and impatient with infant	Teenage pregnancies are at high risk for low birth weight and perinatal and infant mortality; close spacing of pregnancies increases risks to physical health of both mother and fetus	Teenage mother remains at high risk of becoming pregnant; such a pregnancy would be at high risk of complications; additional infant would increase pressures on mother and her parents and disrupt family interactions, creating a high-risk environment for child abuse	Counsel mother regarding birth control options and referral to family planning center Teach mother regarding normal behavior and growth and development of infant, effective ways of caring for infant
No short-term or long-term goals	Low socioeconomic status and multiple pressures are risk factors for child abuse		Assess plans for future; counsel grandparents regarding helping role; refer for family counseling if indicated; contact school nurse for counseling with mother and referral to community adolescent mothers group
Grandmother			
Heavy smoker; obese with shortness of breath; family history of coronary heart disease	Smoking and obesity are risk factors for coronary heart disease (CHD); side-stream smoke can increase risk of other family members for CHD and of premature infant for respiratory infection; family history is also associated with elevated risk for CHD	Grandmother is at high risk for developing CHD and/or emphysema; she is experiencing additional stress because of demands for infant care; stress also is a risk factor for CHD	Check blood pressure; refer to physician for physical examination; counsel regarding risk factors for CHD and measures for personal and family risk reduction and techniques of stress reduction; reduce infant exposure to cigarette smoke by smoking only outside infant's room if she continues to smoke
Cooking meal high in sodium	High sodium diet is risk factor for elevated blood pressure	Nutritional practices may be increasing CHD risk of grandmother and family	Counsel regarding nutrition 1. Calorie and sodium reduction 2. Nutritional needs of adolescents 3. Nutrition and child development
Grandfather			
High blood pressure; stress related to current financial responsibilities and demands of job	High blood pressure and stress are risk factors for CHD, stroke	Grandfather has elevated risk for stroke because of high blood pressure and stress	Counsel regarding stress reduction and low sodium diet to reduce risk of stroke
Pesticide exposure at work—dust on clothing exposes family	Pesticides are associated with increased risk of cancer; infants may be more susceptible than adults; both dermal and respiratory absorption are routes of exposure	Pesticides are introduced into home on clothes; remainder of family is thus exposed; infant may already have had in utero exposure	Counsel grandfather regarding hazards of pesticides, advantages of changing clothes at work; contact occupational health nurse at company regarding possibility of reducing workplace exposures to pesticides and instituting a policy of changing out of dusty clothing at work and having company assume responsibility for cleaning work clothes

pational health nurse at the grandfather's workplace. Knowledge of the epidemiological risk factors and assessment data by nurses in each of these settings facilitates communication of the needs identified for intervention. Facilities such as the family planning center and an adolescent mothers' group are available for referrals because nurses and other professionals engaged in health planning monitored births in the community. Because they observed that the rate of illegitimate births was increasing, particularly among adolescents, they established family planning centers in high-risk neighborhoods. Also, because they were aware of the increased risk among adolescent mothers for child abuse and for continuation of a cycle of poverty, counseling groups for adolescent mothers were organized. Because the health planners were monitoring appropriate epidemiological indicators, the services needed for appropriate intervention with this young mother were available and the nurse providing direct services could make appropriate referrals. Ongoing monitoring of these indicators provides feedback as to the effectiveness of services.

SUMMARY

Epidemiology, the study of the distribution of states of health and of the determinants of deviations from health in populations, is a community health science essential to nursing practice. Epidemiology refers to both the methods used in the study of disease causation and to the body of knowledge that arises from such investigations. Knowledge of the methods of epidemiology is useful to the community health nurse, both as a tool in conducting the investigation to evaluate and to explain phenomena observed in the course of work and as a basis for interpreting and evaluating the epidemiological research literature. Epidemiological methods, such as measures of health, serve on a community level as tools for assessing community needs, monitoring changes in health status of the community, and evaluating the impact of community programs of disease prevention and health promotion.

The body of knowledge derived from epidemiological studies, including the natural history of diseases, patterns of disease occurrence, and factors associated with high risk for developing disease, serves as an information base for community health nursing practice. This knowledge provides a framework for planning and evaluating community intervention programs aimed at primary, secondary, and tertiary prevention, which respectively consist of prevention of illness, early detection and treatment of disease, and minimization of disability. Programs of primary prevention try to keep disease agents away from susceptible hosts, decrease agent viability, increase host resistance, or alter in other ways the established host-agent-environment relationships. Screening and risk factor reduction programs are examples of secondary prevention. Vocational retraining and rehabilitative exercises for the disabled are tertiary prevention.

For the individual nurse, the body of knowledge derived from epidemiological research serves as a basis for assessing individual and family health needs and for planning nursing interventions. It also provides tools for evaluating the success of the interventions.

⟲ KEY CONCEPTS

Epidemiology is the study of the distribution of health and illness in populations.

In the epidemiological approach to illness, the event is described in terms of how it affects the group.

Epidemiologists investigate causality based on relationships between a stimulus and an outcome by using statistical measures of association.

Two kinds of causal associations are direct causal associations and indirect causal associations.

Concepts important to epidemiology are causality, natural history, agent, environment, host, disease process, and levels of prevention.

Natural history is the process by which a disease occurs and progresses in humans. The natural history of a disease involves three factors: a causative agent, a susceptible host, and the environment.

There are three stages to the natural history of a disease: prepathogenesis, or susceptibility; pathogenesis; and advanced disease.

Three levels of prevention are primary, secondary, and tertiary. Primary prevention involves prevention of illness; secondary prevention involves early detection and treatment of disease; and tertiary prevention involves minimization of disability.

Epidemiological methods involve use of data from existing sources, such as census data, and data generated for specific studies. The three types of data required are population statistics, mortality data, and morbidity data.

Rates used in epidemiology include attack rates, incidence, and prevalence. Incidence is a measure of all new cases of illness arising during a given period in a population at risk; prevalence is a measure of the number of existing cases of illness in a population at a given time; and attack rates represent the incidence of illness among an exposed population.

The knowledge derived from epidemiological studies provide a framework for planning and evaluating community health intervention programs.

LEARNING ACTIVITIES

1. Choose one of the major causes of morbidity and mortality, such as cardiovascular disease.
   a. On the basis of current epidemiological research evidence, outline the natural history, including known risk factors.
   b. Based on the natural history, specify interventions for primary, secondary, and tertiary prevention of this disease.

2. Choose one of the interventions identified in activity B of number 1.
   a. Define the parameters of a community population in which such an intervention would be useful.
   b. Decide which measurements of disease would reflect the impact of your intervention on this population, e.g., incidence, prevalence, mortality, survival, complication rates.

3. Decide how the natural history of this disease will affect your own nursing care of patients or families.

BIBLIOGRAPHY

Abramson, J.H.: Re: definitions of epidemiology (letter), Am. J. Epidemiol. 109:99-102, 1979.

Benenson, A., editor: Control of communicable diseases in man, 1985, Washington, D.C., American Public Health Association.

Centers for Disease Control, Follow-up on toxic shock syndrome, Morbidity and Mortality Weekly Reports, 29:441-444, 1980.

Evans, A.S.: Definitions of epidemiology (letter), Am. J. Epidemiol. 109:379-382, 1979.

Frerichs, R.R., and Neutra, R.: Definitions of epidemiology (letter), Am. J. Epidemiol. 108:74-75, 1978.

Friedman, G.: Primer of epidemiology, New York, 1980, McGraw-Hill Book Co.

Gregg, N.M.: Congenital cataract following german measles in the mother, Trans. Ophthalmol. Soc. Australia. 3:35-46, 1941.

Herbst, A.L., and Scully, R.E.: Adenocarcinoma of the vagina in adolescence: report of 7 cases including 6 clear-cell carcinomas (so-called mesonephromas), Cancer 25:745-757, 1970.

Herbst, A.L., Ulfelder, H., and Poskanzer, D.C.: Association of maternal stilbestrol therapy with tumor appearance in young women, N. Engl. J. Med. 284:878-881, 1971.

Kleinfeld, M., Messite, J., and Kooyman, O.: Mortality experience in a group of asbestos workers, Arch. Environ. Health 15:177-180, 1967.

Kuter, B.: The epidemiology of a measles epidemic: suburban Cook County, Ill., 1976-1977, unpublished master's thesis, New York, 1977, Columbia University.

Leavell, H.R., and Clark, E.G.: Preventive medicine for the doctor in his community, New York, 1958, McGraw-Hill Book Co.

Lilienfeld, A., and Lilienfeld, D.: Foundations of epidemiology, New York, 1980, Oxford University Press.

Lilienfeld, D.: Definitions of epidemiology, Am. J. Epidemiol. 107:87-90, 1978.

MacMahon, B., Yen, S., Tuchopoulos, D., Warren, K., and Nardis, G.: Coffee and cancer of the pancreas, N. Engl. J. Med. 304:630-633, 1981.

Mausner, J., and Kramer, S.: Mausner and Baun's epidemiology: an introductory text, Philadelphia, 1984, W.B. Saunders Co.

Morbidity and Mortality Weekly Reports (MMWR), Centers for Disease Control, 30:305-307, 1981.

Morris, J.N.: Uses of epidemiology, ed. 3, London, 1975, E & S Livingstone, Ltd.

National Center for Health Statistics (NCHS), Monthly vital statistics report, 34(suppl) Sept. 20, 1985.

Rich, H.: More on definitions of epidemiology (letter), Am. J. Epidemiol. 109:99-102, 1979.

Smoking and Health: Report of the advisory committee to the Surgeon General of the public health service, USDHEW, Pub. No. (PHS) 1103, Washington, D.C., 1964, U.S. Government Printing Office.

Snow, J.: On the mode of communication of cholera, New York, 1936, The Commonwealth Fund, pp. 1-175.

Valanis, B.: Epidemiology in nursing and health care, East Norwalk, Conn., 1986, Appleton-Century-Crofts.

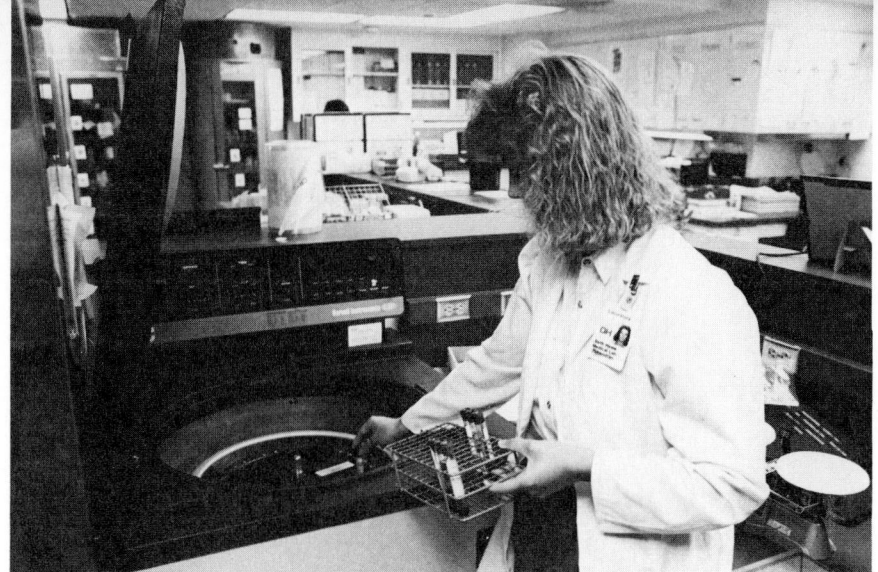

Beverly C. Flynn

9

RESEARCH AS A GUIDE TO COMMUNITY HEALTH NURSING PRACTICE

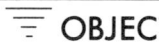 OBJECTIVES

After reading this chapter, the student should be able to:

Discuss priority areas for research in community health nursing with consideration of the WHO and UNICEF (1978) definition of primary health care.

Identify the differences between inductive and deductive approaches to research.

Describe the action research approach.

Interrelate and describe the stages of the research process with the phases of the nursing process.

Describe roles and functions in research.

Identify ways the practicing community health nurse can participate in research.

KEY TERMS

accessibility of health services

action research

appropriate technology

approval

assessment

communication

community involvement

data gathering

deductive approach

elaboration model

evaluation

implementation

inductive approach

multisectoral approach

participatory research

planning

primary health care

random sampling

Research for community health nursing practice is in an early stage of development. Although increasing efforts are devoted to nursing research, much in community health nursing remains largely intuitive and based on tradition. Today, community health nurses need information; they need to know what has worked and what has not worked in similar situations and why. Community health nurses are committed to improving the health of the community and are challenged to search for creative yet scientifically oriented solutions to today's health and nursing problems. Through research, community health nurses will be leaders in developing the knowledge needed to meet the challenge.

This chapter focuses on the development of practice-based research in community health nursing. Primary health care as defined by the World Health Organization (WHO and UNICEF, 1978) is proposed as an appropriate approach to guide research and to develop concepts in community health nursing. An overview of the research process is presented. Research questions that are generated from practice through inductive methods are linked with the key concepts of primary health care. Selected research issues and the roles and functions of the researcher and collaborators are discussed. Examples from community health nursing practice are provided throughout the chapter.

RELATIONSHIP OF COMMUNITY HEALTH NURSING TO PRIMARY HEALTH CARE

The contribution of nursing to the primary health care approach is currently being considered within countries supporting the goal of "health for all by the year 2000" (WHO and UNICEF, 1978). In addition, the International Council of Nurses (ICN) and WHO have provided leadership in supporting national nursing associations in their exploration of contributions nursing can make in primary health care (ICN and WHO, 1979; PAHO, 1977; WHO, 1974; WHO, 1982). In recent years WHO has focused a major effort on issues related to the basic education of nurses and the further training of nurse teachers and managers to orient them to primary health care and community health (WHO, 1984; WHO, 1985).

A link exists between the view of community health nursing delineated in this text and primary health care.

Both incorporate community-based practice, involvement of the community in health care decisions, a focus on disease prevention and health promotion, and use of an interdisciplinary approach in planning and implementing appropriate solutions to health problems. Thus community health nursing and primary health care are complementary; research conducted by community health nurses can make a significant contribution to nursing practice and also to primary health care practice.

DEVELOPING A CONCEPTUAL BASE FOR PRACTICE RESEARCH

The primary health care approach emphasizes conducting research within the context of the community. Some time ago Diers (1970) challenged the profession by claiming such research was possible. She stated, "It is possible to do quite good clinical research if one is deeply enough involved in practice to know what can be controlled and how" (p. 52). Research can help the practitioner find answers to practice issues and in the process help in developing a conceptual base for professional practice.

Considerable agreement exists in nursing literature about the need to develop a body of knowledge through research relevant to nursing practice. Dickoff and James (1975) have criticized nursing research for leaving nursing practice virtually untouched. Nursing research has typically focused on testing research questions that are easily measured and based primarily on a deductive approach. Such an approach leads from the general to the specific. It may be that the deductive approach is too constraining at this stage of the profession's development.

The alternative approach, inductive, focuses on practice problems examined qualitatively within their own context rather than quantitatively from some predetermined theoretical or conceptual basis. The inductive approach, which has been neglected in the past decade, generates concepts and theories from the data collected rather than attempting to fit data to predetermined concepts and theories. For example, the inductive methods of participant observation and open-ended interviews with key informants permit intensive study of clinical practice in its process and context. The concepts generated from the inductive approach come from the data collected rather than having the results reinterpreted from other theoretical perspectives. In this way new theoretical formulations that are more appropriate to the problem under study may result.

ACTION RESEARCH

The primary health care approach is based on the premise that desired changes in health must involve citizens in the creation of their own future. Research suitable for this approach to health care has been neglected by the social sciences. However, based on the approaches and knowledge of community development, health education, and adult education, *action research* has been promoted as an appropriate method for research.

Action research focuses on the process of change in a group or community. In action research, information is fed back into the group and plays an important role in the growth of the group. Since primary health care is a form of community action designed to achieve the goal of "health for all by the year 2000," the relevance of action research to primary health care will be explored.

Some investigators may challenge this concept of research as contrary to the emphasis on scientific rigor that is stressed in nursing research or social science research in general. However, Diers (1970) notes that "research in controlled laboratories has low generality for clinical settings, no matter how rigorous it is" (p. 53). Furthermore, action research encourages the use of research results in practice.

Stinson (1979) reviews several types of action research; one type, participatory research, has gained the most attention in primary health care. Participatory research stems from the field of adult education and has been influenced by Freire (1970) and his concern for liberation of people, particularly the oppressed. Freire's efforts seek to increase people's ability to gain some degree of control over their own lives. Involving people in all stages of the research process supports his goal of increasing awareness of the issue(s) being examined.

Hall (1975) describes a number of key principles of participatory research. First, the community is involved in all phases of the research process. Second, the research team includes persons representing all population groups in the community. Third, the research process is part of the educational experience and involves communication among those participating in the process. Finally, participatory research encourages people to creatively reach solutions to social problems.

A good example of participatory research is Feuerstain's report (1978) on the evaluation of health services by the people of Honduras. In this research the people collaborated in all phases of the evaluation. They identified not only the strengths and weaknesses of the program but also ways to increase the strengths and to remedy the weaknesses, thereby clearly linking research with community practice.

THE RESEARCH PROCESS

The research process is a problem-solving process, much like the nursing process. It involves assessment, planning, implementation, evaluation, and action. The action leads to reassessment, more planning and implementation, and so on. Although the research and nursing processes are similar, they vary in the extent to which scientific principles of inquiry are applied and to which generalizations can be made. The research process is conscious and deliberate; it results from prior planning and decision making.

The stages of the research process are integrated with the phases of the nursing process in the box below. Although the listing is sequential, the researcher actually works back and forth among the various stages of the research process. Decisions made in any one stage must be consistent with decisions made in other stages. All stages are viewed as part of the total study and are arrived at logically and systematically.

Assessment

Assessment involves translating a hunch or a curiosity about a clinical problem into one that can be researched. For example, a community health nurse may be curious about

---

STAGES OF THE RESEARCH PROCESS* BY PHASES OF THE NURSING PROCESS

ASSESSMENT PHASE

Initiating the idea
Initial review of literature
Identifying the purpose of the research
Delineating the population

PLANNING PHASE

Stating specific research problem
Extensive review of literature
Delineating the conceptual framework
Delineating research questions and hypotheses
Selecting research approach and research design
Selecting data gathering method
Developing data analysis plan
Selecting sample
Pilot studies to test instruments and apply data analysis
Human subjects approval process
Identifying assumptions and limitations of research

IMPLEMENTATION PHASE

Inviting sample to participate in research
Implementing data gathering plan
Implementing data analysis plan

EVALUATION PHASE

Analyzing findings
Drawing conclusions
Preparing research reports
Presenting research

ACTION PHASE

Applying results
Taking action for social change

*Selected stages of the research process are modified from Fox (1982), pp. 26-27.

why some elderly in the community are able to live independently while others are institutionalized. The nurse reviews the research and related literature to gain an overview of the problem and its current stage of research. The initial literature review helps the nurse decide on the purpose and population for the study. In our example of the elderly, the community health nurse decides that the purpose of the study is to determine whether or not community health nursing services are assisting the elderly to live in the community. She also needs to decide what ages of the elderly will be studied: all those 65 years and older? 75 and older? Or 85 and older?

Planning

In *planning,* the specific research problem is stated. In our example, the community health nurse decides that the problem to be investigated is a lack of information about the relationship between community health nursing services and living arrangements of the elderly who are 75 years and older.

Next, key terms in the problem are defined. Information obtained from literature reviews can be used to define terms and assist in the further development of a scientific body of knowledge for nursing practice.

Through an extensive literature review the nurse identifies conceptual frameworks and how research and data analyses were done and examines the results of previous research. Of particular concern here is what has and has not worked in previous studies. The nurse is also interested in selecting a conceptual framework that is appropriate for the problem to be investigated. In our example, the nurse selects a conceptual framework that can be adapted from the health services research field, incorporating environmental services, health services, and client characteristics. Next, the nurse delineates specific research questions or hypotheses or both for the research. These statements include the key variables of the study. In our example, the nurse questions if the range of community health nursing services for the elderly is related to the rate of institutionalization of this population.

The nurse next selects a research approach; it may be historical, survey, or experimental. Each approach creates different requirements for a research design. Considerations include whether the data will be collected at one point in time or longitudinally, at various time points, and whether the data will be collected cross-sectionally or across various groups in the population. In our example, the nurse decides that a historical approach, or a review of past information, will not adequately address the problem and that an experimental approach is not feasible because the study cannot be conducted under controlled conditions. Instead, the nurse decides that a survey is the most appropriate approach in which to compare the elderly with different living arrangements. This approach permits a research design for collecting data at one time period among both institutionalized and noninstitutionalized elderly.

The next stage involves selecting a *data gathering* method, such as observing, measuring, or questioning. Specific techniques and instruments are identified in accord with the general method for collecting data. Within the questioning method, for example, the interview or questionnaire technique might be considered and a specific instrument could be selected for the technique. Decisions need to be made about a data gathering method, technique, and instrument for each of the major variables in the research questions or hypotheses. In our example the nurse decides to use the observing and questioning methods. She plans to observe nurses providing services to the elderly to delineate the range of services provided from the perspective of the interaction between the nurses and the elderly. To avoid a situation in which the nurses and the elderly feel uncomfortable about being observed, the observing nurse decides she will be a participant observer and work with the nurses being observed. This allows the nurse researcher to participate in the research situation and to use a natural situation for data collection. In addition to observation, the nurse researcher will use the questioning method and select an interview questionnaire that determines the level of physical functioning of the elderly. This interview may be completed with the elderly person or the elderly person's care giver.

Important in the planning phase is *approval* of the research by the institutional human subjects review committee. Usually an application is submitted to the committee to assure the study subjects will not be physically or mentally harmed by the research. This process also protects the researcher from undue complaints, providing the subject's informed consent is obtained before conduction of the study.

The plan for data analysis is guided by the research questions or hypotheses. If appropriate to the conceptual base for the study, it is useful to identify the statistics to be used and also to delineate sample tables that will contain the data once they are collected. This will help assure the researcher that all the necessary data are being collected to answer the research questions and to test the hypotheses.

The elaboration model of contingency table analysis developed by Lazarsfeld (1972) and further presented by Babbie (1983) is useful in developing a data analysis plan. This model provides a logical framework for the analysis and interpretation of the relationship between two variables through the controlled introduction of other variables. The *elaboration model* clarifies the relationship among three or more variables and is statistically simpler than more refined quantitative methods like covariance and multiple regression techniques. The model can also be used with the deductive or inductive conceptual base for research.

The research questions and plan for data analysis guide sample selection. The statistics to be used direct the sample size. Although many methods of sample selection exist, two will be considered here, random sampling and deliberate sampling. *Random sampling* means that every case or subject has an equal opportunity of being included in the study. Random sampling aims to eliminate the bias of sample selection in that the researcher does not have control over which cases or subjects are included in or excluded from the study. Various procedures can be used to select a random sample. One is the assignment of a number to each case in the entire population. Using a table of random numbers, an unbiased sample from the population can be selected.

In this situation, the researcher is trusting by chance that a representative sample of the population will be selected. Another way to ensure a representative sample is to stratify the population or subdivide cases or subjects on certain characteristics before selecting the sample. In our example, the nurse may wish to first separate the elderly population who live in urban areas from those who live in rural areas. The random techniques can then be applied within each group or stratum to ensure that the sample is representative on these two characteristics. The second method is deliberative selection in which specific cases or subjects are invited to participate in the study. There are very good reasons to use deliberative sampling; for example, the researcher may not know the entire population of cases and therefore cannot use the random method. Or, the researcher may be interested in studying only certain types of cases and the random method is inappropriate to use because all cases, which are few in number, are to be studied.

In our example, the nurse decides to study elderly persons in the county in which she works. She consults a statistician and together they decide that the sample should consist of 20% of elderly persons over 75 years living in institutions and 20% of the same population living outside of institutions. Although the number of elderly persons living in institutions can be identified at any one point in time, it is impossible to know the exact number living in the community. Because of this, it would be possible to take a random sample of elderly persons 75 years and older living in institutions but not for the elderly living in the community. To select a sample of 20% of people 75 years and older living outside of institutions, it is necessary to estimate the total population in this age group. It is decided to use the census data for this purpose. Since random sampling of the elderly living outside of institutions could not be accomplished, a deliberate sample of known elderly 75 years and older is selected until 20% of the estimated number of this population is included in the sample.

Important in the planning phase is approval of the research by the institutional human subjects review committee. Usually an application is submitted to the committee to assure the study subjects will not be physically or mentally harmed by the research. This process also protects the researcher from undue complaints providing the subject's informed consent is obtained prior to the conducting of the study.

Pilot studies can be used to test data gathering methods and to apply the data analysis plan. The nurse researcher decides to pilot test her study and asks a nurse from a neighboring county if she would permit the pilot study to be conducted with at least five of her elderly clients. Client permission is also granted. The actual logistics of the study are worked out in the pilot study. A pilot study is especially important when the data gathering technique is unfamiliar to the researcher, if the instrument is new, if the instrument has not been used with the population under study, and if the study is conducted in an unfamiliar environment.

The assumptions and limitations of the research need to be identified. Assumptions are characteristics of the research situation that are not explored, usually because they have been well demonstrated in previous research, so they are assumed to be true. The limitations are uncontrollable elements of the research, which limit the certainty of the findings or the applicability of the findings to the population in general.

Implementation

Implementation of the research plan refers to carrying out the research procedures. This includes inviting the sample group to participate, obtaining their informed consent, collecting, verifying, collating the data, and analyzing them.

Evaluation

Evaluation includes analyzing the findings and comparing them with previous research results. The conclusions are then drawn, building on a body of previous knowledge. The preparation of research reports should provide a clear documentation of what was done and when. The results of the research are presented for the specific problem, research questions, or hypotheses under study. What was found and what was not found in the study need to be reported. Recommendations for future research should be clear and consistent with the study results. The need for replication studies should be made clear. It is important to support replication studies to validate findings, especially in other samples or populations, because recommendations for practice need to be based on more than one set of study results. The research should be presented to professional colleagues, to persons in decision-making positions such as administrators, policymakers, and legislators, and to the general public, who might be affected by any decisions made. The worth of the research is judged by persons in these groups.

Action

The results of nursing research should increasingly be used in practice. To apply the results, we must take *action* on them beyond the preparation of research reports and formal presentation to professional colleagues. We must make specific recommendations of reliable or valid research findings from nursing practice to improve the health of the community. Because we have control over our own professional practice, we can use our own findings in practice. By applying research results in practice we are taking action for social change. We are demonstrating to community people, professionals, and policymakers that the research findings are relevant and applicable to practice.

In the example of practice-based research about factors that contribute to elderly people's ability to live independently, the nurse may learn that the most significant difference between the groups is the presence of a support person(s). The research may indicate that these clients who live in urban areas and are regularly visited by a community health nurse may be the ones who are able to maintain independent living rather than being institutionalized.

The results of such a study could support the expansion of community health nursing. The economic difference between maintaining an elderly client or married couple in the home vs. placing one or both in an institution could be a compelling argument in support of home health care.

Research documenting the effectiveness of nursing care is vitally needed. Effectiveness is measured in many ways, including cost, quality, and client satisfaction.

PRACTICE QUESTIONS FOR RESEARCH

Significant questions for research can be generated from community health nursing practice and linked with the key concepts of primary health care. A framework for the study of community health nursing practice in primary health care systematically links primary health care concepts, research questions, variables, research indicators, and modes of obtaining information (Flynn, 1984). It can be used to guide practice because it permits the categorization of practice hunches as research questions, and it guides the community health nurse to specify components of these questions through many of the stages of the research process noted earlier, including applying results in practice.

Beginning community health nurses often have difficulty identifying potential research questions arising from their practice. The following discussion focuses on examples of research questions that are generated in practice and linked with primary health care concepts. These concepts are accessibility, community involvement, disease prevention and health promotion, appropriate technology, and multisectoral approach.

Accessible Health Care

Accessibility of health services is an issue concerning persons at the social periphery, including rural, urban, poor, and elderly persons and others who are at greatest risk to health problems. The issue here is the extent to which community health nursing services reach people who need them the most or how equitably these services are distributed throughout the population.

A research question related to this concept is whether the community health nursing services are accessible to those in greatest need. For example, are these services available in both urban and rural areas? Are the services available to groups of people most in need of them, in terms of time, location, and personnel? Other questions related to the use of services include the following: Who uses and who does not use the community health nursing services? What are their characteristics? What are the health care needs of the people who use the service compared with those who do not? What are barriers to the use of services? Are the costs too high? Are the services irrelevant to consumers' perceived needs? Are community health nurses insensitive to the concerns of consumers? Do consumers have transportation to reach the services?

Community Involvement

Community involvement is a key concept of primary health care. It is concerned with the level of citizen or community resident participation in health decision making. To promote the development of the community and the community's self-reliance, residents themselves need to participate in decisions about the health of the community. In primary health care, residents and health providers need to work together in partnership. They each have their own

area and level of expertise that are needed in seeking solutions to the complex problems facing communities today.

Research questions generated from practice relate to the level and mechanism of community involvement in health decision making. For example, to what extent is the community involved in the various stages of assessing health care needs, planning, management, and monitoring community health nursing services? What mechanisms and processes exist to enable people to be actively involved and to take joint responsibility, along with community health nurses, for decisions? In particular, what decisions involving the community have been implemented? Are the community health nursing services better used as a result?

Disease Prevention and Health Promotion

Emphasis in primary health care is directed toward health promotion and prevention of disease rather than being focused on curative services. In primary health care the curative or therapeutic aspects must often be addressed before health promotion and preventive services can be instituted. A common example is the early discharge of hospitalized patients who require highly skilled nursing services in the home. People need to have their illness attended to before they can focus their attention on such future-oriented concerns as prevention of further disease or health promotion activities. The latter is the major focus in primary health care, according to WHO.

Priority questions for research include the following: What are the major preventable health problems in the community? Are there high rates of automobile accidents or high rates of heart disease? Are problems being addressed by preventive and health promotive measures? What measures are being taken to ameliorate or control these problems? Do the community health nursing services include recommendations for infant car seat use, programs to reduce alcohol intake among drivers, and smoking cessation programs?

Appropriate Technology

Appropriate technology refers to health care that is relevant to people's health needs and concerns, as well as being acceptable to them. It includes issues of costs and affordability of services within the context of existing resources, such as the number and type of health professionals and other workers, equipment, and supplies and their pattern of distribution throughout the community. The National Science Foundation's definition (1979, p. 1) of appropriate technology summarizes these considerations: "Appropriate technologies are defined as those which are decentralized, require low capital investment, conserve natural resources, are managed by their users, and are in harmony with the environment."

The overriding questions to be answered by research are: Do the services use the simplest and least costly technology available? Are the services acceptable to the community? Are they affordable? What is the cost effectiveness of alternative approaches or strategies for community health nursing services? Are family home visits as effective as working with families in groups? Are nonprofessionals, such as home health aides, effective in providing some aspects of community health nursing services? What is the most effective management and supervision for nonprofessionals and professionals within a community health nursing agency?

Multisectoral Approach

Primary health care recognizes that the health of a community cannot be improved by intervention within just the health sector. Other sectors are equally important, and in some cases more so, in promoting the community's health and self-reliance. For example, education, environment, industry, housing, and nutrition are interrelated with health. Therefore these sectors need to work together in a *multisectoral approach* to coordinate their goals, plans, and activities to ensure that they contribute to the health of the community and to avoid conflicting or duplicating efforts.

Relevant research questions include the following: What mechanisms exist that promote or hinder intersectoral collaboration? Do the committees or task forces that address community-wide concerns represent various fields, such as education, industry, housing, transportation, and health? What are examples of intersectoral efforts in seeking solutions to community problems? How were successful solutions arrived at? How are conflicting activities across the various sectors resolved? What are the gaps in efforts across the various sectors in solving community health problems? Additional specific questions include these: Why has the birth rate among teenagers increased? Is this increase related to differing opinions among educators, ministers, community health nurses, pediatricians, and parents about offering sex education in public schools? What can community health nurses do to facilitate joint collaboration in seeking solutions to these problems? In establishing an adult day care center as a new service in the local health department, do community health nurses plan with managers of city transportation, physicians, clergy, social workers, nutritionists, and family members?

ROLES AND ISSUES IN RESEARCH

Although some of the roles and functions of the community health nurse researcher are implied in other sections of this chapter, additional aspects are worthy of consideration.

Relationships

The practicing community health nurse may conduct research or work with a researcher within an organization in carrying out a study. The relationship of the practicing nurse, the administrator of nursing services, and the researcher is one of partnership in a joint endeavor. Partners each have their own areas of expertise, yet benefit from the expertise of the others. The community health nurse, as an expert in practice, can identify problems needing to be researched in community work, as well as the feasibility of various research designs. The administrator is an expert in organizational functioning and can help identify policy issues related to the research and can render organizational support, which is often needed. The researcher, on the other hand, is an expert in the research process and can help

develop practice problems into researchable questions, suggest appropriate research methods, and design data analyses.

In conducting practice-based community research, another relationship is also important. It pertains to a partnership with the community group concerned with the research problem. Citizens, professionals, and other persons interested in the health of the community may identify a priority problem needing research. In this case, persons in the group have expertise about the community, and the researcher and the community health nurse have to work as resources to the group in conducting the research. This type of research was referred to earlier in this chapter as participatory research.

Involving others in the research process is not without problems. Perhaps the most difficult for researchers is the sharing of activities usually under their domain. Because community health nursing research is occurring in a dynamic setting in which the chief responsibility is often health care (e.g., a neighborhood clinic), priority may be given to clinical commitments rather than to research. For example, access to records and files may be controlled by others, and client information may be withheld by the agency. As a result, the research itself may become part of the politics of the situation. Researchers will need to be aware of these dynamics and use their expertise to ensure the research is conducted with proper attention to sound principles of research, yet allow for citizen involvement that will foster use of the results. A clear understanding of the different roles of researcher and citizen is necessary.

Communication

Whether research involves the community or not, other issues arise that influence the roles and functions in research. One reason often given for the lack of research findings in practice is the practitioner's lack of receptivity. The reason suggests "victim blaming" rather than addressing a constructive approach to this complex problem. One approach is to ensure good two-way communication between the researcher and the people in the field involved in the research, namely, the subjects or users of the research.

This *communication* can take many forms. The researcher needs to consider the appropriateness of verbal, written, and visual aids in clarifying information being presented. Information needs to be disseminated about the research early in the study and throughout the project. Often the researcher has an academic background and appointment and has been educated differently from practitioners and community citizens. The fact that researchers in nursing are often practitioners first may help close this gap. Even so, the researcher must give careful consideration to how the information is presented, including the level of understanding of the reader or listener, and ensure that attention is given to issues of concern to the audience being addressed. Careful attention to the presentation of negative findings, as well as positive results, also must be made. A focus on concepts rather than on the specific program being studied may facilitate the acceptance of negative findings. The format of presentation will vary depending on whether the audience is a group of academic researchers, practicing community health nurses, policymakers, or community citizens. However, some of the same material is applicable to all groups.

Ethics and the Researcher Role

Ethical issues need careful attention when research of any type is conducted. Examination of these issues begins with the problem identified for study and whether or not it is a priority question for practice. The American Nurses' Association's Cabinet on Nursing Research periodically identifies priority areas for nursing research. Some nurses feel that such priorities impinge on the researcher's freedom to decide what to study (Western Interstate Commission, 1974). The extent to which professional pressures influence the selection of the research problem is a personal decision.

Other ethical issues arise out of conflicting social pressures between the profession and the larger society. For example, in the early 1980s Britain's National Health Service and the British Medical Association were not in support of in vitro fertilization. Ethical questions arose over what to do with fertilized ova; some could be implanted in an infertile mother, whereas another could be frozen for use in other generations. Questions arose over who the parents of the fertilized ova are. This dilemma did not stop the British researchers, who proceeded and found private funding to support their research. Infertile couples were supportive of their efforts even though the medical profession initially was not.

Ethical issues also need to be considered in designing a study. For example, in community health nursing we may wish to investigate the home health agency's policies for the care of AIDS patients to see if they are effective. It would be unethical to assign a group of patients having AIDS as a control group if that meant withholding information about the diagnosis from the community health nurses providing nursing services to these patients.

Dilemmas may arise over ensuring the confidentiality of responses, disclosing the actual purpose of the research to the respondents, or even over disseminating results of the research to the respondents. Research plans are under close scrutiny by human subject review committees in most institutions today. As noted earlier, human subject review committees are groups of representatives of various disciplines or departments brought together for the purpose of reviewing research proposals. Their major concern is protecting human participants in research from physical or mental harm.

The role of the researcher here is to communicate clearly in writing to the review committee what is planned, how subjects will be used in the research, and whether or not they are at risk to injury as a result of participating in the research. The researcher is responsible for carrying out these plans as directed or approved by the committee. Changes that occur in the plans need to be reported to the committee for further sanctioning.

There are also ethical considerations in data analysis. It is hard to believe, but true, that in health-related research fraudulent research data and results have been published. This issue is perhaps more important in nursing research,

as we have few replication studies. The impact of publishing false findings can be widespread, affecting not only the profession but, perhaps more importantly, persons in the community.

Position of Researcher in Employment Setting

The issue of who employs the researcher and potential uncertainties about the authority structure is often a major source of concern for the nurse researcher. In an academic setting the researcher may be a faculty member who also has responsibilities for classroom teaching, clinical supervision of students, academic advising, and committee work. To be involved in a major research effort, the faculty member typically will need to be relieved of some of these responsibilities. Consideration can be given to a semester of full-time research, a reduction in teaching responsibilities and committee work, or some combination of these for the duration of the project.

It may be possible to establish more innovative employment opportunities in research, such as status as visiting scholar or visiting researcher within a community organization or university, shared positions between universities and other organizations, or the promotion of sabbatical leave opportunities between service and university institutions. Whether researchers are hired by community organizations as part-time or full-time workers, questions to be asked in considering their functioning in research include the following: What are the other expectations for this position, for example, service, administration, or other research? Also, how will the results be disseminated if they reflect negative features of a service program or a professional group? If the organization chooses not to publish a research report, what happens to the researcher's work? Does the researcher have continued access to the data? Can the researcher prepare papers for presentation at professional meetings and in the professional literature? In any case, researchers should have a clear understanding with their employers and administrators about the organization and expectations for their work, as well as the organization's authority in relation to publication and the investigator's access to data for professional purposes.

Another aspect that needs to be reemphasized relates to the action phase of the research process. If after completing an investigation, it is concluded that the results are significant for community health nursing practice, the investigator needs not only to use the results in practice but also to see that the findings are clearly understood by relevant others, whether they be administrators, community health nurses, legislators, or community people. The community health nurse researcher may need to lobby for her research conclusions so that appropriate policies or legislation are enacted. At this point the link between research and practice can best become reality.

Funding of Research

A final issue is related to obtaining funds for research. Federal money for research is less available in the 1980s than in the 1970s. Researchers and others need to explore alternative funding sources and to use creative financing options. For example, employers could grant release time from work so that educators, administrators, consultants, and practitioners could conduct research; or joint financing could be arranged between the community group, the service agency, and university for the research. The pursuit of funding from voluntary foundations and organizations should not be overlooked. Likewise, state and local funding should be considered.

In addition to funding for specific research projects, mechanisms for collaborative research need to be established and similarly funded. Research institutes and centers with joint connections between community groups, health care organizations, industries, and universities can facilitate research in community health nursing and primary health care. One example is the National Center for Homecare Education and Research, which is associated with the Visiting Nurse Service of New York. Such institutes can promote interdisciplinary collaboration dedicated to the study of community health problems and practice issues. Responsible persons in these institutes need to publicize potential funding sources for research relevant to these areas. The institutes also provide a unique environment for the delineation and articulation of the various roles in research and afford collaborative opportunities for community residents, students, educators, and service personnel in seeking solutions to community health problems.

CLINICAL APPLICATIONS

Selected examples of research studies are presented here to clarify the types of research proposed in this chapter. These studies were selected because they are generated out of community health nursing practice and represent the basic concepts of primary health care, involve a community health nurse as an investigator, or have implications for the use of research findings in community health nursing practice. Although the first study is over 12 years old, it is a rare example of research relevant to questions of accessibility of health care services and appropriate technology.

The nursing division of the DuPage County Health Department in Illinois undertook a survey of noninstitutionalized older adults to determine their needs for services (Managan et al., 1974). The study described the elderly in terms of their health condition, physical functioning, accessibility of medical care, social isolation, and service needs. The major problems found were functional impairment, lack of a family physician, and social isolation. The results indicated that there was a 10.8% increase in services needed by the elderly population. The services needed were intensive case finding, well-adult conferences, and programs providing friendly visitors. The findings were beneficial because they provided baseline information for evaluation of future services.

A fairly recent analysis of the effectiveness of community health nursing home visits may be related to the concept of appropriate technology (Combes-Orme et al., 1985). Eight studies concerned with maternal and child health were compared on a number of methodological and statistical parameters to determine their reliability and validity. It was concluded that within the studies' methodological limitations there was supporting evidence of the effectiveness of home visits to the maternal child health population. Evidence of effectiveness was based on an increase in health knowledge in high-risk mothers and positive changes in maternal attitudes and parenting practices. These outcomes were also found to be associated with positive changes in infant health and development.

Another interesting study was related to all the major concepts of primary health care. It was an international survey conducted to determine the relationship between nursing and primary health care (Jaeger-Burns, 1981). Chief nurses from 54 countries participated in the survey, representing a 34% response rate. It was found that except for their collaboration with the sanitation sector, nurses did not cooperate with other sectors in promoting improved community health. Nursing faculties were found to be inexperienced in primary health care, and students received little experience in the community. Yet it was also found that nurses were involved in primary health care management and relayed information about community health problems to administrators in their health agencies. Also noteworthy was an association between the presence of primary health care nursing in a country and improved health status. These latter findings suggest the relevance of nursing in primary health care and warrant further study.

SUMMARY

Throughout this chapter examples from community health nursing practice have been provided. This section provides suggestions for the baccalaureate-prepared community health nurse on how to be involved in research. The practicing nurse can participate in each stage of the research process. She is in a key position to identify clinical problems that need research. The nurse can take anecdotal notes about clinical situations that will help in identifying not only key variables for study but also factors that might be controlled. She can also begin to read research on the topic of concern and discuss her observations with other nursing colleagues, including researchers. Frequently, nurse researchers work in universities and are more than willing to collaborate in joint research efforts. The practicing community health nurse has access to populations for study and can assist researchers in securing institutional approval to collect data. She may also be involved in data collection, whether it be for pilot studies, replication studies, or original research. The nurse may be a subject in research, being asked to participate in answering questionnaires and interview questions or being observed in practice. The community health nurse can provide valuable insights into study findings, often explaining relationships, or lack thereof, to researchers. The nurse can use relevant study findings in practice. The nurse can explain or report on findings of research to community people, administrators, policymakers, and others, thus taking action for social change.

The practicing community health nurse works with community members in improving their health. She can help seek and identify scientifically oriented solutions to health and nursing problems; thus she is in a key position for the development of knowledge for practice.

☰ KEY CONCEPTS

Research for community health nursing practice is in an early stage of development. Although increasing efforts are devoted to nursing research, much in community health nursing remains largely intuitive and based on tradition.

Community health nursing and primary health care are complementary; research conducted by community health nurses can make a significant contribution to nursing practice and also to primary health care practice.

Action research focuses on the process of change in a group or community. In action research, information is fed back into the group and plays an important role in the growth of the group.

The research process is a problem solving process, much like the nursing process. It involves assessment, planning, implementation, evaluation, and action.

Significant questions for research can be generated from community health nursing practice and linked with the key concepts of primary health care.

Community involvement is a key concept of primary health care. It is concerned with the level of citizen or community resident participation in health decision making.

The overriding questions to be answered by research are: Do the services use the simplest and least costly technology available? Are the services acceptable to the community? Are they affordable? What is the cost effectiveness of alternative approaches or strategies for community health nursing services? Are family home visits as effective as working with families in groups? Are nonprofessionals, such as home health aides, effective in providing some aspects of community health nursing services? What is the most effective management and supervision for nonprofessionals and professionals within a community health nursing agency?

The issue of who employs the researcher and potential uncertainties about the authority structure are often major sources of concern for the nurse researcher.

Federal money for research is less available in the 1980s than in the 1970s. Researchers and others need to explore alternative funding sources and to use creative financing options.

LEARNING ACTIVITIES

1. Read the newspaper and identify one priority problem that could be researched in the community and has relevance to community health nursing practice.

2. From your community health nursing experiences specify a research question in which you would use the action-research approach in answering the question.

3. Identify a research study relevant to community health nursing in the literature and identify the research approach (inductive or deductive); also indicate the strengths and limitations of the research.

4. Talk with a community member, a community health nurse, a researcher, and an administrator who have been involved in research and ask them about their roles and functions. What were the sources of role strain?

5. Identify from the literature three funding sources for research in community health nursing. From the literature find one research study in which the findings can be used in community health nursing practice.

BIBLIOGRAPHY

Babbie, E.: The practice of social research, Belmont, Calif., 1983, Wadsworth Publishing Co.

Combes-Orme, T., Reis, J., and Dantes, L.: Effectiveness of home visits by public health nurses in maternal and child health: an empirical review, Public Health Rep. 100(5):490, 1985.

Dickoff, J., and James, P.: Research I. A stance for nursing research—tenacity or inquiry, Nurs. Res. 24:84, 1975.

Diers, D.: This I believe about nursing research, Nurs. Outlook 18(11):50, 1970.

Feuerstein, M.: Evaluation—by the people, Int. Nurs. Rev. 25(5):146, 1978.

Flynn, B.C.: An action research framework for primary health care, Nurs. Outlook 32(6):316, 1984.

Fox, D.J.: Fundamentals of research in nursing, ed. 4, Norwalk, Conn., 1982, Appleton-Century-Crofts.

Freire, P.: Cultural action for freedom, Cambridge, Mass., 1970, Center for the Study of Development and Social Change.

Hall, B.: Participatory research: an approach for change, Convergence 8(2):24, 1975.

ICN and WHO: Report of the Workshop on the Role of Nursing in Primary Health Care, Geneva, 1979, World Health Organization.

Jaeger-Burns, J.: The relationship of nursing to primary health care internationally, Int. Nurs. Rev. 28(6):167, 1981.

Lazarsfeld, P., Pasanella, A., and Rosenberg, M., editors: Continuities in the language of social research, New York, 1972, Free Press.

Managan, D., et al.: Older adult: a community survey of health needs, Nurs. Res. 23(5):426, 1974.

National Science Foundation: NSF announcements for December, NSF bulletin, 1979, Washington, D.C.

Pan American Health Organization: The role of the nurse in primary health care, Washington, D.C., 1977, World Health Organization.

Stinson, A.: Action research for community action. In Chekki, D.A., editor: Community development theory and method or planned change, New Delhi, 1979, Vikas Publishing House.

Western Interstate Commission for Higher Education: Dephi survey of priorities in clinical nursing research, Boulder, Colo., 1974, The Commission.

WHO and UNICEF: Primary health care: a joint report, Geneva, 1978, World Health Organization.

World Health Organization: Community health nursing: report of a WHO expert committee, Geneva, 1974, WHO.

World Health Organization: Nursing in support of the goal health for all by the year 2000, Geneva, 1982, Division of Manpower Development, WHO.

World Health Organization: Education and training of nurse teachers and managers with special regard to primary health care, Technical Report Series, 708, Geneva, 1984, WHO.

World Health Organization: A guide to curriculum review for basic nursing education. Orientation to primary health care and community health, Geneva, 1985, WHO.

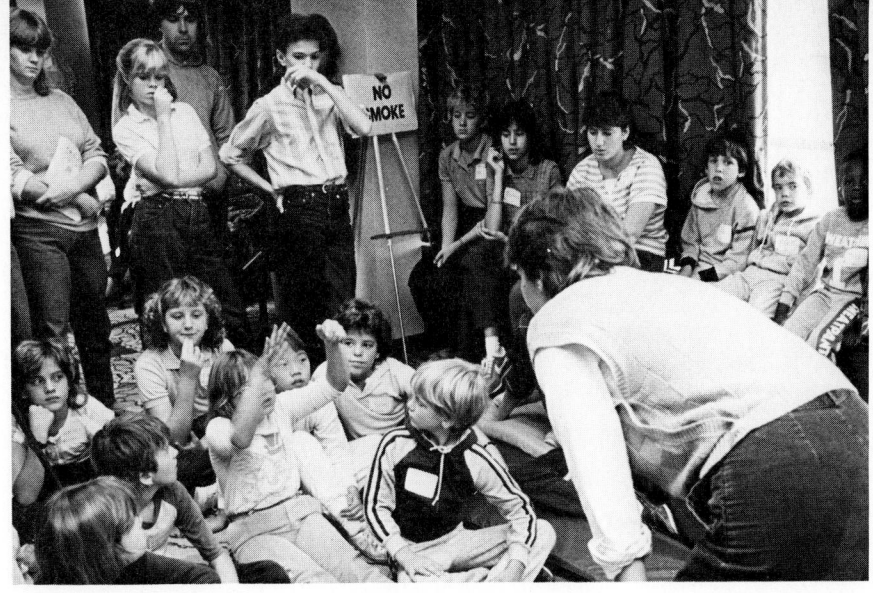

EDUCATION MODELS AND PRINCIPLES APPLIED TO COMMUNITY HEALTH NURSING

Jeanette Lancaster

10

OBJECTIVES

After reading this chapter, the student should be able to:

Summarize the following general theories of learning: stimulus-response, cognitive-discovery, Gestalt, and humanistic.

Differentiate each of the three domains of learning.

Describe at least three characteristics of adult learning that necessitate learning strategies different from those used with children.

Develop a plan for assessing the learning needs of a group of community health clients.

Identify at least 10 factors that facilitate effective teaching.

Identify at least four advantages of group education in community health nursing.

Describe three concepts to consider in organizing learning experiences.

Discuss proper selection of audiovisual materials to enrich learning experiences in community health nursing.

KEY TERMS

accommodation

affective domain

andragogy

assimilation

client centered therapy

cognitive discovery
   theory

cognitive domain

connectionism

equilibration

field theory

Gestalt

humanistic theory

interiorization

learning

operant conditioning

phi phenomenon

psychomotor domain

selective inattention

stimulus generalization

stimulus-response (S-R)
   theory

tabula rosa

third force psychology

■ Special thanks go to Nannette Worel, who developed some components of Chapter 10 for edition 1.

Health education is a vital part of community health nursing, since the promotion, maintenance, and restoration of health rely on the client understanding health care requirements. Early nursing leaders, such as Florence Nightingale and Lillian Wald, demonstrated creativity, initiative, and understanding of the educational needs of their clients. Today health education is equally vital, and community health nurses are in key positions to enact such a role, since they see clients in multiple settings and with varying needs and abilities.

To effectively teach people to care for themselves, nurses must be familiar with key theories of learning, how learning takes place, and principles and concepts of teaching and learning. This chapter focuses on the nursing role in client education and is primarily directed toward adult learners. However, many of the theories and principles presented are also applicable to students and children. The first section of this chapter discusses selected theories of learning with particular application to community health nursing. Succeeding sections present the nature of learning, principles of teaching learning, assessment of learner needs and interests, definition of learning purposes and objectives, and strategies for effective health education, including sources for, barriers to, and evaluation of learning.

THEORIES OF LEARNING

The study of learning is a critical area of investigation for community health nurses. To promote the health of individuals, families, and communities it is necessary to teach the requisite self-care and health-promotion skills. Generally one person cannot promote the health of another. People are responsible for working toward higher levels of health status through their behavior as individuals, as well as in groups. To understand the skills needed to teach concepts of health promotion, it is first necessary to briefly summarize selected learning theories.

Learning is defined in a variety of ways; most definitions include a change in behavior that persists over time, is practiced, and is repeatedly reinforced. Though innumerable theories of learning are potentially applicable to community health nurses, only a sample of the most prominent ones is included. To enrich understanding and promote clarity, the selected theories are grouped into three general

categories: stimulus-response (SR), cognitive-discovery, and humanistic.

SR Theories

SR theorists believe that students should learn in a structured, systematic manner with stimulus situations planned to arouse specific types of responses. This theory builds on the *tabula rosa* (blank slate) view of the mind proposed by John Locke in 1690 (Biehler, 1978). According to Locke, the mind comprises ideas that come from experience. Infants are born with a blank tablet for a mind, on which experiences leave their imprints.

Ivan Pavlov

One of the early SR theorists, Ivan Petrovich Pavlov, left an indelible mark on learning theories primarily by demonstrating SR effects with involuntary reflex actions. His work served as a precursor for later SR theories, although it was not directly applicable to adult learning. His original experiments dealt with digestion; he performed surgery on dogs so that gastric juices were allowed to flow through a fistula to the outside of their bodies where the juices were collected. While carrying out this procedure, he noted that the sight of food caused the dogs to salivate as did the sound of the experimenter's footsteps (Hergenhohn, 1982). Based on what he originally considered a "psychic" reflex, Pavlov demonstrated that dogs can be taught to behave in certain ways when they associate a response with a specific stimulus.

In his most famous experiment, Pavlov taught a dog to salivate when a bell was rung by correlating the ringing of the bell with food. By presenting food immediately after the bell was rung, the response was reinforced. He further determined that if food was not consistently supplied, the response was extinguished. In addition, he demonstrated that generalization from one stimulus to another could occur. For example, if a dog that was conditioned to salivate at the sound of a bell heard a whistle, it experienced what Pavlov labeled *stimulus generalization*. However, such generalized responses could be overcome by supplying reinforcement after the bell was rung but never after a whistle was sounded. When this occurred, he said that discrimination had taken place (Biehler, 1982). Over the years it has been recognized that Pavlovian conditioning is successful only for involuntary reflex actions, such as salivating or responding with fear, and requires periodic reinforcement.

John Watson

Another early SR theorist, John B. Watson, was a behaviorist who believed that psychologists should base their conclusions on their observations of overt behavior. In a classic experiment Watson showed how human behavior could be conditioned. To do this he had an 11-month-old boy play with a white rat. When the child began to enjoy this activity, Watson hit a steel bar with a hammer so that the sudden noise would frighten the boy. The child soon began to associate not only his previously enjoyable rat but everything white and fuzzy with the frightening sensation (Watson and Rayner, 1920).

Edward Thorndike

Some authors consider Edward L. Thorndike to be the "greatest learning theorist of all time" (Hergenhohn, 1982). Thorndike's contributions ranged from comparative psychology, intelligence testing, transfer of learning, educational practices, and application of quantitative measures to sociopsychological phenomena. Thorndike is especially well-known for his theories of connectionism, the law of exercise, and the law of effect.

Thorndike called the association between a sense impression and the impulse to respond a connection. Earlier theories of association linked ideas to actions, whereas Thorndike made a radical departure by linking sensory impulses to actions. *Connectionism* means that the connection is the neural joining between stimulus and response. He believed trial and error was the most basic form of learning.

The law of exercise states that connections between a stimulus and a response are strengthened as they are used. Strengthening means that there is an increased probability that a response will be made when the stimulus recurs. If a bond between a stimulus and a response is strengthened, the likelihood is greater that the response will take place when the stimulus occurs again. Further, connections between situations and responses are weakened when practice is discontinued.

The law of effect originally was conceived as the strengthening or weakening of a connection between a stimulus and a response as a result of the consequences of the response. However, this law was attacked as being circular in logic. Thus after 1930 Thorndike described the law of effect as stating that "reward increases the strength of a connection, whereas punishment does nothing to the strength of the connection" (Hergenhohn, 1982, p. 74). This law has numerous implications for the way in which the behavior of people, especially children, is shaped.

B.F. Skinner

Burrhus Frederic Skinner began his career as a writer, but when this proved unsuccessful, he pursued the study of psychology at Harvard University. His work is similar to Thorndike's since both emphasize the effect of a stimulus on a response. Skinner, like Thorndike, believed that re-

wards influence the probability of a response recurring, whereas punishment does not. Skinner differentiated between respondent behavior (elicited by a known stimulus) and operant behavior (not elicited by a known stimulus but simply emitted by the organism). Examples of respondent behavior include jerking the hand when jabbed with a pin, raising the knee when the reflex is tapped, and constriction of the eye in response to a bright light. Operant conditioning is not associated with known stimuli and appears to occur spontaneously. Examples of operant conditioning include beginning to whistle, discarding one book and picking up another, and starting to tap fingers on a desk or table.

According to Skinner, reinforcement is the key to controlling behavior. To test this view Skinner worked with rats and pigeons to demonstrate that actions followed by a reward are likely to be repeated, whereas those that go unrewarded are not likely to recur. The apparatus for conducting these experiments became known as the Skinner box. The original box was a small enclosure containing only a bar and a small tray. There is a hopper outside the box that contains a supply of food pellets that are dropped onto the tray when the bar is pressed under specific conditions, such as a tone being sounded. A hungry rat can be placed in the box: while exploring its new environment, it bumps into the bar and is rewarded with food. From this experiment Skinner coined the term *operant conditioning* to describe the way the rat operates on the environment. This type of learning also includes instrumental conditioning, since what the animal does is instrumental in securing reinforcement.

Based on his success in controlling the behavior of animals, Skinner decided that his techniques would also work on people. His novel *Walden Two* (1948) described a scientific utopia in which children were taken from their parents immediately after birth and cared for by trained experts who systematically strengthened desirable traits and eliminated undesirable traits (Biehler, 1982).

As Skinner was writing *Walden Two,* he observed the education his daughter was receiving in a public school. From his observations he concluded that children turned in homework and studied to avoid negative consequences such as embarrassment, poor grades, or punishment. However, considerable time passed between the time the child turned in the homework and the grading and return of the work to the child. Skinner became convinced that the principles of operant conditioning held great promise for education. Out of this concern he developed programmed instruction in which learners received instant grading of their work. Essentially, programmed learning is a type of instruction in which material is organized into a series of small steps (frames) and feedback is given after the response to each frame.

Summary of SR Theories

Critics concerned that SR approaches give instructors excessive power and control and that such an approach requires the instructor to determine what is right and reward that behavior. Further operant conditioning or behavior modification can be used to guide learner behavior not only to increase learning but also to make the instructor's job easier. Programmed learning and computer-assisted instruction have applied SR concepts to aid adult learners by giving them immediate feedback on their learning needs.

Cognitive-Discovery View of Learning

In the early to middle 1900s a substantial number of American psychologists, dissatisfied with the pragmatic views of SR explanations of behavior, turned to European theorists for guidance in their thinking. Historically, European scholars have been more inclined to ponder nonobservable and nonmeasurable forms of behavior rather than to observe overt behavior and attempt to change it without grasping the thoughts and feelings motiviating the behavior. Sigmund Freud proposed that people are influenced by behavior that is not only nonobservable but also unconscious. Similarly Jean Piaget devoted his entire career to investigating children's thinking.

Jean Piaget

Many of the assumptions of the cognitive-discovery view are illustrated by the principles derived by Piaget in his theory of cognitive development. After devoting over 50 years to the study of children's minds, Piaget concluded that people have an innate tendency (equilibration) to bring stability and coherence to their perception of the world. Because every child has unique life experiences, each one conceives the world in a highly personalized way.

In his early career Piaget determined that the thought processes of younger children are basically different from those of older children and adults. In evaluating thought processes, Piaget found that children of the same age tended to make the same mistakes, whereas the errors of children of other ages were qualitatively different. Based on these observations, Piaget opposed the definition of intelligence as the number of correct answers on a test. Instead he proposed that an "intelligent act is one that allows the organism to respond effectively to the environment." He believed that organisms are born with two basic processes; organization, or the tendency to systematize and, combine processes into coherent systems (Biehler, 1982), and adaptation, or the tendency to adjust to the environment.

Concepts that assist in explaining how people respond to their environment are assimilation, accommodation, equilibration, and interiorization. *Assimilation* is the process of responding to surroundings in accordance with a person's cognitive structures so that elements in the environment are incorporated into the child's cognitive structure. In contrast, *accommodation* refers to the ways children modify their conception of the world as they have new experiences that influence their response. Further, Piaget believed that intellectual processes seek a balance through *equilibration.* Young children respond in a reflex fashion to the environment. As they have more experiences, they become capable of thinking and thereby are able to respond to more complex situations. This merging of reflex and cognitive processes as a response to the environment is known as *interiorization.* As this process develops, the child's adaptive reactions become more covert and include internal and external actions. Piaget called these internal covert actions *operations* and basically equated them with thinking (Piaget, 1952).

Although Piaget thought that intellectual development was continuous throughout childhood, he established four stages as seen in Table 10-1. Piaget's work significantly influenced the education of children, especially his conclusion that children should be allowed to organize and adapt information in their own ways.

Gestalt Theory

According to Piaget, children are innately motivated to learn by built-in desires to make sense of what they see and

---

TABLE 10-1

Piaget's stages of cognitive development

Age	Name	Major tasks or abilities
Birth to 2 years	Sensorimotor	Thinking centers on mastery of symbols (such as words), which permits child to benefit from past experiences; unable to mentally reverse actions
2 to 7 years	Preoperational	Acquires understanding primarily through sensory impressions and motor actions
7 to 11 years	Concrete operational	Capable of mentally reversing actions but generalizes only from concrete experiences
11 to 14 years	Formal operational	Able to deal with abstractions, form hypotheses, engage in mental manipulation

Modified from Biehler, R.F.: Psychology applied to teaching, ed. 4, Boston, 1982, Houghton Mifflin Co.

experience. His work explains much about the cognitive aspect of learning, which is discussed in the next section, whereas Gestalt theory helps to explain discovery in learning and in many ways can be likened to affective learning. *Gestalt* is the German word for configuration or organization. Gestaltists believe that people experience the world in meaningful wholes; they do not see isolated stimuli but rather stimuli gathered together into meaningful configurations or Gestalten (pleural of Gestalt). We see people, animals, and furniture rather than lines and patches of color. The key principles of Gestaltists became "the whole is more than the sum of the parts" and "to dissect is to distort" (Biehler, 1978).

Max Wethmeimer is considered the founder of Gestalt psychology. The entire Gestalt movement was conceived as Wethmeimer observed two blinking lights while riding a train. He realized that if two lights blink on and off at a certain rate, they give the observer the impression that one light was moving back and forth (Hergenhohn, 1976). He purchased a toy stroboscope and conducted numerous experiments to determine whether or not an illusion of motion would occur if the eye sees stimuli in a certain way. He called this apparent motion the *phi phenomenon.*

Gestalt theorists were interested in the way in which people interpreted what they sensed and observed. When individuals were asked to look at illusions of various kinds, they interpreted what they saw in terms of the arrangement of stimuli. For example, Figure 10-1 depicts two different arrangements of lines the same length; however, the line on top appears longer than the one on the bottom because of the converging lines at the ends of the first line.

Gestaltists also decided that perceptions are influenced by both past experiences and current interests. For example, people generally conjure up different interpretations of the word *joint,* depending on their background and experiences. For some this word means a place; others think of a body part, and still others think of a joint as something to smoke.

To explain how various kinds of physical forces operate, physicists developed the concept of a field of forces that can be illustrated by placing iron fillings and magnets on a table and then tapping the table. The fillings are attracted to the magnets in different and symmetrical ways. Early German psychologists, including the Gestaltists, believed that this

same basic idea, termed *field theory,* explained behavior.

KURT LEWIN. Kurt Lewin, one of the foremost developers of field theory, developed a system for diagramming how behavior is influenced by positive and negative forces (valances) and by the direction of these forces (vectors). He also developed the life-space concept, which means that the life space of a person consists of all that is needed to be known about a person to understand his behavior (Biehler, 1982). Essentially the life-space concept says that it is not always possible to draw accurate conclusions about a person's behavior by simply observing the person's actions. Lewin demonstrated this concept by placing a group of children in a room with several old, well-used toys. The children selected toys and played peacefully. After a few minutes a partition was removed, and the children found themselves in a room with new and shiny toys. They ecstatically delved into these new toys and played happily until they were led back to the old toys. On their return to the old toys, the children were not content with them as they had been previously, and their behavior regressed to a less constructive form. An observer seeing the children for the first time at this point and not realizing the sequence of events might consider these children as immature. Hence behavior is not always what it appears on the surface. Health educators must search for underlying feelings, values, beliefs, and past experiences, all of which influence and guide behavior.

GESTALT PRINCIPLES OF PERCEPTION. Although Gestalt psychologists have identified over 100 principles of perception, only a few of the more vital ones to learning theory are summarized in the box below. In addition, they devised the notion of *perceptual constancy,* which means that an object is seen in the same way under varying circumstances. A door is seen as a door when it is open and when it is closed.

GESTALT PRINCIPLES OF LEARNING. Because of the Gestalt emphasis on perception, it is not surprising that learning was viewed as a special problem in perception. "They assumed that when an organism is confronted with a problem, a state of cognitive disequilibrium is set up and continues

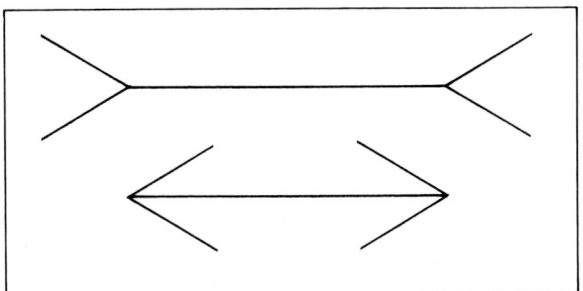

FIGURE 10-1

Different arrangements of lines of identical length alter perception. (From Biehler, R.F.: Psychology applied to teaching, ed. 4, Boston, 1982, Houghton Mifflin Co. p. 247. By permission.)

SELECTED PRINCIPLES OF PERCEPTION

Principle of continuity. Elements that seem to flow in the same direction or follow the same pattern stand out from the background as a figure.

Principle of proximity: When stimuli are close together, they tend to be grouped in our perceptual field.

Principle of inclusiveness: The figure most likely seen is the one that includes the greatest number of stimuli.

Principle of similarity: Similar objects tend to be grouped together in our perceptual field.

Principle of common fate: Elements are grouped together if they move simultaneously or in a similar manner.

Principle of closure: We have a tendency to complete incomplete experiences.

Principle of perceptual constancy: An object is seen in the same way under varying circumstances.

From Hergenhahn, B.R.: An introduction to theories of learning, ed. 2, Englewood Cliffs, N.J., 1982, Prentice-Hall Inc., pp. 250 and 252.

until the problem is solved" (Hergenhahn, 1982, p. 248). A major motivational emphasis came from cognitive disequilibrium. Thus learning is a cognitive phenomenon whereby the individual "comes to see" the solution after pondering the problem. The ingredients are assembled in a variety of ways until the problem is solved. The problem can exist only as solved or unsolved with no in-between state possible.

SUMMARY OF GESTALT THEORY. Gestalt theory is useful in community health nursing because of its emphasis on perception and individual differences and needs. From this perspective, learning needs are uniquely assessed for each learner who occupies a specific life space and sees the world from a personal view. In the next section humanistic learning concepts are summarized, and it is seen that the humanistic view is not totally in opposition to Gestalt thinking.

Humanistic View of Learning

More diversity exists within the humanistic view of learning than in either the SR or cognitive-discovery view. Humanistic theorists come from varying backgrounds, and their concepts are based not on experimental data but instead on observations, impressions, and speculations. In many respects humanistic views resemble those of the cognitive-discovery view. Humanists agree with cognitive-discovery theorists that observing behavior is not sufficient to explain and predict responses; however, they place greater emphasis on the importance of feelings, emotions, and personal relationships in determining behavior.

Humanistic thinkers contend that it is a mistake to separate actual classroom behavior into categories such as cognitive, psychomotor, and affective. They agree that such categorizations are useful when discussing complex topics but should be avoided in dealing with actual behavior. They also believe that learners should be encouraged to explore their feelings and engage in varying forms of self-expression. Additionally, humanists support the belief that people need to become aware of and able to clarify their values. Notable among humanistic thinkers who have influenced education are Maslow, Rogers, and Combs.

Abraham Maslow

Abraham Maslow concluded from studying and working with animals and people that healthy children seek fulfilling experiences. The first two major forces in psychology were SR and psychoanalysis. Maslow (1968) devised what is known as *third force psychology,* which purports that if people are given free choice, they will do what is best for themselves. Thus educators are urged not to be overly controlling and restrictive with learners but rather to help them grow and develop according to their natural inclinations.

In his book *Toward a Psychology of Being* (1968) Maslow described 43 basic propositions that summarized his views. Some of his key assumptions were that all people are born with an essential inner nature. This inner nature is shaped by experiences and unconscious thoughts and feelings but is not dominated by such forces. Maslow believed that people have the ability to control their own behavior, thus educators should assist learners in satisfying their needs for physiological resources, safety, love, belonging, and self-esteem. Specifically Maslow described a hierarchy of human needs starting with physiological requirements that have the highest strength and must be satisfied before people can look at ways for meeting their other needs. The hierarchy does not necessarily follow the pattern just described, but Maslow believed that this was a typical pattern that operated most of the time.

Carl Rogers

Like Maslow, Rogers was a psychotherapist who previously used psychoanalytic techniques but later enthusiastically embraced and contributed to the development of humanistic thinking. He decided that psychoanalysis encouraged dependency, and over a period of years Rogers developed a new, nondirective mode of therapy that he called *client-centered.* In this mode the client is the central figure rather than the therapist. What Rogers found most successful on the part of the therapist was to be warm, positive, accepting, and able to empathize with client's feelings and thoughts. He believed that when clients are so treated, they become more accepting of themselves.

Rogers (1969) transferred his beliefs about therapy to the learning situation and proposed that learning be learner-centered. The outcome of learner-centered education is that students become more self-directed and capable of guiding their own education.

Arthur Combs

Arthur Combs arrived at some of the same conclusions about human behavior as Maslow and Rogers. However, rather than beginning with motivation (Maslow) or psychotherapy (Rogers), Combs began with the cognitive view of behavior. He assumed that "all behavior of a person is the direct result of his field of perceptions at the moment of his behaving" (Combs, 1965, p. 12). Combs advocated that educators should try to understand learning situations by seeing them from the learner's point of view. To help students learn it is necessary to assist them to modify their beliefs and perceptions so that they see things differently and thus behave differently.

He also said that a person's self-concept is critical to learning. A basic purpose of teaching is to help learners develop a positive self-concept. Combs proposed that all human behavior is the result of the need for adequacy. The role of the teacher is to provide a learning situation in which students can be encouraged and aided to develop a feeling of competence or adequacy. He identified six characteristics of good teachers that have relevance for community health nursing educators: (1) They are well-informed about their subject. (2) They are sensitive to the feelings of students and colleagues. (3) They believe that students can learn. (4) They have a positive self-concept. (5) They believe in helping all students to do their best. (6) They use many different methods of instruction (Combs, 1965, pp. 20-23).

◆   ◆   ◆

Humanistic psychologists and educators propose that learners should not only acquire knowledge and psychomotor skills (discussed in the next major sections of the chapter) but also should "examine their emotions, explore their feelings, learn how to communicate with others, engage in many forms of self-expression, and clarify their attitudes and values" (Biehler, 1978, p. 339). As is seen in the following sections, humanistic beliefs are consistent with Bloom's taxonomy of learning needs.

Humanistic beliefs are not universally applauded. Some contend that they convey a "holier-than-thou attitude." Others say that they make too much use of games and also at times lapse into providing therapy and not learning. However, despite these criticisms, humanistic concepts of teaching and learning play key roles in nursing. As a profession, nursing is humanistic in orientation and focuses on the needs of individual learners. Although we may not subscribe to the entire humanistic view and all the methods of implementation, the notions should not be discounted without review.

NATURE OF LEARNING

The goal of all teaching is learning. It is discouraging to labor over the preparation of an educational unit and at the conclusion have a participant say, "I'm sorry, but I did not understand much of what you said; could you repeat your key points?" Giving information does not guarantee that

learning takes place. To understand the nature of learning it is helpful to discuss three domains of learning: cognitive, affective, and psychomotor (Bloom, 1969). Each domain has specific behavioral components that are arranged in hierarchical levels with each level building on the one before and requiring greater cognitive, affective, and psychomotor abilities.

Cognitive Domain

The *cognitive domain* deals with the "recall or recognition of knowledge and the development of intellectual abilities and skills" (Bloom, 1969, p. 7). It is divided into a hierarchical classification of behaviors that Bloom refers to as a taxonomy. Learners master the first and each succeeding behavior in the following order of difficulty; knowledge, comprehension, application, analysis, synthesis, and evaluation. Table 10-2 describes the sequential levels of mastery in the cognitive domain.

For health education to be effective it is important to assess the cognitive abilities of the client so that the nurse's expectations and plans are directed toward that level. Teaching above or below the client's level of understanding may lead to frustration and discouragement if the client perceives that his needs are not clearly understood.

TABLE 10-2
Cognitive domain: levels of mastery

Level	Description	Examples of verbs used to write objectives in domain	Clinical example
Knowledge	Recalling facts, methods, procedures	Cite, name, define, record, identify, state, list, write	Teach diabetic person to recognize symptoms of hypoglycemia
Comprehension	Combining recall and understanding; to grasp the meaning of the information	Classify, distinguish, compare, explain, contrast, interpret, describe, predict, differentiate, report, discuss, restate	Client lists signs of hypoglycemia and describes relationship among hypoglycemia, diet, and insulin
Application	Using information in new, specific and concrete situation	Apply, predict, calculate, relate, complete, report, demonstrate, restate, examine, review, interpret, solve, practice, utilize	Client describes 1200 calorie diabetic diet and specifies foods to use based on personal preference
Analysis	Distinguishing between parts of information and understanding relationship among them	Analyze, differentiate, contrast, distinguish, criticize, question, debate, summarize	Determine factors causing hypoglycemic reaction
Synthesis	Putting the parts of information together in a unified whole	Assemble, integrate, compose, organize, construct, plan, design, prepare, formulate, prescribe, generalize, specify	On experiencing hypoglycemic reaction, client can describe precipitating factors and design a new way to handle such a situation
Evaluation	Judging the value of ideas, procedures, and methods by using appropriate criteria	Assess, measure, choose, rank, critique, recommend, determine, revise, evaluate, test	Diabetic client would judge how effectively and quickly 4 oz. of orange juice relieves symptoms of hypoglycemia

Affective Domain

The *affective domain* describes "changes in interest, attitudes, values, and the development of appreciations and adequate adjustment" (Bloom, 1969, p. 7). This domain is particularly called for in the cognitive-discovery view of learning, the Gestalt theory, and the humanistic view.

Learning in the affective domain is more difficult to assess, since affective behavior is often internalized and hence not readily measurable. In this type of learning nurses influence what clients, families, and students think, value, and feel. The values and attitudes of nurses may differ from those of clients; thus careful, astute listening and willingness to teach what clients are willing and ready to learn is essential. For example, food preferences differ from one culture to another. Counseling about a diabetic diet would be unique for clients who have different cultural backgrounds, such as Mexican, Italian, American Indian, and black and should take into account cultural diet preferences.

Just as with cognitive learning, a series of steps is involved in the affective domain. First, it is important to realize that affective learning occurs on varied levels as learners respond with varying degrees of involvement and commitment (Spradley, 1981). At the first level the learner must simply be willing to *receive* the information. This level coincides with knowledge in the cognitive domain and includes willingness to listen, pay attention, and show awareness of what is being discussed (Krathwohl et al., 1971).

At the second level of affective learning the participant *responds* (or comprehends as in the cognitive domain) to what is being taught by reacting first with compliance and later more willingly and with greater satisfaction. The behavioral tasks expected during this stage include obeying, complying with, enjoying, willingly doing what is required, and accepting responsibility. During this level the diabetic might agree to read educational materials on diets, keep a diet record, and voluntarily seek further assistance and/or information.

During the third level the person begins to *value* the information being taught by accepting the worth of what is being presented, responding to the information, and developing a commitment to change behavior. This level corresponds to application in the cognitive domain. The behavioral tasks expected at this level include choosing from alternatives, stating or demonstrating a preference, desiring to behave in a specific way, and conveying a new level of commitment to what is being espoused. The diabetic black woman might listen to the information about dietary control of her disease, evaluate her diet habits, and select several alternatives to make her diet conform more closely to the recommended standards. She might agree to try cooking her greens in chicken bouillon, broiling rather than frying meats, and limiting her sweets to fruit, sponge cake, or pound cake.

The fourth level, *conceptualization*, corresponds to analysis and synthesis in the cognitive domain (Krathwohl et al., 1971). At this point learners make sense of the values encountered and try to find out more about them.

The fifth level of affective learning occurs when learners *organize* the information by adopting behavior to fit their modified value system. Corresponding to the evaluation level, practice at this stage is crucial to reinforce the modified value system.

Because of the elusive nature and difficulty in modifying such deep-seated qualities as values, attitudes, beliefs, and interests, affective learning is difficult to measure and concretize. Without support, encouragement, and feedback clients can easily step back into old ways of doing things. Praise is useful, since people are often asked to give up cherished habits. Group support can be important because the physical evidence of attitude and behavior change is often only slowly noticed. For example, the visible outcome of conscientious adherence to a diet and exercise regimen may take weeks; thus reinforcement of compliance and devotion to the goal is extremely important.

Psychomotor Domain

The *psychomotor domain* includes observable performance of skills that require some degree of neuromuscular coordination. Community health nursing clients are taught a variety of psychomotor skills, including injecting oneself, determining blood pressure, bathing infants, changing dressings, and walking on crutches. The psychomotor domain can be found in other areas of learning, which have been previously discussed, depending on the task to be learned.

Three conditions must be met before psychomotor learning can take place: (1) the learner must have the necessary ability, (2) he must have a sensory image of how to carry out the skill, and (3) there must be opportunities for practice (Spradley, 1981). Further, there are three prerequisites for skill learning. First, the learner needs to see the process either in person, with video resources, or through clear, pictorial illustrations. Second, there must be a desire, willingness, and need to report the process, and third, there must be an evaluator who will correct any deficits in the return demonstration of the process (Stevens, 1976).

In assessing a client's capability to learn the skill, physical, intellectual, and emotional ability must be evaluated. A tremulous person with poor eyesight may not be capable of seeing well enough or of being sufficiently steady to accurately learn insulin self-injection. To teach a procedure requiring considerable precision to such a client could disrupt health. Similarly, some clients do not have the intellectual capability to grasp all the details of a complex procedure. The steps in teaching the skill should be presented in a manner consistent with the client's physical and intellectual capabilities. It is not desirable to teach above the level of the client's comprehension or to demean the person's ability by oversimplifying the explanation.

Instances exist in which clients are perceived to be both intellectually and physically capable of learning a skill, but their emotional status causes questions to be raised about the wisdom of such teaching. Some people are highly anxious and frightened about self-injections. They may know the process but fear fainting if they see a drop of blood. In such a situation an attempt is made to slowly help the person overcome these fears, but in the meantime a family member may need to be taught the procedure. The behavioral tasks to be used in assessing readiness or ability to learn a skill include determining whether or not clients are able and ready to perform the skill and are aware of the steps required for mastery.

The second condition prerequisite to psychomotor learning is the person's ability to visually construct an image of the procedure. Once clients have observed the process, paying careful attention to the steps or techniques, can they visualize themselves actually doing the same thing? To help people acquire this ability, the steps should be explained and demonstrated slowly, one point at a time, and repeated (or the entire process repeated) until they can picture the sequence in logical progression.

Clients must practice new skills with supervision until they have mastered the steps and have become comfortable with and confident of their ability. They observe, imitate, and practice what has been demonstrated. During practice sessions the teacher should provide feedback immediately regarding the accuracy of the skill. Any errors should be corrected promptly so that only correct behaviors are reinforced. When teaching skills in the psychomotor domain, the nurse must be alert to capability and readiness to learn, and the teaching should match this assessment.

◆ ◆ ◆

Each of the three learning domains must be taken into account in effective health education. Teaching strategies must be based on an assessment of learner needs, abilities, beliefs, values, and readiness to learn.

PRINCIPLES OF TEACHING AND LEARNING

Community health clients vary in age, background, learning needs, and ability to learn. The varying needs, goals, and abilities of potential learners necessitate that nurses have broad knowledge bases from which to select instructional content and teaching strategies. Since a considerable amount of the teaching done by community health nurses is directed toward adult learners, emphasis is placed on the unique characteristics and needs of this group.

Characteristics of Adult Learners

Knowles (1980) contends that most of what is known about learning has been derived from the study of animals and children. Further, much of this information has been generated by experiences with children whose attendance at the learning event was compulsory. Knowles (1980) attributes the current problems with adult education as having derived from this early view of education as an activity for children.

A further problem is the belief that the purpose of education is the transmittal of knowledge. In past generations this premise held true, but with the current rapid advances in knowledge and technology information becomes obsolete in a relatively short time. Hence education cannot be defined as the process of transmitting what is known but rather as a lifelong process of discovering what is not known. A new technique for the education of adults has been developed called *andragogy,* derived from the Greek stem *andr-,* meaning man. Broadly translated, **andragogy** means helping people learn. According to Knowles, andragogy is based on

four assumptions that differentiate it from techniques directed specifically toward children. These assumptions are that as people grow older their concept of self shifts from one of dependency to one of self-direction; they accumulate an enlarging supply of experiences that serve as resources for their own learning; their readiness to learn increasingly becomes consistent with their developmental milestones; and their orientation to learning shifts from future to present and from subject to problem. Adult learners tend to have a greater investment and interest in what they are learning; they see immediate relevance in the information. Hence they want to learn it now in the most painless way possible. Nurses attending continuing education programs exhibit this tendency toward eagerness to have information presented *now*.

Self-Concept

As mentioned, children are initially highly dependent creatures. Their feelings of self-esteem are derived from satisfaction and security in having their needs met. Society defines the normal role of the child as being that of a learner. As children mature, their self-concepts move from the dependency of childhood to the self-direction of adolescence. Adults, in contrast to children, view themselves as doers rather than passive receivers of information. The adult role is one of productivity, self-sufficiency, and independent decision making. The adult self-concept is enriched when the person is treated with respect, allowed to make his own decisions, and seen as a unique person. Adults tend to resist situations in which they perceive that they are being treated like children and are being told what to do.

Consistent with Knowles' beliefs about adult learners, Knox (1977) postulates that adults are more interested in changing their performance level than in learning information. Most adults come to the educational situation with some expectations in mind. As is discussed more fully later, effective learning approaches begin with an assessment of learner needs, drives, resources, and abilities.

Experience

The vast amount of experience and knowledge of adults affects their learning needs. The concept of experience is different for children vs. adults. For children an experience is something that happens to them, whereas to an adult, "his experience is him" (Knowles, 1980). Experience defines who adults are, establishes their unique identity, and represents a vast investment of the person. Adults are more likely than children to contribute to their own learning because of their rich reservoir of personally acquired information. However, because of their experiences, adults are often less open-minded than children. They have felt inconvenience and discomfort from some of their experiences, which may have dulled their desire to try new things.

Because adults are rich resources for learning, greater emphasis can be placed on approaches that draw on their unique experiences, such as group discussions, case presentations, projects, and seminars. Knox (1977) recommends three approaches for assisting adults in acquiring a more positive attitude toward education. These approaches include encouraging learners to participate in the establishment of their own learning objectives and specific activities for obtaining them; assisting adults in identifying people who have met similar goals and using these people as role models; and providing educational settings that are flexible and encouraging the exploration of a variety of educational goals and objectives. The experiences of adults may also require the use of "unfreezing" techniques in which activities are directed toward helping adults look at themselves more objectively and freeing their minds from misconceptions derived from previous experiences.

Readiness to Learn

It is well accepted that children learn best in accordance with their developmental tasks. That is, there are specific times and stages when learning is easier for people because of their developmental readiness. Like children, adults have "their phases of growth and resulting developmental tasks, readiness to learn, and teachable moments" (Knowles, 1980). In contrast to children, whose developmental readiness largely depends on physiological and psychological maturation, adult readiness relates to the evolution of social roles. Havighurst (1961) identified specific adult milestones. A person in early adulthood is much more interested in learning what is essential to a specific job rather than learning the skills of supervision. Adults also need to learn ways to cope with job demands while they are simultaneously learning how to perform expected job functions.

Hence the timing of learning is as important for adults as it is for children. The teachable moment for adults is when the content and skills to be taught are consistent with the developmental tasks. An example would be a community health nurse's decision on when to commence a weight reduction class devoted to instruction in exercise and nutrition. Immediately before Christmas might be a good time in terms of people needing to carefully monitor their weight. However, many potential members would most likely prefer to focus their attention on which pastry to bake, what new candy recipe to try, and how many casseroles are needed for the holiday meals, rather than to concentrate on a new diet. Similarly, many may believe that they get sufficient exercise shopping for holiday gifts, cleaning the house, and getting ready for guests. A health promotion program might be much more successful immediately after the first of the year.

Assumptions about Learning and Teaching

Knowles (1980) believes there are three additional assumptions about learning and teaching that form the basis for an andragogical approach. First, he emphasizes the fact that adults can learn; he refutes the myth "you can't teach an old dog new tricks" by countering that the unimpaired basic ability to learn remains throughout life. If people do not perform well in learning situations, it is not that they are unable to learn but rather that learning conditions are not consistent with their needs, motivation, or style of learning.

For example, because of inexperience with the learning process, adults may doubt their ability to learn. They may avoid attending classes or group sessions devoted to edu-

cation for fear of embarrassing themselves. Likewise, methods of teaching may have changed since adults were in a learner's role, and they must adjust to the new situation. Adults do experience some physiological changes that influence the learning process. For example, visual acuity may decline, necessitating larger visual aids. Adults also tend to have a reduced speed of reaction so that health educators need to pause and provide learners with an opportunity to assimilate information or redirect their attention to a new activity.

Second, Knowles contends that learning is an internal process. Contrary to popular opinion, the most useful type of learning is not the "sponge approach" where learners sit quietly with fixed smiles on their faces while educators pour out the facts for the learners to soak up. In contrast to this view, learning involves the total person, including intellectual, emotional, and physiological functions. Adults are motivated to devote their energies to those things perceived as priority learning needs. The most critical part of adult learning is the interaction between the person and the environment. The critical function of the teacher is to create a rich environment in which students are motivated to learn. Because of the internal nature of learning, most adults do best in self-paced situations where they have the freedom to choose the type of method best suited to their needs (Roberts, 1981).

The third assumption of andragogical learning is that superior conditions of learning and principles of teaching exist. In accordance with a belief in adult stages of development, certain conditions are more supportive to learning than others. These conditions as described by Knowles are summarized in the box on p. 191, at right.

The general purpose of andragogy is to help people realize their full potential. To do this adult learners should be involved in assessing their own needs, formulating their learning goals and objectives, participating in the learning activity, and evaluating their progress toward goal attainment followed by ongoing reevaluation of learning needs. Adults learn better in situations in which they are treated with respect and their experience in life is viewed as a rich resource. Moreover, learning experiences that build and make use of previous learning are the most meaningful (Rosendahl, 1974). However, learning is affected by degree of illness and fear of possible illness. Sensitivity to a client's ability to incorporate new information is essential. If a person is in acute pain, there will be little interest in learning about exercise as a health promotion activity.

Motivation

Adults come to new learning situations with many experiences that influence their motivation to seek additional learning. If past experiences were rewarding and if the learning event made them feel better about themselves, they will bring a far more positive attitude than if they were previously bored, angered, or embarrassed. For example, if a young woman previously attended a preparation for childbirth class in which she perceived the leader thought she was dumb and clumsy, she is not likely to be highly motivated to attend parenting classes provided by the same agency.

SUPERIOR CONDITIONS OF LEARNING AND PRINCIPLES OF TEACHING

It is becoming increasingly clear from the growing body of knowledge about the processes of adult learning that there are certain conditions of learning that are more conducive to growth and development than others. These superior conditions seem to be produced by practices in the learning-teaching transaction that adhere to certain superior principles of teaching as identified below:

CONDITIONS OF LEARNING

The learners feel a need to learn.

The learning environment is characterized by physical comfort, mutual trust and respect, mutual helpfulness, freedom of expression, and acceptance of differences.

The learners perceive the goals of a learning experience to be their goals.

The learners accept a share of the responsibility for planning and operating a learning experience, and therefore have a feeling of commitment toward it.

The learners participate actively in the learning process.

The learning process is related to and makes use of the experience of the learners.

The learners have a sense of progress toward their goals.

PRINCIPLES OF TEACHING

1. The teacher exposes students to new possibilities for self-fulfillment.
2. The teacher helps each student clarify his own aspirations for improved behavior.
3. The teacher helps each student diagnose the gap between his aspiration and his present level of performance.
4. The teacher helps the students identify the life problems they experience because of the gaps in their personal equipment.
5. The teacher provides physical conditions that are comfortable (as to seating, smoking, temperature, ventilation, lighting, decoration) and conducive to interaction (preferably, no person sitting behind another person).
6. The teacher accepts each student as a person of worth and respects his feelings and ideas.
7. The teacher seeks to build relationships of mutual trust and helpfulness among the students by encouraging cooperative activities and refraining from inducing competitiveness and judgmentalness.
8. The teacher exposes his own feelings and contributes his resources as a colearner in the spirit of mutual inquiry.
9. The teacher involves the students in a mutual process of formulating learning objectives in which the needs of the students, of the institution, of the teacher, of the subject matter, and of the society are taken into account.
10. The teacher shares his thinking about options available in the designing of learning experiences and the selection of materials and methods and involves the students in deciding among these options jointly.
11. The teacher helps the students to organize themselves (project groups, learning-teaching teams, independent study, etc.) to share responsibility in the process of mutual inquiry.
12. The teacher helps the students exploit their own experiences as resources for learning through the use of such techniques as discussion, role playing, case method, etc.
13. The teacher gears the presentation of his own resources to the levels of experience of his particular students.
14. The teacher helps the students to apply new learnings to their experience, and thus to make the learnings more meaningful and integrated.
15. The teacher involves the students in developing mutually acceptable criteria and methods for measuring progress toward the learning objectives.
16. The teacher helps the students develop and apply procedures for self-evaluation according to these criteria.

From Knowles, M.S.: The modern practice of adult education: andragogy versus pedagogy, ed. 2, Chicago, 1980, Follett Publishing Co., pp. 57-58.

What can be done if it is perceived that some of the learners have had poor experiences in the past? Initially an attitude of warmth and acceptance helps learners feel that their presence is valued and their needs are important to the leader. Also, begin the first session by asking partici-

pants what they hope to obtain from the class(es), what format they prefer (if the leader is willing and able to be flexible) and also what kind of educational programs they have participated in previously. An attitude of acceptance and interest in meeting learner needs can be built by responding honestly to their questions even when the answer is, "I don't know, but I'll check for you."

Setting attainable goals and objectives helps people feel confident and successful in their accomplishments. It may also be important to pace the educational program to the group's ability to move. Each group of learners has a cumulative personality and an ability to grasp information. It should be determined if the learners need detailed, slow, repetitive instruction consistently or only on some topics or whether they are continually one step ahead of you so that the teaching can be paced to their tempo if possible.

Adults have a different time perspective for learning than children. For children the application of what they learn seems distant, whereas adults can generally perceive an immediate application. Though children enter the learning situation with a subject-centered orientation, adults tend to be problem centered. Adults engage in learning largely in response to stimuli or pressures they feel at the moment. The goal of adult educators is to help them learn what is most relevant at the time. Adults, because of their problem-centered orientation, are motivated by immediate application of the learning. Immediate application provides direct feedback and reinforcement of learning. Errors are corrected as soon as possible, and accurate information or skills are provided (Tarnow, 1979).

Individual Differences

People vary not only in their experience, motivation, and level of readiness but also in perceptions, culture, and language, all of which influence learning deficits. How people view the opportunities available to them affects their learning. Many times potential learners simply are unaware of needs or refuse to learn information or skills that would assist them in promoting or at least maintaining health. It is not rare for diabetics to refuse to learn to inject insulin themselves. It is as if they were saying, "If I don't take insulin, I must not have diabetes." Denial often interferes with accurate perception.

Many factors affect perception, including values, culture, age, past experiences, education, emotional status, religion, and socioeconomic level. Rarely do two people perceive a situation exactly the same way. For example, if while walking down a busy city street on a cold day, a man suddenly fell against the building and slumped to the ground, what would seem to be the problem? Would the conclusion be that he had been drinking and was a degenerate, or would his heart be checked to see if it was beating and whether or not cardiopulmonary resuscitation was indicated?

Clients often use what Sullivan (1953) referred to as *selective inattention*. They simply screen out the part of the message they do not want to hear. This may not be a conscious process, but rather the person may block out a feared or painful message. For example, after suffering a massive heart attack, a 40-year-old man was told to watch his diet, exercise regularly and moderately, and avoid alcohol and cigarettes. Because he had been a heavy smoker and drinker, liked fried foods, and detested exercise, the message he heard was to drink and smoke moderately, avoid exercise, and not eat cheese. The message was misperceived

to meet what he viewed as his ability to cope at that time. Such potential for misinterpretation accompanies any health education and increases the need for home health care where information provided in the hospital can be monitored and corrected if misperception does occur.

Culture also affects learning. Each cultural group has unique values, beliefs, and perceptions that must be taken into account when planning health education offerings. In particular, diets and health attitudes vary considerably. The specific foods recommended on a 1200-calorie diet would be different for middle-aged women who were black, Mexican, American Indian, or Italian; their preferences would differ as would cooking style. Similarly, cultural groups have specific views about health practices, including the role of endogenous practitioners. For many cultures medicine men still provide health care and should not be disparaged but rather collaborated with to ensure consistent and acceptable health advice and care.

Likewise language varies among clients. Many do not understand medical jargon yet are embarrassed to ask for clarification. Thus it is important to observe signs of recognition such as nods, appropriate questions, and directly asking clients to repeat the meaning in their own words. Simply asking if they understand may be insufficient because of a hesitancy to reveal what they may view as deficiencies on their part.

Barriers to Learning

Several barriers to learning are incorporated into the preceding sections. For example, learning is hindered when the teacher fails to determine the learners' readiness or motivations to learn, as well as when the teaching strategies or level of instruction do not match learner needs or ability. Specifically, learning is affected when learners lack the ability to comprehend the information presented because of factors such as: poor vision or hearing, environmental distractions, emotional factors such as anxiety or preoccupation with other thoughts.

Some learners fail to comprehend the information yet are reluctant to ask questions. They may fear that others will think they are "dumb" if they ask for clarification, or they may be so confused they cannot clearly formulate a question.

Learning is also adversely affected when the teacher lacks sufficient skill to effectively present the content. Behaviors such as talking too rapidly or softly or using terms unfamiliar to learners distract from effective learning. Some teachers use strategies designed to maintain learners in a dependent role. It is important to "do with rather than for" learners.

ASSESSING LEARNER NEEDS AND INTERESTS

The first and often overlooked step in health education program planning is the determination of learner needs. Often health educators enthusiastically conceive an idea for an exciting program and develop it only to have it poorly received by potential learners. This may be the result of many factors, but often such failures occur when the needs-assessment step is short-circuited. Frequently educators fall into the trap of providing what they think learners ought to know rather than what they want to know. This does not negate the reality in the health care sector that there is some crucial information that clients must know to ensure their survival. For example, diabetics must know how to regulate their diet to control their disease and many must know how to inject insulin themselves because of a lack of family.

Nature of Needs

The process of needs assessment is discussed in Chapter 11 in relation to program planning and evaluation. Thus this section addresses needs assessment specific to health education. In general, adult learners have two types of needs: (1) basic or organismic needs and (2) educational needs. Although different theorists conceive of organismic needs in slightly variant ways, the common themes include physical safety, security, love and affection, self-esteem, and recognition.

In contrast, an educational need is "something a person ought to learn for his own good, for the good of an organization, or for the good of society" (Knowles, 1980, p. 88). An educational need represents a gap between what a person knows and what knowledge is needed to perform effectively according to personal, organizational, or social expectations. The goal of health educators is to help people assess their key educational needs and determine ways to secure the needed information.

Nature of Interests

Interests are related to needs in that they reflect personal preferences for learning activities. People may have multiple educational needs, yet only one or two of these are of keen interest. A student may have three papers due at the end of the term. Thus an educational need would be to go to the library and thoroughly research each of the three topics. However, the student is keenly interested in one topic, moderately interested in the second one, and actually finds the third topic boring. How does the student proceed? He would probably go to the library and begin with the interesting topic and save the worst (or most difficult) for last.

As expected, interests are highly personal and vary considerably from one person to another and within a person from time to time. Interests, like needs, change as people move through the life cycle. Eighteen-year-olds generally are not interested in the same areas as are 50-year-olds. The current situation also influences a person's interests in learning.

Assessing Needs and Interests

Three sources of needs and interests should be considered in planning adult education programs: those of the people to be served, the sponsoring agency, and the community or society (Knowles, 1980). According to Roberts (1981), assessment of needs can be done either intuitively or systematically through a conscious evaluation process or a combination of the two. Most people rely on intuition to guide many of their actions; however, health educators must be skilled in the systematic process of needs assessment. Since

community and agency assessment is covered in Chapter 13, this discussion is limited to individual needs assessment.

The importance of needs assessment cannot be overemphasized, for with it lies the answer to the first question in health education, "What should be offered?" There are many ways of gaining information from individuals about their perceived educational needs, including surveys, questionnaires, interviews, task forces, and professional literature and the media.

To elaborate on questionnaire usage, Knowles (1980) describes two variations of the projective questionnaire, which were developed by graduate nursing students. One of these, the card sort, uses situations typed on 3- by 5-inch cards to elicit responses. A graduate student developed cards for 52 typical problem situations often encountered by nurses. Respondents were asked to sort the cards into three stacks: those in which perfect confidence and security could be anticipated, those with potentially great insecurity, and an in-between category. By tabulating the results of these cards, it was possible to identify several educational needs of the respondents. Another student devised a picture sort based on the same procedure as the card sort.

Needs assessment also includes an exploration of participants' backgrounds, including their ability, skill, and experience. Nothing is worse than developing a program that is more complex and sophisticated than the learners' capabilities. Likewise, if a program is too simplistic, learners generally get restless and bored. Hence as in the nursing process, the first step is assessment on which the program plan, implementation, and evaluation are built. Principles of needs assessment apply to developing teaching programs for individuals and for groups. In the following section objectives for educational programs are discussed. Although the discussion uses group examples, objectives also must be established for teaching individuals.

DEFINING OBJECTIVES

The formulation of program objectives is described in detail in Chapter 11. However, the purpose here is to briefly discuss health education objectives, followed by a more detailed elaboration of ways to translate learning needs into objectives and principles for writing learning objectives. Program objectives provide guidance and direction in specifically defining the goals to be established. These objectives help determine what learning activities are indicated for a particular group of learners and what content is presented in each learning activity.

Transformation of Needs into Program Objectives

As expected, the starting point for determining program objectives is to identify the needs that have evolved. Knowles (1980) arranges this process in a series of three steps: (1) organizing needs according to priority, (2) screening the needs through designated filters, and (3) translating the remaining needs into program objectives.

Organizing Needs According to Priority

Once learning needs are identified, they can be arranged according to their perceived importance. In planning group educational programs for an agency, a strong advisory committee can help define priorities. For example, if a staff group wants to plan three different programs yet has the resources to only plan one at a time, the advisory committee can assist in identifying priorities based on its personal knowledge of the needs of the population served by the staff. The staff may want to teach nutrition, well-child care, and exercise. However, if the population is primarily an aging one, the advisory committee might encourage them to focus on either nutrition or exercise, depending on the unique characteristics of the aging persons served by the agency.

Also, the frequency with which certain programs are mentioned in an assessment of learning needs indicates the need felt for content to be provided in this area. Another factor affecting setting priorities involves the resources available; the facilities, personnel, supplies, and expertise required to meet certain needs may determine the feasibility at a given time. A specific program may be highly desired in a community, yet no agency has personnel with the needed expertise.

Screening the Needs through Designated Filters

Needs can also be screened to determine whether or not they fit provider goals and purposes. Most health education programs attempt to avoid duplication of other programs in the community; thus identified needs may be referred to the provider who sees that need as a program purpose. For example, most cities have residents who want to participate in smoking cessation clinics. However, if the local chapters of the American Cancer Society and the American Lung Association have frequently scheduled classes, probably the health department does not need to become involved.

Other programs are screened out because of a lack of resources or a lack of interest in moving in a certain direction. No health educator or agency can be all things to all people. Thus priorities must be established regarding program direction. The staff must be knowledgeable about appropriate referral sources. Nothing is more discouraging to a potential learner than to be told "we don't do that, and we don't know who does."

Translating the Remaining Needs into Program Objectives

The next step is to translate the learning needs into objectives that are stated clearly and specifically and define the expected outcomes in measurable terms. Since learning is described as a change in behavior that can include shifts in performance, knowledge, and/or attitudes, objectives are written statements of the intended outcome or change in behavior. Four parts to an objective are addressed in the following questions:

1. Who is to exhibit the behavior?
2. What behavior is expected?
3. What are the conditions?
4. What are the minimally accepted performance standards (criteria)?

The first component, who, refers to the person or group expected to perform the desired behavior. In community

health education, clients, family members, or students are generally the learners.

The expected behavior is a task statement of what the learner can be expected to do following the educational experience. The task statement usually has two components: the actual behavior to be performed in demonstrating mastery of the objective and the result of that behavior. For example, the statement "participants appreciate the need for aseptic technique" is a vague objective and does not contain an observable behavior that can be measured. In contrast, verbs such as define, describe, outline, or demonstrate identify a specific action to be taken by the learner. In a program to teach diabetic clients about their disease and procedures for self-management, a statement such as "each participant can demonstrate the correct technique for insulin self-injection" describes a group learning activity.

The third component refers to the conditions under which the learner is expected to demonstrate mastery of the task. Examples of conditions include the experiences clients are expected to have had before performing a task. For example, "after reading the booklet on insulin injections, clients are able to use aseptic technique in administering the medication." Not all objectives require that conditions be stated, but when they clarify what is expected, they should be included.

The last part includes the criteria or standards for minimal acceptance that the objective has been achieved. Criteria are standards to evaluate whether or not the behavior demonstrated by learners show that they learned what was taught. Criteria may be stated in a variety of ways including the time limit in which learners must accomplish the task to be considered successful (e.g., "clients learn insulin injection technique in 2 weeks"); the amount of information clients are expected to retain (e.g., "clients list four principles of insulin injection technique"); the accuracy of performance (e.g., "clients inject insulin without contaminating surface"); and the degree of consistency with the method taught (e.g., "clients inject insulin using aseptic technique as taught in class"). Regardless of how they are stated, criteria should explain how well learners are expected to perform the task.

Principles for Writing Learning Objectives

A learning objective is a description of an intended outcome rather than a summary of content (Mager, 1975). Objectives must be stated in measurable, behavioral terms. The verbs listed in the box on p. 195, at right help differentiate between words open to few interpretations vs. those open to many interpretations. In general, it is advisable to use the former, since their attainment can be more precisely determined.

MODELS AND STRATEGIES FOR EFFECTIVE HEALTH EDUCATION
PRECEDE Model

Green et al. (1980, p. 7) define health education as "any combination of learning experiences designed to facilitate voluntary adaptations of behavior conducive to health."

DIFFERENTIATION BETWEEN VERBS WITH FEW VS. MANY INTERPRETATIONS

VERBS OPEN TO FEW INTERPRETATIONS

write	contrast
recite	define
identify	outline
differentiate	demonstrate
solve	plan
construct	recall
list	state
compare	classify

VERBS OPEN TO MANY INTERPRETATIONS

know (recall, relate, understand, identify)

understand (realize, know)

appreciate

believe (have faith in)

value

feel

PHASES OF THE PRECEDE MODEL

Phase 1: Consideration of quality of life. What are the major social problems of concern?

Phase 2: Identify specific health problems contributing to the social problem identified in phase 1.

Phase 3: Identify the specific health-related behaviors that seem linked to the selected health problem.

Phase 4: · Sort and categorize into: predisposing factors (attitudes, beliefs, values, perceptions); enabling factors (barriers such as limited facilities, inadequate personnel or community resources, lack of income or insurance or restrictive laws and reinforcing factors (related to the feedback the learner receives from others which may encourage or discourage behavioral change).

Phase 5: Decide which factors make up the three classes on which the intervention will focus.

Phase 6: Develop and implement the program.

Phase 7: Evaluate the program.

Modified from Green, L., et al.: Health education planning: a diagnostic approach, Palo Alto, Calif., 1980, Mayfield Publishing Co.

They contend that the aim of organized health education efforts is to intervene in the process of development and change to maintain positive health behaviors or to interrupt a behavior that predisposes a person to health risks. They have devised a model, or framework, entitled PRECEDE, which is an "acronym for predisposing, reinforcing, and enabling causes in educational diagnosis and evaluation" (Green et al., 1980, p. 11).

The PRECEDE model is outcome-oriented and encourages asking "why" questions before asking "how." Seven phases to the model are shown in the box above, at left. This model is based on four disciplines: epidemiology, social-behavioral sciences, administration, and education. Two basic propositions underscore the model: (1) health and health behaviors are caused by multiple factors, and (2) health education efforts designed to influence these behaviors must be multidimensional.

The PRECEDE model has many characteristics in common with the nursing process. Both are step-by-step problem-solving approaches based upon assessment, planning, implementation, and evaluation. Whereas the nursing process can be applied to individuals, families, groups and communities, the PRECEDE model focuses on the group (aggregate) as the basic unit for planning. PRECEDE focuses primarily on educational needs, whereas the nursing process can focus on a variety of needs such as physical, emotional, or educational. However, PRECEDE, like the nursing process, takes into account a wide range of factors such as physical, emotional, and sociocultural factors in determining educational needs.

Health Belief Model

The Health Belief Model was originally constructed to predict the use of preventive health actions such as obtaining an annual medical examination, seeking tuberculosis or Papanicolaou screening, or making a visit to the dentist for a checkup (Becker, Drachman, and Kirscht, 1974). This model provides a tool for identifying clients' perception of disease and the decision-making process the person uses in seeking health-care services. The Health Belief Model is drawn largely from the work of Kurt Lewin.

The model, formulated by Rosenstock, predicted that people would not attempt to involve themselves in preventive behaviors unless they possessed a minimal level of relevant knowledge and motivation, believed they were potentially vulnerable to health disruption, viewed the potential disruptive condition as threatening, were convinced of the efficacy or usefulness of the intervention, and saw few difficulties in undertaking the recommended action.

The major elements (Rosenstock, 1974) of the Health Belief Model are:

1. Beliefs—perceived susceptibility, seriousness, benefits of taking action, and barriers to action.

2. Cues to action—advice from others, newspaper articles, and forms of information.

3. Modifying factors—demographic variables such as personality and reference groups; structural variables such as knowledge about and experiences with health situations.

Group Versus Individual Education

Although the first portion of this chapter focuses on principles of teaching and learning that can be applied to both individuals and groups, it should be noted that groups do have unique characteristics that must be taken into consideration when planning educational activities. Information on working with groups in the community is given in Chapter 14.

Groups may arise spontaneously and require the assistance of the community health nurse in meeting their common educational needs. For example, adolescent mothers may seek one another in the waiting area of an outpatient clinic. The adolescents may share common concerns regarding parenting, returning to school, and resuming social activities. The social support derived from the group by individual members may facilitate the dissemination of information by the nurse. More commonly, however, individuals are channeled into groups according to disease states, such as hypertension, diabetes, or cancer. As is discussed in Chapter 14, membership in a certain group may also arise from certain characteristics of the individual, such as obesity, age, or use of alcohol or tobacco. Regardless of the input the community health nurse has in the composition of the group of learners, it is helpful to bear in mind the positive aspects of group education for the client and nurse alike.

Planning educational activities for groups of learners offers several advantages to the nurse. First, it may be an economical way to present the same material to more than one individual. By using the same teaching plan for more than one client, resources in terms of time and money are preserved. In addition, by reducing the number of identical individual teaching plans produced, the nurse can greatly increase efficiency in patient teaching. No longer must the nurse "reinvent the wheel" each time client teaching is attempted, but rather groups of learners can be reached with one teaching plan.

Next, group teaching provides the nurse with a mechanism for ensuring that education is incorporated into and implemented through the nursing care plan. Group instruction assists in eliminating the all-too-common practice of providing educational activities only as time allows, thus resulting in "happenstance" teaching. Group activities offer the nurse and client a structured time for the teaching aspect of the nursing role (Evans, 1980).

Group teaching can increase the relevance of educational programs. Because group instruction often allows the nurse to plan the content well in advance, programs are frequently based on identified rather than presumed learning needs. As mentioned previously, programs based on the identified needs of a population group are most likely to be well received by the target group.

Another advantage of group teaching is that people do not feel alone or different. The group setting allows each client an opportunity to talk with others who have similar problems and needs. In groups clients can assume an active role in helping one another and by serving as a role model for changed behaviors (Lorig, 1985).

Teaching Effectiveness

The key to effective teaching lies in planning the approach for the specific situation. Though no "hard and fast" rules exist for effective teaching, the following suggestions provide a guide for implementing the educational aspect of community health nursing (Murray and Zentner, 1985, p. 169-170).

1. Providing consistency and trustworthiness to the learners.
2. Being enthusiastic and letting the learner know there is something of value being offered.
3. Being careful not to discuss one's personal life with the learner.
4. Paying attention to the image presented and the messages given with the posture, clothes, gestures, hair, and tone of voice of the nurse.
5. Being organized, which helps to convey a sense of competence to the learner.
6. Evaluating the effectiveness of teaching methods routinely.
7. Varying teaching strategies and resources as appropriate.
8. Recording teaching experiences, successes, and failures may be helpful to others in similar situations.
9. Expecting good and bad days in teaching and learning; not all educational endeavors have the expected results, so realism is essential.
10. Remembering that the learner is an individual worthy of respect and not a disease process or procedure.
11. Explaining the reason when asking the learner to do something.
12. Never equating intelligence level with educational level. Cultural, religious, and ethnic variables, as well as lack of intelligence, may contribute to misunderstandings.
13. Attempting to motivate the learner through recognition of need, not outward pressure.
14. Learning to sense the appropriate moment for learning and acting on it.
15. Writing instructions legibly.
16. Allowing time for interruptions.
17. Being careful not to overwhelm the learner with technical terms.
18. Providing feedback about learner progress.
19. Correcting errors with information, not judgments.
20. Being careful not to allow racial bias to interfere with the learning process.
21. Not reinforcing destructive thinking but focusing on constructive thoughts.

In addition to these 21 suggestions, creativity enhances teaching effectiveness. Creativity refers to finding ways to provide information that increase the learner's curiosity. The creative educator is open to new ideas, encourages learner input regarding teaching strategies, and is willing to try new ways of doing things. Effective teaching also depends on clear communication, the learning format used, and the climate for learning.

Each person's needs are affected by factors such as knowledge, past experiences, values, priorities, and willingness to change (Miller, 1985).

Sending Clear Messages

Often messages nurses hope to deliver to clients never reach the intended learner because of the use of jargon, cultural influences, or perhaps the present situation of the learner. In presenting educational programs, it is essential to assess learner readiness and to be aware of possible barriers to effective communication. Emotional stress and physical illness are only two factors that may limit the amount of information a learner is able to absorb. The nurse must be

DO'S AND DON'TS FOR EFFECTIVE COMMUNICATION IN TEACHING

DO

- Watch for learner clues indicating the message is unclear.
- Rephrase the message, repeat the content, and ask for feedback until you are certain the learner has received the intended message.
- Be familiar and comfortable with the content before attempting to teach it.
- Speak the learner's language.
- Be specific when giving information.
- Stick to the point and be brief.
- Place key points up front.
- Be careful in teasing and joking with clients.

DON'T

- Be afraid to ask clients to teach you the terms with which they are comfortable.
- Be condescending. Clients quickly pick up such an attitude and resent it.
- Allow language to alienate you from the learner.

Modified from Archer and Fleshman (1979); Narrow, (1979); Miller (1985).

aware of limitations affecting the learner and plan educational activities accordingly.

In addition to ensuring that the material presented is useful to the client, the community health nurse must assume the responsibility for offering information that is understandable. Though medical jargon and technical terms are comfortable for the nurse to use, they may interfere with the clarity of the intended message. For example, in helping clients understand the need for diet control in hypertension, the nurse might use the term *high blood pressure* rather than hypertension to increase clarity for the learner. Thus skill must be developed in fitting the message to the learner. The box above offers do's and don'ts that may be helpful to the nurse in developing communication skills (Archer and Fleshman, 1979; Narrow, 1979; Miller, 1985).

Selecting the Learning Format

Simply stated, the learning format describes the way participants are organized for an educational activity. The variety of formats (or methods) available to the nurse is vast, and selection of the most effective method is at times difficult. To choose the best format the objectives of the teaching program should be kept firmly in mind, and the advantages and limitations of each method must be carefully weighed. Thoughtful consideration of available methods facilitates meeting program objectives, heightens learner interest, and encourages active participation.

Although formats or methods of learning can be divided into individual and group methods, the nurse practicing in the community is most often required to select learning formats appropriate for use with groups. Table 10-3 describes the most commonly used group formats and lists the potential advantages and disadvantages of each.

Setting the Learning Climate

Carefully planned programs quickly lose their effectiveness if the environment is not conducive to learning. The nurse may not have direct control over certain aspects of the learning environment, such as the condition and location of the building or the reputation of the agency. Fortunately, however, the nurse can take simple measures to manipulate the learning climate of the program.

The nurse can first start to set the learning climate for an educational endeavor when the announcment of the program is made. The tone and appearance of the letters, fliers, and media messages that announce the program draw a mental picture for participants of what the activity is apt to be like. By carefully considering the program objectives and information gained in the assessment phase about the culture, beliefs, and educational level of the learners, the nurse can develop preparatory materials appealing to the target population. When advance registration is required, the program announcement may include an activity to encourage participants to think about the subject matter before the program (Knowles, 1980). For example, a request could be made that participants in a stress management workshop complete a physical activity analysis before arrival. The tool could then be discussed in the workshop to provide continuity and feedback.

Creativity can improve the physical setting. For example, chairs can be moved from traditional rows into circles or semicircles to facilitate interaction, or they may be discarded and pillows, mattresses, or sofas used as substitutes. It helps to arrive early to arrange the seating, adjust the temperature, and organize audiovisual materials. Ashtrays, a coffeepot, and soft music often convey to learners that their comfort is important (Knowles, 1980).

The opening session of any educational activity affects the learning climate. Each participant should be greeted cordially and oriented to the objectives. Attention needs to be paid to unique learner characteristics. The degree of formality and privacy created in the learning environment should reflect the information gathered in the needs assessment.

Organizing Learning Experiences

Planning a teaching program requires that the nurse make decisions about the sequence of the learning activities, beginning with consideration of the traits of the learner rather than the nurse's interpretation of a logical organization of the material to be presented. Several principles for organizing learning experiences aid nurses in educational program planning.

First, *continuity* must be incorporated into the teaching plan. The concept of continuity involves placing repeated emphasis on particular components of the educational experience. For example, a community health nurse working with a group of obese people may wish to emphasize the concept of individual responsibility in weight control. Learning activities would then be planned to ensure that the concept was repeated or reinforced as the group progressed.

Second, *sequence* means that each learning experience

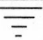 **TABLE 10-3**

Common formats used with groups

Format	Brief description	Materials required	Advantages	Limitations
Open forum	Public meeting in which participants are provided with opportunity to air their views; generally opens with introduction of subject by speaker, panel, or film, a moderator keeps discussion moving	Microphones	1. Allows audience participation 2. Stimulates thought 3. Raises questions 4. Identifies concerns	1. May delay reaching consensus by group 2. Success often rests on ability of moderator
Role playing	Acting out of situations to gain insight by placing oneself in another's position; usually done in front of group with time allotted at conclusion for discussion	None	1. Provides concreteness to learning situation 2. Encourages use of problem-solving skills 3. Requires learner participation	1. Group members may be too shy to participate 2. Intended content (or points) may or may not surface
Skits	Brief, rehearsed, dramatic presentation; usually requires script and more than one actor	Props according to script	1. May evoke emotional involvement 2. Stimulates discussion	1. May distract from intended message 2. Time is required for obtaining necessary props 3. Requires rehearsal time
Field trip or tour	Visit by group to object or place for first-hand observation and study	1. Adequate transportation 2. Advance arrangements	1. Entertains learner 2. Enables learner to view object or place in context of larger community 3. May motivate learners to seek additional learning experiences 4. Sharpens observational skills 5. Traveling time facilitates participant interaction	1. Time is required to make advance arrangements 2. Potential cost may inhibit participation 3. Amount of time required to make trip may not be feasible 4. Finding appropriate agency may be difficult 5. Schedules are difficult to maintain 6. Possibility of injury to participants is ever present
Interview	Presentation in which one or more individuals answer questions posed by one or more interviewers	1. Microphones 2. Seating arrangements so all learners can see and hear individual(s) being interviewed 3. Tape recorder if transcript is desired later	1. Provides common learning experience for all participants 2. Allows audience to hear differing points of view 3. May be used in eliciting audience involvement 4. Requires less preparation time than formal presentation	1. Requires skill on part of interviewer 2. Interviewer must possess knowledge of subject at hand
Lecture	Formal, oral presentation of subject	1. Seating arrangements so all learners can see and hear speaker 2. Podium and any audiovisual materials desired by speaker	1. May be organized easily 2. May be used with groups of any size	1. Requires speaking ability and expertise on subject 2. Audience is passive 3. Feedback is limited

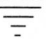 **TABLE 10-3**

Common formats used with groups—cont'd

Format	Brief description	Materials required	Advantages	Limitations
Committee or task force	Small group organized to achieve goal that cannot be efficiently reached by larger group or individual	1. Chalkboard is often helpful for recording ideas or decisions 2. Seating arrangement that facilitates group interaction	1. Relieves members of larger group of tasks at hand 2. Permits variety of interests to be represented 3. Facilitates communication and decision making 4. Provides opportunity for leadership to group members	1. Members of committee may be unable to effectively work together 2. Committee members may not have necessary time to devote to group 3. Larger group may not support actions of committee
Discussion group	Group that meets to discuss predetermined topic; generally governs itself, and may meet as long and as often as is desired by members	Seating arrangement that permits face-to-face interaction of all participants	1. Permits participation of all members 2. Pools abilities and expertise toward reaching common goal	1. Time consuming 2. One member may dominate group 3. Extraneous discussions may divert group's efforts from task at hand
Demonstration	Presentation that shows in detail how to perform certain act or procedure	1. Materials necessary for demonstration 2. Area visible to all group members	1. Learners may be more likely to believe what they see as opposed to what is read or heard 2. Pace is flexible and permits instructor to repeat if necessary	1. Materials needed for demonstration may be expensive, limited, or difficult to transport 2. Number of participants is limited by space and materials available
Brain-storming	Participants "throw out" as many ideas as possible on given subject; ideas are recorded as they are given and are discussed later; all ideas are encouraged without giving thought to practicality of suggestion; requires a moderator	1. Seating arrangement to facilitate group process 2. Blackboard or newsprint on which ideas can be recorded in plain view of entire group	1. Allows participation by all members 2. Allows freedom of expression 3. Encourages creativity 4. May present solutions to previously unsolved problems	1. Suggested ideas may be impractical for implementation 2. Ideas may be criticized during following discussion period 3. Participants may be unable to develop novel approaches to identified problem
Buzz sessions	Large group is divided into several small groups to simultaneously meet for limited time and discuss assigned topic; each group should be small enough to facilitate discussion and may report back to large group at end of session	1. Movable chairs to facilitate formation of small groups 2. Pencils and paper in case notes are desired	1. Allows participation of each member 2. Encourages thought about assigned topic 3. Provides mechanism for generation of "fresh ideas"	1. Reports of small groups may be tedious or contradictory 2. Time may limit contributions each individual may make 3. May be time consuming to organize small groups 4. Small groups may not discuss assigned topic
Case study	Detailed account of one or more events that is presented to group of learners orally or in written form; discussion or written activity usually follows presentation of case study	1. Depends on whether case study is to be presented in written or oral form	1. Assists in developing problem-solving skills 2. Enables learner to consider alternative solutions 3. Presents many concepts on several levels in interesting fashion	1. Learner may not find case study relevant 2. Requires considerable time to prepare 3. Does not require all learners to participate in discussion 4. Requires skill in preparation

Continued

TABLE 10-3

Common formats used with groups—cont'd

Format	Brief description	Materials required	Advantages	Limitations
Mass media	Messages conveyed through television, radio, films, slides, videotapes or audiotapes, as well as charts, books, posters, teaching manuals (see Table 10-5 for further explanation)	Appropriate equipment, supplies, or funds to purchase them	1. Reaches large audience 2. Efficient 3. Low cost per volume	1. Message is not individualized 2. Can be expensive for initial outlay

builds on the previous one and requires a higher level of functioning. This principle is consistent with Bloom's taxonomy of learning domains. For example, when teaching exercises to a weight control group, the learning activities should be sequenced so that participants touch their toes after they touch their knees.

Finally, the concept of *integration* is helpful in organizing learning experiences. Integration of the various components of the teaching plan enables learners to discover how each aspect fits into the "big picture." Participants in a weight control class may find it helpful to understand how proper diet and exercise are related in controlling weight. Thus basic principles of organization allow individualization of the "learning design model" (or plan for accomplishing the program objectives) to the learning situation (Knowles, 1980).

Participative Learning

Learning in either the psychomotor domain or at the application level demands that the instructor use action or participative learning as a teaching strategy. In *participative learning*, learners are responsible for acquiring and actualizing affective, cognitive, and behavioral changes that learning entails whereas the instructor provides the means for this process to take place (Tarnow, 1979). Thus when the objectives of a teaching program require that the learner be actively involved in the learning process, it is the leader's responsibility to structure the learning activities and teaching strategies accordingly. For example, learning the proper technique for injecting insulin requires that the learner have an opportunity to observe a demonstration, practice the procedure, and finally perform a return demonstration for the nurse. The learner's responsibilities can involve observing the demonstration (cognitive domain), practicing the skill (psychomotor domain), and returning the demonstration (psychomotor domain).

The nurse, on the other hand, is responsible for ensuring that proper teaching materials are available (such as alcohol, cotton, insulin, and syringes) and that the learner is provided with adequate information in the demonstration to repeat the procedure. By structuring the learning environment, the nurse is able to allow learner participation, thereby making the learning "more real" than lectures, films, or reading materials (Tarnow, 1979).

Audiovisual Materials

Audiovisual materials are teaching materials, such as printed material, films, videotapes, television, radio, records, and audiotapes.

Selection

When used properly, audiovisual materials can enhance and facilitate learning by creating interest, by motivating and stimulating learning, and by using otherwise nonproductive time, such as in the waiting area of an outpatient clinic. Used inappropriately, however, they are expensive and may inhibit or interfere with learning by overloading the learner with stimuli, for example. Proper selection of audiovisual materials requires consideration of the characteristics of the learner, objectives to be achieved, and characteristics of the audiovisual materials.

CHARACTERISTICS OF THE LEARNER. The audience must be considered when selecting audiovisual materials by determining possible physical handicaps, age, educational level, knowledge of the subject, and size of the group. An understanding of the role that vision, hearing, and to a lesser extent touch, taste, and smell play in the learner's ability to comprehend messages from the media enables appropriate selection of materials to enhance rather than inhibit learning. Any sensory deficit must be carefully considered when selecting educational media. For example, learners with poor vision require different audiovisual aids than those with hearing deficits.

In view of the increasing number of people over 65 years old, nurses need to be aware of sensory changes that occur with the aging process so that they can adapt teaching strategies and media presentations to the target population. Table 10-4 demonstrates ways in which the community health nurse can select audiovisual aids appropriate to clients with physical handicaps.

An often overlooked aspect of any teaching endeavor is the amount of reading the learner is asked to do. Films, slides, pamphlets, videotapes, and filmstrips often require learners to read to obtain the full impact of the message. Unfortunately, many clients with whom community health nurses come into contact are unable to read the messages in the educational media. Although an individual's level of completed formal education is one guide to the level of reading comprehension, such an indicator may be mislead-

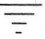 **TABLE 10-4**

Suggested guidelines for selection of audiovisual materials for use with handicapped clients

Deficit	Suggested guidelines
Auditory	Use of visual and tactile techniques in teaching; films, demonstrations, printed materials, and slides enable learner to rely on senses other than hearing to receive messages
Visual	Use of auditory and tactile techniques in teaching; audiotapes, demonstrations with verbal explanations, and specially prepared printed materials, such as large type, boldface lettering, and generous spacing, assist in allowing client to learn in spite of physical handicap

ing. In misjudging the reading ability of the learner, the nurse risks not only embarrasing the client but also closing the door to any future teaching. Thus the community health nurse must be constantly alert for client feedback indicating an inability to comprehend the material presented.

When selecting audiovisual aids requiring reading for a group, the task becomes more complex. The educational level and the occupations of group members provide some estimations of the reading level the presentation should contain. If unfamiliar with group members, another excellent estimation of their reading level is the local newspaper. Learning at what reading level the local newspaper is written and which portion of the community subscribes to the paper enables educators to determine with some degree of accuracy the level on which the program should proceed.

Readability can be determined in a variety of ways including the Fry Readability Formula (1977), the Smog Readability Formula (Miller, 1985) or the Fog Index developed by Gunning (1968).

The readability of educational materials can be affected by the legibility of the printed words, as well as by illustrations. The size of the type used, the shape of the letters, the amount of space between letters, and supplemental illustrations can enhance the readability of printed materials.

OBJECTIVES TO BE ACHIEVED. Earlier in this chapter, writing behavioral objectives was discussed. Well-written objectives are invaluable to the nurse when selecting audiovisual materials. Behavioral objectives specify the learning domain and relative complexity of behavior and therefore are an effective tool in selecting educational media.

CHARACTERISTICS OF AUDIOVISUAL MATERIALS. Audiovisual materials are often selected on the basis of what the instructor is comfortable using or what is currently available rather than by considering the specific advantages and disadvantages of each material. Table 10-5 outlines the various audiovisual materials available and compares the advantages and limitations of each type.

It is beyond the scope of this text to discuss methods of preparation of audiovisual materials. However, the nurse should be aware of the resources available in the agency and the community for production and loan of audiovisual materials. Whether the nurse develops, borrows, or purchases audiovisual aids, no presentation should begin until the material has been previewed, the equipment has been checked to ensure that it is in working order, and the nurse is familiar and comfortable with using instructional media.

In selecting audiovisual aids for a specific presentation, the following questions should be asked:

1. Is audio and/or visual necessary? If so, why?
2. Is color or motion necessary? How will it help the presentation?

Because of the cost and time involved, audiovisual materials should be used only when they are essential to convey a message.

Mass media (radio, television, and newspapers) is especially effective in community health. The same process is used in preparing information for dissemination through the mass media as for selecting media for individual presentations. Characteristics of the intended audience must be assessed, objectives written, and a vehicle for the message selected before teaching begins. The nurse must recognize that, "while the use of the media in community settings is no panacea . . . it can be effective in delivering new information, in setting agendas, and in producing simple behavior changes" (McAlister and Berger, 1979). Improper use of mass media, as with any audiovisual aid, may not only fail to communicate to the target audience the intended message, but may also deter any future participation in desired health-related activities.

RESOURCES FOR COMMUNITY HEALTH NURSING

Resources for planning and implementing educational programs include libraries, health departments, and chapters of national organizations (i.e., the American Cancer Society and the American Heart Association). Such agencies have books and printed materials as well as films, filmstrips, and slide presentations that can be borrowed. It is essential that the community health nurse keep abreast of the audiovisual materials available for use and the means for obtaining them. This can be done by maintaining a file of index cards on which various commmunity resources are indicated. On each card the name, address, and telephone number of a potential resource is recorded along with specific information regarding the types of materials available, potential costs, and persons to contact for the materials. On page 203 is an example of such a resource card.

Keeping the file of community resources updated saves many hours of searching for just the right resource. Each card enables the nurse to know at a glance if a particular agency has the desired materials at a cost that is within budgetary limitations. Many agencies maintain a mutual agreement that says essentially, "our materials are yours as

TABLE 10-5

Advantages and limitations of selected audiovisual materials

Audiovisual material	Advantages	Limitations
Books and other printed material	1. May be used for individual instruction 2. Allow learner to proceed at individual pace 3. Require no special equipment or setting for use 4. May be used to supplement other media	1. Useful only with literate learners 2. Reading level of printed material must match that of learner 3. Not suitable for use with groups 4. Useful only when in language of learner
Chalkboard	1. May be used for audiences of up to 100 members 2. Requires no advance preparation 3. Enhances verbal communication 4. Is inexpensive 5. Is reusable	1. Learner cannot control pace of presentation 2. No way of preserving images
Photographic print series	1. Is inexpensive 2. Is widely available 3. Is easily manipulated 4. Permits close-up study 5. Allows learner to progress at individual pace 6. Requires no equipment for use 7. May be used for self-study	1. Black and white pictures may limit proper interpretation 2. Sizes and distances may be distorted 3. Difficult to use with large groups 4. Photographic skill and equipment required for preparation
Slide series	1. May alter sequence to meet specific needs 2. Can be easily revised 3. Is convenient to handle, store, and use 4. Is appropriate for individual or group instruction 5. Is easily prepared with 35 mm camera 6. May upgrade presentation over period of time by gradually replacing single slides 7. Provides sharp image to learner	1. Special equipment is required for preparation and projection 2. Slides may get out of sequence and be inappropriately projected
Filmstrips	1. Are in same sequence 2. Can be held on screen as long as desired 3. Handle easily; compact 4. May be used for individual or group instruction 5. Projected with simple equipment 6. Learner controls projection rate	1. Fixed sequence limits revision 2. Difficult to produce
Audiotapes	1. Can be used in individual or group instruction 2. Prepared and played back easily with simple inexpensive equipment 3. Economical to duplicate 4. Can be used alone or in conjunction with video materials 5. Stored easily 6. Selected easily (reel-to-reel tapes)	1. Fixed rate for information giving 2. Possible to erase recording if tape is mishandled 3. May be difficult to locate specific portions of tape for playback purposes
Overhead transparencies	1. May be used in front of room, thus permitting eye contact between instructor and learner 2. Prepared easily and inexpensively 3. Operated and maintained easily 4. Are especially effective with large groups 5. Require limited planning; can be written on during presentation 6. May highlight, reinforce, or supplement verbal presentation 7. May be used in lighted or semidarkened room 8. Can be produced for minimal cost 9. Can be used repeatedly 10. Instructor can control speed of presentation 11. May be easily filed for future reference	1. Storage of equipment may be problematic 2. Equipment may block learner's view 3. Ordinary typewriters may produce images too small to be seen

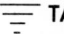

TABLE 10-5

Advantages and limitations of selected audiovisual materials—cont'd

Audiovisual material	Advantages	Limitations
Films or videotapes	1. May be used with individuals or groups 2. May be used in demonstrating motion or relationships 3. Ensure consistency of presentation 4. Enable learner to transcend limitations of time, space, and human body 5. Provide realism in terms of shapes and structures	1. Expensive to prepare, maintain, and purchase 2. Difficult to revise 3. Expense may limit accessibility and cause material to be dated 4. Subject to damage with each use 5. Projection equipment may be cumbersome or difficult to operate 6. Different sizes of reels require special projectors (i.e., 8 mm, 16 mm) 7. Difficult to keep updated

---

COMMUNITY RESOURCE CARD

Date:

Agency name:
Address:
Telephone: Hours:
Contact person(s)
Materials available

Cost:
Comments:

---

long as we may have access to your selection of resources."

Some communities publish a community resource directory that would supplement the previously suggested card file. Such directories often provide information about the purpose of an agency, the services offered, eligibility requirements, and referral procedures. Tools such as a resource card file and community resource directory provide nurses with handy overviews of resources that are available for assistance in planning educational programs.

BARRIERS TO IMPLEMENTING THE EDUCATIONAL ASPECT OF COMMUNITY HEALTH NURSING

Historically nurses in the community have played a large role in client education. Individual teaching was done by visiting nurses, and preventive measures were taught by nurses in a variety of settings. The educational aspect of nursing's role in the community has become widely accepted and is now an expected component of the nursing care plan.

Successful implementation of the educational aspect of community health nursing requires that the nurse be aware of and plan for potential barriers. Such barriers include lack of time, money, space, energy, confidence, organizational support, and equipment.

In planning a teaching program there is rarely enough time to adequately plan and implement the activities. The nurse must establish a schedule that allows flexibility yet ensures that deadlines are met. A good rule is to allow an extra 2 weeks in any schedule to accommodate unforeseen delays. Time management is essential to successful program planning.

Lack of money to implement a desired program is an obstacle that is constantly faced. Organizations, businesses, and industries in the community may grant funds for educational projects if benefits to them in terms of employee health can be demonstrated. The assessment phase of the educational process provides nurses with valuable information regarding individual learners' willingness and ability to pay for educational activities.

The amount and type of space available for teaching projects present another barrier to the nurse. Consideration must be given to the size of the group, or if individual instruction is to take place, the need for privacy should be taken into account. Problems with space limitations can be resolved through several means. Teaching strategies that consider the lack of space can be used. Room size may necessitate that programs are repeated to accommodate all interested learners. Nurses must become increasingly assertive in negotiating for space. The educational aspect of nursing's role is so inherent in the nursing process that to eliminate it because of space limitations is to shortchange the nursing profession and clients. Finally, nurses must become involved when possible in the planning of new facilities to meet the educational needs of the community.

Team management is essential to successful program planning. Likewise, most programs require considerable energy and the nurse must have sufficient personal energy to devote to the task without feeling overwhelmed by the magnitude of the program. Self-confidence is also required for a successful program. Community health nurses must believe they have a message to convey and the ability to provide information in a useful, interesting manner.

With the present push for cost-effectiveness, the nurse may encounter a lack of organizational support in implementing teaching projects. Many agencies are forced because of economic pressures to encourage staff members to see as many clients as possible within a fixed period of time. The educational component of care is often viewed as a nice extra that is to be included only if time permits. The nurse must devote careful attention in the assessment phase to demonstrating the need for educational endeavors. For example, if an industry were reluctant to grant employees time from work to participate in preventive or health-promotion activities, the nurse could gather information to demonstrate to management that such activities would be not only beneficial to the individual employees but also would be cost-effective in terms of fewer days lost as a result of illness. The nurse could involve key people from each agency in the planning process. Such participation often helps to soften negative attitudes and promotes support of educational endeavors.

A final barrier nurses frequently encounter is the lack of necessary equipment for implementing programs. The nurse should be aware of organizations in the community willing to loan or donate the needed equipment. Grants are often available for the purchase or development of audiovisual materials, and the nurse should be familiar with application procedures. In any event, the planning phase of the teaching project must include taking into account the equipment available and developing teaching strategies accordingly.

Teaching and program effectiveness must be evaluated if an educational program is to succeed.

EVALUATION OF TEACHING EFFECTIVENESS

Never take for granted that because an individual has attended an educational program, learning has taken place! All too often nurses and other health professionals assume that because the information has been transmitted to the learner, all program objectives have been met. Unfortunately, this is not generally the case. Evaluative and feedback mechanisms are necessary throughout the teaching-learning process to ensure final attainment of the program objectives.

Ongoing feedback and evaluation are valuable to the learner and teacher alike. For the learner feedback reinforces desired behaviors and allows for the correction of misinformation. Feedback to the instructor allows for modifications in the teaching process so that the learner can be assisted in meeting the program objectives. Because feedback is most effective when it is immediate, it can be considered a learning tool for both the instructor and the learner (Tarnow, 1979).

Evaluation of the teaching process occurs continuously to assist in redirecting teacher and learner activities. The instructor may receive feedback from the learner (about teaching effectiveness) in written form, such as a test or evaluation sheet; verbally in the form of questions asked or responded to; or nonverbally as in return demonstrations and expressions on the faces of the learners. If evaluation is done as teaching is in progress, the nurse will be able to predict with a large degree of accuracy the extent to which the program objectives will be met and the time required

for their attainment. By waiting until the end of the teaching session to obtain feedback, the nurse may miss opportunities to correct misinformation, dispel confusion, or alter the instructor to enhance learning. Redman (1980) suggests that it is unwise to teach for a long period of time without requiring learners to respond so errors can be corrected.

If for some reason evaluation reveals that the desired learning objectives have not been met, the nurse must consider several questions to try to determine the basis for the ineffectiveness of the teaching. How familiar and comfortable was the instructor with the subject matter? Often the learner may perceive the instructor as not understanding the subject, which in turn may leave the learner hopelessly confused. The client may think that the nurse could not understand this, how could he?

The nurse must next ask, "How motivated was the learner?" Factors that influence learner readiness and motivation have already been discussed in this chapter and must be reassessed if teaching seems to be ineffective. Finally, the nurse must ask if the desired behavior change is really necessary. Such a question inevitably leads back to the original learning objectives and encourages the nurse to rethink the practicality and merit of each of the unattained objectives (Redman, 1980).

EVALUATION OF PROGRAM EFFECTIVENESS

Before a nurse or other educator can determine the extent to which teaching programs are evaluated, the individual must determine the view of the educational process. For example, if making changes in a human being is viewed as the major responsibility, the evaluation would be concerned with the measurement of behavioral changes within a specified time frame. On the other hand, if the facilitating of self-development of the learner is viewed as the major responsibility, the focus of the evaluation would be on the involvement of the learner.

It is helpful for the nurse to become familiar with the purpose of program evaluation before attempting to judge the effectiveness of a teaching endeavor. Knowles (1980) identifies two main purposes of program evaluation: (1) to improve the organization of the operation, which includes such aspects as the physical facility, personnel, planning process, and decision-making process, and (2) to improve the actual program, which involves the objectives, teaching strategies, and materials. Both purposes serve to stimulate the learner and promote growth and improvement.

Once the purpose and focus of the program evaluation are determined, the evaluation process follows in a series of several simple steps. First, the questions to be answered must be developed and if possible, pretested. Then data must be collected to answer the questions, and third, the data must be analyzed. Finally, the teaching program must be modified as a result of the findings of the evaluation. The preceding steps require that decisions are made repeatedly in regard to when the evaluation should take place and who should participate in the process.

The importance of ongoing evaluation to the learner and the nurse is discussed previously in this chapter. The nonverbal cues and unsolicited complaints or compliments often result in spontaneous changes or improvements in the teaching program. Though such informal evaluation is important, it does not take the place of systematic, preplanned evaluations. By building in an evaluation mechanism at the end of predesignated program units, the nurse is able to determine the overall morale and satisfaction of the learners as well as suggestions for improvements in the program. In addition, a continuous evaluation process aids in detecting trouble spots before a crisis occurs (Knowles, 1980).

The frequency of evaluation depends on the subject matter, the amount of time available, the amount of material to be presented, and the nature of the learners. For example, a nurse wishing to assess the effectiveness of teaching insulin injection skills may include different evaluative "check points" in the teaching plan than would a nurse attempting to teach the physiology of human reproduction. Whatever form of evaluation is used, the nurse is responsible for communicating to the learner in advance how and when evaluation is to take place (Narrow, 1979). Many times the nurse chooses not to use the word *evaluation* when talking to clients but instead may say something like, "I'll demonstrate a breathing exercise, and then you can show me how to do it."

Outcomes To Be Evaluated

Evaluation of educational programs is one of the most difficult problems encountered in community health nursing. When the program is being planned, decide which outcomes will be measured. Rankin and Duffy (1983, p. 62) enumerate a variety of outcomes that may be selected in patient education programs. These are:

1. Patient compliance with treatment plan
2. Cessation of certain behaviors (e.g., smoking)
3. Knowledge acquisition
4. Patient satisfaction with health care and/or health care provider
5. Reduction in certain emotions such as patient anxiety, fear, or feelings of helplessness
6. Increased confidence levels (e.g., of ability to self-administer insulin)
7. Ability to present self at most propitious time for early diagnosis and treatment

This list, while not inclusive, does give examples of possible outcomes to consider in developing the evaluation plan. Chapter 11 provides in-depth discussion of program evaluation.

Who Should Do the Evaluation?

Every person in a position to make a judgment regarding a program should be included in the evaluation process. The learners and instructors, the program director and management personnel, outside experts, and community representatives provide unique observations, perceptions, and suggestions about the program. The nurse seeking to determine the adequacy of a program for a given community would do well to collect data from as many sources as possible and to include the evaluators in the process of analyzing the data and modifying the program accordingly.

Evaluative Questions

As has already been pointed out, the first step in the evaluation process is to develop questions. The nurse can develop questions to be answered in the evaluation process from the program objectives. For example, an objective of a teaching program may be to provide a physical environment conducive to adult learning. Such an objective lends itself to the formation of such questions as the following: Is the room large enough for the group? Does the room have adequate ventilation and lighting? Can the chairs be rearranged to facilitate group process? These and similar questions provide the nurse with a starting point from which to determine how well program objectives are attained.

Methods of Data Collection

A variety of data collection methods are available to the nurse, and the specific method used is determined by the objectives of the program being evaluated, the variables to be measured, and the time and cost involved (Shortell and Richardson, 1978). The most common methods of data collection have been summarized in Table 10-6 along with some identified advantages and disadvantages of each. Because each method is subject to error and bias, an ongoing evaluation program requires a combination of methods.

Whichever method of evaluation the nurse chooses to use to determine teaching and program effectiveness, a helpful concept to keep in mind is that of the curve of normal distribution (Figure 10-2). In any group of learners about 2% will be extremely negative, and 2% will be extremely positive in their evaluation of the program. Another 14% will be fairly negative with 14% quite enthusiastic. The majority of participants (68%) will be somewhat neutral in their responses (Knowles, 1980). Therefore even though the nurse should consider the extremely negative responses, alarm or discouragement should not appear until the proportion of extremely negative criticism goes above 16%.

CLINICAL APPLICATION

A primary goal of community health nurses is to promote the health of client groups. Often the aim of such health promotion is to reduce the risk of a health-disrupting incident. One such target group for health education would be clients attending a cardiac rehabilitation clinic.

Assume there are ten clients who had cardiac surgery several days earlier. These clients range in age from 39 to 64; all are white males who were employed full-time before their surgery. Each has a good chance of recovery and should be able to resume a reasonably normal life, assuming that careful attention is paid to diet, exercise, stress, physical activity, and medication.

In planning a teaching program for these clients, several factors must be kept in mind including attitudes, beliefs, values, knowledge, motivation, family support, aspirations, readiness to learn, and type of job previously held. Before beginning a teaching program, it is important to find out what past experience the individuals have had with heart disease. For example, if one person in the group knew one person who had ever had heart disease and died, this person would have a different attitude toward health education than

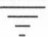
TABLE 10-6

Advantages and disadvantages of common data collection methods

Method	Advantages	Disadvantages
Direct observation of behavior	1. Product and process of learned behavior can be observed	1. Time consuming 2. Does not evaluate cognitive skills underlying psychomotor acts
Interview	1. May be formal or informal, structured or unstructured 2. Data obtained from structured interview may be uniform and easy to analyze 3. Allows for full range of views	1. Time consuming 2. Unstructured may be difficult to analyze 3. May have interviewer bias in results
Questionnaires	1. Obtain reliable information from specific questions 2. Avoid interviewer bias	1. May be misinterpreted by respondent 2. May interfere with activity 3. Time consuming 4. Answers may be misinterpreted by evaluator
Standardized tests	1. Provide an opportunity to compare data from one group with national norms	1. May remind adult learner of childhood schooling 2. Group may not be representative of national norm
Tailor-made tests	1. Produce data about changes for which tests were designed 2. May demonstrate student progress	1. May lack validity and reliability

another group member whose contacts with cardiac patients had all been positive. One method for eliciting this type of background information is to use the initial one or two group meetings to set goals. For example, members might be asked to develop a list of eight concerns they wish to discuss. The group then can set priorities within the list. If crucial content seems to be excluded from the group-oriented list, the nurse can suggest its addition.

Once the content list is generated and the nurse has determined that all key information will be included, the next step is to plan the format and style for offering the classes. The way in which the course is operationalized will depend upon the characteristics of the group. Some groups will respond to lecture, others to lecture and discussion, and still others can benefit from a question and answer format. Regardless of the format chosen, the leader will watch to make certain all members seem to be grasping the information and that content is clear, concise, and understandable.

SUMMARY

This chapter has described several components of the educational aspects of the community health nursing role. Since the major aim of community health nursing is directed toward health promotion and disease prevention, the value of educational strategies is inherent. To provide effective educational offerings to students, clients, and colleagues, it is imperative for community health nurses to understand the nature of learning. Not all learning experiences require that participants be able to synthesize the information provided. In a number of instances it is appropriate for learners to comprehend or apply information without being accountable for higher levels of cognition. Learning also has

cognitive, affective, and psychomotor components. It is insufficient to simply give clinic clients a sheet of diet instructions without paying some attention to their ability to cognitively understand the material and affectively accept the implications of the instructions.

Planning effective health education programs necessitates drawing on theories of learning. People learn in different ways, and beliefs vary about how learning occurs. In some situations the most effective mode for health education follows SR tenets. Other learners and educators are more comfortable with cognitive-discovery, Gestalt, or humanistic views of learning, or some combination thereof.

Effective health education programming takes into account a variety of principles of teaching and learning. The majority of clients seen by community health nurses are adults; hence special characteristics of adult learners have been noted as have other learner qualities such as self-concept, experience, readiness to learn, assumptions about learning and teaching, motivation, and individual differences.

Assessment of learner needs and interests followed the section on principles of teaching and learning. Without a careful assessment, how can educators plan? Historically educators have often tended to develop splendid programs albeit of no interest to learners. Whose time is wasted? To develop educational programs suited to learner needs and wants, a thorough assessment is required. What do learners want or need? How can these needs and desires be most efficiently and effectively met? Who, when, where, and how can an effective program be developed? These questions are answered through careful assessment, planning (including development of purposes and objectives), implementation, and evaluation.

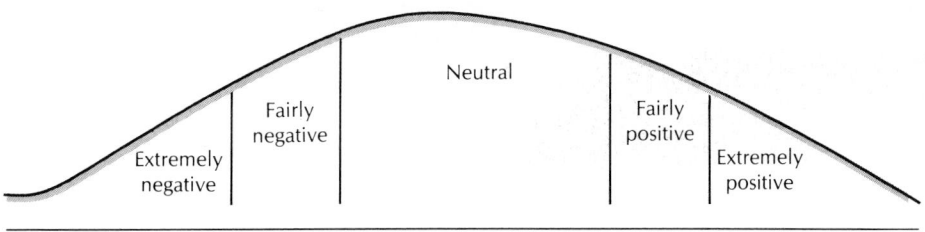

FIGURE 10-2

Curve of normal distribution.

A primary tool of health education is effective teaching. This ability is not inborn. Some people do seem to have a flair for holding the attention of audiences; all people can learn the skills of effective teaching. Many strategies are available to arouse the interest of participants; the careful program planner matches the teaching method to the resources available, the information being presented, and the needs and abilities of the learners. Creativity is an ingredient of health education, which sparks the attention of participants and livens the format of most programs.

In planning health education programs it is necessary to determine whether individual or group strategies will be used. As budgets are cut, emphasis on education often drops noticeably. Thus group approaches are emphasized, since they tend to be less expensive than individual counseling. The value of group education need not be discounted just because it is less costly than other methods.

Any health education offering should ensure clear communication so that learners accurately grasp the message being conveyed. A variety of do's and don'ts for communication were given. For example, educators should know their material before they attempt to teach it. The learning format should be appropriately selected to meet the needs of participants and to be consistent with educator preferences and resources available. The learning climate is also an important consideration. People learn more effectively when their attention is not diverted by being cold, cramped, and unable to hear or see the speaker. Attention to small comfort details yields big dividends in learner satisfaction with programs.

Additionally, learning experiences cannot be simply "thrown together" to be maximally effective. Audiovisual aids must add to and not detract from the learning experience, which can be enhanced by appropriate films, videotapes, or other materials, but each must be selected with the program objectives in mind.

Finally, evaluation methods must be incorporated into the learning process. Without evaluation the nurse has no means by which to judge the effectiveness of the teaching. In addition, evaluation assists the learner in determining the extent to which program objectives have been met by the teacher and the learner. In short, the educational aspect of the community health nursing role has several components. Each is a vital part in ensuring that every educational endeavor produces maximal learning.

⸗ KEY CONCEPTS

Health education is a vital component of community health nursing because the promotion, maintenance, and restoration of health rely on the client understanding health care requirements.

One person cannot promote the health of another. People are responsible for working toward higher levels of health through their behavior both as individuals and in groups.

The most prominent theories of learning applicable to community health nursing are stimulus-response (SR), cognitive discovery, and humanistic theories.

Stimulus-response theorists believe that students should learn in a structured, systematic manner with stimulus situations planned to arouse specific types of responses.

Gestalt theory and Piaget's theory of innate motivation toward stability and coherence in perception are the major cognitive discovery theories in use today.

According to Piaget, the thought processes of a young child are different from those of older children and adults. His work significantly influenced the education of children.

Gestalt theorists believe that people experience the world in meaningful wholes; they do not see isolated stimuli but rather stimuli gathered into meaningful configurations.

LEARNING ACTIVITIES

1. After reviewing the four general types of learning theories, select two and debate their worthiness.

2. Write a brief (two- to three-page) self-evaluation of learning style that identifies your assessment of the most useful learning theory.

3. Review your previous interactions with clients (can be in any clinical area). Identify an example in which the nurse (may have been you or someone else) misunderstood the level of cognitive learning of the client and either provided health instruction at a level that was too advanced or too elementary.

Continued

Field theory describes how behavior is influenced by positive and negative forces and by the direction of these forces. It is an important part of Gestalt theory.

Humanistic theorists believe that learners should not only acquire knowledge but also should examine their emotions, clarify their attitudes and values, and learn to communicate with others and express themselves in a variety of ways.

The most effective technique for teaching adults is *andragogy,* which means helping people learn. In this technique, education helps the learner discover what is not known.

The key to effective teaching is planning the appropriate approach for the specific situation. Effective planning necessitates drawing on theories of learning.

Evaluation is a vital part of the learning process. It helps in determining the effectiveness of the teaching and in determining the extent to which program objectives have been met.

4. Once you have described the misappreciation of the client's level of cognitive learning, reconstruct the situation using the appropriate level.

5. Evaluate a learning experience that has been provided to you regarding its effectiveness in evaluating the learner's readiness to learn, level of reading and general aptitude, motivation, and interest in the topic.

BIBLIOGRAPHY

Adcock, M., et al.: Community health education: the development of effective program strategies. In Lazes, P., editor: The handbook of health education, Germantown, Md., 1979, Aspen Systems Corp.

Archer, S., and Fleshman, R.: Community health nursing: patterns and practice, ed. 2, North Scituate, Mass., 1979, Duxbury Press.

Barrett, N., and Schwartz, M.D.: What patients really want to know, Am. J. of Nurs. 81:1642, 1981.

Bavaro, J.A.: Questioning: the key to learning, Superv. Nurse 11(6):26, 1980.

Biehler, R.F.: Psychology applied to teaching, ed. 3, Boston, 1978, Houghton Mifflin Co.

Biehler, R.F.: Psychology applied to teaching, ed. 4, Boston, 1982, Houghton Mifflin Co.

Bloom, B.: Taxonomy of educational objective. Handbook 1: cognition domain, New York, 1969, David McKay Co., Inc.

Carpenter, W.L.: Twenty-four group methods and techniques in adult education. Unpublished, Florida State University, Tallahassee, 1967.

Cassidy, S.: The ins and outs of presenting a program, Superv. Nurse 11(4):66, 1980.

Combs, A.: The professional education of teachers, Boston, 1965, Allyn Bacon, Inc.

Cooper, S.S.: Methods of teaching—revisited. Field trips and study tours. Part II, J. Contin. Educ. Nurs. 11(3-4):50, 1980.

Cooper, S.S.: Methods of teaching—revisited. The incident process. J. Contin. Educ. Nurs. 11(3):56, 1980.

Cooper, S.S.: Methods of teaching—revisited. Role playing. Part 10, J. Contin. Educ. Nurs. 11(1):36, 1980.

Cooper, S.S.: Methods of teaching—revisited. Films and videotapes, J. Contin. Educ. Nurs. 12(1):34, 1981.

Cooper, S.S.: Methods of teaching—revisited. The incident process, J. Contin. Educ. Nurs. 12(6):22, 1981.

Cooper, S.S.: Methods of teaching—revisited. The interview. J. Contin. Educ. Nurs. 12(4):34, 1981.

Cooper, S.S.: Methods of teaching—revisited. Open forum: buzz session, J. Contin. Educ. Nurs. 13(1):38, 1982.

Evans, L.K.: Health education from a group perspective, Top. Clin. Nurs. 2(2):45, 1980.

Frantz, R.A. Selecting media for patient education. Top. Clin. Nurs. 2(2):77, 1980.

Fry, E.: Elementary reading instruction, New York, 1977, McGraw-Hill Book Co.

Gerlach, V.S., and Ely, D.P.: Teaching and media: a systematic approach, ed. 2, Englewood Cliffs, N.J., 1980, Prentice-Hall, Inc.

Green, L., et al.: Health education planning: a diagnostic approach. Palo Alto, Calif., 1980, Mayfield Publishing Co.

Gunning, R.: The technique of clear writing, rev. ed., New York, 1968, McGraw-Hill Book Co.

Havighurst, R.J.: Developmental tasks and education, New York, 1961, David McKay Co., Inc.

Hergenhahn, B.R.: An introduction to theories of learning, ed. 2, Englewood Cliffs, N.J., 1982, Prentice-Hall Inc.

Hochbaum, G.M.: Patient counseling vs. patient teaching, Top. Clin. Nurs. 2(2):1, 1980.

Kemp, J.E.: Planning and producing audiovisual materials, ed. 3, New York, 1975, Thomas and Crowell Co., Inc.

Knowles, M.S.: The modern practice of adult education: adragogy versus pedagogy, ed. 2, Chicago, 1980, Follett Publishing Co.

Knox, A.B.: Adult development and learning: a handbook on individual growth and competence in the adult years for education and the helping profession, San Francisco, 1977, Jossey-Bass Inc., Publishers.

Krathwohl, D.R., Bloom, B.A., and Masia, B.B.: Taxonomy of educational objectives. Handbook 2: affective domain, New York, 1971, David McKay Co., Inc.

Krawczyk, R.M.: Well persons: their importance to nursing education and practice, Nurs. Forum 18(3):220, 1979.

Lewin, K.: Field theory in social science, New York, 1951, Harper & Row Publishers.

Lorig, K.: Health education: beyond health teaching. In Archer, S.E., and Fleshman, R.P., editors: Community health nursing, ed. 3, Monterey, Calif. Wadsworth Health Sciences, 1985.

Mager, R.F.: Preparing instructional objectives, ed. 2, Belmont, Calif., 1975, Pitman Learning, Inc.

Maslow, A.: Toward a psychology of being, ed. 2, New York, 1968, Van Nostrand Reinhold Co., Inc.

McAlister, A., and Berger, E.: Media for community health promotion. In Lazes, P., editor: The handbook of health education, Germantown, Md., 1979, Aspen Systems Corp.

Miller, A.: When is the time ripe for teaching? Am. J. Nurs. 85(7):801, 1985.

Murray, R., and Zentner, J.: Nursing concepts for health promotion, ed. 3, Englewood Cliffs, N.J., 1985, Prentice-Hall, Inc.

Narrow, B.W.: Patient teaching in nursing practice, New York, 1979, John Wiley & Sons, Inc.

Piaget, J.: The language and thought of the child, London, 1952, Routledge & Kegan Paul of America Ltd.

Piaget, J.: Psychology of intelligence, Totowa, N.J., 1966, Littlefield, Adams & Co.

Pohl, M.: The teaching function of the nurse practitioner, Dubuque, Iowa, 1973, Wm. C. Brown Group.

Rankin, S.H., and Duffy, K.L.: Patient education: issues, principles, and guidelines, Philadelphia, 1983, J.B. Lippincott.

Redman, B.K.: The process of patient teaching in nursing, St. Louis, 1980, The C.V. Mosby Co.

Roberts, F.B.: A model for parent education, Images 13:86, Oct. 1981.

Rogers, C.: Freedom to learn, Columbus, Ohio, 1969, Charles E. Merrill Publishing Co.

Rosendahl, P.: Self-direction for learners, Nurs. Forum. 13(2):136, 1974.

Schultheis, J.G., and de Wolfe, Z.: From academia to practice—realities of delivering nursing education in a medical center, J. Contin. Educ. Nurs. 13(1):21, 1983.

Shortell, S., and Richardson, W.: Health program evaluation, St. Louis, 1978, The C.V. Mosby Co.

Shropshire, C.O.: Group experiential learning in adult education, J. Contin. Educ. Nurs. 12(6):5, 1981.

Spradley, B.W.: Community health nursing: concepts and practices, Boston, 1981, Little, Brown & Co.

Starpoli, C. and Waltz, C.: Developing and evaluating educational programs for health care providers, Philadelphia, 1978, F.A. Davis Co.

Stevens, B.J.: The teaching-learning process, Nurse Educ. 1:9, 1976.

Sullivan, H.S.: The interpersonal theory of psychiatry, New York, 1953, W.W. Norton & Co., Inc.

Tarnow, K.G.: Working with adult learners, Nurse Educ. 4:34, 1979.

Watson, J.B., and Rayner, R.: Conditioned emotional reactions, J. Exp. Psychol. 3:1, 1920.

Wingert, W.A., and Grubbs, J.P., and Friedman, D.B.: Why Johnny's parents don't read, Clin. Pediatr. 8(11):655, 1969.

Wise, P.: Adult teaching strategies, J. Contin. Educ. Nurs. 11(6):15, 1980.

Wise, P.: Methods of teaching—revisited. Character play and role play, J. Contin. Educ. Nurs. 11(1):37, 1980.

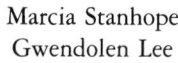

Marcia Stanhope
Gwendolen Lee

11

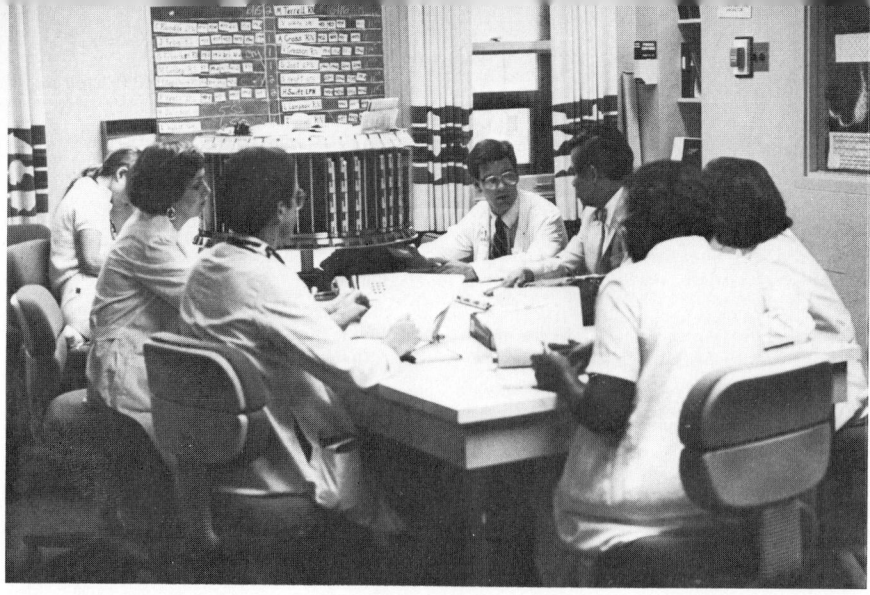

MODELS FOR PROGRAM PLANNING AND EVALUATION

OBJECTIVES

After reading this chapter, the student should be able to:

Analyze the program planning process and application to community health nursing.

Compare and contrast program planning methods and their usefulness in community health nursing practice.

Identify the benefits of program planning.

Analyze the components of program evaluation and application to community health nursing.

Identify evaluation models and techniques.

Name program evaluation sources.

Describe types of program evaluation measures.

KEY TERMS

assessment of need

case register

case studies

census data

community forum

community resident survey

Critical Path Method

estimation of risk

evaluation

evaluation of program effectiveness

evaluative research

formative evaluation

goal attainment

health index

health planning

health systems agency

key informants

Multi-Attribute Utility Method

outcome

planning

Planning, Programming, and Budgeting System (PPBS)

process

program

Program Evaluation and Review Technique (PERT)

program evaluation

Program Planning Method (PPM)

statistical indicators

strategic planning

structure

structure-process-outcome evaluation

summative evaluation

systems model of evaluation

tracer method

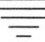

Many of the authors of chapters in this text have referred to the importance of *planning* before *implementing* nursing activities for clients in homes, clinics, groups, and communities. These same authors have talked about the need for the nurse to *evaluate* activities engaged in on behalf of clients. To do this, say the authors, the nurse must have measurable objectives that evolve from the *assessment* of the needs of the client population. In other words, all community health nurses should be applying the total nursing process to all activities in which community health clients participate.

These questions may be asked: "Why is there so much emphasis on planning and evaluation in nursing today? Do nurses constantly need to be reminded that these activities are essential to the delivery of nursing care? Do all nurses not engage in these activities as an integral part of their day-to-day practice?"

Planning and evaluation are essential elements of a quality assurance program for the health care system and the nursing subsystem. As economic resources become scarce, nurses must be able to show their value in providing care to the consumer, show the responsiveness of their services to consumer needs, and show their concern for professional accountability.

Previous history indicates that with seemingly unlimited resources, health care services and nursing services developed in a primarily unplanned manner in reaction to actual or perceived crises or needs. Nurses continue to be told that they "react instead of act," implying that perceived crises or needs continue to be the basis for nursing care delivery instead of "planning to act" based on assessed needs for nursing care delivery, which clients actually need.

With more emphasis on accountability for nursing actions toward clients and the introduction of prospective payment systems, the focus of nursing is changing. Planning for nursing services is essential today if the nursing discipline is to survive in health care delivery.

This chapter examines how nurses can "act" instead of "react" by planning programs that can be evaluated for their effectiveness and efficacy in meeting their social purpose. This discussion focuses on the historical development of health planning and evaluation, program planning and evaluation models and methods, the benefits of planning and evaluation, and the elements of planning and evaluation.

PROGRAM PLANNING AND EVALUATION
Definitions and Goals

A *program* is an organized response designed to meet the assessed needs of individuals, families, groups, or communities by reducing or eliminating one or more health problems. Examples of specific programs in community health nursing are home health programs for individuals and families in the home, immunization programs for children in the school, health risk screening programs for workers in industry, and family planning clinic programs. These specific programs are usually conducted under the direction of the total program plan of the local health department. Broader-based group and community programs are the community school health program, the occupational health and safety program, the environmental health program, and community programs directed at specific illnesses through special interest groups (e.g., American Heart Association programs, the American Cancer Society programs, and the March of Dimes).

Planning is defined by Fox and Fox (1983, p. 11) as the "art of formulating beforehand a detailed scheme for accomplishing one or more goals." Nutt (1984, p. 1) says planning is the "use of a detailed method to create a basis for action." The goal of planning is the organized development of health (nursing) care resources to assure the equitable, efficient, and effective provision of services to the client; or it is an organized response to eliminate or reduce one or more problems where the response includes one or more objectives, performance of one or more activities, and expenditures of resources (Kane et al., 1974).

Evaluation may be defined as "a collection of methods, skills, and sensitivities necessary to determine whether a human service is needed and likely to be used, whether it is conducted as planned, and whether the human service actually does help people in need" (Posavac and Carey, 1980, p. 6). Evaluation for the purpose of assessing the degree to which objectives are met or planned activities are conducted is referred to as *formative evaluation*. This type of evaluation begins while assessing the need for the program. Evaluation to assess program outcomes or as a follow-up of the results of the program activities is called *summative evaluation*.

Program evaluation is an on-going process from the initial planning phase until the program is terminated. The major goals of program evaluation are to determine the relevance, progress, efficiency, effectiveness, and impact of program activities to the clients served (Veney and Kaluzny, 1984).

HISTORICAL OVERVIEW OF HEALTH CARE PLANNING AND EVALUATION

As the health care delivery system has grown in the past 60 years, emphasis in health planning and evaluation has increased. Factors that have fostered increased interest in planning and evaluation are advances in health care technology, consumer education and increased health care expectations, third-party payers, budget pressures, increased professional conflicts, focus on preventive care, new focus on health care as a business, unionization of health care workers, urbanization, increased health risks, manpower shortages, and increasing health care costs.

In the 1920s the American Public Health Association's Committees on Administrative Practice and Evaluation emphasized the need for public health officers to engage in better program planning to change the "topsy-turvy" method by which public health programs were begun (Hanlon and Pickett, 1984). During this same period, the Committee on the Costs of Medical Care, established after a national conference of physicians, social scientists, public health practitioners and consumers, was charged with studying the economic and social aspects of health services. The committee recognized the need for comprehensive health care planning, citing the rising costs and the inequitable distribution of health services across the nation (Anderson, 1966; Committee on Costs of Medical Care, 1970). As a result of the committee report, a few states began to coordinate medical services for area residents. However, regionalized planning for health services nationwide was not attempted until the American Hospital Association established its Committee on Postwar Planning in 1944.

The post-World War II era also brought an interest in evaluating program effectiveness. As government and third-party payers began to finance health care services and money became more plentiful, public demand for health services grew. As demand grew, numbers and kinds of health agencies increased; legislation was passed to increase the scope and control over health care, and the health care delivery system was beginning to be held accountable for its actions (Hanlon and Pickett, 1984). The federal government's first attempt to legislate health planning was the passage of the *Hospital Survey and Construction Act* in 1946 (Hill-Burton Act).

The 1960s were marked by the Great Society programs of President Johnson. The social, economic, and health programs that grew out of the Great Society concept were designed primarily to meet people's needs and to show that the federal government could efficiently deliver services to the population. For example, the *Community Mental Health Centers Act* of 1963 (P.L. 88-464) provided authority to state governments to plan for mental health programs to meet population needs. This legislation clearly delineated the roles of consumers and professionals as advisors in the planning process for all future health planning legislation.

In 1965 the Regional Medical Program legislation (P.L. 89-239) was passed to upgrade the quality of tertiary health care services to consumers. The phrase "partnership for health" was coined because this legislation required health providers and consumers to work together in planning groups to address a number of issues in health care, such as establishing regional medical services for heart disease, cancer, kidney disease, and cerebrovascular accidents. However, a major problem grew out of the regional medical programs; because planning groups were established that included the influential consumer and professional whose cooperation and expertise were criteria for membership. The decision to involve these powerful groups may have been the beginning of the end for the national health planning effort.

During this time the Office of Health Planning was established in the Department of Health, Education and Welfare (now the Department of Health and Human Services, or DHHS). Because the scope and functioning of the Office of Health Planning was limited and had no direct line authority for national health planning, the eighty-ninth Congress, in an attempt to develop a national health planning system, passed the *Comprehensive Health Planning* (CHP) and *Public Health Services* amendments in 1966 (P.L. 89-749) (McCarthy, 1977; McCarthy and Jonas, 1986).

The CHP legislation was intended to establish comprehensive planning for each state and for designated regions within the state. The law provided formula grants and project grants for planning, development, and implementation of a variety of public health services. However, there were many problems with the CHP amendments of 1966. The legislation did not provide legal enforcement power or money to support the administrative functioning of the agencies. As a result, hospitals and other health care facilities were free to build new facilities or expand services without the approval of the health planning agencies. Although the law required 51% consumer membership on the CHP boards, poor training of staff, volunteers, and the consumers led to less than adequate input from these persons into the planning process. Poor orientation of board members resulted in continued provider control over the health plans. The CHP law also exempted "private professional practice of medicine, dentistry and related healing arts" and the principals of the federal government, such as veterans' hospitals, from the health planning system. The actual responsibilities of the CHP agencies were unclear, and although the agencies were asked to "review and comment" on projects submitted for funding under 13 different federal programs, their authority to reject a project was nonexistent. In other words, the Comprehensive Health Planning amendments of 1966 were less than comprehensive.

However, the CHP amendments did provide a format for the development of future planning legislation. From the CHP experience, the states and federal government developed a method for organizing planning agencies. Data on existing needs and resources were collected, procedures for reviewing facilities and program changes were established, and methods for interorganizational cooperation were developed.

Although the CHP legislation proved inadequate for comprehensive health planning, the strengths of the planning legislation led Congress to pass the *National Health Planning and Resources Development Act* (P.L. 93-641) in 1974. P.L. 93-641 is a landmark in health care legislation because of its specificity regarding the structure, process, and functions of a national health planning system. Usually Congress writes legislation that is broad in scope, leaving the writing of specific regulations to the regulatory agencies such as DHHS. Perhaps because of the problems with past health planning legislation, notably the CHP amendments, Congress saw a need to provide some regulations within this new legislation. To give direction to planners of health services, P.L. 93-641 established a national health planning structure that required state governors to designate health services areas to include a population of 250,000 to 3,000,000 to be approved by the DHHS secretary. The health services areas were to be the major planning bodies of the national system, and each area was to have a *health systems agency* (HSA) accountable to the secretary for establishing a local health plan and for adhering to the national health priorities and standards.

P.L. 93-641 stipulated that each HSA was to develop a health systems plan for its health services area and an annual implementation plan. The plans were to be submitted to a statewide health coordinating council (SHCC), composed of representatives from each HSA, who would review (and coordinate) all of the states' HSA plans to reflect one state health plan. The councils also had the responsibility of reviewing and commenting on HSA budgets and state applications for federal health funds.

Although P.L. 93-641 provided a more comprehensive structure and more power over federal program funds than the CHP amendments of 1966, the HSAs had limited authority to carry out some of the more critical tasks of improving the health of residents, increasing accessibility and quality of services, restraining costs, and preventing unnecessary duplication of services. Power over the private health care sector continued to be essentially nonexistent.

As "new federalism" became the catch phrase of the 1980s and emphasis was placed on cost shifting, cost reduction, and more competition in the health care system, President Ronald Reagan proposed the abolition of the federal government's role in health planning. In 1981, with cutbacks in federal funding, states began the takeover of the HSAs and establishment of their own health systems or dismantling of their health systems as established under P.L. 93-641 (Institute for Health Planning, 1981). In 1982 President Reagan recommended only 2 million dollars in the federal budget to continue the closing of HSAs. Today the national health planning system has come to a halt. The macrolevel federal, state, and consumer partnership for health is nonexistent.

From the beginning of the federal government's involvement in national health planning, the structure emphasized external planning and evaluation. The purpose of the national health planning system remained in question throughout the life of the system. Some thought the sole purpose was cost containment, others thought the purpose was to improve health care access to all people, and others emphasized the role of the consumer in health planning at the community level. There were rumors of a DHHS national health policy agenda of extending and improving the health and services to all, conducting a well-designed research program, and promoting health and preventing illness (Hanlon and Pickett, 1984). Perhaps the confusion over the purposes of the planning process, as well as the political issues paramount in the system, led to its eventual demise.

Today there are two predictions about the future of national health planning. The first suggests that communities will again become more involved in meeting the health care needs of their citizenry. The second suggests that the DHHS will develop more control over services offered throughout the nation. Regardless of the outcome of the national health planning effort, which is often influenced by the political party in power, the community health nurse must be concerned about the most important aspect of health planning, the internal planning that must occur for agencies to meet goals and objectives of providing efficient, effective health care services to the consumer at reasonable cost. Hanlon and Pickett (1984) emphasize the responsibility of community health personnel to participate in internal planning and evaluation once they are given the charge to resolve the problems of a client population.

ELEMENTS OF PLANNING

Health planning is described as a continuous social process by which data about a client(s) are collected and evaluated for the purpose of creating "a plan." Such planning generates new ideas, meets identified client needs, solves health problems, and guides change in health care delivery (Ruybal, 1978). Within an agency the data are used to write or revise policy, delete or enhance existing services, develop new services, change staffing patterns, and evaluate the quality of staff performance to meet client needs satisfactorily and efficiently.

Health program planning is affected by governmental control over licensure and funding, by the social structure, and by the cultural and belief system in which the program must function. Program planning is essential to meet federal, state, and local government mandates for funding, philanthropic organization funding guidelines, and internal organizational planning requirements. Program planning is equally essential for the health care organization's rational, effective, and efficient functioning.

To develop quality programs, planning should include four essential elements (Figure 11-1): (1) problem diagnosis—assessment of need, (2) identification of problem solutions, (3) analysis and comparison of alternative methods, and (4) selection of the best plan and planning methods.

Nutt (1984) describes a basic planning process that is reflected in the steps of most planning methods. The basic planning process includes five planning stages for program development as follows. The *formulation stage* defines the problem and assesses the need. This stage in the planning process can be "preactive," projecting a future need; "reactive," defining the problem based on past needs identified

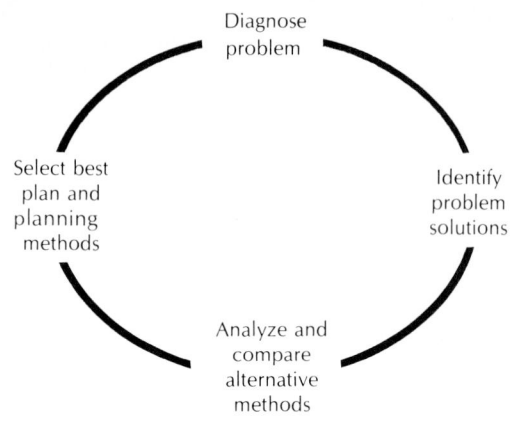

FIGURE 11-1

Essential elements of program planning.

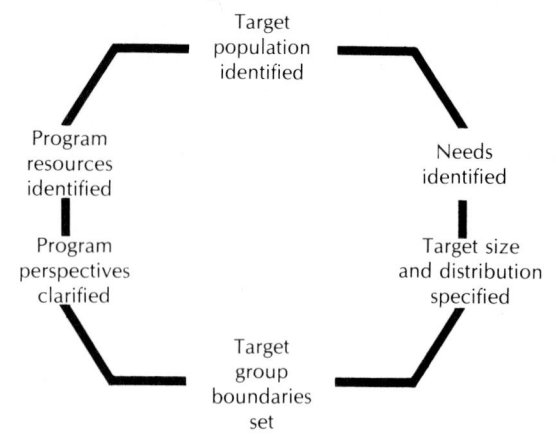

FIGURE 11-2

Steps in needs assessment process.

by the consumer or the sponsoring agency; "inactive," defining the problem based on the existing health state of the population to be served; or "interactive," describing the problem using past and present data to project future population needs (Achoff, 1982). The *conceptualization stage* of the planning process is the point at which problem solutions are identified and explored. The *detailing stage* is used to analyze and compare alternative methods of problem solution. The implications of the choice of each method are considered, including an exploration of the efficiency, effectiveness, and acceptability of each method. The *evaluation stage* focuses on the identification of the costs and benefits of each alternative and the adoption of the best plan and planning methods to be used. Finally, the *implementation stage* of the planning process involves the presentation of the plan to the agency who will sponsor the program or to the client group who is expected to benefit from the program or to both. This stage of planning is omitted from most discussions of planning processes found in the literature. However, it is a most important stage. Although a clear need may exist, unless acceptance of a program plan is attained and funded, all planning effort is lost. Clearly articulated rationale for such a program plan is essential to future development of health care programs.

Assessment of Need

The initial and most critical step in planning for a health program is the assessment of client need. Program planners must verify the existence of a current health problem that is being ignored or being unsuccessfully treated in a client group. These data will provide the rationale to establish a new program or revise existing programs to meet the needs of the client group. The *assessment of need* is defined as a systematic appraisal of type, depth, and scope of problems as perceived by clients or health providers or both.

Six basic steps exist in the needs assessment process (Figure 11-2): (1) identify the client population, (2) identify the needs to be met, (3) specify the size and distribution of the client population, (4) set boundaries for the client group, (5) clarify the perspectives on the program target, and (6) identify the program resources (Posavac and Carey, 1980; Rossi and Freeman, 1985).

The *client population* may be identified as a community or group, as families or individuals. The client population should be defined specifically by its biological and psychosocial characteristics, by geographical location, and by the problems to be addressed. For example, if the client population is a community with a large number of preschool children who require immunizations to enter school, the client population may be described as all children between the ages of 4 and 6 years who reside in central county who have not had up-to-date immunizations by the start of the school year.

The *needs to be met* for the client population must be identified by the client and by the health provider. *If the client population does not recognize the need, the program will usually fail regardless of the amount of assessing and planning before program implementation.* To assist the population toward awareness of the existing need, a health education program may be necessary before a program is implemented. In the example of the need for immunization of preschool children, public service announcements on television and radio and in newspapers may be used to alert parents to laws requiring immunizations, to the continued existence of communicable diseases, and to the communicable diseases successfully eradicated by immunization programs, such as smallpox.

Specifying the size and distribution of a client population for a program involves not only the counting of the number of persons in the community who may be eligible for the program but also finding out the number of persons with the problem who are unserved by existing programs and the numbers of eligible persons who have and have not availed themselves of existing services. In planning the preschool immunization program, the estimates of numbers of preschool children in the county may be obtained from census data. One must then decide if the program will serve all children in the county, children of one school district, or only children who do not attend existing health facilities. The decision will be based on the program's overall goal.

Boundaries for the client population are primarily established by defining the size and distribution of the client population. The boundaries will stipulate who is included and who is excluded in the health program. If the immunization program was designed to serve only preschool children of low-income families, all other preschool children would be excluded. If the program was designed to serve all children without immunization, children partially immunized may be referred to the health care facility that initiated the child's immunization program. If the community is composed largely of middle-class families, limiting the program to low-income children may make the population size so small that the program would not be cost efficient.

Perspectives on the program may be found to differ among health providers, organizational administrators, policymakers, and potential clients. Collecting data on the opinions and attitudes of all persons directly or indirectly involved with the program's success is essential to deciding on the program's feasibility, the need to redefine the problems, or the decision to abandon a new program or expand an existing program. For example, in 1982 in one state all funding for prenatal programs was cut from state, district, and local health budgets. The policymakers had determined that prenatal care was no longer a health priority in spite of existing research that correlates prenatal care with reduction in maternal and infant health problems. A program planner working on expansion of prenatal programs found all work had become meaningless when budgetary requests for program funding were refused. Similarly, policymakers in the 1970s, who determined that neighborhood health clinics were the answer to providing service for low-income residents, found that their perspectives were not the same as most health providers or clients. The neighborhood health clinic concept failed as a viable program.

Before implementing a health program, one must also *assess available resources*. Program resources include manpower, facilities, equipment, and financing. The numbers and kinds of personnel available to implement a program must be determined. The availability of supplies and up-to-date equipment is as essential a resource for implementing a program as are the source and amount of funds to implement the program. If one of the essential resources is unavailable to the program, it likely will be inadequate to meet the needs of the client population.

Needs Assessment Tools

A number of tools exist to assist the program planner in the needs assessment process. The major tools used for needs assessment are census data, key informants, community forums, surveys of existing community agencies with similar programs, surveys of residents of the community to be served (client population), and statistical indicators (Posavac and Carey, 1980; Rossi and Freeman, 1985; Jury, 1984).

Census data are considered valid, reliable, and inexpensive data that are available to the public in several forms. The U.S. census data, updated every 10 years, provide excellent composite data on the population of states, local and political jurisdictions, and census tracts in urbanized areas. The census data may be used to locate client populations by age, sex, race, socioeconomic status, and housing conditions. Census data may be used to compare trends in states and the nation or between states and localities. A word of caution is necessary about the use of census data for program planning. If programs are being planned for rapidly expanding localities, census data may be outdated

before they are published. Census data may also be incomplete or otherwise incorrect for such population groups as rural, underserved communities or unincorporated communities because of the difficulties census workers have in tracking populations in such locations.

The use of *key informants* affords the program planner the opportunity to obtain ideas of professional experts, such as nurses, educators, physicians, social workers, the community leaders, the politicians and entrepreneurs who are in touch with the needs of the community and who are in a position to support new community programs. The major problem with the key informant approach is that the planner may obtain biased data from the informants because of bias these persons have about the community problems or because of the informants' interests in directing projects to certain ends. A program planner may avoid some bias by using a structured interview guide when communicating with key informants. The structured interview guide also provides an easy mechanism for collating and summarizing the data gathered from the key informant. When choosing persons to interview, the community health nurse should attempt to find persons who are leaders in the community, have knowledge of the community, are accessible, and represent the client group or will be consumers of the new program.

The *community forum* is another economical approach to gathering data about needs, size, and characteristics of a client group. The community forum is an open meeting for members of a particular community or group. For example, if the community health nurse is interested in assessing the health needs at Apple School, the administration, teachers, parents, and children could be invited to an open forum to provide input about the health needs of the school children. Of course, being specific about the topic at a forum meeting will make the difference in the usefulness of the data. If the program planner wishes to assess the need to provide an eye screening program in the school, the participants would direct their input to eye problems and eye screening only. The discussion could be focused on the size, extent of need, and characteristics of the population in need of an eye care program. A discussion of all health needs would provide valuable information but may not be as helpful for program planning as a more specific topic.

The disadvantages of the forum are these: (1) a population cross-section may not attend the meeting, thereby biasing the data with the interests of those in attendance, (2) the forum may become a political arena for a few and may limit the kinds of information offered by others who do not feel free to speak out. The forum is valuable in obtaining the perceptions of the participants and the client population about specific problems and about methods of health service delivery.

Surveys of existing community agencies providing similar services are essential to the development of a new program or expansion of an existing program. The nurse may also conduct a survey of services offered in a similar community to get an idea of the best methods of setting up the program and the amount and resources that might be needed. If the community health nurse had identified a need for a home health care program for the elderly population of the community, the nurse should initially conduct an inventory of the number of facilities within the community providing home health services. Once the number of agencies providing services has been identified, the number of personnel employed by the agencies and the number of persons served by the agencies should be determined. These data can usually be obtained through direct requests of the provider agencies.

The program planner may be interested in determining the following: the kinds of persons served by the existing agencies by disease category, age, socioeconomic level, payment mechanism, and so on; the ratio of persons served to the estimated numbers that could be served by the agencies; and the number of persons referred to other agencies for service. This information will provide the planner with data to compare with the population identified in need of home health care. The data may suggest that the client population could potentially be served by all existing agencies, that existing agencies are not employing enough personnel to serve the population and thus a new program may be warranted, that existing agencies are not providing services to certain segments of the client population, and that a new program directed toward the identified population would have more potential for success.

The *community resident survey* assesses the need of a community for a service, the acceptability of the service to the community, and the willingness of the people to use and pay for a program or service. The community resident survey may be conducted by surveying the total population of a community or by surveying a sample of the community. The community health nurse may want to elicit the assistance of a statistician to choose the appropriate sample and size for the resident survey. The community resident survey should be directed to the specific population the program intends to serve.

Statistical indicators of disease incidence, prevalence, and mortality, and other rates such as case-specific, age-specific, and adjusted rates are useful in estimating the nature of the problem, size of the problem, and need for a program within a client population. *Estimation of risk* is also useful in determining the preventive program needs for specific population (see Chapter 8 for additional information about statistical indicators). Statistical data about a community are readily available through local and state health departments and from the publication, *Health Statistics of the United States.*

When assessment of the program needs of the client population is begun, the nurse should consider that a program based on need does not guarantee program success. The demands of the client population for the planned program must be considered. Thus the use of several of the tools just discussed is essential (1) to estimate the need and (2) to assess the demand within the client population to validate that the need is real and a program is desired. Table 11-1 provides a summary of the definition, advantages, and disadvantages of needs assessment tools.

TABLE 11-1
Summary of needs assessment tools

Name	Definition	Advantages	Disadvantages
Community forum	Community, group, organization, open meeting	1. Low cost 2. Learn perspectives of large number of persons	1. Limited data 2. Limited expression of views 3. Discourages less powerful 4. Becomes arena to discuss political issues
Key informant	Identify, select, and question knowledgeable leaders	1. Provides picture of services needed	1. Bias of leaders 2. Community characteristics may be incorrectly perceived by informants
Indicators approach	Existing data used to determine problem	1. Excellent data on problems and location of client groups 2. Observations made at regular intervals show trends 3. New problems can be identified	1. Data may be obsolete 2. Growth and change in population may make data outdated
Survey of existing agencies	Estimates of client population via services used by similar community	1. Easy method to estimate size of client group 2. Know extent of services offered in existing programs	1. Records and data may be unreliable 2. All cases of need may not be reported 3. Exaggeration of services may occur
Surveys/census	Measurement of total or sample client population by interview or questionnaire	1. Direct and accurate data on client population and their problems	1. Expensive 2. Technically demanding 3. Need large number of interviews or observations

PLANNING METHODS

The need and demand for a program have been determined through the needs assessment process. The next step in the development of the program is to choose a procedural method that will assist the community health nurse in planning the program to be offered.

Five planning methods are discussed in this section: (1) the Planning, Programming, and Budgeting System, (2) the Program Planning Method, (3) the Program Evaluation Review Technique, (4) the Critical Path Method, and (5) the Multi-Attribute Utility Method.

Planning, Programming, and Budgeting System

The Planning, Programming, and Budgeting System (PPBS) is a procedural tool initially developed for use by the Department of Defense and other governmental agencies. PPBS is an outcome-oriented accounting system, the extent of which is to determine the most efficient method of resource allocation to attain measurable objectives (LaPatra, 1975; Rakich et al., 1977).

The steps involved in PPBS are (1) setting program goals, (2) defining measurable program objectives, (3) identifying and evaluating alternatives to accomplish program objectives, (4) choosing the method for accomplishing the objectives, and (5) developing a program budget with justification for minimizing costs while maximizing program benefits (Figure 11-3).

PPBS is an economic method of expressing a program plan. In PPBS, *planning* represents formulation of objectives and conceptualization or identification of alternatives and methods for accomplishing objectives, *programming* represents detailing of resources (manpower, facilities, equip-

ment, and financing) for each identified alternative, and *budgeting* represents the assignment of dollar values to resources required for the program implementation, the evaluation of program costs and benefits.

PPBS is widely used for planning broad-scale governmental programs. It is a system that can also be used to plan programs for an agency or for client groups. For example, PPBS could be used to develop the annual program plan for the local health department or a prenatal program for the local community. A community health nurse could also use this method to develop a health education program for the school population on sexually transmitted diseases. PPBS's use of objectives that are operationally defined by standards or performance criteria is a system that lends itself to effective program evaluation.

Program Planning Method

PPM, or program planning method, is a technique employing the nominal group technique of Delbecq and Van de Ven (1971). It can be used by the community health nurse to involve clients more directly in the planning process. This is a five-stage process that focuses on three levels of planning groups comprised of clients' providers, and administrators to identify program needs. The client or consumer group relays a list of problems to the provider group, who in turn aids the client group in presenting problem solutions to the administrative group (Nutt, 1984).

The stages of PPM are compared with Nutt's planning process in Table 11-2. The *PPM stage one* involves problem diagnosis. Each client in the group develops a written problem list and then shares the list with all other members of the group, one problem at a time. After all problems have been shared and recorded they are discussed by the total client group. Following the discussion, clients select the problems with the highest priority by voting on the ranking of each problem.

In the *second stage* of PPM the expert provider group identifies solutions for each of the problems identified by the clients. In the *third stage* the client and provider groups present their problems and suggested solutions to the administrative group to determine the possibilities of developing a program to meet one or more of the problems, using one or more of the solutions. In this phase clients and providers are seeking acceptance from the administrators who control the program resources. *Phase four* of PPM involves identifying the alternative solutions to the problem and analyzing the pros and cons of each. *Phase five* involves the client, providers, and administrators in selecting the best plan for program implementation. In this phase the link between the planned solutions and the problem are evaluated, pointing out strengths and limitations of the proposed program plan.

The community health nurse may use this technique for developing school health services within the total community or in one school. This method may also be used by the nurse working with a senior citizens group to identify their priority needs for nursing or physician clinic services at the health department. It is important to note that this method is used to get consensus among all persons involved

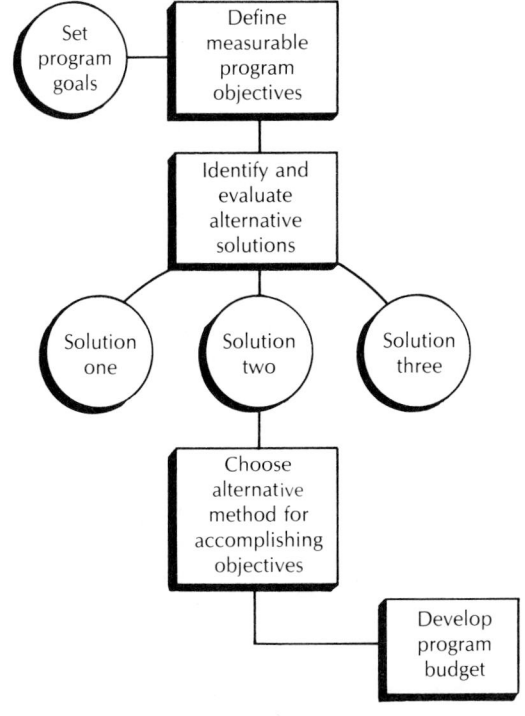

FIGURE 11-3

Planning, programming, and budgeting system.

TABLE 11-2

Planning methods compared with basic planning process

Basic planning	PPBS	PPM	PERT/CPM	MAUT
1. Formulation	Identify goals and define in measurable items	Problems identified by client	Identify program activities	Identify target population and program objectives
2. Conceptualization	Identify alternatives	Provider group identifies solution	Explore time and events required to meet program activities	Identify alternative problem solutions
3. Detailing	Evaluate alternatives for use of resources	Analyze available solutions	Determine sequencing of events and resources to meet activities	Identify criteria for choice; rank, rate, and weight; calculate value
4. Evaluation	Choose method for accomplishing objectives and develop budget to evaluate costs vs. benefits	Clients, providers, administrators select best plan	Select appropriate events	Choose best alternatives
5. Implementation		Best plan presented to administrators for funding		

in the program, clients, providers, and administrators. Consensus is most helpful in providing a successful program.

Program Evaluation Review Technique

The Program Evaluation Review Technique (PERT) is a network programming method developed in the 1950s through a joint effort of the United States Navy, Lockheed Aircraft Corporation, and Booz-Allen and Hamilton, Inc. The method was developed for planning and controlling the program activities involved in developing the Polaris missile.

The PERT method is primarily useful for large-scale projects that require the planning, scheduling, and controlling of a large number of activities. PERT is mentioned here to introduce the reader to the concept of network programming. PERT as a planning method has been used successfully in hospitals to plan for the development of nursing services, by nursing service administrators to plan for new nursing services delivery such as primary care services, and for designing projects such as the installation and use of computers for organizing and providing nursing services.

The major objectives of PERT are to (1) focus attention on the key developmental parts of a program; (2) identify potential program problems that could interfere with movement toward program goals; (3) evaluate program progress toward goal attainment; (4) provide a prompt reporting method; and (5) facilitate decision making (Roman, 1969; Nutt, 1984).

PERT involves the concept of time and events. The basic tool used in the technique is the network or flow plan, which is a series of circles, ovals, or squares representing the program events, or goals, and their interrelationships

with the activities of the program. The program activities are the time-consuming events of the program and are represented by arrows that connect the program accomplishments or goals (Figure 11-4). Note in the flow plan that it may take several activities to attain a program event (goal) and that some events (goals) must be accomplished before other events may be attained. The interrelationship of several program events (subgoals) may be essential to attain the ultimate program event (goal).

Another element in PERT is the estimation of the time it will take to implement activities leading to program goals. In PERT three estimates of activity time are given: the optimistic time it will take to complete activities, given minimal difficulties; the most likely time it will take to complete activities, given past experiences with normal development of said activities; and the pessimistic time it will take to complete activities, given maximum difficulties. From the time estimates a simple formula can be applied to indicate the probability of completing a project in a given time period (Barentson, 1970; Griffith, 1972; Roman, 1969; Wiest and Levy, 1969). The numbers appearing along the arrows in Figure 11-4 are the estimated number of days required for completion of activities leading to a particular event.

PERT embodies three major steps: (1) identification of specific program activities, (2) identification of resources to accomplish the activities, and (3) determination of sequencing activities for the accomplishment of program events.

Critical Path Method

The Critical Path Method (CPM) is a network programming planning method that is described by some authors (Rakich

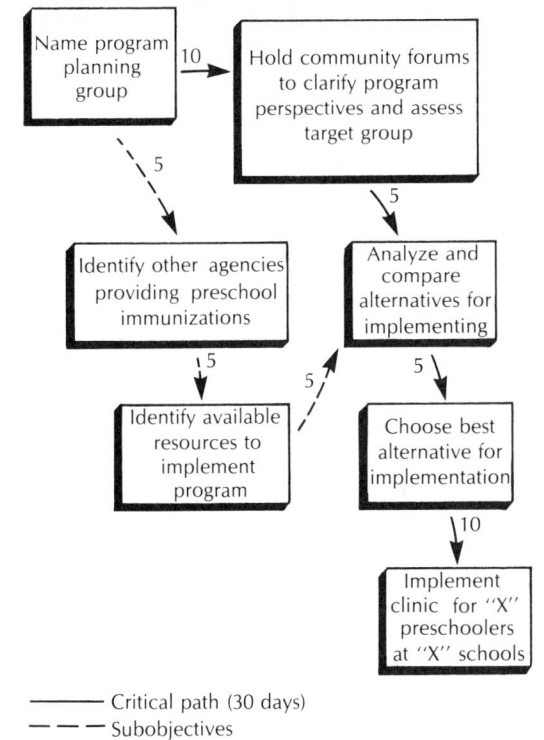

——— Critical path (30 days)
— — — Subobjectives

FIGURE 11-4

Simplified PERT network for planning a preschool immunization program. Numbers represent days required for completion of activities.

et al., 1977; Wiest and Levy, 1969) as a technique in itself and by others (Roman, 1969; Nutt, 1984) as an element of PERT.

CPM is a technique that focuses the program planner's attention on the program activities, the sequencing of activities for the best use of time and resources, and the estimated time it will take to complete the project from beginning to end. Using this method the planner can determine the amount of time it will take to accomplish each activity and can identify those activities that may take longer. The planner can then determine the amounts of resources needed (manpower, money, facilities, and supplies) to accomplish tasks at given points in time along the program's "critical path."

CPM allows for frequent review of progress by program planners. Problems can be identified early in program implementation, and corrective action can be taken or alternative activities can be substituted for activities that are not meeting program requirements. The amount of time and the resources being used during program implementation can be assessed, and time and resources can be increased or decreased as necessary and can be compared to initial estimates of program need.

PERT and CPM embody the five generic stages of planning described by Nutt. However, these two methods focus on specific activities, times, and events essential to program success. The emphasis with these two models is on detailing and evaluation (Table 11-2).

The Multi-Attribute Utility Technique

The Multi-Attribute Utility Technique (MAUT) is a planning method based on decision theory (Edwards, Guttentag, and Snapper, 1975). This method can be adapted for making decisions about the care of one client or for making decisions about the national health care programs. The purpose of MAUT is to separate all elements of a decision and to evaluate each element separately for its impact on the overall decision.

Ten basic steps to MAUT method are described by Edwards, Guttentag, and Snapper (1975):*

1. *Identify the person or aggregate whose utilities are to be maximized.* In other words, who is the client for whom the program is being planned?

2. *Identify the issue(s) or decisions to which the utilities are relevant.* This step involves the identification of the program objectives.

3. *Identify the entities to be evaluated.* The program planner identifies the available options or action alternatives to accomplish the program goals.

4. *Identify the relevant dimensions of value.* The program planner places a value on or identifies criteria to be considered to make a choice between competing options or alternatives.

5. *Rank the value dimensions in order of importance.* The program planner will decide which of the criteria are most important and which are the least important for meeting the program goals.

6. *Rate dimensions in importance.* In this step the program planner assigns an arbitrary rating of 10 to the least important value dimension. In considering the next least important dimension, the planner decides how many times more important it is than the least important dimension. If it is considered twice as important, the dimension will be assigned a 20. If it is only considered half again as important, it will be assigned a 15. If it is considered four times as important, it will be assigned a 40. The process is continued until all dimensions have been rated.

7. *Add the importance weights, divide each by the sum, and multiply by 100.* Edwards refers to this process as "normalizing" the weights. This step is considered a purely mechanical step that provides a clearer picture of the relative values of the dimensions by the program planner. However, if too many dimensions are identified in Step 4, the computational process underestimates the value of some actions and overestimates the value of others. Six to 15 dimensions are recommended to avoid this problem. Therefore, in this initial process the planner can be concerned with only general criteria for choosing action alternatives.

8. *Measure the location of the entity being evaluated on each dimension.* The planner may ask a colleague or expert to estimate the probability on a scale of 0 to 100 that a given option from Step 3 will maximize the value dimensions (criteria) from Step 4. An option thought to have a low probability of meeting the criteria may be assigned a value

*From Edwards, Guttentag, and Snapper: Copyright © 1975 Handbook of Evaluative Research. Reprinted by permission of Sage Publications, Inc.

of 20, whereas an option thought to have a high probability of meeting the criteria may be assigned a value of 80.

9. *Calculate utilities for entities.* The program planner will obtain the utility of each action alternative identified by multiplying the weight for each dimension (Step 7) by the rating of an option for each dimension (Step 8) and adding the products. The sum of the products for each action is termed the aggregate utility.

10. *Decide on best alternative to meet program objectives.* The action alternative with the highest aggregate utility is considered the best decision for meeting the program objectives. If cost was not considered as one of the criteria on which to evaluate the action alternatives, then the utility of each option may need to be considered in relation to cost.

If money is no object, then the option with the highest utility is the best decision. However, if the highest utility option exceeds the budget, then the next highest utility option may be the alternative to choose. An example of the application of MAUT to a program decision in community health nursing is given on pp. 226-228. The steps of MAUT relate clearly to the basic planning process described by Nutt (1984) as shown in Table 11-2.

Steps 1 and 2 of MAUT relate to problem formulation. Step 3 involves conceptualization of the program alternatives, and Steps 4 through 9 focus on detailing and the implications of each option. Step 10 involves the evaluation phase of planning or the choice of the best solution as identified in Steps 4 through 9. Placing quantitative values on solutions to meet program needs is most helpful in the implementation phase of planning, that is, convincing administrators of the need for such a program. However, caution must be taken in using all planning methods since the best solution reflects the bias of the planner.

BENEFITS OF PROGRAM PLANNING

Systematic planning for meeting client needs benefits clients, nurses, and the employing agencies. The act of planning focuses attention on what the organization and the health provider are attempting to do for clients. Planning assists in identifying the resources and activities that are essential in meeting the objectives of client services and directs the attention of the organization and providers toward making sound decisions to attain common objectives. Planning reduces role ambiguity by allowing for assignment of responsibility of the planned activities to specific providers to meet program objectives.

Planning also reduces uncertainty in the internal program environment and enhances the abilities of the provider and the agency to cope with the external environment. All persons involved with the program can anticipate what will occur during program implementation and what will be needed to implement the program and can project the program outcomes. Planning assists the provider and the agency in acting on rather than reacting to events. Finally, planning allows for quality decision making and better control over the actual program results. Today this type of planning is referred to as *strategic planning* and involves the successful matching of client needs with specific provider strengths and competencies and agency resources.

Planning is usually reflective of a desire on the part of the planners to reduce the gap between the program goals and the realities of program implementation and to diminish the unanticipated occurrences that may result during program implementation. Inherent in the planning process is the desire to implement a reality-based program that can be readily evaluated.

PPM and PPBS are more general approaches to program planning, whereas PERT, CPM, and MAUT offer guidelines for identifying and tracking specific program activities essential to program success. All of these approaches establish the basis for program evaluation.

PROGRAM EVALUATION
Planning and the Evaluative Process

As previously indicated, program evaluation begins with the initial program planning phase, a formative evaluation of the assessment of need. The basic questions to be answered, after careful consideration of the data collected from census, key informants, community forums, surveys or health statistics indicators, are: Will the objectives and resources of this program meet the identified needs of the recipients of the health care service? Is the program relevant? Once need has been established and the planning process instituted for designing the program, the community health nurse must plan for program evaluation.

Planning for the evaluative process is an integral part of program planning and should not be considered as something begun after the program has been in operation for several months. This is a common occurrence in health care. As a part of the planning process, Posevac and Carey (1980) describe six steps to use in planning for program evaluation (Figure 11-5):

The *first step* is to identify the relevant people for evaluation. Program personnel, program sponsors, and the recipients of the program should be included in planning for the evaluation.

The *second step* is to arrange preliminary meetings to discuss the questions of whether the group wants an evaluation, and if so, why, what kind, and when. If the program planners and others agree on an evaluation, the resources for conducting the program evaluation must be identified.

The *third step* is to make a decision about whether the evaluation should be carried out. After the relevant people have met and considered the questions in the previous steps, they are ready to decide whether the evaluation should be carried out. The decision to conduct the evaluation may be an administrative one, may be based on availability of resources, or may be determined by the existing circumstances. For example, if a program evaluation were attempted in a situation where program personnel or clients chose to be uncooperative, evaluation efforts would fail.

The *fourth step* is to examine the literature for suggestions about the appropriate methods and techniques and their usefulness in program evaluation. This step is particularly helpful if the organization has chosen an evaluator who is external to the program. If the evaluation is internal, the evaluators may already know the literature.

The external evaluator may make suggestions regarding the questions to be answered in the evaluation process. If

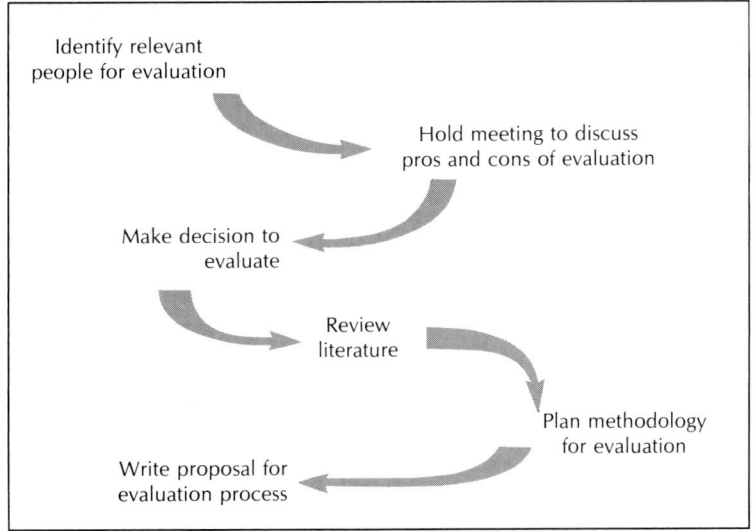

FIGURE 11-5

Six steps in planning for program evaluation.

the literature has been reviewed by the community health nurse and others affected by the evaluation, they can determine whether the evaluation suggestions are appropriate for their situation.

The *fifth step* is to plan the methodology, which includes decisions about what parameters will be measured, how they will be measured, and on what population the measures will be obtained.

The *sixth* and final step is to write a proposal for the evaluation that outlines the purpose and goals of the overall program, the type of evaluation to be done, the operational measure to be used to evaluate the program goals, the choice of internal or external evaluators, the available resources for conducting the evaluation, and the readiness of the organization, personnel, and clients for program evaluation.

Evaluation Functions

The choice of evaluation depends on the reasons program evaluation is being planned. The kinds of evaluation include the following: (1) evaluation of *relevance*, the need for the program; (2) *progress*, the tracking of program activities to meet program objectives; (3) *efficiency*, the relationship between program outcomes and the resources expended; (4) *effectiveness*, the ability to meet program objectives and the results of program efforts; and (5) *impact*, the long-term changes in the client population (Kalyzny and Veney, 1984).

As indicated, evaluation of relevance should be an important component of the initial planning phase. As money, providers, facilities, and supplies for delivering health care services are more closely monitored, the automatic assumption that all health care delivery programs are needed becomes erroneous. The needs assessment done by the community health nurse will answer the question of program relevance.

The monitoring of program activities, such as hours of services, number of providers used, number of referrals made, and amount of money expended to meet program

objectives, provides an evaluation of the progress of the program. This type of evaluation is an example of formative evaluation and occurs on an on-going basis while the program is in existence. This function provides an opportunity to make effective day-to-day management decisions about the operations of the program. Whereas evaluation of relevance occurs primarily during the planning phase, progress evaluation occurs primarily during implementation. The community health nurse who completes a daily or weekly log of her clinical activities (i.e., number of clients seen in clinic or visited in the home, number of phone contacts, number of referrals made) is contributing to progress evaluation of the nursing service.

Case studies, or written analysis of program development and implementation throughout the life of the program, can be used to assess relevance of the program retrospectively. This approach is used to describe how a program has worked and is an inexpensive method of evaluation. If historical preservation of program events would be useful in planning future programs, the case study is a simplistic method for providing such data. A nurse-managed ambulatory clinic was planned and implemented to provide health care for the homeless population of a metropolitan community. A case history was presented by the clinic nurses which included how it was planned, who was involved, how much it cost, the types of clients, their problems, the kinds of care needed, nursing interventions, and the limitations of the clinic. This data was used to obtain funding from the community to provide much improved services for the population.

The more formal scientific methods of *survey research*, *trend analysis*, and *experimental designs* provide more expensive and precise methods for looking at the efficiency, effectiveness, and impact of a program. However, each of these methods, although providing data for decisions about the future of existing programs or the development of new programs, does not offer short-term solutions for daily program decisions or short-range planning.

Community health nurses will usually find themselves involved in evaluation of program relevance and progress. They should become more involved in the evaluation of efficiency, effectiveness, and impact of these programs; this is an excellent way to show what they are contributing to health care. In the clinic for the homeless, survey research and experimental designs are being used to show that nursing care makes a difference in the health of this population.

If the reason for evaluation is to examine the efficiency of a program, this type of evaluation may occur on an ongoing basis as formative evaluation or at the completion of the program as a summative evaluation. The evaluator may be able to determine whether this program provides better benefits at less cost than a similar program or whether the benefits to the clients or numbers of clients served justify the cost of the program.

An evaluation of effectiveness may help the community health nurse evaluator determine both client and provider satisfaction with the program activities, as well as whether the program met its stated objectives. However, if the evaluation of impact is the goal, then the question of long-term effects, such as changes in morbidity and mortality, is the one to be asked. Both effectiveness and impact evaluations are usually summative evaluation functions primarily performed as end-of-program activities.

The Evaluative Process

As previously stated, the evaluative process should be operational at the onset of the program. The evaluative process as described by Suchman (1967) is modified and explained here, but the reader will find it to be very similar to steps in the planning process.

The first step in the evaluative process is *goal setting,* which is preceded or concurrent with values clarification. The values and beliefs of the agency, the providers, and the clients are all considered at every step of the evaluation process.

The statement that children should not be exposed to the illness and suffering of early childhood diseases and polio because they can be prevented is a value statement. It would be followed by a program goal such as a decrease in the incidence of early childhood diseases and polio in the county where the program is planned.

The second step is *determining goal measurement.* In the case of the previous goal, the recording of disease incidence would be an appropriate goal measurement. The third step is *identifying goal-attaining activities,* and in the same case would include such things as media presentation to encourage parents to have their children immunized. The fourth step is *making the activities operational,* actually administering the immunizations. The fifth is *measuring the goal effect,* reviewing the records and summarizing the incidence of early childhood disease and polio before and after the program. The final step is *evaluation of the program,* or a judgment about whether the program goal was achieved. Keep in mind that only one program goal was used in the example, and the program undoubtedly has more than one goal (Figure 11-6).

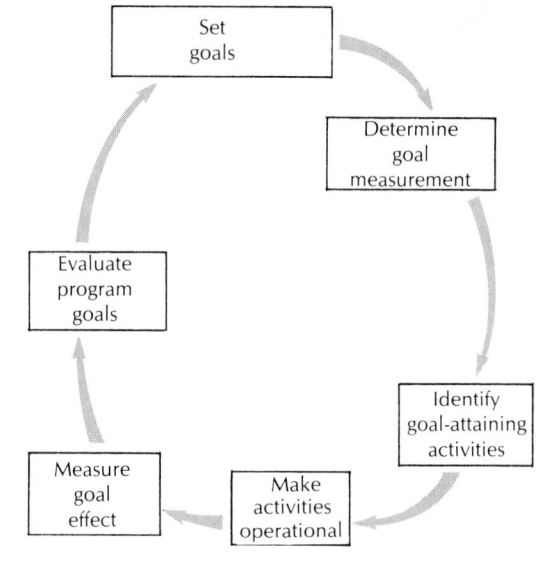

FIGURE 11-6

The evaluative process.

Shortell (1978) divides program evaluation into three steps: (1) the specification of program objectives (goals), which is equated with the program planning phase; (2) organization of resources to conduct the program, which involves program implementation; and (3) the assessment of program performance or the impact of the program. The value structure of the client, provider, agency, and community affect each stage of the evaluation process. Table 11-3 depicts the interrelationship between the evaluative process models of Suchman, Shortell, and the functions described by Veney and Kaluzny. The table includes the steps of the process and the functions and kinds of evaluation that are related to each step of the process. Note that the five evaluation functions described may be conducted at each step in the process, depending on the reason the evaluation is being conducted.

Formulation of Objectives for Evaluation

The most important step in the evaluative process is the formulation of program objectives. The objectives set the stage for the conduct of the program and provide the mechanism whereby the activities and the total program can be evaluated. If the objectives are too general, program evaluation becomes impossible. The objectives must be specific and stated so that anyone reading them could conduct the program without further explanation. The following discussion will help the reader in the development of clear concise objectives. Development of program objectives coincides with the initial phases of program planning.

Specification of Objectives (Goals). According to Mager (1962), objectives should include the specific behavior, the conditions under which the behavior is shown, and the minimum standard of performance. According to Deniston et al. (1969), an objective should specify the following: the *what* or condition to be achieved, the extent or *how much,*

TABLE 11-3

Evaluative process models

Type of evaluation/models	Suchman	Shortell	Veney/Kaluzny
FORMATIVE EVALUATION			
Program planning	Goal setting Determining goal measurement Identifying goal attaining activities	Objective setting	Relevance
Program implementation	Make activities operational	Organize resources to conduct program	Progress
SUMMATIVE EVALUATION			
Total program evaluation	Measure goal effect	Assess program performance	Efficiency Effectiveness Impact
	Judge ultimate program goal		

to whom or what group, *where,* and *when.* The population and geographical area may be included in the general description of the program, but the *when* is an important part of the program objective.

Shortell (1978) indicates that useful program objectives require a statement of the specific behaviors, accomplishments, and success criteria for the program. Each program objective requires a strong action-oriented verb to specify the behavior, a statement of single purpose, a statement of a single result, and a time frame for achieving the expected result. For example, a program objective depicting these criteria may be to decrease (action verb) the incidence of early childhood disease in Center County (result) by providing immunization clinics in all schools (purpose) between August and December of 1988 (time frame).

As objectives are stated, one should consider providing an operational indicator for each objective so the evaluator knows when and if the objective has been met. For instance, an operational indicator for the above objective would be: a 10% to 25% decrease in the incidence rates of the most commonly occurring childhood vaccine-preventable illnesses in Center County. Such indicators provide a target to be reached by all persons involved with program implementation.

Levels of Program Objectives. It is customary for objectives to be stated in levels from low order objectives to higher order objectives. The first level at which the objective is stated is general and broad. Some refer to these as goals. The purpose of the goal or general objective is to focus on the major thrust of the program.

An overall program objective may be to reduce the incidence of low birth weight babies in Center County in 1990 by improving access to prenatal care. The subobjectives or subgoals are more specific; that is, they describe a measurable behavior, the circumstances under which the behavior is observed, and the minimal acceptable standard for the execution of the behavior. A subjective or lower level objective for this program may be to open a prenatal clinic in each health department within the county by Jan-

uary 1989 to serve the population within each census tract of the county.

Some general guidelines for writing objectives follow: (1) they should describe program recipients' behavior, (2) they should be stated as a product or outcome, and (3) they should state only one outcome per objective (Gronlund, 1970).

Program activities are planned to ensure meeting each subobjective or each subgoal; resources are planned for each of the activities. Program assumptions are that attainment of the subobjectives are in sequence and will result in attainment of the general objective, that the planned activity will facilitate or ensure the attainment of the objective, and that the resource will be provided for the planned activity. Remember that several lower level objectives are required to meet an overall program objective (or goal).

Benefits of Program Evaluation

The major benefit of *program evaluation* is that it determines whether the program is fulfilling its purpose. It should answer the question of whether the needs for which the program was designed are being met or whether the problems that it was designed to solve are being solved. Evaluation is a way of demonstrating that the program is fulfilling its purpose. This is critical information for funding agencies, top-level decision makers, accreditation reviews, or the community at large. Evaluation data may be used to justify expanding the program or they may be used to justify reducing the program or even closing it.

Program Evaluation Versus Evaluative Research

Program evaluation collects information in a systematic way to assess the relevance, progress, effectiveness, efficiency, and impact of a program under consideration. The purposes of program evaluation are to provide information to assist in decisions about initiating, continuing, expanding, modifying, terminating, or certifying a program. The evaluation is directed to particular individuals or agencies related in some way to the particular program. Its uses are for problem solving or practical purposes. Community health nurses and administrators engage in data collection for program evaluation on a day-to-day basis to make decisions about program management.

Evaluative research collects information according to the rigors of systematic inquiry. All the steps must be precise and explicit enough to allow replication, the variables must be recognized or controlled, and the findings must be analyzed through appropriate statistical techniques. These steps are aimed at obtaining findings that are generalizable beyond the population under study, and optimally the report is available in the literature to other researchers, the profession, and the public at large (Bloch, 1980; Hegyvary, 1980; Krueger, 1980; Phaneuf, 1980).

Evaluation research designs can be very useful in program evaluation. Such studies may be used to fulfill any of the functions of evaluation; however, they seem to be used more frequently for summative evaluation and to look at the long-term impact of program implementation.

EVALUATION MODELS AND TECHNIQUES
Evaluation of Program Effectiveness

According to the plan for program evaluation formulated by Denniston et al. (1969), programs consist of objectives (including subobjectives), activities, and resources. Assumptions are made that program objectives are met through planned activities (specific for those objectives) and with planned resources (specific for those activities). This plan addresses the question of whether the program is effective. It does not specifically address whether the program is adequate, appropriate, or efficient. The question of effectiveness asks to what extent are the preestablished objectives attained as a result of the planned activity. *Evaluation of program effectiveness* consists of three steps: (1) describing the program, (2) measuring the objectives, and (3) determining effectiveness.

Describing the program consists of naming the program and stating the program objective(s), subobjectives, activities, and resources. Program activities are specified and linked to the objective or subobjective for which the activity was designed. This permits the evaluator to determine the extent to which activities were performed as planned. Resources are specified to determine the extent to which resources were used as planned for the activities.

After the program has been described, the next step is to *measure* whether the objective(s) and subobjectives of the program have been attained. Valid and reliable measuring instruments are essential. The measures must be made at the time specified in the objective(s) and subobjectives. Care must be taken to avoid bias and to use proper sampling techniques.

Effectiveness refers to what extent achievement of the objective(s) can be attributed to the activities of the program. This is accomplished by comparing the program resources, activities, and objectives by using a set of ratios. The first ratio is actual use of resources to planned use of resources, the second ratio is actual program activities to planned program activities, and the third ratio is attainment of the objective attributable to program activity to attainment

desired less the attainment that existed in absence of the program. These ratios answer the question of whether the program was conducted according to the plan and whether the achievement of the objectives was the result of the program or the result of chance.

Structure-Process-Outcome Evaluation

The method for evaluation of programs by Donabedian (1982) was initially directed primarily toward medical care but is applicable to the broader area of health care. He described three approaches to assessment of health care: structure, process, and outcome (see Chapter 12).

Structure refers to settings in which care occurs and includes materials, equipment, qualification of the staff, and organizational structure (Donabedian, 1982). This approach to evaluation is based on the assumption that given a proper setting with good equipment, good care will follow, but this assumption is not strongly supported.

Process refers to whether the care that was given was "good" (Donabedian, 1982), competent, or preferable practice, given a particular client. Use of process in program evaluation may consist of observation of practice but more likely consists of review of medical records. The review may focus on pathology reports to ascertain whether the percentage of surgeries were strongly indicated or questionable. The review could focus on whether documentation of preventive teaching was on the clinical record. Audits using specific criteria are examples of the use of process.

Outcome refers to client recovery and restoration of function and of survival (Donabedian, 1982) but is also used in the sense of changes in health status or changes in health-related knowledge, attitude, and client behavior. Thus program outcomes may be expressed in terms of mortality, morbidity, and disability for given populations such as infants but could be expressed in a broader sense through health promotion behaviors such as weight control, exercise, and abstinence from tobacco and alcohol.

Donabedian (1982) supports the use of the process approach when possible, followed by outcome, and finally by structure. Process and outcome are used more than structure in evaluation of care. Donabedian's model of evaluating program quality is a popular model and is widely used for evaluation in the health care field. It can be useful in evaluating program effectiveness.

Tracer Method

The Board on Medicine of the National Academy of Sciences developed a program to evaluate health service delivery called the tracer method (Kessner and Kalk, 1972). The *tracer method* of evaluation of programs is based on the premise that health status and care can be evaluated by viewing specific health problems called "tracers." Just as radioactive tracers such as iodide are used to study the thyroid gland, specific health problems are selected for use to evaluate the delivery of health and nursing services. Examples of conditions selected as tracers are middle ear infection and associated hearing loss, vision disorders, iron deficiency anemia, hypertension, urinary tract infections, and cervical cancer. This program can be used to (1) compare health status among different population groups, (2) compare health status in relation to social, economic, medical care, nursing care, and behavioral variables, and (3) compare various arrangements for health care delivery. The application of this method for the study of health care for children in Washington, D.C., has been reported by Kessner and Kalk (1973) and is discussed by Palmer (1976) and Veney and Kaluzny (1984).

The tracer method is a useful technique for looking at efficiency, effectiveness, and impact of a program. Stevens (1975) has developed a method for evaluating nursing care that is similar to the tracer method (see Chapter 12).

Goal Attainment

Goal attainment refers to a process for assessing the efficacy of a program by examination or measurement of the predetermined goals (Kiresuk and Sander, 1979). LaPatra (1975) described the components of the *goal attainment* model as setting objectives, setting measures of objectives, collecting data, assessing the effect, and modifying the initial objective on the basis of the data analysis and interpretation. The following model by Shields is an example of a goal attainment model. Shields (1974) applies a process to each goal. For each goal the evaluator examines the categories of wherewithal, structure, operations, and outcomes.

Wherewithal refers to resources, materials, equipment, and physical facilities.

Structure consists of the organizational framework, that is, administrative structure, lines of authority, committee linkages, and patterns of communication.

Operations pertain to the processes and procedures for carrying out the program goals whether they are teaching, treating, or preventing and the performances of the workers doing the processes.

Outcomes refers to whether the goal was attained and to what degree and to other significant events related to the outcome.

The criteria applied to outcomes are: (1) effectiveness—whether the immediate purpose was attained; (2) efficiency—how cost efficient the program was; and (3) impact—whether unexpected and potentially harmful events were associated with the program. If the program has more than one goal, the evaluation process is applied to each goal.

Systems Model

The systems model of evaluation focuses on the process as a working model or a social unit capable of achieving the goal (Schulberg et al., 1969; Shortell, 1978; Liturack, 1985). This *systems model* is concerned with objectives being achieved, subunits functioning in coordination, resources being maintained, and adaptation to the environment (LaPatra, 1975). The systems model examines aspects other than the goal; it recognizes that organizations have multiple goals and considers single goal attainment in relation to its effect on other goals in the system.

Three variables are described and evaluated in the systems model; the input, throughput, and output. *Input* consists of characteristics and conditions of people and the resources.

Throughput refers to the human and nonhuman resources and process. *Output* refers to the products of the system (Baker and Northman, 1979). The systems model is more comprehensive, since it takes more elements into consideration for the evaluation.

Case Register

Systematic registration of contagious disease has been a practice for many years. Denmark began a national register of tuberculosis in 1921 (Horwitz, 1979). Its contribution to the reduction in the incidence of contagious diseases has been widely recognized (Clemesen, 1979). *Case registers* are also used for acute and chronic disease, for example, cancer and myocardial infarction.

Registers collate information from defined groups, and the information may be used for evaluation and planning of services, disease prevention, provision of care, and monitoring changes in patterns and care of diseases (Holland and Karhausen, 1979). The method is described here because of its use in evaluation of services. Information obtained by the community registers in Europe on myocardial infarction is a good example of the way a case register is used (Keil, 1979). The following are questions that were asked about cases of myocardial infarction for the community registers:

1. What is the incidence of disease? What differences in incidence are there between one community and another?
2. What percent recover? Or die?
3. Where does death occur?
4. How long do clients wait before calling a doctor?
5. How long is it before they see a doctor?
6. How many cases are associated with other major coronary heart disease risk factors?
7. How many are associated with environmental factors such as water hardness or air pollution?
8. What happens after clients leave the hospital and when they return to work? Is there a rehabilitation program?
9. How many had been seen by a physician shortly before the infarction?
10. What prevention measures are taken for persons considered susceptible?

The answers to these questions before and after implementation of a given program would give information about the impact of the program. A tuberculosis register indicates the degree to which infection is being controlled. Cancer registers make state, regional, national, and international comparisons possible and provide clues to etiological factors.

Evaluation Indexes

Doster (1979, p. 79) defines a *health index* as a "summary of the health features of a community that enable us to determine health care delivery needs." Doster further categorizes the health index into six headings: definition of community, people, environment, communication, health and illness indicators, and health provider resources and services.

The founder of vital statistics, J. Graunt, was interested

in data on population, births, deaths, and other characteristics for the purpose of urban planning or redevelopment. The collection of vital statistics related to health problems is attributed to the public health movement in the middle of the nineteenth century (Ciocco, 1969).

Today the health and illness indicators such as mortality and morbidity data are probably cited more frequently than any other single indexes not only for program planning but also for program evaluation. Health and illness indicators are useful in evaluating the impact of health care programs.

SOURCES OF PROGRAM EVALUATION

Major sources of information for program evaluation are program participants, program records, and community indexes. The program participants, or consumers of the service, have a unique and valuable role in program evaluation. Whether the clients for whom the program was designed accept and use the service will determine to a large extent whether the program achieves its purpose. Thus their reactions, feelings, and judgments about the program are very important to the evaluation.

The second major source of information for program evaluation is program records, especially clinical records. The most prominent example of the use of clinical records is the Donabedian model for evaluation. According to the model, process and outcomes of care are often examined by review of clinical records. Most recently this has been done in the form of quality assurance (see Chapter 12) and the audit (peer review). Although review of clinical records by professional peers was already being reported in the literature as early as the 1960s (Helbig et al., 1972), legislation in 1972 established the Professional Standards Review Organization to "promote effective, efficient and economical delivery of Medicare and Medicaid health services." For examples of outcome and process criteria the reader is referred to Haussman et al., 1977, and Holland, 1983.

A third major source of evaluation is community indexes, previously described in evaluation indexes (p. 225). However, the evaluator must examine the community indexes in light of other variables or events in the community that may also facilitate or hinder achievement of the program's purpose.

MEASURES OF CONSUMER RESPONSE

To assess the response of participants in a program or consumers of a service, the evaluator may use a written survey in the form of a questionnaire or an attitude scale. Interviews, achievement tests, and observations are other ways of getting feedback about a program. Attitude scales are probably used most often, and they are usually phrased in terms of whether the program met its objectives. The client satisfaction survey is an example of an attitude scale often used in the health care delivery system to evaluate the attainment of program objectives (refer to Chapter 12 for discussion of the pros and cons of the client satisfaction survey).

Morbidity and mortality have been used as indexes to evaluate a plan for community services and also to evaluate the effectiveness of community services. A decline in the morbidity or mortality from one particular cause may indicate the effectiveness or impact of a program, particularly something that has the potential for a dramatic change such as an immunization program. Incidence and prevalence are also valuable indexes used to measure program effectiveness and impact (see Chapter 8 for further discussion of rates and ratios).

CLINICAL APPLICATION

The school health nurse director of the local district was contacted by the president of the local parent-teacher association about an expressed problem by parents regarding the need for hearing screening of elementary school children within the district (client population and need identified by key informants). The community health nurse director was contacted by the school health nurse because such programs for school health are designed as joint efforts between the health department and the school district.

Together the two nurses discussed the number of elementary schools within the district and the issue of the lack of a screening program for 6 years. Based on this data, the nurses decided that all elementary school children within the four schools should be evaluated in the program (size, distribution, and boundaries of client population identified).

At this point the school district superintendent, the four school principals, the local health officer, and the president of the PTA were requested to attend a planning meeting. All agreed that the program was essential to the health of the elementary school population and to the opportunity for a quality education for the same group. Therefore it was decided to proceed with planning (perspective of key persons on the program target).

While at the meeting the group discussed available manpower, facilities, equipment, and financing. It was determined that the number of community health nurses and school health nurses required to perform the screening program would be limited. In addition, the PTA indicated a minimum number of volunteers to assist the nurses with clerical and other duties. The school health infirmaries were considered large enough to handle the program; additional equipment would be supplied by the health department. Monies for the program budget would be jointly pledged by the school district, health department, and the PTA, but the nurses should consider a reasonably economic mechanism for program implementation (available resources assessed).

The two nursing directors proceeded to analyze and compare alternative solutions that would assist them in making decisions regarding the best plan for resolving the community problem. The multi-attribute utility planning method was chosen as a mechanism for arriving at the "best plan" for the community effort. Because of limited resources the nurses arrived at the following overall program goal, and analyzed alternatives for meeting the goal.

The ultimate goal of the hearing screening program is to identify all elementary school children with potential hearing deficits who may require screening within one academic school year. The indicator that the goal was met would be a 50% increase in the number of parents contacted regarding hearing screening for their children.

Step 1: *Identify the person or aggregate whose utilities are to be maximized.* The two organizations involved in the screening program are the local public health department and the school district. The persons representing the organizations are the community health nurses and the school nurses, respectively.

Step 2: *Identify the issue(s) or decisions to which the utilities are relevant.* The major objectives to be met to implement the screening program are to (1) identify the number of elementary school children with diagnosed hearing deficits and (2) identify the number of elementary school children currently requiring hearing screening.

Step 3: *Identify the entities to be evaluated.* The available options considered to accomplish the ultimate goal and the subobjectives were:

1. School health nurse to audit health records of all children to identify client population.
2. Public health nurse to send survey to all parents of elementary school children to identify children with diagnosed hearing deficits and children who have not had prior hearing screening.
3. Teachers be asked to survey children and parents about child's hearing problems during parent teacher conferences.

Step 4: *Identify the relevant dimensions of value.* The nurses identified the following criteria to be considered in making a choice between the alternatives.

	Rank
1. Acceptable cost of surveys.	1
2. Minimal time required of community health nurse, school health nurse, teacher, or parent.	5
3. Parents' acceptance of method chosen to identify children for screening.	2
4. Acceptable level of response to chosen survey method; for example, mailed survey may yield only a 2% to 20% return.	4
5. Minimum time required to schedule parent conferences.	6
6. Children's acceptable reaction to survey.	3

Step 5: *Rank the value dimensions in order of importance.* See Step 4 for ranks. Next the nurses ranked the criteria in Step 4 from the most important to the least important consideration in making a final choice.

Step 6: *Rate dimensions of importance.* (See Step 7.) When the six relevant criteria were considered, the nurses rated #1, cost considerations, as five times more important than #6, conference scheduling; thus cost was assigned the value of 50, and conference scheduling was assigned the value of ten (Table 11-4).

Step 7: *Add the importance weights, divide each by the sum, and multiply by 100* (see Table 11-4). To obtain a "normalized weight" for the six criteria, the raw weights were added and found to total 190. This figure was divided into each of the criteria's raw weights (rate) and multiplied by 100. For example, cost = 50 ÷ 190 = 0.26 × 100 = 26.

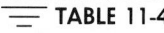

TABLE 11-4

Ranked dimension (5)	Raw weight (6)	Normalized weight (7)
1. Cost	50	26
2. Parents' acceptance	40	21
3. Children's reaction	40	21
4. Survey response	30	16
5. Time	20	11
6. Conference scheduling	10	5
	190	100

Step 8: *Measure the location of the entity being evaluated on each dimension.* Next each nurse asked a colleague to estimate on a scale of 0 to 100 the probability that each of the three alternatives in Step 3 would maximize the value of the six criteria in Step 4. These estimates appear in the worksheet. For example, option one, the school health nurse audit of children's health records, was assigned probability of value estimates on the six criteria as follows in the example in Table 11-5.

Step 9: *Calculate utilities for entities.* See Table 11-6. Finally, the nurses determined the best option based on the value of the six criteria and their relationship to each option (this is termed the aggregate utility of each option). For example, the utility of cost to the school health nurse audit is determined by multiplying the normalized weight of cost, 26, by the probability of cost, .50 = 13.0. When each criteria has been assigned an individual utility, they are summed to obtain the aggregate utility, or the overall value of choosing that option. In this example the total value of Option 1 is *50.9,* which resulted from summing the individual utility of the six criteria.

Step 10: *Decide on best alternative to meet program objectives.* Option 1 identified in Step 3, school health nurse audits children's health records. Option 1 was chosen because its total value based upon the six criteria considered was higher than Options 2 and 3.

The evaluation of the program began with the needs assessment process. The program need was determined to be relevant by all parties involved, providers, administrators, and parents (*formative evaluation*). The initial planning group was again called together to approve the program plan chosen by the nurses (*planning for program implementation*). On acceptance the group (*relevant people*) discussed whether they would like to evaluate the program (pros and cons of evaluation). The nurses provided information to the group on methods of evaluation (*review of literature*).

The decision was made to evaluate the progress of the program (*decision to evaluate*) by monitoring the costs (*costs*), the number of hours of service required by the school nurse to audit the records (*time*), the number of children identified with hearing deficits, the number of children identified who needed screening, and the number of children's records with inadequate data to evaluate (*survey response*), and the numbers

TABLE 11-5

Probability and value estimates assigned to option one, the school health nurse audit of children's health records, by colleagues

Criteria	Probable value	Explanation of rating
1. Cost	50 (average value)	Average cost to agencies. No mailing or printing costs.
2. Parents acceptance	80 (highest value)	Parents will agree because it takes minimal time and effort from parents and problem being solved.
3. Children's reaction	00 (no value)	None—would not be aware of program.
4. Survey response	90 (high value)	High rate of data collection by school nurse.
5. Time	20 (minimal value)	It would take a maximum amount of nurse's time and may take her away from other functions.
6. Conference scheduling	90 (high value)	Not a major factor. Few contacts with parents and teachers required to collect data.

TABLE 11-6

Worksheet for MAUT (4, 5, 6, 7)

Entities to be evaluated (3)	Dimension to be maximized						Aggregate utility (9)	Final rank
	1	2	3	4	5	6		
WEIGHT OF DIMENSIONS	26	21	21	16	11	5		
1. School health nurse to audit children's health records								
Probability (8)	.50	.80	0.00	.90	.20	.90		
Weight × probability (9)	13.00	16.8	0.00	14.40	2.20	4.50	50.90	1
2. Public health nurse to mail parents' survey								
Probability	.20	.50	.50	.20	.80	.50		
Weight × probability	5.20	10.50	10.50	3.20	8.80	2.50	40.70	3
3. Teachers to perform survey during parent-teacher conference								
Probability	.80	.60	.20	.50	.20	.20		
Weight × probability	2.80	12.60	4.20	8.00	2.20	1.00	48.80	2

and types of conferences the nurse scheduled and the reasons for the conferences (*conference scheduling*). With this information collected weekly, the school and health department administrations could make ongoing decisions about the program and the need to make changes in the conduct of the program while it is in progress (*evaluation methods— formative evaluation*).

Finally, the group determined a need to evaluate program effectiveness (*summative evaluation*). Three questions are to be answered in evaluating this program's effectiveness: (1) Did the program meet its stated objectives? (2) Were health department and school health nurses satisfied with program activities? and (3) Were parents of the PTA satisfied with effects of program activities?

To answer these questions the nurse directors, with the assistance of health department and school district statisticians, will develop a satisfaction survey to be administered to nurses and parents involved in the program (*parents' and providers' acceptance and child reaction*). In addition, ratios will be employed to establish the relationships between resources, activities, and objectives to see if the program was conducted as planned. Statisticians will be available to assist the nurses in the development and interpretation of ratios.

Upon completion and evaluation of this program, depending on program outcomes, the planning group projected these areas of consideration for future programming: (1) given the number of children identified who need screening, the school would provide a screening clinic; (2) a health education program would be developed to assist parents with the understanding of the scope of child health deficits and the need for evaluation with private providers; and/or (3) the school would establish hearing screening on an ongoing basis within the school health program.

SUMMARY

Planning programs and planning for the evaluation of programs are two of the most important activities for community health nurses to ensure successful program implementation. Whether the program being planned is a national health insurance program like Medicare, a state health care program like early childhood developmental screening programs, or a local program like vision screening for elementary school children, the essential elements of planning are applicable.

Needs assessment is a key ingredient in the planning process. The target population for any program must be identified and involved in program development. If the client population does not recognize the need for a health services program, that program is designed to fail regardless of the commitment of health providers and the resources of the program.

A number of tools are available for assisting planners in needs assessment. Some of the major tools used for needs assessment are census data, key informants, community forums, surveys of existing community agencies, surveys of community residents, and statistical indicators.

Several procedural methods can be applied to plan program offerings. A few of these methods are the Planning, Programming and Budgeting System, Program Evaluation Review Technique, the Critical Path Method, the Multi-Attribute Utility Method, and the Program Planning Method.

The application of the planning process to program development is an indication that the planners wish to reduce the gap between program goals and the realities of program implementation and the likelihood of unanticipated occurrences during program implementation.

When plans for program implementation are being developed, the plan for program evaluation should also be developed. All persons involved in program implementation should be a part of the plan for program evaluation. The major benefit of program evaluation is to determine whether the program is fulfilling its stated goals. Quality assurance programs are prime examples of program evaluation in health care delivery. Evaluation data are used to justify the continued existence of programs in community health.

Program evaluation focuses on goal attainment and the efficiency and effectiveness of program activities. Many methods of program evaluation are described in the literature. The primary method of evaluation used in health care today is Donabedian's Evaluative Framework. The goal attainment mode, systems model, tracer method, and case register are other methods applied to program evaluation.

Program records and community indexes serve as the major sources of information for program evaluation. Surveys, interviews, observations, and tests are measurements used to assess consumer and participant response to health programs.

Planning for the evaluative process is an integral part of program planning and should not be considered something begun after the program has been in operation for several months. As economic resources become scarce, nursing and the health care system must be able to justify their existence, prove the responsiveness of their services to consumer needs, and show their professional concern for accountability. Planning and evaluation will assist in meeting these objectives.

KEY CONCEPTS

Planning and evaluation are essential elements of a quality assurance program for the health care system and the nursing subsystem and vital to survival of the nursing discipline in health care delivery.

A program is an organized response designed to meet the assessed needs of individuals, families, groups, or communities by reducing or eliminating one or more health problems.

Planning is defined as formulation of a detailed scheme for accomplishing a goal or goals.

Evaluation is defined as a collection of methods and skills to determine if a service is needed and will be used, whether a program to meet that need is carried out as planned, and whether the service actually helps the people it was planned to help.

To develop quality programs, planning should include four essential elements: problem diagnosis and assessment of need, identification of problem solutions, analysis and comparison of alternative methods, and selection of the best plan and planning methods.

The initial and most critical step in planning a health program is assessment of need.

Some of the major tools used in needs assessment are census data, community forums, surveys of existing community agencies, surveys of community residents, and statistical indicators.

LEARNING ACTIVITIES

1. Choose the definitions that best describe your concept of programs, planning, and evaluation.

2. Apply the program planning process to an identified clinical problem for a client group with whom you are working in the community.
   a. Assess client need.
   b. Choose tools appropriate to the assessment of needs.
   c. Apply MAUT to the identified problem.
   d. Analyze the overall planning process of arriving at decisions about program implementation.
   e. Summarize the benefits for program planning that are applicable to your situation.

3. Given the situation just described, choose three to four of your classmates to work with on the following projects.
   a. Plan for evaluation of the above program.

Continued.

The major benefit of program evaluation is to determine whether a program is fulfilling its stated goals. Quality assurance programs are prime examples of program evaluation.

The primary method of evaluation used in the health care system is Donabedian's Evaluative Framework. Other methods are the goal attainment mode, the systems model, the tracer method, and the case register method.

Plans for program implementation and plans for program evaluation should be developed at the same time.

Program records and community indexes serve as major sources of information for program evaluation

Planning programs and planning for their evaluation are two of the most important activities for community health nurses to ensure successful program implementation.

b. Apply the evaluative process to the situation.
c. Choose a model or technique most applicable to what it is you wish to evaluate about your program.
d. Name the measures you will use to gather data for evaluating your program.
e. Name the sources you will tap to gain information for program evaluation.
f. Analyze the benefits of program evaluation, which are applicable to your situation.
4. Talk with a community health nurse (or administrator) about the application of program planning and evaluation processes at the local agency. Compare their answers to your readings.

BIBLIOGRAPHY

Ackoff, R.: Our changing concept of planning, J. Nurs. Adm. 35-40, 1982.

American Public Health Association: Glossary of administrative terms in public health, Am. J. Public Health 50(2):255-226, 1960.

Anderson, O.: Influence of social and economic research on public policy in the health field—a review, Milbank Mem. Fund Q. 44:11, 1966.

Baker, F., and Northman, J.E.: Input-throughout-output evaluation of a school mental health clinic. In Schulberg, H.C., and Baker, F., editors: Program evaluation in the health fields, vol. 2, New York, 1979, Human Sciences Press.

Barentson, P.: Critical path planning: present and future technique, Princeton, N.J., 1970, Brendon Systems Press.

Beatty, W.H., editor: Improving educational assessment and inventory of measures of affective behavior, Washington, D.C., 1969, Association for Supervision and Curriculum Development, National Education Association.

Bice, T.: Health services planning and regulation. In Williams, S., and Torrens, P., editors: Introduction to health services, New York, 1984, John Wiley & Sons, Inc.

Bloch, D.: Interrelated issues in evaluation and evaluation research, Nurs. Res. 29(69):69-73, 1980.

Ciocco, A.: On indices for the appraisal of health department activities. In Schulberg, H.C., Sheldon, A., and Baker, F., editors: Program evaluation in the health fields, New York, 1969, Behavioral Publications, Inc.

Clemmesen, J.: Registration in the study of human cancer. In Holland, W.W., and Karhausen, L., editors: Health care and epidemiology, Boston, 1979, G.K. Hall & Co.

Commission on Hospital Care: Hospital care in the United States, New York, 1947, The Commonwealth Fund.

Committee on the Costs of Medical Care. Medical care for the American people, Chicago, 1932, University of Chicago Press. Reprinted, Washington, D.C., 1970, Department of Health, Education, and Welfare.

Cordes, S.: Assessing health care needs: elements and processes. Fam. Community Health 1:2, 1978.

Cronbach, L.J., et al.: Toward reform of program evaluation, San Francisco, 1980, Jossey-Bass, Inc., Publishers.

Curren, W.: A national survey and analysis of state certificate of need laws for health facilities. In Havinghurst, C., editor: Regulating health facilities construction, Washington, D.C., 1974, American Institute for Public Policy Research.

Davidson, S.: Community nursing care evaluation, Fam. Community Health 1(1):37, 1978.

Delbecq, A., and Van de Ven, A.: A group process model for problem identification and program planning. J. Appl. Behav. Sci. 7(4);:466-492, 1971.

Deniston, O.O.L., Rosenstock, I.M., and Getting, V.A.: Evaluating program effectiveness. In Schulberg, H.C., Sheldon, A., and Baker, F., editors: Program evaluation in the health fields, New York, 1969, Behavioral Publications, Inc.

Donabedian, A.: Evaluating the quality of medical care, Milbank Mem. Fund Q. 44:164, 1966.

Donabedian, A.: The quality of medical care. In Abelson, P.H., editor: Health care: regulation, economics, ethics, and practice, Washington, D.C., 1978, American Association for the Advancement of Science.

Donabedian, A.: Explorations in quality assessment and monitoring, vol. II, Ann Arbor, Mich. 1982, Health Administrations Press.

Dorsey, J.L.: Certificate of need laws, Arch. Surg. 106:765, 1973.

Doster, C.: Health index of a community. In Community health today and tomorrow, NLN Pub. No. 52-1768, New York, 1979, National League for Nursing.

Edwards, W., Guttentag, M., and Snapper, K.: A decision-theoretic approach to evaluation research. In Struening, E., and Guttentag, M., editors: Handbook of evaluation research, Beverly Hills, Calif., 1975, Sage Publications, Inc.

Edwards, W.: Social utilities, The Engineering Economist, Summer Symposium Series 6, 1977.

Finger, K.: Certificate of need procedure under the national health planning and resources development act of 1974, N.Y. State Bar J. 49(4):308, 1977.

Fish, C. (Consultant): Administrators handbook for community health and home care services, New York, Pub. No. 21-1943, National League for Nursing, 1984.

Fox, P., and Fox, R.: Strategic planning for nursing.

Fralic, M.: Using a PERT planning network to manage a nursing service computer system installation, J. Nurs. Adm. 29-31, 1984.

Fuerstein, M.T.: Community participation in evaluation: problems and potentials, Int. Nurs. Rev. 27:187, 1980.

Gordon, M.: Determining study topics, Nurs. Res. 29(2):83, 1980.

Griffith, J.: Quantitative techniques for hospital planning and control, Lexington, Mass., 1972, Lexington Books.

Gronlund, N.E.: Stating behavioral objectives for classroom instruction, New York, 1970, Macmillian Publishing Co., Inc.

Hanlon, J., and Pickett, G.: Public health: administration and practice, St. Louis, 1984, The C.V. Mosby Co.

Haussman, R.K.D., and Hegyvary, S.T.: Monitoring quality of nursing care. III. Professional review for nursing: an empirical investigation, Hyattsville, Md., Aug. 1977, DHEW Pub. No. HRA 77-70, Department of Health, Education and Welfare.

Haussman, R.K.D., Heygvary, S.T., and Newman, J.F.: Monitoring quality of nursing care. II. Assessment and study of correlates, Bethesda, Md., Aug. 1977, DHEW Pub. No. HRA 76-7, Department of Health, Education, and Welfare.

Havighurst, C.C.: Regulation in the health care system, Hospitals 48:65, 1974.

Hegyvary, S.T.: An evaluator's perspective, Nurs. Res. 29:91, 1980.

Helbig, D., O'Hare, D., and Smith, N.: The care component core—a new system for evaluating quality of inpatient care, Am. J. Pub. Health 62:540-546, 1972.

Holland, W.W., and Karhausen, L., editors: Health care and epidemiology, Boston, 1979, G.K. Hall & Co.

Hollard, W.: Evaluation of health care, 1983, Oxford University Press.

Horwitz, O.: Epidemiological parameters for the public health evaluation of a chronic disease. In Holland, W.W., and Karhausen, L., editors: Health care and epidemiology, Boston, 1979, G.K. Hall & Co.

Hyman, H.: Applications of methods of evaluation for studies of encampment for citizenship, Berkeley, 1962, University of California Press.

Institute for Health Planning: A glossary of health care delivery and planning terms, Madison, Wis., 1981, The Institute.

Jelinek, R., et al.: Methodology for monitoring quality of nursing care, Bethesda, Md., 1974, DHEW Pub. No. HRA 76-25, Department of Health, Education, and Welfare.

Jury, J.: Practical tips for establishing a coordinated community wellness program, Health Values 8(5):3-5, 1984.

Kaluzny, A., and Veney, J.: Evaluating health care programs and services. In Williams, S., and Torrens, P., editors: Introduction to health services, New York, 1984, John Wiley & Sons, Inc.

Keil, U.: Community registers of myocardial infarction as an example of epidemiological register studies. In Holland, W.W., and Karhausen, L., editors: Health care and epidemiology, Boston, 1979, G.K. Hall & Co.

Kessner, D.M., and Kalk, C.E.: Contrasts in health status: a strategy for evaluating health services, vol. 2, Washington, D.C., 1973, Institute of Medicine, National Academy of Sciences.

Kiresuk, T.J., and Sander, H.L.: Goal attainment scaling: research, evaluation, and utilization. In Schulberg, H.C., and Baker, F., editors: Program evaluation in the health fields, vol. 2, New York, 1979, Human Science Press.

Knutson, S.L.: Evaluation for what. In Schulberg, H.C., Sheldon, A., and Baker, F., editors: Program evaluation in the health fields, New York, 1969, Behavioral Publications, Inc.

Krueger, J.C.: Establishing priorities for evaluation and evaluation research, Nurs. Res. 29:115, 1980.

LaPatra, J.W.: Health care delivery systems: Evaluation criteria, Springfield, Ill., 1975, Charles C Thomas, Publisher.

LeBreton, P.: Measuring a nursing services department's effectiveness designing the assessment instrument, Nurs. Health Care 1:3, 1980.

Litwack, L., Linc, L., and Bower, D.: Evaluation in nursing: principles and practice, New York, 1985, National League for Nursing.

Lukas, J.: Strategic planning in hospital: applications for nurse executives, J. Nurs. Adm. 11-17, 1984.

Mager, R.F.: Preparing objectives for programmed instruction, San Francisco, 1962, Fearon Publishers, Inc.

McCarthy, C.: Planning for health care. In Jonas, S., editor: Health care delivery in the United States, New York, 1977, Springer Publishing Co., Inc.

McCarthy, C., and Jonas, S.: Planning for health services. In Jonas, S., editor: Health care delivery in the United States, ed. 2, New York, 1981, Springer Publishing Co., Inc.

Mullen, P.D.: Qualitative methods for evaluative research in health education programs, Health Educ. 13:11, 1982.

Munio, B.: A useful model for program evaluation, J. Nurs. Adm.

Nutt, P.: Planning methods for health and related organizations, New York, 1984, John Wiley & Sons, Inc.

Palmer, R.H.: The present range of provider performance in the United States. In Greene, R., editor: Assuring quality in medical care, Cambridge, Mass., 1976, Ballinger Publishing Co.

Phaneuf, M.C.: Future direction for evaluation and evaluation research in health care, Nurs. Res. 29:123, 1980.

Posavac, E.J., and Carey, R.G.: Program evaluation: Methods and case studies, Englewood Cliffs, N.J., 1980, Prentice-Hall, Inc.

Program evaluation, NLN Pub. No. 15-1738, New York, 1978, National League for Nursing.

Public Law 89-749, Comprehensive health planning and public services amendments of 1966, Nov. 3, 1966.

Public Law 79-725, Hospital survey and construction act, Aug. 13, 1946.

Public Law 93-641, National health planning and resources development act, Jan. 4, 1975.

Rakich, J., Longest, B., and O'Donovan, T.: Managing health care organizations, Philadelphia, 1977, W.B. Saunders Co.

Roman, D.: The PERT system: An appraisal of program evaluation review technique. In Schulberg, H., Sheldon, A., and Baker, F., editors: Program evaluation in the health fields, New York, 1969, Behavioral Publications, Inc.

Rossi, P., and Freeman, H.: Evaluation: a systematic approach, Beverly Hills, Calif., 1985, Sage Publications, Inc.

Ruybal, S.: Community health planning, Fam. Community Health 1:9, 1978.

Schulbert, H.C., and Baker, F., editors: Program evaluation in the health fields, vol. 2, New York, 1979, Human Sciences Press.

Schulbert, H.C., Sheldon, A., and Baker, F., editors: Program evaluation in the health fields, New York, 1969, Behavioral Publications, Inc.

Shields, M.: An evaluation model for service programs, Nurs. Outlook 22:448, 1974.

Shortell, S., and Richardson, W.: Health program evaluation, St. Louis, 1978, The C.V. Mosby Co.

Soumelis, C.G.: Project evaluation methodologies and techniques, Paris, 1977, UNESCO.

Stufflebeam, D.L.: Evaluation as enlightenment for decision making. In Educational evaluation and decision making, Itasca, Ill., 1971, Peacock Publishers, Inc.

Suchman, E.A: Evaluative research, New York, 1967, Russell Sage Foundation.

Veney, J., and Kaluzny, A.: Evaluation and decision making for health service programs, Englewood Cliffs, N.J., 1984, Prentice-Hall, Inc.

Welch, L.B., et al.: Program evaluation: an overview, Nurs. Health Care 1:186, 1980.

Wholey, J.S.: Perspective on evaluation from the U.S. Department of Health, Education, and Welfare, Nurs. Res. 29(2):109, 1980.

Wiest, J., and Levy, F.: A management guide to PERT/CPM, Englewood Cliffs, N.J., 1969, Prentice-Hall, Inc.

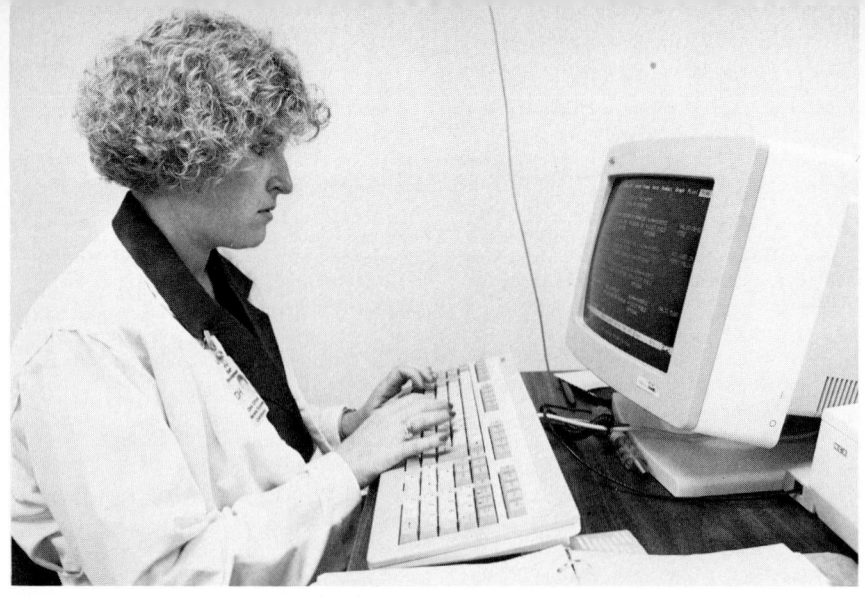

Marcia Stanhope
Kathleen Beckman Blomquist

12

QUALITY ASSURANCE IN COMMUNITY HEALTH NURSING

OBJECTIVES

After reading this chapter, the student should be able to:

Define quality assurance.

State the goals of quality assurance and record keeping.

Discuss the historical development of quality assurance in nursing.

Evaluate approaches and techniques for implementing a quality assurance program.

Describe a model quality assurance program.

Identify the purposes for the types of records kept in community health agencies.

Explain a method of documentation of client care in community health nursing.

KEY TERMS

accountability

accreditation

audit process

certification

clinical record

competitive medical plans (CMPs)

concurrent audit

evaluative studies

health maintenance organizations (HMOs)

institutional licensure

licensure

malpractice litigation

mandatory credentialing

mandatory nurse licensure

permissive licensure

Phaneuf Nursing Audit

Problem Oriented Medical Record System (POMR)

professional review organizations (PROs)

Professional Standards Review Organization (PSRO)

provider service records

quality assurance

quasi-voluntary

reciprocity

retrospective audit

staff review committees

utilization review

voluntary credentialing

Because the health care delivery system has grown into the largest employing industry in the United States, resulting in considerable effect on the total population, society is demanding greater accountability and increased efficiency and effectiveness from the system. Quality assurance, or quality control, is the tool used in industry to assure the public that it is getting top value for money spent.

One may question why a system focused on the delivery of a service needs to be concerned with quality assurance. The major demand for quality assurance programs has resulted because of the vast changes that have occurred in the health care system over time. Some of these changes are increases in third-party insurance coverage, involvement of the federal government in the health care system, demand for service, technological advances, and numbers of health professionals providing care. Other changes include changing consumer expectations for cost, accessibility and equality; changing population demography; rising costs; and the monopolistic character of the system.

Objective and systematic evaluation of nursing care has become a priority within the nursing profession because of prospective payment mechanisms, consumer demands for quality nursing, commitment to direct accountability to the public, nursing evolving as a scientific discipline, concerns about how costs of health services limit access, and the increasing involvement of nurses in shaping both public and individual health agency policies (Lang and Clinton, 1984; Maciorowski, et al., 1985).

Both consumers and providers have a vested interest in the quality of the system. Jonas (1986) indicates that the health care provider has three basic reasons to be concerned about health care quality:

1. The principle of nonmaleficence—above all, do no harm—has been a basic precept of the health care system since the writing of the Hippocratic Oath
2. The principle of beneficence—do good work—is a basic precept of professionalism
3. The strong social work ethic in our culture, which places a high value on "doing a good job in and of itself."

Jonas says that in health care there is a direct link between doing a good job and individual and professional survival.

Records are maintained on all clients of the health care system to provide complete information about the client and to show the extent and quality of care being given the client within the system. Records are an integral part of both the system and the components of a quality assurance program, and of tools and methods for evaluating quality.

DEFINITIONS AND GOALS

Quality assurance is the monitoring of the activities of client care to determine the degree of excellence attained in the implementation of the activities (Bull, 1985). An assessment of quality is a judgment concerning the process of care, based on the extent to which that care contributes to valued outcomes (Donabedian, 1982). The quality assurance or quality control process (1) sets standards for care, (2) evaluates care provided, which is based on the standards, and (3) takes action to bring about change when care does not meet standards (Bull, 1985; Maibusch, 1984).

An implicit factor in quality assurance is the accountability of the provider in the delivery of services. *Accountability* means being responsible for care activities and being answerable to the client for the activities performed (Bergmen, 1980; Hull, 1981).

The goals of quality assurance are (1) to ensure the delivery of quality client care and (2) to demonstrate the health providers' efforts to fulfill their societal responsibility (Jonas, 1986). The process of health care is divisible into two major components: technical, and the management of the interpersonal relationship between practitioner and client. Both are important in providing quality care and both can be evaluated (Donabedian, 1982). A variety of approaches and techniques are used in quality assurance programs. *Approaches* are methods used to ensure quality, and *techniques* are tools for measuring quality (Jonas, 1986). This chapter describes several approaches and techniques used in quality assurance programs.

HISTORICAL DEVELOPMENT OF QUALITY ASSURANCE IN NURSING AND HEALTH CARE

Quality assurance approaches have been evident in nursing since Florence Nightingale in the 1860s called for a uniform format to collect and present hospital statistics to direct efforts to improve hospital treatment. Nightingale was a pioneer in setting standards for nursing care. The impetus for establishing nursing schools in the United States came in the late 1800s from a desire to set standards that would upgrade nursing care. In the early 1900s efforts began to set standards for nursing schools.

From 1912 to 1939 the interest in quality nursing education led to the development of three nursing organizations involved in accrediting nursing programs. The National Organization for Public Health Nursing (1912) accredited programs in colleges and universities preparing public health nurses; the Association of Collegiate Schools of Nursing (1932) required its member schools to meet specific educational standards; and the National League for Nursing Education (1939) accredited basic nursing programs (McCloskey, 1985).

Licensure has been a major issue in nursing since 1892. By 1923 all states had permissive or mandatory laws directing nursing practice. Today revision of nurse practice acts is an ongoing process to assure the public that a minimum level of competence in the expanding practice of nursing will be attained (Bullough, 1981).

After World War II the attention of the emerging nursing profession focused on establishing a scientific method of practice. The nursing process emerged as an identifiable entity with scientific elements, including evaluation of how the activities of nurses helped clients (Maibusch, 1984). Quality assurance is ensured by the evaluative step in the nursing process.

The 1950s brought the development of tools to measure quality assurance. One of the first tools created was the **Phaneuf Nursing Audit** (1952), which has been used extensively in community health nursing practice. This and other tools are discussed later in this chapter.

In 1966 the American Nurses' Association (ANA) created the Divisions on Practice in its bylaws. From this came the charge in 1972 to the Congress for Nursing Practice to develop standards to be used in instituting quality assurance programs. The Standards for Community Health Nursing Practice were distributed to ANA Community Health Nursing division members in 1973. In 1986 the standards were revised; these revised standards can be found in Appendix F1.

Because evaluation of care was not evidenced in health care documentation, Weid (1969) developed the **Problem-Oriented Medical Record System (POMR).** This method is based on the problem-solving process of assessing client problems, developing a plan to resolve client problems, implementing the plan, and evaluating the problems' outcomes. Many forms of POMR have been used since the system was introduced.

In 1972, the Joint Commission on Accreditation of Hospitals (JCAH), already requiring hospitals to develop quality control systems, clearly delineated the responsibilities of nursing in its description of standards for nursing services. JCAH called on the nursing industry to clearly plan, document, and evaluate nursing care provided. During the same year the Social Security Act (Public Law 93-106) was amended to establish the **Professional Standards Review Organization (PSRO)** and to mandate the review of the delivery of health care to recipients of Medicare, Medicaid, and maternal and child health benefits.

The PSRO program was modified to the **Professional Review Organizations (PROs)** by 1983 Social Security Amendments. The purpose of the PROs is to monitor implementation of the prospective reimbursement system based on diagnostic-related groups (DRGs) for Medicare recipients (see Chapter 3). Although PSRO and PROs were primarily designed for medical care evaluation, they have served to make quality assurance a primary issue for all professionals in health care delivery. For example, PROs have the authority to deny payments to health care providers that fail to meet recognized standards of care and to review services that Medicare clients receive in hospitals, **health maintenance organizations (HMOs),** and **competitive medical plans (CMPs).**

In nursing, efforts continue to be directed toward the development of approaches and techniques to assure quality nursing care. These efforts are evidenced in the quality assurance model developed by the ANA (1977), the study by Jacobs et al. (1978) to define critical requirements of safe practice, the ANA study of nurse credentials (1979), and the NLN study of accreditation (1979). Two efforts specifically directed toward strengthening community health nursing practice have been the development of frameworks for community health nursing practice by the ANA (1980) and the APHA (1980). A discussion of these two models and the *Consensus Conference on the Essentials of Public Health Nursing Practice and Education, 1984* can be found in Chapter 7.

APPROACHES FOR A QUALITY ASSURANCE PROGRAM

Two major categories of approaches exist in quality assurance today—general and specific. The *general approach* examines the person's or agency's ability to meet established criteria or standards at a given time. Credentialing mechanisms are general quality assurance approaches often used in the health care system. *Credentialing* is generally defined as the formal recognition of professional or technical competence (Hohman, 1980) and attainment of minimum standards by a person or agency. These mechanisms are used to evaluate the *structure* of the systems through which care is provided and the outcomes of that care. Licensing, certification, and accreditation are all examples of approaches to credentialing.

According to Hinsvark (1981), the credentialing process has four functional components: (1) to produce a quality product; (2) to confer a unique identity, for example, registered nurse; (3) to protect the provider and the public; and (4) to control the profession. Credentialing can be mandatory or voluntary. **Mandatory credentialing** requires statutory law; state nurse practice acts are examples of mandatory credentialing. **Voluntary credentialing** is performed by an agency or institution. Certification examinations offered to nurses by the ANA are examples of voluntary credentialing.

Specific approaches to quality assurance are methods used to evaluate identified instances of provider and client interaction. Examples of specific approaches to quality control are agency staff review committees (peer review), utilization review committees, research studies, PRO monitoring, client satisfaction surveys, and malpractice litigation. The overall goal of the specific quality assurance approaches is to monitor the *process* and *outcomes* of client care (LoGerfo and Brook, 1984). The functional components are (1) to identify problems between provider and client, (2) to intervene in problematical cases, (3) to provide feedback regarding interaction between client and provider, and (4) to provide documentation for interactions between provider and client.

The specific approaches are often voluntarily implemented by agencies and provider groups interested in the quality of interactions in their setting. However, the state and federal governments often call for a mandatory program to be established within public health agencies. For instance, through state departments of human resources and state health laws, regulations are set forth requiring periodic utilization review, peer reviews (audits), and other quality control measures within public health agencies that receive funds from state taxes, Medicaid, Medicare, and other public funding sources.

General Approaches
Licensure

Licensure is one of the oldest general quality assurance approaches in the United States. Licensure exists for both individuals and agencies.

Individual licensure is a contract between the profession and the state, in which the profession is granted control over entry into and exit from the profession and over quality of professional practice. Several disadvantages to professional licensure include: (1) professional self-interest, (2) questionable attention to regulating quality, (3) rigidity in job descriptions, (4) some limits on geographical mobility because of different state law requirements, and (5) discouragement of innovative and creative use of personnel.

When professionals are granted control over their own practice through licensure, questions arise about the profession's interest in safeguarding its own territory or protecting the consumer from unsafe practitioners. Will the profession be interested in regulating quality by setting standards of care and policing the profession to see that standards of care are upheld, or will the profession set standards and provide only a token sanction to those who do not uphold the practice standard?

The licensing process requires that regulations be written to define the scope and limits of the professional's practice. It is from these regulations that job descriptions evolve to set minimum and maximum limits on the functions and responsibilities of the practitioner. Some view the job descriptions as limiting practice to legally defined groups and as precluding people external to this defined group from being assigned duties normally practiced by the legally defined group. It is in this manner that employing agencies are restricted from hiring physical therapists, for example, for registered nurse positions.

Limited geographical mobility of professionals results because of differing licensure requirements from state to state. Although the nursing discipline enjoys *reciprocity,* or the recognition and acceptance of a professional's licensure between certain states, a nurse moving from one state to another could conceivably be required to meet a new set of criteria before receiving licensure in the new state. For example, state continuing education requirements may be different.

The issue over innovative and creative use of personnel led to a movement during the 1970s in favor of *institutional licensure,* that is, allowing the employing agency to be responsible for the competence of the people they employ. This concept was not well received by the nursing and medical professions and to date has not been accepted as the answer to the disadvantages of professional licensure. The concern expressed is that poorly trained persons may be employed at minimum salaries to deliver a lower quality of health care to the consumer.

Licensure of nurses has been mandated by law *since 1903* when North Carolina, New York, New Jersey, and Virginia enacted laws on nurse registration. Today 49 of the 50 states have mandatory nurse licensure. *Mandatory nurse licensure* requires all who practice nursing for compensation to be licensed. One state has a *permissive licensure* law, meaning that a person can practice nursing without a license as long as the term *registered nurse* is not used and the practitioner does not purport to be licensed (Pinkerton, 1985).

Accreditation

Accreditation, a voluntary approach to quality control, is used for institutions, whereas licensure is primarily used for individuals. Since 1954 the National League for Nursing (NLN), a voluntary organization, has established standards for inspecting nursing education programs and community health–home health programs for the purpose of accrediting them. In addition, state boards of nursing accredit basic nursing programs so their graduates are eligible for the licensing examination. The accreditation function may be classified as *quasi-voluntary.* Although appearing to be a voluntary participatory program, accreditation is often linked to governmental regulation that encourages programs to participate in the accrediting process. Examples include the federal Medicare regulations restricting payments to accredited hospitals and home health care agencies, and the federal program funding for nursing that is tied to the United States Secretary of Education's recognition of program accreditation by the NLN, by regional associations of colleges and secondary schools, or by designated state boards of nursing (McCloskey, 1985).

The advantages of accreditation are that it provides a means for effective peer review and an opportunity for an in-depth review of program strengths and limitations (Hawkin, 1984; Hohman, 1980). However, because the accreditation process primarily evaluates physical structures, organizational structures, and personnel qualifications, serious consideration must be given to specific measures of the quality of health care delivery and to educational outcomes to provide more relevance to the accreditation process.

Although accreditation of institutions assumes that certain standards of physical and organizational structure will assure quality health care or quality education at a given time, there are several arguments against the need for accreditation: (1) accreditation has not defined quality health care or education; (2) accreditation does not focus on health or educational outcomes; (3) review by colleagues is suspect, and self-interest may be promoted; (4) innovative and creative programs that deviate from established standards are discouraged; (5) institutional objectives are variable and not subject to standardization, thus making program comparisons meaningless; and (6) federal funding ties have caused accreditation to become quasi-voluntary (LoGerfo and Brook, 1984; McCloskey, 1985).

Certification

Certification, another general approach to quality, combines features of licensure and accreditation. Certification is usually a voluntary process within professions. A person's educational achievements, experience, and performance on examination are used to determine the person's qualifications for functioning in an identified specialty area, such as community health nursing.

In 1958 the ANA began to study reasons for establishing a certification program in nursing. The reasons given for the need for such a program were to provide peer recognition to nurses involved in direct client care and to provide the health care consumer with further evidence of nursing's ability and willingness to accept increasing responsibilities in health care delivery. In 1966, five clinical units were established within the ANA to determine standards of nursing excellence: Medical-Surgical, Geriatric, Community Health, Psychiatric and Mental Health Nursing, and Maternal-Child Health. These units functioned to develop certification criteria, applicant eligibility, and certification mechanisms. In 1985, 17 certification areas existed and 30,429 nurses had been certified by ANA since the program's inception (ANA, 1985). To become a certified community health nurse one must have a baccalaureate degree in nursing and 2 years of practice as a community health nurse immediately before application. Recertification is required every 5 years. In 1985 there were 1388 certified community health nurses in the United States (ANA, 1985).

Certification has become a major issue in health care, as is evidenced by the proliferation of certification programs and the many organizations involved in the certification process. Today there are over 70,000 nurses certified by 13 different organizations. In 1971 the Department of Health, Education and Welfare recommended that certification in health care be studied (ANA, 1979). In 1977 the ANA study of credentialing in nursing was begun. This study resulted in a proposal to establish an umbrella organization for credentialing in nursing so that differences in certification could be eliminated and consistencies could be instituted for all nursing certification programs.

In 1979 a task force on the study of credentialing in nursing was established to act on the report of the initial study. The work on the credentialing issues continues today. Many of the proposals from the initial and continuing study are unresolved. However, one major issue proposed—that only baccalaureate-degree nurses be eligible to apply for licensure to practice professional nursing—is a subject of major debate among the members of the nursing profession.

Although usually a voluntary process, certification can be a quasi-voluntary process. For example, to function as a nurse practitioner in some states, one must show proof of educational credentials and take an examination to be "certified" to practice within the boundaries of the state.

The major concerns about certification as a quality assurance mechanism are that data are lacking about clinical competencies of the practitioner at the time of certification; data are lacking about the quality of the practitioner's work following the certification process; and except for occupational health nurses and nurse anesthetists, certification has not been recognized by employers as an achievement beyond basic preparation, so financial rewards have not occurred. Although the nursing profession has accepted the certification process as a mechanism for recognizing competence and excellence in nursing practice, certifiers must consider the utility and validity of the certification process as it is now set up and must be able to communicate to the public what it means to them to have certified nurses in health care delivery.

Other Approaches

Other general approaches to quality assurance defined in the ANA study of credentialing in nursing involve charter, recognition, and education degrees. *Charter* is the mechanism by which a state government agency, under state laws, grants corporate status to institutions with or without rights to award degrees. The ANA position is that a state government should charter not only university-based programs but also nursing programs outside the university setting, such as hospital schools of nursing. *Recognition* is defined as a process whereby one agency accepts the credentialing status of and the credentials conferred by another. An example of recognition occurs when state boards of nursing accept the credentials of a nurse practitioner when the credentials are awarded by ANA or a specialty credentialing agency. *Academic degrees* are titles awarded to individuals recognized by degree-granting institutions as having completed a predetermined plan in a branch of learning. At present there are four academic degrees awarded in nursing, with some variations at each degree level: Associate of Arts/Science; Bachelor of Science in Nursing; the master's degrees—Master of Science in Nursing and Master of Nursing; and the doctorate degrees—Doctor of Philosophy, Doctorate of Nursing Science, Doctorate of Science in Nursing, and Doctorate of Nursing.

Specific Approaches
Staff Review Committees

Staff review committees are the most common specific approach to quality assurance in the United States. Staff, or peer, review committees are designed to monitor client-specific aspects of care appropriate for certain levels of care. The audit has been the major tool used by peer review committees to ascertain quality of care. Specific kinds of audit instruments are presented later in this discussion. For explicit suggestions for the development of the peer review process, refer to the NLN administrator's handbook (CHHA/CHS, 1985).

The *audit process* (Figure 12-1) consists of essentially six steps: (1) selection of a topic for study; (2) selection of explicit criteria for quality care; (3) review of records to see if criteria for quality care are met; (4) peer review of all cases that do not meet criteria for quality care; (5) specific recommendations to correct deficiencies, such as staff development programs, changes in procedures, or supervisor consultation with staff; and (6) follow-up of the topic to see that problems have been eliminated (LoGerfo and Brook, 1984).

Two types of audits are used in nursing peer review: concurrent and retrospective. The **concurrent audit** is a method of evaluating quality of ongoing care through appraisal of the nursing process. The advantages of the concurrent audit are (1) identification of deficiencies at the time care is given, (2) provision of a mechanism for identifying and meeting client needs during the caring process, (3) implementation of measures for fulfilling professional responsibilities to the consumer, and (4) provision of a mechanism for communicating on behalf of the client. The disadvantages of the concurrent audit are that (1) it is time consuming; (2) it is more costly to implement than the retrospective audit; and (3) because care is ongoing, it does not present the total picture of care the client will receive (Trussell and Strand, 1978).

The *retrospective audit* evaluates quality of care through appraisal of the nursing process after the client's discharge from the health care system. The advantages of the retrospective audit are that it provides (1) for comparison of actual practice to standards of care, (2) for analysis of actual practice findings, (3) a total picture of care given, and (4) more accurate data on which to base corrective action. The

retrospective audit has several disadvantages: (1) the focus of evaluation is directed away from ongoing care; (2) client problems are identified after discharge, when there is no chance to assist that client with the problems; and (3) corrective action can only be used to improve practice for future clients.

Utilization Review

Utilization review differs from peer review in that utilization review is directed toward assuring that care is actually needed and that the cost is appropriate for the level of care provided. LoGerfo and Brook (1984) described three types of utilization review: (1) *prospective*—an assessment of the necessity of care before giving service; (2) *concurrent*—a review of the necessity of services while the care is being given; and (3) *retrospective*—an analysis of the necessity of the services received by the client after the care has been given.

Utilization review grew in the mid-twentieth century out of concern for increasing health care costs. The first committees were developed between insurance companies and professional groups and became mandatory under the 1965 Medicare Law as a control measure for hospital costs (LoGerfo and Brook, 1984).

The utilization review process includes the development of explicit criteria that serve as indicators of the need for services and the length of service. Utilization review has been used primarily in hospitals to establish need for client admission and the length of hospital stay. In community health, especially home health care, utilization review establishes criteria for admission to agency service, the number of visits a client may receive, the eligibility for client services such as a nursing aide or physical therapist, and discharge. Chapter 42 discusses eligibility criteria for home health clients under federally regulated programs. If clients do not meet established criteria or if services are overutilized by the agency on the client's behalf, then the agency is sanctioned or denied reimbursement by third-party payers for services provided the clients.

Utilization review has several advantages: (1) it is designed to assist clients to avoid unnecessary care; (2) it may serve to encourage the consideration of care options by providers, such as home health care rather than hospitalization; (3) it can provide guidelines for staff and program development; and (4) it provides a measure of agency accountability to the consumer. The major disadvantage to utilization review is that not all clients fit the classic picture presented by the "explicit criteria" that serves as the basis for approval or denial of care. For example, an elderly female client was admitted to the home health care agency for management after hospital discharge. The client was paraplegic as a result of a cerebrovascular accident (CVA). After several weeks of physical therapy and speech therapy the client showed little sign of progress. The utilization review committee considered the client's condition to be stable and did not recognize the continued need for management to prevent future complications. Medicare payment was denied.

Appeal mechanisms have been built into the utilization

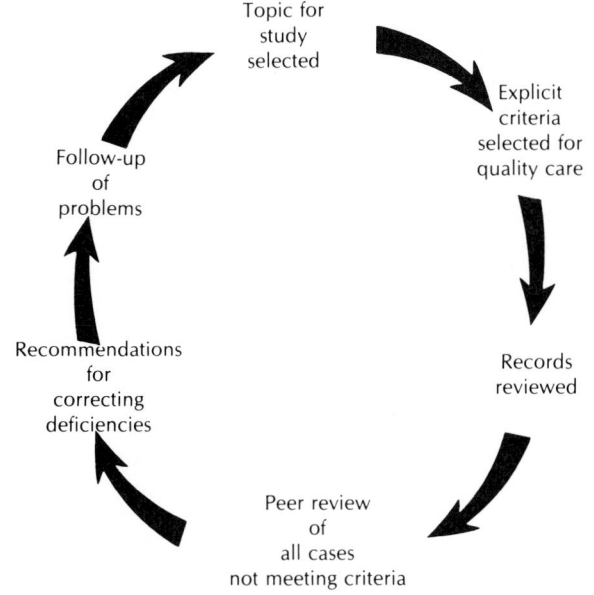

FIGURE 12-1

The audit process.

review process of Medicare and Medicaid. The appeal allows providers and clients to present additional data that may help to reverse the original decision to deny payment.

For explicit suggestions on the development of a utilization review process, refer to the NLN Administrator's Handbook (CHHA/CHS, 1985).

Professional Review Organizations

The *Professional Standards Review Organization (PSRO)* program was established in 1972 in an amendment to the Social Security Act (Public Law 92-603) as a publicly mandated utilization and peer review program. This law provided that medical, hospital, and nursing home care under Medicare, Medicaid, and Title V Maternal and Child Health Programs would be reviewed for appropriateness and necessity and would be reimbursed accordingly.

Community health agencies and nursing services were omitted under the original PSRO guidelines, although the PSRO regulations established an option to include community health agencies at some future date. In 1974 PSRO contracted with the ANA to develop criteria for review of nursing care and guidelines for the participation of nurses in PSRO.

In 1984, as institutions were responding to the prospective payment system (PPS) which instituted diagnostic-related groups (DRGs), Congress passed the Peer Review Improvement Act (PL 97-248), creating Peer Review Organizations (PROs). PROs are directed by the federal government to (1) reduce hospital admissions for procedures that can be performed safely and effectively in an ambulatory surgical setting on an outpatient basis, (2) reduce inappropriate or unnecessary admissions or invasive procedures by specific DRGs, and (3) reduce inappropriate or unnecessary admissions or invasive procedures by specific practitioners or hospitals. Quality measures include reduction of unnecessary admissions caused by previous substandard care, avoidable complications and deaths, and unnecessary surgery or invasive procedures (Gremaldi and Micheletti, 1985).

Institutions contract with PROs for quality reviews. PROs are local (usually state) organizations that establish criteria for care based on local patterns of practice. They can be for-profit or not-for-profit organizations. They have access to physicians or may include physicians in their membership. PROs must define their operational objectives and are required to consult with nurses and other nonphysician health care providers when reviewing activities of those professionals. They monitor access to care and cost of care. Professionals working under the regulation of PROs will want to develop accurate and complete documentation procedures and methods for interdepartmental cooperation to assure compliance with the PROs' criteria.

The federally mandated quality review process has produced much debate regarding limitations and benefits. Professional autonomy is jeopardized as decision making regarding care includes professionals, consumers, and government representatives. This quality control mechanism is costly, and client care activities may be determined by cost rather than professional criteria. The PSRO/PRO system has challenged health care professionals to develop standards and institute peer review mechanisms to increase accountability for care provided (Bull, 1985; Gremaldi and Micheletti, 1985; Lisske, 1985).

In 1985 PRO authority was expanded to include review of services offered by HMOs and CMPs. In addition, the Medicare Quality Assurance Act was passed to strengthen quality assurance programs and to improve access to post-hospital care. This act required hospitals receiving Medicare payments to provide discharge planning, supervised by registered nurses and social workers, to Medicare beneficiaries.

Evaluative Studies

Evaluative studies for quality health care have increased throughout the twentieth century. Three major models have been used to evaluate quality: Donabedian's structure-process-outcome model, the tracer model, and the sentinel model.

Donabedian (1982) introduced three major methods of evaluating quality care. These methods are *structure*—evaluating the setting and instruments used to provide care, such as facilities, equipment, characteristics of the administrative organization, client mix, and the qualifications of the health providers; *process*—evaluating activities as they relate to standards and expectations of health providers in the management of client care; and *outcomes*—the net changes that occur as a result of health care or the net results of health care.

Data for structural evaluations can be obtained from the existing documents of an agency or from an inspection of a facility. For example, if one wants to do an evaluative study of structure in community health nursing, one might look at the ratio of nurses to clients, the educational preparation of nurses, the ratio of nurses to clients with different disability levels, and the defined responsibilities of nurses with different educational preparation in the organizational structure and their actual responsibilities. Two major assumptions relate to structurally oriented studies: (1) if the organizational structure is optimal, better care will be provided; and (2) that quality of organization, physical structure, and staff can be described (LoGerfo and Brook, 1984; Williamson, 1980).

Data for process evaluations can be collected through direct observation of provider encounters and review of records. Examples of process-oriented studies abound in the nursing literature. An audit instrument with established criteria for evaluating nursing performance is an example of a useful method for a process-oriented nursing study. The basis for a process-oriented study can be direct observation of client care using a client encounter protocol, which identifies the nurse's activities relative to history taking, nursing diagnosis, implementing appropriate nursing procedures, providing appropriate illness prevention and health promotion counseling, and record keeping.

The assumptions underlying process evaluative studies are that (1) health care is necessary to prevent illness and maintain or promote health; (2) good health care leads to good outcomes; and (3) the elements of good health care can be defined (Openshaw, 1984).

Both the checklist approach and the criteria mapping approach are used to establish the client encounter protocol. The checklist approach is simply a "laundry list" of activities the nurse should perform to give good care. Table 12-1 illustrates a checklist approach to evaluate the community health nurse working with a hypertensive client. The criteria mapping approach is similar to clinical decision making. In criteria mapping an evaluation of good care depends on the presence or absence of certain signs, symptoms, or client needs in a specific situation. Table 12-1 also illustrates the criteria mapping approach to evaluation.

Data for outcome evaluations can be collected from vital statistics records such as death certificates, in-person or telephone client interviews, mailed questionnaires, and client records. Nurses need to engage in more outcome-oriented studies to show nursing's contributions to health care delivery (Fagin, 1982). Community health nurses could study the outcome of various screening techniques used with clients. For example, when hearing and screening tests are performed on a group of school children, follow-up data could be collected from physicians' records to determine the number of false positive cases identified by the nurses performing the tests. Such a study would provide data about community health nurses' abilities to perform effective screening tests.

Two categories of outcome measures are reflected in the literature: *general health status indicators*, or the physical, emotional, and social aspects of health; and *disease-specific indicators*, which include morbidity and mortality, presence of symptoms, and behavioral disabilities known to occur with a specific disease. The basic assumption underlying outcome studies is that health care interventions will change the person's health status.

The *tracer method* described by Kessner and Kalk (1973) is a measure of both process and outcome of care. This method is more effective in evaluating health care of groups rather than of individual clients and in evaluating care delivered by an institution rather than an individual provider.

To use the tracer method, one must identify a volume of clients with particular characteristics requiring specific health care management. Kessner and Kalk (1973) described the following essential characteristics for implementing the tracer method. A tracer, or a problem, should have a definite impact on the client's level of functioning; well-defined and easily diagnosed characteristics; population prevalence high enough to permit adequate data collection; a known variation resulting from utilization of effective medical care; well-defined management techniques in either prevention, diagnosis, treatment, or rehabilitation; and understood (documented) effects of nonmedical factors on the tracer. Stevens (1985) provided a taxonomy for selecting client groups for tracer outcome studies in nursing: (1) a

---

TABLE 12-1

Comparison of checklist approach and criteria mapping approach for assessing the process of care in a home visit to *selectively* assess client with diagnosed hypertension

Checklist	Criteria mapping
OBSERVE AND ASSESS	**OBSERVE AND ASSESS**
Temperature, pulse, and respiration	Temperature, pulse, and respiration
Blood pressure	Blood pressure—lying, sitting, and standing:
Intake and output	*If pressure variation between three readings is wide:*
Edema	Check side effects of medications
	Check medication compliance
INSTRUCTIONS TO CLIENT	Consult physician
	If orthostatic hypotension is evident:
Taking own blood pressure	Instruct client to stand up slowly and to sit or lie down if dizziness occurs
Accurate measure of intake and	Check known side effects of prescribed medications
output	Edema
	If increase is noted:
	Check client's weight
	Check medication prescribed
	Check medication compliance
	Give client instructions:
	Avoid restrictive clothing
	Tie shoelaces loosely
	Never cross legs
	Elevate legs while sitting
	Avoid salt in foods
	Weigh self same time each day
	Intake and output
	If intake and output are inadequate:
	Instruct client on accurate measuring and recording
	Instruct client on amounts and kinds of fluids to drink for 24 hours

particular disease; (2) similar treatment; (3) similar needs; (4) similar community; (5) similar life-style; and (6) similar illness stage.

The tracer method has been used by physicians and nurse practitioners to identify persons with certain illnesses, such as hypertension, ulcers, and urinary tract infections, and to establish criteria for good medical and nursing management of the illnesses. The criteria have been used by peer review panels to evaluate the actual care given and to evaluate the changes in client status (Brook and Appel, 1973; Sibley et al., 1975). Except in the case of nurse practitioners, nursing has not used this evaluative method. The tracer method seemingly could provide nurses with data to show the differences in outcome as a result of nursing care standards.

The *sentinel method* of quality evaluation is based on epidemiological methods (Rutstein, 1976). This method is an outcome measure for examining specific instances of client care. The characteristics of this method are as follows: (1) cases of unnecessary disease, disability, complications, and untimely death are counted; (2) the circumstances surrounding the unnecessary event, or the *sentinel,* are examined in detail; (3) a review of morbidity and mortality is used as an index to determine a critical increase in the untimely event, which may reflect changes in quality of care; and (4) health status indicators such as changes in social, economic, political, and environmental factors are reviewed, which may have an effect on health outcomes. Changes in the sentinel indicate potential problems for others. For example, increases in encephalitis in certain communities may result from increases in mosquito populations. Chapter 8 discusses the application of epidemiology in community health nursing.

Client Satisfaction

Client satisfaction is another specific approach to measuring quality of care. *Client satisfaction* can be assessed using in-person or telephone interviews and mailed questionnaires. Data from client satisfaction surveys are used to measure structure, process, and outcome of care given. In community health nursing, satisfaction surveys are used to assess care received during a specific agency admission, the client's personal nursing care, or the total care the client received from all services. Satisfaction surveys may measure the technical content of client care, attitudes about the care received and the providers of care, and perceptions of the situation (environment) in which the care was received. A study of client satisfaction conducted by Birch and Wolfe (1975) has indicated that clients are more critical of interpersonal and situational components of care than of the content of care. This may be true because consumers want to be treated as human beings and, given this treatment, trust the provider to have the ability to provide good care; consumers may not understand what is ideal care, or they may fear reprisal if they complain.

Satisfaction surveys are an essential aspect of quality assessment because the survey data give us clues to reasons for client compliance or noncompliance with plans of care. The surveys provide data about health-seeking behaviors, the likelihood of malpractice litigation, and the likelihood of continuing client-provider-agency relationships. The NLN (CHHA/CHS, 1985) provides an example of a client satisfaction survey (Discharged Patient Questionnaire) which can be used in a community health agency (Appendix A1).

Malpractice Litigation

Malpractice litigation is mentioned here as a specific approach to quality assurance imposed on the health care delivery system by the legal system. Malpractice litigation typically results from client dissatisfaction with the provider and with the content of care received. Medical literature abounds with examples of cases of malpractice that flourished through the 1970s and 1980s. Several reasons were given for the increase in malpractice suits: some provider care was of poor or doubtful quality and was recognized as such by the consumers, professions were not showing the capability to police their own ranks and reduce the risk of poor quality care to the consumers, and there was an apparent deterioration in provider and client relationships (Jonas, 1986). Nursing is not immune from malpractice litigation. A discussion of legal issues affecting community health nurses can be found in Chapter 6. If community health nursing establishes a sound quality assurance program, thereby policing its own client care quality, the risk of quality control measures being imposed by an external source such as the legal system can be reduced.

MODEL QUALITY ASSURANCE PROGRAM

The primary purpose of a quality assurance program is to ensure that the results of an organized activity are consistent with the expectations of that activity. To evaluate the total picture of organized activity, the structure, process, and outcome components of health care delivery should be considered. All personnel affected by a quality assurance program should be involved in the development and implementation of the program components, including administration, management, and staff (Decker, 1985; Porter-O'Grady, 1985). If personnel arrive at the agency after the quality assurance program has been developed, then adequate orientation to the program should be provided and personnel acceptance of the program should be assessed.

In 1977 the ANA introduced a schema for a model quality assurance program. Figure 12-2 depicts the model, which identifies these seven basic components of a quality assurance program: identifying values; identifying structure, process, and outcome standards and criteria; selecting measures (techniques) to assess the degree of attainment of the standards and criteria; making interpretations about the strengths and weaknesses of care given; identifying alternative courses of action; choosing courses of action; and taking action.

To use the ANA schema for quality assurance, an organization formulates *objectives* for the total agency. These objectives are used to form *subobjectives,* or level objectives, for each service provided by the agency and for each category of provider in each service (e.g., nursing services and all personnel employed by nursing services in the public health department).

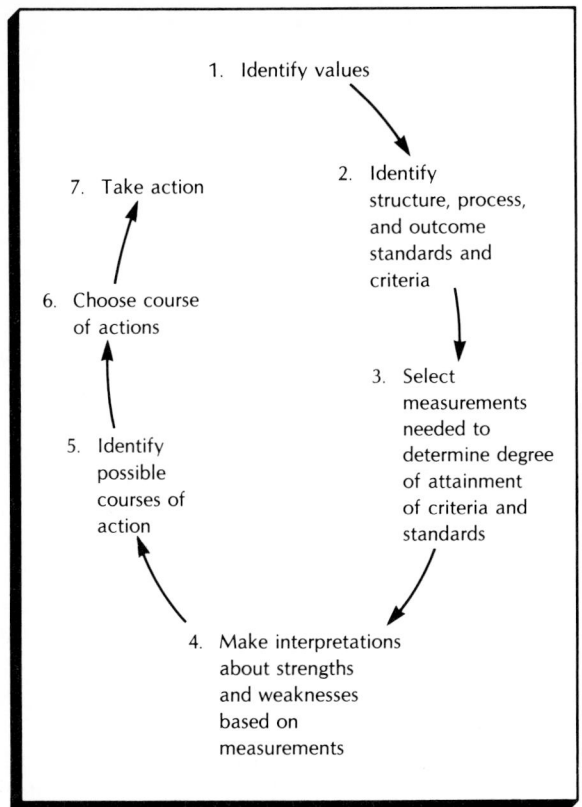

FIGURE 12-2

Model for quality assurance program. (From American Nurses' Association: Quality model: a plan for implementation of the standards of nursing practice, Kansas City, Mo., 1977, The Association. Reprinted with permission of ANA.)

Once objectives are formulated, the required *input resources* are identified to accomplish the objectives. Need for the input resources of manpower, supplies and equipment, facilities, and finances are described. If the required input resources are not available to implement the identified objectives, an organization is restricted in the delivery of a quality service to the consumer. In determining necessary program input, *community resources* and *consumer needs* and *wants* must be examined to plan realistic programs for a community. Consider an example in which the Public Health Department has surveyed the community and identified consumer interest in a new family planning program. The objectives for the program have been written and the nursing services office has been directed to open the clinic by the beginning of the new year. However, the director of nurses has been unable to employ enough nurses for the clinic to begin. Therefore the administration decides that without nurse power the clinic cannot deliver quality services, and the opening of the clinic is postponed until all input resources are available to meet the program objectives.

Once input resources are determined, then *policies, procedures,* and *job descriptions* are formulated to serve as behavioral guides to the employees of the agency. These documents should reflect the essential provider qualifications needed to implement the services of the agency.

Establishing organization objectives, identifying necessary input resources, and formulating policies, procedures, and job descriptions will lead to the development of standards, identification of efficient provider activity, delineation of program costs, and better use of resources.

Values Identification

Values identification, the first step in a quality assurance program, serves to define the beliefs of the agency about humanity, nursing, the community, and health. The development of an agency philosophy describes the nature and the scope of services to be provided by the agency; the clients to be served, such as the individual (across the age span), families, groups, and communities; the services to be offered; and the available resources to provide services. The philosophy will also describe the goals of health care services to be offered by the agency, such as primary, secondary, and tertiary prevention goals. Once the philosophy and objectives are written, Donabedian's framework for evaluating health care programs can be actively used.

Identification of Standards and Criteria

Identification of standards and criteria for quality assurance begins with the writing of the philosophy and objectives of the organization. The philosophy and objectives of an agency serve to define the *structural standards* of the agency. Evaluation of structure is a specific approach to quality appraisal. In evaluating the *structure* of an organization, the evaluator ascertains whether the agency is adhering to the stated philosophy and objectives. Is the agency providing services to populations across the age span? Are primary, secondary, and/or tertiary preventive services offered? Standards of structure are defined by the licensing or accrediting agency, such as the NLN standards for accrediting home health agencies (NLN, 1980). Another standard of structure includes the organizational chart, which shows supervisory methods, communication patterns, staffing patterns, and sometimes staff assignments. How assignments are made, the client mix, and staff qualifications are also standards of structure used to evaluate the quality of an agency. Several questions the evaluator can ask about the standards of structure are: Does the agency use the methods of supervision described in the policies and procedures? Do the nurses function within the scope of their job descriptions? Do staff members have the qualifications required by this agency? *Review of agency documents* (audit), *self-studies,* and *utilization review* are the techniques employed for evaluating agency structure.

Standards of structure are evaluated internally by a committee composed of administration, management, and staff members for the purpose of issuing a self-study report quarterly, annually, or before an accreditation visit by a state or a voluntary agency. Standards of structure are also evaluated by a group external to the agency. Utilization review committees are often composed of an external advisory group with community representatives for all services offered through an agency, such as a nurse, physical therapist, speech therapist, physician, board member, and administrator from a sister agency.

The evaluation of *process standards* is a more specific appraisal of the quality of care being given by agency providers. Criteria for evaluating the activities of all agency personnel need to be defined to make inferences about the quality of care received by the agency's clients. Agencies use a variety of methods to determine criteria for evaluating provider activities. An agency can choose to develop process standards around one of the conceptual models described in Chapter 7, such as a developmental model. An agency can choose to use the standards of care set forth by the providers' professional organization, such as the ANA community health nursing standards; or the agency can use the nursing process and apply it to the activities of the nurses as the activities correspond to the procedures of care defined by the agency.

The primary approaches used for process evaluation include the peer review committee and the client satisfaction survey. The techniques employed for process evaluation are direct observation, questionnaire, interview, written audit, and videotape of client and provider encounters.

Numerous *audit instruments* can be found in the nursing literature to evaluate the process of care. The instrument most often used in community health nursing is the Phaneuf Nursing Audit (Phaneuf, 1976). This 50-item instrument measures 7 functions of professional nursing as they relate to the nursing process. This instrument is an example of a retrospective audit instrument that presents a picture of the total nursing care received by the discharged client. The instrument has been found to have a measure of internal validity and reliability (Stanhope, 1981; Stanhope and Murdock, 1981). The major disadvantage of retrospective chart reviews is that they are not evaluations of care delivered, but rather of the quality of the documentation of that care, which may not correlate highly with the quality of the care (Maciorowski, et al., 1985; Openshaw, 1984).

Two valid and reliable tools that have often been used in conjunction with the Phaneuf Nursing Audit are the Slater Nursing Competencies Rating Scale and the Quality Patient Care Scale. The Slater Nursing Competencies Scale is an 84-item scale intended to rate nurses' performances in the clinical setting after direct observation of an identified number of nurse and client encounters. The nurse's performance is judged against criterion variables representative of a gamut of nursing responsibilities for providing client care (Wandelt and Stewart, 1975). The Quality Patient Care Scale (QUALPACS) is a 68-item scale intended to measure the quality of care received by a client either through direct nurse-client encounters or interventions with others on behalf of the client (Wandelt and Ager, 1975).

Other nursing audit instruments or methodologies that may be used or adapted to evaluate process are the Rush-Presbyterian-St. Luke's Medical Center-Medicus Methodology for Monitoring Quality Patient Care (Haussmann, et al., 1976; Haussmann and Hegyvary, 1977), the Professional Practitioner's Performance Rating Scale (Dunn, 1970), the CASH Nursing Care Evaluation Instrument (Smith, 1975), the Critical Incident Performance Appraisal System (Brief, 1979), the Professional Nurse Performance Evaluation Method (Bernhardt and Schuette, 1975), and the Standards of Nursing Care by Carter (1976).

The *client satisfaction survey* may also be used to evaluate the process of ongoing care as documented in the literature (Trussell and Strand, 1978). The survey may be conducted by direct interview or by questionnaire.

Once data are collected to evaluate nursing process standards, the peer review committee reviews the data to identify strengths and weaknesses in the quality of care delivered. The peer review committee is usually an internal committee composed of representatives of the nursing staff who are trained to administer audit instruments and conduct client interviews.

The *evaluation of outcome standards,* or the end results of nursing care, is one of the more difficult tasks facing nursing today. To be able to identify net changes in the client's health status as a result of nursing care will give the nursing profession data to show the contribution of nursing to the health care delivery system. Research studies using the tracer method or the sentinel method to identify client outcomes and client satisfaction surveys are approaches that may be used to evaluate outcome standards. Techniques that can be used to evaluate outcome standards are client classification systems that use admission data on the client's level of dependence or problems and discharge data that may show changes in levels of dependence (Daubert, 1977; Martin, 1982; Rosser and Watts, 1972), admission and discharge data, morbidity data, community agency readmission data, community agency referrals to hospitals, and client satisfaction surveys.

Horn and Swain (1977) developed an instrument that measures clients' health status in terms of outcomes of care influenced by nursing. Orem's theory of self-care was used to generate and test quality criteria. The most common measurement methods used are direct physical observations and interviews. The criteria measure nursing care and nursing problems that cut across disease entities and specific body systems and also reflect client health status parameters that nursing is expected to affect and for which nursing should be held accountable (Padella and Grant, 1982).

Rissner (1975) developed a client satisfaction survey to evaluate client attitudes and the content of nursing care in a primary care setting. Decker, et al. (1979) reported the development of criteria sets for evaluating outcome of community health nursing care, and Kline, et al. (1980) reported the development of a process and outcome evaluation program for community health nursing in the state of Georgia. However, community health nursing has been primarily involved in evaluating program outcomes to justify program expenditures rather than in evaluating client outcomes. Outcome evaluation assumes that health care has a net positive effect on client status. The major problem with outcome evaluation is determining which nursing care variables are primarily responsible for causing changes in client status. In community health nursing there are multiple uncontrolled variables in the field that have an effect on client status, such as environment and family relationships, and it is often difficult to determine whether these extraneous variables are the cause of changes in client status, or whether nursing interventions have the most effect.

More sophisticated studies are beginning to consider the interaction of process and outcome, structure and process, structure and outcome, and structure, process, and outcome. Descriptive and comparative studies that consider outcomes of patterns of care will be enhanced by applying decision-making models and conceptual frameworks (Lang and Clinton, 1984; Padella and Grant, 1982; Wright, 1984). Too often, quality assurance activities are fishing expeditions to catch problems after they occur.

Theories and models can be used as frameworks for development of standards and criteria; they direct the evaluation to what is important (Maciorowski, 1985; Wright, 1984).

Criteria and Standards Evaluative Measures

Selection of measures to determine the degree of attainment of criteria and standards has been discussed in the previous section. To summarize, the approaches and techniques used to evaluate structural standards and criteria are utilization reviews, review of agency documents, self-studies, and review of physical facilities. The approaches and techniques for the evaluation of process standards and criteria are peer review, client satisfaction surveys, direct observations, questionnaires, interviews, written audits, and videotapes. The evaluative approaches for outcome standards and criteria include research studies, client satisfaction surveys, client classification, admission, readmission, and discharge data, and morbidity data.

The approaches and techniques an agency uses in a quality assurance program often depend on the state or federal guidelines that must be followed to satisfy credentialing requirements. Regardless of the scope of the governmental requirements, a model quality assurance program should include measures for evaluating structure, process, and outcome standards and criteria. Inferences made about the quality of services delivered by an agency are dependent on evaluating all aspects of the health care agency. The box below summarizes quality assurance measures.

Health Provider Evaluation

Inherent in any quality assurance program should be the individual evaluation of health providers. Although the overall agency structure, the process of care delivered by health provider groups, and client outcome may be evaluated, it is also essential to determine the individual provider's contribution to the overall quality of the agency to protect the clients who are the recipients of the provider's care.

Past history of the evaluative process indicates that *personnel evaluation* has often been based on traditional trait ratings of personality and performance traits. Examples of trait rating measures are personal appearance, leadership, responsibility, accuracy, creativity, and ability to articulate. The problem with these measures is that they are not specific enough to measure concrete behavior and therefore are subject to broad interpretation by evaluators (Robbins, 1982).

The present trend in personnel evaluation is to use appraisals based on specific performance objectives. Porter (1974) describes three methods used to evaluate performance: single global ratings, behaviorally anchored ratings, and objectives-oriented ratings.

The *single global ratings* scale includes a number of behaviors that are all-inclusive of the performance expected of a nurse in community health. Supervisors rate nurses on all the behaviors and assign a total score or single rating for overall job performance. One aspect of the Phaneuf Nursing Audit is the provision of a single global rating of a nurse's delivery of nursing care. The global rating for the Phaneuf audit is obtained by adding the score obtained by the nurse on 50 identified behaviors. Based on the total points received, the nurse is then assigned a quality rating of excellent, good, average, poor, or unsafe.

This type of performance evaluation technique allows for comparison of a nurse with peers and offers a mechanism for effectively attaining agreement among separate supervisor ratings. However, global ratings do not relate directly to specific behaviors of the nurse and do not contribute to motivation for change, planning for staff development, or the development of better job descriptions. For the nurse with a low level of trust in the organization, this type of rating may lead to defensiveness and rejection of the evaluation. This rating scale is often used to make decisions about raises and promotions because of the ease with which supervisors can compare employees and because the rating is seemingly reflective of a number of behaviors included in a total scale.

Behaviorally anchored ratings are evaluative tools that include direct observation of a list of behaviors the nurse should perform in delivering quality care. An example of a behaviorally anchored rating in nursing is the Slater Nursing Competencies Scale. Such a scale allows the supervisor to rate the nurse on a list of behaviors that can be generalized to all nurses. This type of scale provides a better rating method than the single global ratings scale because certain

---

QUALITY ASSURANCE MEASURES

STRUCTURE	PROCESS	OUTCOME
Internal agency committees	Peer review committees	Internal agency
Self study	Prospective audit	Evaluative studies
Review agency documents	Concurrent audit	Survey health status change
	Retrospective audit	
External agency	Client	Client
Regulatory audit	Satisfaction survey	Satisfaction survey
Utilization review		Malpractice suits

nurse behaviors can be assessed. Development of better job descriptions could result from the assessment of nurse behaviors in a specific setting, such as community health. The behaviorally anchored rating scale, however, will not give nurses a rating based on behaviors specific to the individual and may not enhance motivation to develop objectives for future job improvement. This scale may provide data about behaviors that are performed well, performed poorly, or are missing. The data can be used as a basis for staff development programs to improve care delivered by the agency nurses.

The *objectives-oriented rating* tools are developed jointly between the supervisor and the nurse. These tools reflect agreement on specific performance objectives to be met by the nurse as well as on how these objectives are to be measured.

The development of objectives-oriented rating tools allows staff members to have input into their evaluation and also allows the supervisor to collect data specific to the individual about acceptable levels of performance and attainment of specific goals. This type of performance rating is said to be both more objective and explicit to the nurse, and it allows the supervisor to pinpoint specific accomplishments of individuals and allows these persons to say how they have met their goals (self-evaluation). When evaluation focuses on individual accomplishments, the nurse becomes less defensive and is more motivated to attain future goals because of the personal feedback given about job performance.

The objectives-oriented rating is not always the evaluative method of choice; it is difficult to compare groups of nurses because evaluative objectives and measures are specific to each individual. Determining pay raises and promotions based on merit becomes more difficult because it is possible for several persons to meet their objectives but to function at different performance levels.

Instances occur when different performance evaluation measures may be more appropriately used. The advantages and disadvantages of each method are outlined in Table 12-2. The objectives-oriented approach is the most costly to implement because of its individualized nature; the behaviorally anchored ratings are also costly because they require direct behavioral observations by supervisors; and the single global ratings are least costly because data can be collected from client records and do not require direct supervisor observations.

The behaviorally anchored and the objectives-oriented ratings are more useful in pinpointing behaviors specific to groups and individuals respectively and provide better performance ratings, better data for staff development, and better data for developing job descriptions. The behaviorally anchored and the single global ratings provide better comparative measures and are more useful for determining promotions and pay raises. The three behaviorally oriented evaluative approaches are preferable to the trait ratings because of the differences in subjectivity and specificity of the evaluation.

Interpreting Measurement Data

Interpreting measurement data is an essential component of the quality assurance process because it allows for the identification of discrepancies between the quality care standards of the agency and the actual practice of the health providers. Data interpretation allows for the identification of strengths in the implementation of the standards of care.

Once the approaches and techniques to be used in the quality assurance program are determined, the program must be organized and implemented so that patterns of health care delivery can be established for the agency. These patterns must reflect the total agency's functioning over time to generate valid data on which to base decisions about the strengths and limitations in meeting the agency's standards and criteria. The amounts of time and the effects of identifying substandard performance are factors to consider in the evaluation process. Problems with agency structure and client outcome may take a longer time to identify than

TABLE 12-2

Select advantages and disadvantages of health provider evaluation methods

Method	Advantages	Disadvantages
Trait ratings	Inexpensive Less time consuming	Permit subjective interpretation by evaluator Examine nonspecific behaviors
Single global ratings	Provide comparative measures for group Inexpensive Collect data from records Less time consuming	Unable to pinpoint behaviors specific to provider Nonmotivating Unable to pinpoint specific deficiencies Unable to use to develop job descriptions
Behaviorally anchored ratings	Collect data specific to group, such as nurses Give better overall performance rating Pinpoint deficiencies for staff development Provide comparative measures for groups Useful for evaluating merit	Expensive Require direct supervisor observation, therefore time consuming Ratings nonspecific to individual behavior
Objectives-oriented ratings	Pinpoint performance deficiencies Provide self-evaluation Collect data specific to evaluatee Motivate personnel	Expensive Time consuming Difficult to compare groups of providers Evaluation of merit difficult

process performance problems. In process evaluation the time spent may not be long enough when evaluating a process using concurrent audits or when using behaviorally anchored personnel evaluation ratings. The nurse may say that these ratings do not accurately reflect total performance in providing client care and may ignore the evaluation as irrelevant to actual performance. However, if all performance decisions are based on retrospective audit data, the interval between appraisals may be too long and the nurse may ignore the evaluation as irrelevant to present practice performance. Some combination of ongoing and retrospective evaluation is essential to make process evaluation meaningful.

Regular intervals for evaluation should be established within the agency and periodic reports written so the combined results of structure, process, and outcome efforts can be analyzed and health care delivery patterns and problems can be identified. These reports should be used to establish an ongoing picture of changes occurring within the agency and justify community nursing services (Flynn and Ray, 1979).

Action Identification

Identification and choices of possible courses of action to correct the weaknesses within the agency should involve both the administration and the staff. The courses of action chosen should be based on their significance, economic benefit, and timeliness. For example, if there is a nursing problem dealing with the recording of client health education, the agency administration and staff may analyze the problem to see why it is occurring. If the reasons given by the nurses include lack of time to do paperwork properly, case overloads that reduce the amount of time spent with clients, or lack of available resources for health education, it would not be significant to choose to provide a staff development program on the importance of doing and recording health education. It would be more important to assess how to provide the time and resources necessary for the nurses to offer health education to clients. Economically it may be more beneficial to provide dictating equipment and clerical assistance so nurses can dictate notes and other paperwork, thereby providing more client contact time, or it may be economically more beneficial to employ an additional nurse and reduce nurse caseloads.

The timeliness of the courses of action identified and chosen is also critical. If the recording problem has been a recurrent one and has not been shared with the staff, and if administration decides to make unilateral decisions to reduce caseloads or introduce dictating equipment, the decisions may be viewed by the staff as negative and may result in reduced motivation and poorer job performance. However, when time is allowed for staff members to give input into decisions that directly affect their work, they will tend to be more committed to the decisions and more motivated to improve the standards of health care delivery.

Taking Action

Taking action is the final step in the quality assurance model. Once the alternative courses of action are chosen, actions must be implemented for change to occur in the overall operation of the agency. Follow-up and evaluation of actions taken must occur for improvement in quality of care to be assumed. Documentation is essential to the evaluation of quality care in any organization. The following section focuses on the kind of documentation that normally occurs in a community health agency.

RECORDS
Purposes of Records

Records are an integral part of the communication structure of the health care organization. Accurate and complete records are required by law and must be kept by all agencies, governmental and nongovernmental. In most states, the state departments of health stipulate the kind and content requirements of records for community health agencies.

Records provide complete information about the client, indicate the extent and quality of services being rendered, resolve legal issues in malpractice suits, and provide information for education and research.

Community Health Agency Records

Within the community health agency many types of records are kept and used to predict population trends in a community, identify health needs and problems, analyze health trends, plan and evaluate programs, prepare and justify budgets, and make administrative decisions. The kinds of records kept by the community health agency may include *reports* of accidents, births, census, chronic disease, communicable disease, mortality, life expectancy, and morbidity, reports of child and spouse abuse, reports of occupational illness and injury, and reports of environmental health.

Other types of records kept within the agency are *records* used to maintain administrative contact and control of the units (departments) of the organization. Three types of records make up this category: clinical, service, and financial. The *clinical record* is the client health record, or chart, used by all health care providers for the purpose of communicating observations, interventions, and prescribed regimens for client care. The clinical record consists of two major content sections: the client's history, including such information as client demography, admission data, primary provider's name, chief health problem, and financial information; and the clinical history, which includes diagnosis, progress notes, physical examination and health assessment, past history of health or illness problems, consultations and referrals, flow charts of medications, diagnostic studies and vital signs, and discharge summaries (Warren, 1978).

The *provider service records* include information about the numbers of home visits made daily, transportation and mileage, the provider's time spent with the client, and the amount and kinds of supplies used. The service record is completed on a daily basis by each provider, summarized weekly for a record of individual personnel service and payment, and summarized monthly and annually to indicate trends in health care activities and costs relative to personnel time, transportation, maintenance, and supplies. The provider service records are used to correlate with the agency's *financial records* of salaries, overhead, and transportation costs and serve as the basis for the cost accounting system (Hanlon and Pickett, 1979).

Three additional kinds of service records seen in the community health agency are the *central index system,* the *annual implementation plan,* and the *annual summary* of agency activities. The *central index system* is a data filing system that indicates the services requested, services offered, active and inactive clients of the agency, and a profile of the agency's clients. The central index system may be subdivided into a computer file for ready retrieval of the data, and the actual chart files that are centrally located in a records office (library) for easy retrieval by health providers. The central index file serves to organize the ongoing activities of the agency and to summarize the history of the agency's services.

The *annual implementation plan* is developed at the beginning of each fiscal year to set forth the short-term and long-term goals of the agency. The plan includes annual program objectives based on community health problems, methodology for meeting the objectives, the process to be used for evaluating the objectives, and the annual projected budgetary, personnel, and facility requirements. The annual implementation plan usually reflects the plans for the total agency and for each unit of the agency.

The annual implementation plan serves as the basis for the agency's *annual summary.* The annual report reflects the success of the agency in meeting the annual objectives, changes in population trends and health status during the year, the actual versus the projected budgetary requirements, the number of services offered, the number of clients served, and the plans and changes recommended for the future. The annual report, like other service records, is often required by funding agencies and state departments of health. The report is used to justify the continued existence of an agency, the budgetary requirements, the relationship of the agency to the community, and requests for funding from governmental and charitable organizations.

As an outgrowth of quality assurance efforts in the health care system, comprehensive methods are being designed to document and measure client progress and client outcome from agency admission through discharge. An example of such a method is the client classification system developed at the Visiting Nurses Association of Omaha, Nebraska (Martin, 1982). This comprehensive method of evaluating client care has several components: a classification system for assessing and categorizing client problems; a data base; a nursing problem list; and anticipated outcome criteria for the classified problems. Such schemes are viewed as having the potential to improve the delivery of nursing care, documentation, and the descriptions of client care. Briefly, implementation of comprehensive documentation methods will enhance nursing assessment, planning, and implementation and evaluation of client care, and will allow for the organization of pertinent client information for more effective and efficient nurse productivity and communication.

CLINICAL APPLICATION

The community health nurse is a member of the health care team designated to monitor the quality of service provided to the clients and community of the health care agency. As a member of this committee the practicing nurse and the student are interested in identifying the system used to monitor quality.

Major influences on the quality control system are state and federal regulations, which often dictate elements to be included in the system. Before planning or implementing a quality assurance program the nurse will read the regulations to identify those elements.

If the quality assurance program is functional when the nurse joins the team, a review of the program is essential for understanding the structure, process, and outcome components (see box on p. 243). When looking at the structural elements the nurse or student is interested in the relationship between the philosophy and objectives of the agency. Does the philosophy reflect beliefs about the clients to be served by the agency, the type of nursing care and services to be delivered, the population or the community to be served, and, finally, beliefs about health care versus illness care? Are the objectives of the agency reflective of the stated beliefs in the philosophy? For example, does the philosophy indicate beliefs about client education or research? If so, are there agency objectives that address providing health education or enhancing research related to better client care?

Once it has been established from the philosophy and objectives that the agency's goal is to deliver primary health care services to the total population of the community, the nurse is interested in the standards of care used to deliver quality health care. In nursing, are the ANA standards for Community Health Nursing used to evaluate nursing care given? Are the nurses employed by the agency qualified to fulfill their job description through education, experience, or both?

What are the employment criteria of the agency? Do the criteria reflect the beliefs of the agency about nursing and the agency goals? Do the agency's policies and procedures assist the nurse in meeting the stated standards of care?

Given the structure of the agency, how is the process of care evaluated? Does the agency employ prospective, concurrent, or retrospective audits to evaluate the process of care given? Are the audits designed to measure the standards of care used by the agency? How is the data used after it is collected? Is there any evidence that the evaluation makes a difference? Has the process of care changed as a result of the evaluation?

After the structure and process elements are identified, the nurse and student are interested in outcome elements. How is health outcome defined by the agency—client satisfaction, change in health status, number of malpractice suits, or number of Medicare payment denials? How is the data used to make a difference in future quality outcomes?

The nurse and student as contributors to the health care of clients are key ingredients in quality control within the agency. Client care documentation in the records, supervisor observation of care delivered, educational and experiential qualifications brought to the job, the expressed satisfaction of clients, and the client who is able to provide self-care as a result of health teaching all reflect the nurse's and student's contribution to quality health care delivery.

SUMMARY

Quality assurance programs in health care delivery are the mechanisms for maintaining control over the system and for requesting accountability from the individual providers within the system. A quality assurance program consists of varying general and specific approaches and techniques used for the purpose of evaluating the structure, process, and outcomes of client care. The ANA has put forth a model quality assurance program that reflects the components of the nursing process in the evaluation of client care activities.

Records kept by community health agencies are instrumental in identifying elements of health care delivery that establish a total picture of the contribution of the agency to the client community.

The beneficiaries of quality assurance programs are (1) the recipients of care, who receive safe, effective, satisfying service; (2) the providers of care, because evaluation offers opportunity to promote personal and professional growth; (3) the agencies, which obtain data for planning, cost-containment, and legal protection; and (4) the profession, because quality assurance programs promote development of standards and protocols and the generation of new knowledge (Bergman, 1982).

KEY CONCEPTS

The health care delivery system is the largest employing industry in the United States; society is demanding increased efficiency and effectiveness from the system. Quality control is the tool used to ensure that effectiveness and efficiency.

Objective and systematic evaluation of nursing care has become a priority within the profession for several reasons, including the effects of cost on health care accessibility, consumer demands for better quality care, and increasing involvement of nurses in public and health agency policy formulation.

Quality assurance is the monitoring of the activities of client care to determine the degree of excellence attained in implementation of the activities.

Quality assurance has been a concern of the profession since Florence Nightingale in the 1860s called for a uniform format for gathering and disseminating hospital statistics.

Licensure has been a major issue in nursing since 1892.

Two major categories of approaches exist in quality assurance today—general and specific approaches.

Accreditation is an approach to quality control used for institutions, whereas licensure is primarily used for individuals.

Certification combines features of both licensing and accreditation.

Three major models have been used to evaluate quality: Donabedian's structure-process-outcome model, the sentinel model, and the tracer model.

Seven basic components of a quality assurance program are (1) identifying values; (2) identifying structure, process, and outcome standards and criteria; (3) selecting measurement techniques; (4) interpreting the strengths and weaknesses of the care given; (5) identifying alternative courses of action; (6) choosing specific courses of action; and (7) taking action.

An instrument often used in community health nursing is the Phaneuf Nursing Audit.

Records are an integral part of the communication structure of a health care organization. Accurate and complete records are by law required of all agencies, whether governmental or nongovernmental.

Quality assurance mechanisms in health care delivery are the mechanisms for controlling the system and requesting accountability from individual providers within the system. Records help establish a total picture of the contribution of the agency to the client community.

LEARNING ACTIVITIES

1. Write your own definition of quality assurance; compare your definition with the one given in the text. Are they the same or different? Give justification for your answer.

2. List the goals of quality assurance.

3. Interview a nurse who is a coordinator of (or responsible for) quality assurance in a local health agency. Ask the following questions and add others you may wish to have answered.
   a. What is quality assurance?
   b. What are the goals the organization hopes to attain by having a quality assurance program?
   c. How are records used for quality assurance?
   d. Describe the components of the quality assurance program.
   e. Discuss the approaches and techniques that are used to implement the quality assurance program.
   f. How has the quality assurance program changed in the health agency over the past 20 years?
   g. What influence has the quality assurance program had on provider accountability?

4. List and describe the types of records usually kept in a community health agency. Explain the purpose of each type of record.

BIBLIOGRAPHY

Abdellah, F., et al.: Patient centered approaches to nursing. New York, 1960, MacMillan Publishing Co.

Ager, J.: Testing the quality patient care scale. In Wandelt, M., and Ager, J.W., editors: Quality patient care scale, New York, 1974, Appleton-Century-Crofts.

American Nurses' Association Committee for the Study of Credentialing in Nursing: The study of credentialing in nursing: a new approach, vols. 1 and 2, Kansas City, Mo., 1979, The Association.

American Nurses' Association: Quality model: a plan for implementation of the standards of nursing practice, Kansas City, Mo., 1977, The Association.

American Nurses' Association: A conceptual model of community health nursing, Kansas City, Mo., 1982, The Association.

American Nurses' Association: Take the extra step . . . become a certified nurse, Kansas City, Mo., 1985, The Association.

American Nurses' Association Congress on Nursing Practice: Standards of nursing practice, Kansas City, Mo., 1973, The Association.

American Nurses' Association: The measure of distinction among professionals, Kansas City, Mo., 1985, The Association.

American Nurses' Association: Facts about nursing, Kansas City, 1985, The Association.

American Public Health Association: The definition and role of public health nursing in the delivery of health care, Washington, D.C., 1980, The Association.

Bergmen, R.: Accountability—definition and dimension, Keynote address at Second National Conference of Israeli Nurses, Tel Aviv, Oct. 1, 1980.

Bergman, R.: Evaluation of nursing care—could it make a difference? Int. J. Nurs. Stud. 19(2)53, 1982.

Bernhardt, I., and Schuette, L.: P.E.T.: a method of evaluating professional nurse performance, J. Nurs. Adm. 5:18, Oct. 1975.

Blake, B.: Quality assurance: an ethical responsibility, Supervisor Nurse, 12:32, Feb. 1981.

Brief, A.: Developing a usable performance appraisal system, J. Nurs. Adm. 9(10):7, Oct. 1979.

Brook, R., and Appel, F.: Quality of care assessment: choosing a method for peer review, N. Engl. J. Med. 288:1323, 1973.

Brook, R.H., Davies, A.R., and Kamberg, C.J.: Selected reflections on quality of medical care evaluation in the 1980s, Nurs. Res. 29(2):127, March-April 1980.

Bull, M.J.: Quality assurance: its origins, transformations, and prospects. In Meisenheimer, C.G., editor: Quality assurance: a complete guide to effective programs, Rockville, Md., 1985, Aspen Publishers, Inc.

Bullough, B.: The first two phases in nursing licensure. In Bullough, B., editor: The law and the expanding nursing role, New York, 1980, Appleton-Century-Crofts.

Carter, J.: Standards of nursing care, New York, 1976, Springer Publishing Co., Inc.

Council of Home Health Agencies and Community Health Services: Accreditation of homes health agencies and community nursing services: criteria and guide for preparing reports, New York, National League for Nursing.

Council of Home Health Agencies and Community Health Services: Administrator's handbook for the structure, operation and expansion of home health agencies, New York, 1985, National League for Nursing.

Daubert, E.: A system to evaluate home health care services, Nurs. Outlook 25(3):168, March 1977.

Decker, F., et al.: Using patient outcomes to evaluate community health nursing, Nurs. Outlook 27(4):278, April 1979.

Decker, C.M.: Quality assurance: accent on monitoring, Nurs. Manag. 16:20, Nov. 1985.

Donabedian, A.: The criteria and standards of quality, vol. 2, Explorations in quality assessment and monitoring. Ann Arbor, Mich., 1982, Health Administration Press.

Dunn, M.: Development of an instrument to measure nursing performance, Nurs. Res. 19: 502, Nov.-Dec. 1970.

Fagin, C.M.: Nursing as an alternative to high cost care. AJN 82:56, 1982.

Flynn, B.C., and Ray, D.W.: Quality assurance in community health nursing, Nurs. Outlook 27:650, Oct. 1979.

Gremaldi, P.L., and Micheletti, J.A.: PRO objectives and quality criteria, Hospitals 59:64, Feb. 1985.

Hanlon, J., and Pickett, G.: Public health administration and practice, St. Louis, 1984, The C.V. Mosby Co.

Haussmann, R.K.D., Hegyvary, S.T.: Monitoring quality of nursing care: part III, Hyattsville, Md., 1977, USDHEW, PHS, HRA, BH Manpower, Division of Nursing.

Haussmann, R.K.D., Hegyvary, S.T., and Newman, J.F.: Monitoring quality of nursing care: part II, Bethesda, Md., 1976, USDHEW, USPHS, HRA, B of HM, Division of Nursing.

Hawkin, P.L.: Accreditation: one measure of quality, Nurs. Educ. 24:20, 1984.

Health Care Financing Administration: HCF research report: P.S.R.O. program evaluation, Washington, D.C., 1979.

Hinsvark, I.: Credentialing in nursing. In McCloskey, J., and Grace, H., editors: Current issues in nursing, Oxford, England, 1985, Blackwell Scientific Publications, Inc.

Hohman, J.: Focus on nurse credentialing, Chicago, 1980, American Hospital Association.

Horn, B.J., and Swain, M.A.: Development of criterion measures of nursing care, vols. 1 and 2, Final report to the National Center for Health Services Research for HS D1649, Springfield, Va., 1977, National Technical Information Service.

Hull, R.T.: Responsibility and accountability, analyzed, Nurs. Outlook 29:707, 1981.

Jacobs, A., et al.: Critical requirements for safe/effective nursing practice, Kansas City, Mo., 1978, Pub. No. 651, ANA Council of State Boards of Nursing.

Jelinek, A., et al.: A methodology for monitoring quality of nursing care, DHEW Pub.

No. (HRA) 74-25, Bethesda, Md., 1974, Health Resources Administration.

Jonas, S.: Measurement and control of the quality of health care. In Jonas, S., editor: Health care delivery in the United States, New York, 1986, Springer Publishing Co., Inc.

Jones, F.: Certification for specialization. In McCloskey, J., and Grace, H., editors: Current issues in nursing, Boston, 1985, Blackwell Scientific Publications, Inc.

Kessner, D.M., and Kalk, C.E.: Assessing health quality—the case for tracers, N. Engl. J. Med. 288:189, 1973.

Kissinger, C.: Community nursing administration: Quantifying nursing utilization, J. Nurs. Adm. 3:43, Sept.-Oct. 1973.

Kline, M.: Quality assurance in public health, Nurs. Health Care 1(4):192, Nov. 1980.

Krumme, U.: The case for criterion-referenced measurement, Nurs. Outlook 23(12):764, Dec. 1975.

Lang, N.M., and Clinton, J.F.: Assessment of quality of nursing care, vol. 2, Annual review of nursing research, New York, 1984, Springer-Verlag New York, Inc.

Lieski, A.M.: Standards: the basis of a quality assurance program. In Meisenheimer, C.G., editor: Quality assurance: a complete guide to effective programs, Rockville, Md., 1985, Aspen Publishers, Inc.

Lindeman, C.: Measuring quality of nursing care, Part I, J. Nurs. Adm. 6:7, June 1976.

Lindeman, C.: Measuring quality of nursing care, Part II, J. Nurs. Adm. 6:16, Sept. 1976.

LoGerfo, J., and Brook, R.: Evaluation of health services and quality of care. In Williams, S., and Torrens, P., editors: Introduction to health services, New York, 1984, John Wiley & Sons, Inc.

Maciorowski, L.F., Larson, E., and Keane, A.: Quality assurance: evaluate thyself, J. Nurs. Adm. 15:38, June 1985.

Maibusch, R.M.: Evolution of quality assurance for nursing in hospitals. In Schrolder, P.S., and Maibusch, R.M., editors: Nursing quality assurance, Rockville, Md., 1984, Aspen Publishers, Inc.

Martin, K.: A client classification system adaptable for computerization, Nurs. Outlook 30: 515, Nov.-Dec. 1982.

McCloskey, J.: ANA's nursing accreditation. To what end? In McCloskey, J., and Grace, H., editors: Current issues in nursing, Oxford, England, 1985, Blackwell Scientific Publications, Inc.

McCloskey, J.: The state board test pool exam: entrance to professional nursing. In McCloskey, J., and Grace, H., editors: Current issues in nursing, Boston, 1985, Blackwell Scientific Publications, Inc.

Mullins, A.C., Colavecchio, R.E., and Tescher, B.E.: Peer review: a model for professional accountability, J. Nurs. Adm. 9(12):25, Dec. 1979.

National League for Nursing: Historical perspective of NLN's participation in the ANA credentialing study, NLN accreditation update, Report No. 1, New York, Oct. 1979, The League.

National League for Nursing: Criteria and standards manual of NLN/APHA accreditation of home health agencies and community nursing services, New York, 1982, The League.

Office of Professional Standards Review: PSRO Program Manual, Washington, D.C., 1974, Department of Health, Education, and Welfare.

Openshaw, S.: Literature review: measurement of adequate care, Int. J. Nurs. Stud. 21:295, 1984.

Osterweis, M., and Bryant, E.: Assessing technical performance at diverse ambulatory care sites, J. Community Health 4(2):104, 1978.

Padella, G.V., and Grant, M.M.: Quality assurance programme for nursing, J. Adv. Nurs. 7:135, 1982.

Phaneuf, M.: A nursing audit method, Nurs. Outlook 5:42-45, 1965.

Phaneuf, M.: The nursing audit: profile for excellence, New York, 1976, Appleton-Century-Crofts.

Phaneuf, M.C., and Wandelt, M.A.: Quality assurance in nursing, Nurs. Forum 13(4):329, 1974.

Pinkerton, S.: Legislative issues in licensure of registered nurses. In McCloskey, J., and Grace, H., editors: Current issues in nursing, Oxford, England, 1985, Blackwell Scientific Publications, Inc.

Porter, L., Lawler, E., and Hackman, J.: Evaluating work effectiveness. In Bass, E., editor: Organizational practices and social processes, New York, 1974, McGraw-Hill Book Co. (Originally published in 1957.)

Porter-O'Grady, T.: Credentialing, privileging, and nursing bylaws: assuring accountability, J. Nurs. Adm. 15(12):23, 1985.

Public Law 97-248, Tax Equity and Fiscal Responsibility Act of 1982.

Rissner, N.: Development of an instrument to measure patient satisfaction with nurses and nursing care in primary care settings, Nurs. Res. 24(1):45, Jan.-Feb. 1975.

Robbins, S.P.: Personnel: the management of human resources, Englewood Cliffs, N.J., 1982, Prentice Hall, Inc.

Rosser, R., and Watts, V.: The measurement of hospital output, Int. J. Epidemiol. 1(4):361-368, 1972.

Rutstein, D.D., et al.: Measuring the quality of medical care: a clinical method, N. Engl. J. Med. 294(11):528, 1976.

Sibley, J., et al.: Quality-of-care appraisal in primary care: a quantitative method, Ann. Int. Med. 83:46-52, 1975.

Smith, R.L.: Internal properties of the C.A.S.H. nursing care evaluation instrument, Health Serv. Res. 10(2):136, 1975.

Stanhope, M.: A concurrent and retrospective evaluation of the effects of intrinsic and extrinsic motivating factors on nurse performance in home health care setting, unpublished doctoral dissertation, Birmingham, March 1981, University of Alabama.

Stanhope, M., and Murdock, M.: A psychometric measure of the Phaneuf Nursing Audit, Paper presented at the American Public Health Association Annual Meeting, Los Angeles, Nov. 1981.

Stevens, B.: The nurse as executive, 1985, Contemporary Publishing.

Trussell, P., and Strand, N.: A comparison of concurrent and retrospective audits on the same patients, J. Nurs. Adm. 8:33, May 1978.

USPHS: Essentials of public health nursing practice and education consensus conference, 1984, 1985.

Wagner, D., and Cosgrove, D.: Quality assurance: a professional responsibility, Caring 5(1):46, 1986.

Wandelt, M., and Ager, J.: Quality patient care scale, New York, 1975, Appleton-Century-Crofts.

Wandelt, M., and Stewart, D.: Slater nursing competencies rating scale, New York, 1975, Appleton-Century-Crofts.

Warren, D.: Problems in hospital law, Germantown, Md., 1978, Aspen Systems Corp.

Weed, L.: Medical records, medical education and patient care, Chicago, 1970, Year Book Medical Publishers, Inc.

Werner, J.: PSROs and hospital accreditation. In McCloskey, J., and Grace, H., Current issues in nursing, Oxford, England, 1984, Blackwell Scientific Publications, Inc.

Williamson, J.: Information management in quality assurance, Nurs. Res. 29(2):78, March-April 1980.

Wright, D.: An introduction to the evaluation of nursing care: a review of the literature, J. Adv. Nurs. 9:457, 1984.

Young, K.E.: National trends affecting credentials. In credentialing in nursing—design for a workshop. New York, 1980, National League for Nursing.

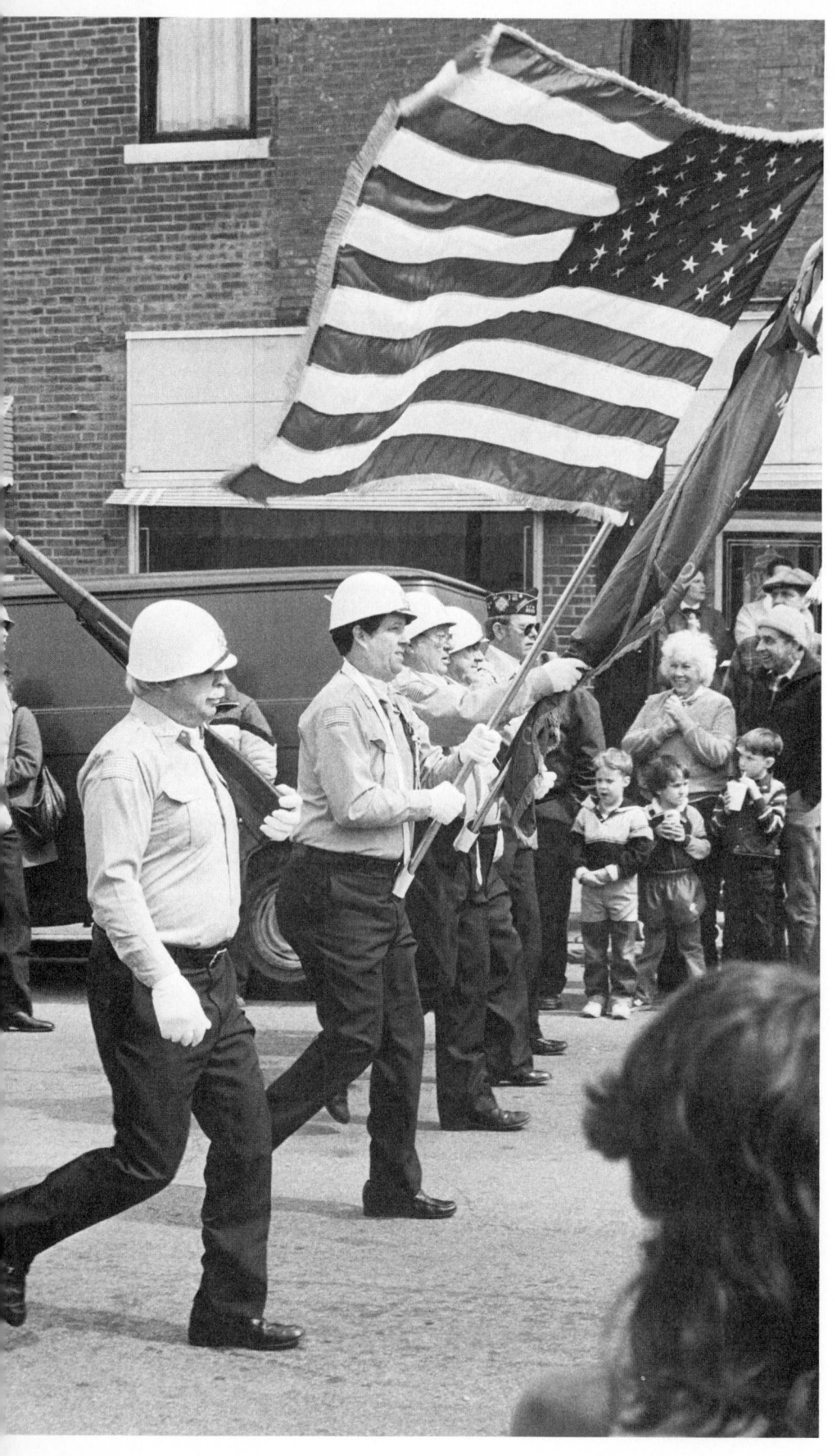

PART THREE

THE COMMUNITY AS CLIENT

The primary orientation of health care delivery through the decades has been one of care and cure of the individual. Today there is increasing evidence that life style and personal health habits influence the health of individuals, families, groups, and communities.

Although it is necessary to identify health-risk factors among individuals and groups in the community, it is of paramount importance that community health nurses learn to identify and work with health problems of the total community. A healthier community life-style and quality of life for the residents can be promoted in this way. Chapter 13 provides conceptual clarity and guidelines for nursing practice with the client community.

The community health nurse may work with the individual and family to promote health behaviors. However, the nurse may find that strategies to introduce health behaviors directed at illness prevention and life-style changes lend themselves to working with groups in the community. Chapter 14 discusses basic group concepts that can be used for promoting health behaviors through groups, identifying community groups and their contributions to community life, and assisting groups to work toward community health goals.

Concern currently exists about a return to environmental and social conditions that may lead to more infectious disease by the year 2000. Community health nurses must be concerned with prevention, control, case finding, reporting, and maintenance strategies as they relate to communicable and infectious processes and environmentally related problems. Technological advances are increasingly influencing the environment and making it a potential threat to many aspects of health maintenance.

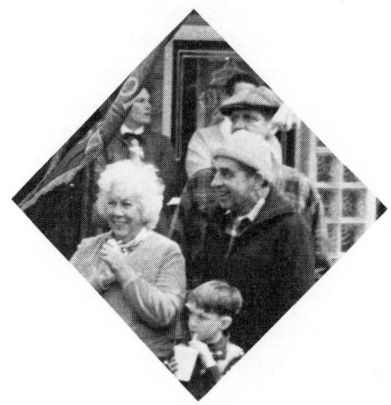

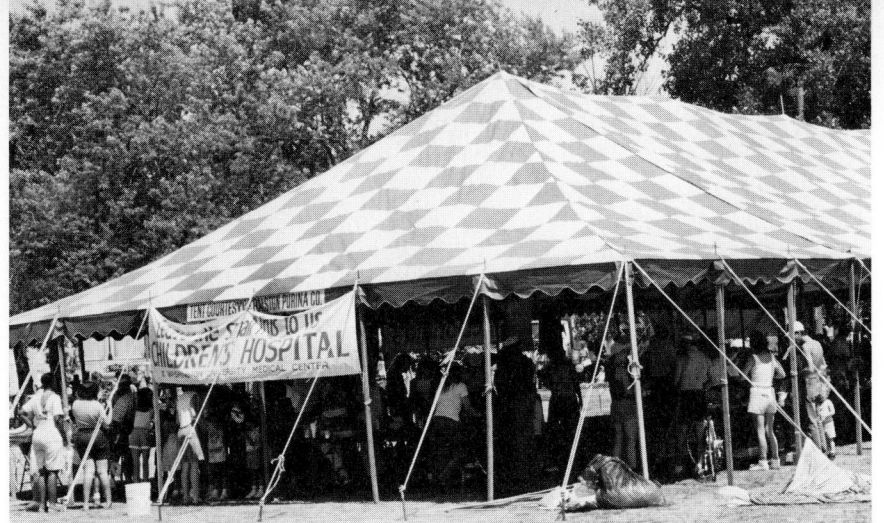

Jean Goeppinger
George F. Schuster III

13

COMMUNITY AS CLIENT: USING THE NURSING PROCESS TO PROMOTE HEALTH

☰ OBJECTIVES

After reading this chapter, the student should be able to:

Decide whether nursing practice is community oriented.

Illustrate selected concepts basic to community-oriented nursing practice—community, community client, community health, and partnership for health.

Understand the relevance of the nursing process to community-oriented nursing practice.

Decide which methods of assessment, intervention, and evaluation are most appropriate in selected situations.

Develop a community-oriented nursing care plan.

☰ KEY TERMS

aggregates

community

community health

community health problem

community health strength

community-oriented practice

confidentiality

data collection

data generation

early adopters

evaluation

goal

health policy

implementation

informant interviews

interacting group

intervention activities

lay advisors

mass media

mediating structures

objective

participant observation

partnership

practice setting

probability

problem analysis

problem prioritization

Program Planning Model

role negotiation

secondary analysis

survey

target of service

triangulation

typology

unit of service

value

windshield surveys

Although nurses have traditionally considered the community as one of their clients, many community health nurses view the community as their most important client. The concept of the community client, however, has never been adequately defined. The development and use of community nursing diagnoses, for example, have been minimal (Hamilton, 1985; Storfjell and Cruise, 1984). As a result, nursing practice deliberately directed to the community has been neglected. The effects of community-oriented nursing practice, to the limited extent they have been documented, have been disappointing. This chapter provides both conceptual clarity and guidelines for nursing practice with the community client, emphasizing the use of the nursing process to promote community health.

COMMUNITY DEFINED

The concept of community has a number of different meanings. Some authors define community very simply. Hanchett (1979, p. 7) defines it as "people in relationship with others." Others define it more elaborately. The Expert Committee Report on community health nursing of the World Health Organization (1974, p. 7) includes this definition: "A *community* is a social group determined by geographic boundaries and/or common values and interests. Its members know and interact with one another. It functions within a particular social structure and exhibits and creates norms, values and social institutions."

Still other theorists and writers present *typologies* rather than single definitions. Turner (1982) describes typologies, or classification strategies, as efforts to organize concepts systematically around formally stated dimensions in which each phenomenon has a place and is a part of a larger "configuration of phenomena."

One such typology of community is particularly well known by community-oriented practitioners. Blum, a health planner, describes types of communities in a typology published in the 1974 edition of his classic text, *Planning for Health*. They are listed at right (see box) and include communities defined by geopolitical, interactional, and problem-solving dimensions. Several other authors (Hanchett, 1979; Shamansky and Pesznecker, 1981; Wellman and Leighton, 1979) have identified and analyzed the common dimensions found among the various definitions and typologies of community.

Wellman and Leighton (1979, p. 365) note that most definitions of community include three dimensions: 1. networks of interpersonal relationships that provide friendship and support to members; 2. residence in a common locality; and 3. "solidarity, sentiments and activities." Hanchett (1979) includes people, place, resources and services, and relationships among the people of the community. Shamansky and Pesznecker (1981) phrase the dimensions, or elements, of community as interrogative pronouns: who, where and when, and how and why. *Who* refers to the people or residents of a community, *where* and *when* to the spatial and time dimensions, and *how* and *why* to the functional dimension.

However, conceptual difficulties with the definition of community are present despite these readily identifiable dimensions of people, place, and function. At least three problems exist. First, the people and function dimensions are often included in definitions of both community and community health; consequently, definitions may overlap. Second, the frequent lack of clear-cut geographical or political boundaries has raised arguments about whether the community has retained a place dimension (Hunter, 1975; Luloff and Wilkinson, 1977; Suttles, 1972). Third, the recent funding shifts to categorical aid programs and block grants raise questions about the continued relevance of the locality-based community. Given these problems, community-oriented nurses need to examine regularly how the

---

THE TYPES OF COMMUNITIES

Face to face community
Neighborhood
Community of identifiable need
Community of problem ecology
Community of concern
Community of special interest
Community of viability
Community of action capability
Community of political jurisdiction
Resource community
Community of solution

From Blum, H.L.: Planning for health, New York, 1974, Human Sciences Press, Inc.

personal, structural, and functional dimensions of community shape their nursing practice. As a general guide, we have found it helpful to define the *community* as a locality-based entity, composed of systems of formal organizations reflecting societal institutions, informal groups, and aggregates that are interdependent and whose function or expressed intent is to meet a wide variety of collective needs (Goeppinger, Lassiter, and Wilcox, 1982). This definition includes the personal, structural, and functional dimensions and recognizes interdependence, or interaction, among the systems within a community. Whenever the term *community* is used throughout this chapter it refers to this interpretation.

THE COMMUNITY AS CLIENT

As discussed in Chapters 1 and 15, the uniqueness of community health nursing has customarily been attributed to its *practice setting.* The idea of health-related care being provided within the community is not new. Indeed, at the turn of the century most city residents in the United States preferred to stay at home during illnesses; consequently, the practice environment for community health nurses was the home rather than the hospital.

As the range of community nursing expanded, many different kinds of agencies were established, and their services often overlapped one another. For instance, both privately established voluntary agencies and official local health agencies fought to control tuberculosis. Regardless of whether the nurses were from voluntary or official health agencies, they practiced in clients' natural environments, their homes, and not in the hospital. Early community health nursing textbooks included lengthy descriptions of the home environment and tools for assessing the extent to which that environment promoted the health of family members. Health education about the domestic environment was frequently a major part of home nursing care.

By the 1930s, visiting nurse associations, health departments, schools, industries, and neighborhood health centers, as well as homes, had all become areas of practice for community nurses. Many of the new community nurses did not consider the environments in which they practiced. Although their practices took place within the community, they focused on the individual patient or family seeking care. The care provided was not community oriented, rather, it was oriented towards the individual or family who happened to live in the community. In other words, because nursing practice located in the community focused only on individuals and family members who were not community residents, the practice was not directed towards the community client. This commitment to direct "hands-on" clinical nursing care delivered to individuals or families in community settings has been and remains a more popular conception of community nursing practice than the idea of the whole community as the target of nursing practice.

Our contention is that a community practice setting is insufficient reason for saying practice is oriented towards the community client. When the location of the practice is in the community but the focus of the practice is the individual or family, then the nursing client remains the individual or family—not the whole community.

Thus the community is considered the client, or *target of service,* when nursing practice, regardless of the geographic setting or unit of service, is community oriented. Community-oriented practice seeks healthful change for the whole community's benefit. The focus is on the collective or common good instead of individual health. The *units of service* may be individuals, families or other *interacting groups, aggregates,* institutions, and communities. Although change may be sought in these various units, change is intended to affect the whole community, including all units of service—not just the individual, family, or specific aggregate. For example, a visiting nurse's target might be an entire work force rather than the single disabled worker in her caseload. In this instance the nurse would provide direct clinical care with the dual goals of returning the worker to his or her job and maintaining a productive work force. The nurse would not only help the individual achieve independence in activities of daily living, but also would become involved with promoting vocational rehabilitation and seeking reasonable employment policies for all disabled workers.

Community Client and Nursing Practice

The community client thus defined is relevant to nursing practice for several reasons. This concept of community client makes direct clinical care an aspect of community health practice. For instance, direct nursing care can be offered to individuals and family members because their health needs represent common community-related problems rather than problems that are unique to their situations. Therefore changes in their health will affect the health of their communities. In such cases, decisions are made at the individual level because of their effect on community health; that is, they affect improved health of the community, which is the overall goal of the nursing intervention. For instance, community health nursing intervention to stop abuse of the elderly and battering of women are two instances where nursing interventions would be undertaken primarily because of the social, not the individual, effects of abuse.

The concept of community client also highlights the complexity of the change process. Change for the benefit of the community client often must occur at several levels, ranging from the individual to the societal. As Ryan (1976) points out, the "victim" cannot always be blamed and expected to correct the deficit without concurrent changes in the helping professions and public policy. For instance, the solutions to lifestyle-induced health problems such as smoking, overeating, and speeding involve not only the individual's choosing health-promoting habits, but also society's facilitating healthful choices. Most individuals cannot alter their habits alone, but require the support of family members, friends, community health care systems that include professional nurses, and relevant social policies.

A commitment to the health of the community client requires a process of change at each of these levels. As a result, nursing roles for each of the units of service are required. Collaborative practice models are also required (Pescznecker and McNeil, 1984). One nursing role emphasizes individual and direct personal care skills. Another nursing role focuses on the family and aggregate as the unit of service. A third nursing role focuses on the community as a unit of service, especially constituent community groups (Goeppinger, 1984).

The definition of community client as the *target of service* includes two key concepts: community health, and partnership for community health, which together are the goal and means of community-oriented practice.

DEFINING GOALS AND MEANS OF COMMUNITY-ORIENTED PRACTICE

Community-oriented practice is targeted to the community, the population group with which healthful change is sought. The practice goal is community health, which is more appropriately considered as an ongoing series of health-promoting changes rather than a fixed state. The major mechanism of facilitating changes for health is partnership; for example, collaboration between the lay public and health professionals and among health professionals themselves.

Community Health

Like the concept of community, community health has three common characteristics, or dimensions: status, structure, and process. These dimensions define community health as the goal of community-oriented practice in different ways.

Status

Community health as defined in status, or outcome, terms is the most well-known and accepted approach. The physical, emotional, and social components of community health are frequently measured by traditional morbidity and mortality rates, life expectancy indices, and risk factor profiles (physical), consumer satisfaction and mental health indices (emotional), and crime rates and functional levels (social). Other status measures such as worker absenteeism and infant mortality rates reflect the effects of all three components.

Structure

Community health as viewed from a structural perspective usually comprises community health services and resources and also attributes of the community structure itself. Those attributes are commonly identified as social indicators, or correlates, of health. Indicators used to measure community health services and resources include utilization patterns, treatment data from various health institutions, and provider/patient ratios. The problems with using these measures are serious. For instance, inequities in access to care and quality of care are well known. Less well known, but still problematic, is the erroneous assumption of a direct causal relationship between the provision of service and improved health (Miller and Stokes, 1978; Mooney and Rives, 1978). Such problems necessitate cautious use of health services and resources.

Measures of community structure attributes include demographic characteristics such as dependency ratios, socio-economic and racial distributions, and educational levels. Their relationships to health status have been thoroughly documented. For instance, health status is inversely related to age and directly related to socioeconomic level.

Process

Community health defined as the process of effective community functioning or problem-solving is the least well-established definition. However, the definition is especially appropriate to community-oriented nursing because it directs the study of community health to the "promotion of effective community action or 'wellness' " (Wilson, 1976), which is an important aim of community-oriented nurses.

We have expanded on this process definition by refining the definition of community competence. Community competence, defined originally by Cottrell (1976, p. 197), is a process whereby the components of a community—organizations, groups, and aggregates—"are able to collaborate effectively in identifying the problems and needs of the community; can achieve a working consensus on goals and priorities; can agree on ways and means to implement the agreed-on goals; and can collaborate effectively in the required actions."

Cottrell (1976) also proposed eight essential conditions of competence. They are commitment, self-other awareness and clarity of situational definitions, articulateness, effective communication, conflict containment and accommodation, participation, management of relations with the larger society, and machinery for facilitating participant interaction and decision making. The conditions are defined in Table 13-1, and Goeppinger and Baglioni (1986) developed indicators of each condition and procedures to gather and/or generate data about them. An integration of status, structural, and process definitions is reflected in the following definition of community health.

Community health as used in this chapter is defined as the meeting of collective needs through identifying problems and managing interactions within the community itself and between the community and the larger society. This requires exercising the eight essential conditions of competence listed above and defined in Table 13-1 (Goeppinger, et al., 1982).

Strategies to improve community health depend, to some extent, on the dimension of community health that is emphasized. If the emphasis is on the status dimension, the most appropriate strategy is usually at the level of primary prevention. The objective is either to prevent a disease—physical, emotional, and societal—or treat it in its presymptomatic stages. Immunization programs for infants, adolescents, and at-risk adults are an example of a primary level nursing intervention that would be reflected in morbidity and mortality measures.

Nursing intervention strategies focused on the structural dimension would be directed to either health services or demographic characteristics. Intervention aimed at altering health services might include program planning, and intervention aimed at affecting demographic characteristics might include community development.

TABLE 13-1

The conditions of community competence

Condition	Definition
Commitment	The affective and cognitive attachment to a community "that is worthy of substantial effort to sustain and enhance" (Cottrell, 1976, p. 198).
Self-other awareness and clarity of situational definitions	The lucid and realistic perception of one's own and the other's community components, identities, and positions on issues.
Articulateness	The technical aspects of formulating and stating one's views in relation to the other's views.
Effective communication	The accurate transmission of information, based on the development of common meaning among the communicators.
Conflict containment and accommodation	The inventive and effective assimilation and management of true, or realistically, perceived differences.
Participation	Active, community-oriented involvement.
Management of relations with larger society	Adeptness at recognizing, obtaining, and using external resources and supports and, when necessary, stimulating the creation and use of alternative or supplementary resources.
Machinery for facilitating participant interaction and decision making	Flexible and responsible procedures, formal and informal, facilitating interaction and decision-making.

From Goeppinger, J., Lassiter, P.G., and Wilcox, B.: Community health is community competence, Nurs. Outlook **30**(8):464-467, 1982.

When the emphasis is on the process dimension, the most appropriate strategy is usually health promotion. For example, if family-life education is precluded because of ineffective communication among families, children, school board members, religious leaders, and health professionals, the most effective strategy may be to open discussion and negotiate a mutually satisfactory resolution. All strategies must include a community partnership because it is the basic means, or key, for improving community health. Its importance in such efforts is emphasized by the following discussion.

Partnership for Community Health

Most changes aimed at improving community health involve, of necessity, partnerships among community residents and health workers from a variety of disciplines. Often, community residents are viewed as data sources and recipients of intervention. This form of partnership is called "passive participation" (Feuerstein, 1980, p. 1). In contrast, the type of lay-professional partnership with which this chapter is concerned emphasizes active participation. Here, power is shared among lay and professional persons throughout the assessment, planning, implementation, and evaluation process.

Historically, nurses have not been influential in initiating community changes. Power for inducing significant changes through assessment and planning has rested with other community workers, particularly physician health officers and health planners. Community health nurses, like the communities they serve, have frequently only been informed of desired changes. However, the nurses have generally been actively involved in the implementation phase. Intervention *by* the nurse, *for* the community's benefit, has been a predominant practice mode. This mode contrasts with a partnership approach, where all involved are assessing, planning, and implementing needed community changes.

The monopoly on the change process previously held by health care providers is now being challenged by an increasingly enlightened public, some assertive community health nurses, and a few health care institutions. For instance, the World Health Organization has made partnership, defined as community involvement, a basic tenent of its campaign, "Health for all by the year 2000" (Mahler, 1981, pp. 8-9).

Partnership Defined

Partnership is often equated with participation and involvement of the community or its representatives in healthful change. We define *partnership* as the informed, flexible, and negotiated distribution (and redistribution) of power among all participants in the processes of change for improved community health. The three main characteristics of partnership are denoted by the adjectives *informed, flexible,* and *negotiated*. First, partnership is *informed;* this is probably the most basic characteristic. Lay and professional partners must be aware of their own and the other's perceptions, rights, and responsibilities. Partnership is also *flexible.* Lay and professional partners must recognize the unique as well as similar contributions each can make to a given situation. Professionals often contribute substantive expertise that lay persons lack. On the other hand, lay persons' definitions of community health problems are often more accurate than those of professionals. Because contributions vary and each situation demands different contributions, the distribution of power must be *negotiated* at every stage of the change process.

Partnership, so defined, is as essential a concept for community health nurses as the concepts of community, community client, and community health. Partnership is important because health is not given, but rather is generated through new and increasingly effective forms of lay-professional collaboration. For example, maternal-child health in both developed and underdeveloped countries is affected more by wise grocery shopping and improvements in home gardening than by the provision and compliant ingestion of vitamin and mineral supplements (Combs-Orme, et al., 1985). Changes in consumer behavior and horticultural practices require active participation of both lay and professional people. Partnership in identifying problems and setting goals is especially important because it engenders the commitment essential to successful change.

The significance and effectiveness of partnership in improving community health is supported by a growing body of literature. Studies document the utility of partnership models involving village health workers (Kingma, 1975), Latina opinion leaders (Lorig and Walters, 1980-1981), health facilitators (Salber, 1981), lay advisors (Salber, 1979; Salber, et al., 1976), and health guides (Warnecke, et al., 1976). The roles of these partners-in-health have included sympathetic listening, offering advice, making referrals, and instituting programs.

Despite supportive data, professional health workers have often challenged the notion of partnership. Partnership involves active collaboration; unfortunately, passive compliance is more frequently sought than collaboration. Also, questions are frequently raised about the health care consumer's ability to determine health needs accurately and to evaluate professional practice.

Conclusions

The meaning of partnership, like the meanings of community, community client, and community health, is not fully understood, nor is any single meaning universally accepted. However, sufficient clarity and agreement do exist to consider these four concepts the basic elements of a conceptual framework for community-oriented nursing practice. In the following sections these concepts form the framework within which the community-oriented nursing process is presented.

Most nurses are familiar with the nursing process as it applies to individually focused nursing care. Using the nursing process to promote community health means applying the nursing process to community-focused nursing care. The steps of the nursing process that directly involve the community client include assessment, planning, implementation of the plan (intervention), and evaluation of the intervention. The process reflects many of the ideas presented in the ANA's recent publication, *A Guide for Community-Based Nursing Services* (1985). Figure 13-1 is a flow chart depicting the nursing process with the community client, providing an overview of the entire process.

Application of the nursing process to the community client is illustrated in the following sections with a case study taken from an actual community health nurse's practice. For clarity, infant malnutrition is the only community health problem used to illustrate application of the nursing process. In reality, several community-health problems besides infant malnutrition were identified. Their relative importance was determined, and infant malnutrition was designated the most important problem before continuing with intervention.

ASSESSING COMMUNITY HEALTH

Assessing community health requires gathering relevant existing data, generating missing data, and interpreting the data base. Gathering of the data and its initial interpretation are the first steps in the assessment phase of the nursing process.

Data Collection and Interpretation

The primary goal of data collection is to acquire usable information about the community and its health. The systematic collection of data about community health necessitates gathering or compiling existing data, which is frequently statistical, and generating missing data, which is often accomplished through participant observation in the community and interaction with key community members. These data are then interpreted, and community health problems and capabilities are identified.

The process of obtaining existing, readily available data is *data gathering.* These data usually describe the demography of a community: age, sex, socioeconomic, and racial distributions; vital statistics, including selected mortality and morbidity data; its institutions, including health care organizations and the services they provide; and health manpower characteristics. Often these data have been collected by others via structured interviews and questionnaires and are available in published reports.

Other data, generally not statistical, are less easily acquired. Frequently such data must be developed by the nurse/data collector through interaction with community members or groups. This process is termed *data generation.* Data that frequently require generation include information about a community's knowledge and beliefs, values and sentiments, goals and perceived needs, norms, problem-solving processes, and power, leadership, and influence structures. These data are therefore more apt to be collected via informant interviews and participant observation and to be qualitative.

A composite data base is created by combining the gathered and generated data. Community health problems and capabilities are then identified from the composite data base through data interpretation. Data interpretation seeks to attribute meaning to the data. First, data are analyzed and synthesized, themes are noted, and *community health problems,* or needs for action, and *community health strengths,* or capabilities, are determined. Next, the resources available to meet the needs are identified. Problems are indicated by differences between the nurse's and community's concepts of community health and the available data. Strengths, on the other hand, are suggested by similarities between the nurse's and community's concepts of community health and available data. The nurse and community, working in a partnership, identify both problems and capabilities for resolving problems. Active community participation is critical for the data interpretation process, particularly in identifying problems.

The *Program Planning Model,* initially proposed by Delbecq and Van de Ven (1971), is a widely accepted technique for encouraging lay participation in problem identification. The model illustrates active community participation in problem identification and program planning. It maximizes the contributions of various groups with diverse interests and expertise. This model depends heavily on nominal groups, "groups in which individuals work in the pres-

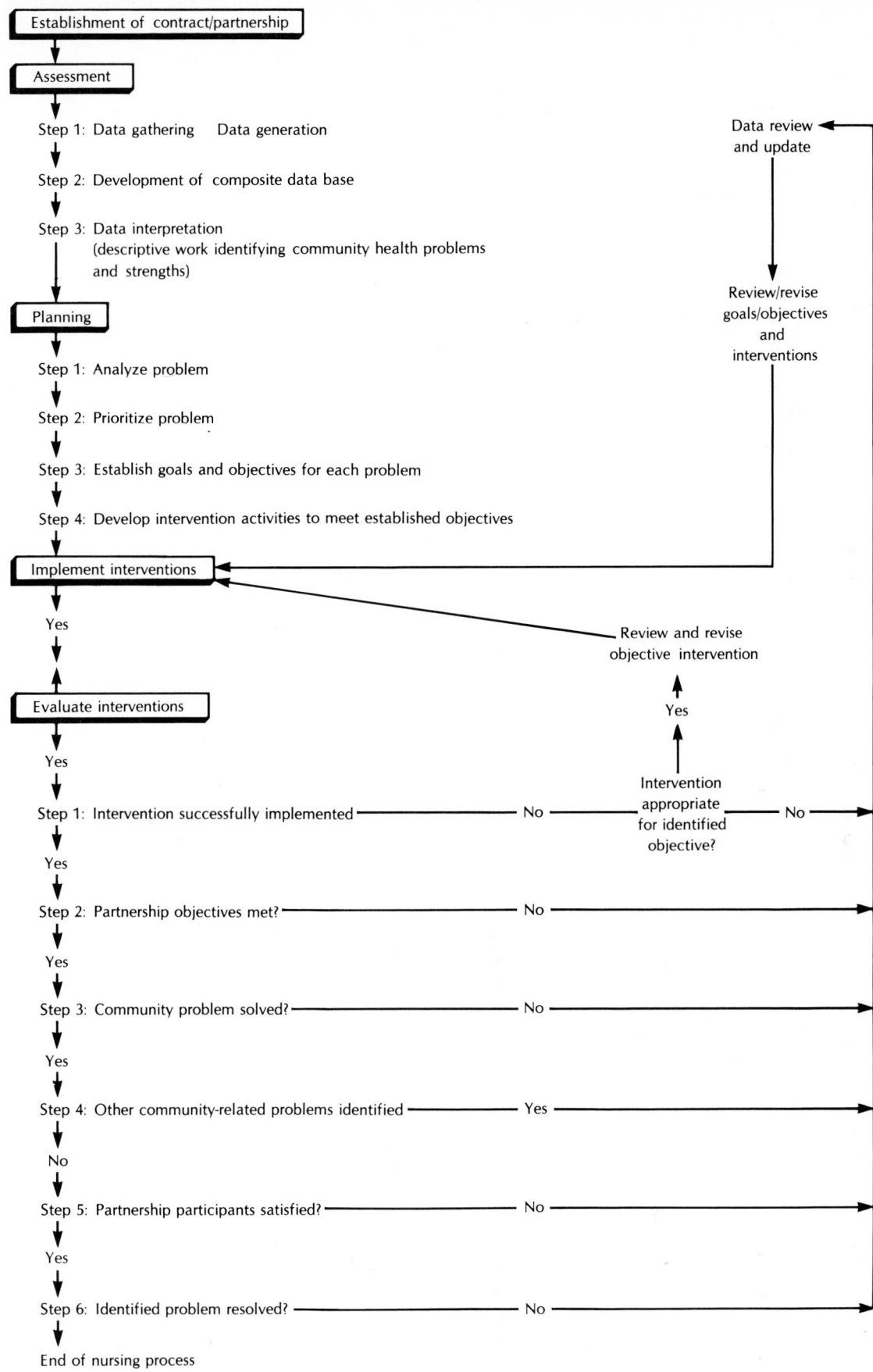

FIGURE 13-1

A flow chart illustrating the nursing process with the community client.

ence of one another but do not interact" (Delbecq and Van de Ven, 1971, p. 467), the separation of personal from collective problems, and a round-robin procedure for listing problems without concurrently evaluating or elaborating on them.

The model, popularly known as the nominal group process, was compared in one study with three other methods for identifying and prioritizing health needs (Scutchfield, 1975). These methods were community diagnosis, random consumer survey, and comprehensive health planning ratings. The health care priorities of the consumer responding to the household survey were the cost of medical care, physician inavailability, and lack of specialty services. Health planning ratings emphasized service gaps and underutilization. The community diagnosis method yielded an emphasis on particular diseases. The nominal group process, which involved consumers as well as health professionals and health planners, resulted in a greater emphasis on lack of services and facilities and financing problems than did the community diagnosis method, which involved only health professionals. Flexner and Littlefield (1977, p. 246) note that the community diagnosis lacks the understanding that "what the consumer feels is important may in fact be important, even though this perspective may be alien to the objective information orientation" of the data gatherer. Conversely, the random consumer survey and comprehensive health planning ratings lack the provider's and planner's perspective. The nominal group process, involving health-care consumers as well as health-care providers and planners, offers the most balanced perspective.

A variety of methods to collect and interpret data are essential. Methods that encourage the nurse to consider the community's perception of its health problems and capabilities are as important as those methods structured to yield knowledge the nurse considers essential. Several of these assessment methods are discussed in the next section.

Data Assessment

Five methods of collecting and interpreting data useful to the community health nurse are informant interviews, participant observation, secondary analysis of existing data, surveys, and windshield surveys. These methods can be clustered into two distinct but complementary categories; methods that rely on what is directly observed by the data collector, and methods that rely on what is reported to the data collector. Informant interviews, participant observation, and windshield surveys are examples of direct data collection; secondary data analysis and surveys represent reported data. The methods are described, the appropriate use of each method is considered, and the importance of multiple assessment methods for triangulation is stressed below.

Among the three methods of directly obtaining data noted above, *informant interviews,* consisting of directed conversation with selected members of a community about community members or groups and events, is basic to effective data collections. Also basic is *participant observation,* or the "conscious and systematic sharing, in so far as circumstances permit, in the life activities, and on oc-

casion, in the interests and affects of a group of persons" (Kluckhohn, 1940, p. 331).

Informant interviews and participant observation are particularly suitable techniques for generating information about community beliefs, norms, values, power and influence structures, and problem-solving processes (Ruffing-Rahal, 1985). Such data can seldom be reported in numbers, thus they are often not collected. Even worse, impressions— intuitive and unverified—are sometimes substituted for data. Yet these data are important.

Using the example of infant malnutrition, informant interviewing with social workers and religious leaders provided data indicating a community with well-defined clusters of persons with low incomes, concerns over adolescent pregnancy, and worries about its babies' health. The data reflecting concerns and worries would have been difficult to acquire without personal interviews.

Windshield surveys are the motorized equivalent of simple observation. Many dimensions of a community's life and environment can be carefully observed through an automobile windshield. Common characteristics of street people, neighborhood gathering places, the rhythm of community life, housing quality, and geographic boundaries are some of the dimensions that can be readily observed. Again, using the infant malnutrition example, the windshield survey suggested the community had a significant unemployed population because adults were observed "hanging out" on street corners during the daytime.

All three of these methods require sensitivity, openness, curiosity, and the ability to listen, taste, touch, smell, and see life as lived in a community at levels far different from those required to understand and cope with most health workers' daily routines. Useful readings on observational methods include Filstead (1972), Glazer (1972), Polit and Hungler (1983), Seaman (1982) and Wilson (1985).

As noted earlier, two methods of collecting reported data are secondary analysis and surveys. *Secondary analysis,* in which the community health nurse uses previously gathered data, such as minutes from community meetings, is extremely valuable because it is efficient and economical. Many sources of data useful for secondary analysis—public documents, surveys, minutes from meetings, statistical data, and health records—are readily available. Major disadvantages of working with existing data, such as missing, inaccurate, or erroneous information, are often not as apparent in community health because demographic and vital statistics are collected in standardized ways that minimize opportunities for error. In the infant malnutrition example, birth records noting low birth weights and health department clinic records of low-weight-for-height children provided information that reflected a higher-than-average rate of infant malnutrition.

Surveys, in which data from a sample of persons are reported to the data collector, are equally useful but somewhat less efficient and economical than observational methods and secondary analyses, because they require time-consuming and costly data collection. Thus the survey method is not often used by the community health nurse. However, surveys are necessary for identifying certain community problems. For example, a lack of accessible personal health service cannot be readily and reliably documented in any other fashion.

Both survey and secondary analysis methods are thoroughly described in *The Practice of Social Research* (Babbie, 1986). In addition, several manuals can help community workers develop, conduct, and analyze a survey. An informative and pragmatic manual is *Needs Assessment: A Model for Community Planning* (Neuber, 1980).

Because no data collection method is without bias, it is best to use several methods with different strengths and weaknesses; this is called *triangulation*. Using multiple complementary methods is essential to and consistent with community health nursing practices.

Nursing assessment of community health—data collection and interpretation—is focused. Focus, or perspective, can be provided by detailed assessment guides, which are built on a conceptual framework consisting of our definitions of community and community health.

Assessment Guides

Concepts stated in behavioral or observable terms can serve as assessment guides. The concepts of community and community health have already been defined in such terms. The concept of community has been specified as presented in Table 13-2. The original definition (see p. 254) includes

three dimensions: place or space, people or person, and function. Each of these dimensions is specified by several indicators. For example, the spatial dimension is represented by indicators such as size and political boundaries. When combined, the indicators for each of these three dimensions constitute a portion of the Assessment Guide included in Appendix E.

The specification of community health—its status, structure, and process dimensions—is presented in Table 13-3. In the infant malnutrition example, status dimension data were gathered from morbidity/mortality data, structural dimension data were gathered from vital statistics and from informant interviews with social workers, and process dimension data were gathered from informant interviews with community religious leaders. In this way the concepts of community and community health provide the framework for the Assessment Guide in Appendix E. Together, the concepts and Assessment Guide constitute the Community Health Assessment Model, the basis of the Community-Oriented Health Record (COHR) (see Appendix E). Data, problems, and capabilities are all organized by using that model.

To assist the community health nurse in collecting and interpreting data about the process dimension of community

---

TABLE 13-2

The concept of community specified

Dimensions	Indicators
Place or space	Geopolitical boundaries
	Local or folk name for area
	Size in square miles, acres, blocks, or census tracts
	Transportation avenues such as rivers, highways, railroads, and sidewalks
	Physical environment such as land use patterns and condition of housing
People or person	Number and density of population
	Demographic structure of population such as age, sex, socioeconomic, and racial distributions; rural and urban character; and dependency ratio
	Informal groups such as block clubs, service clubs, and friendship networks
	Formal groups such as schools, churches, businesses, industries, governmental bodies, unions, and health and welfare agencies
	Linking structures
Function	Production, distribution, and consumption of goods and services
	Socialization of new members
	Maintenance of social control
	Adapting to ongoing and expected change
	Provision of mutual aid

TABLE 13-3

The concept of community health specified

Dimensions	Indicators
Status	Vital statistics—live births, neonatal deaths, infant deaths, maternal deaths, deaths
	Disease incidence and prevalence of leading causes of mortality and morbidity
	Health risk profiles of selected aggregates
	Functional ability levels
Structure	Health facilities such as hospitals, nursing homes, industrial and school health services, health departments, voluntary health associations, categorical grant programs, and prepaid health plans
	Health-related planning groups
	Health manpower such as physicians, dentists, nurses, environmental sanitarians, social workers, and others
	Health resource utilization patterns such as bed occupancy days and patient/provider visits
Process	Commitment
	Self-other awareness and clarity of situational definitions
	Articulateness
	Effective communication
	Conflict containment and accomodation
	Participation
	Management of relationships with the larger society
	Machinery for facilitating participant interaction and decision making

health, researchers at the University of Virginia have developed a guide for assessing community competence (Goeppinger and Baglioni, 1986). This guide, like the Assessment Guide of the COHR, is used to orient community health nurses to community practice.

Another useful assessment guide is the Community Nursing Survey Guide (Tinkham, et al., 1984). The information Tinkham, et al., consider important—data on the community itself, demographic and epidemiological information about the people, data on the environment, knowledge of communication channels, data on health facilities and personnel, and knowledge of community health nursing services and programs—is similar to that specified in the Assessment Guide. However, they do not cover the process dimension of community health as thoroughly.

Connor (1969) has also developed a classic guide, a handbook for community-level personnel. It provides a simple and comprehensive yet flexible approach to understanding the community. The community worker's attention is focused on 12 elements of the community social system, including resources, history, values and sentiments, and goals and perceived needs, and on 11 patterns of social relationships within the community, including the family, government, health, and communication networks. Together these constitute "the social compass applied to the community" (Connor, 1969, p. 25). The social compass provides a systematic, conceptually based approach to gathering information about the community.

Each guide provides a perspective on data collection; each ensures that the data collected are comprehensive and consistent with the community health nurse's conceptual framework. But they also determine whether the data are collected at all and how they are interpreted. As a result, it is essential to remember that the community's perception of its health may vary markedly from that of the nurse. It is critical to remain open to any data and data interpretations, despite the comfort of a highly structured assessment guide.

Assessment Issues

Gaining entry or acceptance into the community is perhaps the biggest challenge in assessment. The community health nurse is usually an outsider and often represents an established health care system that is neither known nor trusted by community members, who may react with indifference or even active hostility. In addition, the community health nurse may feel insecure about her skills as a community worker, and the community may refuse to acknowledge its need for those skills.

Because the nurse's success in collecting and interpreting data and then in planning, initiating, and evaluating intervention largely depends on the way she is viewed, entry into the community is critical. Often the nurse can gain entry by participating in community events, looking and listening attentively, visiting people in formal leadership positions, employing an assessment guide, and using a peer group for support.

Once the nurse gains entry at an initial level, *role negotiation* often becomes an issue. The concept of role involves the values, behaviors, or goals that govern an indi-

vidual's interactions with others. In this instance, the nurse must decide how long to separate the roles of data collector and intervenor. Effective implementation of the nursing process requires initial identification of an objective and collection of an adequate data base, but the dangers of overinvolvement and premature response to health needs and social injustice are great. Role negotiation can be aided by a thoughtful and consistent presentation of the reasons for one's presence in the community and by sincere demonstrations of one's commitment to the community. Keeping appointments, stating the importance of getting the community members' perceptions of health needs, and respecting persons' rights to choose whether they will work with the nurse are often useful techniques.

Maintaining *confidentiality* is also important. Nurses must scrupulously protect the identity of community members who provide sensitive or controversial data. In some cases the nurse may consider withholding data; in other situations she may be legally required to disclose data.

The issues of gaining entry, role negotiation, and confidentiality are of a more personal nature than the issue of small-area analysis. This issue concerns the inappropriateness of making conclusions from data gathered from small areas. For example, calculation of mortality rates when the denominator is as small as 5000 may be skewed. This issue frequently compromises the validity of many identified health problems. It reinforces the usefulness of triangulation, because if similar health problems are identified using several assessment methods, the nurse can be more confident of their validity.

Nursing intervention to assist a community in healthful change depends on understanding the community and its health; that is, on a deliberate, systematic, and informed nursing assessment in partnership with the community. Nursing intervention at the community level includes planning, implementation, and evaluation phases, just as it does at individual and familial levels. Though the intervention process is similar at the various levels, intervention strategies differ. Planning, implementation, and evaluation phases are presented in the following sections. Nursing roles, activities, and issues especially significant to community-oriented practice are highlighted.

PLANNING FOR COMMUNITY HEALTH

The planning phase includes analyzing and establishing priorities among community health problems already identified, establishing goals and objectives, and identifying intervention activities that will accomplish the objectives.

Performing Problem Analysis and Prioritization

Problem analysis seeks to clarify the nature of the problem. The nurse identifies the origins and impact of the problem, the points at which intervention might be undertaken, and the parties that have an interest in the problem and its solution. Analysis often requires the development of a problem matrix, in which the direct and indirect precursors and consequences are identified and interrelationships among problems and their precursors and consequences are mapped. The matrix is important because the nurse can anticipate that several of the same precursors and consequences underlie many of the problems. Among the common precursors and consequences may be the problem of highest priority.

Problem analysis should be undertaken for each identified problem. It often requires organizing a special group composed of the nurse, persons whose areas of expertise relate to the problem, persons whose organizations have the capabilities to intervene, and representatives of the community experiencing the problem. Both substantive and process specialists must participate. Together they can identify the problem correlates and explain the relationships between each correlate and the problem.

This process is seen in the Problem Analysis Sheet of the COHR (Figure 13-2). Problem correlates (precursors and consequences) are listed in the first column. Correlates are sought from all facets of community life. Social or environmental correlates are as appropriate as those oriented to the individual. For example, teenage pregnancy is a social correlate of infant malnutrition, and the lack of home gardening is an environmental correlate. In the second column the relationships between each correlate and the problem are noted. The third column will contain data from the community and the literature that support the relationship, to be written in capsule fashion. The suspected infant malnutrition example and a few of its correlates are given. Infant malnutrition is thought to be correlated with inadequate diet, ignorance, poverty, and disturbed mother-child relationship.

Remember that infant malnutrition represents only one among several community-related problems identified by the community assessment. Each problem identified was put through a ranking process to determine its relative importance. This ranking process, in which problems are evaluated and priorities established according to predetermined criteria, is *problem prioritization.* It involves the contributions of community members, substantive experts, and administrators and resource controllers.

Using predetermined criteria can facilitate problem prioritization. Criteria we have found helpful in ranking problems include: (1) community awareness of the problem; (2) community motivation to resolve or better manage the problem; (3) nurse's ability to influence problem solution; (4) availability of expertise relevant to problem solution; (5) severity of consequences if the problem is unresolved; and (6) speed with which resolution can be achieved. These criteria are listed in the first column of the Problem Prioritization Sheet of the COHR (Figure 13-3). Again the suspected infant malnutrition is used. Although other sets of existing criteria may be used (Dever, 1980, p. 361 or Blum, 1974, pp. 155-156) or be developed by the nurse, it is important to remember that the criteria need to be

Problem Analysis

Name of community: _____ *Jefferson County* _____

Problem/statement: _____ *Suspected infant malnutrition in Jefferson County* _____

Problem analysis

Problem correlates	Relationship of correlates to problem	Data supportive to relationships (refer to appropriate sections of Data Base and relevant research findings in current literature)
1. Inadequate diets	Diets lacking in required nutrients contribute to malnutrition.	
2. Ignorance	The norm is to bottle feed rather than breast feed.	
3. Lack of money	Infant formulas are expensive.	
4. Disturbed mother-child relationship	Poor mother-child relationship may result in infant's failure to thrive.	
Column 1	Column 2	Column 3

FIGURE 13-2

Problem analysis: suspected infant malnutrition in Jefferson County.

Problem prioritization

Criteria	Criteria weights (1-10)	Problem	Problem rating (1-10)	Rationale for rating	Problem significance (weight X rate)
1. Community awareness of the problem	5	Suspected infant malnutrition in Jefferson County	10	Health service providers, teachers, and a variety of parents have mentioned problem.	50
2. Community motivation to resolve the problem	10		3	Most feel this problem is irresolvable as majority of those affected are indigent.	30
3. Nurse's ability to influence problem resolution	5		8	Nurse skilled at consciousness raising and mobilizing support.	40
4. Ready availability of expertise relevant to problem resolution	7		10	WIC program, nutritionists available. County extension agent interested.	70
5. Severity of consequences if problem is left unresolved	8		5	Effects on marginal malnutrition not too well documented.	40
6. Quickness with which problem resolution can be achieved	3		3	Time to mobiline rural community with no history of social action length.	9
					Total - 239
Column 1	Column 2	Column 3	Column 4	Column 5	Column 6

FIGURE 13-3

Problem prioritization: suspected infant malnutrition in Jefferson County.

agreed on by a variety of reference groups before intervention.

Given an acceptable and comprehensive set of criteria and a list of community health problems, the process of assigning priorities is rather simple. The criteria are weighted on a scale ranging from a low score of one to a high score of ten (column two). Then the significance of each relative to the problem is rated according to the preestablished criteria, resulting in a problem rating (column four). The rationale for the problem rating is noted (column five), and the significance of the problem is computed by multiplying each criterion weight score (column two) by the problem rating score (column four) and adding the sums to get a total, the problem significance score (all recorded in column six). This process is repeated separately for each identified problem. Then the significance scores of the problems are compared, and priorities are established. The most significant problems, those with the highest priority scores, are selected as the focus for intervention.

Establishing a priority score for each identified problem can appear complicated; however, it helps to recall that the

criteria were established (column one) and weighted (column two) by participants in the community partnership before prioritization began. Also, problem rating (column four) and the rationale for rating (column five) are also established via the participation of all members in the community partnership. Although the numerical scores are subjective, the active involvement of the nurse and representatives of different community interests and using triangulation help ensure that the data used to establish the rationale are relevant as well as accurate. Community participation also helps ensure that the ranking score established for each problem reflects its importance relative to other community health problems.

The process of establishing a significance score for the problem of suspected infant malnutrition is depicted in Figure 13-3. Community motivation to resolve the problem was the criterion weighted as most important to problem resolution. Yet as most community residents believed the problem was irremediable because of the poverty of those affected, the relative significance of this criterion when applied to the problem of infant malnutrition was low. A

Goals and Objectives

Name of community: _____ *Jefferson County* _____

Problem/concern: _____ *Suspected infant malnutrition* _____

Goal statement: _____ *To document and, if appropriate, reduce the incidence* _____

_____ *and prevelance of infant malnutrition* _____

Present date	Objectives (number and statement)	Completion date
1-87	No. 1 80% of infants seen by health department, neighborhood health center, and private physicians will have their developmental levels assessed.	8-87
1-87	No. 2 WIC program eligibility will be determined for 80% of infants seen by health department, neighborhood health center, and private physicians.	5-87
1-87	No. 3 An outreach program will be implemented to identify at-risk infants not now known to health care providers.	8-87
1-87	No. 4 WIC program eligibility will be determined for 25% of at-risk infants.	1-88
1-87	No. 5 75% of all infants eligible for WIC food supplements will be enrolled in the program.	12-88
1-87	No. 6 50% of the mothers of infants enrolled in WIC will demonstrate 3 ways of incorporating WIC supplements into their infants' diets.	5-88

FIGURE 13-4

Goals and objectives: suspected infant malnutrition in Jefferson County.

similar process with the remaining five criteria yields a total significance score of 239 for the suspected infant malnutrition problem. Assuming 239 is the highest significance score among the several identified community health problems, infant malnutrition is justified as the priority problem for intervention.

Establishing Goals and Objectives

Once high-priority problems are identified, relevant goals and objectives are developed. The *goal,* generally a broad statement of desired outcome, and *objectives,* the precise statements of the desired outcome, are carefully selected.

An example of a goal and objectives relevant to the suspected infant malnutrition problem is depicted in Figure 13-4. The goal presented is to document and, if appropriate, reduce the incidence and prevalence of infant malnutrition. The objectives are more precise and are behaviorally stated, incremental, and measurable. They pertain to assessing infant developmental levels, determining Women, Infants and Children Program (WIC) eligibility, implementing an

outreach program, enrolling infants in the WIC program, and incorporating supplemental foods into existing diets.

As noted earlier, establishing these goals and objectives involves collaboration between the nurse and representatives of the community groups affected by both the problem and the proposed intervention. In discussing the collaborative process, Archer, et al. (1984) point out that collaboration involves the mutual selection of goals and objectives. This often requires considerable negotiation among all participants in the planning process. One important advantage offered by the continuous active involvement of people affected by the outcomes is that they have a vested interest in those outcomes and therefore are supportive and committed to the success of the intervention. Once goals and objectives are established, intervention activities to accomplish the objectives can be identified.

Identifying Intervention Activities

Intervention activities, the means by which objectives are met, are the strategies that clarify what must be done to achieve the objectives, the ways change will be affected, and the way the problem cycle will be interrupted. Because alternative intervention activities do exist, they must be identified and evaluated. Sketching out possible interventions and selecting the best set of activities for each objective is often done unconsciously and intuitively. To make the process deliberate, the Plan Sheet of the COHR was developed. Examples of identifying and evaluating alternative activities to achieve the goal of documenting and reducing infant malnutrition are depicted in Figures 13-5 and 13-6.

In Figure 13-5, five intervenor activities are listed in the second column, each relevent to the first objective in Figure 13-4. The first two activities involve WIC program personnel as the principal change agents. The last three involve the community nurse practitioner (CNP), WIC program personnel, and the staff of the health department, neighborhood health center, and private physicians' offices as the change partners.

The likely effectiveness of each of the activities is considered in the third and fourth columns. The *value,** or the likelihood that the activity will foster achievement of the objective and eventual resolution of the problem, is noted in column three. Clearly it is more valuable to educate others in how to assess infant development (activity four)

---

*The value and probability scores of intervenor activities may range from one (low) to ten (high). The range of one to ten was arbitrarily determined.

Plan: Assess Infants' Developmental Levels

Name of community:___ *Jefferson County* _____

Objective number 1.___ *80% of infants seen by health department, neighborhood health center, and* _____

and statement: ___ *private physicians will have their development levels assessed.* _____

Plan

Date	Intervenor activities/means	Value (1-10)	Probability (1-10)	Activity/means selected for implementation
1-87	1. WIC program supplies	1	10	Insufficient personnel and
	personnel to assess infant			time. Existing community
	developmental levels.			resources (potential)
			Total 10	ignored.
1-87	2. WIC program provides in-	5	5	Antipathy between WIC per-
	service education to staff			sonnel and other health
	on assessment of infant			workers high. Need for
	development.			education must be assessed
				first and enthusiasm for
			Total 25	objectives created.
1-87	3. CNP provides in-service	3	10	CNP can't do it alone!
	education to staff in			
	assessment of infant			
	development.		Total 30	
1-87	4. CNP assists WIC personnel	8	8	Most likely to build
	to identify in-service			on existing community
	educational needs of area			strengths. CNP skilled in
	health care providers			needs assessment and inter-
	about assessment of			personal techniques needed
	infant development.		Total 64	to decrease antipathy.
1-87	5. CNP assists WIC personnel	10	8	Without this, change
	to identify driving and			effort likely to fail.
	restraining forces rela-			
	tive to implementation of			
	objective.		Total 80	

FIGURE 13-5

Plan: assess infants' developmental levels.

than to do it for them (activity one). It is also valuable to analyze the change process necessary to accomplish the objective (activity five). Consequently, activities four and five have higher value scores than activity one.

On the other hand, the *probability,** or the likelihood that the means can be implemented, is highest when only the CNP is involved, because the nurse has more control over her own behavior than over the behavior of others. Therefore activities one and three have higher probabilities than activities two, four, and five. Probability is recorded in column four. Conditions explaining the numerical scores

---

*The value and probability scores of intervenor activities may range from one (low) to ten (high). The range of one to ten was arbitrarily determined.

are noted briefly in the fifth column. The activities with the highest scores, computed by multiplying the value by the probability, are selected because it is important to be able to both affect the objective (value) and carry out the means (probability).

A second example of plan development is depicted in Figure 13-6. The activities relate to objective three in Figure 13-4—implementation of an outreach program—and involve using lay advisors, hospital nurses, public health nurses, and WIC program personnel.

IMPLEMENTING INTERVENTION FOR COMMUNITY HEALTH

Implementation, the third phase of the nursing process, is the *work/activities* aimed at achieving the goals and objec-

Plan: Implement an Outreach Program

Name of community: *Jefferson County*

Objective number 3. *An outreach program is implemented to identify at risk infants*

and statement: *not now known to health care providers*

Plan

Date	Intervenor activities/means	Value (1-10)	Probability (1-10)	Activity/means selected for implementation
1-87	1. CNP identifies and trains lay advisors in community as case finders.	8	6	Lay leaders already known, proven to be effective change agents; can't
			*Total 48	however, be paid.
1-87	2. Local hospital administrators alter job descriptions of nurses in maternity and pediatrics to include case finding and referral.	8	5	All babies in Jefferson County born in hospital since 1978. Administrator interested in community. Administration powerful can alter nurses' job descriptions. Nurses hate
			*Total 40	student nurses.
1-87	3. CNP encourages public health nurses to do better job of case finding.	8	2	Public health nurses have historic role in case finding. CNP not well known by PHN's. PHN's re-
			Total 10	ported to be overworked.
1-87	4. WIC personnel devote 1 evening/week to case finding.	1	10	One nurse (non-resident) eager to do this. Doesn't develop existing community
			Total 110	resources.
Column 1	Column 2	Column 3	Column 4	Column 5

*Means selected.

FIGURE 13-6

Plan: implement an outreach program.

tives. Implementation efforts may be made by the person or group who established the goals and objectives, or they may be shared with or even delegated to others. The issue of centralizing implementation efforts is important, and the community health nurse's position on this issue can be influenced by a variety of factors. Several of these factors, as well as four important implementation mechanisms, are considered next.

Factors Influencing Implementation

Implementation is shaped by the nurse's chosen roles, the type of health problem selected as the focus for intervention, the community's readiness to participate in problem resolution, and the characteristics of the social change process. The nurse participating in community-oriented intervention has a key position and commands knowledge and skills not possessed by the other intervenors. The question is how the nurse should use the position, knowledge, and skills.

Nurse's Chosen Role

Nurses can act as content experts, helping communities to select and attain task-related goals. In our example of suspected infant malnutrition, the nurse used epidemiological skills to determine the incidence and prevalence of malnutrition. The nurse also served as a process expert by increasing the community's own capabilities in documenting the problem rather than by merely contributing her substantive expertise.

The roles of fact gatherer, analyst, and program implementor differ from those of enabler-catalyst, teacher of problem-solving skills, and activist-advocate (Rothman, 1974b). Bodenstein (1974) considers the former as change agent roles and the latter as change partner roles. Community health nurses, like other health professionals, are often taught to impose change, to act as change agents rather than as change partners. We can, however, respond with more flexibility.

The role the nurse chooses also depends on the nature of the health problem and the community's decision-making ability as well as on professional and personal preferences. Some health problems clearly necessitate certain intervention roles. If a community lacks democratic problem-solving abilities, the nurse may select teacher, facilitator, and advocate roles. Problem-solving skills must be explained and modeled. A problem with ascertaining the status of community health, on the other hand, frequently requires fact-gatherer and analyst roles. Some problems, such as the example of suspected infant malnutrition, require multiple roles. In that case, managing conflict among the involved health care providers demanded process skills; collecting and interpreting the data necessary to document the problem required both interpersonal and analytical skills.

The community's history of participation in decision making is a critical factor. In a community skilled in identifying and successfully managing its problems, the nurse may appropriately serve as technical expert or advisor. Quite different roles may be required if the community lacks problem-solving skills or has a history of unsuccessful change efforts. The nurse may have to focus on developing problem-

solving capabilities or achieving one successful change so that the community becomes empowered to assume responsibility for promoting change on its own behalf.

The nurse's role also depends on the social change process. Not all communities are receptive to innovation. Innovation is often inversely related to the extent to which a community adheres to traditional norms and directly related to high socioeconomic status, a perceived need for change, the presence of liberal, scientific, and democratic values, and a high level of social participation by community residents (Rogers, 1983, Rothman 1974a).

The innovation itself affects its acceptance. Innovations with the highest adoption rates are those perceived as relatively more advantageous than the other alternatives, compatible with existing values, amenable to a limited trial before full-scale adoption, easily explained or demonstrated, geographically accessible, and simple (Rogers, 1983, Rothman, 1974a). For example, community residents might go to an immunization clinic rather than a private physician if the clinic is nearby and less expensive and if the physician is not available when needed.

The final variable in the social change process is the diffusion and adoption process. Innovations are accepted more readily when the diffusion and adoption process is compatible with the community's norms, values, and customs and when information is relayed through the appropriate communication mode (the mass media for early adopters and face-to-face for late adopters), other communities support the change efforts, opinion leaders are identified and used, and communication about the innovation is clear and unambiguous (Rogers, 1983, Rothman 1974a).

Because the factors that shape implementation are multiple and their effect on the change process complex and varying, the community health nurse must be adaptable. The roles used to initiate change may differ from those used to maintain or stabilize it. And the roles required to initiate, maintain, and stabilize change may vary from community to community and from one intervention to another within the same community. Thus the nurse must be skilled in a variety of implementation mechanisms, which are considered in the following section.

Implementation Mechanisms

Implementation mechanisms are the vehicles, or modes, by which innovations are transferred from the planners to the units of service. The community health nurse *alone* is never considered an implementation mechanism, for change on behalf of the community client requires *multiple* implementation mechanisms. The nurse must identify and use appropriately all aids relevant to intervention. Some important implementation mechanisms, or aids, include small interacting groups, lay advisors, the mass media, and health policy.

Small *interacting groups,* formal and informal, are essential implementation mechanisms. Many of the formal groups in the community—families, legislative bodies, health-care recipients, and service providers—are fully considered elsewhere in the text. Some of the informal groups, such as neighborhoods and social-action groups, have also been discussed. The common tie among these diverse groups is their location between the community and individual levels. Because of their intermediate position, they can and do act both to support and to constrain change efforts at the community and individual levels. They are potentially powerful simply because they are mediating structures (Berger and Neuhaus, 1977).

Consequently the community health nurse needs to ascertain which groups view the proposed change as beneficial and which do not. New small groups may need to be formed to facilitate the change, and accommodations may be necessary in the innovation or in the diffusion process to increase receptivity. Initially the innovation may have to be directed to groups with a majority of *early adopters* (those with broad perspectives and abilities to adopt new ideas from mass media information sources) and to groups whose goals are like those of the intervention plan (Rothman, 1974a).

Lay advisors, individuals who are influential in approving or vetoing new ideas and from whom others seek advice and information about new ideas (Rothman, 1974a), often perform a similar function to that of early adopters. Lay advisors, or opinion leaders, are characterized by conformity to community norms, heavy involvement in formal service organizations and informal social groups, specific areas of expertise, and a slightly higher social status than their followers (Rogers, 1983; Warnecke et al., 1976). In community-health literature they are frequently referred to as health facilitators (Salber, 1981; Salber et al., 1976), village health workers (Kingma, 1975), health guides (Warnecke et al., 1976), opinion leaders (Lorig and Walters, 1980-1981), and lay advisors (Salber, 1979; Service and Salber, 1977). These persons are also called gatekeepers and key informants.

Irrespective of their title, lay advisors are helpful in community-oriented intervention. In one study, they increased breast self-examination practices among Latina women by about 40% (Lorig and Walters, 1980-1981). In another study, rural blacks in North Carolina received more arthritis care from lay advisors than from physicians (Salber, 1981).

Both small interacting groups and lay advisors are particularly useful in instituting change among late adopters. But groups dominated by early adopters and lay advisors can be reached through the mass media. *Mass media* is typically an impersonal and formal type of communication and is useful in providing information quickly to large numbers of people. Using mass media is efficient because the proportion of resources expended to population covered is low and populations can be targeted. For example, information about teenage pregnancy is more efficiently disseminated through rock music stations than through classical music stations.

In addition to being efficient, the mass media are effective aids in intervention. The Stanford Heart Disease Three Community Program showed that community residents subject to media-only intervention increased their knowledge about cardiovascular risk factors and improved their dietary patterns. Community residents subject to the mass media campaign and face-to-face intervention also, obviously, reduced their cardiovascular risk (Maccoby et al.,

1977). Similar findings have been reported from the North Karelia study in Finland (McAlister et al., 1982).

Health policy can also play a critical part in the adoption of healthful community-oriented change (Milio, 1981). The major intent of a public policy in the health field is to address collective human needs, and it frequently serves to constrain individual choice for the public good. For instance, drivers have been urged for several years to wear automobile seatbelts. However, the incidence of automobile fatalities was not reduced until recently, when drivers were required to observe lowered speed limits and, in some states, to wear seat belts and use special restraining seats for children. Obviously health policy can facilitate interventions that promote community health.

If public policy that will encourage or even simply allow health-generating choices is to be enacted, the community health nurse must actively lobby for it. The nurse must also use small groups, lay advisors, and the mass media as aids to implementation. Working with naturally occurring small groups like the family and with lay advisors is familiar to most community health nurses. Working with legislators and the mass media is less familiar. Yet all resources must be used to achieve healthful change in the community client.

Using a small group to initiate community-oriented change is illustrated in the Progress Notes of the COHR (see Figure 13-5). A plan using lay advisors is outlined in the Plan Sheet of the COHR (see Figure 13-6).

All implementation efforts, no matter what mechanisms are used, must be documented. The Progress Notes of the CNP's interventions to document infant malnutrition are displayed in Figure 13-7. Evaluation is also important to determine and improve the effectiveness of community-oriented nursing practice and thereby increase our knowledge base and improve our success in competing for funds.

EVALUATING INTERVENTION FOR COMMUNITY HEALTH

Simply defined, *evaluation* is the appraisal of the effects of some organized activity or program. It may involve the design and conduct of evaluation research, in which social science research methods are used to determine program effectiveness, efficiency, adequacy, appropriateness, and unintended consequences (Kane, et al., 1974). Evaluation may also involve the more elementary process of assessing progress by contrasting the objectives and the results. Because Chapter 11 is devoted to program planning and evaluation in community health, and because comprehensive references are readily available (American Nurses' Association, 1976; Rossi and Freeman, 1985), this section deals with the basic approach of contrasting objectives and results.

Evaluation began in the planning phase, when establishing goals and measurable objectives and identifying goal-attaining activities was achieved. After implementing intervention, only the accomplishment of objectives and the effects of intervention activities have to be assessed. The Progress Notes of the COHR direct the nurse to perform such appraisals concurrently with implementation. In assessing the data recorded there, the nurse is requested to evaluate whether the objectives were achieved and whether

Progress Notes

Name of community: _____ *Jefferson County* _____

Goal: _____ *To document and, if appropriate, reduce the incidence and* _____

_____ *prevalence of infant malnutrition* _____

Date	Narrative, Assessment, Plan (NAP)	Budget, Time
	(Record both objective and subjective data. Interpret these data in terms of whether the	
	objectives were achieved and whether the intervenor activities used were effective. The plan is	
	dependent on the assessment and may include both new or revised objectives and activities.)	
2-14-87	*Objective 1, Means 4*	
	Narrative: Meeting to develop needs assessment was attended by CNP, 2 WIC personnel,	
	and physicians from health department, neighborhood health center, and local medical	
	society. Consensus rapidly achieved among 5 of 6 participants that goal, objectives, and	
	means (especially Objective 1, Means 4) were appropriate. Physician representing medical	
	society consistently objected, stating vehemently that private sector had long provided	
	adequate medical care for area youngsters. One WIC staff member angrily questioned how	
	physican could document "adequacy." Physician responded that federal aid created more	
	need than disease did. He would not recommend that medical society support the effort. CNP	
	cowered, afraid that this would jeopardize entire effort. Eventually, however, physician left, and	
	plans were made to develop and conduct needs assessment, with or without the medical	
	society's help.	
	Agenda: CNP to develop needs assessment tool with WIC personnel and health systems agency	
	planner. Physicians to develop list of providers to be contacted. Neighborhood health center	
	physician to get a place on medical society agenda and attempt to clarify our plans. WIC per-	
	sonnel to contact nonphysician health workers to introduce plan and develop provider list.	
	Assessment: Plans made to proceed with needs assessment and partner support essential	*$100 2 hours meeting*
	to accomplishment of objective. Group process problematical, and CNP ineffective due to	*and 2 hours*
	discomfort with conflict between physician and WIC staff member.	*preparation*
	Plans: Meeting scheduled for 2-28-87 to deal with agreed-on agenda.	
	* Before 2-28 meeting, CNP will discuss ways of better handling conflict with consultation*	
	group, collaborate in drafting needs assessment, and telephone others by 2-21 to determine	
	their progress.	
	* J. Goeppinger, RN, CNP*	

FIGURE 13-7

Progress notes.

the intervention activities used were effective, and to decide whether the costs in money and time were commensurate with the benefits. This process is depicted in Figure 13-7. Here the nurse has noted progress toward the needs assessment and difficulties encountered in handling conflict among the group members.

Such an evaluation process is oriented to community health because the intervention goals and objectives are derived from the nurse's and the community's conceptions of health. Simplistic as it appears, it is not without problems. The lack of a control community or even adequate baseline information casts doubts about attributing success, or failure, to the intervention. Nursing interventions may also have such diffuse and therefore weak effects that our crude measures do not discern them. Models for the practitioner to use in determining cost-benefit and cost-effectiveness figures are not commonplace. And, finally, the lay role in evaluation has never been fully accepted. Professionals have adopted partnership in assessment and implementation more readily than in evaluation. The issue of who has the power to define, judge, and institute change in professional activities is by no means resolved.

CLINICAL APPLICATION

The problem of suspected infant malnutrition has been used to illustrate the application of the nursing process to promote community health. Examples of the COHR worksheets have been included to depict most stages of the process.

The community-oriented nursing process has also been used in a wide variety of other situations. Several case studies that depict both community-oriented assessment and intervention have recently been published. Muecke (1984) describes the diagnosis of a Laotian refugee community's health problems. She and her students used a thought process much like the one we have described to identify several health risks, including the risks of having accidents and being vandalized, robbed, or raped. Risk identification was the initial step towards achieving the goal of primary prevention. Nursing interventions to reduce the risks were not presented, but might very well have included working with Mein community leaders, the landlords, and the police and fire departments. Follow-up at the household level was mentioned.

Likewise in a case study of Bolton, a small town in northeastern Pennsylvania, Rogers (1984) discusses how a community risk profile was developed. She describes population characteristics such as age profiles, education levels, unemployment rates, and vital statistics. She also presents an analysis of community systems, such as government, communication, religion, and recreation systems. Assets and liabilities; that is, community-health strengths and problems, are identified, and community-health diagnoses

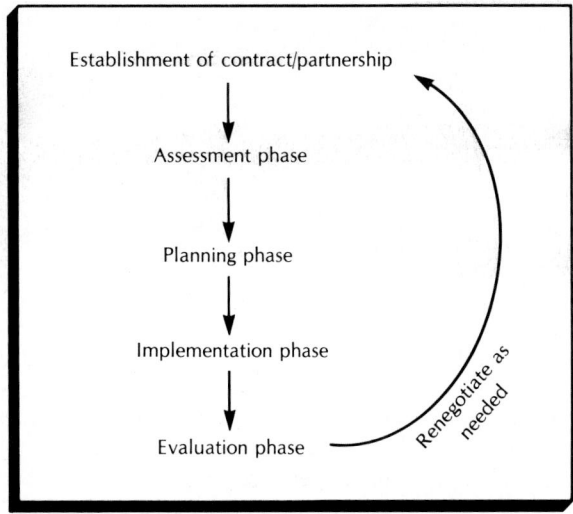

FIGURE 13-8

Summary flow sheet illustrating the nursing process with the community client.

formulated. The rationale for identifying one problem, wife abuse, is described. Changes initiated are listed, and results delineated. They involve using community groups and leaders.

SUMMARY

This chapter has described and illustrated the definition of community client as the target of service; the key concepts of community, community health, and partnership for health; and the nursing process of assessment, planning, implementation, and evaluation to promote community health. This entire process is summarized in Figure 13-8.

Community-oriented nursing practice emphasizes the community as the nurse's client. Healthful change is sought with and for the community client. Community health is the goal of practice and partnership the chief means of practice.

Using the nursing process as a tool for community-oriented practice includes assessment, planning, implementation, and evaluation. Assessment of a community uses a variety of techniques, including interviews, observation, analysis of existing data, and surveys. A variety of assessment guides, such as the one in Appendix E, guide this process. The planning stage of the community nursing process includes performing problem analysis and prioritization, establishing goals and objectives, and identifying implementation alternatives. Several factors affect implementation, including the nurse's chosen role and the mechanisms available for implementation. The final stage of the community-oriented nursing process is evaluation.

≡ KEY CONCEPTS

Most definitions of community include three dimensions: (1) networks of interpersonal relationships that provide friendship and support to members; (2) residence in a common locality; and (3) "solidarity, sentiments, and activities."

A community is defined as a locality-based entity, composed of systems of formal organizations reflecting societal institutions, informal groups, and aggregates that are interdependent and whose function or expressed intent is to meet a wide variety of collective needs.

A community practice setting is insufficient reason for saying practice is oriented toward the community client. When the location of the practice is in the community but the focus of the practice is the individual or family, then the nursing client remains the individual or family—not the whole community.

Community-oriented practice is targeted to the community, the population group with which healthful change is sought.

Community health as used in this chapter is defined as the meeting of collective needs through identifying problems and managing interactions within the community itself and between the community and the larger society.

Most changes aimed at improving community health involve, of necessity, partnerships among community residents and health workers from a variety of disciplines.

Assessing community health requires gathering existing data, generating missing data, and interpreting the data base.

Five methods of collecting data useful to the community health nurse are informant interviewers, participant observation, secondary analysis of existing data, surveys, and windshield surveys.

Gaining entry or acceptance into the community is perhaps the biggest challenge in assessment. The community health nurse is usually an outsider and often represents an established health care system that is neither known nor trusted by community members, who may react with indifference or even active hostility.

The planning phase includes analyzing and establishing priorities among community health problems already identified, establishing goals and objectives, and identifying intervention activities that will accomplish the objectives.

Once high-priority problems are identified, broad relevant goals and objectives are developed.

The goal, generally a broad statement of desired outcome, and objectives, the precise statements of the desired outcome, are carefully selected.

Intervention activities, the means by which objectives are met, are the strategies that clarify what must be done to achieve the objectives, the ways change will be affected, and the way the problem will be interrupted.

Implementation, the third phase of the nursing process, is transforming a plan for improved community health into achievement of goals and objectives.

Simply defined, evaluation is the appraisal of the effects of some organized activity or program.

LEARNING ACTIVITIES

1. Observe an occupational health nurse, community health nurse, school nurse, family nurse practitioner, or emergency room nurse for several hours. Determine which of the nurse's activities are community-oriented and state the reasons for your judgment.

2. Using your own community as a frame of reference, develop examples illustrating the concepts of community, community client, community health, and partnership for health.

3. Read your local newspaper and identify articles illustrating the concepts of community, community client, community health, and partnership for health.

4. Using any two of the conditions of community competence given in the chapter, analyze your own community briefly. Give examples of each condition.

BIBLIOGRAPHY

American Nurses' Association: A guide for community-based nursing services, Kansas City, Mo., 1985, The Association.

American Nurses' Association: Issues in evaluation research, Kansas City, Mo., 1976, The Association.

Anderson, E.T.: Community focus in public health nursing: whose responsibility? Nurs. Outlook 31:44-48,

Anderson, E., McFarlane, J., and Helton, A.: Community-as-client: a model for practice, Nurs. Outlook 34:220-224, 1986.

Archer, S.E.: Community nurse practitioners: another assessment, Nurs. Outlook 24:499-503, 1976.

Archer, S.E., and Fleshman, R.P.: Community health nursing: a typology of practice, Nurs. Outlook 23:358-364, 1975.

Archer, S.E., Kelly, C.D., and Bisch, S.A.: Implementing change in communities: a collaborative process, St. Louis, 1984, The C.V. Mosby Co.

Babbie, E.: The practice of social research, ed. 4, Belmont, Ca., 1986, Wadsworth Publishing Co.

Berger, P.L., and Neuhaus, P.J.: To empower people, the role of mediating structures in public policy, Washington, D.C., 1977, American Enterprise Institute for Public Policy Research.

Blum, H.L.: Planning for health, New York, 1974, Human Sciences Press, Inc.

Bodenstein, J.W.: The role of health professionals—Africanization in mission hospitals, Contact 21:3-10, 1974.

Buhler-Wilkerson, K.: Public health nursing: in sickness or in health? Am. J. Public Health 75:1155-1161, 1985.

Combs-Orme, T., Reis, J., and Ward, L.D.: Effectiveness of home visits by public health nurses in maternal and child health: an empirical review, Public Health Rep. 100:490-499, 1985.

Connor, D.M.: Understanding your community, Oakville, Ontario, 1969, Development Press.

Cottrell, L.S.: The competent community. In Kaplan, B.H., Wilson, R.N., and Leighton, A.H., editors: Further explorations in social psychiatry, New York, 1976, Basic Books, Inc., Publishers.

Delbecq, A.L., and Van de Ven, A.H.: A group process model for problem identification and program planning, J. Appl. Behav. Sci. 4:466-492, 1971.

Dever, G.E.A.: Community health analysis: a holistic approach, Germantown, Md., 1980, Aspen Systems Corp.

Feuerstein, M.T.: Participatory evaluation—an appropriate technology for community health programmes, Contact 55:1-8, 1980.

Filstead, W.J.: Qualitative methodology, firsthand involvement with the social world, Chicago, 1972, Markham Publishing Co.

Flexner, W.A., and Littlefield, J.E.: Comment on alternative methods for health priority assessment, J. Community Health 2:245 and 246, 1977.

Freeman, R.B.: The dilemma of public health nursing today, redesigning nursing education for public health, Bethesda, Md., 1973, United States Department of Health, Education and Welfare, Division of Nursing.

Glazer, M.: The research adventure, promise and problems of fieldwork, New York, 1972, Random House, Inc.

Goeppinger, J.: Primary health care: an answer to the dilemmas of community nursing? Public Health Nurs. 1:129-140, 1984.

Goeppinger, J., and Baglioni, A.J., Jr.: Community competence: a positive approach to needs assessment, Am. J. Community Psychol. 13:507-523, 1986.

Goeppinger, J., Lassiter, P.G., and Wilcox, B.: Community health is community competence, Nurs. Outlook 30(8):464-467, 1982.

Hamilton, P.: Community nursing diagnosis, Adv. Nurs. Sci. 5:21-36, 1985.

Hanchett, E.S.: Community health assessment: a conceptual tool kit, New York, 1979, John Wiley & Sons, Inc.

Hunter, A.: The loss of community: an empirical test through replication, Am. Sociol. Rev. 40:537-552, 1975.

Kane, R.L., Herson, R., and Deniston, O.L.: Program evaluation: is it worth it? In Kane, R.L., editor: The challenges of community medicine, New York, 1974, Springer Publishing Co., Inc.

Kark, S.: Epidemiology and community medicine, New York, 1974, Appleton-Century-Crofts.

Kark, S.L.: The practice of community-oriented primary health care, New York, 1981, Appleton-Century-Crofts.

Kingma, S.J., ed.: Primary health care and the village health worker, Contact 25:4-12, 1975.

Kluckhohn, F.: The participant-observer technique in small communities, Am. J. Sociol. 46:331-343, 1940.

Lorig, K., and Walters, E.G.: Cuidaremos: the HECO approach to breast self-examination, Int. Q. Community Health Educ. 1:125-134, 1980-1981.

Luloff, A.E., and Wilkinson, K.P.: Is the community alive and well in the inner city? Am. Sociologist 42:827-828, 1977.

Maccoby, N., Farquhar, J.W., Wood, P.D., and Alexander, J.: Reducing the risk of cardiovascular disease: effects of a community-based campaign on knowledge and behavior, J. Community Health 3:100-114, 1977.

Mahler, H.: The meaning of "health for all by the year 2000," World Health Forum 2:5-22, 1981.

McAlister, A., Puska, P., Salonen, J.T., et al.: Theory and action for health promotion: illustrations from the North Karelia project, Am. J. Public Health 72:43-50, 1982.

Milio, N.: Promoting health through public policy, Philadelphia, 1981, F.A. Davis Co.

Miller, M.K., and Stokes, C.S.: Health status, health resources, and consolidated structural parameters. Implications for public health care policy, J. Health Soc. Behav. 19:263-279, 1978.

Mooney, A., and Rives, N.W., Jr.: Measures of community health status for health planning, Health Serv. Res. 2:129-145, 1978.

Muecke, M.A.: Community health diagnosis in nursing, Public Health Nurs. 1:23-33, 1984.

Neuber, K.A.: Needs assessment: a model for community planning, Beverly Hills, Cal., 1980, Sage Publications, Inc.

Pesznecker, B., and McNeil, J.: Collaborative practice models in community health nursing, Nurs. Outlook 30:298-302, 1984.

Polit, D.F., and Hungler, B.P.: Observational methods. In Nursing research, principles and methods, Philadelphia, 1983, J.B. Lippincott Co.

Rogers, E.: Diffusion of innovations, ed. 3, New York, 1983, Free Press.

Rogers, S.S.: Community as client: a multivariate model for analysis of community aggre-

gate health risk, Public Health Nurs. 1:210-222, 1984.

Rossi, P.H., and Freeman, H.E.: Evaluation, a systematic approach, Beverly Hills, Cal., 1985, Sage Publications, Inc.

Rothman, J.: Planning and organizing for social change, action principles from social science research, New York, 1974a, Columbia University Press.

Rothman, J.: Three models of community organization practice. In Cox, F., et al., editors: Strategies in community organization: a book of readings, Itasca, Ill., 1974b, F.E. Peacock Publishers, Inc.

Ruffing-Rahal, M.A.: Qualitative methods in community analysis, Public Health Nurs. 2:130-137, 1985.

Ryan, W.: Blaming the victim, New York, 1976, Vintage Books.

Salber, E.J.: Where does primary health care begin? The health facilitator as a central figure in primary care, Isr. J. Med. Sci. 17:100-111, 1981.

Salber, E.J.: The lay advisor as community health resource, J. Health Polit. Policy Law 3:469-478, 1979.

Salber, E.J., Beery, W.L., and Jackson, E.J.R.: The role of the health facilitator in community health education, J. Community Health 2:5-20, 1976.

Scutchfield, F.D.: Alternative methods for health priority assessment, J. Community Health 1:29-38, 1975.

Seaman, C.C., and Verhonick, P.J.: Research methods for undergraduate students in nursing, New York, 1982, Appleton-Century-Crofts.

Shamansky, S.L., and Pesznecker, B.: A community is, Nurs. Outlook 29:182-185, 1981.

Sills, G.M., and Goeppinger, J.: The community as a field of inquiry in nursing. In Werley, H.H., and Fitzpatrick, J.J., editors: Annual review of nursing research, New York, 1985, Springer Publishing Co., Inc.

Skrovan, C., Anderson, E.T., and Gottschalk, J.: Community nurse practitioner: an emerging role, Am. J. Public Health 64:847-853, 1974.

Spero, J.: Issues and concerns in graduate education in public health nursing, Unpublished paper presented at American Public Health Association Convention, Washington, D.C., 1977.

Storfjell, J.L., and Cruise, P.A.: A model of community-focused nursing, Public Health Nurs. 1:85-96, 1984.

Suttles, G.D.: The social construction of communities, Chicago, 1972, University of Chicago Press.

Tinkham, C.W., Voorhies, E.F., and McCarthy, N.C.: Community health nursing, evolution and process in the family and community, New York, 1984, Appleton-Century-Crofts.

Turner, J.H.: The structure of sociological theory, Chicago, 1982, Dorsey Press.

Warnecke, R.B., Mosher, W., Graham, S., and Montgomery, E.B.: Health guides as influentials in central Buffalo, J. Health Soc. Behav. 17:22-34, 1976.

Wellman, B., and Leighton, B.: Networks, neighborhoods, and communities: approaches to the study of the community question, Urban Affairs Q. 14:363-390, 1979.

Williams, C.A.: Community health nursing—what is it? Nurs. Outlook 25:250-254, 1977.

Wilson, H.S.: Research in nursing, Menlo Park, Cal., 1985, Addison-Wesley Publishing Co., Inc.

Wilson, R.N.: Editorial note to the competent community. In Kaplan, B.H., Wilson, R.N., and Leighton, A., editors: Further explorations in social psychiatry, New York, 1976, Basic Books, Inc., Publishers.

Wood, J., and Ohlson, V.: Graduate preparation for community health nursing practice. In Miller, M.H., and Flynn, B.C., editors: Cur-

rent perspectives in nursing: social issues and trends, St. Louis, 1977, The C.V. Mosby Co.

World Health Organization: Community health nursing: report of a WHO expert committee, Tech. Rep. Series No. 558, Geneva, 1974, World Health Organization.

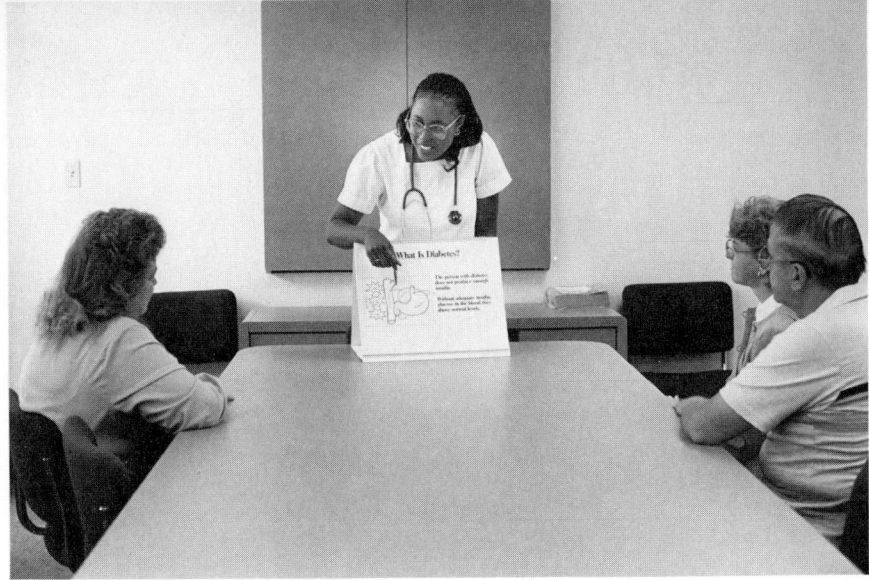

Peggye Guess Lassiter

14

WORKING WITH GROUPS IN THE COMMUNITY

OBJECTIVES

After reading this chapter, the student should be able to:

Describe member interaction and group purpose as the major elements of a group.

Describe the effect of cohesion on group effectiveness.

Identify the influence of group norms on group members.

Appreciate the usefulness of groups in promoting individual health.

Describe nursing behaviors that assist groups in promoting health for individuals.

Identify the groups constituting a community and illustrate links between them.

Describe the role of the community health nurse working with established groups toward community health goals.

KEY TERMS

cohesion

communication structure

conflict

established groups

group purpose

group structure

informal groups

leadership

maintenance function

norms

role structure

selected membership groups

subsystems

task function

Working with groups is an important skill for community nursing. Groups are an effective and powerful vehicle for initiating and implementing healthful changes for individuals, families, organizations, and the community. Community health nurses work with groups because individuals naturally form groups in their home setting and because the community's health is dramatically influenced by the groups composing the community. A deliberate use of groups for health should be based on an understanding of group concepts, practice in group work, and appreciation of the utility of group process.

All nurses have group experience. In daily practice nurses routinely plan and implement health-focused action with clients, other nurses, and other health care workers. Nurses often participate in groups in which they are encouraged to observe their own responses to the membership and leadership. Such study and experience enrich a person's knowledge of group concepts and application to groups of clients, work groups, and community groups.

Additionally, groups are often an inexpensive mode by which information is communicated, decisions made, and issues and concerns handled. As discussed in Chapter 10, community health nurses often use groups to communicate health information to a group of clients who can come together once or on a regular basis to receive the same type of assistance, rather then repeating the information several times to individuals. In an era of decreasing resources, groups are becoming an increasingly popular format for community health nursing intervention.

Groups hold power for individuals and communities, and this power lies in the ability to bring about change. Changes are often needed to improve health and well-being for individuals and communities. Groups are crucial for the development of individuals, and some individual changes for health are possible to achieve with group support and encouragement; these changes would be difficult or impossible to attain without that support. The attitudes that individuals have are developed in kin and friendship groups; continued membership throughout life in other groups influences thoughts, choices, behaviors, and values. People tend to find their social needs met through association with others, and groups are a natural vehicle meeting for these needs.

Groups form for varied reasons; they may form to address a clearly stated purpose or goal, or the purpose may seem somewhat vague. They may form naturally as individuals are attracted to each other by shared values, interests, activities, or personal characteristics. On the other hand, people may come together to accomplish a task and become a group even when personal attraction is low.

Community groups represent the collective interests, needs, and values of individuals; they provide a link between the individual and the larger social system. Through groups people may express personal views and relate them to those of others. Groups serve the whole community as communication networks and may be viewed as an organization of community parts. Identifying groups, their goals, member characteristics, and their place in the community structure is an important first step toward understanding the community and assessing its health. Through community groups nurses assist people to identify priority health needs and capabilities and implement community changes.

GROUP CONCEPTS

The basic group concepts described in this section may be used in nursing practice to promote individual health through group work, to identify community groups and their contributions to community life, and to assist groups in working toward community health goals.

Group Definition

A group is a collection of interacting individuals who have a common purpose or purposes. Each member influences and is in turn influenced by every other member to some extent. The members' characteristics bring a composition to the group that in part determines the degree and kind of influence among them. Key elements in this definition of group are member interaction and group purpose (Figure 14-1).

The following examples illustrate member interaction and group purposes. First, families are a unique example of community groups and the most familiar group form. Family purposes are numerous, including psychological support, and socialization of their members. Usually families share kinship bonds, common living space, and economic resources. Interactions are diverse and frequent because of the multiple ties between members and the particular functions delegated to families by society. Group concepts offer one study approach to family groups.

A second example is groups formed in response to par-

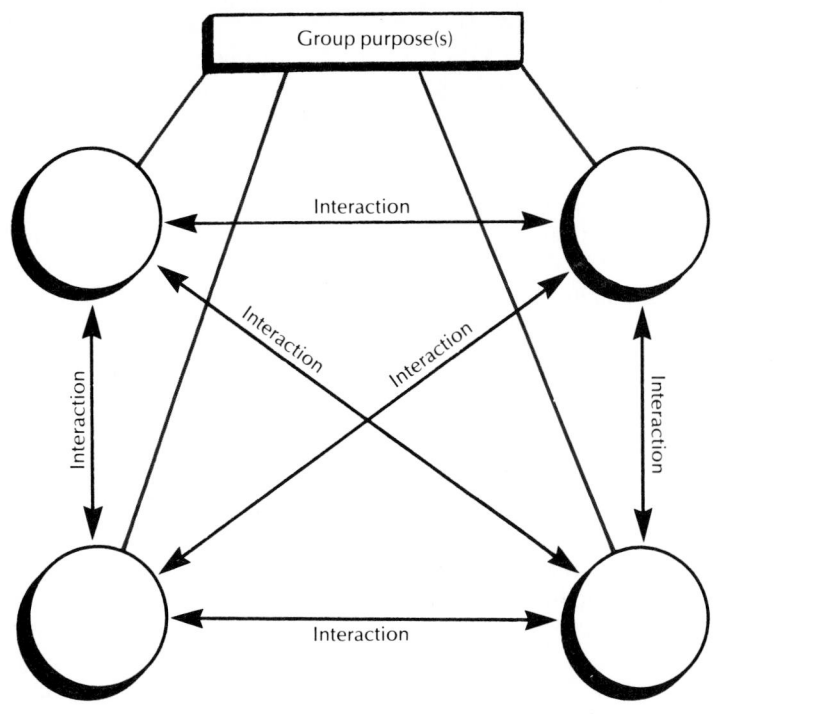

FIGURE 14-1

A group is a collection of interacting individuals who have a common purpose or purposes.

ticular community needs. The purpose of such community groups is to address specific problems or opportunities. For example, in one community residents banded together to form a neighborhood association to protect their health and welfare. This neighborhood of upper middle-class homes was located in an unincorporated area. Over a period of 3 years the residents were threatened with multiple environmental hazards, including forest fire (fire hydrants had been overlooked in developing part of the area), establishment of a small airport near the homes, and construction of an interstate highway adjacent to the homes. To protect their interests residents formed a neighborhood association and elected officers to represent their interests in a constructive manner.

Groups in the community often occur spontaneously because of mutual attraction between individuals and obvious and keenly felt personal needs. Young and single adults sharing similar desires for socialization and recreation are likely to form loosely structured groups. Through parties and other social meetings the young adults establish themselves in new ways of behaving and relating. They select partners, test ideas and attitudes, and establish their identity within a group of people with similar developmental needs. The unstated purpose is to test and become familiar in adult roles. Interactions between members serve to establish relationships appropriate to developing adult needs.

A fourth example is health-promoting groups, which are formed as individuals meet in the community and health care settings and discover common challenges to their physical and emotional well-being. The purposes of health-promoting groups are to improve health for the members and to master specific threats to health. Chapters of Alcoholics Anonymous, Parents without Partners, and La Leche League illustrate such health-promoting groups. Interactions between members are personally supportive and include group problem solving and education. Like other groups organized in response to community issues, health-promoting groups usually organize around particular purposes, and member interactions facilitate work toward those purposes. These groups may be either of two types; established groups or selected membership groups, both of which are discussed later in this chapter.

How do purpose and interaction vary in these four examples? For some groups purpose is obvious and may be easily stated by members. This is true for groups organized to address specific community needs or health challenges. For families, social groupings, and many spontaneously formed groups the purposes are unstated. However, the purpose for the groups can be determined by studying their activities as a group over a period of time. Highly personal and multipurpose groupings serve individual and collective needs in concrete, function-oriented ways and in subtle, less obvious ways.

Purpose and member interaction are important components of all groups, but the expression of purpose, the manner of member interaction, and the intensity of the interaction vary. Group purposes and member interactions help distinguish the group's function for its members and the community.

Group Purpose

When the need for particular health changes is established and group work is selected as the most effective intervention, a purpose or goal for a proposed group must be stated. Clear statement and presentation of this purpose are essential in establishing criteria for member selection. A group purpose clearly stated facilitates recruitment of prospective members to the group.

Such a clear statement of purpose facilitated new group formation in one housing development (in Xeona.) There were numerous reports of child abuse and neglect according to the local department of social services. Routine home visits for well-child care documented high stress between parents and their offspring, and some parents requested guidance from the community health nurse in child discipline. The community health nurse thought that a parent group would best address this community need. Nurses who were involved selected the following purpose for the group: "Dealing with kids for child and parent satisfaction." The purpose showed process, to help parents deal with kids, and the desirable outcome, satisfaction for parents and children. As potential members were approached, this statement of purpose for the group helped the individuals decide whether or not they wanted to join.

Appeals for membership may be public, with all who elect to join accepted. In such situations the membership is self-selected, based on the stated group purpose. In this type of recruitment adequate publicity must be available to those in need of particular health changes. Prospective members often wish to discuss the purpose with leaders or clarify questions concerning the purpose at the first group meeting. Their commitment to the health group is partly based on individual goals and how well the group goal satisfies their personal objectives.

Cohesion

The measure of attraction between members and to the group is called *cohesion.* This pull to each other, to the group, and to its purposes operates for an overall group valence or attraction measurement. Individuals in a highly cohesive group identify themselves as a unit, work toward common goals, are willing to endure frustration for the sake of the group, and defend the group against outside criticism. Attraction is increased when members feel accepted by others, see like qualities in each other, perceive that others like them, and believe they share similar attitudes and values (Figure 14-2). Some individual attributes that influence attraction between members include physical and interpersonal characteristics, behaviors, skills, knowledge, beliefs, and values. Members' traits that increase group cohesion and productivity include (1) congruence between personal goals and those of the group, (2) attraction to group goals, (3) attraction to other selected members, (4) distribution of leading and following skills, and (5) existence of problem-solving skills.

Functions of members that facilitate movement toward the group purpose are termed *task functions.* These task-directed abilities of any member improve her attractiveness. These traits include cognitive ability in problem solving, access to material resources, and skills in directing. Of equal importance are abilities to provide affirmation and support for individuals in the group; these functions that help members to stay with the group and feel accepted are termed *maintenance functions.* The ability to help people resolve conflicts and ensure social and environmental comfort is also a maintenance function. Task and maintenance functions are

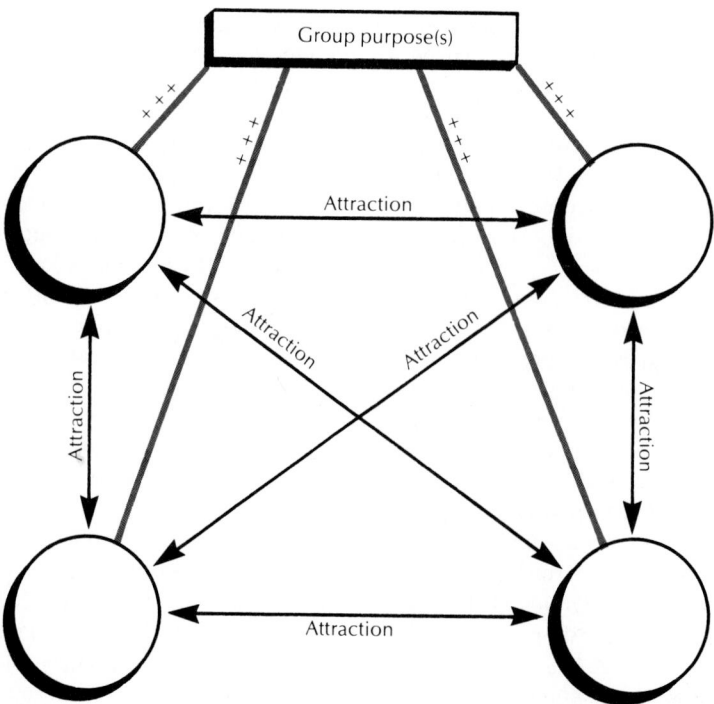

FIGURE 14-2

Cohesion is the measure of attraction between members and member attraction to group purpose(s).

necessary to group progress. Naturally, those members who supply such group requirements are attractive, and an abundance of such traits within the membership tends to increase group cohesion.

Members' attributes held in low regard or judged as personally repulsive or threatening decrease attraction toward those members and the group. Behaviors and attitudes that are poorly understood by others in the group also tend to decrease group cohesion.

Commonly shared characteristics usually contribute to the group attraction for members, whereas differences tend to decrease attractiveness. Members' perceptions of differences can create marked competition and jealousy. However, differences in members' characteristics increase group cohesion if they support complementary functioning or provide contrasting viewpoints necessary for decision making. Cohesion factors are complex; multiple influences affect member attraction to each other and to the group goal. Group productivity and member satisfaction are positively affected by high group cohesion. Two group examples illustrate factors that influence group cohesion and result in effectiveness.

A community health nurse initiated and provided beginning leadership for a group of clients who had been treated for burns. Ten residents, all from one town, had been discharged in 3 months from the local burn unit. The stated purpose for the group was to assist members in the difficult transition from hospital to home. Each individual had been treated for extensive burns in an intensive care treatment center; had relied heavily on health workers for physical, social, and emotional rehabilitation; and had faced the challenge of resuming work and family roles. Individuals shared some similar experiences and hopes for the future. The individuals varied in the amount of trauma and stress experienced, and they differed widely in psychological readiness for return to ordinary daily routines. One woman was able to return quickly to her job as cashier in a large supermarket. The strength of her determination to overcome public reaction to her scars, coupled with an ability to "use the right words" and empathy for others, distinguished her from others in the group. These differences proved very attractive to other members, inspiring them to work toward a return to their own roles in life. Her differences were perceived as attainable by other members. The cohesion for this group was in the member attraction to the common purpose of returning, after hospitalization, to successful life patterns, including work, and managing relations with others. Each member also believed that others with similar burn experiences could facilitate goal attainment. This example shows that certain member experiences, such as crises or traumas, although they are not highly valued by group members, may help individuals define their life situations as similar to each other and may increase member attraction.

Being different from the general population and like the other group members is for some a compelling force for the group. (For others, conversely, it repels them from the group because they cannot tolerate the thought of their own likeness to some aversive characteristic such as disfigurement.) Empathy for another's pain, learned only through mutual experience, may provide each individual with a required perspective for problem solving or validation of reality. The nurse in this example helped members use common experiences and learn from their differences.

Differences created tension in one self-help group for victims of spouse abuse; in this group nurses met a severe challenge stemming from the differences they presented as nonvictims. The community health nurses had been invited by professional staff to assist the group in its process and to provide health information as needed. Victim members of the group felt that the nurses could not truly understand the intensely personal and devastating injury each had experienced and told the nurses so. They initially isolated the nurses from membership but tolerated their presence. Attraction of the group diminished, and attendance at meetings fell. Discussion of superficial issues occupied group time as the victim members avoided topics of member safety and violence in general. The nurses encouraged all the members to describe experiences seen as threatening to self-respect in their family and work roles. The nurses revealed some of their own struggles for responsible self-direction and control. Group members supported one another to assert individual rights for safety, to locate employment, to make living arrangements necessary for independence from the abuser, and to identify needs for personal interactional changes. Cohesive forces for responsible status and the clear purpose of maintaining member safety contributed to successful group work.

Members' attraction to the group depends also on the nature of the group. The group programs, size, type of organization, and position in the community are influencing factors. When goals are perceived clearly by individuals and group programs or activities are believed to be effective, attraction to the group is increased.

The concept of cohesion helps to explain group productivity. Some cohesion is necessary for people to remain with a group and accomplish the set goals. Attractiveness positively influences member motivation and commitment to work on the group task. Cohesion for groups may be increased as members better understand the experiences of others and are able to identify common ideas and reactions to various issues. Nurses facilitate this process by pointing out similarities, contrasting supportive differences, or helping members redefine differences in ways that make those dissimilarities compatible.

Norms

Norms are standards that guide, control, and regulate individuals and communities. The group *norms* represent the standards for group members' behaviors, attitudes, and even perceptions. All groups have norms and mechanisms whereby conformity is accomplished, and group pressures are brought to bear on members to conform to these norms (Sampson and Marthas, 1981). Group norms serve three functions: (1) to ensure movement toward the group purpose or tasks, (2) to maintain the group through various supports to members, and (3) to influence members' perceptions and interpretations of reality.

The *task function* means that certain norms keep the

group focused on its task or direct movement toward the end on which members have agreed. Diversion from a steady focus is permitted only to the extent that members respect central goals and feel committed to return to them. This compelling force to return to agreed on work is the task norm, the strength of which determines the intensity that the group has in keeping to its work.

In the *maintenance function,* maintenance norms create group pressures to ensure affirming actions for members and to help in maintaining comfort. Individuals in groups seem most productive and at ease when their psychological and social well-being is nurtured. Attention to social and psychological tension of members and the resulting steps to support them at high stress points are maintenance behaviors. Healthy maintenance norms may lead a group to pay attention to conditions such as temperature, space, and seating, which ensure the physical comfort of the group during meeting times. The group is maintained by those arrangements that minimize physical tension for members, and this attention to arrangements may include meeting in places that are easily accessible and comfortable to the participants, providing refreshments, and scheduling meetings at convenient times.

A third function of group norms relates to members' perceptions of reality and is of equal importance to group performance. Daily behavior is largely based on the way each aspect of life is understood. Through socialization individuals learn how to gather information, assign meaning to that information, and react to situations in a way that satisfies needs. Decision-making and action-taking processes are influenced by the meanings ascribed to reality. Individuals need validation of their interpretations of reality and look to others to reinforce or to challenge and correct their ideas of what is real. Groups serve to examine the life situations confronting individuals. As individuals gather information, attempt to understand that information, make decisions, and consider the facts and their implications, they can take responsible action not only in relation to self and group but also for the community.

A group culture, or composite of the norms, develops, and though norms dictate behaviors and perceptions, it is important to know that the nurse cannot dictate them. The nurse can implicitly and explicitly support rules, attitudes, and behaviors, which in turn can lead to certain norms. Only when the rules, attitudes, and behaviors become part of the life of the group, independent of the nurse, are they norms.

Figure 14-3 shows that group norms affect members, tending to pressure them to see relevant situations in the same way that others view them. Strong normative pressure may develop to provide support for members considering change. Benne, describing the function of small groups for planned change, pointed out that individuals develop their value orientations through internalizing the norms of small groups on which they depend, notably families. "Changes in value orientations of individuals may be accomplished by seeking and finding significant membership in a small group with norms that are different in some respects from the normative orientation these individuals bring to a group" (1976, p. 76).

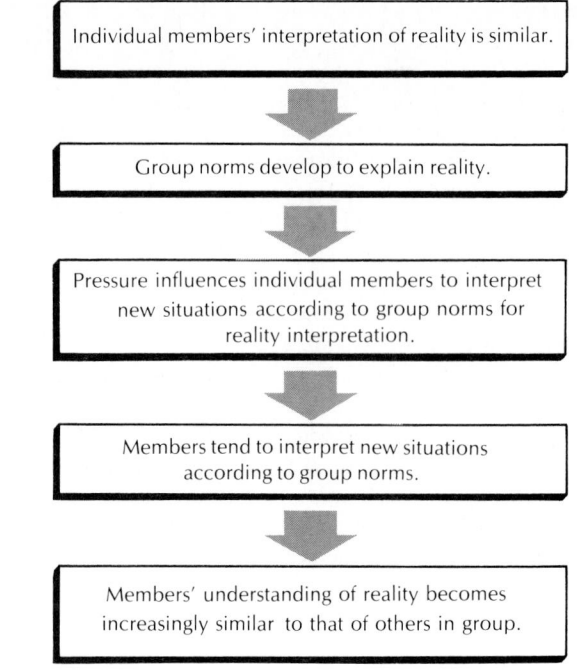

FIGURE 14-3

Influence of group reality norms on individual members.

To illustrate, if a group of people who have diabetes defines uncontrollable diet as harmful, they will direct their efforts toward influencing each other to maintain diet control. The role of the nurse in such a group would involve providing accurate information about diet and the disease process, including cause and effect relationships between food intake and disease, and continually displaying a belief that health through diet control is attainable and desirable.

When members of any group have similar backgrounds, their scope of knowledge may be limited. For example, female members in a spouse abuse group may believe that men are exploitive and harmful based on common childhood and marriage experiences. Such a stereotyped view of men could be reinforced by members' similar perceptions and might lead to continuing anger, fear of interactions with men, and a hostile or helpless approach to family affairs. Nurses or group members who have known men in loving, helpful, and collaborative ways can describe their different and positive perceptions of men, thereby adding information and challenging beliefs based on more limited experiences. Thus the group functions to influence members' perceptions and interpretations of reality. The health and condition of the individual improves as members' perceptions of reality become based on a full range of data, and cause-and-effect factors are understood. Nurses bring an important perspective to groups in which similar backgrounds limit the understanding and interpretation of personal concerns.

Leadership

Leadership in groups is an important and complex concept that involves guiding or directing a course. In a group the members' behaviors that lead include all of those actions that determine and influence the group movement. *Leadership* behaviors and definitions are listed in the box above. Members who have a strong influence over others are identified as leaders.

Sources of leader influence are knowledge, ability, access to needed resources, personal attractiveness, status or position in the community or organization, and ability to control sanctions for others. Leadership behaviors may be concentrated in one or a few persons, or they may be dispersed and shared by many. Effective leadership is necessary for positive group functioning. Leadership is often described as patriarchal, paternal, or democratic, and each of these has a particular effect on members' interaction, satisfaction, and productivity. Some groups reflect a combination of leadership styles.

When the final authority for group direction and movement is vested in one person, the leadership style is patriarchal or paternal. Patriarchal leadership may control members through rewards and threats, often keeping them in the dark about the goals and rationale behind prescribed actions. Paternal leadership wins respect and dependence from followers by parentlike devotion to members' needs at the leader's own expense yet controls group movement and progress through interpersonal power vested in singular leadership. Patriarchal and paternal styles of leadership are authoritarian. For groups in which immediate task accomplishment or high productivity is the goal, these styles are effective. This is especially true for efforts that are technical rather than interpersonal. However, group morale and cohesiveness are typically low under these styles of leadership; members may fail to learn how to function independently, and issues of authority and control disrupt productivity whenever the followers tire of submission to the one leader.

A paternal style was effective in the following situation. Mary Jones, a community health nurse, called her neighbors together to alert them to the threat of undesirable drug traffic in the neighborhood. The residents agreed with Mary that several recent drug-related arrests in the area signaled

a need for community concern. No one knew what to do, but all felt quick action was desirable. Mary had experience in organizing people to work quickly, knew local resources, and thought that information, education, and residents' collaboration with police could substantially control the drug traffic problem locally. She organized the neighborhood group, assigned and monitored their tasks, and praised them highly as progress was made toward the goal of keeping the area free of drug sales. This leadership approach was effective for several weeks but required Mary to maintain a high level of activity.

A different style of leadership, democratic, is characterized by a cooperative structure that promotes and supports members' functioning in all aspects of decision making and planning. Members influence each other as they explore goals, plan steps toward the goals, implement those steps, and evaluate progress.

The previous situation also serves to illustrate the democratic style of leadership. As Mary Jones' neighbors became knowledgeable about controlling drug use and working with educators and police, they began to share the daily responsibilities to keep the project going and to generate new ideas and activities. Bob Smith realized that control of drug sales in one neighborhood failed to address the problem for the larger community. He organized a larger task force to look into the problem in other neighborhoods. Various members served in leadership roles as the project evolved. The change in leadership styles broadened the effectiveness of this community group as the members brought their collectively greater resources to bear.

A more common experience for nurses is illustrated in the following example. A committee of nurses for a small community health organization met weekly to improve nursing services. Tom initiated a revision of written standards. Several members of the group felt threatened that their daily work would change and that a resulting evaluation using new standards would find them inferior or necessitate that they alter familiar procedures. Jane supported the work of updating standards. She also recognized the necessity of continuing support and affirmation of each nurse's worth on the committee. She often interrupted Tom's drive toward stating and refining standards by asking members to respond to suggestions, noting to the group the excellent contributions. Sara provided a touch of humor whenever group tension became high. Amber provided a critical, questioning support to the decision-making process and led the members to evaluate each step. In these and other ways group members shared leadership tasks. Some served predominately to push the group toward its objective, whereas others facilitated that movement by maintaining member involvement through support. For this group the chairperson served as convener but did not dominate in leader activities. The members accomplished the work of writing and implementing an audit for new nursing standards in a democratic leadership style.

Generally speaking, shared leadership in groups increases productivity and cohesion, resulting in friendly interactions between members. It builds appreciation for the work of leadership and inhibits power seekers. Shared leadership supports an idea of group wholeness, flexibility, and freedom. It might be hypothesized that a group in which the leadership is established in one effective and knowledgeable member would benefit from stability in its structure, predictability in its movement, and efficiency in its expenditure of energy. Follower roles would be clear and expectations explicit. Such an arrangement is efficient for groups of short duration, for those with a clearly defined purpose, and for those for which quick action is urgent. Such a leadership arrangement would be efficient for a disaster team but not for a planning committee.

Leadership abilities reside in members as well as health care workers. Nurses use varied leadership styles and exercise executive roles according to their assessment of member leading capabilities, their beliefs about how groups learn and change, their flexibility in leading behaviors, and the group's pressures for autonomy and control. Leadership is a dynamic concept, and although the nurse is active in all stages of group development and usually initiates and aggressively promotes group establishment she facilitates leadership development within and among members, frequently stepping down from control activities to permit membership composition and engagement for work toward group goals to determine the pattern of leadership and ultimate structure of the group.

Group Structure

Structure describes the particular arrangement of group parts that help to describe the group as a whole. *Communication structure* and *role structure* are two such descriptive frameworks. A communication structure identifies the parts according to message pathways and member participation in sending and receiving messages. Such communication structures can be mapped from observation of groups in action. People who are active in receiving and sending messages and who serve as channels for messages because of their verbal skills, personal attractiveness, or spatial position are important in the structure. These "central" individuals derive influence in the group from their access to and interpretive control over communication flow. Communication and role structures are interrelated.

Role structure for a group describes the expected behaviors of members in relation to each other as the group interacts (see box at right). The role assumed by each group member has certain functions, or behaviors, that are displayed in the group and serve a purpose in the life of that group. Examples of roles are leader, follower, task specialist, maintenance specialist, evaluator, peacemaker, and gatekeeper. Members' roles in the group may be described by their predominate actions. Identification of a group's role structure can be accomplished by observation of members' behavior as the group operates. Identification of communication patterns helps also to determine roles, since people occupying particular roles are characterized by certain kinds of communication.

Group structure emerges from various member influences, including members' understanding and support of the group purpose. Nurses assess the group structure as it relates to goal accomplishment. Many groups also consider their structure, assess its usefulness to member comfort and

---

EXPECTED BEHAVIORS DEFINING GROUP ROLES

Leader—guides and directs group activity.
Follower—seeks and accepts the authority or direction of others.
Task Specialist—focuses or directs movement toward the main work of the group.
Maintenance Specialist—provides physical and psychological support for group members, thereby holding the group together.
Evaluator—analyzes the effect or outcome of action or the worth of ideas according to some standard.
Peacemaker—attempts to reconcile conflict between members or takes action in response to influences that disrupt the group process and threaten its existance.
Gatekeeper—controls outsiders' access to the group.

---

productivity, and then plan for a different division of tasks that are agreeable to the whole.

In the earlier example of nurses working on standards of nursing service, Tom served a role as task specialist, Jane as maintenance specialist, and Amber as evaluator. These members occupied particular roles repeatedly and were expected by others to maintain their behavior to serve the purposes of the group.

A person occupying a gatekeeper's role controls outsiders' access to the group. Because gatekeepers are active in deciding issues of outsider entry, they use influence to either facilitate or block communication between outsiders and group members. Identification of those in gatekeepers' roles is crucial in community work when established groups are used for community health. The gatekeeper usually comes forward to confront the nurse after beginning contacts are attempted. An invitation to communicate further with group members is extended only after the nurse and gatekeeper determine mutual benefits and possible risks from continued contact between the nurse and the group.

Conflicts in groups may develop from competition for roles or member disagreement about the role ascribed to them. Struggles between members often result more from disagreement over dominance or out of competition for a favored position than from a conflict regarding group goals or steps in decision making. When group structures are considered from role and communication perspectives, the nurse and members of the group can more clearly understand the pressures affecting conflicting behavior and can work to resolve matters productively.

The following is an illustration of structure analysis leading to conflict resolution. A small church in the rural town of Cookville initiated a project for youth recreation. The teens of Cookville had little opportunity for recreation, aside from driving around the countryside; the roadway was frequently used as a speedway by the restless youths. The church enlisted the high school principal and the community health nurse to work with a project group. All supported the development of a local youth center and worked energetically toward that goal.

After 2 months of smooth work together, many arguments erupted at meetings. Conflicts about the supervision of the proposed center, the site for the physical plant, and numerous smaller concerns seemed to dominate planning time. The group had active, aggressive members; four of these individuals seemed to talk the most and to resist argument resolution. After several frustrating meetings, the nurse asked the group to consider their roles in decision making. She suspected that the disagreements were related to members' functions in the group rather than their ideas. The nurse was supportive to each person as the roles and expectations of each member of the project group were explored. The four most talkative individuals expressed personal wishes to direct the planning and displayed aggravation when these attempts were thwarted. Other members described supportive and task functions but did not seek dominance in leadership functions. The open analysis of role structure made clear to the members that arguments grew out of competition for directing roles rather than from true disagreements about the recreation project. The open discussion in this situation also resulted in an agreement to divide the project work into several task areas to be led by separate area directors. Members expressed relief that basic agreement about the purpose remained intact, and they were able to modify their role expectations to accommodate all members. They joked together about being a collection of bosses and renewed their productive work.

PROMOTING INDIVIDUAL'S HEALTH THROUGH GROUP WORK

Health behavior is influenced greatly by the groups to which people belong and for which they value membership. Individuals live within a social structure of significant others such as family, friends, workers, and acquaintances. The patterns and directions of everyday activities are learned in a family, and these are later reinforced or challenged by new sets of important others. These groups form the context in which values, beliefs, and attitudes are formed; individuals usually consider the responses of others in all types of decisions regarding personal welfare.

The following example illustrates the effects of a person's social network on health behavior. Mary Berton worried about a lump recently discovered in her breast. She first asked her husband, Lew, to confirm its presence, which he did. He agreed that she should arrange for a diagnostic evaluation, and an appointment was arranged. Mary talked with Lew about the possible consequences of malignancy, and she noted Lew's concern for her safety. She was fearful of radical surgery and its impact on her relationship to Lew, but she did not discuss that with him. Mary telephoned two close friends from her workplace and asked them to meet her for coffee. Even though they felt it was premature to fret about the lump being malignant, they discussed all they knew about treatment for breast cancer, including the trials, defeats, and successes of three mutual friends who had had surgery for breast cancer. Each of the experienced friends had reacted differently to her own situation, and Mary's friends retold familiar details. The retelling seemed important in grasping the current situation and helping

Mary sort out her feelings. She was assisted in facing the reality of risk, recognizing the need to follow through with diagnostic procedures, selecting able medical sources, and managing her emotional stress.

Mary's friends' and husband's responses to her situation influenced her assessment, decision making, and subsequent behavior. The work done by Mary and her friends in response to her health need is important business. It illustrates a common mechanism among individuals and the groups to which they belong. The groups described in this example are Mary's family group, which includes Mary and Lew, and Mary's friendship group, of which those who met for coffee are a subset.

Groups supportive of individual health changes are unavailable to some people because of their social or emotional isolation. Also, existing groups sometimes work contrary to health goals. Individuals isolated from supportive groups or hindered by their group connections may find movement toward health difficult, and they may benefit greatly through newly organized groups established for specific purposes. Isolated individuals may have low self-esteem, be mentally ill, or occupy positions of low status in their family or community. They may be disadvantaged, gifted, or deviant, or they may simply live in a rural area or be engaged in solitary work.

As community nurses increase their knowledge of group concepts, develop skills in working with varied groups, and become aware of the power in groups for individual changes, they will become available, visible, and sought for group work. At times community health nurses work with existing groups, and at other times they select members for new groups. A decision about whether to work in established groups or to begin new ones is based on the clients' needs, the nature of existing groups, the purpose of the groups, and the membership ties in existing groups. A typology of established and selected membership groups is shown in Table 14-1.

Choosing Groups for Health Change
Established Groups

There are advantages to using *established groups* for individual health change when membership ties already exist and the people can use the structure already in place. Some beginning work of selecting and making the group attractive has already been done. Membership ties in established groups influence individuals, and even in newly formed groups people bring emotional and social ties from previous and parallel group memberships. People are influenced by the interaction in one particular group and by their alliance with other important groups to which they belong. Memory serves to keep the norms and role expectations from one group present in a person as he moves from group to group. Individual behavior is then influenced not only by the membership, purpose, attraction, norms, leadership, and structure of the established health group but also by those processes remembered from other valued group memberships. Consideration of the multiple influences on members helps to determine an appropriate grouping for each situation and its peculiar dimensions.

TABLE 14-1

Typology of groups

Group type	Examples of established groups	Examples of function by group
1. Established groups (existing groups; membership is linked through multiple connections and for multiple purposes)	Family	Socialization; support
	Friendship group	Recreation
		Psychological and social support
	Social networks	Communication among smaller groups
		Support
	Civic clubs	Promote well being
	Standing committee	Implement organizational or community change
		Conduct work assigned by organizations
	Citizen board	Examine and monitor local services
	Neighborhood organization	Assess local community needs
		Communicate plans to residents
	Worker units	Test and implement ideas or work
		Produce product
	Great books club	Critique books
	Gardening club	Learn and teach new skills
	Governing body	Representative collective needs of individuals
		Establish regulations
	Spiritual growth groups	Establish identity; promote religious ideas
	School group	Support education
	Church group	Provide link between individuals and the larger social system
		Social communication
2. Selected membership groups (composed of persons brought together for purposes of health assessment, intervention and promotion in behalf of individuals, families, organizations and/or communities)	Rehabilitation group	Help members examine perceptions and orientation to health and disability
	Alcoholics Anonymous	Examine and alter value orientations
	La Leche League	Learn new skills for parenting
	Weight Watchers	Promote individual health, teach new daily living practices
	Parents Without Partners	Learn new skills for parenting
	Crime watchers group	Protect safety
	Nursing practice committee	Evaluate professional practice
	Social action group	Speak out for social justice
		Utilize developing opportunities
	Community concerns group	Address community health problems
	Consultation groups	Group problem solving
	Ad hoc committee	Identify and contract for needed resources
	Self study committee	Examine and change work procedures
	Task force	Market new products

Before deciding to work with established groups, the nurse must judge whether or not introducing a new focus is compatible with existing group purposes. In some cases individual health goals enhance existing group purposes, and the nurse may be seen as an important resource for bringing information for health, behavior, and group process. Nurses observe collective needs based on client contacts and assessment of other community data. Just as other nursing interventions are based on assessment of need and knowledge of effective treatment, groups are similarly formed from assessment of priority community needs for individual health change and considerations of group effectiveness in working toward those changes.

How can the community nurse enter existing groups and direct their attention to individual health needs? One nurse employed by an industrial firm noted the deleterious effect of managerial stress on several individuals. They had elevated blood pressure, stomach pain, and emotional tension. The nurse learned that the stressed adults were members of a jogging team that met weekly for conversation in addition to regular parallel workouts. The joggers readily accepted the offer to work together on individual stress management, seeing the need of their fellow members caught in high-stress circumstances and the accompanying danger to health. High-level health had been a shared value by all team members, and though jogging was seen as an enjoyable and health promoting activity, they had never talked about a shared purpose for improved health. In this circumstance the nurse observed a need for stress reduction, thought that the individuals at risk would be able to achieve stress reduction if supported through a group process from valued friends, and proposed that a new purpose be added to the jogging team's activities.

Selected Membership Groups

Nurses are familiar with group work in which members are selected because of the nature of their individual health needs. For instance, individuals with diabetes are brought together to consider diet management and physical care and to share in problem-solving remedies; community residents are brought together for social support and rehabilitation following treatment for mental illness; or isolated elderly persons are brought together for socialization and hot meals.

Members' attributes are an important consideration in composing a new group. As noted earlier, members are attracted to others from similar backgrounds, with similar experiences, and with common interests and abilities. This suggests selecting members so that common ties or interests balance out dissimilar traits. When the nurse is able to arrange it, the membership for *selected membership groups* should contain one or more individuals with expressive and problem-solving skills and some who are comfortable in supportive roles. Many people show ability in task and maintenance functions, and others have undeveloped potential for such functions. Support and training for group effectiveness within the unit build cohesion. As members perform increasingly valuable functions for the group, they become more attracted to it and more attractive to others.

The size of the group influences effectiveness; generally 8 to 12 people are considered a good number for small group work focused on individual health changes. Groups of up to 25 members may be effective when their focus is on community needs, such as the group discussed previously that formed a neighborhood association. Large groups often divide and assign tasks to the smaller subgroups, with the original large groups meeting less frequently for reporting and evaluation.

Recruitment and selection among candidates for optimum group membership require judgment based on knowledge of group concepts. Selection can be facilitated by setting member criteria for specific groups. The criteria usually suggest a mixture of member traits, allowing balance for the process of decision making and growth.

Beginning Interactions

Once a group forms, work begins on the stated purpose. Early meetings require further clarification of both individual and group goals. Members with varying degrees of openness present themselves and their backgrounds. They begin to interact with each other by seeking and giving information about themselves and their circumstances and at the same time demonstrating their capabilities in problem solving and group participation. The nurse assists by supporting ideas and feelings, inviting participation, giving information, clarifying thoughts, and suggesting structure. The method for proceeding toward the purpose varies not only according to the nurse's skill and preference but also to group composition and the skills brought by members.

Nurses in beginning groups should place priority on helping members interact with a degree of satisfaction. This requires close attention to maintenance tasks of attending, eliciting information, clarifying communication when needed, and recognizing contributions of members. At-tending includes simple responses to people, such as listening carefully to their speech and noting their mood, dress, and informal conversation as they enter the meeting. Attending behavior communicates recognition and acceptance of the person and his presentations to the group.

A beginning format that focuses on whatever brought each member to the group provides recognition and helps the individual acknowledge similar and different perspectives. Members may be asked to describe what each hopes to accomplish in the group and what experiences each has previously had in groups. Member-to-member exchanges are encouraged; individuals are recognized and supported as they take on leadership functions.

Even in beginning sessions of groups, some patterns of work are formulated. Members try out familiar roles and test their individual abilities. Those approaches to member support, leadership, and decision making, which are comfortable and productive for the members, become normative ways for the group to work. The nurse enters into such models creatively, evaluating style and productivity according to appropriateness for the members and nurse. The work of the group is begun even as the goals for health change are examined carefully and are realistically accepted. During this early period, members' attractions to each other and to the group begin to develop.

Conflict

Groups at work experience *conflict*. Members come with unique personalities and often disagree about many aspects of the group's work and the part that each member plays. Open discussion of differences and disagreements can promote individual and group growth. The nurse should promote such openness, though making it clear that respect for each person and point of view is necessary. This lays the groundwork for a group norm that supports member esteem during conflict and resolution.

Conflict in groups may grow from unspoken or generally unrecognized issues. These conflicts are sometimes communicated subtly in themes such as control and dependence. Often the conflict regarding status in the health group represents concerns of members who experienced similar problems in other important groups such as their families (e.g., one person's struggle for leadership and dominance is mirrored in a similar struggle at home). For example, persons in victim roles may have integrated low esteem and self-accusation into their views of themselves. The replay of problematic interpersonal transactions in the group allows critical examination by supportive members and leads to healing, understanding, and rejection of low self-evaluation and to the practice of presenting a healthier self.

Problem Solving for Health Change

Work toward established health goals is facilitated by community health nurses through their considerable knowledge of health and health risks for individuals, groups, and communities. Problem-solving and decision-making skills and strategies for change are part of the nurse's resources for such group work.

Basic teaching is sometimes used as an early method.

Members benefit from understanding facts and cause and effect links, the known associations between environment, body response, wellness, and pathology that are pertinent to the health change goal. Participation in formal learning may help people focus on the reality of the problems faced and ways to understand them. The potential of a group for effecting individual change is only addressed fully when members work actively and directly through discussion and other approaches to problem solving. Expectant parent groups illustrate a type of community group in which teaching is a highly appropriate method. Participants need to understand facts concerning pregnancy, labor and delivery, self-care and infant care, parenting, and adjusting to change. Along with factual understanding, they need an opportunity to practice the skills required in anticipated tasks and to explore their attitudes and emotional responses to the anticipated family changes. Specific learning activities in the group might include practice for baby baths and situation enactment of family activity after the baby comes home. Such experiential learning activities, which require interaction between members and use of materials highly relevant to the change goal, are useful.

One way to consider change for health is through analysis of motivating and restraining forces for individuals and groups. For this analysis the group considers major factors that influence the particular change proposed for health. Included are the encouraging and supportive forces for change and the interfering and resistive influences that each person experiences from all sources, including important individuals within the family, work, and community groups. These forces are identified during group meetings, where others help to plan action steps for overcoming interferences and promoting facilitative factors. The group members learn from each other and the nurse to deal effectively with multiple outside influences as they relate to the individuals' desired health goals.

Relationships within the group become increasingly important because of the shared understanding of the what, how, when, and where of health needs and changes. Normative pressures within the group keep members engaged in the agreed-on work and support the progress made by each individual.

Describing and listing the supportive forces and resistive influences for change help people clarify the multiple factors operating in any change. The study of factor sources, whether they arise within the individual, the work group, other valued groups, or the community at large, reveals areas requiring action. Such an analysis encourages consideration of diverse influences.

For the Xeona group at high risk for abusive parenting, eight parents showed up for the first meeting. Some came because they knew the nurse calling the meeting and thought she could help them with discipline problems. Two came only because it was strongly advised by their spouses, and others came because of the stated and publicized purpose of dealing with children for parent and child satisfaction. Offering child care during meetings encouraged parents to attend.

During the first two group meetings they described their children and some of the satisfying and frustrating experiences of parenting. Frustrations in work and family relations also surfaced, along with stress regarding finances and housing. Central to the concern of each parent was an expressed wish to be a better and happier parent. Neglect and violence were not mentioned in early group sessions.

As parents became acquainted, they noticed that they had similar frustrations about discipline. They described their anger, which sometimes erupted in slaps and beatings. They also expressed shame and confusion about these angry expressions of frustrations. After about 3 months, they felt strength from their mutual support and were able to face some changes that were expressed as "finding and using better ways to discipline kids."

What happened in the group to enable recognition of needs and plans to change abusive behavior? The people felt care and respect first from the nurse and later from each other. They recognized comparable frustration in parenting and failure to deal well with anger. Empathy for others in similar circumstances and with shared needs motivated them to work together on their parenting problems. They were encouraged by the nurse's and other group members' belief in each one's ability to change to a healthier parenting position with accompanying responsible behavior. The group helped each parent plan action steps toward individual goals. Progress on individual steps was reported each week with resulting support and reinforcement. The result was a reduction of the abuse and neglect of children by group members. This example illustrates the power of group intervention for change, which could not be accomplished through individually focused methods.

Evaluation of Group Progress

Evaluation of individual and group progress toward health goals is important. (A Guide for Evaluation of Group Effectiveness is shown in Appendix I). Action steps toward the goal are specified from the earliest planning. These small steps may be suggested in response to learning objectives, from listed action steps designed to support facilitative forces and deal with resistive forces, or from whatever problem-solving plan the group designs. These action steps and the indicators of achievement are articulated in discussion and written in a group record. Celebration is built into the group's evaluation system to help individuals recognize and reinforce each step toward the health goal. Celebration may include concrete rewards such as special foods and drinks, or it may be personal expression of joy and member-to-member approval. Celebration for group accomplishments marks progress, rewards members, and motivates each person for continuing work.

Identifying Community Groups

An understanding of group concepts provides a (beginning) basis for identifying community groups, their goals, member characteristics, and group norms. Because individuals develop, refine, and change their ideas within the context of the groups to which they belong, the community health needs and desires for change may also be understood according to the group structure of the community. Nurses may begin community assessment by identifying community subsystems and the formal groups within them. This formal community structure is mapped from data in public documents, such as a community comprehensive plan, and from local communications media (newspapers, television stations, magazines). Community residents, especially those in leadership positions, may provide additional information about the various formal groups and their functions and position in the community. It is important to note the harmony among the goals of various formal groups; the overlap, cooperation, or competition in function; the differences and similarities between member characteristics; and the congruence or lack thereof between formal group standards.

The membership in formal groups can be determined by noting membership lists. The demarcation between subsystems and for formal groupings within them is determined by the statements of community residents about who belongs, works with, or affiliates with particular groupings.

Informal groups are usually identified through interviews with key spokespersons. Informal groups also become distinguished by action or service in the community that is recognized in the news media. Informal groups include friendship, neighborhood, and social network groupings.

Groups are ranked in the community on the basis of characteristics such as social prestige or power. Power in turn is associated with the hierarchies of position in the community subsystems of economics, government, education, religion, health, and welfare. Those in high level positions have greater capacity for influencing community-wide matters than those in relatively lower positions. The nurse should consider the extent to which formal or informal groups are linked through family and friendship ties.

After the community *subsystems,* formal groups, and representative informal groups are identified and links between them are mapped, the nurse may further study the community group structure through observation of each group's goals and their appropriateness to overall community goals. Both stated and unstated goals are identified in this process.

Goals for the community and for various groups are studied through media sources and community informants. In community health assessment the nurse documents needs, resources, and vision for change as perceived by the people living and working in the community. The data may be organized according to the opinions and behaviors of the groups identified.

Interlinking Subsystems

Edwards and Jones (1976) described the community according to differentiated and interlinking subsystems such as family, economy, government, religion, education, health, and welfare. These community subsystems are linked to the larger society and to each other through various communication and cooperative exchanges. Functioning within and between subsystems of the community are individual persons, informal groups such as friendship and other spontaneous groups, and formal groups such as schools, churches, and businesses.

The interrelatedness among individuals is built partly on the network of roles and status levels that exist in the various formal and informal groups in the community's social structure (Edwards and Jones, 1976). Informal groups are linked to the extent that their members have connections with formal groups that are in turn part of the community subsystems. The informal and unofficial channels of interaction that develop between status levels (formal and informal groups) serve to link groups, thus contributing to the community integration. For example, the relationships and patterns of influence existing in local extended family groups are likely to influence the many other groups to which those family members belong. Members of a family in Goff County actively participate in the board of county directors, the school board, the protestant mission council, the youth advisory commission, and the county rescue squad. This family's conservative political views, especially those related to local management of financial affairs, are reflected in the conservative fiscal posture of these five separate community groups.

The various group norms regarding member communication and interaction with others and the degree of harmony between group goals influence the overall harmony and free exchange between individuals and groups in the community. Links between formal groups depend on the degree of coordination, cooperation, and competition between community subsystems. Many communities sanction various cooperative links by means of coordinating groups, such as interagency councils. Links to county, state, and national subsystems exist to a large extent as local groups are increasingly controlled by special community organizations and events.

The small group is potentially able to influence and change the larger social community of which it is a part. The social system depends on groups for governing, making policy, determining community needs, taking steps to alleviate those needs, and evaluating program outcomes. The small group is a mechanism for interrelatedness between community subsystems, certain subsystems and their counterparts in the larger social structure, and factions within subsystems. Change in the composition and function of strategic small groups may produce change also for the wider social system that depends on small groups for direction and guidance (Benne, 1976).

WORKING WITH GROUPS TOWARD COMMUNITY HEALTH GOALS

Community health nurses may use their understanding of group principles to work with community groups to make needed health changes. The groupings appropriate for this work include both established, community-sanctioned groups and groups for which nurses select members representing diverse community sectors.

Existing community groups formed for community-wide purposes such as elected executive groups, health planning groups, better business clubs, women's action groups, school boards, and neighborhood councils are excellent resources for community health assessment, since part of their ongoing purpose is to determine and respond to community needs. These types of groups are powerful actors for community health because they are already established as part of the community structure. When a group representing a community sector is selected for community health intervention, the total community structure is studied. Data about family ties, experiences with resource centers, and lifelong contacts to other sector groups are obtained. Groups are subject to existing community values, strengths, and normative forces.

How might community health nurses help established groups to work toward community goals? The same interventions recommended for groups formed for individual health change are beneficial to community health-focused groups. Such interventions include building cohesion through clarifying goals and individual attraction to groups, building member commitment and participation, keeping the group focused on the goal, maintaining members through recognition and encouragement, maintaining member self-esteem during conflict and confrontation, analyzing forces effecting movement toward the goal, and evaluating progress. On entering established groups, nurses seek to assess the leadership, communications, and normative structures. Knowledge and activity resources of the nurse facilitate involvement in the group planning, problem solving, action, and evaluation steps. The steps for community health change parallel those of decision making and problem solving in other methodologies.

One community health nurse joined the Oswald neighborhood group after several client families recounted stories of multiple gunshot injuries to youths in the neighboring homes. Seven young males aged 14 to 21 had been injured in separate shoot-outs during recent months. The neighbors, mostly parents, formed a concerned parent group to discuss the dangers for all residents and especially for their sons. The clients knew that Ms. Brown, the nurse, knew how to help groups "get their act together" and take action on problems. They had worked with Ms. Brown for the neighborhood health fair. Her assessment was that the Oswald neighborhood could improve their relations if the adults and youths recognized and redirected some emerging problems.

Ms. Brown attended the first few group meetings, taking a back seat as Mrs. Knight, a local resident and parent, recounted the recent violent occurrences, and others added details about the shootings. Feelings ran high and everyone wanted to speak out about the threats to themselves and their families. Urgency for action kept people task directed. Soon they focused on two action goals: (1) to limit youths' access to firearms by getting the weapons out of neighborhood homes and (2) to establish a supervised youth recreation center to provide alternative activities for youth. Both goals were reasonable, partial solutions to the problem of teenage violence in Oswald; they required commitment and action from the majority of the neighborhood residents. Ms. Brown offered to help the group consider action steps toward the goals that were possible, economical, efficient, and productive. She helped the group identify factors that facilitated their work toward goals and other factors that hindered progress. To accomplish the first goal, limiting

youths' access to firearms, the group analyzed facilitative and hindering forces. This analysis led to action steps that would increase residents' awareness of danger from firearms, identify homes where firearms were kept, determine household regulations over these firearms, and launch a person-to-person communication that supported strict control for all guns. Commitment to this community intervention was heightened by the group's fear of violence; thus they spent many hours within a 2-week period to implement steps toward the goal. Their action produced a dramatic effect in the community, culminating in a neighborhood rally, during which most residents spoke on record for strict gun control.

The second goal for a supervised youth center took longer for accomplishment. Although shoot-outs no longer occurred in the community and Oswald became a safer place to live, the youths previously involved in the neighborhood violence remained dissatisfied and conflicts between them and outside gangs continued. Plans to address the continuing needs of local youths included a support group for management of conflict, vocational training classes for young people, service activity projects in a local church, and youth representation on the newly formed neighborhood council. Because adults and youths in Oswald realized that gang action and violence were problems in adjoining neighborhoods, they began linking with citizens in those neighboring areas to promote concern about guns and violence. They recognized that safety in Oswald depended on wider community exchanges and continued work.

Community groupings, because of their interactive roles, seem to be logical and natural ways for people to join to work for community health change. As the decision-making and problem-solving capabilities of community groups are strengthened, the groups become more able representatives of the whole community as well as its sectors. Community health nurses improve the community's health through work with groups toward that goal.

CLINICAL APPLICATION

A rural community health nurse was troubled about the large case load of chronically ill individuals served by the health department. The rate of chronic diseases was much higher than for the neighboring urban county and while individuals and their families received medical supervision from the clinic and public health nurses visited the involved families at home, the judgment of the nursing staff was that chronically ill persons were not managing their pain and mobility problems to their own satisfaction. The nurse set up an initial group meeting inviting all of the persons with chronic illness in the rural town of Afton. The invitation was published in the county newspaper and all local church bulletins. Free transportation was provided by the auxiliary club at the community church. Thirty individuals came to the first meeting indicating great dissatisfaction with their health and interest in working with the nurses on a better approach to their chronic diseases. The first meeting was used to organize three groups which would meet regularly for 6 weeks each. Members selected a group based on their scheduling needs and friendship ties. The nurse met then with each group to facilitate their process in setting goals, selecting a variety of group work steps toward the goal; she served as resource specialist for each group.

One group decided to review each member's individual health care plan and assist in finding needed resources, thereby encouraging members.

Another group thought that stress related to their chronic condition was their biggest concern. They requested a course in stress management, which a community resident taught. Group learning experiences were facilitated by the community health nurse.

The third group was primarily concerned that many residents with chronic disease failed to use existing health care services. Because they believed that lack of transportation was a key causative factor for underuse of services, they decided to find voluntary transporters through the Ruritan Club. Because the group had strong family links to the Ruritans and because their arguments were convincing they were able to establish a car pool at no cost to the needy residents needing rides to health care services.

These group meetings didn't change the rate of chronic illness. They did successfully intervene to address specific health concerns that the people wanted and needed. The nurse working alone or with individuals could not accomplish these interventions as effectively or as efficiently. This nursing intervention was a powerful method for needed changes for individuals and for the rural community.

SUMMARY

The concepts presented in this chapter—member interaction, group purpose, cohesion, norms, leadership, and structure—provide a basic framework for understanding group behavior. The concepts appear deceptively simple, but their application to real groups reveals their complexity for individuals wishing to influence group behavior. Though each group concept is initially considered in isolation, the combination of concepts provides a multidimensional structure for group analysis. Group behavior is complex because of the many factors influencing individual members, member interaction within the group, and the group's community environment.

The examples of group work throughout this chapter show multiple ways that community health nurses apply knowledge of group concepts in their assessment of individuals' and communities' needs. A group perspective of behavior is more comprehensive than one based on individual dynamics alone. Examples show that group factors affect behavior, at times influencing health risks and the needs for healthful changes; they show that group influences may facilitate or hinder health-seeking action. Community health nurses should apply group knowledge in the assessment of health and assist clients in this assessment process.

Group intervention examples show community health nursing approaches to needed healthful changes. Community health nurses work with groups frequently and to excellent advantage. The client group may be persons with comparable health information needs, a group of friends responsive to a sick member, a family who works together to manage a crisis, or a committee that organizes health resources and services. Nurses lead others in using established groups or selecting and recruiting new groups to address both individual and community health needs. Nurses also demonstrate these intervention and evaluation skills as they serve as members of community action groups. These skills are not an addition to nursing—they *are* nursing. Such nursing group skills are based on knowledge and are developed in community practice.

A serious student will want to study different groups, analyzing the various dimensions presented by these group concepts. Such study illustrates the interplay of influences on groups and their members and allows observation of what works and does not work in groups. Discussion and analysis of observed groups in conjunction with experienced teachers enrich the student's study of groups.

The group is both a natural phenomenon affecting everyday life and a deliberate organization for influencing change for health, which is the essence of nursing practice.

The examples in the chapter describe real group situations. However, it is impossible to describe every feasible combination of elements in a cookbook fashion. The nurse must use creativity in the application of knowledge in unique situations. A series of questions to guide the implementation of concepts should be asked. What is the problem? Who are the people involved? Are group methods the best route to accomplish the objectives with these particular people? If so, at what level—individual member focused or community focused? Will the problem be best addressed by an established group, or should members be selected for forming a new group? What is the nursing role in establishing the new group? What strategy is suitable for entering an existing group?

Interventions are products of established knowledge, techniques, and personal attributes such as life experience, personality, and personal style. Ability to work in a group context may vary according to all of these factors along with group members' attributes and needs.

Supervision or consultation assists in self-evaluation and development of group strategies. Such feedback is essential to developing self-awareness in a group practice. Literature describing specific interventions with particular problems or types of groups is available (see bibliography).

Through knowledge of group behavior, skill in group practice, and appreciation of the power that groups have, community health nurses may substantially increase their impact on health for individuals and communities. Community health nurses are challenged to use the opportunities for change through work with groups—an instrument of power for health.

≡ KEY CONCEPTS

Working with groups is an important skill for community health nurses. Groups are an effective and powerful vehicle for initiating and implementing healthful changes.

A group is a collection of interacting individuals with a common purpose. Each member influences and is influenced by other group members to varying degrees.

Group cohesion is enhanced by commonly shared characteristics among members and diminished by differences among members.

Cohesion is the measure of attraction between members and the group. Cohesion or the lack of it affects the group's function.

Norms are standards that guide and regulate individuals and communities. These norms are unwritten and often unspoken and serve to ensure group movement to a goal, to maintain the group, and to influence group members' perceptions and interpretations of reality.

Some diversity of member backgrounds is usually a positive influence on a group.

Leadership is an important and complex group concept. Leadership is described as patriarchal, paternal, or democratic.

Group structure emerges from various member influences, including members' understanding and support of the group purpose.

Conflicts in groups may develop from competition for roles or member disagreement about the roles ascribed to them.

Health behavior is greatly influenced by the groups to which people belong and for which they value membership.

An understanding of group concepts provides a basis for identifying community groups and their goals, characteristics, and norms. Community health nurses use their understanding of group principles to work with community groups toward needed health changes.

LEARNING ACTIVITIES

1. Consider three groups of which you are a member. What is the stated purpose of each one? Are you aware of unstated but clearly understood purposes? What is the nature of member interaction in each group? How do purpose and interaction differ in the three groups?

2. Observe two work groups in session from the community, a health care agency, or a school. Notice the overall attractiveness of each group through the eyes of its members.
   a. List actions that nurses may take to assist groups in various aspects of their work such as member selection, purpose clarification, arrangements for comfort in participation, and group problem solving.
   b. Observe a nurse working with a health promotion group. Does he or she function in the way you anticipated? What nursing behavior facilitated the group process?

3. List the areas of skill and knowledge most likely to be expected of the nurse by the community residents.

BIBLIOGRAPHY

Alinsky, S.D.: Rules for radicals, New York, 1971, Vintage Books.

Anderson, B., and Hrycak, N.: Video—a teaching strategy for learning group process, Nursing Papers: Can. J. of Nurs. Res. 18:5, Spring 1986.

Benne, K.D.: The current state of planned changing in persons, groups, communities, and societies. In Bennis, W.G., et al., editors: The planning of change, ed. 3, New York, 1976, Holt, Rinehart, & Winston.

Bennis, W.G., et al., editors: The planning of change, ed. 3, New York, 1976, Holt, Reinehart, & Winston.

Bertcher, J.H.: Group participation: techniques for leaders and members, Beverly Hills, 1979, Sage Publications, Inc.

Callahan, J., et al.: Processing a task group: a continuing education committee at work planning a conference, J. Cont. Educ. Nurs. 11:8, Sept. 1980.

Corbin, D.E.: Self-help groups: what the health educator should know. Health values, 7:10, 1983.

Cottrell, L.S.: The competent community. In Kaplan, B.H., et al., editors: Further explo-rations in social psychiatry, New York, 1976, Basic Books, Inc., Publishers.

DelBueno, D.J.: Power and politics in organizations, Nurs. Outlook 34:124, 1986.

Dombeck, M.T.: Faculty peer review in a group setting, Nurs. Outlook 34:188, 1986.

Doyle, M.A.T., and Brunk, S.E.: Bone up on arthritis: arthritis self care goes to the country, Fam. Commun. Health 9:45, 1986.

Edwards, A.D., and Jones, D.: Community and community development, The Hague, 1976, Mouton Publishers.

Flynn, B.C.: Public health nursing education for primary health care, Pub. Health Nurs. 1:36, 1984.

Forsyth, D.M., et al.: Preventing and alleviating staff burnout through a group, Psychosoc. Nurs. Ment. Health Serv. 35:8, 1981.

Gorman, S., and Clark, N.: Power and effective nursing practice, Nurs. Outlook 34:129, 1986.

Henkel, B.O.: Solving health problems through small group action. In Spradley, B.W., editor: Contemporary community nursing, Boston, 1975, Little, Brown & Co.

Hogan, R.: Gaining community support for group homes, Commun. Mental Health J. 22:117, 1986.

Kagey, J.R., et al.: Mental health primary prevention: the role of parent mutual support groups, Am. J. Pub. Health 71:166, 1981.

Krawczyk, R.M.: Peer participation conferences: a dynamic method of nursing instruction, Nurs. Ed. 17:5, 1978.

Lassiter, P., and Goeppinger, J.: Education for rural community health nursing practice, Fam. Commun. Health 9:56, 1986.

Lipson, J.G.: Consumer activism in two women's self-help groups, West. J. Nurs. Res. 2:393, 1980.

Lorig, K., Laurin, J., and Gines, G.: Arthritis self management: a five-year history of a patient education program, Nurs. Clin. North Am., 19:637, 1984.

Mallick, M.J.: A community-based support group for families and patients with acute coronary disease, Pub. Health Nurs. 2:43, 1985.

McGrath, B.B.: The social networks of terminally ill skid row residents: an analysis, Pub. Health Nurs. 3:192, 1986.

Michael, M.M., et al.: Symposium on the self-care concept of nursing: use of the adolescent peer group to increase the self-care agency of adolescent alcohol abusers, Nurs. Clin. North Am. 15:157, 1980.

Nix, H.: Why Parents Anonymous? J. Psychiat. Nurs. 18:23, 1980.

Pesznecker, B.L., and Zahlis, E.: Establishing mutual-help groups for family-member care givers: a new role for community health nurses, Pub. Health Nurs. 3:29, 1986.

Politser, P.E., et al.: Social climates in community groups: toward a taxonomy, Commun. Ment. Health J. 16:187, 1980.

Sampson, E.E., and Marthas, M.: Group process for the health professions, ed. 2, New York, 1981, John Wiley & Sons, Inc.

Shamansky, S.L., and Pesznecker, B.: A community is . . ., Nurs. Outlook 29:181, 1981.

Smith, L.L.: Finding your leadership style in groups, Am. J. Nurs. 80:1301, 1980.

Spradley, B.W., editor: Community health nursing concepts and practice, Boston, 1981, Little, Brown & Co.

Veninga, R.: Are you a successful communicator? Can. Nurse 74:34, 1978.

Walsh, S.: Parents of Asthmatic Kids (PAK): a successful parent support group, Pediat. Nurs. 7:28, 1981.

Yalom, I.D.: The theory and practice of group psychotherapy, New York, 1975, Basic Books, Inc., Publishers.

Zinober, J.W., et al.: Another role for citizens: variations of citizen evaluation review, Commun Mental Health J. 16:317, Winter 1980.

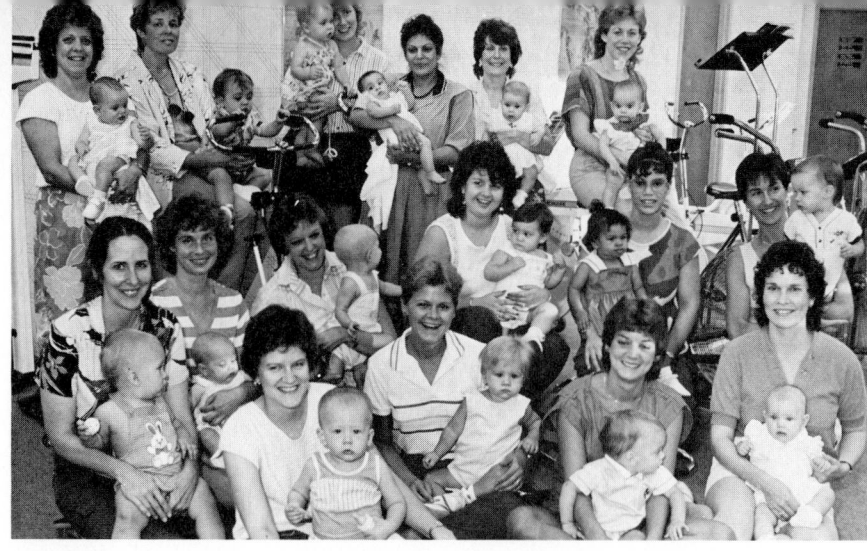

Carolyn A. Williams

15

POPULATION-FOCUSED PRACTICE: THE BASIS OF SPECIALIZATION IN PUBLIC HEALTH NURSING

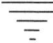 **OBJECTIVES**

After reading this chapter, the student should be able to:

Describe two concepts of community health nursing practice and the practice goals of each.

Contrast clinical community health nursing practice with population-focused practice.

Describe the confusion and ferment surrounding population-focused practice.

Define population-focused community health nursing practice.

Name the barriers to acceptance of population-focused community health nursing.

Analyze the dilemmas and challenges to population-focused practice.

KEY TERMS

aggregates

body of knowledge

community nurse practitioner

conceptual model

Consensus Conference of 1984

epidemiology

noninstitutional population

nursing process

nursing roles

population

population-focused practice

public health nurse

In this chapter issues of concern to those interested in the specialties of community health nursing and public health nursing are discussed. The chapter begins with an overview of the nature of community health nursing and public health nursing and then considers how these two areas of specialization interface. The second part of the chapter examines the importance of *population-focused practice,* suggesting that the population focus is what distinguishes public health nursing from other specialties. Further, it is argued that population-focused community health nursing is consistent with a public health philosophy and is scientifically desirable. Barriers that mitigate against such practices are also considered.

The chapter concludes with a discussion of three dilemmas that occur as a result of the adoption of population-focused practice. Questions considered in this section include: What is the arena for public health nursing practice? Is it limited to populations outside of institutions? Is it useful to talk about the role of the public health nurse? How does one prepare for population-focused practice?

COMMUNITY HEALTH NURSING TODAY: VIEWS AND PROBLEMS

Diverse opinions abound as to what public health nursing and community health nursing are. However, it is important to distinguish between population-focused nursing and clinical nursing delivered in community settings. As an introduction to the topic of the nature of community health nursing, two contemporary but different views of community health nursing are described.

Provision of Personal Nursing Services in Community Settings

The notion that the focus of community health nursing is ". . . the provision of health services among people of the community and the encouragement of health promoting behavior," is one held by many nurses and was proposed in a paper by de Tornyay (1980, p. 85). de Tornyay emphasized that community health nursing places particular attention on the maintenance of health, the provision of service extending over time as opposed to episodic services, and the prevention of disease. She described the responsibilities of community health nurses in the area of long-term care, in primary care, in work with certain population

groups, and in provision of a range of services for people living in a specific area. In each of the descriptions the emphasis is on the direct care services provided by the nurse. Although population groups variously defined are mentioned, the basic message is that a community health nurse is primarily a direct care clinician, providing services to the members of various groups in the community. In de Tornyay's discussion only brief mention was made of the administrative and supervisory responsibilities of community health nurses.

Much of the material in current textbooks reflects a perspective similar to that of de Tornyay's. The emphasis on providing clinical services in community settings is also the predominant focus of the American Nurses' Association's statement, A Conceptual Model of Community Health Nursing, developed by the Division of Community Health Nursing (1980).

Several distinctions relevant to this discussion are set forth in the ANA *conceptual model.* First, the statement identifies two categories of nurses in community health— generalists prepared at the baccalaureatte level who practice in community health settings and specialists in community health nursing who have master's level preparation or beyond. The statement does not refer to the generalist as a specialist or even as a community health nurse, although the latter is implied. The practice of the generalist is described as follows (ANA, 1980, p. 9):

> The nursing process is applied to the client, who may be an individual, family, group, or community. While working with individual clients, the nurse keeps the community perspective in mind.

In describing the scope of practice for community health nursing, the major objectives of the community health nurse are stated as "the preservation and improvement of the health of a community" (ANA, 1980, p. 11). These are accomplished through what are referred to as "two major modes or roles" (ANA, 1980, p. 11). The first mode is the direct care of individuals, families, and groups in a specified community; in the second mode the community is the client. It is interesting that the direct care mode is discussed first as opposed to the second mode, which is more consistent with historical understanding of public health practice.

Serious limitations of the conceptual model include the emphasis given the clinical focus, the lack of an in-depth treatment of the second mode (which perhaps should have been the focus of the statement), and the resultant failure to clearly identify what differentiates community health nursing from other specialty areas. The statement's declaration that "the distinguishing characteristic of community health nursing is primary health care, with emphasis on prevention of illness and promotion in maintaining and restoring maximum health" (ANA, 1980, p. 13) does little to set community health nursing apart from other nursing specialty areas.

Community Nurse Practitioner

A different conceptualization of community health nursing is reflected in descriptions of the *community health nurse practitioner,* a term sometimes used to refer to nurses who work with individuals and families in providing direct care services outside of institutional settings, as was the case in the paper by de Tornyay (1980) cited earlier. Use of the term in this discussion is different and refers to a role first developed in the early 1970s by faculty members associated with the School of Public Health at the University of Texas (Skrovan et al., 1974). The intent of the master's level program at the University of Texas was to develop a nursing role in which the nurse would focus on the community as the client. The approach was innovative and had a number of positive features.

A major strength was the serious effort to translate into practice terms the community component of community health nursing that was so seriously neglected in many other programs during that period. As stated by the program's originators, "it is the emphasis upon community self-help and the focusing upon the health of the total community as one's caresphere which differentiates the CNP role from others today" (Skrovan et al, 1974, p. 849). Much attention was placed on determining health care needs and priorities from the perspective of the community and working with the community to develop acceptable and effective approaches to the problem. Philosophically, the approach to make operational the community component was based on understanding community development processes as a foundation for working with communities. Students were prepared to assess communities through observation, participation in various action groups, and use of secondary data sources; work with community members as facilitators and collaborators in the formulation of health-related goals and plans for implementation; and monitor and evaluate progress with appropriate feedback to the community (Skrovan et al., 1974).

At the end of the grant period the community nurse practitioner training program at the School of Public Health was phased out; however, the key idea of developing a master's level practitioner with a clear focus on working with communities to improve health status did not die and has been adopted in varying degrees by several other graduate programs (Flynn et al., 1978; Goeppinger, 1979, Woods and Ohlson, 1977).

Confusion Regarding the Focus of Community Health Nursing Practice and Public Health Practice

The central distinguishing feature that sets apart the two conceptualizations of community health nursing just discussed is the clear effort on the part of those who worked with the community health nurse practitioner role to focus on what it means to have the community as a client instead of simply providing nursing service in a community setting. In both conceptualizations, emphasis is placed on practice rather than management and administration.

The effort to develop a community nurse practitioner program, to facilitate such practice, and to see the outcomes that have followed from that original endeavor represents some of the most interesting and refreshing developments in the field of community health nursing. Yet the attempt to implement the community focus in practice has been extraordinarily difficult for many nursing schools. In struggling with the basic idea of community as client, which underlies the community nurse practitioner role, the following questions have been repeatedly asked:

To what extent should the community nurse practitioner have a direct care clinical role?

Should preparation for the role include those direct care assessment and management skills associated with other practitioner roles, such as the family nurse practitioner or the pediatric nurse practitioner?

If advanced preparation in the direct care role is to be provided, will there be sufficient time in a master's curriculum for the development of the community skills?

Is a conceptualization of community health nursing with emphasis on skills such as community development a focus that nursing should adopt?

Can other groups provide such services?

Where does a community nurse practitioner fit into the present delivery system?

These questions reflect the present confusion surrounding community health nursing. There is also confusion as to how this specialty is distinct from other areas of nursing practice, the lack of clarity regarding what it means to have a community focus for practice, and the ambivalence many nurses who identify with community nursing have about moving from a direct care orientation to dealing with the concept of population groups, or *aggregates.* *

Because of this confusion, the American Public Health Association (1981) and the Community Health Nursing Division of the American Nurses' Association (1980), have developed the position statements mentioned above to clarify the scope of the specialty. These statements are summarized in Chapter 7 and similarities and differences between them are noted. However, the lack of consistency in the content of the two statements has led to further debate because of concern and confusion regarding the absence of guidelines for the many roles being developed in community health nursing as well as questions about preparation for

---

*The terms *population, population groups,* and *aggregates* are used interchangeably.

practice in the field. To address all of these concerns, the Consensus Conference on the Essentials of Public Health Nursing Practice and Education, sponsored by the Division of Nursing and held in Washington in September of 1984, brought together representatives from a wide range of community health/public health groups. This conference resulted in a number of recommendations (U.S. Dept. of Health and Human Services, 1985).

One of the most interesting outcomes was the consensus on the use of the terms *community health nurse* and *public health nurse*. It was agreed that the term "community health nurse" could apply to all nurses who practice in the community, whether or not they have had preparation in public health nursing. Thus nurses providing tertiary care in a home setting, a school nurse, a nurse in a clinic setting, in fact, any nurse who does not practice in an institutional setting falls into the category of "community health nurse." Nurses with a master's degree or a doctorate who are practicing in community settings can be referred to as "community health nurse specialists" regardless of the area of nursing in which the degree was earned! According to the conference statement, "the degree may be in any area of nursing, such as maternal-child health, psychiatric-mental health, or medical-surgical nursing or some subspecialty of any clinical area" (p. 4).

In contrast to the focus on the setting as the key variable in defining the community health nurse, public health nurses were defined in terms of their educational preparation. The participants of the consensus conference agreed "that the term 'public health nurse' should be used to describe a person who has received specific educational preparation and supervised clinical practice in public health nursing" (p. 4). At the basic, or entry, level a public health nurse is one who "holds a baccalaureate degree in nursing that includes this educational preparation; this nurse may or may not practice in an official health agency but has the initial qualifications to do so" (p. 4). Specialists in public health nursing are defined as those who are prepared at the graduate level, either master's or doctoral, "with a focus in the public health sciences" (p. 4).

How Do Community Health Nursing and Public Health Nursing Differ?

If one takes seriously the definitions of community health nursing and public health nursing agreed to in the 1984 consensus conference, it is clear that the setting is viewed as the feature distinguishing community health nursing apart from other nursing specialties. Unfortunately, the way community is equated with "noninstitutionalization" leads to further confusion. According to the statement, an individual who has received preparation in any clinical or subclinical area and who practices in a noninstitutional setting can be seen as a community health nursing specialist! Such a broad view may indeed be consistent with the way things have been perceived, but it is not clear that the distinction of setting is very meaningful. For example, two nurses could have completed a master's program in medical-surgical nursing with a subspecialization in nephrology.

They could both be providing the same clinical services to similar populations, including home visits. But the one who is employed in a dialysis center would be viewed as a community health nursing specialist and the one in the hospital-based dialysis center would not be seen as such a specialist.

Another problem with the use of setting as a distinguishing feature is that there is so much shifting and reorganization occurring in the health care system, that the institutional/noninstitutional distinction made in the consensus statement is outdated. Is a hospital-linked HMO an institutional setting? How does one define a hospital-based home care agency? Are not the more important distinctions the care needs of the populations or subpopulations being served and the types of decisions required by the professional nurses involved? For these reasons the use of setting as a meaningful way of making distinctions that imply an area of specialization for the nurse with graduate preparation has serious problems.

What is special about public health nursing? At present there is serious interest and concern about the preparation of practitioners for public health nursing practice. It seems clear that the preparation being recommended is that of Master's level graduates prepared for population-focused practice. In the consensus statement it was specifically pointed out that the public health nursing specialist "should be able to work with population groups, and to assess and intervene successfully at the aggregate level" (p. 11). Key content areas deemed essential for the preparation of such specialists were "Epidemiology, Biostatistics, Nursing theory, Management theory, Change theory, Economics, Politics, Public health administration, Community assessment, Program planning and evaluation, Interventions at the aggregate level, Research, History of public health, and Issues in public health" (p. 11).

The above discussion leads to several conclusions. First, public health nursing seems to be seen as a subset, a specialty in the broad arena of community health nursing. Secondly, population-focused practice is clearly the focus of specialization in public health nursing. Thirdly, defining community health nursing in the manner agreed to in the consensus statement is problematic if community health nursing is to be seen as a specialty area.

Population-focused Nursing: A Primary Focus of Public Health Nursing

Elsewhere it has been argued that the primary focus of public health nursing practice should be on defining problems (assessment) and proposing solutions (treatment) for population groups or aggregates (Williams, 1981). Such a focus entails decision making that is categorically different from the decisions nurses and other direct care providers have been prepared to make in the process of giving direct care to individuals or families. In other words, basic professional education in nursing, medicine, and other clinical disciplines focuses primarily on developing competence in decision making at the level of the individual client—assessing health status, making management decisions (ideally with

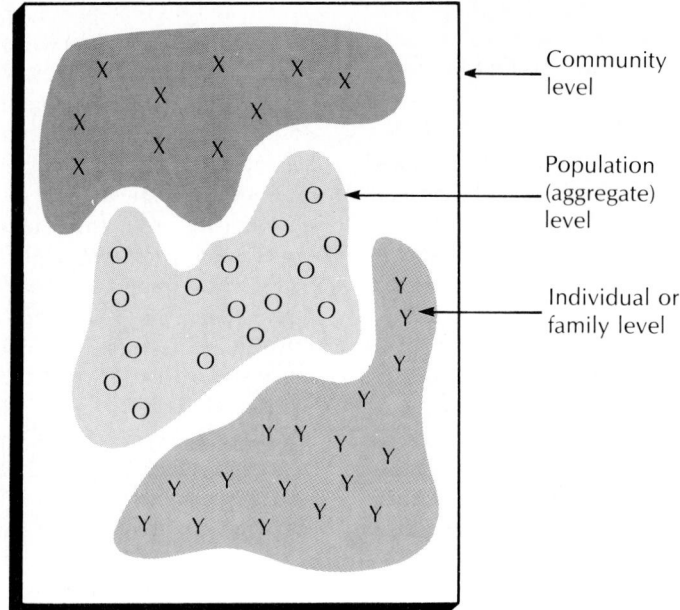

Community level

Population (aggregate) level

Individual or family level

FIGURE 15-1

Levels of practice.

the client), and evaluating the effects of care. This is at the level of the individual X's, O's, and Y's in Figure 15-1. Little attention is given to defining problems and proposing solutions at the population or subpopulation level, the groups of X's, O's, and Y's in Figure 15-1. Population level decision making is different from that which occurs in clinical care. For example, in a clinical direct care situation the clinician may determine if a client is hypertensive and if so explore with the person options for intervention. At the population level the questions are different and might include the following:

What is the prevalence of hypertension among various age, race, and sex groups?

Which subpopulations have the highest rates of untreated hypertension?

What programmatic options are there for reducing the problem of untreated hypertension and thereby lowering the risk of further cardiovascular morbidity and mortality?

The fundamental factor that should distinguish public health nursing from other specialties in nursing is a population focus. Not only is a population focus historically consistent with public health philosophy but it is necessary if one is to deal with public nursing needs in a scientific manner. It is therefore gratifying that the population focus is in accord with the definition of public health nursing developed by the Public Health Nursing Section and officially adopted by the American Public Health Association (APHA, 1981). That statement defines the goal of public health nursing as "improving the health of the entire community" (p. 4). Of particular significance to this discussion is the following quote from the APHA statement: "Identifying subgroups (aggregates) within the population which

are at high risk of illness, disability, or premature death and directing resources toward these groups is the most effective approach for accomplishing the goal of public health nursing" (p. 4).

Meaning of a Population Focus

At this point it may be useful to elaborate on the meaning of the term *population.* A basic definition of population is a collection of individuals who share one or more personal or environmental characteristics. Thus those who are members of a community defined either in terms of geography or special interests can be seen as constituting a population or an aggregate. Frequently it is useful to identify subpopulations within the larger group. Examples include high risk infants under 1 year, unmarried pregnant adolescents, and school age children. The group of X's, O's, and Y's in Figure 15-1 are meant to denote such subpopulations.

It is important to recognize that the specialty of public health nursing involves more than a focus on one subpopulation. Although individual professionals and some agencies or other health organizations may limit their attention to one subpopulation, those concerned with the health of a given community must ultimately give attention to the health of many subpopulations. Therefore specialization in public health nursing necessitates attention to multiple and sometimes overlapping subpopulations. Further, in contrast to the usual clinical approach, a population focus requires that public health specialists not limit their concern to individuals who seek care but extend attention to those who may need particular services and who are not in the care system (e.g., untreated hypertensive patients [Williams and Highriter, 1978]).

Population-focused Practice: A Must for Scientific Public Health Nursing

No one would want to have as a primary care provider an individual (e.g., a family nurse practitioner) who makes recommendations regarding therapy without first obtaining information from the client. A minimum assessment should include data on health status, characteristics of life-style, and preferences regarding the management of identified problems. No less should be expected when the client is the community. To obtain information that is valued and provides a clear picture of the status of the community, one must take a population focus. For example, looking only at the health status of those clients who happen to come to a particular clinic is likely to produce a biased, unrepresentative picture of the community's health status.

A systematic process analogous to what is referred to in clinical nursing as the *nursing process* should be used in making assessment and management (programming) decisions regarding the community's health status. However, the process has two major differences. First, rather than an individual (an X, O, or Y in Figure 15-1), the unit of analysis is a population or perhaps several subpopulations (a group of X's, O's, and Y's as in Figure 15-1). Second, the type of data obtained and the sources are different. In other words, rather than directly obtaining information through one's own assessment of a client, the nurse may have to use data gathered by others. Examples include the use of vital statistics and data gathered in surveys. Or if the nurse does actually gather data, they are not only obtained on one individual but from all people in the population or a representative sample, and the data are obtained in a systematic and consistent manner.

A scientific approach to public health nursing practice requires that assessment and management decisions be based on solid data obtained through the use of objective techniques. Two types of information are necessary. One type is generally referred to as the *body of knowledge* or the *epidemiology* of a given problem and represents what is known about specific health problems and potential solutions. Included in this body of knowledge is information on etiological factors, groups at highest risk, and treatment methods and their relative effectiveness. This type of information, usually obtained from the literature, has been generated by basic epidemiological studies; community health nursing research; and research in clinical nursing, clinical medicine, and other fields.

The second type of information must be obtained from the populations in the community of interest and is usually more difficult to obtain than the first type. Information on the community should include demographic data, the health status of various subpopulations, the services given to defined subpopulations, and the effectiveness of the services. Ideally, for public health nursing to be scientific, there should be ongoing mechanisms for assessment at the population level, which are systematic, objective, and would allow a continuing surveillance of both the population's health status and the services given. Such surveillance would be analogous to the monitoring of an individual client but should include the entire population and not be limited to those who seek care (Williams and Highriter, 1978).

An excellent example of such an approach to surveillance, developed by community nursing specialists, is the computerized monitoring information system for high-risk infants in the Gaston County Health Department, in North Carolina. Through the use of birth certificates of infants possessing a selected group of high-risk characteristics, the nursing unit of the health department defines a target population. All infants who meet the criteria for high risk are entered into the system and monitored for information about health status and services rendered. The system is set up to expect information on each infant at ages 3, 6, 12, and 24 months, and if data are not submitted at the appropriate times, the names of those infants who may need to be located are printed out. In addition to providing for the tracking of individual infants who are members of the target population, this system allows for the generation of population-level data. Examples of the latter include the proportion of infants born in a specified time period who are receiving care from the health department and the proportion receiving care from private physicians; the proportion of infants cared for by the health department who received initial DPT injections by 3 months of age; and the proportion (and names) of infants who have a specified deviation from the norm (e.g., low hemoglobin or underweight). A fuller description of this pacesetting project can be found in Highriter (1981).

If a population focus is taken seriously and strategies for implementing assessment, intervention, and evaluation activities at the population level are considered carefully, the nurse must think of organized approaches. The one-to-one care of individual clients by clinicians is a necessary part of any care system that deals with a population or subpopulation. However, with a population focus the emphasis should be on the interrelationship between the health status of the population, factors that influence health status, and the responses and effectiveness of the care system in dealing with the population's health. Therefore public health nursing specialists who adopt a population focus should have the following as priority practice responsibilities: developing and maintaining organized mechanisms for the provision of care to defined populations; collaborating with clients in the identification of needs and the development of solutions; participating actively in system-level decisions; and influencing other decision makers to enable such development.

Adoption of this understanding of public health nursing has an important implication for the specialty. For such practice to take firm root it is necessary for more public health nurses to be at high level positions in structures within the community that have the authority and funding to provide such services. Though roles like the community nurse practitioner may be viable ones, additional attention must be given to the development of nurses with high-level management skills—nurses who can be involved in the decisions associated with top echelon leadership—"developing policy, setting priorities, allocating resources, and modifying and manipulating organizational structure" (Milbank, 1976, p. 39). Many of the roles nurses currently occupy in organizations are at lower levels at which policy making is limited and carrying out policy is emphasized.

BARRIERS, DILEMMAS, AND CHALLENGES
Barriers to Acceptance of Population-focused Public Health Nursing

There are several barriers to the fuller development of population-focused community health nursing. One of the most serious is the "mind set" of many nurses that the only role for a nurse is at the bedside or at the client's side, the direct care role. Clearly, the heart of nursing is the direct care provided in personal contacts with clients. On the other hand, two things should be clear to the observant nurse. The first is that whether a nurse is able to provide direct care services to a given client is contingent on a number of decisions on the part of individuals within and without the care system, and second, nursing needs to be involved in those fundamental decisions. Perhaps the one-to-one focus of nursing and the cultural expectation of the "proper role" of women has influenced nursing's hesitancy in viewing positively more indirect modes of contributing, such as administration, consultation, and research. Unfortunately, this mindset on the part of many nurses is reinforced and adopted by others.

A case in point is a discussion of the roles of the community nurse and the community physician presented in a monograph by Kark (1981) on community-oriented primary health care. In that discussion community nurses were described as having major clinical roles in a unified practice of community medicine and primary health care. Not only were comments made about their direct care roles in the community setting but also it was mentioned that their roles should go beyond the nurse-client relationship to include skills in community diagnosis and action directed to meeting community health problems. All the comments were positive; however, it was interesting that in the discussion of community physicians there was a clear indication that community physicians would assume a major responsibility for community diagnosis and evaluation of health care. Because of this major responsibility, it was stated that physicians would need to have preparation in the principles and methods of epidemiology and its use in primary care. There was absolutely no comment about the need for nurses to have such preparation. The clear implication is that physicians would assume leadership in the scientific aspects of making operational the community-oriented primary care being described.

Another barrier to the type of practice implied in population-focused public health nursing is the structures within which nurses work and the process of role socialization that occurs within those structures. The fact that a particular role might not exist within the nursing unit may suggest that it is undesirable or impossible for nurses. For example, nurses interested in using political strategies to effect changes in health-related policy, an activity clearly within the practice domain of public health nursing, may

run into a number of barriers if their goals disrupt the agendas of other groups within the health care arena. Such groups may use subtle but effective maneuvers to lead nurses to conclude that involvement takes them from the client and is not in their own or the client's best interests.

There is also the barrier of relatively few nurses receiving graduate level preparation in the concepts and strategies of disciplines basic to community health (e.g., epidemiology, biostatistics, community development, service administration, and policy formation). One of the problems mentioned earlier in the discussion on the community health nurse practitioner, which continues to be a problem in master's level preparation for public health nursing, is that in many programs the skills necessary for population assessment and management are not given the in-depth treatment accorded other components of the curriculum, particularly the direct care aspects. In short, with few exceptions within the graduate programs in public health nursing there is no aggressive effort to develop population-focused skills commensurate with the need. The bias of many nurses seems to be that these skills are less important than clinical skills. However, these skills are as essential as direct care skills; they are just as difficult to develop and they should be given more attention in public health nursing graduate programs.

In discussing population-focused skills, selected analytical and measurement skills from the disciplines of epidemiology and biostatistics as they relate to population surveillance and programming for the delivery of personal health services are especially important. It must be clarified that epidemiological and biostatistical skills represent only two of many important skills for population-focused community health practice. A 1976 report of the Milbank Memorial Fund Commission on Higher Education for Public Health suggested that there were three elements that were central and generic to public health: ". . . the measurement and *analytical* sciences of epidemiology and biostatistics; social policy and the history and philosophy of public health; and the principles of management and organization for public health" (Milbank, 1976, p. 74-75). Noticeably absent from this general list is a clear identification of community development processes cited in the discussion of the community nurse practitioner. The issue is not to enumerate all of the areas that might be important to population-focused practice but rather to focus attention on the reality that those concerned about the future of community health should place more effort on developing public health nursing specialists with advanced skills in one or more of these arenas. Unless such attention is given, the lack of knowledge and skills represents a serious barrier to further development of the specialty.

Dilemmas and Challenges from Acceptance of Population-focused Public Health Nursing
What is the Arena for Practice?

If the premise is accepted that the distinctive feature of public health nursing is a focus on populations and the interplay between the health status of populations and other characteristics of the community, an important question is whether the only populations that should be considered are those outside of institutional settings. To answer "no" to this question implies that all of nursing practice can be subsumed under public health nursing practice. Although this might not appear to be a satisfactory conclusion for those who do not define themselves as community health nursing specialists, a broad understanding of public health should include all populations within the community. Further, a broad approach should also consider the match between the health needs of the population and the health care resources in the community, including services offered in institutional settings.

However, to say that all populations and health-related services within a geographically defined community should be of concern to public health specialists is not to say that everybody who provides direct care services within a community is a public health specialist. All direct care providers may contribute in their individual ways to the community's health in the broad sense, but not all are primarily concerned with the population focus, the "big picture." Thus all nurses in a given community, including those in hospitals, physicians' offices, and health clinics, should theoretically be contributing positively to the health of the community. However, the special contribution of public health specialists is to look at the community as a whole and raise questions about its overall health status and factors associated with that status.

The prevalent view of public health nursing at present

and historically has been to provide direct care services, including health education, to persons or family units outside of institutional settings. Such practice falls into the upper right quadrant in Figure 15-2, where the Hx appears. To adopt the arguments made earlier for population-focused practice would mean at least that public health nursing should be moving toward the upper left quadrant, a population focus outside of institutional settings. What about populations within institutional settings? Should population approaches be considered there? Would the nursing services of a given hospital be more appropriately developed if systematic mechanisms were in place to identify clinical subpopulations with particular nursing needs and target services to those subpopulations? Are some of the assessment and management decisions analogous to those necessary in dealing with subpopulations outside of institutional settings? Clearly, there are important conceptual, analytical, and methodological commonalities between noninstitutional populations and those within institutions. A key example is the common need for computerized information systems.

Within the field of epidemiology there is an emerging subdiscipline that attracts mainly physicians who identify themselves as clinical epidemiologists and who concentrate on subpopulations within clinical settings. In working with these clinical populations, the same epidemiological strategies are applied as are used with free-living populations

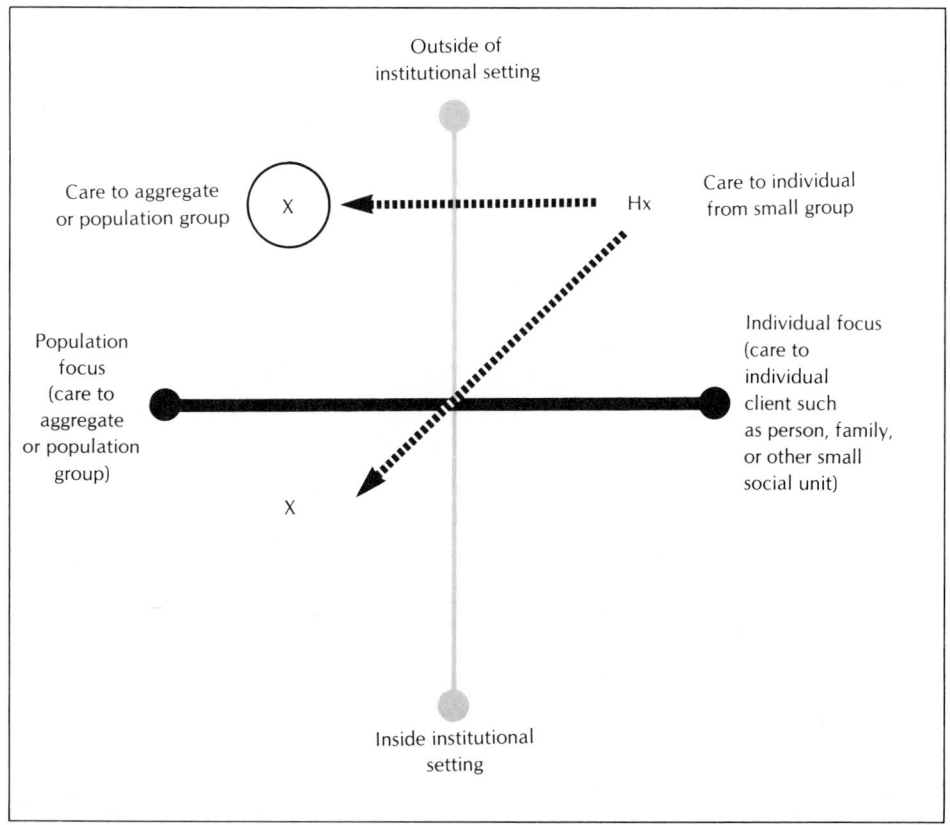

FIGURE 15-2

Arenas for practice.

more traditionally associated with epidemiology, the major difference is in the questions being pursued.

Should the specialty of public health nursing claim as its arena for practice a population focus regardless of where the population is located? An affirmative response makes more sense than a negative one particularly in terms of the knowledge and skills needed for decision-making versus the way health services are being reorganized within the United States.

Elsewhere an argument has been made for a new synthesis between selected aspects of what has been thought of as nursing administration and specialization in public health nursing (Williams, 1985). The basis of the argument is the need for nursing administrators, regardless of setting (in hospitals or in environments usually thought of as "community-based") to possess those skills described as necessary for population-focused practice. In fact, with the recent changes in the restructuring of health care settings (Starr, 1982, Ginzberg, 1984) now more than ever there is a critical need for strong, well-prepared, creative nursing leadership.

In response to the major changes in structuring the organizations through which care is given and how it is paid for, those in positions of leadership in the medical community are saying some very interesting things. In one commentary it was suggested that physicians should consider taking the responsibility for health plans so they could influence what happens. And, in the same commentary, it was pointed out that "assuming responsibility for a health plan means assuming financial, organizational, and clinical responsibility for the health of a population" (Kralewske et al., 1986, p. 342). In another commentary Hillman and his associates (1986) argued that physicians should become more involved in the design and management of care systems and that they should receive additional training for roles as physician-executives. The emergence of such interests in medicine presents a new challenge to nursing leadership and makes it urgent that we move forward in preparing nurses who can design nursing services that can effectively identify and respond to the needs of the many subpopulations in the community.

When responsibility for population-focused decisions regarding nursing needs is assumed, the nurse is practicing in the arena of community health nursing. In Figure 15-2 this is represented by the upper and lower left quadrants. However, whether the practice is seen as public health nursing or nursing service administration is not crucial. The important thing is that we concentrate more attention on preparing nurses for such responsibilities.

There are, however, three reasons the upper left quadrant in Figure 15-2 should be the most important practice arena for health nursing. First, in dealing with noninstitutionalized populations, which represent the majority of a community most of the time, preventive strategies can have the greatest impact. Second, the major interface between health status and the environment (physical, biological, sociocultural) occurs in the *noninstitutional population.* Third, for philosophical, historical, and economic reasons it is in organizational structures that serve noninstitutionalized pop-

ulations (health departments, health maintenance organizations, health centers, etc.) that population-focused practice is most likely to flourish.

The Need to Deemphasize Focus on the "Role" of the Public Health Nurse and Expand Possibilities

Within community nursing circles there has been a tendency to talk about community health nursing from the point of view of a role, such as the public health nursing role or the community health nursing specialist. This is viewed as limiting. In discussing such roles there is an enormous preoccupation with a direct care provider orientation. Even in discussions about how a population perspective can be made operational in practice, it is interesting that the focus is frequently on how an individual practitioner, such as a staff nurse in an agency, can adopt such a practice focus. Rarely is attention given to how nurse administrators might reorient their practice to be concerned with a population focus, which is more critical, useful, and possible for an administrator than for the staff nurse. This is because in many agencies nursing administrators, supervisors, or others (sometimes program directors who are not nurses) make the key decisions about how staff nurses will spend their time—what types of clients will be seen and under what circumstances. To what extent are such decisions based on the types of data described earlier?

With regard to administrators, those who are prepared to practice in a population-focused manner are more effective than those who are not prepared. On the other hand, staff nurses would benefit from having a clear understanding of population-focused practice for three reasons. First, it would give them professional satisfaction in being able to put their own clinical activities into perspective, to see how what they do clinically contributes at the population level. Second, it would help them understand and appreciate the practice of their associates who are population-focused specialists. Third, it would give them a firmer basis for providing clinical input to decision making at the programmatic or agency level, a necessary contribution to effective and efficient population-focused practice. Clearly it is desirable that staff nurses have a population focus, but the reality is that their ability to make decisions at that level is more limited than that of the nurse with some administrative responsibility.

Another problem with thinking in terms of nursing roles is that present role conceptualizations are frequently too limited to allow for population-focused practice. Also, roles that might include the type of decision making being suggested may not be defined as nursing roles. Examples of the latter include directorships of health departments, state or regional programs, and units of health planning and evaluation. If population-focused public health nursing is to be taken seriously and strategies for its implementation (assessment, intervention, and evaluation) at the population level are to be applied, more consideration must be given to organized systems for assessing population needs and managing care. Such a view of public health nursing clearly places those who specialize in this area in the position of dealing with health care policy. In other words, public health nurses must move into situations in which policy formation is a recognized component, but to do so some may have to assume positions outside of what is usually thought of as a nursing position or a nursing role. This is true because at present much of the policy making that directly affects whether nursing services are provided to certain populations and what services are rendered occurs outside of the range of what are normally referred to as *nursing roles.*

Too much attention on defining nursing roles, particularly defining them in such a manner that they would fit into the present way of structuring nursing services, may have unfortunate limitations. For the immediate future it may be more useful to concentrate on the identification of skills and knowledge necessary for the type of decision making suggested as being inherent in population-focused practice. The question can be raised of where in the broader community and health care system such decisions are made and given the answers, the strategy should be to develop nurses with the substantive knowledge, skills, and political finesse necessary for success in such positions. Some of these positions are within nursing settings, particularly roles such as the administrator of the nursing service and top level staff nurse administrators, but as suggested earlier, other such positions may be outside of what are traditionally viewed as nursing roles.

Can a Viable Balance Be Achieved Between Clinical and Population-focused Skills in Graduate Preparation?

Whether or not a balance between clinical and population-focused skills can be achieved is a question that public health nursing educators and service people have asked in contemplating a more serious effort in developing aggregate and community skills, as was undertaken in the community nurse practitioner program discussed earlier. There are several issues that need to be considered in dealing with this question. First, there is the issue of appropriate preparation. Second, there is the question of what is possible in the practice world following preparation, discussed in part earlier.

To date most of the discussion regarding preparation for public health nursing has been limited to thinking in terms of baccalaureate and master's level preparation. One problem with present-day master's preparation is the fact that there is not sufficient emphasis in most curricula to lead to an in-depth understanding and reasonable level of skill in those areas basic to population-focused practice. Much of this has been the result of the fact that master's programs in community health nursing and public health nursing have tried to include a component of direct care. In only a few exceptions has there been a strong emphasis on population-focused skills. If master's level programming concentrated on such a perspective, and started with students who were well prepared at the undergraduate level and experienced in direct care, it would be possible to go further in the development of population skills. Clearly master's programs might be profitably strengthened by refocusing objectives, but such developments should not detract from

the serious attention that must be given to doctoral study as a basis for the further development of community health nursing practice.

Doctoral work could be concentrated in one of the areas identified by the Milbank report (1976) cited earlier. With regard to the health assessment of populations and the evaluation of outcomes, there is a high level of congruence between the skills necessary for such functions and research skills, for which there is wide consensus that doctoral study is essential. This should not be taken to mean that all assessment and evaluation activities of public health nursing specialists should be viewed as research; the objectives are different, but the knowledge and skills necessarily overlap to a high degree, particularly in the use of content from epidemiology and biostatistics. It is important to remember that the use of such skills in population-focused practice has as its primary objective obtaining a sound knowledge base of the population being served as opposed to a primary concern of developing generalized knowledge, the goal of research. There are some circumstances in which both goals can be met, and a challenge for the future is to work toward creating more of them.

Achieving a balance between preparation, advanced clinical skills, and population-focused skills should not be an objective of a graduate program in public health nursing. At the graduate level a choice needs to be made so that advanced preparation in one area does not suffer at the expense of the other. Those who want graduate preparation in both areas should consider two separate programs of study. For example, a sequence that may become increasingly familiar is a clinical master's degree (direct care-focused) and a population-focused doctorate.

CLINICAL APPLICATION

This chapter has described the controversy that surrounds the definition of the community health and public health nursing specialists. The thesis of this chapter is that population-focused nursing practice is different from clinical nursing care delivered in the community. If one accepts the thesis of this chapter that public health nursing is population-focused and encompasses a unique body of knowledge, then it is useful to debate where nurses practice public health nursing.

In your community, health class, debate with classmates whether the following categories of nurses who typically function in the community are practicing population-focused public health nursing:

1. School nurses
2. Home health nurses
3. Discharge planners
4. Nurses in a health maintenance organization
5. Nurses in public health clinics
6. Nurses working in nursing homes

Which are (are not) public health nurses? Why are they considered (not considered) public health nurses?

Interview three nurses working in one of the settings on the list. Determine what their scope of practice is. Are they carrying out population-focused practice? Could they? How?

SUMMARY

Arguments for population-focused public health nursing have been offered, and it has been suggested that preparation for practice would include graduate study in areas such as epidemiology, biostatistics, community development, policy formation, and administration. Further, the relationship between the type of position held in an organizational structure and the potential to practice with a population focus has been discussed. The central point is that those in administrative roles in settings providing personal care services make decisions affecting aggregates or populations; thus population-focused public health nursing is more directly relevant and applicable to their situation. Such administrators would profit from being prepared to practice in a population-focused manner and from having staff associates who are also prepared (e.g., specialists in planning, evaluation, and community development).

In view of the previous comments, the question of how baccalaureate level preparation fits in can be raised, and there are various opinions on this topic. One is that at the baccalaureate level there ought to be two types of learning objectives. First, undergraduate students ought to be introduced to the earlier mentioned key concepts and strategies of the disciplines basic to community health. Second, baccalaureate students ought to be provided opportunities to understand how (a) decision making on the part of those responsible for population-level decisions differs from clinical decisions made by individual providers but (b) influences the latter in a variety of ways (i.e., population-focused decisions determine what kinds of providers are hired, nurse practitioner or physician, what patients can be seen; what range of services are offered; and in what type of settings).

A key distinction between the focus of preparation at the baccalaureate level as opposed to the intent of master's and doctoral preparation is that preparation at the baccalaureate level should be directed to providing beginning insight into what population-focused practice is—its benefits and some understanding of the knowledge and skills necessary for such practice. Preparing graduates to assume primary responsibilities as public health nursing specialists should be left to graduate programs.

For several reasons it is important to emphasize that undergraduate programs introduce students to population-focused practice. First, as professionals, all baccalaureate graduates entering first-level staff positions should have an appreciation of the context of their practice—how what they do as clinicians relates to the populations served by the settings in which they work. Second, such preparation should facilitate a better understanding of the reciprocal relationship that is desirable between direct care clinicians and population-focused specialists. Such reciprocity might lead to better collaboration and more effective and efficient nursing services. Finally, a good foundation in public health nursing at the undergraduate level can be extremely important in attracting students to this practice specialty. Without such preparation they might be lost to other areas of specialization.

☰ KEY CONCEPTS

The community health nurse practitioner is sometimes described as a nurse who works with individuals and families in providing direct care outside of institutional settings.

The notion that the focus of community health nursing is "the provision of health services among people of the community and the encouragement of health-promoting behavior" is one held by many nurses. Another way to view the community health nurse practitioner is as a nurse who focuses on the community as client.

According to the 1984 Consensus Conference sponsored by the Nursing Division of the Department of Health and Human Services, a public health nurse is one who "has received specific educational preparation and supervised clinical practice in public health nursing."

Setting is viewed as the feature that distinguishes community health nursing from other nursing specialties. Unfortunately, the equation of the term community with the term noninstitutionalized leads to further confusion. Further, the present reorganization of the health care system has made the institutional/noninstitutional distinction outdated.

Public health nursing is seen as a subset or specialty of community health nursing.

Population-focused practice is the focus of specialization in public health nursing. This focus on population is the fundamental factor that distinguishes public health nursing from other nursing specialties.

Population is defined as a collection of individuals who share a common one or more personal or environmental characteristics.

LEARNING ACTIVITIES

1. Define for your personal understanding (a) the community health clinical nurse practitioner and (b) the community health nurse population-focused practitioner.

2. State your opinion of the similarities and/or differences between the clinical role and the population-focused role of the community health nurse practitioner.

3. Review the models of Community Health Nursing Practice of the ANA and APHA as described in Chapter 7.

4. With three to four of your classmates debate the issue of clinical nurse role versus population-focused practice.

One of the most serious barriers to the fuller development of population-focused community health nursing is the mindset of many nurses that their proper role is the direct care role at the client's bedside.

An important question regarding population-focused practice is whether the only populations that should be considered are those outside of institutional settings.

5. With your instructor invite two community health nurse practitioners with opposing views to present a discussion and debate on the issue stated in number 4.

BIBLIOGRAPHY

Acheson, R.M.: Epidemiology: the training of community physicians in Great Britain. In White, K.L., and Henderson, M.M., editor. Epidemiology as a fundamental science, New York, 1976, Oxford University Press, Inc.

American Nurses' Association, Division on Community Health Nursing: Conceptual model of community health nursing, Pub. No. CH-10, Kansas City, Mo., 1980, The Association.

American Public Health Association: The definition and role of public health nursing in the delivery of health care: a statement of the public health nursing section, Washington, D.C., 1981, The Association.

Consensus Conference on the Essentials of Public Health Nursing Practice and Education, Rockville, Maryland, 1985, U.S. Department of Health and Human Services, Bureau of Health Professions, Division of Nursing.

deTornyay, R.: Public health nursing: the nurse's role in community-based practice, Ann. Rev. Public Health 1:83, 1980.

Flynn, B.C., et al.: One master's curriculum in community health nursing, Nurs. Outlook 26:633, 1978.

Ginzberg, E.: The monetarization of medical care, N. Engl. J. Med. 310:1162, 1984.

Goeppinger, J.: Community health nursing: primary nursing care in society. In Flynn, B.C., and Miller, M.H., editor: Current perspectives in nursing, II, St. Louis, 1979, The C.V. Mosby Co.

Highriter, M.E.: A computerized nursing management information system for identification and community follow-up of high-risk infants. In Werley, H.H., and Grier M.R., editors: Nursing information systems, New York, 1981, Springer Publishing Co., Inc.

Hillman, A.L., et al.: Managing tthe medical-industrial complex, N. Engl. J. Med. 315:511, 1986.

Kark, S.L.: The practice of community-oriented primary health care. New York, 1981, Appleton-Century-Crofts.

Kralewski, J.E., et al.: The physician rebellion, N. Engl. J. Med. 316:339, 1986.

Milbank Memorial Fund: Commission on higher education for public health, (Cecil G. Sheps, Chairman), New York, 1976. Prodist.

Skrovan, C., Anderson, E.T., and Gottschalk, J.: Community nurse practitioner, an emerging role, Am. J. Public Health 64:847, 1974.

Starr, P.: The social transformation of American medicine, New York, 1982, Basic Books, Inc., Publishers.

Williams, C.A.: Nursing leadership in community health: a neglected issue. In McCloskey, J.C., and Grace, H.K., editors: Current issues in nursing, Oxford, England, 1981, Blackwell Scientific Publications, Ltd.

Williams, C.A.: Population-focused community health nursing and nursing administration: A new synthesis. In McCloskey, J.C., and Grace, H.K., editors: Current issues in nursing, ed. 2, Boston, 1985, Blackwell Scientific Publications, Ltd.

Williams, C.A., and Highriter, M.E.: Community health nursing: population focus and evaluation, P.H. Reports, Public Health Reviews 7:197-221, 1978.

Woods, J., and Ohlson, V.: Graduate preparation for community nursing practice. In Flynn, B.C., and Miller, M.H., editors: Current perspectives in nursing: social issues and trends, St. Louis, 1977, The C.V. Mosby Co.

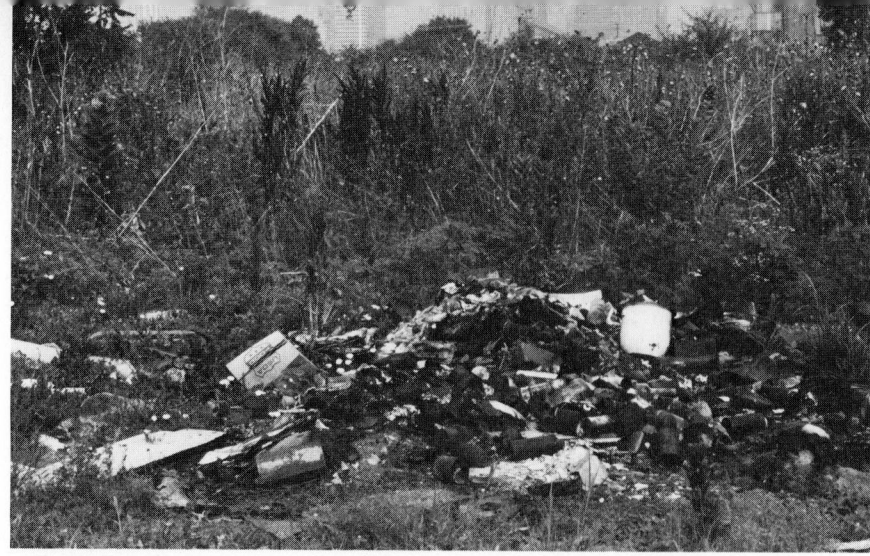

Jeanette Lancaster

ENVIRONMENTAL HEALTH AND SAFETY

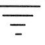 OBJECTIVES

After reading this chapter, the student should be able to:

List the major environmental health hazards and describe why and how they pose a serious threat to the general quality of life.

Briefly discuss the science that provides a model for looking at the human/environmental interaction and name the theory underlying this science.

List several environmental health disasters and the environmental hazards associated with each.

Name the major types of environmental hazards and the specific types of physical hazards affecting the environment.

Define environmental health and identify three primary routes of entry.

Identify the federal agency with primary responsibility for regulating the safety and health of workers.

Describe the assessment role of community health nurses in dealing with environmental health and safety.

Plan an intervention strategy complete with an evaluation schedule to deal with one environmental health problem noted in the community.

KEY TERMS

biosphere

carbon monoxide

chemical additive contamination

chlorine

Commoner's "laws of ecology"

ecology

ecosystem

environmental health

Environmental Protection Agency (EPA)

eutrophication

host-agent-transmission model

hazard

microbiological comtamination

molds

natural radiation

naturally occurring chemicals

ozone

pneumoconiosis

pulmonary irritants

radioactivity

suboptimal food handling

synthetic radiation

threshold limit values (TLVs)

toxicity

vector control

water pollution

Environmental problems are as old as history itself; over the centuries some have increased in severity, others have diminished, and discouraging new problems have emerged. Issues identified decades ago have not been solved; the problems have increased and the issues remain, although in increasingly complicated forms. Some are merely eyesores, others are serious enough to make the simple act of breathing a difficult task. Nurses play a key role in detecting environmental health hazards and in developing and implementing health promotion and treatment programs.

Environmental degradation and deterioration have been concerns of environmentalists for many years; however, public awareness remained low until the 1960s, when it began to increase dramatically. Since the 1960s environmental groups have become more active. Early in the 1980s several leading U.S. environmental groups criticized the Reagan administration's environmental policies. Criticism was aimed at the weakening of the Clean Air Act, failure to act on acid rain and toxic air pollutants, loosening of controls on hazardous wastes, and subsidizing of nuclear energy. Critics still contend that safeguards to prevent threats to environmental health have yet to be fully implemented.

In 1970 the United States Environmental Protection Agency (EPA) was formed and given primary responsibility for controlling pollution and dealing with threats to life and the environment. The EPA has been accused of being lax in meeting deadlines, and some programs have never been initiated. Under the Reagan administration the agency encountered large reductions in personnel, authority, and budget.

Even with EPA regulations and achievements, some environmental hazards have reached critical levels, posing a threat not only to health but also to the general quality and fabric of life. Newspaper, radio, and television repeatedly offer horror stories of chemical spills and exposures, acid rain, asbestos in city water, contaminated fish, and deterioration of the ozone level. Acid rain caused by ozone pollution is responsible for billions of dollars of damage to crops annually. Ozone depletion will result in increased susceptibility to skin cancer.

The production and maintenance of a healthy, stimulating, and enjoyable environment will require a combination of increased litigation, vigorous enforcement of existing laws, increased cooperation by business, and greater public awareness and education. Community health nurses can make significant contributions to this process.

There are four basic ways in which hazardous substances enter the environment and are transmitted to people:

1. Direct exposure to the source—for example, lead in paint, insecticides such as DDT, or chemical compounds such as Tris flame retardant in children's sleepwear.
2. Direct discharge into air or water such as through smokestacks or via automobile exhaust or untreated sewage into waterways.
3. Inadequate landfills that result in runoff (rain carrying hazardous substances to rivers and lakes which provide water for people); leaching, in which the hazardous wastes seep into groundwater or travel through the food chain and are incorporated into plants, which are eaten by animals, which are eaten by people.
4. Dumping—for example in Byron, Illinois, 1500 drums filled with chemical waste and buried for many years allowed the leakage of cyanide, heavy metals, and other toxins into both surface and groundwater (Blumenthal, 1985).

Each of these problems are discussed in the sections that follow.

HISTORICAL PERSPECTIVE

The environment played a key role in early community health measures. In biblical times many customs, taboos, and religious practices were derived from interactions between people and environmental conditions. Moses' Law satisfied both religious and sanitary conditions. As people became aggregated or urbanized, problems such as an adequate supply of water and the removal of wastes were apparent. As early as 3000 to 1500 BC, the Minoans and Egyptians built flood dikes, drainage, and irrigation systems and had public water systems (Hanlon and Pickett, 1984). The Romans built impressive aqueducts, drainage systems, gutters, and public baths and paved the streets. As cities developed in the Middle Ages, communicable diseases evolved. Pandemics of cholera associated with polluted water and bubonic plague (Black Death) carried by rats drastically reduced the population of Europe. Leprosy probably started in Egypt and was spread by the Crusaders.

In the United States the development of the colonies led to the establishment of textile and paper mills. The demand for an endless number of products increased, and the nation's transition from a farm economy to early industry was underway.

Another historical change was the replacement of flatboats with railroads as a means of transportation. Railroads pushed their way across the American frontier, linking two oceans. Hastily constructed steel mills with their numerous emissions provided the tracks on which the trains ran, and newly dug coal mines provided their fuel. Factories still depended on workers' skills; as technology increased, so did the demand for workers.

Environmental health in the United States was seriously questioned after 1850 following publication of the *Report of the Sanitary Commission of Massachusetts* (Rosen, 1957). This report, although largely ignored at the time of publication, is regarded today as a landmark document because of the implications for environmental health. Recommendations specific to environmental health included the development of a systematic plan for observing atmospheric phenomena, smoke prevention, measures to ensure pure air and water, adequate drainage, sewage, and pest control. Other recommendations dealt with occupational health, housing, pest control, food, drugs, and schools. Ironically, many of the problems addressed in the report exist today.

The Industrial Revolution brought new hazards to people and the environment. The use of machinery and suboptimal work methods led to stress, physical injuries, and chemical exposures. Cities doubled in size. Knowledge of sanitation and personal hygiene was unavailable for the poor and the hundreds of immigrants who flocked to this country in search of jobs.

Conditions in the mines and the steel mills were deplorable in the early twentieth century. In the large cities sweatshops were a constant threat to life and health for many workers. Men, women, and children put in 70- and 80-hour work weeks in factories. Tuberculosis and other diseases were common among workers. The early 1930s brought badly needed legislation that changed working hours for children and adults. New automated machines and techniques replaced the old. Sophisticated mechanization led to mass production, and cities became increasingly overcrowded. Emissions from industries and automobiles polluted the air. Factories discharged industrial wastes into the air and waterways.

World War II brought an increasing number of women into the labor force. Women worked with chemicals and gases, such as benzidine and vinyl chloride, both of which are now considered to be carcinogenic. After the war men replaced a large majority of women in the work force and continued to work with these and other carcinogenic substances. The use of amines such as benzidine has now been banned in foreign countries; they are not used in the United States either but were until the 1970s. Many of the women workers during World War II have since developed bladder cancer.

As the demand for supplies and products increased, so did the pressures to keep costs down and production up.

The results were increased accidents, injuries, and deaths. Legislation regulating workplace hazards was passed in 1970 with the enactment of the Occupational Safety and Health Act (OSHA). The law requires employers to comply with specific standards promulgated by the Department of Labor. In addition to OSHA, the act created the National Institute for Occupational Safety and Health (NIOSH) within the Department of Health and Human Services (DHHS) to conduct research on occupational hazards and recommend new standards to OSHA. Both agencies have tended to be understaffed and underfunded. The effectiveness of OSHA and NIOSH has also been diminished by the lengthy process involved in setting standards.

People are currently experiencing the most varied and intense life stressors in the history of humanity. Tremendous advances in science, technology, education as well as the social and behavioral sciences are altering the ability of individuals, families, groups, and communities to maintain balance and stability. Not all of these changes are positive. Despite considerable knowledge about the relationship between health and the environment, waterways are increasingly polluted, the air is filled with noxious substances and pesticides, and radiation and nuclear power threaten livelihood. Each attempt to make life more comfortable and pleasant leads to new sources of pollution and stress.

Past models of environmental influences on health are no longer effective for the complex problems of the twentieth century. Although some water, air, or noise pollution in isolation may not disrupt homeostasis, when all three are present in combination with factors such as crowding, interpersonal stress, and chemical or biological hazards, their cumulative impact can disrupt the ability to cope successfully with environmental stimuli.

ECOLOGY AND ENVIRONMENTAL HEALTH

Ecology, the age-old study of living organisms in interaction with the environment, provides a model for looking at environmental health. Ecology is concerned with the broad conceptualization of the interrelationships between living and nonliving things. The term *ecology* was first proposed by German biologist Ernst Haeckel in 1869; the word is derived from the Greek root *oikos,* meaning house. Ecology literally means the study of organisms at home. Ecology is concerned with both structure and functioning of the organism; it attends to the surroundings as well as that which is surrounded.

Ecology, in order to study the interrelationships within an environment, is action oriented and focuses on what can be rather than ending its conceptualization of the human/environment relationship with either what has been or what is. The term **biosphere** refers to the world of living things and is made up of numerous ecosystems. Each **ecosystem** represents all living and nonliving parts that support a chain of life within a selected area (Wilner et al., 1978) and is the sum total of all existing subsystems.

In each ecosystem, nature provides specific conditions essential for supporting plant and animal life. Each ecosystem is a "circle of life" comprising four principal types of components: (1) sunlight, water, oxygen, carbon dioxide, organic compounds, and other nutrients for plant growth; (2) plants, which convert carbon dioxide and water into carbohydrates through photosynthesis; (3) consumers of the products of plants: herbivores (for example, cows and sheep) and carnivores (man and other meat-eating animals); (4) decomposed organisms such as bacteria, fungi, and insects.

Barry Commoner's "laws of ecology" help to explain the scope of environmental health. Commoner (1971) organized an informal series of laws of ecology, with the first one holding that "everything is connected to everything else" and stating that sunlight, water, oxygen, carbon dioxide, organic compounds, and all organisms are interconnected. The second law, "everything must go somewhere," stipulates that one organism's excretion or waste is taken up by another organism as food. The third law "nature knows best," holds that human changes within a natural system do not always improve that system and may prove to be detrimental. The fourth law, "there is no such thing as a free lunch," stipulates that anything removed from the natural environment by human effort must be replaced and anything added to the natural environment must be removed if the environment is to be preserved. The extent to which these laws are violated or obeyed determines the status of the environment. These laws call attention to the interrelated nature of the human environment and support the need for using an ecological perspective in viewing environmental health.

In studying ecosystems it is also necessary to consider people as part of, not separate from, a life support system composed of the atmosphere, water, soil, plants, and animals that function together to keep the system viable. When people are considered a part of their environment, it is essential to consider attitudes, values, and perceptions. The behavior of people is influenced by their values and attitudes about themselves, others, and the world around them. Similarly, one's perception of reality is usually more influential in determining behavior than the reality itself. People act in accordance with what they perceive, think, feel, and cherish.

From an ecological perspective the environment is a multifaceted system made up of biophysical and sociocultural components. The interrelationships between the person and the environment are dynamic. Each makes demands on the other, as people try to adapt to the environment or adapt their needs and desires to meet the current state of the environment. Adaptation is a process, not an event. For any organism to survive, it must learn to adapt. Nothing remains fixed or constant in a living system; rather, living systems are in a constant state of adaptation as organisms continually accommodate to new stressors. Not all adaptations are smooth or positive in outcome. A system can be overloaded so that it cannot adapt to the stimuli. For example, people can be temporarily placed in a noisy situation that is intolerable but over time they may adjust, for example, to the sound of large airplanes landing near their homes, or the sound may decrease. However, if the noise overload is too great or is constant, a person can experience psychotic symptoms caused by continuous sensory overload.

People often overlook the multiple interactions required to maintain a stable relationship among living and nonliving parts of the environment. A classic example of the lack of an orientation to planning occurred in Borneo with a World Health Organization mosquito control program (Harrison et al., 1969). After a community was heavily sprayed with DDT, the mosquitoes were controlled, but roofs began to be eaten by caterpillars, which were unaffected by DDT. The spray also killed wasps that previously ate the caterpillars. The problem was complicated after indoor spraying to control houseflies. Previously, a small harmless gecko lizard ate the houseflies. However, when the lizards ate the diseased flies, the lizards become debilitated and were easily captured by their predators, the cats. As cats disappeared due to the consumption of DDT, which was passed from one animal to another in the chain, the rat population boomed, invading houses and threatening Borneo with the plague (Hanlon and Pickett, 1984). This example shows how easily, with the help of people, an ecosystem can be thrown out of balance. Throughout the remainder of the chapter consider how each of the environmental hazards could ultimately lead to an equally undesirable outcome.

Not only do people contribute to the status of their environment, but also they are products of that environment; therefore the environment is a determinant of health and well-being. *Environmental health* may therefore be defined as that aspect of community health which is concerned with these forms of life, substances, forces, and conditions in the surroundings of people that may exert an influence on their health and well-being. Environmental health embodies the absence or presence of illness, health maintenance, human efficiency, and the enjoyment of life.

Many parts of the environment can produce health hazards; biological organisms, toxic chemicals, radioactivity, ineffective waste disposal, noise, and other physical and psychosocial forces.

IDENTIFICATION OF ENVIRONMENTAL HAZARDS

Many contemporary changes disrupt the circle of life. Hanlon and Pickett (1984) propose two contexts for describing the human and environment relationship. The first includes elements of the natural environment hazardous to health such as biological agents of disease or injury, including microorganisms, plants, and animals; weather; radiation, naturally occurring chemicals; and geological perturbations such as earthquakes and volcanoes. The second context consists of health hazards brought on by the actions and maladaptations of people to their environment and includes suicide, accidents, genetic damage, poisoning, and health threats from pollution.

The modern environment is hazardous in at least two ways: it contains noxious and stressful events and it changes so quickly that people are unable to adapt. As discussed in Chapter 30, the rate of change offers phenomenal stress caused by rapid and often novel requirements for human adaptation. Even small doses of a contaminant over a long period of time can disrupt health. Factors within the environment often work together to reinforce one another (synergism) or act in opposition (antagonism). Problems, because of their interactive nature, cannot be considered in isolation but rather must be viewed from an ecological perspective. Community health nurses are called on to provide information to consumers and agencies about the effect of the environment on health as well as to carefully assess for environmental hazards and plan appropriate interventions. To do this, an understanding of contemporary environmental contaminants is needed.

Biological Hazards

Biological hazards include disease-producing agents that can enter the human body. They consist largely of bacteria, viruses, and other microorganisms and parasites (Hanlon and Pickett, 1984). As discussed in Chapters 8 and 17, for a disease to be transmitted, a host source, causative agent, and means of transmission must be present. The following outline depicts selected environmental aspects of the host-agent-transmission model.

Environmental Impact Analysis Areas*

Potential impacts to the physical environment
- Air
    - Climate
    - Air emissions
    - Air quality
- Water
    - Water requirements
    - Water availability
    - Water quality
- Physiography
    - Soils
    - Geology
    - Topography
    - Drainage modifications
- Solid wastes
    - Quantity
    - Disposal
- Mineral resources
    - Consumption
    - Depletion

Potential impacts to the biological environment
- Flora
    - Terrestrial
    - Aquatic
    - Endangered species
- Fauna
    - Terrestrial
    - Aquatic
    - Endangered species
- Ecological relationships
    - Ecological balance
    - Critical species in food chain
    - Productivity
    - Diversity

Potential impacts to human environment
- Socioeconomic impacts
    - Population and demographic changes
    - Economic conditions
    - Employment
        - Wages
        - Tax base
    - Social conditions
        - Noise
        - Pressure on services such as police, fire, schools, and hospitals and on utilities and transportation
    - Changes in daily living patterns
    - Land use
    - Water use
    - Aesthetics
    - Special interest points
        - Archaeological
        - Paleontological
        - Historical
        - Recreational
    - Human health effects
        - Air emissions
        - Water residuals
        - Solid wastes

Biological hazards are primarily concerned with entry of disease-producing infectious agents into the body (Purdom, 1980). Many biological hazards are described in detail in Chapter 17. In general, biological hazards are transmitted either through the escape of an agent from a source or reservoir to a susceptible host.

Some people are more seriously affected by communicable disease than others, depending on their state of health, level of immunity, heredity, and environmental and other prevailing conditions at the time of exposure (Purdom, 1980). Common forms of invading pathogens are bacteria, fungi, and mold.

Water

As discussed in Chapter 1, water has served as a waste disposal mechanism since early recorded history. Rome channeled its sewage into the Tiber River through aqueducts. Epidemics of typhoid fever, cholera, and dysentery occurred during the Middle Ages when the same bodies of water were used for waste disposal and for drinking. In the last century oceans, lakes, and rivers have become dumping sites for sewage and industrial wastes. Health hazards come from ingesting polluted water from one of the following sources: waterborne viruses and bacteria, waste heat, radioactivity, industrial pollutants, oil spills, and underground pollution from dumping.

Drinking water is obtained either from surface sources such as lakes or streams or from underground. Surface sources are more susceptible to contamination with infectious organisms. Drinking water can be contaminated in one of four ways: if untreated; when deficiences exist in the treatment system; when deficiencies exist in the distribution system, for example, if sewage and water lines get crossed; or when a properly functioning treatment system is unable to remove contaminating agents or chemicals (Blumenthal, 1985).

Contaminants that currently pose major problems for water sources include fertilizers, herbicides, fungicides, irrigation residues, detergents from homes and industry, radioactive wastes from power plants and industrial and research facilities, heavy metals, and salts. Many of these are

---

*From Golden, J., et al.: Environmental impact data book, Ann Arbor, Mich., 1979, Ann Arbor Science Publishers, Inc.

not readily broken down and are unaffected by usual treatment methods, so they build up in the water.

Increasing concern in recent years has revolved around the contamination of drinking water. Previously, groundwater was thought to be reasonably free from pollution. However, evidence now indicates that this water source is often contaminated by industrial and agricultural chemicals. Most of these chemicals take years, even decades, to clean up because they disintegrate slowly. The effects of these contaminants in small doses in water remains unknown; hence, consumers living in such areas must decide whether to take a chance that the water is safe, buy bottled water, or install a purifying device in the home water system. Once contaminated water becomes known in an area, housing prices drop and residents are often captive in the area.

Waterborne viruses and bacteria require moisture, a food medium, and proper temperature and pH to survive any length of time; therefore, water is an excellent medium for cultivating bacteria. Bacteria is normally filtered out of water as it moves through soil; waste that follows passageways along fissures in rocks, coarse gravel, or limestone conveys bacteria. Shallow wells may become contaminated when the distance the water travels through the soil is insufficient to filter out bacteria. Most communities have wells 450 to 1400 feet deep.

Bacteria or viruses may enter wells through surface water, by the use of contaminated water to prime pumps, through contamination of ropes, by buckets handled with unclean hands, or by cross connectors between water pipes and waste piping. Most outbreaks of waterborne diseases occur in private supplies, but contaminated public supplies affect more people.

Waterborne bacteria diseases include typhoid and paratyphoid fevers, dysentery, and cholera. Waterborne viral diseases include infectious hepatitis and poliomyelitis. The pathogens responsible for these diseases are found in the intestinal and urinary tracts of infected people.

The *temperature of water* directly influences the toxicity of many pollutants and the growth of bacteria and viruses. Aquatic life is damaged when industry dissipates heat in circulating water. As aquatic life is harmed, the circle of life or food chain is disrupted. Many factories use cooling towers to lower water heat; however, only a fourth to two thirds of the heat can be dissipated by this method.

Small amounts of toxic chemicals in water threaten all forms of life. For example, mercury has for many years been discharged from both industrial and agricultural sources. As it increases in concentration in the food chain, mercury can result in serious or even fatal poisoning, neurological disorders, or birth defects (Spath and Crook, 1985). Not only are food sources poisoned by chemicals in water, but recreation is also affected. Swimming in contaminated water can increase the incidence of gastrointestinal disease.

Radioactivity has been introduced into water in areas such as mining or milling, which use radioactive substances. In addition, industries making and testing atomic bombs release radioactive substances.

Water pollution can be broadly defined as the addition of something that changes the natural qualities of water.

Industry has altered water quality for years by dumping industrial waste into rivers and seas. Industrial wastes primarily consisting of paper, chemicals, primary metal, or petroleum are derived from the manufacturing process. These pollutants deplete the dissolved oxygen, causing fish to die and odors to develop. Contaminants, although not lethal to fish and shellfish, do render them inedible to humans.

Certain pollutants, such as phosphates, promote excess growth of nutrients in lakes. The nutrient, in a process called *eutrophication,* promotes the growth of algae, which cause cloudy, odorous water and produce deposits. These deposits are incompatible with most forms of aquatic life.

Oil spills and discharge from onshore and offshore facilities threaten marine life. Oil spills kill fish and certain birds and make beaches unusable for recreation. Onshore and offshore oil spills at the Atlantic, Pacific, and Gulf shores have killed fish and birds and made beaches undesirable recreation areas. Lakes are polluted also; almost all fish species in Lake Ontario have been found to be contaminated. Fish have been tainted with DDT, mercury, toxaphene, and other chemicals dumped by industries. Chlorinated hydrocarbons that remain poisonous for years have accumulated. The lake itself, once pleasing to look at, now poses an eyesore. Waterways leading to the lake often serve as dumps containing radioactive debris (Brown, 1982).

Moreover, oil-laden sediment can move with bottom currents and contaminate unpolluted offshore areas. As a result, the sea floor near an oil spill remains toxic to animals for long periods following the initial spill.

The National Community Water Supply Study of 1970 made numerous recommendations about the delivery of safe water. The study led to the enactment of the Safe Drinking Water Act of 1974. This act falls short of meeting the need for water safety because it fails to address the problem of small public water supplies or poor quality and large systems that obtain their water from sources polluted by synthetic organic chemicals not affected by the treatment processes being used (Hanlon and Pickett, 1974).

Food

An estimated 2 to 10 million people in the United States contract a foodborne disease annually. These diseases rank second only to the common cold as the most frequent cause of illness (Wilner et al., 1978). Environmental hazards related to food are of three main kinds. The first consists of *microbiological contamination* and usually occurs as a result of deposits of toxins on food. Contaminated foods may cause salmonellosis and shigellosis, illness from *Clostridium perfingens, Vibrio,* and viruses, and food poisonings from *Staphylococcus* and *Clostridium botulinus* toxins. Food poisoning from microbiological contamination is caused by the transfer of an organism through food to a human victim after which internal growth of the organism occurs.

A second environmental problem related to food is *chemical additive contamination.* Most Americans consume 5 pounds of chemical additives in food each year (Wilner et al., 1978). Chemical food additives fall into two categories: intentional additives and incidental additives. Intentional additives are deliberately used in food processing to enhance or conserve nutritional value or to improve or maintain flavor, color, texture, or consistency. The use of these additives is sanctioned by the Food and Drug Administration under the GRAS list (Generally Recognized As Safe). Typical GRAS additives include vitamins A_1, D_2, D_3, carotene, ascorbic acid, riboflavin, and others. A complete listing of such additives may be found in the *Federal Register*.

Incidental additives enter and remain in food as a result of their use as pesticides or herbicides, after addition to animal food, from packaging material, or through chemical changes brought about by processing methods. In these cases the levels in food must not exceed the tolerances set by the FDA.

A third environmental hazard relates to *suboptimal food handling*. Careless food handling, inadequate pretreatment, a contaminated environment, a high bacterial count, and poor food storage have negative influences on food safety and quality. A major community health nursing role in regard to food is that of education. Both consumers and other health care providers need to be well informed about the potential adverse effects of food contamination, additives, and improper handling. Education can be conveyed in a variety of ways including direct provision of facts to individual clients or groups, classes on the effects of environmental hazards, and a variety of public service announcements.

Air Pollution

Air pollution has always been present in the forms of volcanic eruptions, tree and grass pollination, and swamp gas. Today the majority of air pollution comes from industrial activities. Air pollution affects human health, property, animals, and plants. The control of air pollution is costly; thus the challenge is to determine what level of pollution can be tolerated.

Air is a mixture of gases, including nitrogen (78%), oxygen (21%), and a combination of carbon dioxide, helium, argon, neon, and others (1%). Air can contain water vapor and particulate material such as dust, haze from chemical reactions, and smoke (Reist, 1985). Air is continuously circulating because of energy from the sun and the rotation of the earth, and this atmospheric circulation influences the extent and concentration of pollutants in the air. In the broadest sense, air pollution results from the presence of foreign materials in the air and is either natural or manmade. Air pollutants are categorized as particulates (aerosols), inorganic gases, and organic gases.

The toxic action of a pollutant is rarely the same for any two individuals because of varying human factors (Purdom, 1980). Athough all three forms are present in the atmosphere simultaneously, gases constitute about 90% of all pollutants. A pollutant exerts its effect by either depressing or stimulating normal functioning within an organ (see Figure 16-1).

No discussion of air pollution would be complete without a brief review of selected classic disasters that have shaped many contemporary environmental health practices. Between December 3 and 5, 1930, several thousand people

in the densely populated Meuse River Valley west of Liege, Belgium, were stricken, and 60 died as a result of industrial air pollution. In this narrow strip of land, barometric pressures were high, temperatures at or below freezing, and no wind was blowing. Factory smoke combined with fog to create a "soupy" mixture that settled on the grounded. Victims became hoarse, short of breath, and nauseated. Deaths were the result of heart failure in the elderly or others already weakened by other causes (Waldbott, 1978).

The Belgian disaster did not motivate other countries to take precautions against air pollution. The greatest air pollution disaster occurred in the United States in October, 1948, at Donora, Pennsylvania. Circumstances similar to those in the Meuse Valley led to the Donora disaster. Many factories, including zinc smelters and producers of wire, steel, and sulfuric acid, lined the river front, and freight trains emitted great clouds of smoke that rose to 350 feet. When a high pressure front moved in, rainfall added fog and moisture to the air. On October 26, an inversion began in cold weather with a wind velocity near zero. A constant smog blanket produced a virtually air-tight chamber, day and night, for more than five days, during which the air was permeated by an odor of sulfur (Waldbott, 1978). Twenty persons died and 5910 persons, or 42% of the population, suffered from irritation of the eyes, nose, and throat, pain and chest constriction, cough, labored breathing, severe headaches, nausea, and vomiting.

A different type of disaster occurred in London, England, on December 4, 1952. As a high-pressure mass of cold air moved across the English Channel toward the Thames Valley, people used fireplaces extensively. With practically no wind, the city became engulfed in a heavy cloud of smoke that condensed in the moisture of London's fog. The greatly reduced visibility for trains and automobiles and for boats on the waterways led to many accidents. Although impossible to assess the death toll caused by respiratory and heart problems from the fog, 2851 persons over the usual death rate for 1 week (between December 4 and 13, 1952) died and during the following week another 1224 deaths were attributed to the presence of the fog. London suffered a second fatal fog in 1956 which claimed 1000 lives (Waldbott, 1978).

Virtually all human activities bring people into contact with some form of air pollution. Indoors, people are exposed to vapors in the kitchen, fumes from cleaning detergents, particulates in cosmetics, aerosols in spray cans, tobacco smoke, fibrous particles from rugs, draperies, blankets, and clothes. In homes and commerical establishments, central heating and air conditioning circulate dust continuously.

Outside, people are exposed to particles from insects, animal and human excretion, odors, gases from marshes, and dust from fields and streets. During spring and summer, pollen adds to the burden of particles to be inhaled, while spores, constitutents of decaying plants and animals, bacteria, and viruses permeate the air throughout the year. The terrain affects air pollution. For example, fumes are more easily concentrated in one area in hilly sites, particularly when people settle in a valley.

Five main classes of human-generated air pollution are

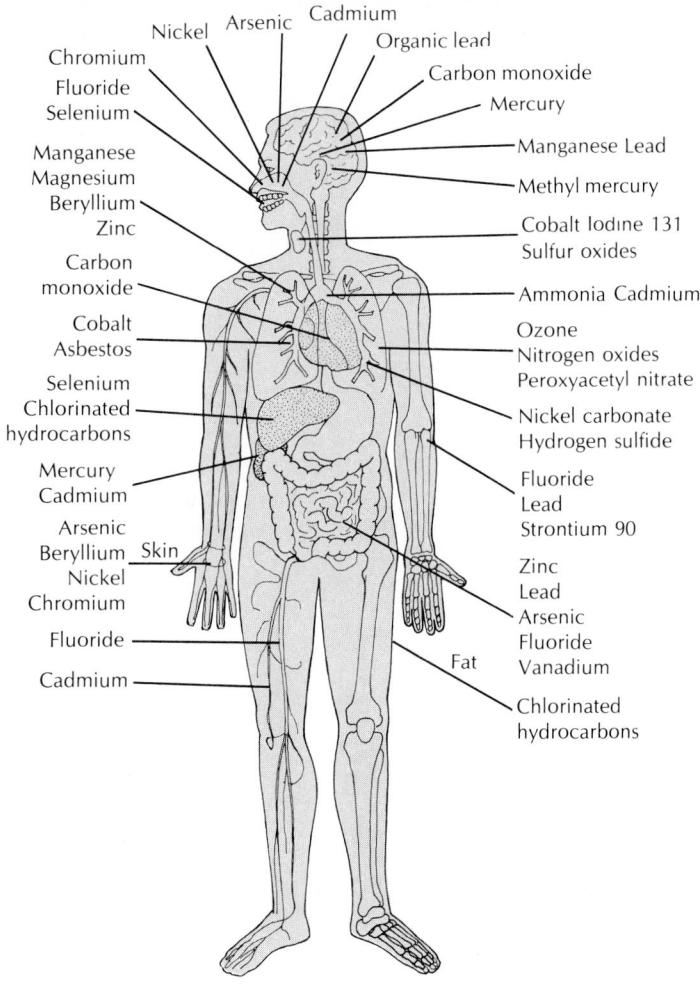

Figure 16-1

Main targets of major air pollutants. (From Waldgott, G.L.: Health effects of environmental pollutants, ed. 2, St. Louis, 1978, The C.V. Mosby Co.)

(1) carbon monoxide, a significant element in motor vehicle exhaust; (2) sulfur oxides, produced mostly by the combustion of coal, fuel oil, and natural gas; (3) hydrocarbons, a family of compounds containing carbon and hydrogen; (4) nitrogen oxides, mainly emitted by power plants and in transportation vehicle exhausts; and (5) particulate matter such a dust, soot, or ash.

At present, limited information is available concerning the possible health effects of many chemical compounds. The immediate cause for concern arises from the number of chemical compounds available, their versatile use, and the adverse effects associated with some chemicals (see Table 16-1).

Air pollution emissions from the burning of fuel for automobiles, trucks, buses, ships, railroads, and airplanes are 25 times greater in cities than in rural areas. Exhausts from transportation vehicles produce about 60% of the total air pollutants and as much as 90% in certain urban areas. These emissions result from the burning of gasoline, diesel fuel, distillates, and residual oils.

Emissions from transportation vehicles may be calculated

from the total gallons of fuel consumed for each source. Standard emission factors and fuel consumption data are used to obtain the weight of pollutants discharged. Standard emission factors are determined from a statistically valued sample and are established by the Department of Health and Human Services. Ajustments are calculated and are made to account for pollution-reduction devices.

Burning of coal, gas, and oil constitutes the principal source of sulfur oxides and nitrogen oxide. Coal is burned in power plants, in many industrial processes, as well as for domestic and commercial heating purposes. Coal, oil, and gas are used for space heating and gas and oil for heating of water; gas is used for cooking. Public utilities are a major source of sulfur oxide, nitrogen oxides, and particulate matter.

Industrial processes produce 56% of particulates. Certain kinds of industry produce more particulates than others. These types of industry include power plants that emit carbon, silica, aluminum, and iron oxide; the construction industry, which emits various kinds of dust; cotton ginning industry, a major source of trash, dust, and lint; and the

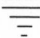

TABLE 16-1

Examples of specific effects of pollutants

Groups	Agent	Principal affected organs
Respiratory pollutants		
Pulmonary irritants	Sulfur oxides	Lining of the respiratory tract
	Nitrogen oxides	
	Ozone	
	Chlorine	
	Ammonia	
Dusts	Quartz	Pulmonary interstitial tissue
	Silica	
	Carbon	
	Asbestos	
	Cobalt	
	Iron oxides	
Granuloma-producing agents	Beryllium	Lungs
Fever-causing agents	Zinc	Alveoli
	Manganese	
	Hemp, cotton	
Asphyxiating pollutants	Carbon monoxide	Hemoglobin
	Hydrogen sulfide	Respiratory center
Systemic pollutants	Lead	Nerve tissue
	Mercury	Brain, bowels
	Fluoride	Bones, teeth
	Cadmium	Blood vessels, kidneys
	Chlorinated hydrocarbons	Fat tissue, liver
	Organophosphates	Nerve-muscle synapsis
Host-specific agents		
Allergenics	Thiocyanate	Respiratory tract
	Formaldehyde	Skin, lungs
Carcinogenics	Strontium 90	Bones
	Iodine 121	Thyroid
	Nickel carbonate	Lungs, sinuses
	Chromium	Nose
	Asbestos	Pleura
	Selenium	Testicular tissue
	Arsenic	Skin
Mutagens	Most systemic pollutants; organic mercury, lead, chlorinated hydrocarbons, arsenic, fluoride, cadmium	

From Waldbott, G.L.: Health effects of environmental pollutants, ed. 2, St. Louis, 1978, The C.V. Mosby Co.

feed and grain industry, a source of dirt (silicates), grain dust, and chaff.

Excluding diseases directly associated with high concentrations of specific pollutants, illnesses related to air pollution include chronic and acute respiratory disease, cancer of the lung, heart diseases, and increases in asthma attacks.

Control

It was not until 1963, with passage of the Clean Air Act, that the federal government got involved in setting air pollution standards. Two types of standards were considered: (1) Ambient Air Quality Standards to apply to outside air in a town, city or other defined region, and (2) emission standards to apply to industrial emissions. The Air Quality Act of 1967 mandated the establishment of criteria for six major pollutants: sulfur oxides, total suspended particu-

lates, hydrocarbons, carbon monoxide, photochemical oxidants, and nitrogen oxides. The Amendments of 1970 and 1977 constitute the Clean Air Act currently in effect. The Act established Ambient Air Quality Standards based on health and welfare, and states are required to develop implementation plans to be approved by the Environmental Protection Agency.

Just as with the detection of potential health problems resulting from food sources, community health nurses often assess the presence of air pollution. Frequently the community health nurse is the one individual who recognizes the total type and amount of pollution with which clients come in contact. For example, a person working in an industry that emits noxious fumes and living in an area polluted by a different type of substance is particularly at risk for developing a pollution-related health problem.

Also, nurses have many opportunities to assess the hazards of air pollution in the home and instruct families in proper ventilation, cleaning techniques, and use of pollutants.

Physical Hazards

Physical hazards can cause death, disease, or disability (Purdom, 1980). Historically, the effects of earthquakes, volcanic eruptions, floods, and tidal waves have been dramatic. In recent years, synthetic physical hazards have joined the ranks of naturally occurring hazards. Among the more widespread physical hazards are radiation, noise, solid waste, insects and rodents, and accidents.

Radiation

People have been exposed to radiation from the sun and minerals since the origin of our species. The extent and effect of *natural radiation* are unknown. However, currently, natural radiation accounts for about 55% of the total radiation for the average American. Of the natural sources, cosmic radiation emanates from the sun and other parts of earth and consists of many types of particulate and electromagnetic radiation. It increases during solar flares and is greatest at high altitudes. Cosmic radiation accounts for about 30 millirem (0.03 rem) per year (Silberstein and Silberstein, 1985).

Natural radiation also comes from the soil and certain rocks. Although radioactivity is low in most sedentary rocks, it is high in volcanic rocks. Some natural materials release small amounts of radiation. Living in a brick or stone house adds about 30 millirems of exposure annually compared with living in a wooden house (Silberstein and Silberstein, 1985). "One millirem is one one-thousandth of a rem; rem stands for 'roentgen equivalent man' and reflects the amount of radiation absorbed in human tissues" (Wilner et al., 1978, p. 255). The radioactivity in residential dwellings depends on the composition of the dwelling as well as local geological formation.

A third source of natural radiation comes from normal body potassium. A radioisotope known as potassium 40 constitutes about 0.01% of the potassium in the body. People receive between 15 and 20 millirems per year from potassium 40 and about 0.7 from carbon 14, which is formed within the atmosphere by the action of cosmic radiation and then incorporates in body tissues.

An additional natural form of radiation involves the possible loss of protection from ultraviolet rays of the sun. Released gases may be destroying the stratospheric protective layer of ozone, thereby permitting more of the sun's ultraviolet radiation to reach earth. An increased dose of ultraviolet radiation is linked to skin cancer in light-skinned people. The hazardous gases are fluorocarbons known by the trademark Freon. This gas is often used in spray can repellants and in refrigerators, freezers, and air conditioners. Fluorocarbons are highly stable, and instead of breaking down over time, they accumulate and move upward into the stratosphere, interrupting the ozone layer (Wilner et al., 1978).

Radioactive minerals also present serious hazards for miners. According to Hanlon and Pickett (1984) a group of 907 uranium miners with 3 years of underground experience has 17.8 times the normal death rate for heart disease, 5 times the rate for respiratory cancer, and 4.5 times the rate for nonautomotive accidents.

Uses of *synthetic radiation* include x-rays and radioisotopes in clinical diagnosis and treatment; radioisotopes in industry for measuring, testing, and processing; electric power generation; lasers in science, industry, and medicine; and electronic devices at home (Wilner et al., 1978). At present, between one third and one half of all critical medical decisions are based on radiology (Hanlon and Pickett, 1984). Medical uses account for about 94% of all exposure to synthetic sources of radiation, or about 40% of the total radiation exposure for a person (Wilner et al., 1978). Numerous devices serve to decrease the amount of radiation in medicine. The size of the x-ray beam has been reduced to limit exposure to only the required areas. Lead-containing aprons shield the gonadal region, and a variety of techniques are used to filter the beam.

The effects of radiation depend on the dose, type of radiation, and the sensitivity of various organs to the particular radiation. Some side effects of high levels of radiation are disruption of bone marrow, ulcers of the skin, diminished kidney function, pulmonary edema, and a diminished concentration of red and white blood cells and platelets. Other side effects have been linked to genetic damage to cells, causing mutations that may be passed on to subsequent generations. Unborn fetuses are at risk from radiation exposure. Irradiation of the mother immediately before conception or at the time of conception results in a high incidence of prenatal deaths. Nurses must caution clients about the possible effects of radiation and instruct them to inform all other health care providers treating them if they have undergone radiography.

The interest in nuclear energy as a source to generate electric power has increased because of declining oil reserves. The dilemma that arises in nuclear power production is how to dispose of the reactor wastes. Waste is produced as a result of activation of extraneous products found in coolants and as a result of nuclear fission.

The most outstanding potential source of radioactive pollution is the testing of nuclear weapons. The product of instantaneous and delayed fallout may be carried around the world several times with a number of years required before the bulk of the radioactive material is deposited on the ground.

A community's proximity to a source of fissionable material such as a nuclear reactor or its importance as a military target should be known to community health nurses. A nuclear reactor accident could leave an area larger than Louisville, Kentucky, uninhabitable for a year. Unprepared citizens exposed to radioactive fallout may die or develop radiation sickness or cancer years after exposure.

A 1-megaton nuclear warhead exploding with the force of one million tons of TNT could kill from a few hundred to several million people, depending on the target's population density. Fallout radiation would leave 8000 square miles unfit for human habitation for at least a year (Fetter, 1981).

A growing industry is based on the production and use of artificial radionuclides and compounds in research establishments and in hospitals. Through injection of radioisotopes into the body, organs have been scanned to determine the presence or absence of certain diseases. Industry, biology, and agriculture make use of radioisotopes as tracers. These procedures become hazardous to the environment as radioactive materials are discharged with the sewage into the waterways, thus affecting aquatic life and humans through drinking water and the food chain.

A relatively new potential source of environmental pollution is the use of nuclear energy as a power source for rocket propulsion and satellites. The hazard in this use of nuclear energy stems from the possibility of a satellite failing to go into orbit at the point of launching. At this point, isotopic power devices have the potential to liberate radioactive substances into the atmosphere.

Noise

Noise is defined as any unwanted sound within the environment. *Noise pollution* is concentrated in cities, with urban areas becoming steadily noisier. The sources of noise include construction activity, aerospace vehicles, diesel trucks, power mowers, radio and television sets, and people. Noise is particularly difficult to deal with because it is highly subjective.

Noise is a health hazard according to its level, frequency, and length of exposure. Depending on these three factors, noise reaction falls into the categories of annoyance, disruption of activity, loss of hearing, and physical or mental deterioration (Hanlon and Pickett, 1984).

The magnitude or level of noise is measured in decibels (dB). The dynamic range of the ear, or the difference between the loudest and the faintest sound, is about 120 dB (Bruce, 1985). Generally, the danger level for hearing loss for most people is about 80 dB, and the current standard for workplace exposure is 90 dB averaged over 8 hours. The Environmental Protection Agency (EPA) defines 75 dB as a long-time range goal for workplace exposure (UAW Sound Security Department, 1979). The dB scale is based on powers of 10. Each increase in 10 dB is equivalent to multiplying the intensity by 10; in other words, 30 dB is 10 times as intense as 20 dB and 40 dB is 10 times as intense as 30 dB.*

Noise can affect a person's psychological and physical well-being. Communication is disrupted by increasing noise, particularly in industries where people must shout to communicate. The quality of work is diminished in the presence of noise. Physiological responses to noise include vasoconstriction of the peripheral blood vessels, slow and deep breathing, skeletal muscle tension, and galvanic skin responses. People exposed to loud noises of long duration have an increase in urinary output, an increase in urinary catecholamines, and an increase in blood pressure.

Various forms of wildlife are also affected by noise pollution. Generally animals adapt to a predictable, regular noise or to continuous noise. A grizzly bear will run when disturbed by the noise level of 81 dB. When sound reaches a level of 165 dB, it can kill small animals; the energy of the sound wave is converted to heat within the animal's body (Wilner et al., 1978).

An individual's length of exposure to noise is largely determined by socioeconomic status, life style, and occupation. Essentially how people spend time determines their exposure to noise. How people react to noise is largely determined by their perception of the noise. Some people are more sensitive to noise than others. Several specific ways in which noises either annoy or disrupt health are described in the following section.

NOISE AS AN ANNOYANCE. Annoyance is the most widespread reaction to noise. The noise level, frequency, and length of exposure influence how annoying a noise is. A major characteristic of environmental noise is unpredictability; noise often startles people, disrupting their physiological and psychological stability. An annoying noise can aggravate existing physical disorders, disrupt sleep, lower the body's resistance to disease or physical stress, interrupt concentration, and generally disturb feelings of well-being. As noted, noise interferes with communication because people instinctively speak louder when the noise level increases (Bruce, 1985). Noise from machinery can interfere with instructions or the hearing of safety signals. Workers continuously exposed to high-intensity noises show an increased incidence of nervous complaints, nausea, headaches, instability, argumentativeness, sexual impotence, mood changes, and anxiety (Cohen, 1981).

The greatest physiological effect of noise is temporary or permanent hearing loss. Temporary impairment, or auditory fatigue, occurs after a short exposure to an intense noise. Exposure to a continuous high sound level with no recovery time between exposures can cause permanent hearing damage (Hanlon and Pickett, 1984).

METHODS OF NOISE CONTROL. Bruce (1985) proposed the source-path-receiver concept of noise control. For example, the source may be a machine, the highway, neighborhood children, or pets. The receiver is the recipient of the unwanted sound, and the path is the route the noise takes between the source and the receiver. Control of the source includes use of quieter equipment, relocation of source, or better maintenance of equipment.

Interference in the path can take the form of a barrier such as trees between houses and a highway or an enclosure such as a shed for noisy equipment. Wrapping or muffling the sound, acoustical absorption materials, surface damping, or application of a coating to lightweight panels can reduce noise radiations.

Receiver controls include such tactics as use of earplugs or relocation of the receiver. Each form of control should fit the situation and the people involved. Nurses can assess noise sources and help clients plan suitable methods of interruption of noise pollution.

Waste Disposal

SOLID WASTES. The traditional methods of disposing of these wastes included the open burning dump or the poorly designed smoking incinerator. Incinerators and dumps vi-

---

*Sound frequencies are measured in hertz (Hz), or units of frequency representing cycles per second. The audible range of frequencies for the human ear is between 20 and 20,000 Hz.

olated air pollution regulations and were breeding grounds for rats, flies, and other rodents. The most commonly used solid waste disposal methods today are sanitary landfills and incineration.

In sanitary landfills, waste is disposed of in canyons, swamps, and ravines and then compacted by heavy machinery and covered with earth before rodent infestation can occur. By filling the undesirable plot, the site can be integrated into the surrounding lands for public or private use.

Even though it is the best known method of waste disposal, landfilling is not without fault. When rainfall infiltrates the landfill surface or when the groundwater table saturates a part of the landfill, matter can be leached by the water moving through the system. As the water drains from the landfill, it carries debris or dissolvent matter with it. As a result, the possibility exists for contamination of underground waters and surface water supplies. Most urban areas have no remaining sites for landfill.

Unlike a sanitary landfill, incineration of solid wastes can be located on the premises of apartments, department stores, hospitals and similar establishments. On-site incineration reduces the volume and weight of wastes, which must be removed for final disposal. Incinerators are used in hospitals for destruction of pathological waste because heat destroys most pathogens.

Incineration of solid wastes yields a high percentage of volume reduction; however, the total weight reduction achieved depends on the amount of glass, metal, and other noncombustible materials. The volume reduction is generally between 70% and 85% and the weight reduction is between 50% and 80%. It is this volume and weight reduction that gives incineration its appeal as a method of solid waste disposal. The hazards of incineration result from the environmental nuisances of noise, dust, and air pollution. The average American discards 3 to 5 pounds of trash daily incurring an annual cost for collection and disposal of wastes of $6 billion (Geller, 1986).

Disposal of wastes is both costly and difficult. Each of the methods just described has advantages and disadvantages. New methods of waste disposal are being tried. One method grinds waste and subjects it to jets of air to separate paper from metals and plastics. Iron and steel can be removed by magnets. In two other methods, once the material is ground, it is incinerated and produces a glasslike slag used in bottles, building materials, or highway aggregate. The second method suspends and centrifuges the ground waste into various components (Hanlon and Pickett, 1984).

Approximately two thirds of the cost of solid waste disposal comes from pickup and transfer to a collection site. Compactors can reduce cost by providing a smaller mass for collection. There are at least five reasons for more effective management of solid wastes (Chanlett, 1985).

1. Decrease pathogen transmission
2. Reduce discarded toxic and infectious materials
3. Increase esthetic effect of areas previously used for waste disposal
4. Recover materials and energy
5. Maintain costs

Solid waste provides fertile areas for pathogen transmis-

sion resulting from its attraction for flies and rodents. Mosquitoes breed on water accumulated in bottles, cans, and other containers in open dumps. Mosquitoes are associated with the transmission of yellow fever, dengue, or hemorrhagic fever.

OTHER WASTES. Other wastes include toxic materials such as poisons, inflammables, infectious contaminants, explosives, and radionuclides (Chanlett, 1985). Hazardous materials make up about 10% of industrial waste output. Disposal of such wastes is difficult. Some can be neutralized, others burned, and still others buried or distilled. Although few cases of human injury are documented, the example of Love Canal has caused concern about the potential for disaster. A rising water level at Love Canal at Niagara Falls, New York, caused by excessive rainfall, brought chemical wastes to the water surface. The site was about a mile long, following an old canal previously used as a chemical dump. Later the area was filled and used for a school and 100 homes. Problems became apparent in 1978. Alleged health hazards included a high miscarriage rate, increased birth defects, children being burned on contact with the oozing liquid, and several cancer deaths. Tests demonstrated the presence of 82 chemicals, 11 of which are on the suspected carcinogenic list. The economic loss in depreciation of homes and the emotional loss from fear are quite high (Chanlett, 1985), but the actual human injury at Love Canal has yet to be established.

Nuclear shipments are an area of concern because of the risks posed from transporting the wastes from power plants to disposal sites. People opposed to transporting the wastes cite leaky casks or the possibility of a truck accident. To date there have not been any accidents, but some near accidents have occurred. If an accident occurred in New York City and just 1% of leaking radiation found its way into the city, the predicted results would be 1300 deaths immediately or within days or weeks, followed by 170,000 delayed cancer deaths (Holzer, 1982). Currently New York City is leading the nation's opposition to ban nuclear shipments.

The chemical industry is the major source of hazardous wastes. Since 1958 the 53 largest chemical manufacturers have disposed of over 750 million tons of unwanted byproducts. Industry, transportation, and agriculture are also major contributors of hazardous chemical wastes. Many chemicals in liquid waste effluents make their way to water supplies, industrial and transporation vehicle exhausts permeate the air, pesticides are often found concentrated in humans and animals, with many containing high levels of residues from agricultural pesticides.

PROBLEMS OF WASTE DISPOSAL. The esthetic offenses of irresponsible waste discard must be emphasized. Dumping of refuse along streets and on vacant land is a tribute to the lack of value some Americans place on the cleanliness and beauty of their homeland. Many counties have effectively dealt with unsightly dumping by installing the "green box." The green box is a large metal box with a capacity of 4 to 12 cubic yards; it is placed at road intersections near service stations and grocery stores (Chanlett, 1985). Conveniently located, these boxes serve residents and travelers alike. The contents are collected regularly and transported to a sanitary landfill. This disposal method has reduced open dumping by 70% to 75% in the southeastern United States.

In recent years it has become increasingly apparent that natural resources, if used at the present rates, will not sustain the same quality of life for an indefinite period. Recycling is one effective method of waste disposal; 25% of the 200 million tons of major metals, rubber, glass, and textiles processed annually are recycled materials. Copper, stainless steel, nickel, aluminum, lead, steel, and zinc are particularly valued. Currently the federal government supports several recycling efforts, and both states and private enterprise are active participants in this process. As an example, private efforts have established 1300 recycling centers that process 1 million of the 4 million cans produced annually. Recycling these cans saves $300 per ton, since the electricity required to reprocess the cans in only 5% of that needed to refine bauxite ore.

Solid wastes as sources of energy yield mixed reviews. The best method equips incinerators with heat recovery equipment to generate steam that can heat or produce electricity.

As mentioned, the largest costs associated with waste disposal come from collection. The cost for public or private disposal efforts runs about $45 per person per ton of solid waste a year (Chanlett, 1985). Management skills are being applied to the business of solid waste collection, since costs for the United States approach $4 billion annually. Collection routes, hauling times, and methods of containing waste (bag or can) are being evaluated to improve cost effectiveness.

Essentially, two choices exist for the disposal of waste; "burn it" or "bury it." Both methods are currently in use; however, the latter will become more difficult as population increases and less land is available for waste disposal.

An increasingly popular goal is "transform it" and this includes composting. However, in the United States composting has been less successful than in other countries. Basically, composting is an aerobic process whereby bacteria, especially fungi, feed on organic material. A carbon/nitrogen ratio of 30:1 is needed to provide the nitrogen for forming new protoplasm. If the pile is stirred regularly to renew its oxygen supply, it becomes an excellent soil conditioner, but it is not a complete source of fertilizer, since compost is low in phosphorous and potassium. Composting has been effective in many countries including Switzerland, Japan, Thailand, South Africa, Israel, West Germany, The Netherlands, England, Scotland, France, and Mexico (Chanlett, 1985).

In the future there will be new methods of solid waste disposal. Poor burial sites of the past have later posed far-reaching dangers. Sites used in the past are yet to be identified. Subsequently, in later years homes, schools, industry, and recreational areas were built on these sites. It is not known how the contents of solid waste affect people. It can be anticipated that refillable bottles will be used more extensively, new packaging efforts will reduce the volume of discardable paper and plastics, and more materials will be repaired rather than discarded.

Vector Control

Insect and rodent control is commonly referred to as *vector control* because of the disease transmission potential. "The rodent is the host for the flea, which is the vector, or carrier, of plague and endemic typhus; anopheles mosquitoes transmit malaria" (Wilner et al., 1978, p. 264).* Vector control is most effectively carried out by modifying and regulating the environment to reduce or prevent propagation. Vectors of community health concern are rodents and arthropods. Among rodent vectors, rats, ground squirrels, and prairie dogs are most important, since they spread the plague. Of the arthropods certain mosquitoes, flies, fleas, roaches, lice, mites, and ticks are important sources of disease. (Hanlon and Pickett, 1984).

Vector control has become a reality in recent decades, since the life cycles of many organisms have become known. However, control requires the cooperation of many groups, organizations, and the public. Buildings must be constructed to keep rodents from entering, kept in good repair, and maintained free of food wastes. Pest control measures must be carefully carried out so that unsuspecting people and animals are safe. Nurses must consistently assess for the presence of vectors as they make home visits and see clients in clinics, schools, work sites, and other community health settings. Once the presence of vectors are noted, nurses can provide relief measures through education of clients or referral to agencies that might provide vector control services.

Trapping is often used in rodent control, although it is a slow and difficult process. Poisons, while effective for rodents, do pose new hazards for people, especially children. One material, red squill, kills rodents because they cannot regurgitate but only acts as an enteric for humans, poultry, and other animals (Wilner et al., 1978). In the United States, plague-infected wild rodents have spread eastward from the West Coast at a rapid rate. The ecological distribution of plague is not clearly understood. However, murine typhus is endemic in several southeastern and some western states where rats and mice infest households. Many health departments are launching programs to tackle the rodent problem but challenges still exist.

Because *mosquito* "eggs hatch and the larvae and pupae develop only in quiet water and under certain conditions, mosquito control is most effectively accomplished by eliminating or modifying these waters" (Wilner et al., 1978, p. 265). Each species prefers one type of water. Anopheles mosquitoes prefer clean, shallow water, whereas *Aedes aegypti,* which transmits yellow fever and dengue, prefers water near people, including rainwater. *Culex tarsalie,* the vector for encephalitis, breeds in a variety of nonsalty waters such as surplus irrigation waters. *Aedes,* a vicious daytime biting mosquito, prefers salt marshy areas, whereas *Culex fatigans,* the cause of urban filariasis, prefers water heavily contaminated with human wastes.

Mosquito control includes draining and filling marshes

---

*A vector is an agent that actively carries a germ to a susceptible host. Vectors are considered animate vehicles for the transmission of pathogenic organisms and include birds, beasts, bugs, or people.

and low areas, stocking larvae-eating fish, varying water level to cause larvae and pupae to be exposed to waves and currents, spraying, improving irrigation practices, providing better drainage systems, and conducting public education on control methods.

Accidents

Accidents are a major cause of death in the United States. The major causes of accidental injury and death result from carelessness or ignorance; many accidents are preventable. The top categories of accidents are motor vehicle accidents, falls, drownings, and fires. It is difficult to accurately report the number of annual accidental injuries because many do not require medical care and hence go unreported.

Injuries occur most frequently in boys between the ages of 6 to 16 and men age 17 to 44. In the over-65 age group, women have the higher rate. As income increases, the rate of accidents decreases. Teenage boys, because of their activities and often daring and risk-taking behavior, are a high-risk category. Contact sports, motorcycling, high-speed driving, and the use of firearms increase the accident rate for this age group.

Because community health nursing emphasizes prevention and health education, it is important to review several common, preventable causes of accidents. Community health nurses during home visits should assess home safety and educate clients about reducing or eliminating actual or potential hazards.

In the home, injuries result from fires, falls, poisoning, and lacerations, abrasions, and fractures from tools or equipment. A home survey would look for fire hazards such as unprotected sources of fire; combustive materials, including curtains, rugs, rags, and loose clothing worn near a fire; access to matches by children; malfunctioning smoke detectors; and improper use of heaters such as poorly installed wood-burning stoves or lack of screens or doors on fireplaces to prevent sparks from igniting combustible materials.

Falls can be prevented by securing loose rugs or cords, removing furniture from walkways which might cause people to trip; putting rails on stairs and keeping stairs and steps free from slippery rugs, toys, and other objects; putting a gate at the top or bottom of stairs if small children or confused adults are present. Toys and pets should be kept out of walkways, especially when elderly people whose balance may be poor live in the home.

Bathtubs and showers should have nonslip bottom surfaces or rubber mats. Handrails are useful if someone in the family has poor balance or vision problems.

Sharp instruments such as razors and knives should be kept out of reach of children. Likewise, medicine and chemicals such as bleach, cleaning materials, and liquid plumbing solutions, should be safely secured. Small, inexpensive locking devices can be attached to cabinets to prevent access by small children or adults who may be confused and unaware of potential danger.

Yard and farm equipment should be used as intended and kept away from children. Tools, fertilizers, and insecticides should be safely stored.

The same principles of safety should be maintained in schools, businesses, and particularly health care facilities as well as in the home.

Chemical Hazards

Chemical hazards, though by no means new, are increasing annually. In addition to chemicals occurring in nature, an estimated two million other chemicals are currently known. Of these 30,000 are synthetic; approximately 1000 new synthetic chemicals are introduced annually (Hanlon and Pickett, 1984). At present limited information is available concerning the possible health effects of many chemical compounds. One problem with chemicals is that they abound in the workplace, existing in the form of gases, dusts, mists, and vapors. Industrial gases affect the body directly or indirectly; some cause an acute effect, whereas others can be linked to chronic effects occurring from repeated low-level exposures. Nitrogen dioxide, sulfur dioxide, and hydrogen sulfide are extremely irritating to the eyes and upper respiratory tract. Cyanide presents itself in various forms in industry. One form, hydrogen cyanide, a side product from blast furnaces, coke ovens, and gas works, interferes with the body's use of oxygen. Some mild symptoms of cyanide poisoning include headache, weakness, nausea, and vomiting. Higher doses result in cessation of breathing and death. Repeated insults from exposure to gases may result in chronic cough or bronchitis in mild cases. In more severe cases the result may be emphysema or pulmonary edema.

The use of chemicals has increased remarkably since World War II. These chemicals include pesticides, food additives, drugs, other household materials, and many industrial wastes. A particularly striking use of chemicals occurred during the Vietnam War when dioxin, known as agent orange, was sprayed on jungles, trails, and rice paddies in Southeast Asia for many years to make it difficult for North Vietnamese and Viet Cong troops to move through the jungles undetected. An estimated 11 million pounds of agent orange containing 220 pounds of dioxin were sprayed. To date the only health effect linked to dioxin is chloracne. However, other effects, including skin rashes, fatigue, decreased fertility, emotional disorders, cancer, liver disorders, and nervous disorders are being investigated as possibly related to dioxin (Drotman, 1985).

Dusts

Dusts, extremely common in the workplace, involve many different kinds of substances. The lung disease associated with dusts is called *pneumoconiosis.* One problem with dusts results from the size of the particles. Some are so small (visible only through a microscope) that they can easily enter the nasal passages and remain in the lungs. The classic example of exposure to a certain type of dust particle that has been linked to cancer is exposure to asbestos. Asbestos, a fibrous mineral, has been used widely for insulation and fireproofing, in textiles, drywall compounds, cement, and thousands of other products. For years scientists knew that exposure to asbestos caused asbestosis, a severe and sometimes fatal scarring of the lungs, but it was not until the 1960s that asbestos was recognized as the cause of mesothelioma. This type of cancer is associated with the membranes that surround the lungs and line the abdominal cavity. Asbestos has also been linked with cancer of the larynx and the gastrointestinal tract. It is difficult to estimate the number of workers and consumers who have been exposed to asbestos. Increasingly asbestos has been found in the insulation material in public buildings; asbestos removal is necessary; however, it is expensive.

In the past many employees working with asbestos brought the fibers home on their clothes, thus exposing their families. A worker exposed to asbestos for 1 day may develop cancer in later life as a result of the exposure. The asbestos entering the nasal passages remain deposited in the lungs. It is estimated that hundreds of thousands of asbestos workers will die as a result of exposure. This estimate does not include family members or consumers who have been exposed.

Other types of dusts affecting workers are coal, silica, and wood. Sandblasters and tunnel workers exposed to silica dust have contracted silicosis, which results in massive fibrosis of lung tissue with increased susceptibility to tuberculosis and infection. Silicosis is also associated with pulmonary hypertension and cor pulmonale.

Coal miners, exposed to coal dust, may develop large, solid, black lung masses as a result of black dust deposited in the lungs. This disease is referred to as simple pneumoconiosis, or more appropriately as "black lung." Carpenters, foresters, loggers, and pulp mills, paper mill, and plywood mill workers are among those exposed to wood dusts. Some of these workers are showing an abnormally high rate of cancer of the stomach, lymph, and blood-forming tissues.

Byssinosis, another type of lung disease, has been identified among workers in cotton mills. The disease is similar to nonoccupation bronchitis and has been confused with emphysema.

Organic Chemicals

Organic chemicals are substances containing carbon. Thousands are used in industrial processes as solvents, intermediates, and starting materials. Carbon tetrachloride, a common solvent, is used as a drying agent for spark plugs, a dry cleaning agent, a fire extinguishing agent, a fumigant, and an anthelmintic agent. Excessive exposure may result in depression of the central nervous system, whereas acute exposure causes kidney damage. The vapors from perchlorothylene, another organic chemical, have toxic effects on the liver.

Exposure to various forms of ether may cause dermatitis, lung disease, eye irritation, or kidney or liver damage. For years, hospitals used ethyl ether as a general anesthetic. Most hospitals have discontinued using it, preferring other anesthetics, but women working in operating rooms where ethyl ether is still used have an increased risk of miscarriage, birth defects in their children, liver and kidney disease, and cancer.

Aromatic hydrocarbons such as benzene, toluene, xylene and northalone irritate the skin, eyes, and upper respiratory tract. Benzene, once the most commonly used solvent in the industry, has been linked to leukemia. Aldehydes and ketones, organic compounds containing carbon, are widely used in industry and chemical synthesis. Excessive exposure to ketones may result in coma, respiratory depression, or death in severe cases.

Naturally Occurring Chemicals

Many naturally occurring chemicals are hazardous to humans. For some of these, trace or small amounts are beneficial, whereas excesses or deficiencies cause health problems. For example, excesses or deficiencies of metals such as cadmium, selenium, chromium, lead, copper, zinc, and lithium may be related to major degenerative disease such as heart disease, muscular dystrophy, diabetes, multiple sclerosis, cancer, mental illness, or congenital malformations (Hanlon and Pickett, 1984). Previously mentioned, asbestos has carcinogenic properties because of its composition of trace metals and chemical compounds such as benzpyrene. *Benzpyrene* is also found in tobacco smoke, and asbestos workers who smoke have up to 30 times greater risk of lung cancer than their nonsmoking counterparts. In addition, trace metals such as nickels, chromium, and iron are associated with certain types of asbestos fiber. Cancer may be activated by a reaction among benzpyrene compounds, an enzyme, and the particular trace metals.

The trace element *cadmium* has been found in the kidneys of people dying from hypertensive complications. The chief sources of cadmium are foods grown in soils containing cadmium from fertilizers, beverages in containers coated with galvanized zinc, and vegetables, drinking water, coffee, and tea.

Chromium is associated with cardiovascular disease, and *lead* has many harmful properties. In addition to numerous industrial uses, lead is found in the environment. Occupational safeguards have limited many of lead's harmful effects; however, tetraethyl lead used as an antiknock and power-increasing gasoline additive still presents health problems. Not only does this compound pollute the environment, but it also is highly toxic when inhaled or absorbed through the skin, largely leading to cerebral or central nervous system symptoms (Hanlon and Pickett, 1984).

Inorganic *nitrites* and *nitrates* contaminate drinking water and are especially dangerous for infants up to 6 weeks who have not yet developed certain metabolic enzymes. Infants also have a more readily reactive hemoglobin level and a small blood volume relative to fluid intake.

Molds

Another group of toxic chemicals, often classified as a biological hazard, includes fungi called *molds*. Mold deteriorates food fiber, induces plant disease, and can cause pulmonary and invasive diseases in people. Some food molds produce toxic metabolites known as mycotoxins. The oldest mycotoxin, ergot, infects cereal grasses, especially rye, and can cause serious epidemics. The last outbreak of ergotism was reported in 1951 in southern France. Many victims showed central nervous system symptoms such as hallucinations, depression, and self-destructive mania (Hanlon and Pickett, 1984).

Other mycotoxins include the aflatoxins, produced by mold on peanuts and other agricultural products. Even in low doses, aflatoxins can cause acute intoxication, liver damage, and cancer of the liver in animals. The entire effect on humans is not known. Reaction to chemicals depends on the toxicity and concentration of the chemical, individual susceptibililty, and the duration of exposure. The effect is often related to the body weight of the person as well as the chemical's state (solid, liquid, gas) at the time of exposure.

Pulmonary Irritants

Some substances pass rapidly through the respiratory system whereas others remain in the lungs for extended periods of time. Prolonged or continuous exposure to certain gases, vapors, and fumes can lead to chronic inflammatory or neoplastic changes as well as lung fibrosis. Gases and vapors of low water but high fat solubility pass through the lungs to the blood and are carried to organ sites for which they have affinity.

The principal respiratory diseases induced by pollutants are bronchiectasis, emphysema, pulmonary fibrosis, pulmonary edema, and partial collapse of lung tissue. Although the range and list of pulmonary irritants is endless, some are particularly common and exhibit diverse effects.

Sulfur oxide has been extensively researched; its presence is an indicator of pollution because it gives off bluish-white plumes and reduces visibility. This substance is generated by burning wood, coal, and petroleum products. The degree of irritation depends on the concentration in the atmosphere and the size of the particles (Waldbott, 1978). Sulfur oxide interacts with a variety of other pollutants. For example, January 22, 1970, in Detroit, salt was used to melt snow and ice on the streets. Droplets of sulfuric acid coalesced with the sodium chloride (salt) to form the highly irritating hydrochloric acid, leaving a residue of sodium sulfate (Kellogg, et al., 1972).

Nitrogen oxide (N_2O) come primarily from automobile exhaust and almost all forms of combustion; it is a byproduct of many industries and is used in making explosives. In high concentration nitrogen oxide reduces the oxygen-carrying capacity of blood by increasing the blood level of methemoglobin. In contrast, nitrogen dioxide is about four times as toxic as nitrogen oxide. Insoluble in water, nitrogen dioxide passes through the trachea and bronchi into the alveoli of the lungs where it forms nitrous and nitric acid. Both are highly irritating to the mucous lining of the lungs. Both short- and long-term exposure to nitrogen dioxide increases susceptibility to infection by decreasing the ability of the lungs to clear inhaled infectious organisms.

Acute nitrogen dioxide poisoning can occur in farmers filling silos. During the early weeks when a silo is being filled, nitrogen dioxide is generated from moldy silage. Similar incidents occur in power plants as people work with boilers and industrial gases. Symptoms of chronic poisoning range from slight irritation, burning and pain in the throat and chest, to violent coughing and shortness of breath. Nitrogen oxide reacts with alkali in lung tissue, causing

edema. Nitrogen dioxide interacts with tobacco smoke, causing smokers to be at higher risk for developing health problems. This gas has poor warning qualities because it smells good.

Ozone (O_3) is an unstable colorless gas with an oxidizing power surpassed only by fluorine. Originally viewed as beneficial because it was believed to have bacterial action and to assist in the oxygenation of blood, ozone is now recognized as one the the most dangerous irritants to eyes, throats, and lungs (Waldbott, 1978). It is found in smog created by the interaction of hydrocarbons, nitrogen oxides, and sunlight. In the air it can be a threat to aviation personnel at altitudes over 30,000 feet (Werthamer et al., 1970).

Synthetic sources of ozone include high-voltage electrical equipment such as electrical insulators, x-ray and ultraviolet ray equipment, quartz lamps, and electrostatic air cleaners. Ozone is used as a commercial bleaching compound and sterilant. Ozone impairs the functioning of pulmonary macrophages by thickening the walls of small pulmonary arteries, resulting in chronic pulmonary disease, emphysema, and right heart failure (P'an, A.Y.S. et al., 1972). Because it depresses respiration and causes lung edema, ozone interferes with normal lung ventilation.

Chlorine, a common toxic gas, is frequently used in the chemical industry for preparation of organic and inorganic agents such a trichlorethylene, vinyl chloride plastics, pesticides, herbicides such as DDT, refrigerants and propellants such as Freons, detergents, and pharmaceuticals (Stahl, 1969). It is also used in the paper industry.

Acute epidemics have occurred repeatedly from accidents associated with the handling or emptying of liquid chlorine cylinders. In March, 1961, while supposedly empty chlorine cylinders were being handled, the main valve of one slipped off, causing 156 people to be immediately stricken. Some had lung hemorrhages; others experienced asthmalike wheezing and pneumonia-like lung infiltration for as long as 35 months (Kowitz et al, 1967). Other episodes of chlorine spillage have led to congestive heart failure, pulmonary edema, and pneumonia.

Only one other gas, *carbon monoxide,* is discussed here, although many more affect health. Carbon monoxide (CO), because it deprives the hemoglobin of its oxygen-carrying ability, is a common asphyxiant (Waldbott, 1978). It is a poisonous gas produced by incomplete combustion and is particularly dangerous since it cannot be seen, smelled, or tasted by potential victims. Carbon monoxide is considered the greatest single, nonindustrial hazard. It is responsible for half of all fatal poisoning in the United States; often the engine of a running car or an open, unlighted gas burner is used in suicide. Oceans are a major source of CO (Coburn, 1970), as are automobile exhausts, cigarette smoke, and gas and coal heating systems.

When CO replaces oxygen in the blood, the functioning of lungs, brain, and heart is impaired. Initial symptoms range from dizziness, headaches, nausea, and general fatigue to impairment of memory and loss of muscular control (Waldbott, 1978). It is a deceptive gas because of its poor warning characteristics and because people affected by it may appear drunk and act belligerent. Smokers are affected at lower concentrations, although less seriously.

Chemical Pesticides

Chemical pesticides vary considerably and include insecticides, fungicides, herbicides, rodenticides, arachnicides (spider killers), and nematocides (worm killers). Over the past 20 years the use of these chemical substances to destroy unwanted insect, animal, or vegetable life has increased tremendously. Spraying, dusting, baiting, drenching, dipping, and painting are used to eliminate pests. In an attempt to avoid one hazard to health, other hazards are often invited—air pollution, water pollution, and consumption of these chemicals through food products. Not all noxious material acts on the desired target. A portion of the applied chemical contaminates the air, water, soil, plant life, wildlife, and humans.

Pesticides remaining in the air are quickly diluted in large masses of air to what would appear to be harmless concentrations. The "harmless concentration" in air must be questioned, however, when concentrations of chemicals are found in migrating animals thousands of miles from its use. Pesticides settling on soil may be carried into larger bodies of water by runoff. Pesticides in water are concentrated in fish, which in turn are consumed by humans. Pesticides falling on plant surfaces may be consumed by animals or harvested with crops, or leaves may be carried away by wind or waters. In any event, the pesticide is eventually consumed by people either by consumption of the crop or of animals grazing on the crop.

DDT, the most widely used and best known chlorinated hydrocarbon, is a matter for great environmental concern. Most uses of DDT have been barred since 1972 (Wilner et al., 1978). Three properties render DDT one of the most dangerous chemical pollutants: (1) it is extraordinarily stable with the half-life of the residues ranging up to 20 years (Woodwell et al., 1971); (2) its high solubility in fat and low solubility in water enables it to penetrate into animal food products; and (3) the high vapor pressure of DDT causes it to evaporate from soils and plants and to circulate widely in the atmosphere.

Unlike the chlorinated hydrocarbons, the organophosphates produce no chronic effects on the ecosystems. In fact, some organophosphates, such as malathion, which are extremely poisonous to insects, have relatively little effect on mammals. However, other organophosphates such as parathion, have caused serious illness among humans.

Pesticides do present a problem. In Dade County, Florida, roughly 2 million pounds of pesticides are used each year. That averages out to more than 1 pound of pesticide per person. Questions about the safety of pesticide use in Dade County arise because only three quarters of an ounce is needed to spray an entire acre for mosquito control. Migrant farmworkers are especially at risk and are frequently sprayed while working in fields. Many farm workers have not been adequately trained to work with pesticides, and problems have occurred because restricted-use pesticides have been applied by inexperienced applicators. The EPA requires that certain information be included on every pesticide label, including directions for use, first aid instructions, storage and disposal guidelines, and rules for general or restricted use; ironically many migrant workers are unable to read. Pesticide poisonings have resulted from workers entering fields recently sprayed or from pesticide drift. To further compound the problem, working conditions in the fields are often intolerable; because of the lack of toilets, washing facilities, and drinking water, migrant workers have a high rate of infectious diseases and kidney and bladder problems. Very few pesticide poisonings are reported.

The EPA is responsible under the Federal Insecticide, Fungicide, and Rodenticide Act (FIFRA) for protecting human health and the environment from unreasonable harm from pesticides. The agency has been accused of being extremely lax regarding its responsibililty to protect workers. OSHA has recently developed standards for migrant farm workers.

Chemical Effects on Fetus

Another area of concern is the effect of a chemical on the unborn fetus. Environmental hazards enter the body through inhalation, skin contact, and ingestion. These three routes will be presented in more detail later in this chapter. Important questions can be raised regarding the potential health effect a toxic substance may have on the fetus.

For example, there is a possible correlation between dioxin and birth defects in Vietnamese children. To date, scientists cannot accurately predict exactly how much of a toxic substance will reach the fetus, or at what concentration the fetus can be exposed without resultant adverse effects.

The primary way a chemical or other hazardous substance reaches the unborn child is through the placenta. Most chemicals or toxins cross the placental barrier and enter the circulatory system of the developing fetus. After these chemicals enter the expectant mother's body, through one or more of the routes mentioned earlier, they eventually find their way into the mother's circulation and then into the child's. Some chemicals are rapidly transported across the placenta. The mother's liver will detoxify some substances, and the kidneys will excrete others. Because the tissues of the fetus are developing rapidly, they are more susceptible to adverse effects than are adult tissues.

Areas of Concern

The immediate cause for concern arises from the number of chemical compounds available, their widespread use, and the adverse effects associated with some. Exposure to low levels of these chemicals may produce or aggravate chronic disease. These chronic diseases are not associated with the workers' environment, so identifying the specific cause of a disease is sometimes difficult. Many workers change jobs frequently and are exposed to various chemicals at different times. The onset of a chronic disease may not appear for several years, thereby making it difficult to determine the source. Other diseases may result from cumulative exposures.

Threshold limit values (TLVs) are the maximum concentration to which workers can be exposed for 8 hours a day without developing disease. Because they are based on average exposure, workers may conceivably be exposed to higher levels at certain times. Although TLVs have been established for many chemicals, it is virtually impossible for the government to establish TLVs for all chemicals because of the vast numbers of the chemicals in use. Problems arise because monitoring of TLVs is left up to industry. Often industries do not have the necessary monitoring equipment. OSHA has the broad responsibility for monitoring chemical exposure in the workplace, but because of understaffing, they cannot do the work that is necessary. The existing TLVs have been established without regard to individual susceptibility or the cumulative effects of chemicals.

The three primary routes of entry of chemical hazards are inhalation, skin contact, and ingestion, The adult human being has a large gas-tissue interchange (90 square meters of total surface, 70 square meters of alveolar surface). This large surface combined with the blood capillary network (surface of 140 square meters) with its continuous blood flow allows for a rapid absorption of many substances from the air into the alveolar portion of the lungs and on into the bloodstream. See Chapter 17 for additional information on entry and modes of action.

Chemical Effects on Body Systems

The inhalation of pollutants affects not only the respiratory and cardiovascular systems and the brain but also the gastrointestinal tract, kidneys, and many other target organs. Fig. 16-1 illustrates the health effects of several environmental pollutants on target organs. Table 16-1 presents examples of specific effects of several pollutants.

Hazardous substances affect people not only through inhalation but also through skin contact. A major purpose of the skin is to serve as a barrier against the entry of foreign substances; however, substances do penetrate the skin or react with substances on the skin surface to cause a primary irritation (dermatitis). The main routes of skin absorption are through epidermal cells, hair follicles, and sebaceous glands. Toxic substances are absorbed more rapidly when the person is sweating or wearing wet clothes or when the skin is abraded.

Ingestion of environmental hazards is easier to monitor and control than inhalation and skin contact. Toxicity by mouth is generally of a lower order than that by inhalation because of poor absorption into the blood stream, the high acidity as the substance goes through the stomach, as well as subjection to the alkaline medium of the pancreatic juice on passing through the small intestine. Exceptions to these characteristics are arsenic, cadmium, lead, and mercury (Waldbott, 1978).

Psychosocial Hazards

Sociological and psychological variables in the environment are more difficult to define than are biological, chemical, and physical hazards. However, any consideration of the environment must take into account psychosocial influences that are hazards. Many of these hazards are described in Chapters 30, 32, and 34 which deal respectively with community mental health, violence and human abuse, and the recognition and management of stress. So that redundancy will be avoided, this section is somewhat briefer than preceding ones, but this should not be interpreted as a minimization of the health hazards associated with the psychosocial components of the environment.

Dubos (1969) contends that mental characteristics are shaped by the environment, and genes only determine responses to stimuli. Environmental stimuli affect people from the time of conception. Survival depends on a variety of environmental stimuli, but often it is the amount and rapidity of stimuli that determine a person's ability to adapt. Although people can adapt to psychosocial stressors, they often experience stress that ultimately leads to disorders of the body and mind.

Noise, overcrowding, lack of privacy, lack of opportunity for social interaction, lack of space, boredom, excessive leisure, tedium, traffic, crowds, and feelings of estrangement from the mainstream of life can be psychosocial hazards.

Change constitutes a psychosocial hazard for nearly everyone. Both positive and negative changes require human energy for adaptation. Change, inevitable for most people, is more tolerable if it occurs at a reasonable rate and does not conflict with previously held values or beliefs.

Many societal changes result in potential psychosocial hazards such as increasing mechanization and automation, mobility, and dehumanization of societal institutions. People must adapt to new jobs, new homes, and new social groups, often without assistance from friends, family, or social support networks. Other psychosocial stressors and potential health hazards come from changing female and ultimately family roles as described in Chapter 32.

The United States has increasingly becoming a country of many cultures. When people holding highly divergent beliefs and attitudes live in close proximity, the potential for stress and often conflict arises. Chapter 15 describes key social and cultural variables affecting community health nursing.

COMMUNITY HEALTH NURSING AND ENVIRONMENTAL HEALTH

Community health nurses must have an understanding of the biological, physical, chemical, and psychosocial hazards affecting both men and women, elderly persons, and children as well as potential health effects on the unborn fetus. Community health nurses may be actively involved in the control of communicable diseases. Therefore nurses must be aware of the many factors that influence the spread of disease. Nurses who work in the community should be aware of the types of environmental hazards. They must also know where to locate sources of information identifying the specific effects a hazard may have on an individual or an entire community. Currently there are many environmental health resources available. These might include programs offered by universities, public health departments, medical centers, community health centers, or information obtained from federal agencies such as the EPA, OSHA, NIOSH, Centers for Disease Control (CDC), and the National Institutes of Health (NIH).

Voluntary agencies are excellent sources, because they are involved in health maintenance and disease prevention. The American Heart Association, the American Lung Association, the National Association for Mental Health, and the Arthritis Foundation are some of the voluntary agencies. These organizations have pamphlets that are excellent resource material both for the nurse and for the consumer.

Newspapers are excellent resources. In some cities articles that discuss the effects of environmental degradation and deterioration appear daily or weekly. Some articles address current research, while others discuss the role of the federal government.

A major nursing activity is health education. As with all types of health education, the first step is assessment of environmental hazards and worker or occupational team member educational needs, which includes both employee and health team in-service programs on health and safety as well as one-to-one counseling of workers. The Occupational Safety and Health Act of 1970 requires that workers be told about any possible hazards in the workplace, and the nurse is often given this responsibility.

Health education includes both formal and informal teaching. During each encounter with a worker, nurses can provide health education related to the worker's needs. For example, hypertensive employees often benefit from diet counseling, especially with regard to preparing foods with low salt content. Group and individual teaching are used to provide information needed to maximize employee health. Health education also includes interpreting health and welfare benefits to workers so they know what is available through both the employer and the community. The nurse can make appropriate referrals and procure a variety of services unavailable within the occupational health unit.

Employee health educational programs can include a wide range of topics. Possible topics might deal with alcoholism, cancer, obesity, exercise, nutrition, stress management, coping effectively with retirement, and so forth. Programs can also be developed around safety measures, avoidance of hazards in the workplace, and other topics specific to a work setting.

Another responsibility of the occupational health nurse is to act as a resource person for the community. The nurse should have current knowledge pertaining to community health resources. Community health nurses working in clinics or public health departments should have an understanding of the occupational health nurse's role and strive to work together in complimentary ways. The community health nurse may be involved in the establishment of a disaster plan for a hospital, a plant, or a factory. The establishment of such a plan will require coordinated efforts.

The industrial hygienist is the professional who is most often identified with the recognition and control of toxic substances in the workplace. If the company does not have an industrial hygienist, the safety specialist may be charged with this responsibility in addition to establishing and maintaining a safety program. The nurse working in the clinic may be the first to detect a potential health problem stemming from the work setting. The community health nurse has the responsibility for notifying the industrial hy-

gienist, the occupational health nurse, the physician, or the safety specialist so appropriate methods for identifying and controlling the toxic substance can be undertaken.

Community health nurses come in contact with many workers who do not benefit from the services of these occupational health specialists. Therefore, the nurse must be able to advise the worker on the recognition of health hazards. Workers should be advised that any abnormal eye irritation, especially on entering the workplace, may be a warning that exposures or TLVs are too high. Some chemicals produce mild eye irritations, whereas others can be more damaging. Therefore, early detection is important. If irritation occurs, the worker should report it to the appropriate authorities in the workplace as this may be an indication of a potential health hazard. Detecting an odor may indicate exposure to a dangerous chemical. Many chemicals have a distinctive odor. Sulfur dioxide has a strong suffocating odor, hydrogen sulfide has a characteristic rotten egg odor, and chlorine has a distinct odor similar to that of household bleach.

An excess of dusts or fumes may indicate a nonexistent or a poorly functioning ventilation system. For noise exposure, the general rule is that if a worker must yell to be heard at a normal conversation distance, then the noise levels may be too high and permanent damage may result over a period of prolonged exposure. The other health effects resulting from noise have been discussed. Careful handling of chemicals and the proper handling of chemical spills are important in the workplace.

Recurring symptoms or prolonged illness may indicate a potential problem and workers should be advised to consult a physician. Because symptoms may occur gradually, workers sometimes assume that frequent headaches or a constant cough are nothing to be alarmed about; however, those symptoms may be the initial indicators of a chronic progressive disease that, if detected early, may be preventable.

For the most part, physicians and nurses are involved in the practice of curative medicine, the "hands on" healing practice. However, preventive medicine is gaining interest, and it has practical application with regard to environmental health. The mechanisms responsible for the degenerative disease process (for example, cancer, heart disease, and diabetes) remain somewhat obscure, but the causes of some environmentally induced diseases are relatively accessible.

A key community health nursing role is assessment of the environment: home, school, recreational area, work site, or community as a whole. Community health nurses, especially those involved with home health care, must do a careful assessment of the safety of the home. Electrical cords should not be hidden under throw rugs. This is especially true in situations where elderly people might trip. Cleaning agents contain chemicals, and if not used and stored properly, these agents may be hazardous. Elderly people with poor eyesight are at risk. One example involved an elderly woman who mixed several cleaning agents, which led to unconsciousness and severe respiratory irritation. Improper food storage in the home has resulted in many cases of food poisoning. Children who have ingested cleaning agents or plant fertilizers are taken to emergency departments. For some, ingestion has been fatal.

Schools present many hazards. Accidents occur on playgrounds, gyms, grandstands, and bleachers. High schools have laboratories with chemicals that may result in burns to individuals or fires from explosions. Machinery in shops pose a threat. Poor lighting, littered floors, and narrow or broken stairs are other areas of concern. Improper playground equipment has caused numerous injuries to children.

In assessing the environment, community health nurses should consider the degree of potential toxicity present or proposed through an introduction of some substance or activity and should determine whether a health hazard will be likely. From the perspective of physical, chemical, and biological hazards *toxicity* refers to the ability of a substance to cause injury to biological tissue. The *hazard* associated with the substance is the likelihood that it will cause injury in a given environment or situation.

Both recognition and interaction are important. The person who drove to work in heavy traffic or walked down a busy street is exposed to carbon monoxide. This exposure may be greater than carbon monoxide exposure in the workplace. The person who smokes a pack of cigarettes a day may be exposed to higher levels of carbon monoxide than those associated with the workplace. People who consume excess amounts of alcohol are more susceptible to the effects of carbon tetrachloride. Similarly, exposure to silica increases the susceptibility of tuberculosis. People with asthmatic conditions should not be placed in dusty work areas. Consequently, both an assessment of the individual and the environment is necessary.

Community health nurses must be aware of the hazards that exist in the community. This information is gained by careful observation as the nurse travels through the community. Observations might include the presence and characteristics of trash collection sites, standing water, the quality of the air as determined by sight and smell, the level and type of noise, and the conditions of housing, including their closeness to one another. The environmental analysis outline on p. 308 presents many areas for assessment.

Community health nurses use the nursing process to assess the quality and safety of the environment and to plan and implement interventions. Because other health and safety providers often have greater designated responsibility for environmental control, the nursing role in many areas includes assessment and reporting to the appropriate agency as well as being health educator and advocate or catalyst for environmental change.

Upon observing potential or actual environmental hazards, nurses report them to the appropriate regulatory or intervening authority or citizen action groups. In some cities, the health department, county commission, housing authority, or other agency maintains responsibility for some aspect of environmental safety. It is important to know which local agencies handle specific environmental problems so quick and accurate referrals can be made. Frequently, citizen action groups are vital forces in instigating environmental change. The nurse alerts such groups to health hazards and works with them as they establish an intervention plan.

Another nursing action is education of environmental health and safety to school children, health providers, fire and police personnel, and the general public. These groups must be informed about environmental issues such as pollution, vehicular safety, product safety, and the presence or potential for additional physical, chemical, biological, and psychosocial hazards.

Nurses must often serve as catalysts to see that actions are taken. It is not always easy to persuade individuals and groups that an occupational or environmental health factor is potential. Interventions may be designed but may never get implemented. The nurse serves as a vital force to see that people follow through on the plans and commitments they make.

ROLE OF GOVERNMENT IN ENVIRONMENTAL HEALTH AND SAFETY

The decades of the 1960s and 1970s, especially the last half of the latter 1970s, will be known in environmental history as the Age of Realization. People finally recognized how badly they had fouled up their own nests with multiple forms of pollution. Over the years standards for control of emission of air pollutants were established and the Environmental Protection Agency (EPA) was created.

Early local governmental efforts dealt with services such as water supply, sewage collection and deposit, refuse collection and disposal, control of rodents and pests, and regulation of housing and recreation. Some of the earliest efforts at environmental control were performed by the official health departments in Philadelphia, New York, Baltimore, and Charleston. They directed activities toward community sanitation and the prevention of filth and oral disease. Often separate departments tended to specialize in specific entities such as food sanitation and housing sanitation. In some instances, the specialization was extreme with food sanitation divided into milk, meat, and food divisions. The state health department and other statewide environmental health and safety agencies are responsible for ensuring that all people within the state receive comprehensive services. Few, if any, direct services are performed at the state level, and the pattern of organization among states varies.

The national level is primarily charged with establishing regulations. The initiative to clear up the environment began slowly in the 1960s with the passage of five pieces of environmental legislation dealing with air and water pollution (Sandhu, 1981).

The trend over many years has been to look carefully at the way people influence the environment and vice versa. In 1967, a task force was established by the Secretary of Health, Education, and Welfare to assure that all Americans could live in a healthy environment "by controlling pollution at its source, reducing hazards, converting waste to use, and improving the esthetic value of man's surroundings" (Hanlon and Pickett, 1984, p. 628). Since that time, the Task Force on Environmental Health and Related Problems has struggled for a coordinated environmental health protection system. The struggle bore fruit with the National

Environmental Policy act of 1969, which declared a national environmental policy, established a Council on Environmental Quality, and paved the way for the formation of the EPA in 1970. Creation of the EPA consolidated the federal environmental efforts into one agency and gave it far-reaching authority to control air and water pollution, including noise, radiation, and toxic substances (Sandhu, 1981). One of the highest priorities of the EPA is the identification and assessment of toxic substances.

Other agencies besides the EPA involved in controlling hazardous materials include the Food and Drug Administration (FDA), OSHA, NIOSH, the Consumer Product Safety Commission, and the Food Safety and Quality Service. In addition, the Toxic Substances Strategy Committee Group (1977) and the Regulatory Council (1978) promote and improve coordination of regulatory activities.

The focus of the government's role in toxic substances is to reduce exposure.

Legislative Acts

The federal government has been involved in environmental legislation since the 1800s. The first federal legislation to regulate pollution of waters was the Rivers and Harbors Act of 1899.

In 1960 the passage of five pieces of environmental legislation spurred the regulatory initiative to make the en-

vironment more livable. Early environmental legislation addressed air and water pollution. Later Congress looked at food additives. The FDA believed that food additives containing any carcinogenic hazard should be banned. The EPA has been responsible since 1970 for controlling and abating pollution in the areas of air, water, noise, pesticides, solid waste, toxic substances, and radiation. The agency has regulatory authority in all matters pertaining to air, water, noise, and pesticides under specific federal laws (Your Guide, 1980). The major legislative acts pertaining to these subjects have been summarized (see Table 16-2).

Criticism of EPA

The EPA conducts extensive research in an effort to control and abate the nation's pollution problems. EPA's Office of Research and Development has 15 laboratories throughout the nation for the purpose of conducting such research.

In recent years there has been much criticism and controversy regarding the federal regulatory attempts. The EPA, accused by some of being understaffed, recently experienced additional personnel losses. Attempts to reduce inflation by tightening economic controls forced the agency to operate under much tighter budget constraints.

Environmentalists criticize EPA standards as being lax. They cite polluted rivers and streams, dead water birds, and fish kills as examples of environmental degradation.

TABLE 16-2

Selected examples of major environmental legislative acts involving the Environmental Protection Agency

Subject	Legislative act	Purpose
Air pollution	Air Quality Control Act, 1970; amended, 1977	The act grants EPA authority to establish national air quality standards to protect community health and welfare. The act also calls for states to examine air quality more closely and, if standards are not being met, to revise state plans.
Water quality	Water Pollution Control Act Amendments, 1972	The act imposes on EPA the task of restoring and maintaining the chemical, physical, and biological integrity of the nation's waters.
Water quality	Safe Drinking Water Act, 1974; amended, 1977	The act requires that EPA issue regulations that set national standards to protect drinking water.
Ocean dumping	Marine Protection Research and Sanctuaries Act, 1972	The act authorizes EPA to establish a dumping permit program and site for dumping. The Army Corps is authorized to control dredged material.
Noise	Noise Control Act, 1972; amended, 1978	The act calls for EPA to establish standards and promulgate regulations concerning major sources of noise. The act further requires EPA to conduct research into the effects and control of noise and to help states and local assistance programs.
Solid waste	Solid Waste Disposal Act, 1965; Resource Conservation and Recovery Act, 1976	The acts provide for the establishment of regulations and devise EPA programs to ensure safe disposal of wastes, i.e., toxic substances, pesticides, explosives. They also require states to look at existing waste disposal sites and develop plans.
Toxic substances	Toxic Substances Control Act, 1976	The act compels industry to develop adequate data on the effect of chemical substances on health and the environments and to regulate and ban substances when necessary.

However, state and local governments blame EPA standards for keeping new business from entering their states. Throughout the years some state legislators, in an effort to appease industry, have attempted to weaken environmental enforcement. Chemical manufacturers have criticized EPA efforts at more stringent control, although chemicals found to be extremely dangerous have been banned. Workers suffering from chronic disease attributed to the use of such chemicals are calling for stricter controls. EPA is not the only agency concerned with the control of toxic substances; five agencies have formed the Interagency Regulation Liason Group (IRLG). The IRLG comprises the EPA, the Occupational Safety and Health Administration, the Food and Drug Administration, the Consumer Product Safety Commission, and the Food Safety and Quality Service of the Department of Agriculture.

ROLE OF PRIVATE SECTOR IN ENVIRONMENTAL HEALTH AND SAFETY

Some manufacturers of pesticides, farmers, and citrus growers question the approach the government has taken to regulate pesticide use and want less stringent controls. Migrant farm workers and advocate groups point to the lack of federal involvement regarding personal protective equipment. They cite unsanitary field conditions, lack of drinking water, and an increasing number of unreported pesticide poisonings each year.

Environmentalists and some scientists have expressed concern about pollutants such as trihalomethanes in water, whereas other researchers and scientists point out that a direct causal link between drinking water quality and cancer incidence has not been established. The controversy goes on and on. As health care professionals, nurses must objectively assess the effect of the environment on health. As new legislation is passed and old legislation amended, they must continue to ask questions, attempt to remain objective, and weigh the evidence of both sides. They must be able to comprehend the complexity of each problem as well as the ramifications involved in possible alternatives, bearing in mind that the best approach toward solving any environmental problem is an informed one.

CLINICAL APPLICATION

Assume you are a community health nurse who is making a home visit to the home of a young couple with a 6-month-old child. The mother asks you to assist her in completing an environmental survey of the home to make it a safe place for a child who will soon be crawling and walking. Knowing that mothers and young children spend a considerable amount of time in the kitchen, you decide to start the survey there.

Your investigation would include the following:

1. Paint—make sure that it is not lead-based; even if not lead-based be sure that it is not cracking. Young children like to pick and pull at loose items, including peeling paint.

2. Check the dishes for cracks and chips. The family could cut themselves, and the dishes could harbor bacteria in the cracks.

3. Look for loose rugs, which might cause tripping.

4. Suggest that the parents install locks on cabinets that the child can reach. The mother might choose to leave one or more cabinets open and place plastic bowls and pans in that location. Young children like bowls and pans and occupy themselves for long periods with such harmless items.

5. Suggest that matches, cleaning supplies, glass items, sharp items such as razors, knives, forks, and so on be in high places or in locked cabinets.

6. Remind the mother to turn the handles of pans away from the edge of the stove or cabinet so the child cannot grab them.

7. Suggest that pet food be kept out of reach of the child.

8. Electric outlets should have caps on them if the child has any tendency to poke fingers or things into the outlets.

9. Plants that are dangerous to eat should be discarded or put in inaccessible locations.

10. If the child sits in a high chair, suggest that the parents always securely strap the child in to prevent falls.

These same ideas can be used to guide an inspection of the remainder of the house. Remind the mother that young children soon become skilled climbers; they can grab curtains, chairs, and tables to assist them in their explorations.

SUMMARY

The challenge of maintaining environmental health and safety is tremendous. Each innovation seems to exact a price in terms of destruction or threat of pollution to the environment. This chapter discussed significant biological, chemical, physical, and psychosocial hazards and the governmental role in maintaining and regulating environmental health and safety.

Community health nurses are in key positions to detect environmental hazards. Although nurses do not always directly combat these hazards, they monitor, report, and serve as action-oriented catalysts. Community health nurses must recognize potential hazards in the communities they serve and aid clients in protecting themselves against these health risks. Water, air, soil, and food are only a few possible health hazards. To implement an ecological approach to community health, nurses must be constantly aware of the interaction among people and the environments in which they live. This human and environment interaction and its effect on health have been sources of concern since early recorded history. Many problems have been solved, but new and often more challenging and resistant ones continually arise.

KEY CONCEPTS

Nurses play an important role in detecting environmental hazards and in developing and implementing health promotion and treatment programs.

The production and maintenance of a healthy environment will require a combination of increased legislation, vigorous enforcement of existing laws, increased cooperation by business, and greater public awareness and education. Community health nurses can make significant contributions to this process.

Ecology, the study of living organisms in interaction with the environment, provides a model for looking at environmental health.

Two contexts have been proposed for describing the human and environmental relationship. The first includes elements of the natural environment hazardous to health, such as biological agents of disease or injury. The second context consists of health hazards created by actions and maladaptations of people to their environment.

Community health nurses must have an understanding of the biological, physical, chemical, and psychosocial hazards affecting both men and women, the elderly, and children as well as potential health effects on the unborn fetus.

A major community health nursing activity regarding environmental hazards is education.

Assessment of the client's environment is also an important community health nursing role.

The federal government has been involved in environmental legislation since the 1800s. However, the biggest nationwide effort at pollution control began in the 1960s.

The modern environment is hazardous in at least two ways: it contains noxious and stressful events and it changes so quickly that people are unable to adapt.

LEARNING ACTIVITIES

1. Read the local newspaper to determine information about major environmental hazards in a given community.

2. Describe one real or potential chain of events in a community that could have negative ecological results.

3. Review one environmental hazard that has occurred in the last 10 years and discuss three potential long-range consequences.

4. Drive through the community of residence or select a community and identify potential disasters. You may have to assume that certain weather conditions prevail.

5. Drive through a community and identify the quality of environmental health and safety.

BIBLIOGRAPHY

Banks, H.O.: Comprehensive health planning in relation to environmental problems, Am. J. Public Health 61:1972-1979, 1971.

Blumenthal, D.S.: Introduction to environmental health, New York, 1985, Springer Publishing Co.

Brown, M.: The forgotten great lake, Audubon 84(1):88-95, Nov. 1982.

Bruce, R.D.: Noise pollution. In Jarvis, L.L., editor: Community health nursing: keeping the public healthy, ed. 2, Philadelphia, 1985, F.A. Davis Co., pp. 817-833.

Chanlett, E.T.: Solid waste management. In Jarvis, L.L., editor: Community health nursing: keeping the public healthy, ed. 2, Philadelphia, 1985, F.A. Davis Co., pp. 847-867.

Coburn, R.F.: Biologic effects of carbon monoxide, Ann. NY Acad. Sci. 174:1-43, 1970.

Cohen, S.: Sound effects on behavior, Psychology Today 15:38-46, Oct. 1981.

Commoner, B.: The closing circle: nature, man and technology, New York, 1971, Alfred A. Knopf, Inc.

Drotman, D.P.: Chemicals, health and the environment. In Blumenthal, D.S.: Introduction to environmental health, New York, 1985, Springer Publishing Co., pp. 47-78.

Dubos, R.: The crisis of man in his environment, Proceedings of Symposium on Human

Ecology, Pub. No. 1929, 1968, Department of Health, Education, and Welfare.

Fetter, S., and Tsipis, K.: Catastrophic releases of radioactivity, Sci. Am. 4:41-47, 1981.

Geller, E.S.: Prevention of environmental problems. In Edelstein, B.A., and Michelson, L.: Handbook of prevention, New York, 1986, Plenum Press, pp. 361-383.

Golden, J., et al.: Environmental impact data book, Ann Arbor, Mich., 1979, Ann Arbor Science Publishers, Inc.

Hanlon, J.J., and Pickett, G.E.: Public health: administration and practice, ed. 7, St. Louis, 1979, The C.V. Mosby Co.

Hanlon, J.J., and Pickett, G.E.: Public health: administration and practice, ed. 8, St. Louis, 1984, The C.V. Mosby Co.

Harrison, G., Gates, D., and Halling, C.S.: Ecology: the great chain of being, Ekistics 27:161, March 1969.

Holzer, H.: A doomsday scenario on 59th Street, New York, 15:21, May 24, 1982.

Kellogg, W.W., et al.: The sulfur cycle, Science 175:587-596, 1972.

Kowitz, R.A., et al.: Effects of chlorine gas upon respiratory function, Arch. Environ. Health 14:545, 1967.

Lancaster, J.: Community mental health nursing: An ecological perspective, St. Louis, 1980, The C.V. Mosby Co.

Nelson, K.W.: Government regulations—environmental and occupational health, Am. Ind. Hyg. J. 42:633-636, Sept. 1981.

P'an, A.Y.S., Beland, J., and Zygmunt. J.: Ozone-induced arterial lesions, Arch. Environ. Health 24:229-232, 1972.

Purdom, P.W., editor: Environmental health, New York, 1980, Academic Press, Inc.

Reist, P.C.: Air pollution. In Jarvis, L.L.: editor, Community health nursing: keeping the public healthy, ed. 2, Philadelphia, 1985, F.A. Davis Co., pp. 805-816.

Rosen, G.: A history of public health, New York, 1957, M.D. Publications.

Sandhu, S.S.: Regulation of environmental pollutants: introductory remarks 37:1-3, Jan. 1981.

Silberstein, C.A., and Silberstein, E.B.: Ionizing radiation and community health. In Jarvis, L.L., editor: Community health nursing: keeping the public healthy, ed. 2, Philadelphia, 1985, F.A. Davis Co., pp. 869-881.

Spath, D.P., and Crook, J.: Water pollution. In Jarvis, L.L., editor: Community health nursing: keeping the public healthy, ed. 2, Philadelphia, 1985, F.A. Davis Co., pp. 835-846.

Stahl, Q.R.: Air pollution aspects of chlorine and hydrogen gas, Litton Systems, Inc., Bethesda, Md. 1969, Pub. No. 188087, Department of Commerce, National Bureau of Standards.

United Auto Workers Sound Security Department: What every representative should know about health and safety, Pub. No. 449, Detroit, 1979, UAW, p. 6.

Waldbott, G.L.: Health effects of environmental pollutants, ed. 2, St. Louis, 1978, The C.V. Mosby Co.

Werthamer, S, et al.: Ozone-induced pulmonary lesions, Arch. Environ. Health 20:16-21, 1970.

Wilner, D.M., Walkley, R.P., and O'Neill, E.J.: Introduction to public health, ed. 7, New York, 1978, MacMillan Publishing Co., Inc.

Woodwell, G.W., Graig, P.P., and Johnson, H.A.: DDT in the biosphere: where does it go? Science 174:1101-1107, 1971.

Your guide to the Environmental Protection Agency, Washington, D.C., Dec. 1980, Office of Public Awareness, EPA.

Joan Turner

17

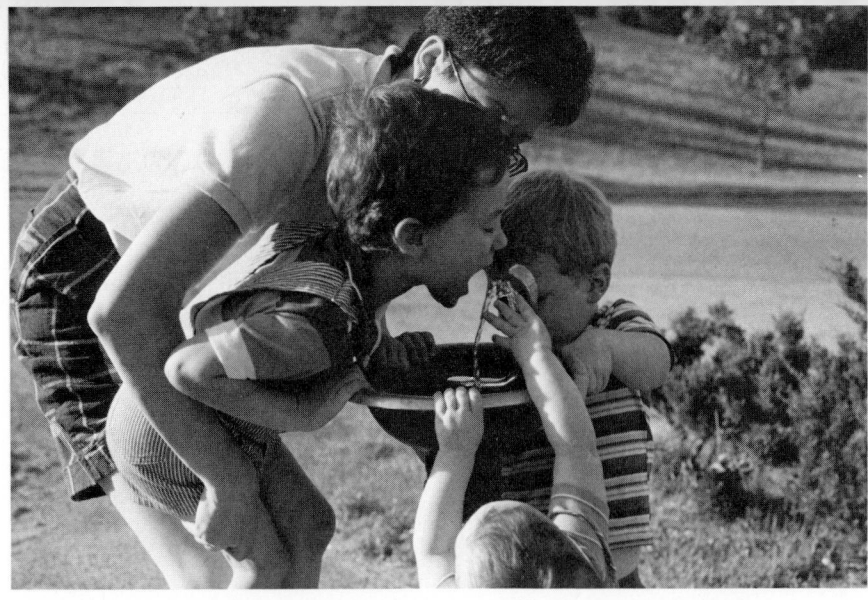

COMMUNICABLE DISEASES AND INFECTION CONTROL PRACTICES IN COMMUNITY HEALTH NURSING

OBJECTIVES

Explain the host, agent, environment triad and how these factors may interact to cause infectious disease.

Explain the process and goal of surveillance activities in infectious and communicable disease.

Discuss the impact of communicable and infectious diseases in terms of morbidity and mortality.

Explain the difference between active and passive immunity and give several examples of each.

Discuss the indications and/or contraindications and untoward effects of active and passive immunity.

Explain the ramifications of antibiotic-resistant organisms to community health nursing practice.

Name the diseases included within "sexually transmitted diseases" and state their comparative incidence and identify the age groups at greatest risk.

Explain the treatment for pediculosis and helminth infections.

Describe AIDS as a major communicable disease.

KEY TERMS

acquired immune deficiency syndrome (AIDS)

agent

anaphylaxis

botulism

communicable disease

delta hepatitis

dosage

drug resistance

endemic

enzyme-linked immunosorbent assay (ELISA)

epidemic

haemophilus influenzae

host

immune globulin

immunization

infectivity

invasiveness

legionellosis

nationally notifiable conditions

nosocomial infections

pandemic

passive immunization

pediculosis

salmonellosis

sexually transmitted diseases

temporal patterns

vaccines

virulence

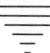

In recent decades the impact of *communicable diseases* on contemporary society has been drastically reduced and altered by the combined efforts of pharmacology, sanitary engineering, public health, medicine, and nursing. The declining mortality associated with communicable diseases is illustrated in Table 17-1. The vast majority of persons who succumb to communicable or contagious diseases contract them in the community and are cared for at home throughout minor illnesses or periods when the disease process can be managed on an outpatient basis. This chapter discusses the role of the community health nurse in prevention, control, case finding, reporting, and maintenance strategies as they relate to communicable and infectious diseases. This chapter also discusses aspects of communicable disease and infection control, including surveillance mechanisms, temporal and geographic patterns, realized and potential effects of current and past immunization programs, the emergence of new communicable or infectious processes, and the increasing appearance of drug-resistant diseases and antibiotic resistant organisms. Incidence, mortality, and morbidity data are used to explore these phenomena.

HISTORICAL PERSPECTIVE

Communicable diseases are primarily infectious and require interaction between a host agent, direct or indirect transmission from the agent reservoir and a host that supports

adequate living conditions. Communicable diseases have shaped human life since earliest times. Because humans are the only reservoir for many diseases, microbiologists ponder questions such as "which came first, human beings or infectious organisms?" Evidence gathered by anthropologists indicate that humans who lived in the Paleolithic period (18,000 to 6000 BC) were susceptible to tapeworms and roundworms as well as tetanus and gas gangrene. However, the occurrence of *epidemics,* or outbreaks involving large numbers of people, was not evident until approximately 5000 to 4000 BC. Before then, family groups were largely nomadic and isolated from similar social groups. As the first large cities came into existence and great numbers of persons lived in close proximity, the stage was set for innumerable epidemics of communicable diseases. Occasionally these epidemics came close to exterminating organized society.

Some of history's most notorious and lethal epidemics were the Black Death in Europe in 1345, smallpox among the North American Indians in 1633, dysentery during the Crusades, and influenza pandemics of 1889 and 1918. In a few days, an epidemic of yellow fever left Napoleon with 3000 survivors out of 25,000 troops. Such mortality figured heavily in his ultimate defeat at Waterloo (Hare, 1955).

Communicable diseases played a significant role in the death and illnesses of people during the colonial period in the United States, and they were still leading causes of death in 1900. In fact, the need to control the spread of communicable diseases rather than the concern for infected individuals stimulated the first health legislation in the United States, including the establishment of health departments in colonial America. Nevertheless, the antibiotics of the 1940s, the vaccines of the 1950s, 1960s, and 1970s, and the general improvement in nutrition and sanitation gradually brought many of the traditional killing and crippling communicable diseases under control in the United States and other industrialized nations. However, in the developing Third World countries of Asia and Africa, communicable diseases are still a major public health threat. But with the 1980s came *Acquired Immune Deficiency Syndrome (AIDS).* Dubbed "the most complex problem of the century" (Silverman & Silverman, 1985, p. 22), AIDS has produced a virtual renaissance in worldwide concern with communicable diseases.

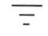

TABLE 17-1

Deaths attributed to common communicable diseases in the United States in 1900, 1935, and 1983

Communicable disease	1900	1935	1983
Influenza and pneumonia	202.2	103.9	30.9
Tuberculosis	191.2	55.1	1.7
Diptheria	40.3	3.1	*
Typhoid	12.0	2.7	*
Meningococcal infections	12.0	2.1	0.3

All statistics represent rates per 100,000 persons.
*None or few deaths.

CURRENT PERSPECTIVE

Some infectious diseases, such as smallpox, have been completely eliminated throughout the world, and most traditional communicable diseases can be therapeutically managed so that often death can be prevented. Although some communicable diseases such as cholera still occur in epidemic proportions in some parts of the world, the incidence is low in the United States. Regardless of these advances, there are four reasons why community health nurses must appreciate the real and potential effects that communicable and infectious diseases have on society.

First, the types and causes of communicable diseases are not static, but are constantly being changed and updated by new knowledge. For instance, in the past decade agents such as various herpesviruses, including cytomegalovirus (CMV), played a role in the causation of innumerable perinatal and adult diseases previously attributed to a noninfectious or nonspecific etiology. Additionally, several infectious diseases have been documented for the first time in recent years. Examples of these "new" diseases are shown in Table 17-2.

Increasingly, communicable diseases fail to respond to previously successful treatments due to a phenomenon known as *drug resistance* (antibiotic resistance). Drug resistance is discussed in more detail later in this chapter; it has been documented in a wide range of communicable diseases such as tuberculosis, malaria, salmonella, and gonorrhea.

The scope of communicable diseases is changing as standard immunization schedules are modified when new information and new vaccines become available. Information of this sort is vital to community health nursing practice.

Secondly, community health nurses must be knowledgeable about communicable diseases so they can effectively counsel parents, family, or friends about the care of potentially exposed or frankly infected persons. Often community health nurses are in the position to recognize signs and symptoms of actual or impending disease and make appropriate referrals for diagnosis that leads to treatment and control of spread.

Third, communicable disease plays a tremendous role in the economic viability of both specific communities and the nation. The U.S. Department of Health, Education, and Welfare estimated that the total economic loss from the 1968-1969 Hong Kong influenza in the United States alone was $46 million (Beveridge, 1978). The cost of treating persons with AIDS was estimated to be 45.6 billion dollars through the end of 1986 (Volberding & Abrams, 1985). In addition, acute respiratory disease (i.e., the "flu" or a "cold") is the most common human illness and the principal reason for people to consult a physician. Approximately 156 million workdays are lost annually at a cost of $24 billion as a result of communicable and infectious diseases (Healthy People, 1979).

Fourth, failure to enforce the recommended schedule for communicable disease control (see Tables 17-7 through 17-10) or a break in community sanitation or water purification can result in an epidemic at any given time. An epidemic is not the only threat; communicable diseases also result in chronic disability and irreversible disease processes every year. For instance, it is estimated that the occurrence of measles (rubeola), a disease that is 95% preventable by immunization, resulted in 600 cases of mental retardation as recently as 1975 in the United States (Brown, 1975).

Factors Influencing Infection
Agent Factors

The following discussion describes various *agent* characteristics that are influential in disease causation (Ramsay and Edmond, 1979).

Infectivity is the ability of the organism to spread rapidly from one *host* to another. High infectivity is not necessarily associated with the severity of disease. For example, chickenpox virus is believed to be one of the most infectious agents in contemporary times but the disease is generally self-limited in that there are usually no permanent effects from it.

Invasiveness refers to the agent's ability to spread within the host. An example of this characteristic is the organism *Treponema pallidum*, which is capable of spreading throughout the body.

Virulence is the ability to produce severe disease. An example of this agent characteristic is the influenza-A virus, which is capable of producing more severe disease than the influenza-C strains.

Dosage refers to the fact that multiple organisms invading the host are more apt to overwhelm host defenses, whereas small numbers of the same organisms are frequently suppressed or tolerated without disease actually occurring. For instance, a host eating a hearty portion of salmonella-infected food would be more likely to get food poisoning than one who ate sparingly of the same food. Also, a mixed or multiple-agent infection often produces more serious effects than separate invasion by the components. For example, the onset of bacterial pneumonia in addition to a generalized influenza syndrome greatly increases the threat to the affected host.

Host Factors

In general, most disease processes produce the greatest morbidity and mortality in the very young and the very old in any given population, but there are some important exceptions. Many viral diseases produce much less disturbance (are less virulent) in the young. For instance, mumps are generally tolerated better by young children than middle-

---

TABLE 17-2

Incidence of AIDS, legionellosis, Reye's syndrome, and toxic shock syndrome (TSS), 1982-1984

	1982	1983	1984
AIDS	—	—	4445
Legionellosis (legionnaire's diseases (LD))	654	852	750
Reye's syndrome	222	198	190
TSS	400	502	482

From CDC: Annual Summary, *MMWR*, 1984.

aged adults. However, chickenpox in a newborn, although rare, is frequently life-threatening. Other host factors that influence the incidence of communicable diseases are:

Sex and sex hormones

Hereditary resistance

The host's local and systemic responses (immune response)

General health status, including adequate nutritional intake or status

Environmental Factors

Some factors of the host's ability to ward off infection are interdependent with environmental factors such as humidity, temperature, and crowding. Other environmental factors that influence the incidence of communicable diseases are:

Atmospheric conditions (pollution and smoke)

Availability of nutrients (protein and vitamins)

Contamination of food and water supplies

Efficient transmission of most communicable diseases requires that large numbers of people interact. In addition, when people come into contact with animals or their byproducts, the risk of contracting certain communicable diseases is increased. For instance, veterinarians are particularly susceptible to brucellosis and rabies, hunters who prepare animal hides are susceptible to anthrax, and bird fanciers are susceptible to psittacosis, or parrot fever.

The quality and safety of any community's drinking water is usually assured by some municipal authority that has designed its system to meet community needs. Additionally, community building codes usually require that plumbing be designed, installed, and maintained so as to avoid contamination of the water supply. However, in times of natural disasters such as in flooding, individual and community plumbing systems can be overwhelmed, causing sewage to mix with drinking water. Because sewage contains numerous microbiologic pathogens (such as the hepatitis B virus and salmonella), the potential for community-wide epidemic exists if inhabitants consume contaminated water.

Surveillance Systems

Trends in the occurrence of communicable diseases are monitored nationally by the Centers for Disease Control (CDC) in Atlanta, Georgia. Each week the CDC publishes the *Morbidity and Mortality Weekly Report* (MMWR). These reports include weekly and cumulative totals of reported communicable diseases by geographic region and individual state. The MMWR provides enlightening, authoritative, and up-to-date information on many facets of communicable disease occurrence, prevention, and control. Additionally, various topics of public health interest such as unusual cases of disease, communicable disease outbreaks, and environmental and occupational hazards are discussed.

Notifiable and Non-notifiable Conditions

Federal law requires that occurrence of certain communicable disease (*nationally notifiable conditions*) be reported to the CDC by all states on weekly, monthly, and annual bases. Examples include *sexually transmitted diseases,* tetanus, and rabies. Other diseases may be classified as "op-

tionally reported"; these are diseases that states may choose to report based on their statewide health regulations. In addition to the nationally notifiable communicable diseases, the MMWR and the national surveillance program also monitor the occurrence of other conditions (non-notifiable conditions) of interest to community health nurses and others. Such communicable disease phenomena are optionally reported by state health departments and include conditions such as giardiasis, histoplasmosis, infectious mononucleosis, meningitis, Reye's syndrome, strep throat, scarlet fever, toxoplasmosis, and influenza. In some instances, these diseases are reported only when they are believed to be occurring in epidemic proportion (in excess of expectations). At other times, a given disease is reported in a particular state because it is believed to be *endemic,* or continuously present in the area, and therefore an ongoing public health problem. For instance, histoplasmosis is believed to be endemic to the Ohio Valley region.

Morbidity and Mortality Associated with Communicable Disease

As can be seen in Table 17-3, the total number of deaths attributed to communicable diseases in the representative year of 1983 was 92,549. That figure makes infectious and communicable phenomena the fourth leading killer in the United States for 1983 (National Center for Health Statistics, 1985, p. 152). The data in Table 17-3 are undercounts in that the total figure for infectious diseases would be 152,549 if *nosocomial infections* that *contributed* to death were counted. One can also understand that deaths attributable to AIDS would certainly inflate annual counts of deaths due to infectious diseases since 1983.

Tables 17-4 and 17-5 also illustrate the impact of communicable disease. It should be noted that the seven communicable diseases with the highest incidence are those diseases for which there is no effective active *immunization* with the exception of hepatitis B.

TEMPORAL PATTERNS. Certain communicable or infectious disease processes occur more frequently during one season

---

≡ **TABLE 17-3**

Number of deaths in the United States attributable to infectious or communicable diseases, 1983

Cause of death	Number of deaths
Specific notifiable communicable disease	3592
Fungal infections	892
Respiratory infections	56,771
Miscellaneous infectious processes*	1394
Nosocomial infections	30,000-90,000†
TOTAL:	92,549-152,549

Data compiled from Centers for Disease Control, Annual Summary, *MMWR,* 1984.

*Miscellaneous infectious processes include herpes, meningitis (excluding meningococcal and tuberculosis), mononucleosis, streptococcal sore throat, scarlet fever, and toxoplasmosis.

†Nosocomial infections *contributed* to 90,000 deaths. Nosocomial infection was the direct cause of 30,000 deaths.

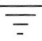

TABLE 17-4

Incidence of notifiable communicable diseases in
the United States, 1984

Disease	Number of cases reported
Gonorrhea	878,556
Chickenpox	190,894
Syphilis (all stages)	69,888
Hepatitis (all types)	52,026
Salmonellosis (excluding typhoid fever)	40,861
Tuberculosis	22,255
Shigellosis	17,371
Measles (rubeola)	2587
Mumps	3021
Aseptic meningitis	8326
TOTAL:	1,283,950

Data from Centers for Disease Control (September 27, 1985, *MMWR*).
These data do not include estimates of the common cold nor do they
include pneumonia and influenza, which are not mandatory reportable
diseases.

TABLE 17-5

Deaths from specified notifiable diseases,
United States, 1983

Cause of death	Number of deaths reported in 1983
Tuberculosis (all forms)	1937
Hepatitis (all forms)	862
Menigococcal infections	459
Encephalitis	164
Syphilis	136
TOTAL	3558

Data from Centers for Disease Control (1984 Annual Summary, *MMWR*).

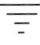

TABLE 17-6

Temporal patterns in communicable or
infectious diseases

Type of disease	Season of peak occurrence
Polio	Spring
Roseola infantum	Spring
Rubella	Late winter and spring
Meningococcal infections	Winter and spring
Rubeola (measles)	Late winter and early spring
Diptheria	Autumn and winter
Rocky Mountain spotted fever	Summer
Legionellosis	July through October
Reye's syndrome	December through March

DISEASES FOR WHICH ACTIVE IMMUNIZATION IS AVAILABLE

Adenovirus (types 4 and 7)
Anthrax
Botulism
Cholera (vaccine has only limited value)
Cytomegalovirus (experimental attenuated CMV vaccines are under evaluation)
Diptheria
Haemophilus influenzae (Type B)
Hepatitis B
Influenza
Measles (rubeola)
Meningitis (cased by *Neisseria meningitidis*)
Mumps
Pertussis
Plague
Pneumococcal infections
Polio
Rabies
Rocky Mountain spotted fever
Rubella
Salmonellosis (typhoid immunization afford protection in approximately 70% to 90% of subjects)
Smallpox
Tetanus
Trachoma conjunctivitis (temporary and limited protection study)
Tuberculosis
Tularemia
Typhus
Yellow fever

of the year (see Table 17-6). Awareness of these *temporal patterns,* seasonal fluctuations, can alert the community health nurse to what disease phenomenon might be expected at any given time of year.

PANDEMICS. The term *pandemic* refers to a worldwide outbreak of the same epidemic disease phenomenon. Contemporary pandemics of communicable diseases have been essentially limited to the type-A influenzas. In this century there has been the Spanish (swine) influenza pandemic 1918-1919, the Asian influenza pandemic of 1958-1959, and the Hong Kong influenza pandemic of 1968-1969. In the case of influenza, virologists restrict the definition of pandemic to mean a worldwide epidemic caused by a new subtype of influenza type A. It is believed that the characteristic of being a new subtype is important in that people are far more susceptible to a subtype that has not been demonstrated in the population previously than they are to those subtypes that are present at frequent intervals.

COMMUNICABLE DISEASES AND IMMUNIZATION PRACTICES

Although immunizing agents, or *vaccines,* are available for about 25 disorders (see box above) only 7 are recommended for routine use (Appendix D). The remaining 18 vaccines

DISEASES FOR WHICH PASSIVE IMMUNIZATION IS AVAILABLE

Botulism (but administration carries with it a great danger of sensitivity reaction)
Hepatitis type A (ISG)*
Measles (rubeola) (ISG)
Mumps
Rubella (ISG)
Smallpox
Tetanus
Varicella-zoster virus infection
Mycoplasma pneumoniae infections
Otitis Media
Parainfluenza virus infections
Pediculosis
Psittacosis
Primary amebic meningocencephalitis
Rhinovirus infections
Rickettsialpox
Roseola infantum
Scabies
Schistosomiasis
Shingellosis
Staphylococcal infections
Streptococcal infections (including pharyngitis, scarlet fever, and erysipelas)
Syphilis
Tapeworm disease
Tinea capiti, corporis, cruris, pedis
Toxoplasmosis
Trichinosis
Viral gastroenteritis

*ISG, immune serum globulin.

COMMUNICABLE DISEASES FOR WHICH NO ACTIVE OR PASSIVE IMMUNIZATION IS AVAILABLE

Actinomycosis
All arboviruses except yellow fever
Amebiasis caused by *Escherichia* species
Ascariasis (roundworm infection)
Aspergillosis
Balantidiasis
Blastomycosis
Brucellosis (undulant fever)
Candidiasis (moniliasis, thrush)
Cat-bite fever
Cat scratch disease
Chlamydial infections
Coccidioidomycosis
Clostridium perfringens food poisoning
Coxsackie virus
Cryptococcosis
Echoviruses
Enterobiasis (pinworm infection)
Erythema infectiosum
Escherichia coli diarrhea
Gas gangrene
Genital herpes
Giardiasis
Gonoccal infections
Hemorrhagic fever
Herpes virus hominis (simplex infections)
Histoplasmosis
Impetigo
Larva migrans
Leprosy
Leptospirosis
Listeriosis
Lymphocytic choriomeningitis
Lymphocytosis
Malaria
Molluscum contagiosum
Mononucleosis

are not recommended for routine use because the diseases are sufficiently rare to preclude routine immunization except to special high-risk people. Examples of these special health status situations are shown in Table 17-14. Usually vaccines are recommended for either general or specific use. Vaccines recommended by the American Academy of Pediatrics for general use as well as immunization procedures to be followed for children not immunized in early infancy are shown in Appendix D.

Active Immunization

Active immunization is discussed in Chapter 8. The community health nurse should realize that an artificial acquired immunity or vaccination is not without some risks to the host. Risks or side effects associated with vaccination depend on the nature of the specific vaccine; that is, whether it has bacterial or viral antigens and if antigens are killed whole organisms or live attenuated organisms. In general, the vaccine label explains its composition. Table 17-7 describes some side effects of administering recommended childhood immunizations and corresponding nursing actions. There are several contraindications and special circumstances for which the routine immunization administration schedule may be temporarily interrupted (Table 17-8).

Special Considerations for DPT Immunization

DIPHTHERIA. Although diphtheria was once common in the United States, its current rarity is due primarily to the fact that an estimated 96% of all children entering school have received three or more doses of DPT vaccine (CDC, July 12, 1985). Primarily because an immunized host is still capable of carrying *Corynebacterium diphtheriae* in the nasopharynx, there is always a ready reservoir and therefore a potential for outbreak among the unimmunized and the inadequately immunized.

Adequate immunization is thought to protect the individual from diphtheria for at least 10 years. The ages of hosts infected with diphtheria over the last few years suggest that many American adults are not protected. Thus it is currently recommended that adults receive a combination tetanus-diphtheria (Td) toxoid every ten years. Because Td contains much less diphtheria toxoid than other diphtheria

TABLE 17-7

Possible side effects and nursing responsibilities of recommended childhood immunizations

Immunization	Reaction	Nursing responsibilities
Diptheria	Fever usually within 24-48 hours; soreness, redness, and swelling at site of injection.	Instructions for DPT: Advise parents of possible side effects; may be recommended prophylactic use of aspirin or acetaminophen if fever occurred following previous DTP immunization; recommend its use if fever occurs following present immunization; advise parents to notify physician immediately of any unusual side effects, such as those listed under pertussis.
Tetanus	Same as for diphtheria but may include urticaria and malaise; all may have delayed onset and last several days; lump at injection site may last for weeks, even months but gradually disappears.	
Pertussis	Same as for tetanus but may include loss of consciousness, convulsions, and thrombocytopenia.	
Poliovirus (TOPV)	Essentially no side effects; vaccine-associated paralysis usually occurs within 2 months of immunization.	See general comment to parents.*
Measles	Anorexia, malaise, rash, and fever may occur 7 to 10 days after immunization; rarely (estimated risk 1 in 1 million doses) encephalitis may occur.	Advise parents of more common side effects and use of antipyretics for fever; if a persistent high fever with other obvious signs of illness occurs, have them notify physician immediately.
Mumps	Essentially no side effects other than a brief, mild fever.	See general comment to parents.*
Rubella	Mild rash that last 1 or 2 days within a few days after immunization; arthralgia, arthritis, and/or paresthesia of the hands and fingers may occur about 2 weeks after vaccination and is more frequent in older children and adults.	Advise parents of side effects, especially of time delay before joint swelling and pain; assure them that these symptoms will disappear may recommend use of mild analgesics for pain.

Modified from Whaley, L.F., and Wong, D.L.: Nursing care of infants and children, ed. 2, St. Louis, 1985, The C.V. Mosby Co.
*General comment to parents regarding each immunization: The benefit of being protected by the immunization is believed to greatly outweigh the risk from the disease.

combinations such as DPT, reaction to the diphtheria component is much less likely to occur.

PERTUSSIS. Even though the routine use of pertussis vaccine has resulted in a substantial reduction in the incidence of and mortality from pertussis, the number of cases has changed relatively little in the past 10 years. For those years, an average of 1835 cases and 10 fatalities have occurred (CDC, July 12, 1985). Moreover, several documented outbreaks in 1984 produced the largest annual total since 1974. Examination of these 2464 cases revealed that children under 6 months of age were at greatest risk of disease morbidity and mortality. Because most of those infants under 6 months of age had not received their third DPT booster, they were in effect inadequately immunized (CDC, July 5, 1985). Of interest is the fact that nearly half of the victims in one pertussis outbreak in 1985 were 7 years of age or older, but the disease was very mild and may have not been diagnosed at all under ordinary circumstances.

Pertussis is a good example of a disease that is usually underreported because many cases are not recognized or are inaccurately diagnosed. In fact, many microbiology laboratories do not possess the proper equipment or expertise in personnel to correctly identify *Bordetella pertussis.*

Because the incidence and severity of pertussis decreases with age, and because the vaccine may cause side effects and adverse reactions (see Table 17-7), routine pertussis

immunization is neither needed nor recommended for persons who are 7 years of age or older, except under unusual circumstances.

TETANUS. Tetanus occurs almost exclusively in unimmunized or inadequately immunized individuals. In 1983, 91 cases of tetanus were reported from 29 states, and in 1984, 74 cases were reported. The relationship between age of the host and subsequent mortality is illustrated by the fact that no deaths occurred in persons under 30 years of age, but 52% of persons over 60 years of age died of tetanus (CDC, October 4, 1985).

Because tetanus occurs most often and most lethally in adults, CDC has suggested that one method to ensure adequate protection is to routinely provide booster doses of Td at mid-decade years; that is, 15 years of age, 25 years, 35 years, etc. In fact, Td is the only universally recommended immunization for individuals of all ages.

SIDE EFFECTS AND ADVERSE REACTIONS FROM DPT IMMUNIZATION. Local reactions, generally erythema and induration with or without tenderness, are common after the administration of vaccines containing diphtheria, tetanus, or pertussis antigens. These reactions occur in approximately 40% to 70% of all DPT immunizations, are usually self-limited, and require no therapy. Mild systemic reactions such as fever, drowsiness, fretfulness, and anorexia occur quite frequently. Fever and other systemic symptoms are much less

TABLE 17-8

Contraindications to routine immunizations

Contraindication	Immunization	Rationale	Nursing considerations
Acute febrile illness or chronic debilitating diseases	All	Masks febrile reactions from the immunization, decreases body's natural defense mechanisms	Explain reason for postponing immunization to parent and reschedule it at earliest return visit For chronic diseases, check with physician before administering any immunization
Gastroenteritis	Live poliovirus vaccine	May interfere with colonization of the viruses in the intestines, which is essential for the immune response to occur	Explain reason for postponing immunization and reschedule it as soon as possible
Altered immune system Immunologic disease Generalized malignancy (leukemia, lymphoma) Immunosuppressive therapy (steroids, antimetabolitics, radiation)	All live viral vaccines (measles, mumps, rubella, and polio)	Depressed immune defenses may result in extreme reactions to the immunizations	Emphasize to parents the need to prevent their children from exposure to any of these childhood diseases, since they cannot be artificially protected from them
Recently acquired passive immunity Blood transfusion or immune serum globulin within last 6 weeks Maternal antibodies during first year	Measles, mumps, and rubella vaccines	Presence of passive immunity prevents formation of antibodies to the vaccine	Inquire during the history concerning recent blood transfusions or injections of immune serum globulin; wait recommended 6 weeks before administering the immunization; follow suggested schedule for measles, mumps, and rubella (15 months)
Allergy to substances in vaccine, for example, egg protein, neomycin	Live virus vaccines grown on chick embryos, treated with neomycin	Known hypersensitivity to substance will also result in reaction to substance in vaccine	Check manufacturer's product information for specific contraindications and screen child for known allergies to potential foreign substances
History of nervous system disorders Reaction of high fever, somnolence, or convulsions following a DTP immunization	Pertussis vaccine	Danger of serious reaction to pertussis vaccination is greatly increased	Take a detailed neurologic history, including past convulsions, fainting spells, tremors, or twitching and specific reactions to DTP; report any such findings to a physician before administering the pertussis vaccine
Pregnancy	All live virus vaccines except for poliovirus	Potential risk to fetus, especially from rubella	Take a careful history of all women of childbearing age regarding the possibility of pregnancy or conception within the next 2 months

From Whaley, L.F., and Wong, D.L.: Nursing care of infants and children, ed. 2, St. Louis, 1985, The C.V. Mosby Co.

common after administration of preparations that do not contain pertussis vaccine (CDC, July 12, 1985).

Because severe systemic reactions such as generalized urticaria or **anaphylaxis** have been reported, epinephrine should be accessible during the immunization process. The exact frequency of severe events following pertussis vaccination is unknown, but reported ranges for some of these adverse phenomena are shown as follows:

1. Collapse or shocklike state (60 to 300 per million doses).
2. Persistent screaming episodes—prolonged periods of peculiar crying or screaming that cannot be controlled by comforting the infant (70 to 2000 per million doses).
3. Isolated convulsions with or without fever (40 to 700 per million doses).
4. Encephalopathy, with or without convulsions and manifested by a bulging fontanel with changes in the level of consciousness or focal neurological signs; the encephalopathy may lead to permanent neurologic deficit (1.3 to 30.0 per million doses) (CDC, August 21, 1984).

It is important for community health nurses to be aware of these and subsequent findings so that they may intelligently counsel clients. Such findings sometimes cause generalized panic when presented to lay people in a biased fashion by the media. The community health nurse should encourage reporting of adverse reactions by parents and clients. Reports of severe or unusual reactions that seem to temporally correspond with immunization procedures should be forwarded to local or state health departments.

Tuberculosis Immunization and Testing Practices

In 1984, 22,255 cases of tuberculosis were reported to CDC. Compared with 1983, this was a 6.7% decrease in the number of cases reported. In 1984, as in previous years, individual cases of tuberculosis cases occurred in all 50 states. Persons living in cities with population of 250,000 or more had twice the national rate of cases than smaller cities (CDC, May 31, 1985).

When antituberculosis drugs were first introduced over 35 years ago, there was hope that the disease would soon be eliminated in the United States, even though over 100,000 new active cases and about 40,000 deaths from tuberculosis were reported annually. Given the current rate of decline, the elimination of tuberculosis appears unlikely in the next 100 years.

Control of tuberculosis has been hampered by a number of factors. One of the major problems involves noncompliance with prescribed therapy. Most clients require a minimum of 9 months treatment, including ongoing monitoring for drug toxicity and response to therapy. Some of these individuals are unwilling or unable to complete such a long course of therapy, and when they interrupt the drug regimen, they frequently become reinfected or symptomatic again.

A second obstacle to effective control of tuberculosis is the emergence of tuberculosis organisms that are resistant to antituberculosis drugs, especially isoniazid and streptomycin. And although this type of drug resistance was once limited to persons from Asia, Africa, and Central and South America, resistance to antituberculosis drugs has recently been documented in persons residing in Mississippi, Montana, New York, Massachusetts, and North Carolina (CDC, May 31, 1985). When resistance occurs, drugs and dosages have to be promptly manipulated to avoid exacerbation of disease and infectivity.

Further compounding the problem of tuberculosis control is the fact that an estimated 10 million persons in this country are infected with the tubercle bacilli and thus carry a lifelong risk of developing tuberculosis. Even if health departments could identify all the infected individuals in the country who are at high risk of developing disease and then provide them with preventive therapy, tuberculosis would still continue to occur in some infected individuals over the age of 35 in whom preventive therapy is not recommended because of the risk of isoniazid toxicity, which outweighs the benefit of therapy.

Regardless of the inherent problems in tuberculosis control, it is believed that it is possible to accelerate the decline in active cases by (1) full implementation of existing prevention and control methods, (2) development of new treatment, diagnostic, and prevention technologies, and (3) rapid implementation of these new technologies in all areas of the country as they are developed (CDC, May 31, 1985).

ADMINISTRATION OF TUBERCULIN SKIN TEST. Community health nurses need to be aware of several factors that influence tuberculin skin testing: (1) reactivity to tuberculin skin testing may be depressed or suppressed for up to 4 weeks by viral infection or live virus vaccines such as measles, polio, rubella, and mumps; (2) a reactive skin test indicates exposure to the causative agent for tuberculosis; (3) read all instructions carefully before skin testing and perform the test in the specified manner; (4) do not skin test a known tuberculin-positive reactor.

Measles (Rubeola), Mumps, and Rubella

MEASLES (RUBEOLA). The number of reported cases of measles in 1984 was 2534, which was a 69.3% increase over the 1497 cases reported in 1983. But even though reported cases of measles increased significantly, it must be remembered that the 1984 figure was still far lower than the 525,000 cases annually in the prevaccine era from 1950 through 1962 (CDC, May 31, 1985).

Of the 2543 cases of measles in 1984, 1184 (46.6%) had been vaccinated; 999 (33.3%) had been vaccinated on or after the first birthday; and 185 (7.3%) had been vaccinated before the first birthday. A total of 1359 (53.4%) of victims were either unvaccinated or of unknown vaccination status (CDC, May 31, 1985).

Because of the 5% to 15% susceptibility level among college students, the American College Health Association adopted a Preadmission Immunization Policy stating that by September 1985, all colleges should require students to present documentation of immunization to measles and other vaccine-preventable diseases as a requisite to graduation. However, many colleges have been reluctant to respond; thus the college-age individual remains a significant reservoir for measles infection and transmission.

Measles vaccine produces a mild or unapparent noncommunicable infection. A single subcutaneous dose of live measles vaccine provides durable protection against measles illness in approximately 95% of persons and extends probably for a lifetime. Combined measles, mumps, and rubella vaccine (MMR) is preferable for children and adults if recipients are likely to be susceptible to rubella or mumps as well as to measles. Although mild side effects do occur, vaccination with MMR in persons who were previously immune to one or more of the components is not associated with significant adverse effects (CDC, September 28, 1984).

MUMPS. The occurrence of reported mumps cases in the United States has decreased steadily since the introduction of live mumps virus vaccine in 1967. In 1984, 3021 cases were reported to CDC and that figure represented a 98% decline from the 185,691 cases reported in 1967 (CDC, September 28, 1984).

Although mumps is generally self-limiting, meningeal signs of severe headache, vomiting, pain, and neck stiffness may appear in up to 15% of cases, and orchitis, or inflammation of the testes, may occur in up to 20% of clinical cases among postpubertal men. Sterility is a rare sequelae of mumps orchitis among men. Another disability associated with mumps is deafness, which occurs in 1 of 15,000 cases of mumps.

Live mumps vaccine has been available in the United States since 1967. A single dose of live mumps vaccine administered subcutaneously provides long-lasting levels of antibody in over 90% of recipients. As with measles vaccine, MMR is the vaccine of choice as opposed to a single mumps vaccine. The vaccine should be given at least 14 days before or deferred for at least 6 weeks, and preferably 3 months, after a person has received immune globulin (IG), whole blood, or other blood products containing antibodies. Further, the vaccine should not be given to persons who are immunocompromised or who have generalized malignancies. Serologic surveys have indicated that most individuals have been infected with mumps by the twentieth birthday and most adults can be considered immune, even if they did not have clinically recognizable mumps disease. However, persons who received killed mumps vaccine that was available from 1950 until 1978 might benefit from vaccination with the now-available live mumps vaccine (CDC, September 28, 1984).

RUBELLA. Although the incidence of rubella continues to decrease, 745 cases were reported in 1984 in the United States. Several accounts of rubella outbreaks have involved young adults in universities, among hospital employees, and in office workers. These outbreaks not only led to disruption in the workplace and time lost through illness but also provided potential infection in women of childbearing age who may have been pregnant. Despite efforts to date, several studies have shown that the rubella susceptibility rate for adolescents and young adults continues to be 10% to 20%. Because of that 10% to 20% susceptibility level, congenital rubella syndrome (CRS) continues to be reported at low endemic levels in the U.S. (CDC, July 26, 1985).

A nationwide initiative to hasten the elimination of rubella has recently begun. As with measles elimination, efforts are aimed at (1) achieving and maintaining a 95% immunization level in susceptible persons, (2) intensifying surveillance of rubella and CRS, and (3) promptly controlling outbreak. Specific activities will focus on further increases in the delivery of vaccine to women of childbearing age and enhancement of the lay and medical communities' awareness of the current problem. Considering the economic impact of CRS and other outcomes of rubella infection during pregnancy, any effort that can hasten the elimination of rubella should be undertaken (CDC, February 8, 1985).

As a part of the initiative to eliminate rubella and to reduce the number of susceptible young adults, it is further recommended that nonpregnant susceptible women of childbearing age should be provided with rubella vaccine (1) during routine internal medicine and gynecologic outpatient care, (2) during routine care in a family planning clinic, (3) following premarital screening, (4) before discharge from a hospital for any reason, and (5) after childbirth or abortion. In essence, any contact with the healthcare system should be used as an opportunity to vaccinate susceptible women (CDC, September 28, 1984).

Because of the theoretical risk to the fetus, reasonable precautions should be taken before women of childbearing age are immunized with MMR vaccine. These precautions include (1) asking the woman if she is pregnant, (2) excluding those who say they are, and (3) explaining the possible risks of the vaccine and counselling them not to become pregnant for 3 months after vaccination. If a pregnant woman is vaccinated or if a woman becomes pregnant within 3 months after vaccination, she should be counseled about risks to the fetus. Instances of vaccination of known susceptible women who are pregnant or become pregnant within 3 months should be reported through state health departments to the Division of Immunization, Centers for Disease Control (CDC).

Rubella vaccine contains trace amounts of neomycin, to which patients may be allergic. Persons with a history of anaphylactic reaction following receipt of neomycin should not receive rubella vaccine.

Haemophilus Influenzae

Haemophilus influenzae is a leading cause of serious systemic bacterial disease in the United States, and approximately 1 in 1000 persons under the age of 5 will develop a systemic disease caused by the organism each year without immunization. *Haemophilus influenzae* is the most common cause of bacterial meningitis and is credited with causing 12,000 cases a year among children 5 years of age or younger. Meningitis caused by *H. influenzae* has a case fatality rate of 5%, and neurologic sequelae are observed in approximately 25% to 35% of survivors. Although type B accounts for only 1 of 6 known species, it causes virtually all cases of *H. influenzae* meningitis among children. Type B (Hib) is also responsible for other invasive diseases, including epiglottis, sepsis, cellulitis, septic arthritis, osteomyelitis, pericarditis, pneumonia, and occasionally otitis media (CDC, April 19, 1985).

Approximately 35% to 45% of associated disease occurs among children 24 months of age or older. Children who are at high risk for *H. influenzae* include native Americans (Indians) and Eskimos, blacks, persons from low socioeconomic backgrounds, persons with asplenia, sickle cell disease, Hodgkin's disease, or antibody deficiency syndromes, and those under 5 years of age who attend day care centers (CDC, April 19, 1985).

Currently, it is recommended that Hib vaccine be administered to all children at 24 months of age. It is thought that immunization at 24 months will protect the child from 18 to 40 months, and no additional vaccination is recommended. It is also recommended that children in high riskgroups be immunized at 18 months. These clients should receive a second dose of Hib vaccine within 18 months of the initial dose to ensure protection. At present, there is insufficient data on which to base recommendations for vaccination of children older than 2 years and adults who have never been immunized.

Immunization Under Special Circumstances
Pneumococcal Polysaccharide Vaccine

Precise data on the occurrence of pneumococcal disease in the United States is not available, partly because it is not a nationally notifiable disease. However, the annual incidence of pneumococcal pneumonia is estimated to be 68 to 260 cases per 100,000 population. The incidence of pneumococcal pneumonia, which causes a number of deaths annually, increases in those over 40 years of age and shows a twofold increase in those over 60 years of age. Mortality from pneumococcal disease is highest among clients who develop bacteremia or meningitis, persons with underlying medical conditions, and elderly persons (CDC, September 28, 1984).

Persons at increased risk for developing severe pneumococcal disease include those with sickle cell anemia, multiple myeloma, cirrhosis, alcoholism, renal disease, splenic dysfunction, diabetes mellitus, chronic pulmonary disease, or conditions associated with immunosuppression.

Licensed in 1978, the pneumococcal polysaccharide vaccine currently available provides protection against the various types of *Streptococcus pneumoniae* that is responsible for 87% of recent bacteremic pneumococcal disease in the United States. Most healthy adults who receive the vaccine demonstrate rises in titer that indicate immunity.

About half of the persons given the vaccine experience mild side effects, but severe adverse effects such as anaphylactic reactions have rarely been reported. Although it is unknown how long vaccine-induced immunity lasts, booster doses are not recommended because of increased adverse reactions associated with second doses of the vaccine (CDC, September 28, 1984).

Community health nurses often administer the vaccine to high-risk or elderly clients. Pneumococcal vaccine should be given subcutaneously, and the client or parent should be informed that mild side effects such as low-grade fever, mild erythema, and induration at the injection site may be experienced from about 4 hours after inoculation up to 4 days afterward. Typically, mild reactions subside within 24 hours.

Meningococcal Vaccines

N. meningitis causes both endemic and epidemic disease and is the second most common cause of bacterial meningitis in the U.S. Bacterial meningitis affects between 3000 and 4000 persons each year.

The case fatality rate associated with meningococcal meningitis is 10% and rises to 20% for meningococcemia despite therapy with antimicrobial agents such as penicillin.

As noted in Table 17-6, the incidence of meningococcal disease peaks in the late winter to early spring. Incidence is highest among children, particularly those age 6-12 months; after 1 year of age incidence steadily declines. By age 5, the incidence among children approximates that for adults. Serogroup B, for which a vaccine is not yet available, accounts for 50% to 55% of all cases. Even though serogroup A causes only a small portion of endemic meningitis disease in the United States, it is the most common cause of meningitis epidemics elsewhere in the world (CDC, May 10, 1985).

The recently licensed quadrivalent A, C, Y, W-135 is the formulation currently available in the United States. The serogroup A polysaccharide has been shown to induce antibody in some children as young as 3 months of age,

although a response comparable to that seen in adults is not achieved until 4 or 5 years of age. Antibodies formed after a single dose of vaccine decline markedly over the first 3 years after a single dose of vaccine, although the antibody decline is more rapid in infants and young children than in adults.

Routine vaccination of civilians is not recommended because the risk of infection in the United States is low, and because the serotype B that causes most cases of meningococcal infection in the United States cannot be combated with the present vaccine. However, routine immunization with the quadrivalent vaccine is recommended for particular high-risk groups, including individuals with terminal complement component deficiencies and those with anatomic or functional asplenia. When indicated, the vaccine can be given at the same time as other immunizations. Subsequent antibody titers are achieved within 10-14 days after vaccination (CDC, May 10, 1985).

Antimicrobial chemoprophylaxis of persons in intimate contact with individuals having meningococcal disease remains the chief preventive measure in sporadic cases of *N. meningitidis* disease in the United States. Examples of "intimate contact" include household members, daycare center contacts, and anyone directly exposed to the patient's oral secretions, such as through mouth-to-mouth resuscitation or kissing.

Hepatitis B Virus Vaccine (HBV Vaccine)

CDC estimated that hepatitis B virus (HBV) infections occurred in at least 200,000 Americans each year before hepatitis B vaccine was available. Further, it was estimated that at least 4000 persons would die of chronic effects of HBV such as cirrhosis, acute hepatitis, and liver cancer each year. Treatment costs for those 200,000 annual cases was estimated at $365 million (Dowdle, 1983).

HBV vaccine was licensed in 1981, and in 1984, a total of 26,115 cases were reported to CDC (CDC, September 27, 1985). The majority of cases occurred in individuals 20 years of age or older, and between 6-10% of these adults became chronic carriers of the disease. CDC estimates that the United States has between 400,000 and 800,000 carriers of hepatitis B. The estimated risk of acquiring HBV infection in the U.S. is approximately 5% for the population as a whole but may reach 100% for the highest risk groups (CDC, September 28, 1984).

Persons may be at increased risk of HBV by virtue of occupational, social, family, environmental, or illness-related reasons. For instance, health care workers are considered at high risk because of their potential exposure to blood and body fluids. Groups at increased risk of contracting the HBV are: (1) immigrants/refugees and their descendants from areas where there is a high endemic rate for HBV, (2) actively homosexual men, (3) users of illicit injectable drugs,* (4) inmates of prisons (who may have a history of prior parenteral drug abuse), (5) patients and staff in custodial institutions for the mentally retarded, (6) class-

---

*Users of illegal injectable drugs are at risk because usually the needles are dirty and are shared by several drug users.

room contacts, teachers of some deinstitutionalized carriers, (7) household contacts and sexual partners of HBV carriers, (8) hemodialysis clients, (9) health care workers who have contact with blood, (10) inmates of long-term care or correctional facilities, and (11) international travelers (CDC, June 7, 1985).

To administer HBV vaccine, a series of three 1.0 ml doses containing 20 units/ml of HBs Ag protein should be given intramuscularly in the deltoid muscle. Completion of the series of three such injections provides protective antibodies in over 90% of healthy adult recipients for at least 2 years. A course of three doses at 10 units/ml induce antibody formation in virtually all infants and children aged day of birth to 9 years of age. The first two doses should be given 1 month apart, and the third dose, 5 months after the second. For susceptible hemodialysis clients, three 2 ml doses should be given at the above stated schedule (CDC, June 7, 1985).

HBV vaccine is recommended for most individuals who are members of high risk groups. Because some areas of the world, such as eastern Asia and sub-Saharan Africa, have high endemic rates of HBV, travelers who plan to have close contact with the local population should complete the series of 3 immunizations before leaving the United States. HBV vaccine is primarily intended for pre-exposure prophylaxis; however, when exposure to HBV occurs in a high-risk person with no pre-exposure immunization, the vaccine may be administered in combination with hepatitis B immune globulin (HBIG). When HBV vaccine and HBIG are given in combination, they provide sustained protection levels of antibody and obviate the need for a second dose of HBIG, although the series of HBV vaccine should be completed (CDC, September 28, 1984).

Unlike live-virus vaccines such as rubella, pregnancy is not a contraindication for use of HBV for persons otherwise eligible (CDC, June 7, 1985). In fact, one of the most efficient modes of HBV transmission is from the mother to infant during birth. Because HBV in a pregnant woman may result in severe disease for the mother and chronic infection or even fulminant hepatitis in the neonate, all pregnant women should be serotested for the presence of hepatitis antibodies.

Influenza Vaccine

Influenza viruses have repeatedly demonstrated the ability to cause major and excess morbidity and mortality. Fifteen times in the years 1957-1984, epidemics of influenza have been associated with 10,000 or more excess deaths annually. In the 1984-1985 flu season, influenza type A viruses were isolated in every state in the United States, and these viruses were associated with the highest ratio of pneumonia and influenza deaths (as a percentage of total deaths) since 1976 (CDC, July 19, 1985).

The greatest impact of influenza normally occurs when new strains appear against which most of the population lacks immunity. In those circumstances, (e.g., 1957, 1968), pandemics occur. Only influenza type A, which is generally more severe than either types B or C, is capable of causing pandemics.

The two groups most often and most severely affected are chronically ill persons and persons over 65 years of age. Because these two groups are increasing in size, the toll of influenza may increase further unless control measures are used more vigorously than in the past.

Several groups of persons have been identified that would benefit from annual influenza vaccination. These groups are (1) adults and children with chronic disorders of the cardiovascular or pulmonary systems that are severe enough to have required regular medical checkups or hospitalization during the preceding year; (2) residents of nursing homes and other chronic-care facilities; (3) physicians, nurses, and other personnel who have extensive contact with high-risk clients; (4) otherwise healthy individuals 65 years of age and older; and (5) adults and children with chronic metabolic diseases, renal dysfunction, anemia, immunosuppression, or asthma severe enough to require regular medical follow-up or hospitalization during the preceding year. Influenza immunization is also recommended for otherwise healthy children and adults who wish to reduce their chances of acquiring influenza infection.

When target or risk groups overlap for influenza and pneumococcal vaccination, both may be given simultaneously at separate anatomical sites. In contrast to influenza vaccine, which should be administered annually, pneumococcal vaccine should be given only once.

The occurrence of influenza, like some other communicable diseases, is temporal, occurring from October to February and declining in March. The vaccine should be administered from mid-October through December since, if given earlier, protection may be waning when there is still widespread influenza activity. Influenza vaccine may be given to pregnant women after the first trimester. In fact, it is thought that immunization during the third trimester when it occurs from October to December of any given year may provide antenatal protection to the mother and the fetus (CDC, October 18, 1985).

It is necessary to obtain an adequate history before immunizing for influenza because persons who are allergic to eggs or those with acute febrile illness should not be immunized. As with any vaccine, clients should be advised of possible reactions. Reactions to influenza vaccines may be either local or systemic. Approximately one-third of those immunized will develop local redness or induration at the injection site. Systemic reactions have been of two types. The first type consists of fever, malaise, and myalgia. Although these reactions are infrequent, they do tend to occur most often in children and those who have had no exposure to the particular viral antigen. The second type of systemic reaction is immediate and anaphylactic in nature. Anaphylaxis occurs very rarely and is presumably attributed to egg allergy. Of interest is the fact that unlike the 1976 swine flu vaccine, subsequent vaccines have not been associated with an increased frequency of Guillian-Barré Syndrome.

Amantadine is an antiviral agent that works by interfering with the uncoating step in the viral replication cycle. It also acts to reduce viral shedding and therefore helps prevent person-to-person transmission of diseases such as influenza. Unlike the influenza vaccine, amantadine does

TABLE 17-9

Vaccines and toxoids indicated or specifically contraindicated for special health status situations

Health situations	Indicated	Vaccines or toxoids contraindicated
Pregnancy	Diphtheria and tetanus toxoids (TD)	Live virus vaccines
Immunocompromised	Influenza Pneumococcal polysaccharide	Live virus vaccines
Splenic dysfunction, anatomic asplenia	Influenza Pneumococcal polysaccharide	
Hemodialysis	Hepatitis B (double dose) Influenza Pneumococcal polysaccharide	
Deficiencies of factors VIII or IX	Hepatitis B	
Chronic alcoholism	Pneumococcal polysaccharide	
Diabetes and other high-risk diseases	Influenza Pneumococcal polysaccharide	

NOTE: Refer to text on specific vaccines or toxoids for details on indications, contraindications, precautions, dosages, side effects and adverse reactions, and special considerations.

not prevent actual infection, but it does reduce the duration of fever and other systemic symptoms. Amantadine is in no way a replacement for vaccination, but it is useful to supplement the protection afforded by the vaccine. It is also used in individuals with impaired immune responses, who may have a poor antibody response to the vaccine, and in those who are unable to take the vaccine (CDC, October 18, 1985).

Immunobiologics Recommended for Special Occupations, Lifestyles, Environmental Circumstances, Foreign Students, and Refugees

Persons in certain occupations or who practice certain lifestyles may be at increased risk of exposure to vaccine-preventable illness. Specific recommendations for these persons may be found in Table 17-9 and Table 17-10.

Passive Immunization for Hepatitis A and B

Although hepatitis A is not associated with high mortality, it does cause significant morbidity. Hepatitis A, unlike hepatitis B, is primarily transmitted by person-to-person contact. Also unlike hepatitis B, no carrier state is associated with hepatitis A. Transmission is facilitated by poor personal hygiene, poor sanitation, and household or sexual contact. Common-source epidemics from contaminated food and water also occur. Hepatitis A has occurred at an endemic level for the past 15 years in the United States; in 1984, 22,040 cases were reported.

The passive immunization for both hepatitis A and B can both utilize *immune globulin (IG)*. IG is essentially a sterile solution of antibodies from human plasma that contain anti-HAV (hepatitis A virus) and anti-HBV antibodies. The only difference between IG and HBIG is that HBIG contains higher titers of antibodies to hepatitis B (CDC, June 7, 1985).

IG should be given as soon as possible after exposure to HAV because it is much more effective when given very early in the incubation period. The index case (see Chapter 8) in any outbreak should be serologically tested for infection by HAV before that person receives IG. However, serologic testing of contacts for anti-HAV before giving IG is not recommended after the index case is established because the screening tests are more costly than IG and delay administration. Giving IG more than 2 weeks after exposure is not recommended. Specific recommendations for prophylaxis of HAV depend on the nature of the HAV exposure. Those recommendations are listed in Appendix D and are adopted from recommendations by CDC (CDC, June 7, 1985).

TRENDS IN INFECTIONS AND COMMUNICABLE DISEASE

The following discussion explores the role and impact of selected communicable diseases on contemporary society. In some instances these phenomena are relatively new and therefore less understood than more familiar communicable diseases. In other instances the communicable phenomena discussed have relevance for community health nursing practice and warrant exploration.

Drug Resistance

Microorganisms, like all living things, occasionally undergo genetic mutations as a result of alterations in the enzyme production of mutant cells. For example, when mutation occurs in a cell of a given species of microorganism that is multiplying in a host being treated with penicillin, the subsequent change occasionally alters a few cells in such a way that they are no longer susceptible to the action of penicillin. These microorganisms are then said to be antibiotic resistant, or drug fast. A similar resistance pattern may develop in any number of microorganisms in response to chemotherapeutic drugs. The resistant cells grow and ultimately replace sensitive cells.

In the preceding description, resistance occurred osten-

TABLE 17-10

Immunobiologics recommended for specific life situations

Indication	Immunobiologic(s)
Occupation	
Hospital, laboratory, and other health care personnel	Hepatitis B Polio Influenza
Staff of institutions for the mentally retarded	Hepatitis B
Veterinarians and animal handlers	Rabies
Selected field workers	Plaque
Lifestyles	
Homosexual males	Hepatitis B
Illicit drug users	Hepatitis B
Environmental situation	
Inmates of long-term correctional facilities	Hepatitis B
Residents of institutions for the mentally retarded	Hepatitis B
Travel	Measles Rubella Polio Yellow Fever Hepatitis B Rabies Meningococcal polysaccharide Typhoid Cholera Plague Immune globulin
Foreign students, immigrants and refugees	Measles Rubella Diphtheria Tetanus

NOTE: Refer to text on specific vaccines or toxoids for use by specific risk groups, details on indications, contraindications, precautions, dosages, side effects and adverse reactions, and special considerations.

sibly in a person taking a therapeutic dose of penicillin, but that is usually not the case. The situation that is most often credited for the phenomenon of resistant organisms is overuse or abuse of antibiotics. This abuse by physicians includes prescribing excessive doses, prescribing antibiotics prophylactically in preoperative or postoperative situations or in the presence of presumed viral infections, and prescribing antibiotics without the aid of culture and sensitivity reports. Other examples of real or potential antibiotic use include the practice of adding various antibiotics to cow, pig, and poultry feed and over-the-counter sale of antibiotics in countries such as Mexico.

Antibiotic resistance has been of great concern to infection control practitioners in episodic settings for over two decades, but resistance patterns are increasingly affecting a broader range of microbiological agents, including com-municable diseases. Some of the best known and most notorious drug-resistant communicable diseases are tuberculosis and gonorrhea.

Staphylococcus aureus and pneumococci organisms are also frequently penicillin resistant; instances of full drug resistant pneumococci were reported in 1985 (CDC, September 6, 1985). In recent years, reports of infections with methicillin-resistant staphylococcus organisms have increased. When methicillin, a member of the penicillin family, was first developed, all strains of staphylococcus were believed to be sensitive to this antibiotic. Although that is no longer true, most of these methicillin-resistant strains seem to be occurring at large hospitals affiliated with medical schools. If such infections are truly more common in these institutions, it may be because they usually include burn and trauma units, which provide a source of periodic reintroduction of the organisms. For this reason, CDC recommends that people who are known to be colonized or infected with this particular strain of staphylococcus not be transferred to other medical facilities whenever possible or be discharged home for treatment. At this point, the potential risk of spread to healthy family contacts is not known but is probably very small.

In 1984, there was a documented outbreak of drug-resistant salmonella in four Midwestern states that was ultimately traced to consumption of meat from animals who were fed antimicrobial agents. Until that 1984 outbreak, it had been difficult to document the relationship between mixing antimicrobials into animal food and clinically important infections in humans. But the study done as a result of the outbreak of salmonella demonstrated empirically that antimicrobial-resistant organisms of animal origin cause serious human illness. Such findings emphasize the need for more prudent use of antibiotics in both human beings and animals (Holmberg, et al., 1984).

It is difficult to accurately predict where resistance patterns will end or what the full ramifications of drug-resistant strains are for the future. Some predictions are frightening, but at present it seems that research and development of new treatment alternatives stay just a little ahead of the microorganism's amazing ability to form resistance patterns.

Unfortunately, in many countries of the world, antibiotics may be obtained without a prescription, and this is believed to account for the high rate of chloramphenicol resistance in populations of such countries. It would be helpful if worldwide agreement could be reached on the principles of antibiotic use. For instance, antibiotics important for treating human infections should be excluded from animal feeds. In fact, all antibiotics should be excluded from animal feed in the United States, as they are in Great Britain. Also, no disease should be treated with antibiotics unless positively indicated by clinical and laboratory data. Even topical gentamicin should be avoided if possible because pathogens such as *Pseudomonas aeruginosa* may acquire resistance in its presence. In essence, every animal or person taking an antibiotic (therapeutically or subtherapeutically) becomes a factory producing resistant strains of microorganisms (Levy, 1984).

Sexually Transmissible Diseases

According to the CDC (1980), the term *venereal disease* is now inadequate because it is too limited; hence the term *sexually transmissible diseases (STD)* is now used. The scope of STD includes the following estimates worldwide:

Chlamydial infections—3 to 4 million cases annually

Gonorrhea—2.5 million cases annually

Nongonococcal urethritis (NGU, caused by organisms such as chlamydia and mycoplasm)—2.5 million cases annually

Genital herpes—500,000 cases annually

Syphilis—80,000 new cases annually

AIDS—15,000 to 30,000 cases annually

Three sexually transmitted diseases, including AIDS, are discussed in more detail because they are comparatively new and have wide-ranging public health effects.

Chlamydia Infections

Infections caused by *chlamydia trachomatis* are now the most frequent occurring of all STDs. Men, women, and infants are affected, but women bear an inordinate burden because of their increased risk for adverse reproductive consequences. Although *C. trachomatis* infection is currently not a reportable disease on the national level in the United States, data obtained from metropolitan STD clinics suggest sharp increases in incidence during the period 1975-1985 (CDC, August 23, 1985).

Most *C. trachomatis* infections among women are asymptomatic, but account for one quarter to one half of the 1 million recognized cases of pelvic inflammatory disease in the United States each year. Maternal infection during pregnancy has been associated with postpartum endometritis and with increased maternal mortality. Infants with infected mothers can acquire chlamydial infection at birth from exposure to cervicovaginal secretions. The more than 500,000 infants born to chlamydia-infected mothers each year are at high risk of developing inclusion conjunctivitis, pneumonia, otitis media, and bronchiolitis. In fact, chlamydia is the most common cause of neonatal eye infections and of afebrile interstitial pneumonia in infants less than 6 months of age (CDC, August 23, 1985).

Several risk factors for chlamydial infections have been identified. For instance, sexually active women less than 20 years of age have chlamydial infection rates 2 to 3 times higher than those for women over 20 years of age. Similarly, the rates of urethral infection among teenage boys are higher than those for men over 20 years of age. Risk of chlamydial infection, like the risk for virtually all STDs, increases with the number of sex partners. Although homosexual men are at high risk for STD, they have one-third the rate of urethral chlamydial infection of heterosexual men. However, 4% to 8% of homosexual men seen in STD clinics have rectal chlamydial infection. Chlamydial infection also sometimes accompanies infection with other STDs.

All persons sexually exposed to *C. trachomatis* infection should be examined for other STDs and treated promptly. The effective management of chlamydial infection includes counseling of patients; such counseling should be designed to influence specific behavior that will contribute to successful therapy, disease intervention, and prevention. For instance, pamphlets designed for easy comprehension are one way of conveying basic information. These messages should be reinforced by community health nurses through discussions with patients that are tailored to provide an opportunity for questions. Patients must clearly understand that they must continue to take medication according to schedule, despite abatement of symptoms, and it should be suggested that the individual abstain from sexual activity until medication is completed. Both sexual partners are treated in most cases. If this is not possible, clients should be encouraged to use condoms until treatment is completed (CDC, August 23, 1985).

Genital Herpes Infection

Data compiled by the CDC support the notion that an epidemic of genital herpes infection occurred in the United States from 1966 to 1979 and that the disease continues to occur in epidemic proportions. The number of consultations with physicians for genital herpes infection increased from a reported 29,560 visits in 1966 to 260,890 in 1979. In contrast, the same survey showed less than a twofold increase in the rate of consultation for oral herpes infection (CDC, March 26, 1982).

The increased incidence of genital herpes infection is particularly noteworthy for community health nurses for several reasons: (1) there is an association between genital herpes infection and development of cervical cancer; (2) infections acquired during passage through the birth canal are often life-threatening to the newborn; and (3) although a relatively new drug, acyclovir, is available for treatment of *initial* genital herpes infection, there is no specific treatment for *recurrent* or chronic genital herpes. These recurrences are common and are physically painful and emotionally distressing.

According to CDC, social, demographic, and behavioral changes within the U.S. population during the past decade have placed an increased proportion of people at risk for STDs such as genital herpes (March 26, 1982). However, because of the AIDS phenomenon, surveillance in cities such as San Francisco show that other STDs have declined in incidence. For example, in San Francisco the incidence of gonorrhea has decreased 50% since 1986. Presumably, the gonorrhea incidence is down because both homosexual and heterosexual persons are practicing "safe sex." Guidelines for safe sex are designed to reduce the incidence of all sexually transmissible diseases and may be found in Appendix A. The most important role for the community health nurse in relation to bringing STDs under control continues to be public education aimed at prevention when feasible, and early diagnosis and treatment when disease does occur.

Acquired Immune Deficiency Syndrome

In the United States, Acquired Immune Deficiency Syndrome (AIDS) has predominantly affected users of intravenous drugs and the homosexual community. However, through the efforts of the WHO it is known that AIDS occurs worldwide and that the epidemiology of AIDS in some countries differs from that seen in the United States.

For instance, although 79% of AIDS cases have occurred among homosexual or bisexual men in the United States, AIDS is primarily transmitted heterosexually in Central Africa (CDC, November 8, 1985).* The widely publicized morbidity and mortality associated with the disease have forced the health care community to operate under the glare of media attention and public scrutiny. Every American knows at least a little about the disease, and thousands of families have been forced to deal with the consequences of this deadly disease. Aside from actual cases of AIDS and AIDS Related Syndrome (ARS), an estimated *2-3 million* persons in the United States are believed to be infected with the causative virus. It is unknown how many of these individuals will become symptomatic in the coming months or years.

Persons identified at high risk of being infected with human T-lymphocytic virus type III (HIV), the virus that is believed to cause AIDS, include homosexual men, intravenous (IV) drug users, persons transfused with contaminated blood or blood products, heterosexual contacts of persons with HIV infection, and children born to infected mothers. HIV has been isolated from blood, semen, saliva, tears, breast milk, and urine and is likely to be isolated from some other body fluids, secretions, and excretions, but epidemiological evidence has implicated only blood and semen as significant in terms of transmission (CDC, November 15, 1985).

Numerous studies of nonsexual household contact of AIDS patients have shown that casual contact with saliva and tears does not result in transmission or infection. It is also important to note that the kind of nonsexual contact that generally occurs among workers and clients or consumers in the workplace does not pose a risk for transmission of AIDS. Because AIDS is not transmitted through preparation or serving of food and beverages, CDC has recommended that persons with AIDS not be restricted from the work environment unless they have another infection or illness for which such restriction *would* be warranted (CDC, November 15, 1985).

The AIDS phenomenon has raised many unique questions regarding client confidentiality, civil liberties, ethics, and liability. For instance, in 1985, a serology test called the *enzyme-linked immunosorbant assay (ELISA)* was made available in the United States. In essence, a positive ELISA (or a series of two positive ELISAs) could be interpreted to mean that the individual in question had been infected with HIV/LAV. Even though the ELISA was originally developed primarily as a mechanism to protect the nation's supply of blood and blood products from contamination with the AIDS virus, guidelines stated that it could also be used to screen individuals for AIDS under specific medical circumstances. The United States Public Health Service guidelines

that accompanied distribution of the ELISA stated that this was not a diagnostic tool and that the ELISA should not be used as a condition for employment, as a determinant of insurability, or as a criterion to determine fitness for military service. Ethical and legal parameters were not specifically delineated, but confidentiality of test results was urged.

At this point in our understanding of the disease process and its impact on clients and their families and significant others, community health nurses play vital roles in prevention, control, and informed care of persons with AIDS. Until an effective vaccine is developed or other effective treatment is introduced, the only means available to stop the transmission of AIDS is education. We must educate everyone about the hazards of intravenous drug use and the advantages of practicing safe sex when sexual relationships are not mutually monogamous. Additionally, it is likely that a greater number of people will endorse and practice sexual abstinence in reaction to the AIDS phenomenon.

Moreover, community health nurses need to understand that infection control practices relative to AIDS are quite similar to those used for control of HBV. The rationale for both is simple: "Because the hepatitis B virus is also blood-borne and is both hardier and more infectious than HIV/LAV, recommendations that would prevent transmission of hepatitis B also will prevent transmission of AIDS" (CDC, November 15, 1985). Both lay and professional people need to be educated as to how to take reasonable precautions without subjecting clients with AIDS to human and environmental isolation. Guidelines for home care of clients with AIDS are listed in Appendix I. Health care personnel in institutional settings should use infection control guidelines published by CDC.

It has always been important for community health nurses to possess indepth knowledge of community resources, but a disease such as AIDS that affects not only individuals but also their families and friends seems to underscore the importance for such knowledge. When clients with AIDS are homosexual, it may be helpful to refer them to one of the numerous gay outreach groups that offer services such as workshops and support groups for persons with AIDS and their families or significant others.

The treatment of the topic of AIDS in this text is necessarily brief. The reader is urged to consult pertinent literature such as the *MMWR* and other periodic literature because the body of knowledge germane to AIDS is growing rapidly.

Other Diseases of Special Concern
Pediculosis

Pediculosis, or lice infestation, occurs worldwide, and outbreaks are common among school-children and other groups. *Pediculosis* refers to infestations of the head or hairy parts of the body or clothing with adult lice, larvae, or nits (eggs), leading to severe itching and excoriation of the scalp or scratch marks on the body.

From a public health standpoint, the louse is not only a human nuisance but also transmits epidemic typhus, trench fever, and louse-borne relapsing fever (Benenson,

---

*For the first time ever all developed countries, including the Union of Soviet Socialist Republics and Yugoslavia, have joined together under the umbrella of the WHO to form a framework for international cooperation relative to AIDS research. This Collaborating Centre of AIDS exists to provide training, provision of reference regents, evaluation methods, and epidemiological surveillance of AIDS.

1980). The mode of transmission is direct contact with an infected person and indirect contact with the personal belongings of an infected person, especially clothing and headgear. Pediculosis is communicable as long as lice remain alive on the infected person, and until eggs in the hair and clothing have been destroyed. Diagnosis of pediculosis is accomplished by finding either lice or nits on hairy surfaces of the body.

Pediculosis is treated with lindane (Kwell). Kwell comes as a lotion and a shampoo and contains lindane 1% as its active ingredient. The client should be instructed to apply a sufficient quantity to cover only the affected and adjacent hairy areas. The lotion should be rubbed into the scalp and hair and left in place for 12 hours, after which a shower should be taken.

For head lice, the shampoo is used. The client should be instructed to use enough to thoroughly wet the hair and skin of the affected area and adjacent hairy areas. When the hair and skin are thoroughly wet with shampoo, small quantities of water should be added, with the shampoo worked into the hair and skin until a good lather forms. Shampooing should be continued for 4 minutes, and then the hair should be rinsed thoroughly. When the hair is dry, any remaining nits or nit shells (debris) may be removed with a fine-toothed comb. One application is usually curative. Some people do suffer persistent pruritus after treatment; however retreatment should not be instituted unless living mites are seen. Measures that can be instituted to prevent spread, aside from specific treatment, include (1) avoiding physical contact with infected persons or their belongings or clothing and (2) educating the public on the value of laundering clothing and bedding in hot water (55° C or 131° F for 20 minutes) or dry cleaning to destroy nits and lice.

Botulism

Fortunately, the incidence of adult *botulism* in the United States is quite low, because when it occurs, it causes severe morbidity and sometimes mortality. Although botulism outbreaks are most commonly associated with consumption of improperly prepared home-canned foods, it is important to know that *Clostridium botulinum* can also contaminate fresh foods. Not only can fresh foods, especially those harvested from the ground, contain *C. botulinum;* when these foods are initially cooked and then held at ambient temperatures for 14 to 16 hours, toxin from the spores is released just as it is in improperly prepared home canning.

Three different botulism outbreaks in 1985 involved foods that are not usually associated with botulism because they did not involve canning or preserving. For instance, one outbreak involved turkey loaf made from fresh ingredients and then stored in a gas oven with the pilot light on overnight. Another outbreak involved consumption of a beef stew made from fresh ingredients and then left overnight at room temperature. Outbreaks prior to 1985 reportedly involved commercial pot pies, sauteed onions, and in one instance, a baked potato (CDC, March 22, 1985).

Two key factors affect community health nursing practice concerning botulism. First, clients should be taught that fresh foods can be a source for botulism poisoning, and therefore foods initially heated for serving should either be eaten hot or refrigerated and later reheated thoroughly (since the botulism toxin is heat labile). Second, when botulism poisoning is suspected, requests for stool and serum for botulinial toxin, and for trivalent botulism antitoxin, can be obtained through state health departments.

Salmonellosis (Salmonella gastroenteritis)

Salmonellosis is a disease that is usually accompanied by nausea, abdominal pain, abdominal cramping, and diarrhea. It is thought that *salmonellosis* is greatly underreported, so the 20,000 to 30,000 cases reported each year probably represent only 1% to 10% of those that actually occur. The overall mortality is very low, probably less than 1%, although the death rate is much higher in infants and among elderly persons (Tortora, Funke, and Case, 1982).

The normal habitat for *salmonella* organisms is the intestinal tract of humans and some animals. Prevention of salmonellosis depends on good sanitation practices to avoid initial contamination or inoculation of food with the organism. Another practice that prevents outbreaks is refrigeration of foods that may be mildly inoculated with organisms to prevent further growth. Salmonellosis is a good example of the concept of dosage discussed earlier in the chapter because the severity and incubation time of the disease depend on the number of *salmonella* organisms ingested.

Poultry, eggs, and egg products have been implicated in salmonellosis outbreaks. The organisms are generally destroyed by normal cooking that heats food to an internal temperature of about 68° C (145° F). However, foods can become contaminated and mishandled after cooking (Tortora, Funke, and Case, 1982).

Several unusual outbreaks of salmonellosis were reported in 1985. One of those involved the largest number of culture-confirmed cases ever associated with a single outbreak of salmonellosis in the United States. This outbreak occurred in early spring and involved residents of Indiana, Michigan, Illinois, and Iowa. *S. typhimurium* was isolated from unopened lots of milk produced by the same dairy plant. The dairy plant subsequently stopped producing milk, but by then 5770 cases had been reported (CDC, April 19, 1985). Salmonella is sometimes found in dairy cattle and raw milk but pasteurization kills the organism. Because the implicated milk had been pasteurized, it was either inadequately pasteurized or contaminated after pasteurization. This outbreak serves as an alarming reminder of how quick to develop and far-ranging communicable diseases can be in this era of mass production and rapid transit.

Legionellosis

Legionnaire's disease (later called LD, or *legionellosis*) is caused by *Legionella pneumophila,* a newly recognized gram-negative bacillus. Contrary to popular belief, the outbreak that occurred in Philadelphia at the fiftieth annual convention of the American Legion in 1976 was not the first recorded outbreak. The bacillus was isolated as early as 1947, and the first well-documented outbreak of the disease occurred in 1957 (Edelstein and Meyer, 1984). However, legionellosis was recognized as a distinct clinical entity in 1976 during the outbreak involving American Legionnaires.

Much more is now known about legionellosis, its distribution, and clinical presentations. For instance, a nonpneumonic form of disease associated with *L. pneumophila* (Pontiac fever) has been described, and at least nine other species of the bacillus have been discovered or rediscovered.

Environmental risk factors associated with legionellosis include contaminated potable water and water fixtures and contaminated heat-exchange apparatuses in large buildings. Host risk factors associated with legionellosis include advanced age, underlying chronic cardiopulmonary disease, chronic renal failure, or diabetes mellitus. In addition, legionellosis is more common in men, in those who smoke, and in those who are immunosuppressed from either primary disease or medication(s) that affect cellular immunity. Person-to-person transmission does not occur; instead the disease is transmitted airborne from the environment (Edelstein and Meyer, 1984).

In 1984, 750 cases of legionellosis were reported to CDC, but one must remember that legionellosis is probably greatly underreported (CDC, September 27, 1985). The occurrence of legionellosis is generally categorized as either community or nosocomially acquired. Whenever clusters of legionellosis appear, investigations should be undertaken to locate the reservoir and then modify the environment in question to eliminate that reservoir. In some instances, different institutions have had to stop taking immunocompromised clients until the environmental reservoir for *L. pneumophila* was located and modified to prevent further serosoling the organism. The overall case fatality rate is affected by drug therapy and the client's underlying disease, with death rates up to 80% in the immunosuppressed patients not treated; overall, the case fatality rate is about 15% to 20% (Edelstein and Meyer, 1985).

Literature to date estimates the incidence of legionellosis seen in nonhospital settings to range between 1% and 15% of all community acquired pneumonias. Community health nurses should be aware that the sputum of clients with legionellosis is usually nonpurulent and watery, but it may be grossly bloody. Thick green or yellow sputum is almost never observed with legionellosis. If a sputum specimen is obtained for gram stain only, it is unlikely *L. pneumophila* can be identified. To diagnose legionellosis, it is necessary to submit a sputum specimen for *L. pneumophila* identification by direct immunofluorescent examination. In some instances in which laboratories have the capability, urine specimens may be collected and tested for soluble antigens. Besides sputum and urine testing, blood can be drawn for serologic examination (Edelstein and Meyer, 1984).

The importance of specifically identifying pneumonias caused by *L. pneumophila* is that effective treatment with erythromycin or a similar drug can be started. Additionally, the client treated at home should be observed for signs of respiratory failure or hypotension that are common in legionellosis. If the client is receiving immunosuppressive agents, including corticosteroids, they should be stopped or the dosage reduced whenever possible.

Delta Hepatitis

A new form of hepatitis, delta hepatitis, has been detected in all areas of the United States and is thought to affect 200 million persons worldwide. Delta hepatitis results from a virus that cannot cause infection by itself; however, when it "piggy backs" with the virus that causes HBV, the result is an illness more severe than that caused by HBV alone (Altman, August 28, 1984).

Although it is known that the virus that causes delta hepatitis may be transmitted by blood transfusion or parenteral drug use, other mechanisms of spread are unclear at this time. Many cases probably go undiagnosed because there is presently no diagnostic test available. Experts agree that delta hepatitis may be avoided in large part by widespread use of HBV vaccine, which has been available since 1981. However, there is no mechanism available to protect persons who have already been infected with HBV from the delta virus.

Delta hepatitis is another example of an old disease that has only recently been detected. But discovery of the delta virus has provided health professionals with a new perspective on a condition usually called chronic active hepatitis since it now appears that some of these relapses are caused by infections with the delta agent (Altman, 1984).

CLINICAL APPLICATION

The majority of communicable disease occur in children, who are usually cared for at home. For this reason community health nurses need to teach parents and daycare workers proper care of infected children. Although the discussion is geared toward infants and children, many of the general principles, such as those related to adequate hydration and general comfort measures, are readily applicable to the adolescent and adult.

Adequate management of the individual suffering from a communicable disease can result in earlier treatment of untoward effects such as high fever, sepsis, or pulmonary infiltration. Generally it is helpful to advise the parents of the expected course of the illness, including possible high fevers. If parents are aware of usual symptoms, when unexpected signs such as unconsciousness or seizure occur, they will be more likely to seek immediate medical attention. It is helpful to go over various treatment settings that are available to the parent for emergency treatment before the need arises.

The incubation period is of particular concern to parents who have other children at home or who have not had the disease or have children in day care because they wonder when their children might develop disease. Frequently it is necessary to counsel parents about preventive measures, particularly when their own children have been exposed to children who subsequently become ill. Most communicable diseases are transmissible before the onset of rash or other definitive symptoms. The boxed material on pp. 332 and 333 and Tables 17-7 to 17-9 assist in making decisions about when to advise immunization and when to defer such intervention. Helpful too is a personal or office copy of a standard reference on communicable diseases, such as the *Report of the Committee on Infectious Diseases* (frequently called simply *The Red Book*), which is updated every 4 years by the American Academy of Pediatrics.

When antibiotics are prescribed, the community health nurse should emphasize the importance of taking the recommended dosage for the entire time prescribed, regardless of signs of improvement. Taking antibiotics any less than the amount prescribed not only may result in a recurrence of infection but also may cause recurrence by an organism that has become resistant to the original antibiotic. Antibiotics prescribed for one member of the family should never be saved and then administered to another family member or friend, no matter how similar the symptoms. Antibiotics should be purchased in amounts sufficient to complete a prescribed regimen of treatment and the remainder disposed of safely. Though nurses may understand this concept quite well, lay people tend to save unused medications for any number of reasons, including their cost.

Some general tips to share with parents include the following. First, fever can usually be relieved by antipyretics, liberal fluids, and tepid water baths. The choice of antipyretics should be left up to family preference, assuming no allergies exist. The child should be dressed lightly and kept well-sheltered from the elements while febrile. Second, itching associated with chickenpox and measles can be relieved by oral antihistamines (if the physician does not object), which can be purchased over the counter. The pharmacist can advise as to appropriate dosage when the drug is purchased. The parent should be told that antihistamines may cause drowsiness. Baths with 2 to 4 tablespoons of bicarbonate of soda also may be helpful in relieving itching. Third, although a cough may be controlled with an over-the-counter cough supressant, parents should be warned about the potential for "double dosing" children with a cough mixture containing antipyretics and antihistamines.

Adequate hydration and nutrition during the acute and convalescent periods are essential. Often the patient has mouth or throat lesions in addition to a generally poor appetite. Some of the more acidic fruit juices may be poorly tolerated for this reason. The parent should be encouraged to offer small feedings at frequent intervals rather than two or three large meals a day. Also, the parent needs to be alerted to the dehydration effects of diarrhea that may accompany influenza syndromes.

As children begin to feel better there is a tendency to become too active. Bedrest is important throughout the acute and convalescent stages but may be mixed with other quiet activities consistent with the child's developmental level and tolerance. The child suffering from a communicable disease should not be isolated from family contact any more than is absolutely necessary.

SUMMARY

Although communicable diseases are no longer the most frequent cause of morbidity and mortality, they still represent a major health problem. The nature and sometimes the name of communicable processes change over time, but they nonetheless retain a sinister ability to weaken, disable, and kill.

A good deal of irony surrounds our relationship with the microorganism. Any student of microbiology understands our reliance on this basic life form. At the same time, clinical microbiologists and infectious disease experts struggle to retain some margin of control over these rudimentary organisms.

The effort to monitor and control communicable disease phenomena is worldwide. However, the effectiveness of larger surveillance systems depends on astute individuals on the local level who must find cases and implement preventive, control, and maintenance strategies. Because of the practice arena involved, the community health nurse occupies a position of responsibility for all these functions. There are few other instances in which the opportunity to contribute in an intradisciplinary fashion for the common good is so operative.

≡ KEY CONCEPTS

The vast majority of persons who succumb to communicable or contagious diseases contract them in the community and are cared for at home throughout minor illnesses or periods when the disease process can be managed on an outpatient basis.

Some infectious diseases, such as smallpox, have been completely eliminated throughout the world, and most traditional communicable diseases can be therapeutically managed so that often death can be prevented.

The types and causes of communicable diseases are not static, but are constantly being changed and updated by new knowledge.

Community health nurses must be knowledgeable about communicable diseases so they can effectively counsel parents, family, or friends about the care of potentially exposed or frankly infected persons.

Communicable disease plays a tremendous role in the economic viability of both specific communities and the nation.

Failure to enforce the recommended schedule for communicable disease control or a break in community sanitation or water purification can result in an epidemic at any given time.

Infectivity is the ability of the organism to spread rapidly from one host to another.

Invasiveness refers to the agent's ability to spread within the host.

Virulence is the ability to produce severe disease.

In general, most disease processes produce the greatest morbidity and mortality in the very young and the very old in any given population, but there are some important exceptions.

Some factors of the host's ability to ward off infection are interdependent with environmental factors such as humidity, temperature, and crowding. Other environmental factors that influence the incidence of communicable diseases are atmospheric conditions, availability of nutrients, and contamination of food and water supplies.

According to the U.S. Centers for Disease Control, social, demographic, and behavioral changes within the U.S. population during the past decade have placed an increased proportion of people at risk for sexually transmissible diseases.

LEARNING ACTIVITIES

1. Write a paper covering the stage of susceptibility of the Natural History Model on a communicable and/or infectious disease (student's choice, subject to faculty approval). Host, agent, environment factors should be clearly delineated, and nursing strategies relative to primary prevention should be included.

2. Ascertain the mechanism for reporting various types of infectious and /or communicable diseases in the county.

3. Instructors may plan a clinical rotation for students in local sexually transmitted disease (STD) clinics. Local and state statistics on STD should be compared with the national incidence.

4. Survey health and/or nursing personel in local schools to ascertain when the last outbreak of pediculosis occurred in the community.

BIBLIOGRAPHY

Altman, L.K.: Mysterious form of hepatitis seen as widespread threat, the *New York Times,* August 28, 1984, pp. 19, 22.

American Adademy of Pediatrics: Report of the committee on infectious diseases, ed. 20, Evanston, Ill., 1986, The Academy.

Benenson, A.S., editor: Control of communicable diseases in man, ed. 13, Washington, D.C., 1980, American Public Health Association.

Beveridge, W.I.: Influenza: the last great plague, New York, 1978, Prodist Publishers.

Brown, M.S.: What you should know about communicable diseases and their immunizations: a guide for nurses in ambulatory settings, Nursing 9(5):72, 1975.

Centers for Disease Control: Annual summary, MMWR, Atlanta, 1984.

Centers for Disease Control: Diphtheria, tetanus, and pertussis: guidelines for vaccine prophylaxis and other preventive measures, MMWR, Atlanta, Aug. 21, 1984, pp. 392-407.

Centers for Disease Control: Meticillin-resistant *Staphylococcus aureus*—United States, MMWR, Atlanta, March 26, 1982, pp. 557-559.

Centers for Disease Control: Genital herpes infections—United States, 1966-1979, MMWR, Atlanta, March 26, 1982, pp. 137-138.

Centers for Disease Control: Adult immunization: recommendations of the Immunization Practices Advisory Committee (ACIP), MMWR (supplement), Atlanta, Sept. 28, 1984, pp. 125-145.

Centers for Disease Control: Elimination of rubella and congenital rubella syndrome—United States, MMWR, Atlanta, Feb. 8, 1985, pp. 65-66.

Centers for Disease Control: Botulism from fresh food—California, MMWR, Atlanta, March 22, 1985, pp. 156-157.

Centers for Disease Control: Update: Milkborne salmonellosis—Illinois, MMWR, Atlanta, April 19, 1985, pp. 215-216.

Centers for Disease Control: Vaccine for prevention of *Haemophilus influenzae,* MMWR, Atlanta, April 19, 1985, pp. 201-205.

Centers for Disease Control: Meingococcal vaccines, MMWR, Atlanta, May 10, 1985, pp. 255-259.

Centers for Disease Control: Measles—United States, 1984, MMWR, Atlanta, May 31, 1985, pp. 308-312.

Centers for Disease Control: Tuberculosis—United States, 1984, MMWR, Atlanta, May 31, 1985, pp. 293-308.

Centers for Disease Control: Recommendations for protection against viral hepatitis, MMWR, Atlanta, June 7, 1985, pp. 315-335.

Centers for Disease Control: Petussis—Washington, 1984, MMWR, Atlanta, July 5, 1985, pp. 341-342.

Centers for Disease Control: Diphtheria, tetanus, and pertussis: Guidelines for vaccine prophylaxis and other preventive measures, MMWR, Atlanta, July 12, 1985, pp. 405-426.

Centers for Disease Control: Drug-resistant tuberculosis among the homeless—Boston, MMWR, Atlanta, July 19, 1985, pp. 429-431.

Centers for Disease Control: Influenza—United States, 1984-1985 seasons, MMWR, Atlanta, July 19, 1985, pp. 440-443.

Centers for Disease Control: Measles on college campuses—United States, 1985, MMWR, Atlanta, July 26, 1985, pp. 445-449.

Centers for Disease Control: *Chlamydia trachomatis* infections: Policy guidelines for prevention and control, MMWR (supplement), Atlanta, August 23, 1985, pp. 535-745.

Centers for Disease Control: Isolation of multiply antibiotic-resistant pneumococci—New York, MMWR, Atlanta, Sept. 6, 1985, pp. 545-546.

Centers for Disease Control: Tetracycline-resistant *Neisseria gonorrhoeae*—Georgia, Pennsylvania, New Hampshire, MMWR, Atlanta, Sept. 20, 1985, pp. 563-570.

Centers for Disease Control: Final 1984 reports of notifiable disease, MMWR, Atlanta, Sept. 27, 1985, pp. 590-595.

Centers for Disease Control: Tetanus—United States, 1982-1984, MMWR, Atlanta, Oct. 4, 1985, pp. 602-611.

Centers for Disease Control: Prevention and control of influenza, MMWR, Atlanta, Oct. 18, 1985, pp. 633-649.

Centers for Disease Control: Acquired immunodeficiency syndrome: Meeting of the WHO collaborating centers on AIDS, MMWR, Atlanta, Nov. 8, 1985, pp. 678-680.

Centers for Disease Control: Recommendations for preventing transmission of infection with HTLV-III/LAV in the workplace, MMWR, Atlanta, Nov. 15, 1985, pp. 682-694.

Dowdle, W.R.: Surveillance and control of infectious diseases: Progress toward the 1990 objectives, Pub. Health Rep. 98(3):210-217, 1983.

Edelstein, P.H., and Meyer, R.D.: Legionnaires' diseases: a review, Chest 85(11):114-120, 1984.

Hare, R.: Pomp and pestilence, New York, 1955, Philsosophical Library, Inc.

Healthy people: the Surgeon General's report on health promotion and disease prevention, DHEW Pub. No. (PHS) 79-55071, Washington, D.C., 1979, U.S. Department of Health, Education and Welfare.

Holmberg, S.D., Osterholm, M.T., Senger, K.A., and Cohen, M.S.: Drug-resistant salmonella from animals fed anitmicrobials, N. Engl. J. Med. 311(10):617, 1984.

Levy, S.B.: Playing—antibiotic pool: time to tally the score, N. Engl. J. Med. 311(10):663-664, 1984.

Physician's desk reference, ed. 35, Oradell, N.J., 1981, Medical Economics Books.

Ramsay, A.M., and Emond, R.T.: Infectious diseases, London, 1979, William Heinemann Medical Books, Ltd.

Tortora, G.J., Funke, B.R., and Case, C.L.: Microbiology: an introduction, Menlo Park, Calif., 1982, The Benjamin/Cummings Publishing Co., Inc.

Turner, J.G., and Pryor, E.R.: The AIDS epidemic: risk containment for home health care providers, Fam. Commun. Health, 8(3):25-36, Nov. 1985.

Volberding, P., and Abrams, D.: Clinical care and research in AIDS, *Hastings Center Report,* pp. 16-18, August 1985.

Whaley, L.F., and Wong, D.L.: Nursing care of infants and children, ed. 2, St. Louis, 1985, The C.V. Mosby Co.

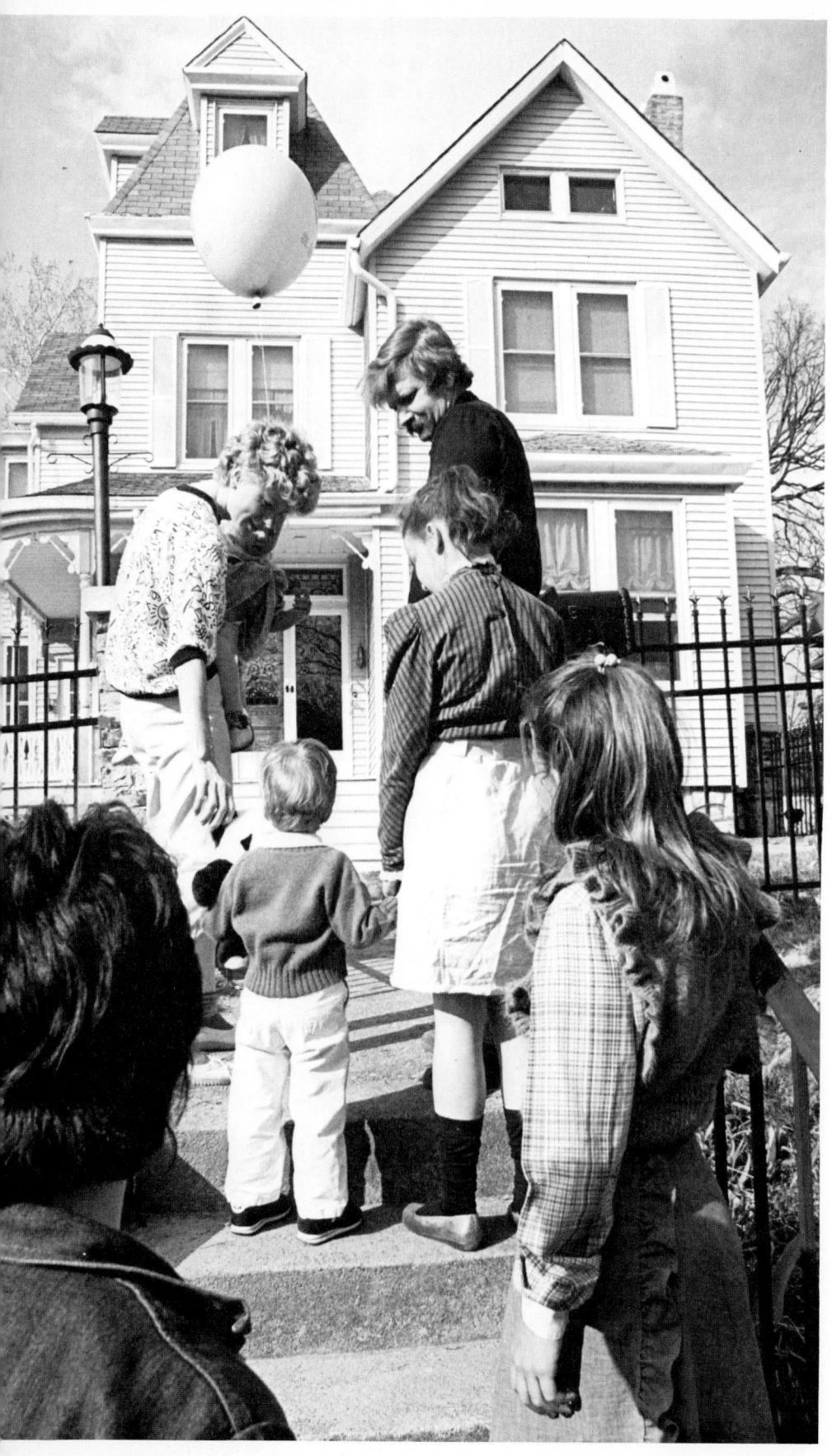

THE INDIVIDUAL AND FAMILY AS CLIENT: A DEVELOPMENTAL APPROACH

The family is a major influence on the individual's concept of health and illness. It influences the action taken by or for the person with a health problem. The environmental, social, and economic factors, as well as the resources of the community to meet health needs, influence the family's health risks and reactions to health.

The community health nurse has the opportunity to influence the actions and reactions to health of all individuals of the community from birth through senescence. The community health nurse may influence the health of the neonate and infant by introducing healthy parenting behaviors, risk factor appraisal, and interventions at this stage of life. Likewise the community health and/or school health nurse is in a position to introduce illness prevention and health promotion activities to the school-age and adolescent populations. Appropriate influences during these developmental stages have the potential for changing the future outlook for the nation's health.

Young and middle-aged adults are faced with many life changes and challenges that they may find rewarding or demanding. Previous life-styles and increases in stress from social, environmental, and economic constraints often result in risk for major health problems during this life stage.

The community health nurse's primary function with persons of all ages should be to promote quality, as well as quantity, of life. As the elderly population continues to increase (grow), the health care delivery system and nursing must address and plan strategies to cope with increasing longevity, chronic health problems, and technological advances, as well as twentieth century economic, social, and health issues.

Major health problems of individuals can be identified and related to their developmental phase. This factor becomes evident when age-specific morbidity data are reviewed. Chapters 18 through 20 explore family theories, the nursing process applied to family health and to the health of individuals in the family system, and family health promotion issues. Chapters 21 through 26 explore the major developmental tasks, health needs, risk factors, and issues for individuals from birth through senescence.

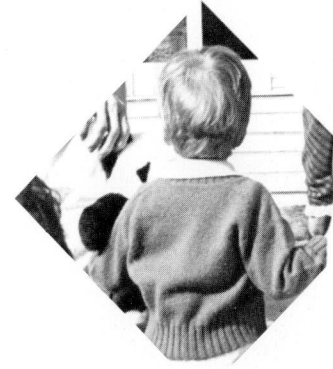

Rosemary Johnson

18

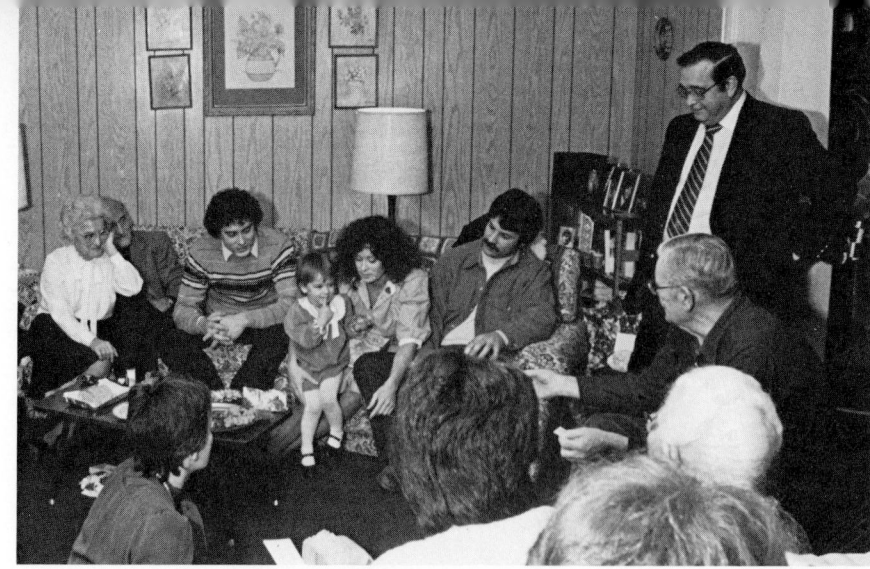

FAMILY DEVELOPMENTAL THEORIES

OBJECTIVES

After reading this chapter, the student should be able to:

Analyze various approaches to defining the family.

Discuss the various types of family structures.

Identify trends in marriage and the family that have implications for family focused community health nursing practice.

Identify and discuss family adult roles.

Identify and discuss the functions performed within the sibling interactional system.

Identify and discuss functions common to most families.

Identify and discuss family health functions and tasks.

Analyze the developmental conceptual approach to studying families.

Discuss the application of the developmental framework to community health nursing practice with single parent, remarried, and vulnerable families.

KEY TERMS

age pattern

demographic trends

developmental approach

ethnicity

family developmental task

family functions

family roles

family structure

Mills' model for stepfamily development

nontraditional family

nuclear family

plurality patterns

Rodgers' developmental framework

remarried family (stepfamily)

role position

role sequence

sex pattern

sibling relationship

single parent families

spacing pattern

traditional family

One theoretical framework used to study families is that of family development. This approach emphasizes how families change over time and focuses on interactions and relationships among family members. This chapter examines issues relevant to family development and discusses the developmental conceptual framework from a general perspective and in relation to variations in family structures. Other concepts related to the developmental framework are discussed, such as family structures, roles, and functions.

The reader is encouraged to draw from the many chapters in the text that have direct application to the study of the family. Especially relevant are the chapters focusing on family health (Chapters 19 and 20) and the chapters emphasizing individual developmental stages (Chapters 21 through 25).

DEFINING THE FAMILY

Definitions of the family abound in the literature and frequently are expressed in relation to the discipline represented by the definer. For example, a biological approach may view the family as a unit with the biological function of perpetuating the species. A psychological approach emphasizes the family as a basic unit for personality development and the development of subgroup relationships, such as the parent-child relationship. The discipline of economics focuses on the family from the perspective of standard of living, socioeconomic status, economic conditions of the society, and consumer behavior and motivation (Rice, 1966). Various definitions of the family include aspects of different disciplines.

In the past, the family was defined in relation to the *nuclear family* (mother, father, and young children) in which the original parents remained together throughout the family life cycle. The nuclear family, as a continuing unit with original parents, is no longer as predominant. Today, the family as an intact social unit is more transient. This transient nature has resulted in changes in family structure, membership, goals, and, in some instances, the family's reason for being.

A consequence of family changes and the emergence of variant family forms is the increased difficulty associated with defining the family. The importance of defining the family is that the way one defines the family determines to some extent how one describes the family's function and role in society. Several definitions of the family are:

1. Two or more individuals who reside in the same household, who can identify some common emotional bond, and who are interrelated by performing some social tasks in common, for example, socialization of children (Baranowski and Nader, 1985)
2. A special human group held together by meaningful emotional bonds, rather than as a purely legal, economic, biological, or genetically circumscribed entity (Leavitt, 1982)
3. Two or more persons comprising a group in which the persons (a) are related by blood, marriage, adoption, or mutual consent; (b) interact with each other through designated or assumed familial status, positions, and roles; (c) create and maintain a common subculture (Stevenson, 1977)
4. A semiclosed system of actors occupying interrelated positions, defined by the society of which the family system is a part, as unique to that system with respect to the role content of the positions and to ideas of kinship relatedness (Rodgers, 1973)
5. A group of two or more persons related by blood, marriage, or adoption and residing together (U.S. Bureau of Census, 1975)

The author defines the family as two or more individuals, coming from the same or different kinship groups, who are involved in a continuous living arrangement, usually residing in the same household, experiencing common emotional bonds, and sharing certain obligations toward each other and toward others. This definition is applicable to both *traditional* and *nontraditional family* structures and addresses the phenomenon of commuter marriages.

Definitions of the family range from viewing the family as one structure exclusively to perceiving the family as a household unit representing various types of family structures. A broad definition of the family is needed in community health nursing because community health nurses work with families that represent both traditional and nontraditional structures.

FAMILY STRUCTURES

The family, society's most significant unit of social behavior, has experienced considerable changes that have affected the family's development in relation to structure, functions, and interactions, both within the family and in the community. Recent trends affecting marriage and the family are becoming well established, whereas others are more tenuous.

Traditional and Nontraditional Families

The social significance of the family has been founded in its mediating function within the larger society by which it "links" the individual family member to societal structures. This linking process serves society's needs through motivating individuals' participation in the production and distribution of food; protection of the young, old, and sick; and socialization of the young (Goode, 1964; Leslie, 1973). Although all family units do not fit the definition of the *traditional family* (i.e., nuclear family), each family, regardless of its structure, has the potential for serving societal needs in one way or another. In addition, families tend to be similar in relation to needs such as affectional interchange; reasonable stability; financial resources for food, clothing, and shelter; educational opportunities; and the availability and accessibility of health services.

Families with which the community health nurse works represent a variety of structures and living arrangements. The community health nurse is responsible for assisting the family to promote its health, to meet family health needs, and to cope with health problems within the context of the existing family structure and life-style. Thus community health nurses must be knowledgeable about family structures, functions, processes, and roles; in addition, they must be aware of and understand their own values and attitudes pertaining to the family and varying family life-styles.

Family structure (configuration) refers to the characteristics (gender, age, number) of the individual members who comprise the family unit. There are increasing variations in family structures, and an individual may participate in a number of different family structures over a lifetime.

One attempt at developing a typology of family structures is reflected in the works of Sussman and Cogswell. Sussman (1971) initially developed a classification of traditional family structures, as outlined in the box above.

Cogswell and Sussman's examination (1972) of the increasing variations of the traditional family resulted in the further development of a typology that included experiments with traditional marriages, experimental family forms, and experimental marriages (unions). This typology focuses on the positions or roles present in each family type and identifies the most salient and predominant patterns of relationships and activities. A taxonomy of experimental families and marriages is found in the box on the facing page.

The group marriage families are considered to be "experimental" families, since procreation and childrearing are involved. The procreation of children and their socialization may be involved in some of the experimental marriages (unions), but for the most part the alliances focus on adult members' needs for identity, intimacy, and interaction (Cogswell and Sussman, 1972).

Macklin (1980) proposed including the binuclear family

TRADITIONAL FAMILIES

1. Nuclear family—husband, wife, and offspring living in a common household
   a. Single career (husband only working)
   b. Dual career
      1. Wife's career continuous
      2. Wife's career interrupted
2. Nuclear dyad—husband and wife alone: childless, or no children living at home
   a. Single career
   b. Dual career
      1. Wife's career continuous
      2. Wife's career interrupted
3. Single parent family—one head, as a consequence of divorce, abandonment, or separation (with financial aid rarely coming from the second parent) and usually including preschool and/or school-age children
   a. Career
   b. Noncareer
4. Single adult living alone
5. Three generation family—may characterize any variant of family forms 1, 2, or 3 living in a common household
6. Middle aged or elderly couple—husband as provider, wife at home (children have been "launched" into college, career, or marriage)
7. Kin network—nuclear households or unmarried members living in close geographical proximity and operating within a reciprocal system of exchange of goods and services
8. "Second career" family—the wife enters the work force when the children are in school or have left the parental home

Reprinted from Sussman, M.B.: Family systems in the 1970's: analysis, policies and programs, vol. 396, The annals of The American Academy of Political and Social Science." Copyright © 1971 by The American Academy of Political and Social Science.

(joint child custody and coparenting) and reconstituted, blended, family (stepfamily) among the alternative family structures. Also included in Macklin's proposal were alternative family relationship options for the elderly: (1) a quasi-family structure of nonrelated aged persons sharing a communal arrangement that involved a common household and divided expenses, (2) an "affiliated" family relationship in which the older nonkin member was integrated into a younger family unit, and (3) nonresidential affiliations through which the relationships between the older kin member and other extended family members could be maintained.

Community health nurses should continue to develop their knowledge and understanding of different family structures. This knowledge will assist the nurse to intervene more effectively with each family on an individual basis to promote and protect the family's health.

Trends in Marriage and the Family

Historians have reported that by the end of the 1700s numerous demographic and economic factors had altered social

EXPERIMENTAL FORMS OF FAMILIES AND MARRIAGES

GROUP MARRIAGE FAMILIES

Form A: Common residence or compound of households
  1. Composed usually of three or more monogamous couples
  2. Practice sexual exclusivity
  3. Members have ready access to one another for social interactions
  4. Share resources, common facilities, and socialization of children
  5. Some communes take this form
Form B: Similar to form A
Sexual swapping within group is practiced
Form C: Mixture of formerly married couples and singles
  1. May be composed of all singles
  2. With or without sexual swapping
Form D: Multilateral marriage similar to form B
  1. Usually involving fewer than six members
  2. Most frequently two-family monogamous couples
  3. Sometimes only three persons

EXPERIMENTAL "MARRIAGES"

Form A: Nonrelated adults sharing a common household
  1. Involving a division of labor
  2. With or without sexual accessibility
Form B: Heterosexual cohabitation where there is a de facto marriage with recourse to legal requirements
Form C: Homosexual unions involving same sex pairings in a single household
  1. Sharing roles, intimacies, experiences, and resources
  2. In some instances more than two members may form a colony or commune
Form D: Affiliated family usually involving unrelated members of different generations
  1. For example, aged woman and a single parent and offspring
  2. A division of labor appropriate to needs and capabilities of participants

Adapted from Cogswell, B.E., and Sussman, M.B.: Fam. Coord. 21:506-507, 1972. Copyrighted 1972 by the National Council on Family Relations. Reprinted by permission.

relationships within the American family, as well as in society. Demographic factors reflecting structural changes in the family were people living longer, families having fewer children, and the age range between siblings being narrower. As the economic system of industrial capitalism became established during the nineteenth century, new social roles and opportunities for social mobility developed. As a consequence of these changes, the family changed from a self-sufficient, functional unit consisting of kin and nonkin members to a smaller child-centered nuclear unit (Hiestand, 1982). Demographic and socioeconomic changes have continued with increased rapidity throughout the twentieth century, resulting in further changes in the family structure.

Demographic Trends

Demographic trends affecting the family's structure and development are related to age at the time of first marriage; fertility patterns and birth rates; increases in the number of individuals engaging in singlehood, divorce, and remarriage; increases in the number of dependent children experiencing divorce in the family or living with a never married parent; and an increase in the number of elderly.

CHANGING PATTERNS OF MARRIAGE. Presently, over 90% of Americans marry, but it is predicted that by the year 2000 this percentage may drop to 85%. The national marriage rate fell 0.3% between 1984 and 1985 from 10.5 to 10.2 per 1000 population. The 1985 marriage rate is the lowest since 1977 (NCHS, 1986c); as a result of the weakening of religious, social, and legal norms, greater sexual freedom may promote the continued growth of cohabitation, single person households, unwed single parent families, and homosexual couples. The traditional nuclear family (husband as wage-earner, wife as homemaker, and two or more dependent children) will continue, but its role will diminish.

Presently, this type of family structure accounts for less than 10% of all households, mainly because of the increased number of women in the labor force (Family Service of America, 1984).

In 1981, 60.3 million of the 82.4 million households in the United States were comprised of families (Table 18-1). Between 1970 and 1981, there was an increase in single parent families headed by both men and women, but the greater increase was for women. Nonfamily households maintained by men increased by over half a million households, but nonfamily households maintained by women more than doubled. The number of unmarried couples, defined as two unrelated adults of the opposite sex sharing a household with or without the presence of children under 14 years of age, doubled also (Population Reference Bureau, 1982).

In 1979 the median age at time of marriage was 22.1 years for women and 24.1 years for men. Fifty percent of the women aged 20 to 24 years were still single, and twenty percent of the women aged 25 to 29 were single. Black women comprised the largest number in each age group. By 1982, 58% of females 20 to 24 had never married. It is predicted that in the future 12% of all females may never marry (Population Reference Bureau, 1982).

DIVORCE. National divorce statistics include absolute divorces, annulments, and dissolutions of marriages (NCHS, 1986a). In 1982, the rate of divorce dropped for the first time in 20 years (Table 18-2). The rate continued to decline until 1985, at which time it started to increase. During 1984, divorcing couples, on the average, were married for 9.5 years. The largest percentage (33.6%) of divorces granted was to couples married 1 to 4 years. The pattern for divorces in relation to duration of marriage depicted a gradual decline each year after the fourth year of marriage (NCHS, 1986a).

TABLE 18-1

Households in the United States
in 1970 and 1981

	1970 (millions)	1981 (millions)
Families (TOTAL)		60.3
Female headed	5.5	9.1
Male headed	1.2	1.9
Unmarried couples	.52	1.35
Nonfamily households		
Female maintained	7.9	12.8
Male maintained	4.1	9.3

Adapted from Population Reference Bureau: Where we are and where we're going, Pop. Bull., 37, Washington, D.C., 1982, Population Reference Bureau, Inc.

TABLE 18-2

Divorces in the United States
1981 through 1985

Year	Rate*	Number†
1981	5.3:100	
1982	5.1:1000	
1983	4.9:1000	1,158,00
1984	4.9:1000	1,155,000
1985	5:1000	1,187,000

*Per total population.
†Couples divorced.
Adapted from National Center for Health Statistics: Advance report of final divorce statistics, 1984, Mo. Vital Stat. Rep., 35, 1986, U.S. Department of Health and Human Services National Center for Health Statistics: Annual summary of births, marriages, divorces, and deaths: United States, 1985, Mo. Vital Stat. Rep., 34, 1986, U.S. Department of Health and Human Services.

The divorce rate for women in 1984 was 21.5 per 1000 married women, and the average age was 33.6 years, up from 32.4 years in 1980. The 1984 divorce rate for men was about the same as that for women, and the average age for divorcing men was 36.2 years, as compared with 35.1 years in 1980. The highest rate of divorce for women was for those 15 to 19 years of age—45.5 divorces per 1000 married women. Divorce rates fell steadily for each successive age group. Women aged 35 to 39 years were only half as likely to divorce as their teenage counterparts, and women aged 45 to 49 years were only one quarter as likely to divorce. Men aged 15 to 19 years experienced a rate of 42.9 divorces per 1000 married men. The rate for men aged 20 to 24 years was 48.2 divorces per 1000 married men. The rates for men declined steadily with age thereafter. The percentage of divorces in which the husband had married as a teenager decreased from 19.5% in 1974 to 14.9% in 1984. By comparison, the percentage of divorces for women who had married as teenagers fell from 43.8% in 1974 to 34% in 1984 (NCHS, 1986a).

REMARRIAGE. About 75% of divorced people remarry; one of seven divorced persons remarries during the first year after divorce. Four of ten men and slightly fewer divorced women remarry within 3 years. Eventually five of every six divorced men and three of four divorced women remarry; approximately 25% of divorced persons never remarry (NCHS, 1986a).

CHILDREN OF DIVORCE. In 1984, 1,081,000 children under the age of 18 years were affected by divorce. The number of children involved in divorce per 1000 children under 18 years of age increased from 6.3 in 1950 to 18.7 in 1981. In 1984 the rate fell to 17.2 per 1000 children under 18. The average number of children per divorce decree granted has been falling since 1964, from 1.36 to 0.92 children per decree. In 1984, 47% of the divorcing couples had no children, 20% had one child, 20% had two children, and 8% had three or more children (NCHS, 1986a).

SINGLE PARENT FAMILIES. As noted previously, in 1981 there were 9.1 million single parent families headed by women and 1.9 million such families headed by men. One third of the families headed by women had cash incomes below the poverty level. Presently, 50% of all black dependent children and 20% of all Hispanic dependent children are being raised in single parent families. White single parent families represent 15% of the families with dependent children. It has been predicted that by 1990, 30% of all dependent children will be living in single parent families, and 50% of all children will have spent some time in a single parent family before reaching age 18 (Family Service of America, 1984).

FERTILITY PATTERNS AND BIRTH RATES. The fertility rate (number of births to women of childbearing age) declined from 65.8 live births per 1000 women 15 to 44 years of age in 1983 to 65.4 live births per 1000 women (15 to 44 years of age) in 1984. The fertility rate was predicted to decline further to 65.1 live births per 1000 women during 1986. In 1984, the birth rates for teenagers 15 to 19 years of age dropped to the lowest levels observed in the United States since 1940, although the actual number of births in this age group continued to remain high. The birth rates increased from 1.1 to 1.2 births per 1000 women aged 10 to 14 years between 1983 and 1984 and remained unchanged for women 45 to 49 years of age. Women 20 to 24 years of age experienced the lowest birth rates ever observed for that age group, and birth rates for the age group 25 to 29 years were lower than for any year since 1976. The birth rate for women aged 30 to 34 years increased by 5% between 1983 and 1984, and for women aged 35 to 39 the increase was 11%. First births to women in their early thirties increased by 27% between 1980 and 1984 and increased by 58% for women aged 35 to 39 years. The rate for second births increased by 1% overall between 1983 and 1984, but there were increases of 5% for women aged 30 to 36 years and 11% for women aged 36 to 39 years.

The tendency for women to delay the start of their families is becoming an established pattern for many American families. The increase in first births for women in their thirties is largely a consequence of delayed marriages and the postponement of starting families. The birth rates in relation to men (live births per 1000 men aged 15 to 54 years) tended to decline for all groups except for men aged 30 to 44 years and 50 to 54 years. There was a 1% increase for men 30 to 39 years of age and a 3% to 4% increase for men in the age groups 40 to 44 years and 50 to 54 years. This pattern in birth rates as related to men is consistent with the trend toward delayed parenting (NCHS, 1986b).

BIRTHS TO UNMARRIED WOMEN. All measures describing the incidence of childbearing by unmarried women rose between 1983 and 1984 to the highest levels observed since 1940. One of every five births in 1984 was to an unmarried mother. Since 1975, the birth rate for unmarried black women has declined, whereas the birth rate for white women has steadily increased. Although the birth rate for unmarried black women remains high, 76.8 births per 1000 women, the 1984 rate was 9% below the 1975 rate. By comparison, the 1984 birth rate of 20.1 births per 1000 white women was 62% higher than the 1975 birth rate for that group. Unmarried postteenage women accounted for 65% of all nonmarital births, compared with 59% in 1980 (NCHS, 1986b).

ELDERLY. The number of elderly is increasing and will continue to increase. In addition, by the year 2000 almost 50% of the elderly will be over 75 years of age, with many women being in their eighties. Elderly couples will probably experience separations and divorces with increasing frequency. Although some of the elderly are experiencing increased financial independence, a large number of them are still living at the subsistence level. More of the elderly have never had children or have no surviving children or spouse and have limited financial resources; they are sustained by public and private funds and services. With societal emphasis on self-reliance, competitiveness, "survival of the fittest," and accompanying reductions in funding for human services, it is anticipated that there will be a growing suicide rate among the elderly (Family Service of America, 1984). Thus the final phase of the family life cycle may be extended for some elderly couples, disrupted by divorce for others, or filled with survival problems for the remaining groups of elderly experiencing limited resources and support systems.

Trends in the Family Life Cycle

If the present demographic trends continue, it can be expected that there will be a decline in the proportion of adults experiencing the typical family life cycle. These trends will affect the child's family life experiences also.

The trend toward the postponement of marriage and delayed first and second births, or no children at all, reflects a growing acceptance of adulthood with delayed parenthood or even without parenthood. The effect of delayed parenting on family roles will be older parents who may be better prepared emotionally and economically to provide for the child. There is also the probability that grandparents may be more infirm or deceased.

The trend toward postponement of marriage has been referred to as a new transition stage for continued personal development in the life course between childhood and adulthood. Traditionally marriage marked the transition to adult status. Young adults married, set up housekeeping independent from their parents, and very soon thereafter started their own family. Now a growing number of young adults live apart from their parents and other relatives and delay the start of a family.

It is predicted that divorce and remarriage will continue as an acceptable response to unsatisfactory marriages. Thus changes in patterns of family formation will involve more transitions (e.g., marital breakdown, divorce, remarriage) in the life courses of both children and their parents (Norton, 1983).

Although a large number of divorcing couples remarry, some do not. Those divorced adults who do not remarry frequently find themselves in the position of a single parent responsible for maintaining a family life for their children. Thus the families of divorced single parents join the ranks of the families of never-married single parents. Both of these types of families develop a unique life cycle, which they implement in their own way.

Adults who elect to remain single and childless and adults establishing alternative households will tend to remain outside of the typical family life cycle. Some of the changes that have contributed to singlehood and other types of households have been greater sexual freedom; more flexible, egalitarian roles for men and women; higher education levels for women; more women pursuing careers; and a greater societal acceptance of adults remaining single (Duvall and Miller, 1985; Knox, 1980).

With the increasing number of single people and childless couples approaching old age, one can only estimate the impact this group may have on the development of various family structures and support systems. It is expected that this group, as well as elderly couples, will have the opportunity to work more years of their lives. In addition, the increasing financial independence of the elderly may contribute to further creative family structuring. It can be expected that a certain percentage of the elderly will live with an adult child or in some other type of extended family arrangement.

FAMILY ROLES AND FUNCTIONS

Implicit in the developmental approach to the study of the family are the concepts of family roles and functions. Knowledge in these areas is essential to adequately assess the family and to effectively plan, intervene, and evaluate care with the family. Although there are societal and familial expectations about family roles and functions in general, the current trends in marriage and the family influence the types of roles found in families, the enactment of those roles, and the functions carried out by the family.

Family Roles

Family roles are related to the organizational structure of the family, the division of labor in the family, and family processes. Part or most of one's life is spent in some type of family in which there are defined role relations and defined rights and obligations of each member of the family unit (Goode, 1964). An individual will occupy a *role position* of husband-father, wife-mother, son-brother, or daughter-sister, and certain roles are associated with each position. An example of a set of role behaviors related to the spouse (husband or wife) position is the sexual role. Positions and roles within the context of any family can change over time; this is called *role sequence* (Rodgers, 1973).

There are societal, as well as family, expectations for behaviors associated with certain family roles, and these expectations may not be congruent. Similarly, differences may exist within families. Each family tends to modify family roles and role behaviors in relation to the family structure and forces internal and external to the family unit.

Family Adult Roles

The work of Nye (1976) is used in this section as an example of family adult roles. The enactment of these roles (described here), as well as the behaviors associated with the roles, will vary in relation to the family form, that is, traditional or nontraditional.

1. *Child socialization* encompasses processes and activities in the family that contribute to the development of the child's social and mental capacities.
2. *Child care* involves provision of physical and emotional care to the child for the purpose of developing a healthy individual.
3. *Provider role* includes the production of goods and services needed by the family or the obtaining of them through the exchange of goods and services.
4. *Housekeeper role* involves preparing and maintaining the goods and services for the family's use. This role also includes services in the home that contribute to family members' pleasures and comfort.
5. *Kinship role* includes the maintenance of contact with kin and, in addition, implies assistance during periods of crisis.
6. *Sexual roles* require mutual participation of both partners, with the implicit assumption that both partners enjoy the sexual relations.
7. *Therapeutic role* entails assisting the family member to cope with problems and providing emotional support, as well as handling intrafamilial problems.
8. *Recreational role* implies family recreation, with aspects of relaxation, entertainment, and personal development.

Sibling Roles

As noted previously, one of the positions that may exist within a family is that of sibling (brother, sister). Sibling roles may include involvement in the household division of labor, such as child care tasks. Siblings are also instigators of socialization in the family, as well as participants in the socialization process.

A *sibling relationship* refers to the nature of interaction between brothers and sisters. Schvaneveldt and Thinger (1979, p. 459) listed functions performed on a day-to-day basis within the sibling (sib) interactional system:

1. *Identification:* process by which a sib experiences life vicariously through the behavior of the other sib(s) and learns through the other sib's experiences
2. *Differentiation:* process of a sib defining his own iden-

tity and space in the family rather than fusing with a sib
3. *Mutual regulation:* process whereby sibs serve as "mirrors, sounding boards, and testing grounds" for each other
4. *Direct services:* sibs teach each other skills, "manipulate powerful friendship rewards for each other," control resources, act as buffers for each other, and so forth
5. *Negotiate with parents:* sibs negotiate with parents for one another, form coalitions against adult power, and serve as translators between a sib and parents
6. *Pioneering:* one sib initiates a process, thereby giving permission to other sibs to follow accordingly

The preceding discussion of family roles includes references to various family-related functions associated with specific roles. The following section continues the discussion of family functions from a more general perspective.

Family Functions

All families have certain *family functions* that are performed to maintain the integrity of the family unit and to meet the family unit's needs, individual family members' needs, and society's expectations. Depending on the positions occupied, the family member may have functional responsibilities in relation to a social position (e.g., community leader), as well as functional responsibilities in the family.

One approach to examining family functions is in relation to the family's physical, affectional, and social properties (Murray et al., 1975). Examples of these three types of functions are as follows:

1. *Physical functions:* provision of food, clothing, and shelter; protection against danger; provision for health and illness care
2. *Affectional functions:* meeting emotional needs
3. *Social functions:* provision for social togetherness; fostering self-esteem; supporting creativity and initiative

These three family functions are applicable to both traditional and nontraditional family structures. Duvall (1985, p. 8) identified six family functions that are also generally applicable to all types of family structures:

1. *Generating affection:* affection is generated between spouses, between parents and children, and among members of the generations.
2. *Providing personal security and acceptance:* the family provides a home base with stability that allows the family members to develop naturally in their own way at their own pace.
3. *Giving satisfaction and a sense of purpose:* in the family setting, the family members enjoy life with each other through satisfying activities.
4. *Ensuring continuity of companionship:* in most cases, family associations that provide sympathetic companionship and encouragement can be expected to endure.
5. *Providing social placement and socialization:* the family serves as the transmitter of culture from one generation to the next and prepares family members for their place in the social hierarchy.
6. *Inculcating controls and a sense of what is right:* within

the family, members first learn the rules, rights, obligations, and responsibilities characteristic of human societies.

The family is the primary social system within which the individual develops, is nurtured, and becomes socialized and within which personal growth and autonomy are fostered. The family contributes to individual family members' health through supporting their (members') biophysical and psychosocial development. Within the family system, individual members learn to interact with others and develop social skills. The members learn how to cope with personal, family, and societal problems, and they learn methods for developing external family linkages with community groups and organizations. It is also within the family unit that members develop their concept of health and establish health habits.

The family as a social unit develops a system of values, beliefs, and attitudes about health and illness that are imparted to and demonstrated through the health-illness behaviors of the family members. The family also functions as the primary intermediary for transmitting health-related cultural traits to the next generation. It is through the family that family members learn the beliefs and practices of the larger society concerning health and illness.

A basic family function is to protect the health of its members and to provide supportive, nurturing care during periods of illness. The manner in which the family carries out its health-illness care responsibilities and the ability to do so will be influenced by factors such as the family's structure, division of labor, socioeconomic status, and ethnicity.

The list of health-related functions and tasks in the box below is applicable to most families, but the extent to which these functions and tasks will be observed for every family will vary in accordance with the family character-

---

FAMILY HEALTH FUNCTIONS AND TASKS

Provision of adequate food, shelter, and clothing
Maintenance of health-supporting physical home environment
Maintenance of health-supporting psychosocial home environment
Provision of resources for maintenance of personal hygiene
Provision for meeting spiritual needs
Health education
Health promotion (nutrition, exercise, etc.)
Health-illness decision making
Recognition of developmental disruptions
Recognition of health disruptions
Seeking health care
Seeking illness care
Seeking dental care
First aid
Supervision of medications (prescribed and over-the-counter)
Illness care (short-term and long-term)
Rehabilitation care
Involvement with the community's health

---

istics. The community health nurse supports the family in its ability to perform health-related functions and tasks, contributes through assisting the family in strengthening its resources for carrying out these responsibilities, and intervenes more directly as necessitated by the family situation.

DEVELOPMENTAL CONCEPTUAL FRAMEWORK

A conceptual framework is essential for guiding the community health nurse in the process of assisting families in their health promoting efforts. The framework directs the community health nurse in data collection and assessment, diagnosis, planning, implementation, and evaluation. One framework, generated for studying families, that has been used by community health nurses singularly or in conjunction with other conceptual approaches is the developmental framework.

Family Developmental Theory

Developmental theory focuses on common, general features of family life. It assumes that there are successive distinct and different phases and patterns that occur within the experience of family living over the years. The idea of family life cycle assumes that there is a high degree of interdependence among the family members. As a consequence of this interdependence, families change each time members are added to or subtracted from the family (Duvall and Miller, 1985; Friedmann, 1986). These changes, referred to as critical transition points, also result in changes in the status and roles of family members. The healthy family performs explicit and implicit roles appropriately, according to family members' ages, competencies, and needs during the family life cycle.

The stages in the family life cycle outlined in the box on p. 360 are sometimes referred to as *normative events* and occur regularly in a large number of families. Events that modify the normative development of the family have been referred to as *paranormative* events (Terkelsen, 1980). Paranormative events include miscarriage; marital separation and divorce; severe illness, disability, and death; relocation and dislocation of the family; and changes in socioeconomic status. Although most of the family stages are guided by socially and culturally defined norms, events such as divorce and remarriage constitute aspects of family life lacking clearly defined sociocultural norms. These two events exemplify the consequential shifting of roles and tasks within family systems, as well as alterations in the interaction and roles of the family in relation to the outside world.

The family development framework, as originally formulated, focused essentially on the life cycle of the nuclear family from the wedding, to the birth of children, to the death of the surviving spouse. Over the last couple of decades it has become apparent that not everyone fits into this family life cycle pattern. As stated by Duvall and Miller (1985, p. 21) "Families express their individuality in the distinctive ways in which they proceed through the universal life cycle. Each family history has its own unique design."

The developmental framework encompasses systems theory, the structural-functional approach, and interactional

STAGES IN THE FAMILY LIFE CYCLE

Stevenson (1977)
Family: Emerging
      Crystallizing
      Integrating
      Actualizing

Aldous (1978)
Newly established couple
Childbearing family
Family with schoolchildren
Family with adolescents
Family with young adult
    children
Family in middle years
Aging family

Geyman and Tupin (1980)
Birth of family
Phase of expansion
Phase of dispersion
Phase of independence
Phase of replacement

Terkelsen (1980)
Marriage
Birth of a child
Child enters school
Adolescent period
Child enters adulthood
Birth of grandchildren
Retirement
Senescence

Havighurst (1974)
Married couple
Family with children
Family with adolescents
Children starting own family
Grandchildren arriving
Family of elderly couple

Feldman and Feldman (1975)
Sexual experience career
Marital career
Parental career
Adult-parent career

process (Rowe, 1967). The reader should refer to Chapter 7 for further discussion of these approaches.

Family Developmental Framework

The *developmental approach* to the family has tended to assume that family development followed a series of orderly, sequential changes in the family's growth, development, and dissolution throughout the family's life cycle (Duvall and Miller, 1985). As originally conceived, the family life cycle (also referred to as the family career) consisted of stages related to the child's entry into and exit from the family. Events related to the child's stages in the family were considered to be transitional points for the family because role relationships among family members were significantly altered by those events (Nock, 1979).

Duvall (Duvall and Miller, 1985) has categorized the family life cycle into eight stages: (1) married couple without children, (2) childbearing family in which the oldest child is 30 months of age, (3) family with preschool children (oldest 2½ to 6 years), (4) family with schoolchildren (oldest 6 to 13 years), (5) family with teenagers (oldest 13 to 20 years), (6) family launching young adults (time from first and last child leaving home), (7) middle-aged parents (residing alone to retirement), and (8) aging family members (retirement to death of both spouses). Although Duvall's classification for the family life cycle has tended to be used as the reference point for studying family developmental stages and tasks associated with those stages, there presently exist numerous formulations of the family life cycle, as noted in the box above. All of these classification schemes

involve the presence of children, which has been a point of criticism because all families do not have children. Although it is not clearly emphasized in Stevenson's family development approach, "childbearing" and "childrearing" are associated with the family stages of emerging and crystallizing. The major difference between Stevenson's conceptualization of the family life stages and that of others is that Stevenson's stages focus on the development of adults in the family constellation rather than on the child.

Assumptions of the family developmental framework can be summarized as follows (Aldous, 1978):

1. Families develop and change over time in similar and consistent ways.
2. Humans initiate actions as they mature and interact with others, as well as react to environmental pressures.
3. The family and family members must perform certain time-specific tasks set by themselves, as well as those determined by culture and society.
4. Families tend to have a beginning and an end.

Rodgers' Developmental Framework

The Rodgers' (1973) family interaction and transaction approach to family development encompasses aspects of systems theory, the interactional approach, and the structural-functional approach with emphasis on the complexity of roles throughout the family career. In addition, variations in family structures are taken into account. The *Rodgers' developmental framework* consists of the societal-institutional, group-interactional, and individual psychological facets (Table 18-3). The *societal-institutional facet* views the family as a major social system and stresses how the family system is interrelated with other structures of the society as a functioning whole. As a subsystem of the larger societal system, the family has certain functions that the larger society has determined to be the family's responsibility. Society also defines family roles designed to carry out societal functions. The institutional perspective emphasizes the influence of society on the family structure. Some of the ways in which society affects the family system are outlined in Table 18-3.

The *group-interactional facet* of the developmental framework emphasizes structural conditions in the family, as well as changes in the family system. A given society defines normatively the expectations for a family's structure and specifies family positions with identified role content. Any variations from this pattern constitute an "atypical" family structure as represented by an excess or deficit in the structure, atypical formations, and inability or unwillingness to play roles. When a *deficit* occurs in the family structure, one or more of the normatively defined family positions are vacant, as occurs in divorce, for example. The role content of the deficit position must be accounted for by the family. *Excess* in the family structure results when there are individuals present in the family for whom there normally are no designated positions (e.g., married child and family living in the parental home). The consequences of such an arrangement necessitate the reallocation of the roles to the positions of the extra members.

TABLE 18-3
Rodgers' developmental framework

Facets	Characteristics
Societal-institutional	Functions of the family system for society (reproductive roles, maintenance of biological functioning, socialization of new members, production and distribution of goods/services, maintenance of order, maintenance of meaning and motivation)
	Impact of society on the family system (societal definitions of roles for societal functions; government—legal authority, provision of services, taxing power, military function; education-socialization, economic investment, social mobility; economy—family as producer of workers and consumer of goods and services; religion—variable impact on family; other systems—recreational, health services)
Group-interactional	Family as a semiclosed system (family as system, historical perspective regarding roles)
	Structural conditions (deficit structure; excess structure; plurality; spacing, age, and sex patterns)
	Change in family system
	Changing normative content of positions (variation in family structure, shifting importance of roles, developmental tasks, daily interactional experiences of family)
	Societal change as a source of familial change (long-term and short-term historical changes)
Individual-psychological	Individual as actor (impact of individual on family)
	Individual as reactor (impact of family on individual)

Adapted from Rodgers, R.: Family interaction and transaction: the developmental approach, Englewood Cliffs, N.J., 1973, Prentice-Hall, Inc., p. 23.

TABLE 18-4
Family developmental tasks

Family stages	Developmental tasks
Beginning family	Establishing a marriage Relating to kin network Family planning
Early childbearing family	Stabilizing the family unit Reconciling family members' conflicting developmental tasks Facilitating developmental needs of mother, father, and infant
Family with preschool children	Nurturing and socializing children Maintaining a stable marriage
Family with school-aged children	Socializing children Promoting school achievement Maintaining satisfactory marital relationship
Family with teenager(s)	Balancing teenage freedom and responsibility Maintaining open parent-child communication Maintaining a stable marital relationship Building a foundation for future family stages
Launching family	Releasing children as young adults Readjusting the marriage Assisting aging parents
Middle-aged family	Strengthening the marital relationship Sustaining relationships with parents and children Providing a healthy environment Cultivating leisure-time activities
Aging family	Adjusting to retirement Maintaining satisfactory living arrangement Adjusting to reduced income Adjusting to health problems Adjusting to death of spouse

Adapted from Friedman, M.: Family nursing: theory and assessment, New York, 1981, Appleton-Century-Crofts, p. 50.

The focus on *plurality patterns* emphasizes family size and the pairs of relationships that are a consequence of the number of members in the family. An important aspect of family size relates to fluctuations in which additions and subtractions from the family membership result in role and positional reorganization in the family structure. Three additional structural factors associated with the plurality issue are spacing patterns, sex patterns, and age patterns.

A given *spacing pattern,* as related to the entrance of children into the family (by birth, adoption), places important structural influences on the developing role structure of the family (e.g., several closely spaced births during young adulthood as compared with the postponement of parenting until the age of 35 or later). *Sex patterns* in the family, such as a family with all female children, has quite a different set of role characteristics from a family with all male children. This is important to keep in mind when working with families with children. Role structure in the family is further modified by the *age patterns* existing within the family at any one point in the family career. The age pattern consists of ages of the siblings, as well as the gap between the ages of the children and the parents. Parents who had their children at a young age will probably experience the children as young adults leaving home while the parents are at a relatively young age. Parents who delayed having children until their late thirties will still have children at home in their (parents') later years.

The process of change is an inherent characteristic of the family system. Changing normative content of family positions over time can be attributed to variations in the family structure (e.g., excess or deficit); the shifting importance of roles (e.g., role of wife becoming recessive and role of mother becoming dominant in the wife-mother position); developmental tasks associated with critical periods in the family life cycle (e.g., socialization of child); and the day-to-day interactional experiences of the family (e.g., existing agreements concerning role relationships are abandoned and new ones are developed for the purpose of performing more satisfactorily the daily operations of the family system). In addition to changes arising from within the family, societal changes, such as increased technology and economic depressions, can introduce change into the family.

The final facet of Rodgers' developmental framework is the *individual-psychological* one. From this perspective, individual family members are viewed as actors affecting one another. Individuals, as actors, introduce their own characteristics into a role, particularly in relation to other processes occurring in the family career. For example, while an individual in the late teens is engaged in increasing independence in role behavior, the wife-mother may be facing the roles of middle age and the husband-father may be trying to adjust to the leveling of career aspirations. The general effects a family may have on a family member, as *reactor,* are special definitions for role occupancy, stereotyping the role occupant, special patterning of relationships within the family (e.g., cliques), the development of typical interactive styles (e.g., use of strong moral values), provision of particular emotional climates (e.g., affectionate, hostile), and the provision of facilitating mechanisms (e.g., books, instruction).

Family Developmental Tasks

A *family developmental task* is defined as a "growth responsibility that arises at a certain stage in the life of a family, the successful achievement of which leads to present satisfaction, approval, and success with later tasks." Failure in the task can lead to family unhappiness, societal disapproval, and difficulty with later developmental tasks (Duvall and Miller, 1985, p. 61). The criteria for task accomplishment are satisfaction of the family's biological requirements, cultural obligations, and its own values and aspirations. The developmental tasks basic to most families, such as physical maintenance and socialization of family members, tend to be congruent with the family functions. Examples of family tasks appear in Table 18-4. Some of the developmental tasks outlined are more relevant for the intact nuclear family than for some of the other types of family structures.

The achievement of family developmental tasks at each family stage is interrelated with the accomplishment of developmental tasks by individual family members (see Chapters 21 through 25). Family developmental tasks assist the individual members to accomplish their tasks, which in turn enables the family to complete its task(s). In addition, individual family members have to accomplish many of their individual developmental tasks to be able to adequately fulfill their family roles (Aldous, 1978; Duvall, 1977; Havighurst, 1974; Stevenson, 1977). The box on the facing page exemplifies the interrelationship between individual, sibling, and family developmental tasks in a family consisting of two parents and school-age and adolescent children.

Close examination of the individual, sibling, and family developmental tasks clarifies the interrelationship of the tasks and also demonstrates the complex nature of the family at this stage of its development. For example, when an adolescent becomes pregnant, in addition to working on the developmental tasks common to adolescence, the teenager is confronted with the developmental tasks associated with pregnancy. Pregnancy viewed as a series of developmental tasks implies that the way in which the tasks are accomplished will be predictive of subsequent task accomplishment and adaptation to future parental responsibilities (Valentine, 1982). Developmental tasks associated with pregnancy are (1) development of an emotional attachment to the fetus during the first trimester, (2) differentiation of the self and the fetus during the third trimester, (3) acceptance and resolution of the relationship with the pregnant woman's mother, and (4) resolution of dependency issues in relation to the woman's mother and husband/partner.

Successful accomplishment of these tasks should contribute to the development of a coherent sense of self as a person and parent. Thus the adolescent is confronted with a double set of developmental tasks that are not necessarily compatible. The adolescent is also confronted with premature entry into the parental role and possible premature exit from the educational role. In addition, the tasks of the family, adults, and siblings become more complex because certain role shifts occur for some or all of the family members (e.g., the parents may become grandparents prematurely, and the siblings may become aunts and uncles). If the adolescent

INDIVIDUAL AND FAMILY DEVELOPMENTAL TASKS

Family

Providing a variety of facilities for the family's varying needs

Sharing responsibilities of family living

Maintaining a vital marital relationship

Maintaining constructive, open generational communications

Maintaining contact and communications with relatives

Broadening the social horizons of all family members

Maintaining sound ethical and moral standards

Sibling

Developing an affectional sibling structure

Gender role socialization/learning

Engaging in role-making with each other

Supplying younger sibling with information on content of adolescent tasks

Role modeling heterosexual behaviors among peers

Providing support and understanding to adolescent sibling

Adolescent sibling serves as a mediator within the family and between the younger sibling and the broader community

School age children
(6 to 12 years)

Learning physical skills for valued physical activities

Building healthy attitudes toward one's body and its development

Developing a social personality with peers

Learning appropriate social roles

Developing fundamental intellectual skills (reading, etc.)

Developing concepts necessary for everyday life

Developing inner moral control and a value system

Achieving personal independence from parents and other adults

Developing social attitudes toward social groups and institutions

Adolescents

Achieving new and more mature relations with peers of both sexes

Achieving a masculine or feminine social role

Accepting one's body and using it effectively

Achieving emotional independence from parents and other adults

Preparing for marriage and family life

Preparing for an occupation or career

Achieving an identity and developing an ideology

Desiring and achieving socially responsible behavior

Adults
(30 to 50 years)

Objective: to be responsible for one's own growth and development and that of organizational projects and to assist younger and older generations without controlling them

Developing socioeconomic strength

Evaluating the relationship between one's occupation/career and value system

Helping younger persons to become more integrated

Strengthening/redeveloping intimacy with spouse or significant other

Developing in-depth friendships

Assisting the elderly progress through the later years of life

Assuming responsible positions in occupational, social, and community activities

Maintaining and improving the home

Using leisure time in satisfying and creative ways

Adjusting to biological and/or personal changes

---

decides to keep the baby and remain in the family, the family will experience an excess in the family structure.

SINGLE PARENT FAMILIES. This discussion of the *single parent family* focuses on the separated or divorced woman as head of the household, since that family structure continues to predominate for divorced single parent families. The reader should refer to Chapter 19 for additional discussion of the single parent family.

Aldous (1978) identified six developmental stages for single parent families of divorced women: establishment of the single parent family; the woman continuing, instituting, or reinstituting her occupational career; the family with adolescents; the family with young adults; the woman in middle years; and the woman's retirement from her career and/or assuming responsibilities for parents. Table 18-5 depicts some of the developmental tasks associated with the first two stages of the single parent family. Many of the tasks related to the last four stages are comparable to the tasks that have been identified for most families, with the exception of those related to the spouse.

Many of the tasks delineated for the single female–parent family would apply to the single father–parent family also. The community health nurse working with the single parent family will need to be prepared to assist the parent and child with developmental tasks through the provision of professional support, anticipatory guidance and problem solving, and the development of support systems and social networks. The single parent family represents a family structure with a deficit.

Essential to the satisfactory implementation and achievement of the single parent family tasks is a satisfactory resolution of the divorce. Carter and McGoldrick (1980) identified four steps involved in the divorce process (Table 18-6). Successful passage through the divorce process necessitates the development of prerequisite attitudes involved in the emotional transition process to satisfactorily achieve the related developmental tasks.

The Carter-McGoldrick model also identifies attitudes and developmental tasks for the postdivorce family. One of the major problems for single parent families is task overload. This problem is apparent in the single mother–parent family with young children because the major task of raising children becomes the responsibility of one parent. A problem for the children is not only the absence from the home of one of the parents but also the perceived loss of both parents when the mother seeks employment outside of the home.

REMARRIED FAMILY. There are several synonyms for the term *remarried family:* merging, blended, restructured, reconstituted, synergistic, and stepfamily. The terms *remarried family* and *stepfamily* are used interchangeably in this section because of the selected developmental issues discussed.

TABLE 18-5

Developmental tasks for single mother–parent families

Developmental stages	Tasks
Establishment of the single parent family	Developing new patterns of power, communication, and affection Altering childrearing patterns Developing new social networks Fulfilling physical maintenance tasks Coping with disrupted intimacy and sexual aspects of the marital relationship
Mother continuing, instituting, or reinstituting an occupation	Developing new family physical maintenance arrangements Restructuring relationships with younger children Emphasizing affectional relationship with children Maintaining morale of children Providing children with needed extra nurturance Reestablishing self-esteem (mother) through outside involvement

Adapted from Aldous, J.: Family careers: developmental change in families, New York, 1978, John Wiley & Sons, p. 91.

There is no widely accepted, concrete model of normative behavioral stages related to how a remarried family, with children involved, should function most satisfactorily. Consequently, stepfamilies, as well as community health nurses, tend to develop their ideas about the expected family roles from models of the biological nuclear family. In remarried families that include children, many habitualized family behaviors may no longer apply. As a result, these families must solve problems unknown to other types of families. Some of the major structural elements associated with the stepfamily are (Visher and Visher, 1979):

1. Permeability of the family's boundaries and shifting family membership
2. Presence of family members with interpersonal bonds associated with another previous family constellation
3. Presence of at least two individuals who experienced the rupturing of spousal and/or parent-child bonds
4. Possible presence of another natural parent with power outside of the stepfamily boundary
5. New relationships that are more difficult to negotiate because they do not develop slowly, as in the early stages of the nuclear family life cycle (they possibly begin in the school-age or adolescent period)
6. Family members' rapid engagement in instant multiple roles

The formative steps and the developmental issues out-lined in Table 18-7 provide a format for conceptualizing the development of a remarried family. The developmental steps in the formation of the remarried family build on the successful resolution of the developmental issues involved in the divorce process (Table 18-6).

The Mills' model for stepfamily development (1984) (Table 18-8) can be used as a guide by the community health nurse in assessing, guiding, and evaluating the family's task accomplishments relevant to the stepfamily cycle. An adequate model for the stepfamily should stress the ways in which the stepfamily functions that are unique to that type of family structure. For example, the model should focus on the developmental tasks appropriate for the stepparent-stepchild relationship while taking into account that this relationship will differ with different children. The stepparent may be able to eventually develop a parental role with a young stepchild but may never fully achieve the parental role with a teenager. This may be the result of the lack of a common family history over most of the teenager's life, as well as the teenager's needs in relation to the developmental task of seeking more autonomy from the family. General characteristics of the model are (1) both spouses, working as a pair, should assume conscious executive control of the family; (2) with the cooperation of the biological parent, the stepparent can select from a variety of possible roles (e.g., friend, parent, etc.) the one most appropriate for the stepparent-stepchild relationship; and (3) the stepfamily will need to select that family structure which best satisfies the individual needs of all its members. This structure may change considerably over time.

The developmental tasks in the Mills' model (Table 18-8) are implemented sequentially so that each task can build on the process initiated in the preceding stages. All of the tasks should continue throughout the stepfamily development process.

Throughout this discussion of the remarried/stepfamily, certain themes emerge:

1. There are no clearly delineated sociocultural norms for enactment of family roles in the stepfamily.
2. There are identifiable developmental tasks for the remarried family.
3. The boundaries of the stepfamily are permeable and sometimes changing as family members (i.e., children) move in and out of the family.
4. Most of the concerns related to the stepfamily center around the stepparent-stepchild relationship.
5. The individuals in the remarried family engage in instant multiple roles and relationships.

The child in the stepfamily is an example of this last point. The child may be in a position of interacting with two biological parents, one or more stepparents, biological siblings, stepsiblings, half siblings, as well as a variety of extended family members. The reader may want to follow up on this subject by referring to the various references that address the relationship between the child's and adolescent's development and changing family structures.

Ethnicity in the Family Life Cycle

When assessing the developmental events in the family, one should always consider the family's *ethnicity* in the

TABLE 18-6

Dislocations of the family life cycle

Phase	Emotional process of transition prerequisite attitude	Developmental issues
DIVORCE		
1. The decision to divorce	Acceptance of inability to resolve marital tensions sufficiently to continue relationship	Acceptance of one's own part in failure of marriage
2. Planning the break-up of the system	Supporting viable arrangements for all parts of the system	Working cooperatively on problems of custody, visitation, finances Dealing with extended family about the divorce
3. Separation	Willingness to continue cooperative co-parental relationship Work on resolution of attachment to spouse	Mourning loss of intact family Restructuring marital and parent-child relationships; adaptation to living apart Realignment of relationships with extended family; staying connected with spouse's extended family
4. The divorce	More work on emotional divorce Overcoming hurt, anger, guilt, etc.	Mourning loss of intact family: giving up fantasies of reunion Retrieval of hopes, dreams, expectations from marriage Staying connected with extended families
POSTDIVORCE FAMILY		
Single parent family	Willingness to maintain parental contact with ex-spouse and support contact of children with ex-spouse and his family	Making flexible visitation arrangements with ex-spouse and his family Rebuilding own social network
Single parent (non-custodial)	Willingness to maintain parental contact with ex-spouse and support custodial parent's relationship with children	Finding ways to continue effective parenting relationship with children Rebuilding own social network

Reprinted from Carter, E., and McGoldrick, M., editors: The family life cycle: a framework for family therapy, New York, 1980, Gardner Press, Inc., p. 18. Copyright © 1980 by Gardner Press.

TABLE 18-7

Remarried family formation: developmental issues

Steps	Prerequisite attitude	Developmental issues
Entering the new relationship	Recovery from loss of first marriage (adequate "emotional divorce")	Recommitment to marriage and to forming a family with readiness to deal with the complexity and ambiguity

Conceptualizing and planning new marriage and family	Accepting one's own fears and those of new spouse and children about remarriage and forming a stepfamily
	Accepting need for time and patience for adjustment to complexity and ambiguity of:
	  Multiple new roles
	  Boundaries: space, time, membership, and authority
	  Affective issues: guilt, loyalty conflicts, desire for mutuality, unresolvable past hurts
		Work on openness in the new relationships to avoid pseudomutuality
		Plan for maintenance of cooperative coparental relationships with ex-spouses
		Plan to help children deal with fears, loyalty conflicts, and membership in two systems
		Realignment of relationships with extended family to include new spouse and children
		Plan maintenance of connections for children with extended family of ex-spouse(s)

Remarriage and reconstitution of family	Final resolution of attachment to previous spouse and ideal of "intact" family Acceptance of a different model of family with permeable boundaries	Restructuring family boundaries to allow for inclusion of new spouse-stepparent Realignment of relationships throughout subsystems to permit interweaving of several systems Making room for relationships of all children with biological (noncustodial) parents, grandparents, and other extended family Sharing memories and histories to enhance stepfamily integration

Reprinted from Carter, E., and McGoldrick, M., editors: The family life cycle: a framework for family therapy, New York, 1980, Gardner Press, Inc., p. 19. Copyright © 1980 by Gardner Press.

≡ TABLE 18-8

Mills' model for step family development

Stages	Tasks
Setting goals	Develop desired long-term goals for the family structure based on the needs of all the family members (focus on satisfactions to be gained in the stepfamily)
	Explore possible roles for the stepparent in relation to the stepchildren (the stepparent may or may not work toward a parental role)
Parental limit-setting	Biological parent (in stepfamily) in charge of setting and enforcing limits for biological child
	Stepparent sets limits in accordance with biological parent's rules
	In the family in which both spouses have children, the couple will need to accept the existence of different rules for different children
Stepparent bonding	Allocate time free from limit-setting for stepparent nurturing of the stepchild for the purpose of allowing stepparent-child bonding appropriate to the age of the child
Blending family rules	Stepfamily develops own new rules and traditions
	Negotiate regarding the stepparent parental role (if there is to be one; this begins only after the initial bonding phase is completed)
	Disagreement regarding rules resolved by the biological parent
	Biological parent accommodates to the stepparent regarding rules to the extent that the stepparent contributes positively to the child's development
Stepfamily's relations in the binuclear family	Stepparent supports the child's relationship with the same sex parent in the other household
	Differentiate between the two binuclear households

Adapted from Mills, D.: A model for stepfamily development, Fam. Rels. 33:365, 1984.

sociocultural context. The enactment of family roles and the appropriateness of the accompanying developmental tasks are defined by the family's culture and society's expectations. The timing of the developmental tasks and the meaning attached to the different stages of the family life cycle vary from culture to culture.

The community health nurse can use Rodgers' (1973) developmental framework as a guide in working with families from various cultural backgrounds. The nurse should determine the *societal-institutional* definition of family in the culture or subculture represented by the family(ies) with which one is working. The nurse should identify the culture's definitions for the family structure and family career and the manner in which the definitions of positional role content change over the life cycle of the family. From the *group-interactional* aspect, the nurse should collect information about the normative expectations regarding the role content of family positions, definitions of roles, and so forth, which arise within the context of the family's experiences. The *individual-psychological* perspective assists the nurse in determining the ways in which the occupants of positions within the family system influence the definition of their family roles, as well as the family roles in positions reciprocal to theirs.

Awareness by the community health nurse of cultural variations in the family life cycle has implications relevant for the family assessment process, recognizing family crisis points, differentiating functional from dysfunctional behavior, and selecting nursing interventions that are culturally appropriate (the reader should review Chapter 5 in relation to this section).

CLINICAL APPLICATION

The following discussion of one type of vulnerable family focuses on vulnerable families, generally, who fall into that category, rather than describing a specific family situation. The reader should keep in mind the preceding discussion on the uses of the family developmental framework and make application, as appropriate, to the general discussion of the vulnerable family (for further application, see Chapters 32 through 35).

In every community health nurse's caseload, there are families who have experienced generational poverty, as well as multiple problems of a physiological, psychological, and/or social nature. This is the family (referred to as a vulnerable family) that has never experienced financial stability; has been a long-term client of public agencies; has experienced frequent, if not continuous, states of disorganization; and whose life cycle represents an endless succession of crises. The family members of the vulnerable family usually possess deep-seated assumptions about themselves as related to society: (1) they are not needed or wanted; (2) they really have no right to exist; (3) they are helpless; and (4) they are being destroyed by society itself (Colon, 1980). The adults may develop a conviction that regardless of what they do to get a job or try to keep it, their efforts are useless. For this reason, they may view illegal options as the only opportunity for economic gains and consequently develop a pervasive sense of impotence, rage, and despair; the important struggle is for survival.

There are certain factors related to the vulnerable family that the community health nurse should keep in mind when preparing to work with the family: (1) the family should be viewed across a three generational time frame (members of the immediate family and the extended family); (2) the vulnerable family is subject to a more abrupt loss of membership through desertion, death, imprisonment, etc.; and (3) the vulnerable family seems to have less time in which to experience the various developmental stages. The shortened duration of the family life cycle frequently results in (1) inadequate time to achieve the developmental tasks of each family life stage, (2) more blurring of the boundaries of the family life stages, and (3) difficulty with the subsequent stages because the previous developmental tasks have not been resolved. The community health nurse can assume that the vulnerable family has developed a variant family structure for the purpose of surviving and carrying out essential functions.

If the community health nurse adopts a developmental framework to guide the nursing process with the vulnerable family, a three-stage family life cycle framework will probably be the most appropriate. The three stages are (1) the unattached young adult (includes late adolescence), (2) the family with children, and (3) the family in later life (Colon, 1980).

It is generally assumed for most young adults that during the first stage, the major developmental tasks for the unattached young adult are to develop an identity and make a commitment to work/career and marriage. By contrast, the adolescent (i.e., young adult) in the vulnerable family may not grow away from the family gradually but may be forced to leave the family and become independent. This phenomenon of being forced to leave home prematurely may occur with children as young as 10 to 11 years of age. Another possibility may be that the adolescent/young adult will remain with the family as a source of income. Another developmental problem for the young adult is that without viable work options, it is difficult to make a commitment to work. This is particularly important for the young adult male who may have infrequently observed adult males functioning in a stable work role. Because of limited job opportunities and limited opportunities to see an adult male functioning in a stable parental role, the young adult male may function as a transient participant in heterosexual relationships.

The young adult female tends to perceive her role as a mother and develops her identity with that role. When two such young adults get married or decide to live together for a period, the relationship is generally unstable. There have been few models representative of a stable married couple except those on television, which are difficult for the young adults to identify with. As the couple moves into the second stage of the family life cycle (family with children), the arrival of children, coupled with unemployment, results in additional problems for the family. The family may receive public assistance, with the result that the father becomes more peripheral to the family (or he may have been peripheral to begin with). Another pattern that may develop is that the parents primarily identify with their adolescent peer groups and avoid the adult parenting roles. In contrast, if the adult has not had an opportunity to develop an identity

through the satisfactory fulfillment of the child and/or adolescent roles and developmental tasks, the individual may view the parental role as a source of identity.

Within the vulnerable family, one of the children may emerge as a surrogate parent to assist with the siblings. In addition, the school-age children may not receive adequate attention from the mother and/or father, resulting in the inadequate development of cognitive, affective, and communication skills to benefit adequately from their learning experiences in the school system. As more children are born over a longer period, the childrearing stage tends to be protracted, resulting in the older children frequently being discharged to their peer groups. The older children are displaced by the younger children through competing needs for parental attention and thus turn to their peer groups for needs fulfillment.

During the third stage (family in later life) of the life cycle of the vulnerable family, the forward progress of the generational process may come to a standstill or break down, especially if the household is three generational. The adult daughter's mother may assume the care of the grandchild as one of her children, the adult daughter remains a daughter instead of a mother, and thus family roles become very confused. The family system becomes a system for survival and homeostasis and not for change and growth. The death of the grandmother can have a devastating effect on the family both emotionally and developmentally. It is at this time that the oldest daughter, who was unable to become a mother in terms of fulfilling the role, may be able to move into that role now available because of the death of her mother. Thus the new mother role-occupant begins to repeat the life cycle of the vulnerable family.

The community health nurse can combine theories about the family system's development, family roles, functions, and interactions with knowledge about vulnerable families. The emerging framework should generate a working plan that will serve to guide the assessment of the family, assist the involvement of the family in the planning process, and provide direction for the intervention strategies and evaluation.

The community health nurse should realize that the family members may distrust professionals because of past experiences with public agencies. The nurse should also make clear to the family the type and extent of assistance that can be expected from the nurse and agency. It is important that the nurse retain a flexible perspective on the family and avoid viewing the family within a middle-class family developmental model of structure, roles, and functions. The community health nurse can view the nursing process with the vulnerable family as a socializing experience for the family members in which they participate in problem solving and informed decision making, identify their strengths and resources, plan their care, and evaluate the outcomes of their health care efforts.

SUMMARY

The family, as society's most significant unit of social behavior, has been experiencing considerable changes that have affected the family's development in relation to structure, functions, and interactions, both within the family and in the community. Demographic and socioeconomic changes, which had their beginnings in the late 1700s, have continued throughout the twentieth century, resulting in considerable consequences for families in the United States. Demographic trends that affect the family are age at time of first marriage; fertility patterns and birth rates; increases in singlehood, divorce, and remarriage; larger numbers of children experiencing divorce or living with a never-married parent; and a growing elderly population.

Although there are general societal and familial expectations about family roles and functions, trends in marriage and the family influence the types of roles found in families, the enactment of those roles, and the functions carried out by the family. Each family tends to modify family roles and role behaviors in relation to the family structure and forces internal and external to the family unit. All families, regardless of their structure, have certain functions that are performed to maintain the integrity of the family unit and to meet the family needs, individual family member's needs, and society's expectations.

A conceptual framework is essential for guiding the community health nurse in the process of assisting families in their health-promoting efforts. One framework generated for studying families, which has been used by community health nurses singularly or in conjunction with other conceptual approaches, is the developmental framework. Developmental theory focuses on common, general features of family life and provides a longitudinal view of the family life cycle. The family developmental framework identifies points in the family's development at which changes (i.e., critical transitions) occur in members' status and roles. The developmental framework encompasses systems theory, the structural-functional approach, and the interactional process. Normative events, such as marriage, birth of a child, and children entering adolescence, occur in the majority of families. Paranormative events, which modify the normative development of the family, include marital separation and divorce, disability and death, and changes in socioeconomic status. Increasingly, variations in family structures, such as single parent families, remarried families, and vulnerable families, are being studied from the developmental perspective.

The family developmental framework contributes to the community health nurse's understanding of families at different points in their life cycle. A major strength of this approach is that it provides a basis for forecasting what a family will be experiencing at any period in the family's life cycle, such as role transitions and family constellation changes.

The developmental approach can be used successfully in practice with a variety of family structures, but the nurse must recognize that in every family there are individual and family developmental tasks to be accomplished that are peculiar to that particular family. Implicit in this approach is awareness of the internal and external environmental forces (e.g., psychosocial) that influence the family's development.

Knowledge about family life stages and the accompanying tasks affords the community health nurse a focus for family assessment, intervention, and evaluation. Assessing the family's developmental stage and its performance of the tasks appropriate for that stage provides the nurse with guidelines for analyzing the family's development and health-promotion needs. Anticipatory guidance can be implemented to prepare the family to cope with predictable changes in roles and positions. The developmental approach also identifies periods in the family life cycle when problems may emerge as a result of limited or strained personal, emotional, and financial resources. Consequently, the family may need to be made aware of available support resources in the extended family or in the community.

In summary, the developmental theory as a framework assists the community health nurse to:

1. Keep the family in focus throughout its life cycle
2. See family members interact with one other
3. Observe the ways in which family members and the family unit influence each other
4. Recognize what a given family is experiencing at a particular time
5. Identify critical periods of growth and development for both the individual family members and the family
6. Recognize the commonalities and variations among the life cycles of families
7. Respect the ways in which culture and families influence each other
8. Forecast what a family will be experiencing at any period of its life cycle (Duvall and Miller, 1985)

Although anticipation is inherent in family development, the nurse must recognize that not all families move through the family life cycle in the same way. The nurse can still predict important aspects about the overall pattern of a family's developmental activities by knowing (1) where the family is in its developmental history and life cycle; (2) the number, age, and relationships of the family members in the household; and (3) the family's ethnic, religious, and socioeconomic characteristics.

≣ KEY CONCEPTS

Family development is one theoretical framework used to study families. This approach emphasizes how families change over time and focuses on interactions and relationships among family members.

Demographic trends affecting the family's structure and development are age at time of first marriage; fertility patterns and birth rates; increase in the number of individuals engaging in singlehood, divorce, and remarriage; increase in the number of dependent children experiencing divorce in the family or living with a never-married parent; and an increase in the number of elderly.

Implicit in the developmental approach to the study of family are the concepts of family roles and functions. Knowledge in these areas is essential to adequately assess the family and to effectively plan, intervene, and evaluate care with the family.

Rodgers' developmental framework for the family consists of the societal-institutional, group-interactional, and individual-psychological facets.

A family developmental task is a responsibility for growth that arises at a certain stage in the life cycle of a family. Successful accomplishment of the task leads to satisfaction, approval, and success with future tasks.

Mills' model for stepfamily development can be used to help assess, guide, and evaluate the stepfamily's task accomplishment.

The family's ethnicity affects the enactment of family roles, the timing of developmental tasks, and the meaning attached to the different stages of the family life cycle.

The family developmental framework identifies points in a family's development at which changes occur in family members' status and roles.

Increasingly, variations in family structure, such as single parent families, remarried families, and vulnerable families, are being studied from the developmental perspective.

Normative events in the family life cycle are events such as marriage and childbirth; paranormative events include divorce, disability or death of a family member, and changes in socioeconomic status.

LEARNING ACTIVITIES

1. Select six or more health professionals and other human service workers and ask them to define a family. The health professionals should include community health nurses and physicians, and the human service workers represent social workers and teachers. Analyze the responses for commonalities and differences.

2. Form small groups and discuss the implications of trends in marriage and the family for family-focused community health nursing.

3. As a group project, each student should select several families and interview the family, as a unit, about their (a) perceptions of health-related functions and tasks, (b) health-promotion behaviors, and (c) values and attitudes about health promotion. The families selected should represent different ethnic and socioeconomic backgrounds. Analyze the responses for commonalities and differences in relation to the families as a whole and in relation to the variables of ethnicity and socioeconomic backgrounds.

4. Select a family-focused television program and analyze the family's behavior in relation to the family.

BIBLIOGRAPHY

Ahrons, C.: Divorce: a crisis of family transition and changes, Fam. Rel. 29:533, 1980.

Aldous, J.: Family careers: developmental change in families, New York, 1978, John Wiley & Sons.

Baranowski, T., and Nader, P.: Family health behavior. In Turk, D., and Kerns, R., editors: Health, illness, and families, New York, 1985, John Wiley & Sons.

Carter, E., and McGoldrick, M.: The family life cycle and family therapy: an overview. In Carter, E., and McGoldrick, M., editors: The family life cycle: a framework for family therapy, New York, 1980, Gardner Press, Inc.

Cogswell, B.E., and Sussman, M.B.: Changing family and marriage forms: complications for human service systems, Fam. Coord. 21:505, 1972.

Colon, F.: The family life cycle of the multi-problem poor family. In Carter, E., and McGoldrick, M., editors: The family life cycle: a framework for family therapy, New York, 1980, Gardner Press, Inc.

Duvall, E., and Miller, B.: Marriage and family development, ed. 6, New York, 1985, Harper & Row, Publishers.

Erikson, E.: Childhood and society, New York, 1963, W.W. Norton & Co., Inc.

Eshleman, J.R.: The family: an introduction, Boston, 1974, Allyn & Bacon, Inc.

Falicov, C., and Karrer, B.: Cultural variations in the family life cycle: the Mexican-American family. In Carter, E., and McGoldrick, M., editors: The family life cycle: a framework for family therapy, New York, 1980, Gardner Press, Inc.

Family Service of America: the state of families 1984-85, New York, 1984, Family Service of America.

Feldman, H., and Feldman, M.: The family life cycle: some suggestions for recycling, J. Marr. Fam. 37:277, 1975.

Friedman, M.M.: Family nursing: theory and assessment, New York, 1981, Appleton-Century-Crofts.

Friedman, M.M.: Family nursing: theory and assessment, ed. 2, New York, 1986, Appleton-Century-Crofts.

Geyman, J., and Tupin, J.: Family development. In Rosen, G., Geyman, J., and Layton, R., editors: Behavioral science in family practice, New York, 1980, Appleton-Century-Crofts.

Goetting, A.: The six stations of remarriage: developmental tasks of remarriage after divorce, Fam. Rels. 31:213, 1982.

Goode, W.J.: The family, Englewood Cliffs, N.J., 1964, Prentice-Hall, Inc.

Havighurst, R.: Developmental tasks and education, ed. 3, New York, 1974, David McKay Company, Inc.

Hiestand, W.: Nursing, the family, and the "new" social history, Adv. Nurs. Sci. 4:1, 1982.

Kitagawa, E.: New life-styles: marriage patterns, living arrangements, and fertility outside of marriage, The Annals 453:1, 1981.

Knox, D.: Trends in marriage and the family—the 1980s, Fam. Rels. 29(2):145, 1980.

Leavitt, M.: Families at risk: primary prevention in nursing practice, Boston, 1982, Little, Brown & Co.

Leslie, G.R.: The family in social context, ed. 2, New York, 1973, Oxford University Press.

Macklin, E.D.: Nontraditional family forms: a decade of research, J. Marr. Fam. 42:905, 1980.

McGoldrick, M., and Carter, E.: Forming a remarried family. In Carter, E., and McGoldrick, M., editors: The family life cycle: a framework for family therapy, New York, 1980, Gardner Press, Inc.

McIntyre, J.: The structure-functional approach to family study. In Nye, F.E., and Berardo, F.M., editors: Emerging conceptual frameworks in family analysis, New York, 1967, Macmillan Publishing Co., Inc.

Mills, D.: A model for stepfamily development, Fam. Rels. 33:365, 1984.

Murray, R., Meili, P., and Zentner, J.: The family—basic unit for the developing person. In Murray, R., and Zentner, J., editors: Nursing concepts for health promotion, Englewood Cliffs, N.J., 1975, Prentice-Hall, Inc.

National Center for Health Statistics: Advance report of final divorce statistics, 1984, Mo. Vital Stat. Rep., 35, 1986a, U.S. Department of Health and Human Services.

National Center for Health Statistics: Advance report of final natality statistics, 1984, Mo. Vital Stat. Rep., 35, 1986b, U.S. Department of Health and Human Services.

National Center for Health Statistics: Annual summary of births, marriages, divorces, and deaths: United States, 1985, Mo. Vital Stat. Rep., 34, 1986c, U.S. Department of Health and Human Services.

Nelson, M., and Nelson, G.: Problems of equity in the reconstituted family: a social exchange analysis, Fam. Rels. 31:223, 1982.

Nock, S.: The family life cycle: empirical or conceptual tool? J. Marr. Fam. 41:15, 1979.

Norton, A.: The influence of divorce on traditional life-cycle measures, J. Marr. Fam. 42:63, 1980.

Norton, A.: Family life cycle: 1980, J. Marr. Fam. 45(2):267, 1983.

Nye, F.I.: Role structure and analysis of the family, Beverly Hills, Calif., 1976, Sage Publications, Inc.

Papernow, P.: The stepfamily cycle: an experiential model of stepfamily development, Fam. Rels. 33:355, 1984.

Population Reference Bureau: Where we are and where we're going, Pop. Bull. 37, Washington, D.C., 1982, Population Reference Bureau, Inc.

Pratt, L.: Family structure and effective health behavior: the energized family, Boston, 1976, Houghton Mifflin Co.

Price-Bonham, S., and Balswick, J.: The noninstitutions: divorce, desertion, and remarriage, J. Marr. Fam. 42:959, 1980.

Rice, A.: An economic framework for viewing the family. In Nye, F., and Berardo, F., editors: Emerging conceptual frameworks in family analysis, New York, 1967, The Macmillan Co.

Rodgers, R.: Family interaction and transaction: the developmental approach, Englewood Cliffs, N.J., 1973, Prentice-Hall, Inc.

Rowe, G.P.: The developmental conceptual framework to the study of the family. In Nye, F.I., and Berardo, F.M., editors: Emerging conceptual frameworks in family analysis, New York, 1967, The Macmillan Co.

Schvaneldt, J.D.: The interactional framework in the study of the family. In Nye, F.I., and Berardo, F.M., editors: Emerging conceptual frameworks in family analysis, New York, 1967, Macmillan Publishing Co., Inc.

Schvaneveldt, J.D., and Thinger, M.: Sibling relationships in the family. In Burr, W.R., et al., editors: Contemporary theories about the family: research-based theories, New York, 1979, The Free Press.

Stevenson, J.: Issues and crises during middlescence, New York, 1977, Appleton-Century-Crofts.

Sussman, M.B.: Family systems in the 1970s: Analysis, policies, and programs, Ann. Am. Acad. Pol. Soc. Sci. 396:40, July 1971.

Terkelsen, K.: Toward a theory of the family life cycle. In Carter, E., and McGoldrick, M., editors: The family life cycle: a framework for family therapy, New York, 1980, Gardner Press, Inc.

Turk, D., and Kerns, R.: The family in health and illness. In Turk, D., and Kerns, R., editors: Health, illness, and families, New York, 1985, John Wiley & Sons.

Valentine, D.: The experience of pregnancy: a developmental process, Fam. Rels. 31:243, 1982.

Visher, E., and Visher, J.: Stepfamilies: a guide to working with stepparents and stepchildren, New York, 1979, Brunner/Mazel Publishers.

Wilkie, J.: The trend toward delayed parenthood, J. Marr. Fam. 43(3):583, 1981.

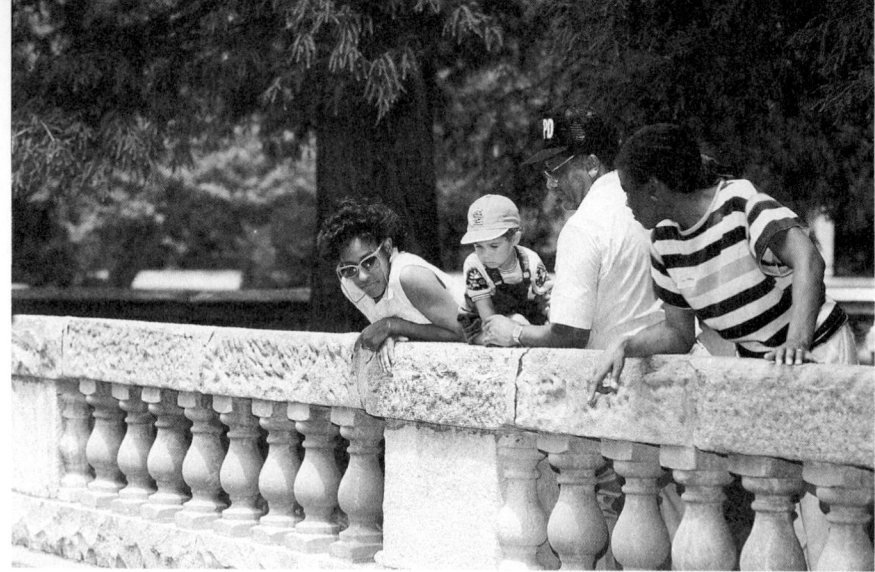

Julia W. Balzer

19

THE NURSING PROCESS APPLIED TO FAMILY HEALTH PROMOTION

⟱ OBJECTIVES

After reading this chapter, the student should be able to:

Discuss family functioning as a continuum from functional to dysfunctional.

Discuss unrealistic beliefs about marriage and family life that can influence successful family functioning.

Identify family dynamics that may affect how work in the family is accomplished.

Explain the application of the nursing process—assessing, planning, implementing, and evaluating—to family health promotion.

Apply the nursing process to families experiencing childbearing loss.

⟱ KEY TERMS

barriers to change
blaming
computing
distracting
dysfunctional family
failed expectations

family dynamics
functional family
leveling
multiproblem family
nursing strategies
placating

problem prioritization
rescue fantasy
scapegoat
systems theory
triangulation

A nurse brings to the practice of community health nursing a wealth of knowledge, skills, and tools to assist in the application of the nursing process to promote family health, but these must be used with realism and humility. The nurse works with the data collected but must always keep in mind the complexities of the family that do not reveal themselves.

Chapter 18 provides a broad definition of family and describes a variety of traditional and nontraditional family forms. References to the development of a family by the marriage of a couple, a traditional family form, are used in this chapter to simplify the discussion of unmet expectations that influence a family's success. Consider the couple who begins a relationship and builds a family with the intent of a life filled with health and happiness. The reality may be quite different.

This chapter provides information about failed expectations of family life, family assessment, and the use of the nursing process as a problem-solving approach to promote family health. A clinical application section on promoting health in a family experiencing childbearing loss is included.

FUNCTIONAL VERSUS DYSFUNCTIONAL FAMILIES

In theory, family functioning exists on a continuum from the highly *functional family* to the severely *dysfunctional family*. In reality, every family has strengths and weaknesses.

Otto provides criteria for assessing family strengths, "those factors or forces that contribute to family unity and solidarity and that foster the development of the potentials inherent within the family" (Otto, 1973, p. 88) (Figure 19-1). This framework has been useful for community health nurses in family assessment and planning family health care programs. The nurses and the family work together to identify and develop its strengths and use them in family problem solving (Otto, 1973) (see box on p.375).

Identification of weaknesses in family functioning is important because they affect the family's ability to promote health. Minuchin and his colleagues (1975) theorized that certain family factors are related to the disease process in children. They studied diabetes mellitus, asthma, and an-

orexia nervosa. Characteristics such as overprotectiveness, rigidity, poor conflict resolution skills, and involvement of a child in conflict between parents were found to be more prevalent in "psychosomatic families." The overprotectiveness adversely affects individual family members' sense of competence and autonomy. This inhibits a sense of personal control and participation in problem solving, which the nurse seeks to encourage in health promotion.

In contrast, Pratt (1976) suggests certain types of families have structural or undetermined patterns that are associated with coping with illness without major disruption. She calls these "energized families," characterized by frequent intrafamily communication, community ties, promotion of autonomy, creative problem solving using family strengths and goals, and flexibility in role changes in the family (Turk and Kerns, 1985). The nurse builds on family assessment skills (discussed later in this chapter) and evaluates problems, strengths, and resources in a variety of areas of assessment. The nurse assists the family to accomplish developmental family tasks that are unmet and assesses which family health functions and tasks are being met and which need to be supplemented to assist in health promotion. Assistance may be needed because family life is not always what the family expects.

FAILED EXPECTATIONS

When family life is not smooth and members are not healthy and happy, the family experiences *failed expectations,* which arise from myths about marriage, the faulty notion that life must be fair, and the belief that the family members will always be healthy.

Myths About Marriage

Relationships in families are complex. In a marriage, to listen to one spouse's point of view without consideration of the other's is to disregard the interaction patterns that may reveal how the family system works. It is impossible to quantitatively measure a healthy marriage. It is helpful, however, to consider some of the false assumptions with which marital systems are begun that lead to the family's inability to perform its functions and tasks. Lederer and Jackson (1968) identified seven false assumptions, discussed below, which they call the "mirage" of marriage.

It is assumed that people get married because they love each other. Love is difficult to define. According to American

---

*This chapter contains excerpts and materials developed and written by Rosemary Johnson for the first edition of this text (pp. 330-360).

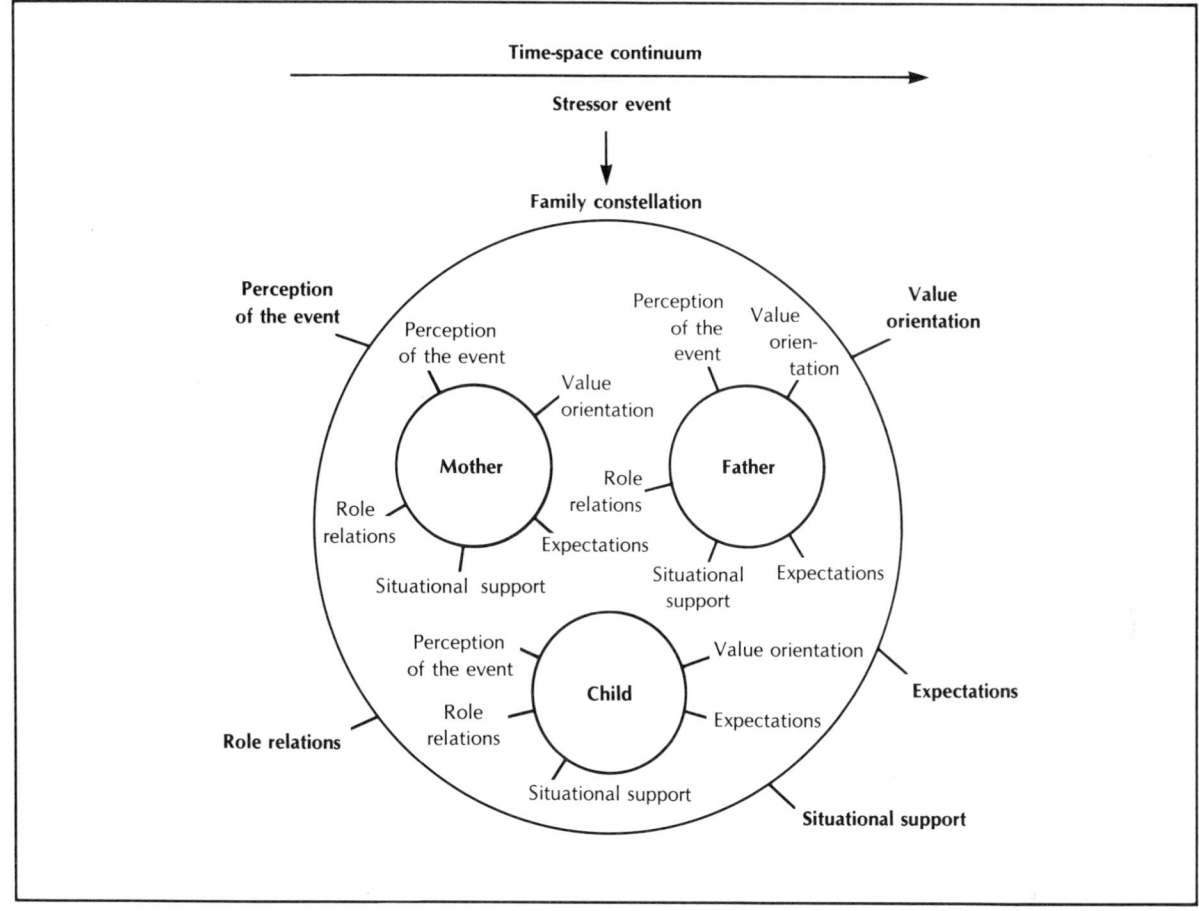

FIGURE 19-1

Family-specific risk factors and related health problems. (Used with permission. From Oehrtman, S.E.: Assessment and crisis intervention: a model for the family. In Hall, J.E., and Weaver, B.R., editors: Nursing of families in crisis, Philadelphia, 1974, J.B. Lippincott Co.)

psychiatrist Harry Stack Sullivan (1953), "When the satisfaction or security of another person becomes as significant to one as is one's own satisfaction or security, then the state of love exists." Although this is possible in marriage, it is hard to achieve. Many partners get together for reasons such as the sexual excitement of courtship, societal pressures, loneliness, a desire to better themselves, or neurotic needs to continue a pattern of relating that may be unhappy but familiar and thus comfortable.

Most married people love each other. Partners may feel they are trying to make a marriage work while actually they are acting destructively in the name of love. Consider the wife who loves to cook and sees this as a way to define what a good wife, mother, and woman she is. The family members are becoming overweight. Although they may try to limit what they eat, in doing so they feel guilty and rejecting of the wife and mother who provides large quantities of rich food as a sign of love.

"Romantic" love is essential for a satisfactory marriage. As reflected in advertising, our culture worships romantic love and fosters the notion that a marriage must sparkle to be successful. Such beliefs contribute to divorce as a substitute for the work, compromise, and problem solving that is necessary to sustain any relationship. Sue Bale, a psychiatric

clinical nurse, describes marriage as "some ups and downs, but mostly plateaus." A relationship based on Sullivan's definition of love is one in which individual idiosyncrasies are tolerated and individual growth is encouraged. An example of such approaches to a relationship is the case of a woman in her thirties who entered into therapy at a mental health center after having several affairs through which she had hoped to regain the "passion" she felt was missing in her marriage. Therapy was directed toward helping her to understand her normal developmental concerns about attractiveness and a more mature understanding of the concept of love, intimacy, and relationship work. Both partners contracted to work on mutual concerns in the marriage.

There are inherent differences between attitudes and behaviors of men and women that cause most marital difficulties. Instead of inherent differences, such as a man assuming to be more fit to lead a family, the real issue is the different roles into which man and woman have been socialized. The notion of the man as the breadwinner is challenged when the woman earns a higher salary. The number of single parents who manage a multitude of roles previously ascribed to the opposite sex falsifies such assumptions. *The Cinderella Complex* (Dowling, 1981) discusses the problems women have had when they operated on the belief that a woman must be dependent on a man to be successful as a woman. Kolbenschloz (1979) and Bettelheim (1977) write about the origin and implications for the family of such a false assumption through the interpretation of fairy tales.

Flexibility is a keynote of a successful marriage. Roles may need to be alternated, depending on the current life-style, and roles may need to be merged in times of illness.

Having children automatically improves a problematic marriage. The attention a child demands for its well-being may serve to take the focus temporarily off a troubled dyadic relationship, but, at best, problems may be postponed. Couples may project their hopes on their children to live the perfect lives they themselves were unable to achieve, thus unrealistic life expectations are transmitted to the future generation.

Loneliness will be cured by marriage. Often two people whose social skills are minimal marry and expect the other to bring satisfaction in the social arena. Each blames the other for bringing inadequacies to the marriage. Such couples seem to be chronically unhappy and socially isolated.

If one spouse expresses open anger toward the other, a poor marriage exists. It is impossible for there to be agreement at all times in a relationship in which two people are growing and changing. When conflict arises, one spouse may need to act in opposition to the other to meet personal needs and then work through the conflict. Consistent agreement is unusual. It is likely in such a relationship that one spouse is quietly giving in to the other and will eventually feel justified at getting even.

Myths in a family can serve as that family's reality. Family members may not have information about how people in other, perhaps healthier, families relate. Children may assume it is their role to mediate in parental conflict. This can drain needed energy from the child's own quest for autonomy and independence. A child may assume that open expression of anger or disagreement is bad. This can prevent the child from developing problem-solving skills in which alternative behaviors must be considered.

Interpreting Life

A family may have the unrealistic expectation that life is and must always be fair; in fact, life is difficult. Even if a person does all the right things, crises occur. Peck (1978), a psychiatrist, writes that once a person accepts this, life is no longer difficult. Peck offers four tools for dealing with the pain of life's problems:
1. Delay of gratification
2. Acceptance of responsibility
3. Dedication to truth
4. Balancing

Some families are able to continue to function in the face of catastrophe without denial of the reality of life's difficulty. In practice, this means one is able to put personal preferences aside, accept responsibility for the task of problem solving and hard work, face life changes, work through denial, and retain a sense of perspective and balance to life.

An example of a family who has been able to use these tools is a family whose 30-year-old son, John, was receiving the services of a home health-care agency. This son was brain damaged after being the victim of an assault 7 years earlier. As a result of the brain damage, John was blind, confined to a wheelchair most of the time, and had limited intellectual ability and a very short attention span. John continued to live with his parents since his wife had sought a divorce. John's father, when discussing the family's situation, advised that one must give up the bitterness. It is this bitterness that is a sign of a family being unable to move beyond the insistence that life has to be fair, that the catastrophe is undeserved and unacceptable.

John's family accepted the fact that life presents unexpected problems. Coping skills included the ability to rely on religious faith, support from friends, continued involvement with community activities, and budgeting of financial resources for the son received from litigation. John's family is prepared to accept responsibility for his care when his parents are no longer able. John's parents look forward to retirement, when they will be able to offer him more environmental stimulation. They are adding ramps and a deck to their home to increase John's mobility.

This family was able to use the tools Peck described to face an unexpected difficulty, " . . . common people, made uncommon by hardship . . ." (Dotson, p. 37, 1985).

Another expectation unlikely to be fulfilled is that all the family members will be healthy. People do not usually plan to be sick and dismiss thoughts of accidents, thinking that such things only happen to other people. Consider a couple who has saved money and planned for an early retirement in which they would travel. The husband is then fatally injured in an auto accident caused by an intoxicated driver. Unrealistic expectations of freedom from disease and catastrophe seem irrational and ridiculous to the experienced nurse; however, people embrace and operate on false assumptions and myths such as these.

The clinical application section on childbearing loss in this chapter discusses the death of a baby to demonstrate an abrupt end to the family's expectation that all family members will be healthy and live a full life.

FAMILY ASSESSMENT

H.E. Otto's criteria for assessing a family's strengths (see box on facing page) provide a framework provides community health nurses with a method for psychosocial assessment. Too often health care providers focus on weaknesses. Otto's work helps nurses to reverse that focus. Selected information about family dynamics and the family as a system and a model for intervention in families in crises are included to assist the community health nurse in the family assessment process.

Family Dynamics

Family dynamics influence the work of the family, its ability to complete its functions and tasks. From research on families and through family therapy, much information about family dynamics has been generated. An understanding of these dynamics assists the community health nurse in both collection and interpretation of data for family assessment.

CRITERIA FOR ASSESSING FAMILY'S STRENGTHS

The ability to provide for the physical, emotional, and spiritual needs of a family

The ability to be sensitive to the needs of the family members

The ability to communicate effectively

The ability to provide support, security, and encouragement

The ability to initiate and maintain growth-producing relationships and experiences within and without the family

The capacity to maintain and create constructive and responsible community relationships in the neighborhood, the school, town, local and state governments

The ability to grow with and through children

The ability to perform family roles flexibly

An ability for self help and the ability to accept help when appropriate

Mutual respect for the individuality of family members

The ability to use a crisis experience or seemingly injurious experience as a means of growth

A concern for family unity, loyalty, and interfamily cooperation

Adapted from Otto, H.E.: Fam. Process 2:333, Sept. 1963.

Altered Family Communication Styles Under Stress

The family experiences stress when failed expectations occur, and this stress can alter the members' communication styles. Patterns have emerged from systematic study of families (Satir, 1972). Four problematic communication styles are *blaming, placating, computing,* and *distracting;* a healthy style is termed *leveling.*

Blaming

For some people, a serious threat to self-esteem arises when something goes wrong. A simplistic example is a man who sees himself as thoroughly organized and responsible yet forgets a dental appointment. This view of himself, which he holds as an important part of being a competent person, is threatened. At some level he says to himself "This is awful. If I have forgotten this appointment I cannot be organized and responsible. I can't have made a mistake. It must be someone else's fault." As the pressure mounts, he reacts, almost automatically, by blaming. He accuses his wife of not reminding him and moves into blaming behavior, acting and speaking in an accusatory manner.

This same blaming behavior may be seen when a family who cannot accept the failure of chemotherapy in the treatment of a family member with cancer accuses the nurse for somehow being at fault. A nurse who does not understand these dynamics may react defensively, denying blame, or retreat from the family, leaving them isolated with their pain. A more helpful response from the nurse is to acknowledge how difficult the situation is and reaffirm her willingness to continue to work with the family. Further experience teaches the nurse that time and patience are often the only possible interventions. The most carefully phrased therapeutic responses of empathy cannot stop the patient from dying. The nurse struggles with feelings of helplessness but continues to offer what one hospital chaplain calls the "ministry of listening."

When persons continue to blame, it protects them from the anxiety that always accompanies change. In the first example, the change needed is in organizational skills. The person may note appointments on a calendar and check it daily or may need to understand and accept that everyone makes mistakes. An appointment can be rescheduled. In the second example, the change needed is in the expectation that life will provide happiness and health for all family members. The family *needs* to be supported while accepting the terminal illness of the family member.

Placating

Some people have such low self-esteem that it seems natural for them to accept blame even for situations in which they could not possibly be at fault. Consider the wife of the man who missed the appointment. A placator moves automatically to accept the blame, to smooth over the event. Suppose the wife does not make dental appointments for the husband and keeps no record of them. It is unreasonable that she would accept blame. It would be more helpful to help the husband figure out how he could prevent the problem from recurring. The placator seeks reinforcement of the view of self as worthless or useless.

This same placating behavior may be seen when a child is injured in a bicycle accident. A mother who placates might focus her energy on self-blame for allowing the child to ride a bicycle. A father who tends to blame under stress might reinforce the mother's guilt. The mother may become more overprotective instead of teaching the child safety rules and the expectation that life will present problems with which the child must cope. At this time, the nurse might intervene to focus on problem solving about specifics, such as how the child will attend school with a leg cast. The nurse understands that communication patterns under stress become familiar ways of coping and are difficult to change.

Computing

For some people to express feelings is a sign of weakness. It is more important to appear in control during times of stress. There is an overwhelming fear of not being able to control one's life. The computer may talk coldly, use big words, and appear rigid and tense. Consider a woman whose husband returns home after hospitalization for treatment of serious heart disease. She focuses on prescribed treatment of the disease, asks questions focused on medical issues, but never seems to express any emotion. An inexperienced nurse might conclude that this woman does not have any feeling for her husband, that she is denying the seriousness of the disease, or perhaps that she is functioning out of a sense of duty rather than love. Observation of communication patterns within the family might reveal that one way the woman copes with stress is to control her responses and thus insulate herself from the overwhelming fears that her husband may die, that she might be left alone, and that she might have to face her complete lack of ability to control life.

Distracting

Some people seem easily overwhelmed in the face of stress. A distractor is someone whose behavioral response to a situation seems irrelevant, completely unrelated to the situation at hand. Consider a woman who receives the result of a breast biopsy and learns that she has a malignancy. A distractor might offer to fix coffee for the nurse or pick lint off her sweater. This person is so unable to focus on the event or its effect on herself or others that she shuts all of it off from her immediate attention. Her conversation may be tangential and her movements actually distracting to the nurse. A nurse might intervene by speaking slowly, calling the woman by name, attempting eye contact, and acknowledging how difficult it must be to hear this information. High levels of anxiety decrease this person's ability to hear and remember details. Knowing this, the nurse can gently reintroduce the subject and spend time with this woman and her family as she attempts to focus her attention on the issue at hand.

Leveling

A healthy communication style under stress is leveling. The goal in communication between family members is for members to be able to say what they feel and believe. No feeling is bad. Feelings are amoral, without morality, neither good nor bad; they simply exist. It is no worse to experience anger, sadness, or boredom than it is to experience happiness or elation. The nurse looks for ways to help family members speak for themselves and not through another member. The nurse helps family members to ask each other for what they need and to not expect that a loved one automatically knows what will offer comfort or expect the others to "mind-read." The nurse models this through personal assertive communication with the family (see Chapter 31).

The Triangle

Triangulation is an important concept in understanding the communication between family members. How a family communicates affects the work of the family, its ability to cope with problems, and its ability to promote health among its members (Bowens, 1971).

Whenever two people form a relationship, the issues of closeness and personal need conflict. How much closeness is enough? How much closeness is too much? The example of magnets of opposite charges demonstrates this tension. As the two opposing poles are pushed closer together, one feels the pressure to force them apart.

A couple trying to live together in the same environment is comprised of two different people with different personal preferences. To compromise and make changes to live harmoniously takes energy and causes anxiety. Change produces anxiety because one is fearful of losing something valuable of self. Sometimes, rather than dealing with this anxiety that comes when conflict resolution is needed, a

third person; two or more persons such as parents or in-laws; an object, such as a pet or boat; or an issue, such as work or alcoholism, will be used.

As a person can turn to or focus on a person, an object, or an issue, there is less need for change. For example, a wife remains silent when she disagrees with her husband but turns to her mother to berate her husband. A husband begins working later and later although it is not necessary but apologizes for never being home with his wife with whom he is in current conflict over future career plans. A mother and father continue to have children they cannot afford financially or emotionally and live in constant chaos without any time to work on their own troubled marriage. The mother, the job, and the children have been brought in to serve as the third point of a triangle, to take the attention and focus away from working on the conflict normally experiencd in a dyad. This tension-reducing mechanism prevents people from working on relationship issues and problem solving needed to promote family health.

Family members may attempt to involve the nurse in triangulation. The wife of a cardiac client may complain to the nurse about her husband's dependency on her and her inability to participate in any activities outside the home. For the nurse to accept this as the complete picture and to intervene with the husband strictly on the data given by the wife is to ignore the complexity of a family system and the concept of triangulation. When the wife complains to the nurse, she feels better, is less anxious, and is less motivated to work out the relationship with the husband. The nurse might listen initially and then redirect the wife to discuss this with the husband, and the nurse might be with her while she discusses it. The nurse will consider the information given by the wife when she offers client education to the husband about his increasing level of activity. The nurse might initiate a discussion of his concerns, knowing that change in the role of any family member affects the roles and lives of all other family members. The nurse must not assume the responsibility to "fix" the relationship between the husband and wife.

The Scapegoat

From the discussion of communication styles under stress, one can see that direct problem solving in the face of family difficulties is not always easy. Other dynamics can be operating of which the nurse is unaware.

Failed expectations in families often produce further problems. What if family members are unhappy and life is not smooth? Some people come to believe that someone must be at fault. Blame can become pervasive in a family and focused on one member. In some families one member is unconsciously chosen as the *scapegoat,* the focus of all family difficulties. It is as if everyone believed that if only this one member were not ill, everything else would proceed smoothly and everyone in the family would live happily ever after. This dynamic may operate in families in which mental illness exists and the family wants an agency or healthcare worker to "do something" or remove the family member. A less severe example is a family in which an elderly woman lived most of her later years with her daughter, son-in-law, and their children. Whenever anything was misplaced or lost, everyone complained "Well, Grandma took it" or "Grandma is always giving our things away." The elderly woman began to have transient ischemic attacks, finally a stroke, and was placed in a nursing home. Then, whenever the family misplaced or lost things, they learned it was not Grandma's fault.

Family dynamics can affect the nurse's ability to collect data and the family's ability to resolve problems. Recognition of communication patterns under stress enables the nurse to assist family members in better problem solving. The nurse can avoid siding with one family member when information about the nature of triangles is applied to family communication. Families that attempt to focus all family problems on one member may be scapegoating and may require assistance from a mental health resource.

The Family as a System

The application of social systems theory to the family unit demonstrates the complexity of family functioning. Some critics of nursing education contend that there is heavy emphasis on the wellness and illness of the individual within nursing curricula, with minimal attention given to the family. Some nurses approach the study of families with some degree of ethnocentricity, assuming that because they were part of a family they already understand all there is to know about families. (Chapter 18 offers several approaches to the systematic study of families to assist in the development of a family approach.) *Systems theory* teaches the nurse to be aware that the health status of any one family member affects that of all the other members. The general health practices of the entire family, bsed on their values, attitudes, and beliefs about wellness and illness, in turn affect the health status of each individual. A family is more than the sum of its parts. Two loving siblings can create more projects of interest and chaos in a home and far more intriguing communication possibilities than just adding the activities of two children playing alone. Any mother can confirm that one plus one equals more than two when it comes to childrearing, which illustrates the progressive complexity that occurs in interaction as each member's behavior influences the behavior of every other member (von Bertalanffy, 1968).

The family does not survive alone; it interacts with its environment, society. Its functioning depends on what is happening in society. Consider a military family faced with the prospect of travel to a foreign country during a time of escalating terrorist activity. The sense of security felt by the children is influenced by interaction from the parents, whose own sense of security is threatened by current world events. A family assessment model useful in clinical practice, and one that illustrates the application of systems theory, is shown in Figure 19-1. The outer circle represents family components for assessment. The inner circles represent family members with the same components. A stressor is an event that could potentially upset the homeostasis, or balance, of the family's ability to cope with life's problems. The five components to be assessed provide information about whether the event is causing a crisis state that would require assistance from outside the family to restore equilibrium.

Aguilera and Messick (1982) suggest three balancing factors that must be assessed to determine if a crisis state exists: whether the person has a realistic perception of the event, adequate coping skills, and an adequate support system. The family as a whole, for example, may be coping adequately with its tasks in the face of acute illness of one of its members, but one family member may be identified as needing additional support.

An understanding of the existing climate in a family, how it communicates, and how it copes with stress can assist in the application of the nursing process.

COMMUNITY HEALTH NURSING PROCESS WITH FAMILIES

The nursing process provides the concrete problem-solving approach necessary to assist the family in its work to promote health. Getting the big picture and not being lost in details require a systematic approach provided by the nursing process, information about families and how they operate, a family assessment tool as a reminder of what data might be useful, and a genuine desire to work with the family as it is at the present time.

Remember that the family is more complex than the nurse will ever be permitted to see. One works with the data at hand, continuing to add data and change plans as a more complete view of the family begins to emerge. Remember also that problems do not get resolved when the family does not accept that the issue is a problem.

The implementation of the nursing process is the foundation of nursing practice. Basic information about its application is found throughout this text and others. The issues discussed in this chapter are how the nurse uses the nursing process to promote health in families and how this is different from work with individual clients.

The nurse works with data from family assessment in addition to data from individual assessment; this makes the process more complex. The nurse also recognizes the effect of family dynamics not only on family life but also on how data are analyzed. She reexamines her own values when confronted with life-styles and value systems that may be unfamiliar or at least easier to minimize in the hospital or clinic setting, the nurse's "turf." It is important to remember that information about health promotion can only be made available to the family: the task of health promotion belongs to the family and can only be facilitated by the nurse (see Appendix C4 on Lifestyle Assessment).

Assessment
Initiating Contact

The nurse begins by clarifying with the referral source the purpose of the contact with the family. The nurse is not a member of the family, and the contact, often involving intimate family business, may be considered an invasion of privacy if it is not clear to the family why the nurse is involved. (See Chapter 20 for a discussion of home visits and contracting.)

Data Collection

An example of a family assessment tool can be found in Appendix B3, Family Health Assessment Guide. See the boxed material on this page for a helpful summary of the assessment categories and three issues to assess in each category used: family problems/stresses, family strengths, and family resources.

The nurse begins the family assessment with the initial reason for contact with the family, the identified client, and the client's health problem. Haley (1978, p. 9), a family therapist, noted that "If therapy is to end properly, it must begin properly—by negotiating a solvable problem." Trainees in family work function "more effectively using a concrete, problem-oriented framework" (Weber, 1985, p. 358). Family assessment initially focuses on how family functioning will affect the progress of the client and how the client's health problem will affect other members, their roles and functioning, and the total family's functioning. Working with the family, the nurse can collect data that may lead to the identification of other health problems and identify areas for family health promotion. (See Chapters 27 to 31 and Appendix C, Health Risk Appraisal Forms.) Table 19-1 presents family-specific risk factors and related health problems in each stage of family development. This information gives the nurse clues to potential problems throughout the life cycle.

Johnson (1984) suggests several approaches for the collection of family data, the interview, the questionnaire, and the participant-observer method. The nurse can use a structured interview in which specific questions are asked from a prepared list. This technique is useful for short-answer factual data. A nonstructured interview allows for elaboration and open-ended questions but requires skill in keeping the interview focused on appropriate content. A typical question might be "What kinds of things do you do in your family to protect your health?"

Questionnaires may be useful to collect data from family members who are not available for interviews. The Lifestyle Assessment Questionnaire in Appendix C4 is an example of a self-report questionnaire. Attention must be paid to the reading abilities of the family members asked to provide data by this method.

The participant-observer method allows the nurse to collect data about family dynamics and problem-solving skills. Cross (1986) provides a lengthy clinical example of verbatim data collection and its analysis. Additional sources of information include contacts with other human service personnel working with the family (Johnson, 1984).

The nurse might look over a list of areas of concern before the contact to help focus thinking during the meeting. The nurse can review developmental tasks appropriate for each age level and observe for evidence of them (see Chapters 21-25 and Appendix A, Individual Assessment Tools) and the tasks and functions appropriate for the current stage of family life development. It is helpful to make anecdotal notes immediately after the meeting. Initially it is difficult to juggle so many concepts at once, but as the nurse gains personal and professional experience she becomes more comfortable and familiar with the signs and symptoms of the

---

FAMILY HEALTH ASSESSMENT SUMMARY TO ORGANIZE DATA COLLECTION

Consider in each category 1. Family problems/stresses
2. Family strengths
3. Family resources

Family composition: socioeconomic information

Family environment: residence, neighborhood, community

Family structure: roles, division of labor, authority and power, values

Family processes: communication patterns, decision making, problem solving

Family functions: physical, emotional, social

Family coping: conflict, life changes, support systems, life satisfaction

Family health behavior: health history, health status, activities of daily living, risk behaviors, health beliefs, self-care, health care resources, community health nursing service (attitudes and expectations)

---

various stages of family life development and is better able to interpret the current stage of the family client.

Planning
Individualized Plans

It is important to remember that the family has its own agenda for how the nurse will be of use. The family or some of its members may prefer to focus solely on the original reason for contact. In these families, the nurse assists the family to meet the identified need. The nurse builds trust and through assessment and education identifies some mutually agreed-on problem to pursue.

Another family or one of its members may be struggling with a more urgent concern, such as needing money to pay their heating bill in a severe winter. The nurse may choose to assist the family with the identified problem by helping the family to contact the appropriate community resource. After this need is met, the family may be ready to return to the problem for which the nursing contact was initiated.

Another family may identify the nurse as a much needed resource and greet the nurse with eager questions. In this case the nurse is challenged to provide assistance and grows professionally with the family as they learn together new ways to promote health.

The community health nurse often is faced with multiproblem families, and because of this it is easy to lose sight of the fact that most families do deal with their problems and rely on the problem-solving skills they have learned from other family members. The nurse learns from these families in her practice and uses this knowledge to help other families cope. A recent newspaper article (Holland, 1986), describing health problems in a subdivision, illustrates the difficulties of working with multiproblem families and some of the environmental hazards that hinder health promotion and limit interventions by community health nurses. This community had no indoor plumbing, no indoor source of water, no paved roads, no central heat, and no regular pick-up of garbage. At the time the sub-

TABLE 19-1

Family-specific risk factors and related health problems

Stage	Risk factors	Health problems
Couple and childbearing family	Lack of knowledge concerning family planning Teenage marriage Lack of knowledge concerning sexual and marital roles and adjustments Lack of prenatal care Inadequate nutrition Underweight or overweight Poor food habits Smoking, alcohol, and drug abuse Unmarried status First pregnancy before age 16 or after age 35 History of hypertension and infections during pregnancy Rubella, syphilis, and gonorrhea Genetic factors present Low socioeconomic status Lack of safety in the home	Premature pregnancies Unsuccessful marriage Low-birth-weight infant Birth defects Birth injuries Accidents Sudden infant deaths
Family with school-age children	Home unsafe Home unstimulating Working parents with inappropriate use of resources for child care Poverty environment Abuse and/or neglect of children Generational pattern of using social agencies as way of life Multiple, closely spaced children Low family self-esteem Child or children used as scapegoat for parental frustration Repeated infections, accidents, and hospitalizations Parents immature, dependent, and unable to handle responsibility Unrecognized or unattended health problems Strong beliefs about physical punishment for obedience Toxic substances unprotected in the home Poor nutrition (overeating and undereating)	Birth defects Behavior disturbances Speech and vision problems Communicable diseases Dental caries School problems Learning disabilities Cancer
Family with adolescents	Racial and ethnic family origin Life-style and behavior patterns leading to chronic disease Lack of problem-solving skills Family values of aggressiveness and competition Socioeconomic factors contributing to peer relationships Family values rigid and inflexible Daredevil risk-taking attitudes Denial behavior Conflicts between parents and children Pressure to live up to family expectations	Violent deaths and injuries Alcohol and drug abuse Unwanted pregnancy Sexually transmissible diseases
Family with middle-aged adults	Hypertension Smoking High-cholesterol diet Diabetes Overweight Physical inactivity Personality patterns related to stress Genetic predisposition Use of oral contraceptives Sex, race, and other hereditary factors Geographic area, age, and occupational deficiencies Habits (diet with low fiber, pickling, charcoal use, broiling) Alcohol and smoking Exposure to certain substances (sunlight, radiation, pollution) Social class Residence Depression Gingivitis	Cardiovascular disease, principally coronary artery disease and cerebrovascular accident (stroke) Cancer Accidents Homicide Suicide Abnormal fetus Mental illness Periodontal disease and loss of teeth

From McCarthy, N.C.: Health promotion and the family. In Edelman, C., and Mandle, C.L., editors: Health promotion throughout the lifespan, St. Louis, 1986, The C.V. Mosby Co.

Continued.

TABLE 19-1

Family-specific risk factors and related health problems—cont'd

Stage	Risk factors	Health problems

Family with older adults	Age
	Drug interactions
	Depression
	Metabolic disorders
	Pituitary malfunctions
	Hypercalcemia
	Cushing's syndrome
	Chronic illness
		Mental confusion
		Reduced vision
		Hearing impairment
		Hypertension
		Acute illness
		  Infectious diseases
		  Influenza
		  Pneumonia
		Injuries such as burns and
		  falls

	Retirement Loss of spouse Reduced income Poor nutrition Lack of exercise Past environments and life-style	Depression
	Lack of preparation for death	Death without dignity

division was built, no zoning laws existed to regulate the area's development. These poor conditions resulted in unusually high rates of intestinal parasites and stomach problems in the residents.

Residents had been frustrated with attempts to get assistance. The article reported that a government grant had been promised to remedy some of the community problems. The residents were skeptical and remained "locked in a living time warp, a community of numbing poverty and neglect . . ." (Holland, 1986, p. A-12).

Community health nurses conducted a study to provide documentation of internal parasites in preschool and school-age children living in the community. Nurses checked these children regularly and treated them for whipworms and round worms. They identified sources of contamination of water by sewage, and concluded that the lack of adequate sanitation contributed to high-risk pregnancies.

Families in this community struggled unsuccessfully to meet the lowest level of needs. Interventions focused on Maslow's hierarchy of self-actualization would have been inappropriate. The community health nurse had to meet these families where they were and support their community's efforts to make progress.

Prioritizing Problems

As the nurse reviews data collected about the family, it is helpful to identify any problems, strengths, and resources in each area of assessment (see box on p. 378 and Family Problem-Solving Guide, Appendix B4, for details).

When a list of problems is developed, the nurse can simplify *problem prioritization* by using predetermined criteria, such as the six criteria that follow:

1. Family awareness of the problem
2. Family motivation to resolve or better manage the problem
3. Nurse's ability to influence problem solution

4. Availability of family or community resources to solve the problem
5. Severity of the consequences if the problem is unresolved
6. Quickness with which resolution can be achieved

Chapter 13 describes a method for rating and ranking problems identified.

As an example, a nurse may be working with the family of a child who will be needing insulin injections. From assessment the nurse learns that the mother works during the hours the injections are needed and is limited intellectually. The mother's sister lives in the home and is willing and able to give the injections. For these reasons, the nurse, with agreement from the mother, instructs the aunt. Short-term goals focus on the aunt's being able to give the injection. This goal is evaluated by a return demonstration. The family needs information about the administration of the medication, its importance, and possible reactions before it can work on the long-term goals of accepting information about the possibility of long-range complications of the illness. The nurse supports the family in its use of various family members for resources. An older sibling of the child tells the aunt and nurse that a friend of his also has diabetes. He contributes that this child's mother said "Pow!" to distract the child when the needle was inserted. The aunt was able to use this suggestion, and the nurse helped the aunt to add this step into the steps for giving the injection.

The nurse works with the family in an ongoing process to implement strategies to promote health. It remains the family's choice as to its desire to work on problems identified, with or without nursing intervention.

The nurse and the family may disagree as to what are health problems that need resolution. For example, cigarette smoking presents a high-risk situation to individual health and to nonsmokers in the environment with the smoker, but it may be seen by the client as a much needed coping device to deal with anxiety.

Rescue Fantasies

The nurse must remember who owns the problem and beware of rescue fantasies. A *rescue fantasy* is a well-intentioned intervention by a helping person who unwittingly attempts to take over the person's problems to solve them for the client. For the nurse, a sign to indicate that rescue fantasies are in operation is feeling an unnecessary sense of urgency about the individual's or family's work on a certain problem. The nurse may become attached to a specific intervention similar to a personal course of action in such a situation, and may be unable to stop insisting on a course of action even when it becomes obvious that the family will not pursue it. Consider a nurse who had made a personal decision to have an abortion when faced with an unplanned pregnancy. The nurse makes the assessment that the client, an unmarried, pregnant teenager, is not physically, emotionally, or financially prepared to parent a child. The nurse becomes attached to this young woman and envisions a different life for her, a better life. She finds herself wanting to advise the girl to have an abortion. The nurse seeks supervision from another community health nurse who helps the nurse recognize that the final decision must be made by the client, her family, and the baby's father. An essential quality for a community health nurse is self-awareness, an understanding of personal strengths and limitations (see the box above for a list of other qualities). All nurses need to be able to seek supervision, a problem-solving and perspective process, when a relationship with a client becomes too intense or too clouded for the nurse to analyze alone.

Implementation of Interventions

Peitze (1984) suggests that family nursing care focus on transitions into parenthood, adulthood, loss from death or disability, and illness from the acute, to chronic, to rehabilitative stages. She describes nursing care as a bridge for the family that provides assistance with problem-solving, coping behaviors, and evaluation of health outcomes. The family is encouraged to see itself as competent to cope with the present and future. Peitze (1984, p. 235) delineates concrete nursing interventions:

1. Discussing behaviors and conversation of family members that demonstrate functional and dysfunctional areas of coping
2. Providing direct care to meet physical and emotional needs
3. Providing education and educational materials
4. Identifying appropriate resources (e.g., agencies, people, supplies, support groups)
5. Providing compassionate support throughout the nurse-patient, nurse-family relationship
6. Clarifying ways family members can and do contribute to individual and family health

Table 19-2 provides examples of interventions for health promotion and disease prevention through each stage of family development.

ESSENTIAL QUALITIES FOR THE COMMUNITY HEALTH NURSE TO PROMOTE HEALTH IN FAMILIES

Holistic approach: looks for ways to promote wellness
Family-centered approach: looks for how illness of one member affects all others
Nonjudgmental: one may never have all the facts that affect another's actions
Accepting of different value system
Self-awareness: continues to increase understanding of personal weaknesses and strengths
Comfortable in nonstructured environment: able to work with distractions
Forgiving of self and client when perfection is not possible
Sensitive, with sense of timing, awareness of another's pain
Flexible: if one tactic fails, try another
Tolerant for the emotions of everyday life
Confident in skills
Independent in nursing judgments
Self-starter
Able to terminate a relationship
Assertive
Able to manage personal stress
Meets personal needs outside of work setting
Common sense

Barriers to Change

Transition in families means change. Change brings anxiety as the family deals with unknowns. The nurse assists the family in problem identification and prioritization, but *barriers to change* in behavior may exist that affect the family's move toward problem resolution.

The family may not understand a need for change in behavior; for example, they may not understand the connection between a low sodium diet and hypertension.

The family may habitually use defense mechanisms such as denial, repression, or rationalization to lessen the threat of change. Although these defenses help the client handle anxiety, they may impede the change process. The nurse can gradually decrease the client's anxiety by providing information about the disease process and ways to cope with it, thus making it possible for the client to give up the initial defense against anxiety.

A *multiproblem family* may feel powerless to control what happens to it and to effect change based on past life experiences. The nurse helps the family set small, attainable goals, in diet changes, for example, and focuses on successes to build the clients view of self as someone who can become more healthy.

The family may value the very behavior the nurse targets for change. For example, the family may be used to serving steak as frequently as possible as a symbol of their prosperity and ability to provide for members. If red meat is to be limited in the father's diet to promote health, the family may be reluctant to give it up.

The client may have unrealistic expectations of life and may not believe that serious illness could strike the family.

TABLE 19-2

Nurse's role in health promotion and disease prevention through stages of family development

Stage	Nursing role	Stage	Nursing role
Couple	Counselor on sexual and marital role adjustment Teacher/counselor in family planning Teacher of parenting skills Coordinator for genetic counseling Facilitator in interpersonal relationships	Family with adolescents	Teacher of risk factors to health Teacher in problem-solving issues regarding alcohol, smoking, diet, and exercise Facilitator of interpersonal skills with teenagers and parents Direct supporter, counselor, or referrer to mental health resources Counselor on family planning Referrer for sexually transmittable disease Participant in community organizations or disease control
Childbearing family	Monitor of prenatal care and referrer for problems of pregnancy Counselor on prenatal nutrition Counselor on prenatal maternal habits Supporter of amniocentesis Counselor on breastfeeding Coordinator with pediatric services Supervisor of immunizations Referrer to social services	Family with young or middle-aged adults	Teacher in problem-solving issues regarding life-style and habits Participant in community organizations for environmental control Case finder in home and community Screener for hypertension, Pap smear, breast examination, cancer signs, mental health, and dental care Counselor on menopausal transition for husband and wife Facilitator in interpersonal relationships among family members
Family with preschool and school-age children	Monitor of early childhood development; referrer when indicated Teacher in first-aid and emergency measures Coordinator with pediatric services Supervisor of immunizations Counselor on nutrition and exercise Teacher in problem-solving issues regarding health habits Participant in community organizations for environmental control Teacher of dental care hygiene Counselor on environmental safety in the home Facilitator in interpersonal relationships	Family with older adults	Referrer for work and social activity, nutritional programs, homemakers' services, and so on Monitor of exercise, nutrition, preventive services, and medications Supervisor of immunization Counselor on safety in the home

From: McCarthy, N.C.: Health promotion and the family. In Edelman, C., and Mandle, C.L., editors: Health promotion throughout the life span, St. Louis, 1986, The C.V. Mosby Co.

The nurse helps the family cope with the diagnosis of disease in gradual steps and if necessary links the family to an appropriate support group (Cobb-McMahon, Williams, and Davis, 1984).

Nursing Strategies

Three *nursing strategies* summarize the community health nurse's use of the nursing process to help the family move toward wellness. *The nurse functions as a health educator* to provide education to assist the family to see how its behavior affects the health of family members. Haggarty (1977, p. 276) states "One's life-style, including patterns of eating, exercise, drinking, coping with stress, and use of tobacco and drugs, together with environmental hazards, are the major known modifiable causes of illnesses in America today."

Based on epidemiological analysis, it is widely believed that the best chance for health promotion lies in decreasing self-destructive habits and increasing sound health practices (McKeown, 1976).

As a health educator, the nurse interprets health information and creates opportunities for the family to participate in health education and related activities (Breckon, Harvey, and Lancaster, 1985). For example, hospitals, competing for the health dollar in this time of change in reimbursement systems, offer health screenings in readily accessible areas, such as shopping malls. Hospitals also offer health education classes such as clinics to help stop smoking. Often these are offered at a nominal fee or at no charge to attract future purchases of health care.

The nurse functions as a problem solver. As the nurse and family formulate a plan for problem resolution, the nurse suggests possible solutions. Part of crisis intervention involves asking the client if such a problem has occurred in the past and, if so, what solutions were used then. *The nurse functions as a resource-linker.* As the nurse assists the family to identify problems, strengths, and resources in each area of assessment, appropriate information is shared about community resources that may be unknown to the family. The nurse demonstrates the process of approaching agencies by writing down a phone number and the name of a contact person when possible. With time, the nurse's personal knowledge of community resources grows. It is helpful to carry a community resource book or an address book in which notations can be added about specific services and helpful contact people. It is also useful to help the family learn how to call a number of agencies, if necessary, to find an appropriate resource.

The support group movement provides community resources for approximately 350 types of health and life-style problems. An estimated 15 million people belong to a half million support groups in the United States (Boberg and Hedrick, 1986). Referrals can be made to groups offering support for such conditions as Alzheimer's disease, arthritis, premenstrual syndrome, ostomy, diabetes, impotence, mental illness, and learning disabilities.

Evaluation

The nurse and family use mutually agreed-on goals to evaluate the success of nursing intervention. The evaluation that occurs throughout the implementation phase is called *formative* evaluation; *summative* evaluation occurs when the nurse and the family decide whether the relationship needs to continue or be terminated (see Family Health Care Plan in Appendix B1).

The nurse cannot expect that at each visit family members will do comprehensive planning and evaluation. It is important for the nurse to end each visit with clarification of goals for the next meeting, a summary of progress already made, and input to formulate future goals. Strategies to consider in evaluation when the established plan is not working are:

1. Seek information about what prevented follow-through with the plan. Is there a family crisis? Is there a problem with resources such as money or transportation?
2. Review the family's understanding of what they had agreed to do and what the nurse had agreed to do.
3. Determine if the problem is a priority with the family at this time.
4. Provide further client education about the problem as appropriate.
5. Ask yourself: Am I operating from a personal value system? Am I aware of a sense of personal urgency about this plan or anger with the family that might indicate rescue fantasies? Discuss these issues with nurse supervisors.
6. Reformulate the plan, if appropriate, incorporating the new data.

Three of the assumptions and beliefs about community health nursing set forth by the American Nurses' Association (1980) summarize the focus of the nursing process with the family (see Chapter 7 for the entire list).

Belief 5: Prevention of illness is essential to promote health

Belief 7: The client is the only constant member of the health care team

Belief 8: Individuals within a community are ultimately responsible for their own health and must be encouraged and taught to be active participants in their own health care

CLINICAL APPLICATION

Childbearing loss is a significant family health problem. In the United States almost one of three women who conceive loses the baby to perinatal death. Perinatal death includes deaths within the first year from an unknown cause (e.g., sudden infant death syndrome); deaths within the first 6 months of life from a known cause, or neonatal death; stillbirth; and prenatal deaths from miscarriage or spontaneous abortion (Peppers and Knapp, 1980).

H.S. Schiff (1977) notes that when two people marry, they seem to believe they become joined together as one. This idea is shattered with the death of a child. Each person must mourn as an individual. Perhaps this brings to consciousness each person's mortality and essential aloneness.

Information from the nurse and from other sources of support assist the family that experiences childbearing loss in coping with its grief. Literature written by families who have successfully coped with a childbirth loss can provide further information about interventions by the nurse. Some families will benefit from bibliotherapy, recommendation of books for the family to read. *When Bad Things Happen to Good People* (Kushner, 1981) and *Man's Search for Meaning* (Frank, 1963) conclude that although a person cannot always control things that happen in life, a person can control what one makes of the event, one's response. Berezin (1982) cites an extensive list of books to help children with the grief process.

The nurse can help the mother understand that the grief she experiences is normal and that although there may be no solution, life cannot remain unchanged. One normal behavior of bereavement that may require reassurance is searching. The mourner, although realizing that the hope is irrational, may peer into baby strollers looking for the dead baby (Berezin, 1982).

Nurses can intervene to encourage the mother to allow herself the privilege to grieve in her own way and to be protective of her time. The mother needs to let friends and relatives know when she needs to be alone. Some people will hesitate to approach her, not wanting to interrupt the grief, or will feel paralyzed for fear of saying or doing the wrong thing. The mother can be encouraged to make the first contact, if necessary, to get the assistance she needs.

The nurse can suggest that the mother look beyond the husband's facade of strength to see his hurt. One useful way of handling hurt feelings or a missed communication is for one family member to ask the other "Can we start over?" When the hurt or angry member is able, they wipe the slate clean, effectively saying they love each other enough to forgive imperfections. If one member is not quite ready to begin again, this person can indicate this and take a cooling-off time before beginning again. Physical contact such as hugging is helpful for adults and children when the words do not come out smoothly. Not every problem can be worked out, and "agreeing to disagree" on some issues clears the air. Members in healthy families do not always agree or see things the same way; that is acceptable.

The nurse can help the father by sanctioning his need to express his feelings. Crying is helpful but not easy; it may be more "manly" to be comfortable with himself than to play the expected role.

The nurse can suggest that the couple plan some time together, even if it is only an hour or two. Children can be helped to understand a parent's need for privacy by explaining to them that children grow from the parents' love. When parents take time to strengthen their love and work on their problems, the children benefit.

Reminders about proper nutrition and exercise at this time may be helpful. In one case, the father of a stillborn child reported that when he returned to a regular physical workout, it gave him more time to focus on his feelings about the death of his daughter (Panuthos and Romeo, 1984). The nurse can address the issue of exhaustion in both parents. Physical exhaustion may be magnified by sleep disturbances at this time. The nurse can suggest that the parents try music or other brief relaxation techniques to aid sleep (see Chapter 38). Slow deep breaths and focusing on a simple word, such as "calm," can be useful. It may be helpful to instruct the parents to try to visualize a familiar tranquil scene, such as woods, a stream, or a beach. The nurse can encourage the person to bring to mind the sights, sounds, smells, and textures of this place. Children can also use this technique by focusing on a happy place.

The nurse may identify a couple's fear of sexual intimacy at this time. Encouraging the couple to focus on caring aspects of their relationship is appropriate. Backrubs, massage, and physical closeness by mutual commitment of the spouses can substitute for intercourse for a while. When the couple is ready to resume intercourse, they may choose to use added contraceptive methods as extra protection against a pregnancy feared at this time. The idea of another pregnancy at this time, when the grief is yet unresolved, can make sexual intimacy a dreaded experience. The passage of time offers much comfort in the grief process (Panuthos and Romeo, 1984).

Rituals of mourning may serve to bring the family together. Difficult days for the family may be Mother's Day, Father's Day, Christmas, or the due date or birthdate of the baby (Berezin, 1982). Memories awaken the grief. On such occasions, a family visit to the cemetery, or, if there is no grave, a memorial service, or asking the minister to remember the family may be helpful (Berezin, 1982). A donation can be made to a favorite charity in the child's name (Schwiebert and Kirk, 1985).

The nurse may need to initiate the discussion of how the parents are helping the other children deal with death. Some families use natural occurrences, such as the death of a pet, to explain death as a natural, although painful, part of the life cycle. Hugging and the parents allowing themselves to cry in front of the children are helpful. Children need to know that life has good and bad experiences that can be shared with others (Berezin, 1982). Furman (1978) notes that how successful parents are in helping their children deal with their bereavement may be an accurate measurement of their own coping success. Prolonged affected behavior and school problems of the children may be indicators that a referral to a mental health resource may be needed (Schwiebert and Kirk, 1985).

The family's healthy resolution of grief requires mutual support and flexibility with work and social and home schedules. Sensitive treatment by caregivers can assist family members to emerge as stronger people. Unhealthy resolution can lead to separation or divorce, psychosomatic illness, or prolonged emotional disturbance (Berezin, 1982).

Life experience is a valuable teacher. Nurses can look to literature written by parents who have survived childbirth loss to find concrete, practical suggestions for families.

Four beliefs that aid in coping and resolution of childbearing losses are offered in *Ended Beginnings,* a book written for parents by parents (Panuthos and Romeo, 1984, p. 121). They suggest that parents need beliefs in:

1. Our drive toward psychological and physical health
2. Our goodness within the human condition
3. Our own inner wisdom as the ultimate guide
4. Our ability to accomplish healing

Emphasis on holistic care and self-care points to the importance of a family's taking responsibility for its own healing in bereavement, with assistance from helping resources. Naisbitt (1982) describes these changing attitudes, people learning to make personal decisions about health care, as a major trend in America. Opinions differ as to the statistical significance of attitude and positive thinking on health promotion, but experience in nurse-client relationships over time points to an enhanced sense of well-being, mastery, and hope in the family in which strengths rather than weaknesses are emphasized.

Health promotion in any aspect of the family is an ongoing process. Healthy grief resolution does not proceed in clear-cut stages as texts may portray but rather follows its own timetable. The effect of resolution of grief on the family's physical and emotional well-being can be profound. The nurse's intervention with clients may produce personal growth for family members of which they may never become aware. For the nurse to communicate trust in the family's strengths and not place a value judgment on the family's progress, the nurse must be involved in relationships and activities outside the nurse-client relationship that confirm the nurse's value as a person.

SUMMARY

The role of the community health nurse in health promotion in families is unique. The nurse has a view of family life to which few professionals have access. The nursing process is used as an organizing framework with which to assist family members to a higher level of functioning.

As the community health nurse applies the nursing process to family health promotion, family strengths and weaknesses become apparent. Application of Otto's criteria for assessing family strengths assists the nurse in helping the family to identify and develop its strengths and use them in family problem solving. The nurse helps the family to identify weaknesses that may be affecting their ability to promote health.

Often persons develop myths about marriage and family life that prevent them from coping with real life events such as illness or loss. Peck provides four tools to assist the family in dealing with life events.

Family dynamics influence the work of the family and its ability to complete its functions and tasks. During stressful events, family communication patterns may be altered.

Four patterns of altered communication are blaming, placating, computing, and distracting.

In some instances families may be able to use the healthy communication style of leveling in stressful situations. However, if the family is unable to communicate effectively, triangulation may occur. The nurse must be aware of this occurrence and avoid becoming involved in triangulation. The nurse must also be aware of scapegoating of one family member by another. These communication patterns can affect the nurse's ability to collect data and the family's ability to resolve problems.

Community health nurses must be able to assess the family as a unit, in addition to assessing individuals who comprise the family system. Systems theory and developmental theories assist the nurse to assess the health status of the family unit and of each family member.

In planning and implementing strategies to promote family health, the nurse functions as problem-solver, resource link, and health educator. The nurse must avoid attempting to rescue families from their problems by imposing her own values and solutions on the problems of the family. Evaluation of the family's problem resolution and the nurse's strategies for intervention occurs throughout the nurse's contact with the family and at the point of terminating the relationship.

The nurse often sees families without the masks and defenses shown to the outside world. The nurse grows with the family through experiences with illness and wellness. Intimate moments, such as a family's response to childbearing loss, demonstrate that the family has as much to teach the nurse as the nurse has to teach the family. Family expectations are not always fulfilled. Often the nurse assists the family in its coping with failed expectations.

Families are complex, and family assessment is a complicated and never completed task. Some families will reveal more of themselves than others. It is a special privilege and a credit to the nurse's skills and genuineness when the family invites the nurse to take a glimpse at its work as a family.

≡ KEY CONCEPTS

In theory, family functioning exists on a continuum from the highly functional to the severely dysfunctional family.

When family life is not smooth and family members are not healthy and happy, the family experiences failed expectations. Failed expectations arise from myths about marriage, the faulty notion that life is or ought to be fair, and the belief that family members will always be healthy.

Family dynamics influence the work of the family and its ability to complete its functions and tasks.

The family experiences stress as a result of failed expectations, and this stress can alter communication styles. Problematic communication styles are blaming, placating, computing, and distracting; a healthy style is leveling.

Triangulation, a tension-reducing mechanism to take the focus away from working on a conflict, is an important concept in understanding the communication between family members. Unconsciously, in some families one member is chosen as the scapegoat, the focus of all family difficulties.

The application of social systems theory to the family unit demonstrates the complexity of family functioning. Systems theory teaches the nurse to be aware that the health status of any one family member affects the health of all the other family members.

The nursing process provides the concrete problem-solving approach necessary to assist the family in its work to promote health.

Three strategies that summarize the community health nurse's use of the nursing process in working with the family are nurse as health educator, problem solver, and resource-linker.

LEARNING ACTIVITIES

1. Using Otto's criteria for assessment of family strengths, discuss your own family's strengths and weaknesses in meeting the tasks of the family.

2. Assume the role of participant-observer at your next family gathering, perhaps at a holiday. Identify communication patterns that you or other family members may demonstrate under stress.

3. Select a family in your clinical practice caseload. Identify risk factors and health problems evident from those listed for each family stage in Table 19-1.

4. Select a family in your clinical practice caseload. Identify and discuss which nursing roles are appropriate for health promotion and disease prevention in this family using Table 19-2.

BIBLIOGRAPHY

Aguilera, D., and Messick, J.: Crisis intervention theory and methodology, ed. 4, St. Louis, 1982, The C.V. Mosby Co.

American Nurses Association: A conceptual model of community health nursing, Kansas City, 1980, The Association.

Aslen, S.P.: Coping with family crisis: intervention with sudden infant death syndrome, Fam. Rel. 29:584-590, 1980.

Benfield, D.G., Leib, S.A., and Vollman, J.H.: Grief response of parents to neonatal death and parent participation in deciding care, Pediatrics 62:171, Aug. 1978.

Berezin, N.: After a loss in pregnancy: help for families affected by a miscarriage, a stillbirth, or the loss of a newborn, New York, 1982, Simon & Schuster.

Bettelheim, B.: The uses of enchantment: the meaning and importance of fairy tales, New York, 1977, Alfred A. Knopf.

Boberg, J.T., and Hedrick, H.L., editors: Support groups: potential roles for health professionals, Allied Health Educator Newsletter 17:1, Jan. 1986.

Bowen, M.: Family and family group psychotherapy. In Kaplan, H.I., and Sadock, B.J., editors: Comprehensive group psychotherapy, Baltimore, 1971, The Williams & Wilkins Co.

Breckon, D.J., Harvey, J.R., and Lancaster, R.B.: Health educator, Rockville, Md., 1985, Aspen Publications.

Cherryholmes, L.G.: The qualities of a home health care nurse. In Stuart-Siddell, S., editor: Home health care nursing: administrative and clinical perspectives, Rockville, Md., 1986, Aspen Publications.

Clemen, S.A., Eigsti, D.G., and McGuire, S.L.: Comprehensive family and community health nursing, ed. 2, New York, 1987, McGraw-Hill Book Co.

Cobb-McMahon, B.A., Williams, D.D., and Davis, J.H.: Changing health behavior of community health clients, J. Community Health Nursing I (1):27-31, 1984.

Cross, J.R.: Nursing process of the family client. In Griffin-Kenney, J.W., and Christensen, P.J., editors: Nursing process: application of theories, frameworks, and models, St. Louis, 1986, The C.V. Mosby Co.

Crowley, C., et al.: Innovations in family and community health: incorporating home health care into the baccalaureate nursing program, Community and Family Health 2:81, Aug. 1985.

Dotson, B.: In pursuit of the American dream, New York, 1985, Atheneum Press.

Dowling, C.: The Cinderella complex: women's hidden fear of independence, New York, 1981, Summit Books.

Edelman, C., and Mandle, C.L.: Health promotion throughout the lifespan, St. Louis, 1986, The C.V. Mosby Co.

Elkins, C.P.: Community health nursing: skills and strategies, Bowie, Md., 1984, R.J. Brady.

Flynn, J.B., and Griffin, P.A.: Health promotion in acute care setting, Nurs. Clin. North Am. 19(2):239, June 1984.

Frank, V.E.: Man's search for meaning, New York, 1963, Washington Square Press.

Friedman, M.M.: Family nursing theory and assessment, New York, 1981, Appleton-Century-Crofts.

Furman, E.P.: The death of a newborn: care of the parents, Birth Family J. 5:4, Winter 1978.

Haggarty, R.J.: Changing life-styles to improve health, Prev. Med. 6:276, 1977.

Haley, J.: Problem-solving therapy, San Francisco, 1978, Jossey-Bass.

Hall, J.E., and Weaver, B.R.: Distributive nursing practice: systems approach to community health, Philadelphia, 1985, J.B. Lippincott Co.

Hall, J.E., and Weaver, B.R.: Nursing of families in crisis, Philadelphia, 1974, J.B. Lippincott Co.

Havelock, R.: Training for change agents, Ann Arbor, Mich., 1972, University of Michigan Press.

Holland, N.: Health hazard is home for Page's people. The Florida Times-Union, Jacksonville Journal, Jan. 12, 1986.

Holmes, T.H., and Rahe, R.H.: The social readjustment rating scale, J. Psychosom. Res. II:213-218, 1967.

Johnson, J., and Parsons, M.: Symposia on health promotion, Nurs. Clin. North Am. 19:2, June 1984.

Johnson, R.: Promoting the health of families in the community. In Stanhope, M., and Lancaster, J., editors: Community health nursing: process and practice for promoting health, St. Louis, 1984, The C.V. Mosby Co.

Johnson, S.H.: High-risk parenting: nursing assessment and strategies for the family at risk, Philadelphia, 1979, J.B. Lippincott Co.

Kastenbaum, R.: The child's understanding of death: how does it develop? In Grollman, E.A., editor: Explaining death to children, Boston, 1967, Beacon Press.

Knapp, R.J., and Peppers, L.G.: Doctor-patient relationships in fetal/infant death encounters, J. Med. Educ. 54:775-780, Oct. 1979.

Kohnke, M.F.: The nurse as advocate, Am. J. Nurse 80(11):2038-2040, 1980.

Kolbenschlag, M.: Kiss sleeping beauty goodbye: breaking the spell of feminine myths and models, Garden City, New York, 1979, Doubleday & Co., Inc.

Klaus, M., and Kennell, J.: Maternal-infant bonding, St. Louis, 1976, The C.V. Mosby Co.

Kushner, H.S.: When bad things happen to good people, New York, 1981, Avon Books.

Lederer, W.J., and Jackson, D.D.: The mirages of marriage, New York, 1968, W.W. Norton & Co.

Lewis, C.S.: A grief observed, New York, 1961, The Seabury Press.

MacVicar, M.G., and Archbold, P.: A framework for family assessment in chronic illness, Nurse Forum XV(2):180-195, 1976.

McCarthy, N.C.: Health promotion in the family. In Edelman, C., and Mandle, C.L., editors: Health promotion throughout the lifespan, St. Louis, 1986, The C.V. Mosby Co.

McCormick, M.C., Shapiro, S., and Starfield, B.: High-risk young mothers: infant mortality and morbidity in four areas in the United States, 1973-1978, Am. J. Public Health 74(1):18-23, Jan. 1984.

McKeown, T.: The modern rise of population, New York, 1976, Academic Press, Inc.

Miller, J.R., and Janosik, E.H.: Family-focused care, New York, 1980, McGraw-Hill Book Co.

Minuchin, S., et al.: A conceptual model of psychosomatic illness in children, Arch. Gen. Psychiatry 32:1031-1038, 1975.

Mundinger, M.: Home care controversy: too little, too late, too costly, Rockville, Md., 1983, Aspen Publications.

Murray, R.B., and Zentner, J.P.: Nursing concepts for health promotion, Englewood Cliffs, N.J., 1979, Prentice-Hall, Inc.

Naisbitt, J.: Megatrends, New York, 1982, Warner Books.

Nelson, E.C., Keller, A.M., and Zubkoff, M.: Incentives for health promotion: the government's role. In Ng, L., and Davis, D., editors: Strategies for public health, New York, 1981, Van Nostrand Reinhold.

Northman, J.E.: Human service program design and the family, Family Community Health 1(2):17-25, July 1978.

Oehrtman, S.E.: Assessment and crisis intervention: a model for the family. In Hall, J.E., and Weaver, B.R., editors: Nursing of families in crisis, Philadelphia, 1974, J.B. Lippincott Co.

Otto, H.E.: A framework for assessing family strengths. In Reinhardt, A.M., and Quinn, M.D., editors: Family centered community nursing: a sociocultural framework, vol. 1, St. Louis, 1972, The C.V. Mosby Co.

Otto, H.E.: Criteria for assessing family strengths, Fam. Process 2:329, Sept. 1963.

Panuthos, C., and Romeo, C.: Ended beginnings: healing childbearing losses, Boston, 1984, Bergin & Garvey Publishers, Inc.

Parkes, C.M.: Bereavement: studies of grief in adult life, New York, 1972, International Universities Press, Inc.

Peck, M.S.: The road less traveled, New York, 1978, Simon & Schuster.

Peitze, C.F.: Health promotion in the well family, Nurs. Clin. North Am. 19(2):229, June 1984.

Pratt, L.: Family structure and effective health behavior: the energized family, Boston, 1976, Houghton-Mifflin Co.

Rhodes, S., and Wilson, J.: Surviving family life, New York, 1981, G.P. Putnam's Sons.

Satir, V.: Peoplemaking, Palo Alto, Calif., 1972, Science and Behavior Books, Inc.

Schiff, H.S.: The bereaved parent, Middlesex, England, 1977, Harmondsworthy Penguin Books.

Spradley, B.W.: Community health nursing: concepts and practice, Boston, 1985, Little, Brown & Co.

Spradley, B.W.: Readings in community health nursing, Boston, 1982, Little, Brown & Co.

Sullivan, H.S.: Conceptions of modern psychiatry, New York, 1953, W.W. Norton & Co.

Turk, D.C., and Kerns, R.D., editors: Health, illness and families: a life-span perspective, New York, 1985, John Wiley & Sons, Inc.

von Bertalanffy, L.: General systems theory, New York, 1968, George Braziller.

Weber, T., McKeever, J.E., and McDaniel, S.H.: A beginner's guide to the problem-oriented first family interview, Fam. Process 24:357, Sept. 1985.

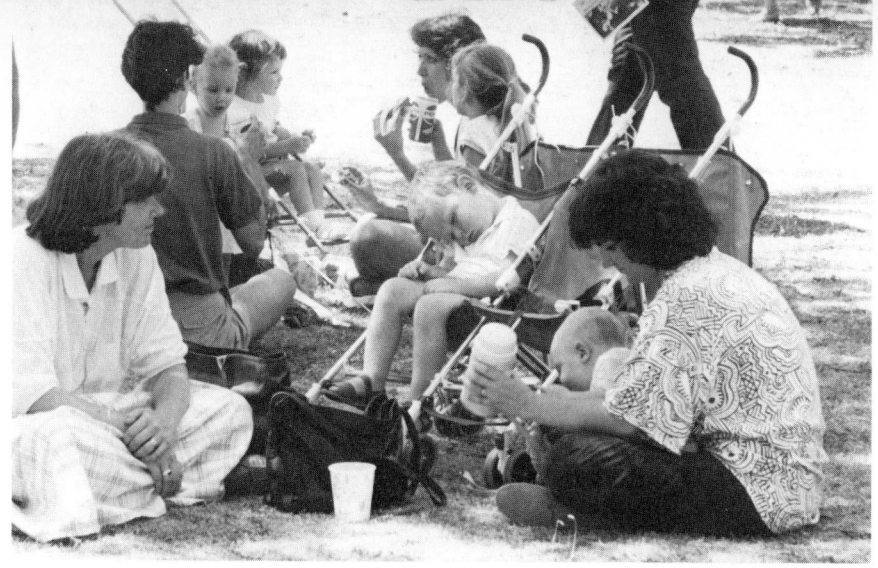

Carol Loveland-Cherry

20

ISSUES IN FAMILY
HEALTH PROMOTION

☰ OBJECTIVES

After reading this chapter, the student should be able to:

Identify factors that interfere with or serve as barriers to implementing a family health promotion focus in community health nursing.

Analyze the interrelationship between individual health, family health, and community health.

Explain the relevance of knowledge about family structures, roles, and functions for the family-focused community health nursing process.

Analyze the various approaches to defining and conceptualizing family health.

Identify and analyze the factors related to family health promotion.

Analyze the relevance of conceptual frameworks (family) for the family-focused community health nursing process.

Explain the application of the nursing process (assessing, planning, implementing, evaluating) to family health promotion.

☰ KEY TERMS

adaptive model	health paradigm	previsit phase
clinical model	home visits	role-performance model
contracting	inhome phase	termination phase
eudaimonistic model	pathogenic paradigm	
family health	postvisit phase	

$\underline{\underline{\underline{\underline{\smile}}}}$

Working with families is a complex task that is both rewarding and frustrating. The importance of the family as a major client system for community health nursing in promoting the health of individuals and populations is well-documented. The family system is a basic unit within which health behavior, including health values, health habits and health risk perceptions, are developed, organized and performed (Litman, 1974; Mauksch, 1974; Pratt, 1976). Further, the interrelationship between health, health behavior, and the family "is a highly dynamic one in which each may have a dramatic effect on the other" (Litman, 1974, p. 495).

Knowledge of family structure and functioning, family theory, nursing theory, and models of health behavior are fundamental to implementing the nursing process with families in the community.* However, community health nurses need to recognize important issues that influence family health promotion. Issues related to family health promotion originate from three major sources: the family system itself; the health care system, which includes the nursing profession; and the social, political, and economic environment within which the family exists.

This chapter examines issues related to family health promotion and presents some approaches to enhance community health nursing intervention with families. The focus is on a systems perspective within a developmental framework.

CONCEPTUAL BASES FOR FAMILY HEALTH PROMOTION

Community health nursing has advocated the promotion of family health, and a closer examination of the components of this goal prompts a number of questions for the nurse to consider in working toward this goal.

Traditionally, community health nursing has been viewed as an integration, or synthesis, of "public health, the humanities, the social and behavioral sciences, epidemiology, and nursing science" (ANA Standards, 1986, p.2). Effective understanding of health promotion in families requires an integration of concepts and theories derived from a number of these areas.

The concepts of *health, health protection* (prevention), and *health promotion* as they relate to individuals have been clar-

---

*See Chapters 7, 8, 18, 19, 21-25, 27-31.

ified within the last decade, with the goal of defining the characteristics or parameters of each (See Chapters 2 and 7). The explication of these terms in relation to families has occurred more slowly and with less clarity. Prevention, or health protection, has been defined as being "directed toward decreasing the probability of specific illnesses or dysfunctions in individuals, families, and communities, including active protection against unnecessary stressors" (Pender, 1987, p.4). Thus for a family with a history of cardiac diseases, nursing interventions directed toward health protection may focus on assisting the family to pattern their eating, exercise, and stress management behaviors in directions consistent with prevention of cardiovascular disease. Health promotion has been defined as being "directed toward increasing the level of well being and actualizing the health potential of individuals, families, communities, and society" (Pender, 1987, p. 4). A nursing intervention emphasizing health promotion may be directed toward meeting a family-identified goal of establishing an appropriate program of physical activity for all members of the family to enhance family interaction and cohesion. Historically, community health nursing has been concerned with both health protection and health promotion (see Chapters 1 and 2). Consequently, this chapter considers both, although recognizing the distinction between the two. To promote family health, it is essential to understand the dimensions of family health.

Defining Family Health

Historically, practice in community health nursing has been characterized by an orientation developed within what has been termed a *pathogenic paradigm,* or model (Laffrey, Loveland-Cherry and Winkler, 1986). Within this model, health is viewed as freedom from disease, and health behavior thus includes behaviors related to preventing or curing disease. Humans are viewed from a machinelike model, composed of parts which may or may not function effectively. The recipient of health services is viewed as a *patient,* one who is relatively passive, dependent, and accepting of treatment by an expert practitioner, in this instance the community health nurse. Interventions are disease-specific and efficient; examples of such services include immunization programs, screening programs, and teaching behaviors designed to prevent specific diseases; for example, dietary practices related to preventing heart disease. The emphasis is on increasing clients' compliance to professionally prescribed regimens.

Within the *health paradigm* (Laffrey, Loveland-Cherry, and Winkler, 1986), humans are viewed as organismic beings characterized by wholeness, ability to initiate action, potential for growth, and both qualitative and quantitative change. Relationships between health professionals and *clients* focus on interactive processes to assess the health situation and to promote higher levels of health. Health is viewed as a dynamic process defined by individuals within their own values and culture. Community health nursing interventions framed within this model emphasize the importance of exploring with clients what health means to them and where it falls in their value system.

To be clear about what community health nurses' goals are in working with families to promote health, they should be aware of which of these two perspectives is most appropriate in the specific situation. Neither is more or less valuable than the other; they are different. If the critical issue is an immediate response for a family in a crisis situation, the family may in its best interest abdicate their control and choice to health professionals for the immediate period. However, a different approach is proposed to be more effective in working with families to reach desired levels of health, one in which the values, desires, and capabilities of the client are not only acknowledged but also promoted in the process of seeking health.

Family theorists refer to healthy families, but generally do not define *family health.* Based on the various family theoretical perspectives (see Chapters 7 and 19), definitions of healthy families can be derived within the guidelines of any one of the frameworks. For example, within a structural-functional framework, family health can be considered as the continuing ability to maintain a family system structure that facilitates meeting of defined functions in interaction with other social, political, economic, and health systems. From the perspective of the developmental framework, family health can be defined as possessing the abilities and resources to accomplish family developmental tasks.

Although the majority of the existing theoretical models developed within nursing were originally directed toward individuals, recent work has focused on clarifying their applicability to families.* Based on several of these discussions of the extension of Orem's self-care model (1985), family health can be defined as a state of wholeness or integrity of the family, its parts, and its modes of functioning. The health of a family can be assessed in terms of its ability to exercise its essential self-care or dependent-care capabilities (Tadych, 1985).

Within Roy's (1984) model, family health can be considered both the state and process of becoming an integrated and whole system. Because the promotion of adaptation is proposed to lead to health in this sense, assessment focuses on adaptation on two levels. First level assessment is an evaluation of the family's current adaptive and ineffective

behavior within the four adaptive modes—physiological function, self-concept, role function, and interdependence. Hanson (1984) has identified guidelines for each of these areas (see box below). Second level assessment would emphasize identification of focal, contextual, and residual stimuli contributing to any behaviors that were identified in the first-level assessment.

Another dimension of family health could be identified by the application of Smith's (1983) four models of health: clinical model, role-performance model, adaptative model, and eudaimonistic model. In the *clinical model* health is viewed as the absence of disease; consequently, family health could be defined in terms of the absence of disease or dysfunction. Assessment includes a family health/illness history; the family's definitions of health and illness; the value the family gives to health; the family's knowledge of health promotion and illness prevention/treatment; family resources for health promotion and illness prevention/treatment; family practices related to nutrition, sleep and rest,

---

FAMILY ASSESSMENT BASED ON ROY'S ADAPTATION MODEL

PHYSIOLOGICAL MODE

Physical maintenance of members—food, clothing, shelter
Allocation of resources for health care needs—emergency care, medical care, dental care, preventive care
Allocation of space and equipment—rest, exercise, aloneness and togetherness
Provision of a safe environment
Provision for cleanliness and sanitation
Accessibility to goods and services

SELF-CONCEPT MODE

Solidarity of the family
Social integration of the family into the community
Understanding the family provides to its members
Companionship the family provides to its members
Moral-ethical values of the family
Future and present orientation of the family
Provision for sexual identity for family members
Family support for its members in conflicts with family or community

ROLE FUNCTION MODE

Decision-making processes
Clarity of roles
Flexibility of roles and tolerance for change
Division of responsibility
Clarity of communication

INTERDEPENDENCE MODE

Family interaction with neighbors and political, social, educational, health, and religious systems
Support systems
Significant others for family

Modified from Hanson, J. In Roy, C., editor: Introduction to nursing: an adaptation model, ed. 2, Englewood Cliffs, N.J., 1984, Prentice-Hall, Inc.

---

*Chin, 1985; Clements and Roberts, 1983; Hanson, 1984; Johnston, 1987; King, 1983; Rogers, 1983; Tadych, 1985; Whall, 1987.

exercise and recreation, use of alcohol, tobacco, and drugs; and processes for determining when a member is ill and whether professional care will be sought and how. A goal is to promote the family's physical, mental, and social health through the use of nursing interventions, to provide comfort to the family, and to prevent deterioration of the family system.

In the *role-performance model,* health is viewed as effective performance of roles; family health then can be defined along the dimensions identified in the structural-functional and developmental frameworks as the effective meeting of family functions and developmental tasks. The nurse assesses how effective the family structure and processes are in accomplishing critical functions and tasks. Areas for assessment include family current developmental stage and developmental history; family role structure; socialization patterns; family resources for meeting family functions and developmental tasks; and family perceptions of family functioning. Nursing goals are to promote effective performance of family functions and the achievement of family developmental tasks through interventions that assist the family to identify and mobilize support systems and resources.

Health in the *adaptive model* is the condition of the whole person engaged in effective and fruitful interaction with the physical and social environment; adaptation is the predominant feature of this interaction (Smith, 1983). The nursing goal in the adaptative model is to promote the family's adaptation and health-directed patterning with the environment.

Health in the *eudaimonistic model* is defined as the "condition of complete development of the individuals' potential for general well-being and self-realization" (Smith, 1983, p. 87). Family health is viewed within this model as the development of the family's well-being and maximum potential, with the goal of promoting the same. This implies a target of mobilizing the full energy level and creativity of the family system. Areas of assessment include the family's values and goals; family interaction patterns; family patterns of recreation and relaxation; family cohesion; and family promotion of autonomy. Interventions include working with families to clarify values; assisting families to identify and prioritize their goals; and working with families to implement plans to meet goals.

Clinical Example

Consider the example of the Russell family. The family consists of Mr. and Mrs. Russell, 6-year-old Ann, 4-year-old Jim, and 1-month-old Karen, who was born prematurely and spent 3 weeks in a neonatal intensive care unit (NICU). The community health nurse has been working with the family as the result of a referral from the NICU stating the parents expressed concern about caring for such a small infant and about her future health. Obviously, in this example community health nursing intervention could be emphasized in any one of the four dimensions of health promotion.

The focus in a clinical health promotion approach might be to work with the family to identify realistic perceptions of health risks for Karen and to teach the parents how to recognize symptoms of distress and appropriate measures to take. Assessment would include determining Mr. and Mrs. Russell's perceptions and knowledge of premature infants, identification of the family's health care resources, and recognition of their concerns regarding caring for a premature infant.

This family is in the developmental stage of families with preschool children, based on the age of the oldest child. Developmental tasks for families in this stage include:

1. Supplying adequate space, facilities, and equipment for the expanding family.
2. Meeting predictable and unexpected costs of family life with small children.
3. Sharing responsibility for household management and care within the young family.
4. Maintaining mutually satisfying intimate communication in the family.
5. Rearing children already present and planning future family size.
6. Relating to relatives on both sides of the family in creative ways.
7. Tapping resources outside the family in the wider community.
8. Maintaining morale in the face of life's changes and dilemmas. (Duvall & Miller, 1985, p. 199.)

Assessment in the *role-performance model* would include exploring with the family their feelings regarding their abilities and resources to accomplish these tasks. Based on the assessment, the nurse can help the family identify areas of strength and areas in which external resources may be necessary to accomplish tasks, for example working with the family to identify ways to mobilize social supports to give the family the flexibility to meet needs for socialization and affection.

Assessment within the dimension of *adaptive health promotion* would focus on identifying with the family the kinds of changes that have occurred since Karen's birth and the different or new demands that have resulted. The nurse would work with the family to adapt to both a new member of the family and to repattern their life to account for the increased and different demands of a premature infant. Pointing out the knowledge and skills the family already has, and ways to adapt them to the changes in the family system, build on family competencies. Another potential intervention would be working with the family to identify parent support groups in the community.

In the eudaimonistic model, the nurse could work with the family in reassessing family goals and ways to meet them. At some point it might be appropriate to discuss with the family ways in which they could offer support to other families in similar circumstances.

Families' Perspectives

From the perspective of the health paradigm, another, less prevalent, approach to identifying dimensions of family health is to examine families' perceptions of their health. As part of a larger study of families and health behavior (Loveland-Cherry, 1983) parents and children were asked to rate their families' health on a six-point scale and to describe what they thought of when asked about family health. Characteristics of family health identified by children and parents included participation in health behaviors (eating healthy foods, getting enough rest, exercising regularly); absence of illness (very little sickness, healthy bodies, mentally healthy); a feeling of well-being (high energy levels, enthusiastic living, happy home, supportive, mutual respect, love, having fun together; having regular health care; and ability to function in usual roles. Knowing what the family identifies as being healthy provides direction for the nurse in working with the family to identify and reach health promotion goals.

Defining the Focus of Family Health Promotion
Promoting Family Members' Health

An important question for the nurse to consider in working with families is the emphasis on the client unit; that is, whether the focus is on an individual family member or on the family unit. Nursing interventions may focus on promoting the health of individual family members in interaction with the family environment. In this instance, the goal, whether from a pathogenic or health paradigm, is to promote the health of the individual by working with the family system unit. The basis for this approach derives from the identification of relationships between specific family characteristics and the health and health-related behavior of family members. Parenting styles characterized by a high degree of autonomy and support for the child, active participation in the community, health training efforts by parents, flexible division of tasks, egalitarian power structure, family cohesiveness, and promotion of autonomy of family members have been found to be positively related to both parents' and children's health beliefs and behaviors (Hanson, 1986; Loveland-Cherry, 1984, 1986; Pratt, 1976). These findings are consistent with the view that competency in managing one's life is a basis for participation in health-promoting behaviors (Loveland-Cherry, 1982; Petze, 1984; Pratt, 1973, 1976). The importance of the family as the primary environment for learning values and behavior and for reinforcing positive behaviors is critical in planning strategies for family health promotion.

Most of the models for understanding health behavior—and consequently interventions based on them—have been developed for individuals or special population groups. A number of the critical variables in the models—for example, cognitive-perceptual factors, including importance of health, definition of health, perceived self-efficacy (Pender, 1987); perceived barriers (Pender, 1987; Becker, Haefner, Kasl, et al., 1977); general resistance resources (Antonovsky, 1979)—are developed and learned within the family environment. Therefore renewed interest in designing family interventions to promote health behavior is evident in the recent literature. Some initial success of a project "encouraging family members to support each other's attempt to alter their diet and exercise patterns" has been reported by Baranowski, Nader, Dunn and Vanderpool (1982). This intervention consisted of using tangible and emotional social support by families to promote dietary and exercise change in family members. The results indicate that promotion of

social support for change among family members encourages changes in diet but not in exercise. Additionally, it was found that families need assistance in learning how to provide support to promote health behavior changes. The work was preliminary to development of the Family Health Project, which focuses on low-income black families with children ages 8 to 10 years (Barnowski, Dunn, Simon Morton, et al., 1986). Other programs have focused on promoting cardiovascular health through family intervention programs in the community (Glueck, Laskorszewski, Rao, et al., 1985; Matarazzo, Connor, Fey, et al., 1982). The viability of family interventions for health promotion has long been advocated (Mauksch, 1974) and is now documented (Simons-Morton, O'Hara and Simons-Morton, 1986).

Promoting Family System Health

In contrast to working with the family system to promote individuals' health, the focus of nursing service can be the health promotion of the family system both internally and in interaction with social, political, economic, educational, physical and health systems. In this instance the goal is to promote the health of the family system. Areas for assessment may not differ markedly in either focus, but in this instance the emphasis is on how the family system interacts as a whole and how capable it is of interacting with other systems. The community health nurse often functions as a facilitator between the family and other systems. For example, the nurse often functions as the link between schools and families in identifying health-related needs of families and assisting school personnel to design programs related to health (see Chapters 39, 40, and 41 for further elaboration).

MODALITIES FOR PROMOTING FAMILY HEALTH
Family Home Visits

Community health nurses work with families in a variety of settings, including clinics, schools, support groups, offices, and the family home. An important aspect of community health nursing's role in promoting the health of populations has been the tradition of providing services to individual families in their homes.

Purposes

Home visits afford the opportunity to gain a more accurate assessment of the family structure and behavior in the natural environment. Home visits also provide opportunities to make observations of the home environment and to identify both barriers and supports for reaching family health promotion goals. The nurse can work with the client firsthand to adapt interventions to meet realistic resources. Meeting the family on their home ground may also contribute to the family's sense of control and active participation in meeting their health needs. The majority of these studies have focused on the maternal-child population.*

A home visit may be more than just an alternative setting for service; it may be an intervention modality. If the home

---

*Barkauskas, 1983; Lowe, 1970; Hall, 1980; Larson, 1980; Siegel, Bauman, Schaefer et al., 1980; McNeil & Holland, 1972.

visit is to be a valuable and effective intervention, careful and systematic planning must occur. Mayers (1973) cautions that the process of home visits may become more a patterned response set, or ritual, rather than a vital exchange with productive outcomes.

In recent years the viability of providing large portions of health promotion services through home visits has been critically reexamined by agencies, including health departments and visiting nurse associations (VNAs). Barkauskas (1983) identified the following advantages and disadvantages of home visits. Advantages include convenience for the client, client control of the setting, option for those clients unwilling or unable to travel, and a natural, relaxed environment for the discussion of concerns and needs. Costs were the major disadvantage identified by Barkauskas; the costs of previsit preparation, travel to and from the home, time spent with one client, and postvisit preparation are high. In a study comparing teaching new mothers in groups versus during home visits, the group approach was found to be more effective in terms of knowledge and cost approximately one third that of home visits (McNeil & Holland, 1972). Many agencies have actively explored alternative modes of providing service to families, particularly group interventions (see Chapter 14). The important issue regarding the value of home visits is determining which families would most benefit from them and how home visits can most effectively be structured and scheduled. With increasing demands for home health care, the home visit is once again becoming a prominent mode for delivery of nursing services.

Process

The components of a home visit are summarized in Table 20-1 and elaborated in the following sections.

INITIATION OF A HOME VISIT. Usually a home visit is initiated as a result of a referral from a health or social agency. However, a family may request services or the nurse may initiate the home visit as a result of casefinding activities. Subsequent home visits should be based on need and mutual agreement between the nurse and the family. Regardless of the impetus for making a home visit, it is essential that the nurse be clear about the purpose for the visit and that the nurse's perceptions or understanding be shared with the family.

PREVISIT PHASE. The previsit phase has several components. First, if at all possible, the family should be contacted before the home visit. A telephone call to the family to introduce oneself, identify the reason for the contact, and schedule the home visit is strongly recommended. Leavitt (1982) suggests that a first telephone contact should be brief, with an outside limit of 15 minutes. The nurse should give both name and professional identity: for example, "This is Karen Smith. I'm a community health nurse from the Middle County Health Department." The family should be informed of how they came to the attention of the community health nurse, for example, a referral or a contact from observations or records in the school setting. If a referral has been received, it is important and useful to ascertain whether or not the family is aware of the referral. This will establish a perspective of valuing the client's input and

TABLE 20-1

Phases and activities of a home visit

Phase	Activity
I Initiation phase	Clarify source of referral for visit
	Clarify purpose for home visit
	Share information on reason and purpose of home visit with family
II Previsit phase	Initiate contact with family
	Establish shared perception of purpose with family
	Determine family's willingness for home visit
	Schedule home visit
	Review referral and/or family record
III In-home phase	Introduction of self and professional identity
	Social interaction to establish rapport
	Establish nurse-client relationship
	Implement nursing process
IV Termination phase	Review visit with family
	Plan for future visits
V Postvisit phase	Record visit
	Plan for next visit

involvement in care. Next, a brief summary of the nurse's knowledge and information allows the family to know the extent of the nurse's information about the family. The nurse might say "I understand that your baby was discharged from the hospital yesterday and that you requested some assistance with caring for her at home." A visit should be scheduled for as soon as is possible and appropriate for both the nurse and the family. Letting the family know agency hours available for visits and the approximate length of the visit as well as the purpose are helpful to the family in determining when to set the visit. Although the length of the visit may vary, depending on circumstances, approximately 45 minutes is usual (Kallins, 1967).

If possible, the visit should be arranged so that as many of the family members as possible will be available for the entire visit. It is also important for the nurse to tell the client about any fee for the initial visit and subsequent visits and potential methods of payment. The telephone call can terminate with a review by the nurse of the time, place, and purpose for the visit and a way for the family to contact the nurse in case they need to verify or change the time for the visit or to ask any questions they may not have asked during the initial phone call. If the family does not have a telephone, another method for setting up the visits can be used. The most obvious are dropping off a note at the family home or sending a letter or postcard informing the family of when and why the home visit will occur, again with a means for the family to contact the nurse if necessary.

Of course, the possibility always exists that the family may refuse to agree to a home visit. Less experienced nurses or students may interpret this as a personal rejection when it is not. Families regulate who and when outsiders are allowed entry into their territory (Kantor and Lehr, 1982). The nurse needs to explore the reasons for the family not wanting a visit; there may be a misunderstanding about the reason for a visit or lack of information about services. If the nurse determines that either the situation has been resolved or services have been obtained from another source, and if the family understands the services available and how to contact the agency if desired, then the contact may be terminated as requested. However, the nurse should leave open the possibility of future contact. There are instances when legal obligations, for example follow-up of certain communicable diseases, mandates that the nurse persist in requesting a home visit.

Before the visit it can be useful for the nurse to review the referral or, if not a first visit, the family record. If there is a time lapse between the contact and the visit, a brief telephone call to confirm the time often avoids a not at home visit.

IN-HOME PHASE. The actual visit to the home affords the nurse the opportunity to assess the family's neighborhood. An issue that may arise either in approaching the family home or once the family has opened the door to the nurse is that of personal safety. Nurses need to examine their own fears and objective threats to determine if safety is indeed an issue. Certain precautions can be taken in known high-risk situations. Agencies may provide escorts for nurses or have them visit in pairs; readily identifiable uniforms may be required; a signout process indicating timing and location of home visits may be used routinely. The nurse needs to use caution; if a reasonable question about the safety of making the visit exists, the visit should not be made.

"Pride, the ethic of self-sufficiency, territoriality, and privacy" are issues for nurses making home visits with families (Leavitt, 1984, p. 288). The nurse needs to be aware that families may feel that they are being "checked up on," are seen as being inadequate or dysfunctional, or that their privacy is being invaded. Nursing services, especially those from health departments, are thought of by the public as being "public services" for needy families or those with insufficient funds to pay for care. These potential concerns underline the needs for sensitivity by the nurse, clarity in information regarding the reason for visits, and the establishment of collaborative, trusting relationships with the family.

The changing nature of the American family can make it difficult to schedule visits during what have been traditional agency hours. The number of working single-parent or dual-wage earner two-parent families is increasing, which means that families have many more demands on their time. Even if one parent is at home during the usual work day, the ideal is to work with the entire family. This is often not possible because of conflict between agency hours and school or work schedules. It may be possible to schedule a visit at the beginning or end of a day to meet with working or school-age members. In some parts of the country agencies are reconsidering traditional hours and Monday through Friday visits.

Families may not be able to control interruptions during the visit. Telephones ring, pets join in the visit, people come and go, televisions are left on. The nurse can ask that for a limited time televisions be turned off or other disruptive activities be limited (Leavitt, 1982). Families may be so used to the background noises and routine activities that they do not recognize them as being potentially disruptive.

The actual home visit includes several components. First, once at the home, the nurse needs to again provide personal identification and professional affiliation. This is part of the introductory phase. Then there should be a brief social period to allow the client to assess the nurse and to establish rapport (Leahy, Cobb & Jones, 1982).

The major portion of the home visit is concerned with establishing the relationship and implementing the nursing process. Assessment, intervention, and evaluation are ongoing. It is important that the nurse be realistic about what can be accomplished in a home visit. In some situations, one visit may be all that is possible or appropriate. In this instance, needs and resources for meeting needs are explored with the family and determination made if further services are desired or indicated. If the latter is the case and the current agency is not appropriate, the nurse can assist the family to identify other services available in the community and help in initiating any referrals. Although it is not unusual to have only one home visit with a family, often multiple visits are made (Guilino & LaMonica, 1986). The frequency and intensity of home visits vary not only with the needs of the family but also with eligibility for services and agency policies and priorities. It is realistic to expect at least the beginning of building a relationship and initial assessment to occur on a first visit.

TERMINATION PHASE. When the purpose of the visit has been accomplished, the nurse reviews with the family what has occurred and been accomplished. This provides the client the opportunity to recognize what has been done and provides a basis for planning any further home visits. Ideally, termination of the visit and ultimately of service begins at the first contact, with the goal or purpose being defined. Frequently, nurses are not sure of the reason for the visit; consequently, the visit is unfocused and either aimlessly comes to a close or abruptly ends. If communication has been clear to this point, the family and nurse can plan for future visits, specifically, the next visit. Planning for future visits is part of another issue—setting goals and planning service. Contracting is a constructive approach to working with clients and is receiving increasing attention by health professionals. The purpose and components of contracting with clients are discussed in the next section.

POST-VISIT PHASE. Even though the nurse has concluded the home visit and left the client's home, responsibility for the visit is not complete until the interaction has been recorded. (See Chapter 12 for a discussion of the purposes of record keeping). Agencies may or may not organize their records by families; that is, the basic record may be a "family" folder, or a record with all members included in one record, or it may be that each family member receiving services has a separate record, with family members' records cross referenced. In reality the concept of a family-focused record often breaks down. History and background are usually given to some extent for the family, but often the focus shifts to individual health histories and consequently nursing diagnoses, goals, and interventions that are directed toward individual family members rather than the family unit. Record systems and formats vary from agency to agency. The nurse needs to become familiar with the particular system used in the agency. All systems should include the following elements: a data base, nursing diagnoses and problem list; a plan, including specific goals; actual actions and interventions; and evaluation. These are the basic elements needed for legal and clinical purposes. The format may consist of narrative, flow sheets, POMR, SOAP or a combination of formats. It is important that all records be current, dated, and signed.

Using theoretical frameworks appropriate to working with families gives direction to the family-centered nursing process. For example, a nursing diagnosis of "Ineffective mothering skill related to lack of knowledge of normal growth and development" is an individual-focused nursing diagnosis. "Inability for family to accomplish stage-appropriate task of providing safe environment for preschooler related to lack of knowledge and resources" is a family-focused nursing diagnosis based on knowledge of the developmental approach to families. To provide family centered nursing care, diagnoses, goals, and interventions need to be family focused. At times the need will also exist to present information for a specific family member. However, the emphasis should be on the individual as a member of, and within the context of, the family.

Contracting in Family Health Promotion

Increasingly, health professionals have come to look toward working with clients in a more interactive, collaborative style. This approach is consistent with a more knowledgable public and the recent self-care movement. *Contracting,* which is an agreement between two or more parties, involves a shift in responsibility and control to a shared effort by client and professional versus that of the professional alone. The ANA Standards of Community Health Nursing Practice (1986) explicitly state the rights of clients to actively participate in planning their own health care and designate that "in partnership with the family and individual" the community health nurse collects, interprets, and analyzes data; formulates and validates diagnoses; formulates plans and implements interventions; and evaluates process and revision of the plan. This active involvement of the client is reflected in several of the existing nursing models, particularly those of Rogers (1979), King (1981), and Orem (1984). Contracting is one strategy aimed at promoting a collaborative working relationship, in this instance, one specifically focused on health promotion.

Contracting is one way of formalizing and explicating the involvement of the family in the nursing process. Some nurses are reluctant to use the term *contracting* but discuss essentially that very process in terms of *mutual goal setting.* Some of this reluctance may be related to the potential legal ramifications of a contract, whether formal or informal.

There may be concern regarding possible liability in terms of services agreed upon versus those delivered or received, or attainment of agreed-upon outcomes. Further, the connection of the term *contracting,* in some instances, with that of compliance may be contrary to a philosophy of an interactive partnership between nurse and client.

Thus an important issue is the purpose and/or philosophy that underlies the nurse's contracting with families. A large body of literature addresses the "non-compliant" client or family. Edel identifies the concept of compliance as applying to relationships between "those who have power and those over whom they exercise it" (Edel, 1985, p. 183). These relationships are described as vertical, with one party dominating the other. This approach is obviously incongruent and inconsistent with the collaborative relationship described above. If contracting is viewed only as another approach to increase compliance, the basic premises of the concept are violated. Contracting addresses the issue of control by client versus control by the professional (Hayes & Davis, 1980).

Purposes of Contracting

The purpose of contracting is to enhance and support the client's active role in health care by defining who will do what to accomplish health-related goals (Herje, 1984). Sloan and Schommer (1975) differentiate between a legal contract and a nursing contract. The former is defined as a written, binding agreement; the latter as a working agreement that is continuously renegotiable and may or may not be written. Further, a nursing contract may be either a contingency or noncontingency one. A contingency contract explicates a specific reward for the client based on completion of the client's portion of the contract; a noncontingency contract does not specify rewards. The implied rewards are the positive consequences of the reaching of goals specified in the contract.

In the instance of family health promotion, it is essential that the contract be made with all responsible and appropriate members of the family. Involving only one individual is invalid if the goal is family health promotion, which requires a total family system effort and change. Scheduling a visit with all family members present may require extra effort; if meeting with the entire family is not possible, each family member can review a contract, give input and sign it. This allows for active participation by all family members without the necessity of finding a time when everyone involved can be present.

The Process of Contracting: Phases and Activities

Contracting is a learned skill on the part of both the nurse and the family. All parties involved need to know the purpose and process of contracting. Leavitt (1982) identifies three general phases: beginning, working, and termination. The three phases can be further specified into seven sets of activities: mutual exploration of problems or needs, mutual establishment of goals, mutual exploration of resources, development of a plan, mutual agreement on division of responsibilities, setting of time limits, mutual evaluation, modification, and renegotiation or termination of contract (Sloan & Schommer, 1975). The phases and activities are summarized in Table 20-2, and an example of a contract is included in Appendix B2.

The first activity involves both the family and the nurse in data collection and analysis of the data. An important aspect of this step is obtaining the family's perspective of the situation and its needs and problems. The nurse can present her observations and validate them with the family and also gain the family's view. Leavitt (1982) suggests that the initial contract be based on the most obvious or concrete of the family's needs; more subtle problems can be added as the family and nurse build their working relationship.

It is important that goals be mutually set and realistic. A pitfall for nurses and clients who are new to contracting is to set overly ambitious goals. The nurse should recognize that there may be discrepancies between professional priorities and those of the client and thus real negotiation is required. Because contracting is a process characterized by renegotiation, the goals are not static.

Throughout the process, the nurse and family need to continually learn and recognize what each can contribute to meeting health needs. This exploration of resources allows both parties to become cognizant of their own and others' strengths and requires a review of the nurse's skills and knowledge, family support system, and community resources.

Developing a plan to meet the goals involves specifying activities, prioritizing goals, and selecting a starting point. Next the nurse and the family need to decide who will be responsible for which activities. Structuring time limits involves deciding on a deadline for accomplishing or evaluating progress toward accomplishing a goal and the frequency of contacts. At the agreed on time, the nurse and family together evaluate the progress to date in both process and outcome. Based on the evaluation, the contract can be modified, renegotiated, or terminated.

Advantages and Disadvantages of Contracting

Contracting takes time and effort and may require a reorientation to roles on the part of both the family and the nurse. Increased control by the family also means increased responsibility. Some nurses may have difficulty relinquishing the role of the controlling expert professional. Contracts will not always be successful. In fact, there are instances in which contracting is neither appropriate nor possible. There are clients who because of a variety of personality characteristics and other reasons do not desire to have this kind of involvement; they prefer to defer to the "authority" of the professional. Included in this group are individuals with minimal cognitive skills, those who are involved in an emergency situation, those who are unwilling to be more active in their care, and those who do not see control or authority for health concerns within their domain (Herje, 1980). Some of these clients may learn to contract; some never will.

The use of the nursing process does not necessarily provide for an active role for the family as a client; it assumes that needs exist based only on professional judgment and that changes should and can be made within the family unit. Contracting is one alternative approach that is predicated upon the value of input from both the nurse and the

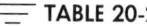

TABLE 20-2

Phases and activities in contracting

Phase	Activity
I Beginning Phase:	Mutual data collection and exploration of needs and problems
	Mutual establishment of goals
	Mutual exploration of resources
	Mutual development of a plan
II Working Phase:	Mutual division of responsibilities
	Mutual setting of time limits
	Mutual implementation of plan
	Mutual evaluation and renegotiation
III Termination Phase:	Mutual termination of contract

family, responsibility on the part of the family, and the dynamic nature of the process, which not only allows for but also requires continual renegotiation. Although it may not be appropriate in all situations or with all families, contracting can give direction and structure to health promotion in families.

Community Resources

Families have varied and complex needs and problems. The community health nurse often mobilizes a number of resources in order to effectively and appropriately meet family health promotion needs. While the specific resources vary from community to community, general types can be identified. A number of governmental resources, such as Medicare, Medicaid, Aid to Families of Dependent Children, Supplementary Security Income, Food Stamps, and W.I.C. (Women, Infants, Children) are available in most communities. These programs primarily provide support for basic needs, i.e. illness/health care, nutritional needs, funds for housing and clothing, based on meeting of eligibility criteria.

In addition to governmental agencies providing health related services to families, most communities have a number of voluntary (nongovernmental) programs. Local chapters of such organizations as the American Cancer Society, American Heart Association, American Lung Association, and Muscular Dystrophy Association provide educational and support services and some direct services to individuals and families regarding specific conditions. These agencies provide primary prevention and health promotion services as well as screening programs and assistance once the disease or condition is diagnosed. Local social service agencies, such as Catholic Social Services, provide direct services such as counseling to families. Other voluntary organizations provide direct service (e.g., shelters for homeless or battered individuals, substance abuse counseling and treatment, Meals on Wheels programs, transportation, clothing, food, furniture).

Health resources in the community may be proprietary, voluntary, or public. In addition to private health care providers, community health nurses should be aware of voluntary and public clinics, screening programs, and health promotion programs.

Identifying resources in a community requires time and effort on the part of the nurse. One obvious and valuable source is the telephone book. Often community service organizations, for example, the Chamber of Commerce, and the local health department publish community resource listings. Regardless of how the resource is identified, the nurse must be familiar with the type of service offered and any requirements or costs involved. If this information is not available, the community health nurse can contact the resource to obtain necessary information. (See Chapter 38 for more discussion of available community resources.)

Locating and using these systems often require skills and patience that many families lack. Community health nurses work with families not only in identifying community resources but also as a client advocate and in assisting families to learn to use resources. This may involve sharing information with families, rehearsing with families what questions to ask, preparing required materials, making the initial contact, or arranging transportation. Finally, the appropriateness and effectiveness of resources should be evaluated with families following referrals.

CLINICAL APPLICATION

The initial referral for community health nursing service to a family provides limited information, and the situation that develops may turn out to be much more complex than anticipated. The following example, based on an actual case, illustrates the issues and approaches outlined in this chapter.

A referral was received at the Middle County Health Department indicating that Amy Cress, age 16, had been referred by the school counselor at the local high school for prenatal supervision. Amy was 4 months pregnant, in apparently good health, in the tenth grade, and living at home with her mother, stepfather, and younger sister. The family lived in a rural area outside of a small farming community. Amy's boyfriend and father of the baby also lived in the community and continued to see her on a regular basis.

The community health nurse phoned the home to make an appointment for a home visit. Amy's mother answered the phone and indicated that Amy was at school during the day. The nurse introduced herself and explained that the counselor at the high school had talked with Amy about the possibility of having a community health nurse from the health department assist her to learn more about her pregnancy, labor and delivery, and caring for a new infant. Amy's mother sounded both relieved and enthusiastic about having the nurse visit. Although Amy was in school during the day, she could arrange to be at home so the nurse could meet her at the end of the agency working day. An appointment was made for within the week to meet with Amy and her mother.

At the first home visit, it became apparent that Amy and her mother were interested in continuing community health nursing service. Amy and her mother identified a number of questions and concerns. How could Amy finish her education and care for a child? What would labor and delivery be like? How could Amy and her boyfriend avoid unplanned pregnancies in the future? How could the family

members be supportive and yet have their own needs met? A second visit was scheduled to include Amy's boyfriend and father. During the second visit, a contract was negotiated to continue visiting with Amy, but the visits would occur at school during a study period. The focus would be on prenatal teaching on the nurse's part, with Amy agreeing to attend a group for pregnant students offered at the school. Additionally, visits were arranged with Amy's mother to discuss her concerns. Over time, the contract was modified and expanded to include well-child supervision during the year following the birth of a healthy baby boy. Additionally, during this time Amy's paternal grandfather, who had been recently widowed, became ill and unable to live alone. The grandfather moved into the family home, and the family became a four-generation unit. Amy's mother discussed a number of conflicts regarding her commitment to caring for her father, assisting with the care of her grandson until Amy finished school and could make other arrangements, having time for her other daughter, and continuing to develop her relationship with her husband in a fairly new marriage (she had been widowed 3 years earlier). The contract was modified to include working with Amy's mother to renew her child care skills, provide health supervision for the grandfather, and identify a schedule for the family that allowed time for the mother and stepfather to have some time alone. The complexity of the family's needs meant that the contract was frequently modified and that not all plans worked. Amy's mother eventually indicated that alternative care was needed for the grandfather and, based on a variety of options identified by the nurse and the mother, an adult foster home was located and a placement made. Conflict arose between Amy's and her boyfriend's individual developmental needs as adolescents and family developmental tasks to be accomplished (see box on p. 363 for a comparison of tasks). Plans and responsibilities had to be renegotiated. With much effort, some pain, and a great deal of commitment to each other, the family moved to a pattern described by Smith (1983) as role-sharing in incorporating the adolescent mother and child into the household. Successful completion of the developmental tasks of confirmation of pregnancy to family, committing to a new system, redefining relationships and role-sharing characterized the evolution of this family into this pattern. The family has yet to deal with whether or not Amy and her son will continue to live in the family home when she finishes the beautician training she enrolled in after high school. Amy's mother has indicated a desire to have Amy, Amy's son, and the baby's father live as a separate unit, with or without marriage.

This family situation is not an unusual one and reflects many of the problems and needs of contemporary families. The skills required of the community health nurse are many and varied. Knowledge of family structure, function, developmental tasks, family support systems, health promotion over the lifespan, and community resources have been essential at various points in working with this family.

SUMMARY

Promoting health in families is a complex process that requires an understanding of family therapy, health promotion, changing family structure, and forces that affect families. This chapter presented an overview of the implications of changing family and health systems for family health promotion.

Although community health nurses come in contact with families in a variety of settings, the home visit continues to be a major modality for providing service to families. The purposes and advantages and disadvantages of home visits were reviewed. The considerations necessary for effective implementation of home visits with families were also presented.

To formalize and effectively implement the nursing process in family health promotion, the concept of contracting with families was identified. Three phases and specific activities provide guidelines for implementing this strategy. Working with families to promote the health of family systems, family members, and ultimately communities will continue to be an important aspect of community health nursing.

KEY CONCEPTS

The importance of the family as a major client system for community health nursing in promoting the health of individuals and populations is well-documented; the family system is a basic unit within which health behavior, including health values, health habits, and health risk perceptions are developed, organized, and performed.

Knowledge of family structure and functioning, family theory, nursing theory, and models of health behavior are fundamental to implementing the nursing process with families in the community. However, community health nurses need to recognize important issues that influence family health promotion. Issues related to family health promotion originate from three major sources: the family system itself, the health care system, which includes the discipline and profession of nursing; and the social, political, and economic environment within which the family exists.

From the perspective of the health paradigm, another, less prevalent approach to identifying dimensions of family health is to examine families' perceptions of their health.

An important question for the community health nurse to consider in working with families is the emphasis on the client unit; that is, whether the focus is on an individual family member or on the family unit.

In contrast to working with the family system to promote individuals' health, the focus of nursing service can be the health promotion of the family system both internally and in interaction with social, political, economic, educational, physical, and health systems.

An important aspect of community health nursing's role in promoting the health of populations has been the tradition of providing services to individual families in their homes.

Home visits afford the opportunity to gain a more accurate assessment of the family structure and behavior in the natural environment. Home visits also provide opportunities to make observations of the home environment and to identify both barriers and supports for reaching family health promotion goals.

Increasingly, health professionals have come to look toward working with clients in a more interactive, collaborative style.

Contracting, which is an agreement between two or more parties, involves a shift in responsibility and control to a shared effort by client and professional versus that of the professional alone.

The purpose of contracting is to enhance and support the client's active role in health care by defining who will do what to accomplish health related goals.

Families have varied and complex needs and problems. The community health nurse often mobilizes a number of resources in order to effectively and appropriately meet family health promotion needs.

LEARNING ACTIVITIES

1. Select one or more agencies in which community health nurses work and examine the agency's and community health nursing's philosophies and objectives with emphasis on individual care, family care, illness care, health promotion, and prevention.

2. Form small groups and discuss approaches that can be used by community health nurses for integrating family health promotion and prevention activities into existing health services.

3. Identify three community health problems in your community and discuss the implications of these problems for the health of families. Identify three health problems common to families in your community and discuss the implications of the problems for the health and/or health care resources of the community.

4. Select three to four families (hypothetically or from actual situations) representative of different ethnic and socioeconomic backgrounds. Compare the similarities and differences in their health promotion behaviors. How are their health promotion behaviors related to the factors of motivation, perceptions, values, and attitudes?

BIBLIOGRAPHY

Antonovosky, A.: Health, stress, and coping, San Francisco, 1979, Jossey-Bass Publishers.

American Nurses' Association, Council of Community Health Nurses: Standards of community health nursing practice, Kansas City, 1986, American Nurses' Association.

Baranowski, T., Nader, P.R., Dunn, K., and Vanderpool, N.A.: Family self-help: Promoting changes in health behavior. J. Communication 32(3):161-172, 1982.

Barkauskas, V.H.: Effectiveness of public health nurse home visits to primarous mothers and their infants, Am. J. Pub. Health 73(5):573-580, 1983.

Becker, M.H., Haefner, D.P., Kasl, S.V., et al.: Selected psychosocial models and correlates of individual health-related behaviors, Medical Care 15:27-46, 1977.

Berg, C.L., and Helgeson, D.: That first home visit, J. Commun. Health Nurs. 1(3):207-215, 1984.

Chin, S.: Can self-care theory be applied to families? In Riehl-Sisca, J., editor: The science and art of self-care, Norwalk, Conn., 1985, Appleton-Century-Crofts. (pp. 56-62)

Clements, I.W., and Roberts, F.B., editors: Family health: a theoretical approach to nursing care, New York, 1983, John Wiley & Sons, Inc.

Duvall, E.M., and Miller, B.C.: Marriage and family development, ed. 6, New York, 1985, Harper & Row, Publishers, Inc.

Edel, M.K.: Noncompliance: an appropriate nursing diagnosis? Nurs. Outlook 33(4):183-185, 1985.

Gluek, C.J., Laskorszewski, P.M., Rao, D.C., et al.: Familial aggregation of coronary risk factors. In Coonan, W., and Bristow, D., editors: Complications in coronary heart disease, Philadelphia, 1985, J.B. Lippincott.

Guilino, C., and LaMonica, G.: Public health nursing: a study of role implementation, Pub. Health Nurs. 3(2):80-91, 1986.

Hall, L.A.: Effect of teaching on primiparas' perception of their newborn, Nurs. Res. 29:317-321, 1980.

Hanson, J.: The family. In Roy, C., editor: Introduction to nursing: an adaptation model, ed. 2, Englewood Cliffs, N.J., 1984, Prentice-Hall. (pp. 519-533)

Hanson, S.M.H.: Healthy single parent families, Fam. Relations 35(1):125-132, 1986.

Hayes, W.S., and Davis, L.L.: What is a health care contract? Health Values: Achieving High Level Wellness, 4(2):82-89, 1980.

Helgeson, D.M., and Berg, C.L.: Contracting: a method of health promotion, J. Commun. Health Nurs. 2(4):199-207, 1985.

Herje, P.A.: Hows and whys of patient contracting, Nurse Educator 5(1):30-34, 1980.

Johnston, R.L.: Approaching family intervention through Rogers' conceptual model. In Whall, A.L., editor: Family therapy theory for nursing: four approaches, Norwalk, Conn., 1987, Appleton-Century-Crofts. (pp. 11-32)

Kallins, E.L.: The textbook of public health nursing, St. Louis, Mo., 1967, The C.V. Mosby Co.

Kantor, D., and Lehr, W.: Inside the family, San Francisco, 1977, Jossey-Bass.

King, I.M.: A theory for nursing: systems, concepts, process, New York, 1981, John Wiley & Sons.

King, I.M.: King's theory of nursing. In Clements, I.W., and Roberts, F.B., editors: Family health: a theoretical approach to nursing, New York, 1983, John Wiley & Sons. (pp. 177-188)

Laffrey, S.C., Loveland-Cherry, C.J., and Winkler, S.J.: Health behavior: evolution of two paradigms, Pub. Health Nurs. 3(2):92-100, 1986.

Larson, C.P.: Efficacy of prenatal and postpartum visits on child health and development, Pediatrics 66:183-190, 1980.

Leahy, K.M., Cobb, M.M., and Jones, M.C.: Public health nursing, ed. 3, New York, 1982, McGraw-Hill, Inc.

Leavitt, M.B.: Families at risk: primary prevention in nursing practice, Boston, 1982, Little, Brown & Co.

Litman, T.J.: The family as a basic unit in health and medical care: a social behavioral overview, Soc. Sci. Med. 8:495-519, 1974.

Loveland-Cherry, C.J.: Family system patterns of cohesiveness and autonomy: relationship to family members' health behavior, Dissertation Abstracts Intern. 43(11B):35-37, 1982.

Loveland-Cherry, C.J.: Family system patterns of autonomy and cohesiveness: relationship to family members' health behavior, Nurs. Res. 33(1):51-52, 1984.

Loveland-Cherry, C.J.: Personal health practices in single parent and two parent families, Fam. Rel. 35(1):133-139, 1986.

Lowe, M.L.: Effectiveness of teaching as measured by compliance with medical recommendations, Nurs. Res. 19:59-63, 1972.

McCubbin, H., and Patterson, J.: Family adaptation in crisis. In McCubbin, H., Cauble, A., and Patterson, J., editors: Family stress coping and social support, Springfield, Ill., 1982, Charles C Thomas, Publisher. (pp. 26-47)

McNeil, H.J., and Holland, S.S.: A comparative study of public health nurse teaching in groups and in home visits, Am. J. Pub. Health 62(12):1629-1637, 1972.

Matarazzo, J.D., Connor, W.E., Fey, S.G., et al.: Behavioral cardiology with emphasis on the family heart study: fertile ground for psychological and biomedical research. In Millon, T., Green, C.J., and Meagher, R.B., editors: Handbook of health care psychology, New York, 1982, Plenum Press.

Mauksch, H.O.: A social science basis for conceptualizing family health, Soc. Sci. Med. 8:521-528, 1974.

Mayers, M.: Home visit—Ritual or therapy? Nurs. Outlook 21(5):328-331, 1973.

Olson, D.H., Sprenkle, D.H., and Russell, C.: Circumplex model of marital and family systems. I. Cohesion and adaptability dimensions, family type, and clinical applications, Fam. Proc. 18:3-28, 1979.

Orem, D.E.: The self-care deficit theory of nursing: a general theory. In Clements, I.W., and Roberts, F.B., editors: Family health: a theoretical approach to nursing care, New York, 1983, John Wiley & Sons. (pp. 205-217.)

Orem, D.E.: Nursing concepts of practice, New York, 1985, McGraw-Hill Book Co.

Pender, N.J.: Health promotion in nursing practice, ed. 2, Norwalk, Conn., 1987, Appleton & Lange.

Pesznecker, B.L., and Zahlis, E.: Establishing mutual help groups for family-member care givers: a new role for community health nurses, Pub. Health Nurs. 3(1):29-37, 1986.

Petze, C.F.: Health promotion for the well family, Nurs. Clin. North Am. 19(2):229-237, 1984.

Pratt, L.: Child rearing methods and children's health behavior, J. Health Soc. Behav. 14:16-19, 1973.

Pratt, L.: Family structure and effective health behavior, Boston, 1976, Houghton Mifflin Co.

Rogers, M.: An introduction to the theoretical basis of nursing, Philadelphia, 1970, F.A. Davis Co.

Rogers, M.E.: Science of unitry human being: A paradigm for nursing. In Clements, I.W., and Roberts, F.B., editors: Family health: a theoretical approach to nursing care, New York, 1983, John Wiley & Sons. (pp. 219-228)

Roy, C.: Introduction to nursing: An adaptation model, ed. 2, Englewood Cliffs, N.J., 1984, Prentice Hall, Inc.

Siegel, E., Bauman, K.E., Schaefer, E.S., et al.: Hospital and home support during infancy: impact on maternal attachment, child abuse and neglect, and health care utilization, Pediatrics 66:183-190, 1980.

Simons-Morton, B.G., O'Hara, N.M., and Simons-Morton, D.G.: Promoting healthful diet and exercise behaviors in communities, schools, and families, Fam. Commun. Health 9(3):1-13, 1986.

Sloan, M.R., and Schommer, B.T.: The process of contracting in community nursing. In Spradley, B.W., editor: Contemporary community nursing, Boston, 1975, Little, Brown & Co.

Smith, J.A.: The idea of health: implications for the nursing professional, New York, 1983, Teachers College Press, Columbia University.

Smith, L.: A conceptual model of families incorporating an adolescent mother and child into the household, Adv. Nurs. Sci. 6(1):45-60, 1983.

Tadych, R.: Nursing in multiperson units: the family. In Riehl-Sisca, J., editor: The science and art of self-care, Norwalk, Conn., 1985, Appleton-Century-Crofts. (pp. 49-55.)

Whall, A.L.: Family therapy theory for nursing: Four approaches, Norwalk, Conn., 1987, Appleton-Century-Crofts.

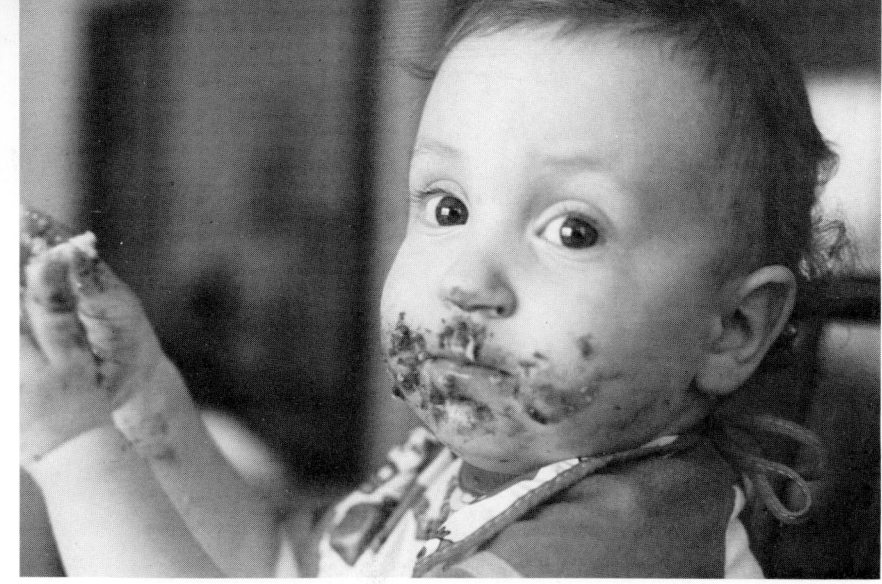

Nancy Dickenson-Hazard

21

THE FIRST YEAR OF LIFE

☰ OBJECTIVES

After reading this chapter, the student should be able to:

Identify and discuss significant factors in the prenatal environment that influence neonatal health.

Describe the characteristic elements of physical and psychosocial growth and development in the first year of life.

Discuss appropriate nursing assessment tools for the child from birth through 1 year.

Identify and discuss major factors affecting growth and development.

Identify and discuss major causes of death and illness in the child from birth through 1 year.

Identify the role of the community health nurse and discuss appropriate nursing interventions that promote and maintain the health of the neonate and infant.

☰ KEY TERMS

allergy

Apgar scoring

bonding

congenital anomaly

critical period of development

dehydration

fetal assessment

gestational age

growth spurts

hyperbilirubinemia

immunity

jaundice

kernicterus

low birth rate

malnutrition

maternal-infant bond

mothering

motherliness

neonatal period

otitis media

parent-child bond

paternal-infant bond

prematurity

Recommended Daily Allowances (RDAs)

reflex activity

sensory function

sudden infant death syndrome

temperament

upper respiratory tract infection (URI)

vomiting and diarrhea syndrome

Children are one third of our population and all of our future . . . their health is our foundation.

The promotion of child health provides society with an opportunity to be well. Since children must learn health practices, the opportunity to teach health promotion and maintenance is greater for children than any other population.

Childhood is the period of life when most behaviors are learned, and parents are the primary teachers of acceptable behavior. The community health nurse has the opportunity to be involved in this learning process by helping parents learn methods of teaching children positive behaviors.

This chapter provides information on the assessment of child health within the community for the child from birth through age 1 year. The content includes age-specific growth, development, definition of major health problems, and the tools and techniques of health promotion activities.

PRENATAL ENVIRONMENT

Assessing the quality of the atmosphere in which a fetus grows is the first step in ensuring a healthy childhood. The community health nurse has the opportunity to make this assessment in a variety of settings. Being aware of the prenatal factors that promote wellness facilitates the nurse's assessment.

Before Conception

At the moment of conception some aspects of wellness are determined. Influential in their effect on fetal health before and at the time of conception are genetic and chromosomal abnormalities, blood group incompatibilities, and maternal age and state of health. The education and counseling of prospective parents about these factors are important aspects of the nurse's role.

Of primary concern is that up to 5% of all births in the United States involve birth defects, the majority of which are inherited (Behrman, 1987). Although prevention of genetic defects is the primary objective when advising the parents at risk, facilitating parental knowledge regarding the disorder becomes a priority once conception has occurred. Nursing's assessment and referral are essential elements of the complex process of genetic counseling. Table 21-1 describes appropriate nursing interventions before and after conception (Williams, 1986).

TABLE 21-1

Nursing implications: facilitating parental knowledge regarding genetic disorders

Before conception	After conception
Identify parents at risk	Identify parents at risk prenatally
Provide educational programs on common genetic disorders	Implement data collection including medical history, family pedigree, and laboratory data
Provide individual explanation sessions for parents at risk	Implement individual counseling session regarding the disorder with parents
Implement data collection, including medical history, family pedigree, and laboratory data	Refer parents for genetic counseling
Implement an education session on the specific disorder	Refer parents to local groups
Refer parents for detailed genetic counseling	Teach family regarding genetic counseling program
	Evaluate family understanding, coping and adjustment
	Be knowledgeable regarding available health care services and resources specific to the disorder

After Conception

Once conception has occurred, fetal growth becomes dependent on the intrauterine environment. The physical and psychosocial well-being of the mother is influenced by many elements such as nutrition, physical health, use of prenatal services, exposure to hazardous substances in the environment, circumstances of conception, and adjustment to pregnancy. The role of nursing at this point is to facilitate good maternal health, thereby ensuring fetal health.

Nursing activities that promote maternal health and the environment after conception include:

Complete data collection mechanism, including pregnancy, maternal health and family history

Physical assessment and appropriate laboratory studies

- Plan of care in collaboration with parents-to-be, focusing on their physical and psychosocial needs, including readiness and ability to parent.

Fetal Assessment and Parent Education

Despite efforts to ensure fetal health through maternal health promotion, fetal difficulties can and do arise. **Fetal assessment** evaluates the fetus's physical environment and the physical and psychosocial environment of the mother. Through knowledge and use of data from modern technologies which detect these difficulties (sonography, amniocentesis, and mechanical fetal monitoring), the nurse can better assess fetal health. Being aware of the indicators of high-risk parents (i.e. adolescent, single, unplanned, history of mental illness, substance abuse or child abuse, previous pregnancy or child loss, no permanent living plan, or a high number of children close together) assists the nurse in the fetal assessment. Further nursing interventions should be based on actions that provide optimal adjustment to the parent role through information sharing, explanations, reassurance, and assisting parents to balance family stresses and support (Miller, 1986).

As the pregnancy progresses, education about the neonate and parenting must begin and monitoring of maternal and fetal physical health must continue. The pediatric prenatal visit is an effective health promotion activity in which expectant parents, with the nurse's help, can lay the groundwork for positive influences on the child's health. The optimal time for the prenatal assessment is at 33 to 37 weeks gestation before parents begin to focus on delivery (Miller, 1986).

PHYSICAL GROWTH AND DEVELOPMENT

The terms *growth* and *development* incorporate two distinct concepts: (1) quantitative or measurable aspects of the increase in the size of individuals (growth) and (2) qualitative or observable aspects of the progressive changes in the individuals as they adapt to their environment (development) (Waechter, 1976).

Human growth and development are orderly, predictable processes that begin with the embryo and continue until death. Individuals progress through definite phases of growth and development in their lifetime. These phases are influenced by a multitude of hereditary and environmental factors.

When assessing the measurable and observable aspects of growth and development, the nurse must be cognizant of the overall process as well as the factors that influence it. In addition, each person progresses through the different phases of growth and development in his own manner and at his own pace, demonstrating behaviors that are clearly individual to him. These individual variations within orderly growth and development processes must also be considered when assessment is implemented.

The Neonate

The period of life from birth to 1 month is commonly referred to as the **neonatal period.** During this phase of life the newborn's functioning and behavior are mostly reflexive. Stabilization of major body functions is the primary task of the neonate and occurs in a definite sequence of physiologic events in the first hours of life. Nurses need to be aware of the normalcy of this sequence and to be alert to the subtle physical changes it produces when making an assessment (see a basic pediatric text for a complete discussion of the neonatal transition period).

Physical Assessment

Physical examination of the newborn is one of the most important tools for assessing neonatal health. Using the data obtained from a physical examination provides the nurse with an opportunity to implement preventive health activities.

With the trend toward early discharge after delivery (within 24 to 48 hours), the community health nurse frequently conducts a *neonatal assessment.* Though the physical examination of a newborn does not differ greatly from the general pediatric physical assessment, the nurse needs to be aware of normal variations and minor abnormalities that may be apparent, especially in the home setting. Appendix J1 provides a compilation of these normal variations and guidance for appropriate anticipatory nursing procedures.*

Though these variants place the newborn in no immediate danger, they are usually a cause of worry and concern for parents. Understanding their origin, presence, and course enables the nurse to facilitate parental coping and should be the basis, along with reassurance and support, for educating parents about these normal variations.

Apgar Scoring

Neonatal physiological function at birth is assessed through observation and scoring of the newborn characteristics of appearance, pulse, grimace, activity, and respirations (Apgar, 1966). (See a basic pediatric text for a complete discussion of *Apgar scoring.*) Although the community health nurse does not perform this assessment, knowledge of the data obtained provides information pertinent to the management of well-infant care.

Gestational Age

Gestational age (GA) is defined as the number of weeks spent in utero to the time of birth (Dubowitz, 1970). Estimates of GA serve as indicators to physical maturity, are an important aspect of evaluating neonatal physical growth and development, and provide a method for identifying potential problems needing preventive action. The community health nurse will find knowledge of GA useful for nutritional teaching, developmental assessment, parent education regarding infant care, and providing referrals for identified problems.

Physiological Changes

The average newborn weighs 7 lb 1 oz (3200 g), is 19½ inches (49 cm) in length, and has a head circumference of 13½ inches (34 cm). At birth, major organ systems are

---

*Brown and Murphy, 1981; Chow et al., 1984; DeAngelis, 1979; Scipien et al., 1979; Tackett and Hunsberger, 1981; Behrman et al., 1983.

functional though not advanced. As the neonate develops physically, an individual and identifiable pattern of growth begins to appear. The normal newborn can lose up to 10% of birth weight in the first few weeks of life, primarily as a result of fluid losses through respiration, urination, defecation, and decreased intake. Generally, birth weight is regained between the second and third week of life. By 1 month the neonate should be beginning a pattern of weight gain of 5 to 7 ounces per week. A gain in length of ½ to 1 inch per month, and an increase of 2 cm per month in head circumference. See Appendix K2 for growth measurement averages.

Physiological stabilization is affected by birth and the rapid growth of the neonate. These physiologic changes are evidenced through the monitoring of vital signs. Community health nurses should be proficient in measuring vital signs and growth and need to be aware of the subtle changes which occur in these indicators during the neonatal and infancy periods, to make an accurate assessment of the newborn's physiological functioning. (See a basic text in pediatric nursing for a review of vital sign values.)

Danger Signs

Although most newborns adjust to functioning outside the uterine environment without incident, the possibility of neonatal difficulty exists. The nurse should therefore be alert to the danger signs indicating a need for referral and management when assessing the newborn (Chow, et al., 1984). These danger signs are presented in the box below.

Reflex Activity

Reflex activity of the neonatal period and early infancy stage is dominated by a large number of primitive reflex patterns. These reflexes are generally present at or shortly after birth. Absence or asymmetry of reflexive response or abnormal persistence of response beyond the time of voluntary motor function is an indication of a serious health problem. Since the newborn, later the infant, is largely dependent on re-

flexive ability, assessment of these response characteristics and their timing of appearance and disappearance becomes vital to the infant's health. (See Appendix K4 for a summary of reflexes and techniques of assessment.)

Sensory Function

Sensory function of the newborn is primitive. The neonate perceives and responds to tactile stimulation that is soothing and painful. Although visual acuity is poor, the newborn can fixate both eyes for a short period of time as well as follow large moving objects and blink in response to bright light. Auditory stimulation evokes changes in motor activity as evidenced by the startled reaction to loud, sudden noises. Taste is also primitively developed in the newborn, demonstrated by a response to sweet and sour stimulation. Additional techniques for screening infant sensory function can be found in Appendix K5.

Family Adaptation to the Neonate

The birth of a child creates changes for the family members. Assessment of how the family is adapting to these changes becomes an essential part of the nursing process and should focus on parenting skills and ability of parents to assume new roles and responsibilities; sibling reaction and behavior; changes in the marital and parent–previous child(ren) relationships and communication patterns; reorganization of daily family functioning and distribution of labor; availability of resources outside the family; changes in extended family and friend relationships; and making family adjustments. Nursing interventions to facilitate these changes are indicated and may include actions such as encouraging parents to go out by themselves; encouraging parents to set aside time alone with older sibling(s); encouraging parents to ask grandparent or friend to babysit; referring parents for financial assistance or other government-sponsored child health programs; and assisting parents in planning their daily activities.

DANGER SIGNS IN THE NEWBORN

A positive family history for major disease or illness	Full, bulging fontanel
Gestational or delivery complications	Small head size
Abnormal positioning of baby	Convulsions, twitching, excessive irritability
Congenital malformations	Lethargy
Rapid or difficult respirations	Fever or hypothermia
Rapid, slow, or irregular pulse	Paralysis
Abnormal cry	Jaundice
Unusual cough	Pallor
Cyanosis	Petechiae
Sweating	Behavior or appearance change
Vomiting of bile	Excess salivation
Delayed or inadequate voiding	Diarrhea
Bleeding, specifically noting cord and circumcision	No meconium passage in first 48 hours
Single umbilical artery	Cord odor or exudate

Adapted from Chow, M.P., et al.: Handbook of pediatric primary care, ed. 2, New York, 1984, J. Wiley & Sons, Inc., pp. 262; and Behrman, R.E., and Vaughan, V.C., editors: Nelson textbook of pediatrics, ed. 13, Philadelphia, 1987, W.B. Saunders Co., pp. 373-385.

The Infant

Infancy extends from 1 month to 1 year, and during this period of time major physical growth is occurring. Generally infants double their birth weight by 6 months and triple it by 12 months of age. By the end of the first year, an infant grows between 10 and 12 inches in length.

Physiological Stability

Physiological functioning becomes more sophisticated at this time. Circulatory and respiratory function matures, as evidenced by stabilization of vital signs. Refinement of physiological ability is also seen in the evolution of patterns of body function.

Sleep

The average newborn sleeps approximately 16 hours a day. During wakeful periods, the baby's attention span is quite short (7 to 10 minutes) and focuses primarily on gratification of needs. The timing and pattern of newborn sleep is generally quite unpredictable and without routine (Table 21-2).

Sleeping patterns become more predictable over the next few months, and by 3 months of age the infant is generally sleeping through the night and taking several naps during the day. By 12 months nighttime sleep is extended to 11 to 12 hours, naps are decreased to 1 to 2 per day, and a quite predictable routine of sleep and activity has developed. The attention span of a 12-month-old also has increased, demonstrated by an ability to remain engaged in an activity up to 30 to 45 minutes versus 15 to 20 minutes at 6 months.

Elimination

The elimination patterns of the infant also change throughout the first year. The first meconium stools are generally passed within the first 48 hours followed by transitional stools about the third or fourth day. Subsequent stool frequency and consistency are dependent on the type and amount of oral intake an infant receives. Breast-fed babies tend to have bright mustard yellow stools that are soft and unformed with curdlike matter and very little odor. Bottle-fed babies tend to have yellow to yellowish green stools that are more formed and odoriferous. Frequency of stool elimination is largely dependent on gastrointestinal absorption and mobility and is thus individualized from infant to infant. In general, breast-fed babies have fewer stools per day (one to three) than bottle-fed babies (four to six) in the first weeks. This pattern reverses after 2 to 3 weeks, and the frequency of stool elimination increases in breast-fed babies and decreases in bottle-fed babies.

Most newborns urinate involuntarily within the first 24 hours and have between six to eight wet diapers per 24 hours in the first weeks. As bladder capacity increases,

TABLE 21-2

Normal sleep patterns

Age	Number of hr/24 hr	Advice about sleeping habits
Newborn	Low: 10 Average: 16½ High: 23 (7-8 short naps)	No child fits into a routinely prescribed sleep pattern.
8-12 weeks	(2-4 naps)	Release into sleep varies with infants. Some are more tense than others.
2-4 months	Low: 8-10/night High: 11-12/night 2-3 naps/day	Although there is no correlation with solid food intake and sleeping through the night, the parent's attitude may make the difference.
6-12 months	11-12/night 2-3 naps/day	There should be an established routine for bedtime. Baby may wake because of illness, teething, or separation anxiety.
12-18 months	8-12/night 1-2 naps/day	There may be waking problems after the mother returns to work, even after several months.
2-3 years	8-12/night 1 nap/day	There is a need for rituals and consistency at bedtime. Active children may not nap after 2½ years.
3-4 years	8-12/night May take 1 nap/day	Some children wake with dreams. (One fifth of the night is spent dreaming.) Many children wake and wander at night. Some children accept a net over the crib or a locked half-door on the bedroom. The habit of sleeping with parents should be discouraged. This is a good time to shift from crib to bed.
4 years	8-12/night	Some dreaming and waking may result.
4½-5 years	8-12/night	There may be an increase in bad dreams and night terrors. The child may need considerable attention to get back to sleep. The child may enjoy reading at bedtime before lights out. Dreams may be at a low peak.

From Chow, M.P., et al.: Handbook of pediatric primary care, ed. 2, New York, 1984, John Wiley & Sons, Inc., p. 264.

frequency tends to decrease, and volume of voiding increases.

Feeding

During the first year of life feeding behavior and patterns become a function of physiological development. The stomach capacity for fluids at birth is 30 to 60 ml (1 to 2 oz). Caloric and fluid requirements of the newborn are 55 kcal/kg/24 hours and 80 to 150 ml/kg. Hence the neonate feeds often in small amounts. As stomach capacity for fluids increases from 90 to 150 ml (3 to 5 oz) at 1 month to 240 ml (8 oz) at 1 year and caloric and fluid requirements stabilize, the feeding frequency of an infant decreases, and the amount per feeding increases.

In general, newborns are unpredictable in regard to how often they want to feed. Some require feeding every 2 hours, whereas others extend to over 4 hours. However, a pattern of feeding every 3 to 4 hours should begin to appear by 12 weeks of age. By 6 months an infant wants to eat 3 to 5 meals per day, and by 12 months most have developed a pattern of 3 meals a day and a snack. (See Appendix J4 for feeding and nutritional guidelines.)

Growth Spurts

Physical growth in the first year is evidenced by periods of time called *growth spurts.* During these spurts patterns of infant behavior change in a chain-reaction type of response to the process of physical maturation. Physiological functioning and subsequent metabolic requirements increase in response to the growing body's demand for increased energy through calories, the infant alters feeding patterns by increasing both the amount and the frequency of feeding. The infant may also become fussy and irritable.

Sleeping patterns may be altered, with some infants requiring more sleep while others may have interrupted or fretful sleep due to hunger. Elimination is also affected and generally decreases in frequency. However, if feeding needs are overmet, elimination patterns may increase or remain the same.

Growth spurts are most frequent and noticeable by parents in the first 6 to 8 months of life but occur periodically until adolescence. The first evident spurt occurs approximately at 6 weeks of age, and growth spurts may recur every 6 to 8 weeks until approximately 6 months of age. The behavioral changes usually last 4 to 7 days. For parents who have not been prepared to expect this normal growth occurrence, the changes in the infant's behavior can be stressful. Nurses can prevent this potential stress for parents and infants by providing (1) early anticipatory guidance and education regarding the origin and course of growth spurts, (2) counseling on how to manage them, and (3) support and reassurance when they do occur.

Neuromotor Assessment

Neuromotor development in the first year occurs in a cephalocaudal direction of head to foot progression. As the infant progresses through this pattern of physical development, he or she gains more voluntary control over the use of his or her body. Activity and behavior by 1 year have become more purposeful and less reflexive. (See Appendix K9 for physical and motor developmental characteristics.)

PSYCHOSOCIAL DEVELOPMENT

A child's growth process includes not only physical development but also emotional and social development. Many variables influence the child's psychosocial growth. Psychological variables generally relate to interpersonal and cognitive characteristics, as well as personality and temperament differences. Social and cultural variables include such factors as family structure, familial attitudes, beliefs, and economic status.

Critical Periods

As with physical development, individual differences must be considered when assessing the child's psychosocial development. The individuality of a child's progression through the developmental phases is also influenced by the concept known as *critical periods of development.* A critical period is a specific span of time during which the environment has its greatest impact on a child's development. The nature of stimuli provided by the environment varies among children. A child's developmental progression depends on the timing and degree of environmental stimuli and his or her readiness to be stimulated by the environment (Sutterly and Donnelly, 1978). For example, an infant cannot learn to ride a bike regardless of the intensity of the stimuli, whereas a 6-year-old has the readiness and ability to learn.

Developmental Theories

Many theories of growth and development have evolved to explain this human process. Most familiar are the theories of Erikson and Piaget. The framework of these developmental hypotheses is used throughout this section.

Erikson

Erikson's theory of psychosocial development is based on the process of socialization. He theorizes life development as a continuous struggle for an emotional-social equilibrium. Though Erikson's theory acknowledges the presence of an id, ego, and superego as defined by Freudian theory, it adds the further dimension of environmental influences on personality development. According to Erikson, each stage of life has its own tasks to be mastered, each has negative counterparts. Equilibrium occurs when the primary task of the stage is mastered. However, Erikson stresses that the negative counterparts are never completely mastered and must be reevaluated at subsequent times throughout life (Erikson, 1963).

Piaget

Piaget's theory of development focuses on cognition, which undergoes a gradual qualitative growth over the childhood years. According to Piaget, a variety of new experiences (or stimuli) must exist for learning to occur. The individual response to these stimuli occurs through assimilation and accommodation. *Assimilation* is the process of incorporating new experiences into current activities or thinking (i.e., experiences are adapted to the individual). *Accommodation* is the process of responding to the environment through a new means of activity and thinking (i.e., the individual is adapted to experiences). The combination of these processes allows the child to organize his or her world by ordering and classifying personal experiences. The end result is adaptation or the balance between the individual and his environment through new and expanded thoughts, behaviors, and problem-solving methods (Piaget, 1951).

Psychosocial Competency

Much of the foundation for psychosocial competency is built during the first year of life. According to Erikson, this first stage of life from birth to 1 year is charged with the task of developing trust versus a sense of mistrust. The newborn enters the world dependent on others for meeting his needs. If basic needs are met through a close, warm, comforting relationship, a sense of trust develops. If needs are not met or are only met sporadically, a sense of mistrust develops, since a child is never certain that needs will be met. The caretaker-infant relationship therefore becomes an important factor in the infant's development of a sense of trust. The quality of this relationship has a direct impact on the infant's sense of well-being as influenced by the behavioral consistency and motivation of the caretaker.

Traditionally, the caretaker in our society is the infant's mother. However, becoming a mother does not necessarily mean being motherly. A *mother* is defined as a biological parent, whereas *mothering* is the means necessary to care for the infant. *Motherliness* is the capacity of the mother to be gratified by the exchange between herself and her infant and to use this gratification for her own growth. Mothering and motherliness are the qualitative characteristics that are necessary for the infant's development of a sense of trust (Klaus and Kennell, 1976). However, these qualities do not spontaneously occur at the moment of conception or birth but are developed as the mother and infant learn to respond to each other. The synchronization of maternal and infant responses, which results in a unique emotional relationship, is termed *bonding* or *attachment*.

Bonding theory has been closely scrutinized and its early research criticized in the past few years. Moderate short-term effects for some parents and their infants have been found, and it has been discovered that bonding is a multifaceted, complex process (Mitchell and Mills, 1983). Only nurses who understand the process and know when to use it can intervene to strengthen the parent-child relationship.

MATERNAL-INFANT BOND. Attachment occurs when mother and infant elicit behaviors from each other that are reciprocal and complimentary. Maternal attachment behaviors are largely centered on a mother's attentiveness to her infant and her maintenance of physical contact. Infant attachment behaviors center on maintaining focus or contact with the mother (Bowlby, 1969). The box below outlines attachment behaviors identified in mothers and infants.

As with any process of human development, the interaction between mother and infant and subsequent attachment are influenced by many factors. These variables include not only maternal and infant characteristics but also environmental factors, such as housing conditions and sleeping arrangements, as well as the mother's cultural and preg-

---

MATERNAL AND INFANT ATTACHMENT BEHAVIORS

MATERNAL BEHAVIORS

1. Prenatal period
   a. Expression of attitude about changing body image
   b. Verbalization about fetus
   c. Response to quickening
   d. Preparations for baby
   e. Degree of anxiety and fear about labor and delivery
   f. Desire for knowledge about labor and delivery
   g. Degree of emotional lability
2. Intrapartum period
   a. Spontaneity of verbal response at delivery
   b. Attempts to see and touch baby
   c. Questions about condition, appearance, and behavior of infant
   d. Reaction to sex of baby
3. Postpartum period: claiming and identification through
   a. Touch—proximal, ventral (close to body), affectionate
   b. Distal contact—talking to and about infant
   c. Eye contact
   d. Recognization of individualization of infant
   e. Performance of caretaking responsibilities in a positive manner

INFANT BEHAVIORS

1. Sucking
2. Rooting
3. Grasping
4. Clinging
5. Regular changes between sleep, wakefulness, activity, and crying
6. Smiling and babbling
7. Normal activity level
8. Response to ministrations by calming
9. Visual alertness
10. Response to sensory stimuli
11. Quiets when presented with mother's face, voice, touch
12. Response to feeding

Adapted from Bowlby, J.: Attachment and loss, vol. 1, Attachment, New York, 1969, Basic Books, Inc., Publishers: Clark, A.L., and Alfonso, D.D.: Childbearing: a nursing perspective, ed. 2, Philadelphia, 1979, F.A. Davis Co.; and Klaus, M.H., and Kennell, J.H.: Maternal-infant bonding, ed. 2, St. Louis, 1982, The C.V. Mosby Co.

nancy experiences, the infant's appearance and responsiveness, and the family's financial and psychosocial support resources. Nurses can facilitate the attachment by assessing the influence these factors have on the process and intervening with support and guidance when appropriate.

FATHER-INFANT BOND. Although the maternal-infant bond is the primary influence on the infant's sense of well-being, the importance of the father-infant bond cannot be negated. This attachment occurs in much the same manner as the maternal-infant bond. Infant and father progress through an acquaintance process. Initially in this process, father and infant acquire information about each other through behaviors and signals. Once signals are received and responded to, each assesses the other's responsiveness to the signals. Finally, as infant and father begin to relate in a reciprocal manner, further aspects of personality become known to each other and serve to validate or negate previous responsiveness.

The father's participation in meeting the demands of child rearing and nurturing is further facilitated when the opportunity for bonding occurs early in the infant's life. A father's image of a baby is one of separateness, contrary to the mother, who views the baby as an integral part of herself; therefore the father's attachment to the infant is not as strong initially. Nursing suggestions which promote early exposure, such as holding the baby in the delivery room, interacting with the baby at home by rocking, talking to, and holding the infant, and participating in the infant's care, provide the needed circumstances for father-infant bonding to begin.

The development of a *paternal-infant* bond is especially important in our society today. Extended families are less available to new parents, thereby increasing the father's support role within the nuclear family. Bonding of father and infant facilitates the development of this paternal role, allowing the father to provide for the emotional and physical needs of the infant (Wieser and Castiglia, 1984).

PARENT-CHILD BOND. In addition to the individual bonds mother and father develop with their infant, they also need to nurture a bond as a parental unit (Duvall, 1977). Working in unison to promote healthy growth and development of their infant needs to be a focus of new parents, but often feelings of insecurity intervene. The nurse can assist parents in developing as a unit by being an empathetic listener, by teaching parenting skills that gratify the infant's and parents' needs, and in understanding normal growth and development.

Cognitive Competency

The development of cognitive competency is rapidly expanding in the first year of life. Piaget views the first 2 years of life as the sensorimotor period. During this period the infant moves from reflexive to symbolic behavior, when expression and communication originate from the infant's body. During the first 24 months a child progresses through six stages toward cognitive competence. Stage 1 from birth to 1 month is characterized by the use of reflexes and random body movements. A neonate has no awareness of self or of a world outside of self. Stage 2 from 1 to 4½ months is characterized by habits of behavior that are learned by chance and repeated for their pleasurable benefit. These new behaviors or habits are the result of physical maturation as well as repetitive use of reflexes and random movements. In stage 3 an infant of 4½ to 9 months achieves eye-hand coordination. New behaviors that were accidentally discovered initially are repeated as a means of making the environment more interesting. Stage 4 brings the coordination of more complex behaviors as perception begins to develop in the 9- to 12-month-old. The infant learns to get around obstacles or to use a new means to get what he wants.

By 12 to 18 months the toddler is demonstrating experimentation behaviors. Through trial and error the toddler discovers different ways to achieve the desired result. The evidence of beginning reasoning, memory, and retention appears in these activities. Between 18 and 24 months the child develops the ability to form mental images, and thoughts are characteristically symbolic. Imitation becomes apparent in this stage, and permanency of objects is a well-developed thought.

Nursing Role

Stimulation of an infant's psychosocial and cognitive environment is an important parenting skill that nurses can teach. The need for visual, sensory, and tactile stimulation in promoting healthy development is as essential for the infant as food. Appendix J3 provides age-appropriate stimulation suggestions that can be used in the first year.

Knowledge and assessment of developmental milestones are also important aspects of infant development. Fine and gross motor skills were previously reviewed in this chapter. An appropriate focus when assessing psychosocial and cognitive development centers on an infant's social and language behaviors. Characteristic behaviors are reviewed in Appendix A3 and K9.

FACTORS AFFECTING GROWTH AND DEVELOPMENT
Mastery

Human growth and development are continuous processes that are complex yet predictable. Although the exact age for accomplishing the specific tasks of each stage varies from child to child, a chronology of events does exist, which involves a wide range of norms, allowing for individual differences. The individual pace of a child through the developmental stages is set by a variety of factors. Of primary importance in this progression from one stage to another is the successful mastery of the tasks and milestones of the preceding stage (Erikson, 1963). Because development is a sequential process, a child must successfully complete, in an individual style, the particular task of the specific developmental stage. For example, a 15-month-old cannot run unless walking occurs first. Similarly a 2-year-old cannot separate easily from mother unless the child has come to trust her. Although a child never completely finishes all the developmental tasks in a given stage, some degree of mastery and comfort must be achieved before proceeding successfully to the next stage (i.e., a child continues to learn to trust other people throughout life but must have developed a basic trust of mother to separate and expand into the world).

Heredity

Hereditary variables must be considered as factors that influence growth and development. In assessing such variables the nurse must be cognizant of the physical and psychosocial results of an individual's genetic makeup. Physical characteristics and diseases are inherited as are some aspects of the individual's behavioral temperament (Chess and Thomas, 1983). Therefore the nurse should assess these genetic forces through an evaluation and history of the genetic makeup of several generations.

Temperament

Children differ in personality temperament. *Temperament,* defined as an individual's behavior style, is usually one of the following three types: easy, slow to warm, and difficult (Chess and Thomas, 1983). Characteristics are shown in Table 21-3. Children have been found to demonstrate temperamental characteristics in the first weeks of life. Though the environment can influence a child's behavior, the basic temperament is unique to each child.

Health and Living Environment

The health of an individual and the quality of the living environment influence growth and development. A child's state of health affects not only his or her responsiveness in the developmental process, but the responsiveness of others to him or her as well. Similarly, conditions affecting health, such as adequacy of nutrition, sleep, rest, and exercise influence the child's development. For example, the infant who does not sleep well at night and has become a picky eater may be unable to meet the developmental task of sociability because of being tired and possibly poorly nourished.

Characteristics of the physical environment also play an important part in this process. These factors include adequacy of housing, socioeconomic status, season and climate of the home, and geographic location.

Family, Peers, and Life Experiences

The family's central purposes are the protection and promotion of its members. Of importance early in the child's life are the nature and adequacy of the bond developed between family members, particularly between parent and child. The quality of the parent-child relationship has been found to affect the child's development.

Second to the family in influencing development are a child's peers. Through and with a peer group, a child learns about self, others and society, accomplishing a wide variety of developmental tasks.

Dealing with and learning through family and peers provides the child with experiences that enable progress developmentally. By applying what has been learned to what needs to be learned the child can use experience to recognize and master further developmental tasks.

Additional nurturing influences that affect development include the ordinal position (oldest, youngest, or middle child), presence and sex of siblings, sex of the child, family structure and societal attitudes, and expectations and culture as interpreted within the child's home.

COMMON CAUSES OF MORBIDITY AND MORTALITY

Major strides have been made over the past 5 years to improve the safety of life for infants. The infant mortality in 1984 was a record low 10.8 infant deaths per 1000 live births. This reduction in infant mortality is attributable to improved nutrition, housing, and prenatal, obstetrical, and pediatric care. Provided current trends continue, the mortality for infants in the United States will be reduced to 8 deaths per 1000 live births in 1990 (Progress Review, 1985).

Despite a drop in the infant mortality over the past 10 years, significant problems still exist. The first year of life is the most hazardous period until age 65. Black infants remain at risk. Nearly twice as many black infants die before their first birthdays than do white infants. Similarly, infants from low-income situations, certain regional areas, and of certain heritages demonstrate higher morbidity and mortality (Progress Review, 1985).

The primary threats to infant health and survival are low birth weight (immaturity), congenital anomalies with associated problems, and *sudden infant death syndrome (SIDS).* In 1982 the leading cause of death in children under 1 year of age was congenital anomalies and the secondary effects of such birth defects. The second leading cause of death in 1982 was SIDS, followed by immaturity (Progress Report, 1985).

Congenital Anomalies

A *congenital anomaly* is any deviant organ or part existing before or at birth in an abnormal form, structure, or location, but not necessarily detected at birth (Behrman et al., 1987). Congenital anomalies involving the heart and circulatory system occur in approximately 8 of every 1000 infants. The chance of a congenital heart defect in the new-

---

TABLE 21-3

Temperament and personality characteristics

Temperament	Characteristic
Easy	Positive mood
	Regular body functions
	Low to moderate intensity of reaction
	Adaptability to new situations
Slow-to-warm up	Low activity level
	Tendency to withdraw on first exposure to new stimuli
	Slow adaptability
	Somewhat negative mood
	Low intensity of reaction to situations
Difficult	Irregular body functions
	Intensity in reactions
	Withdrawal from new stimuli
	Slow adaptation
	Negative mood

Adapted from Chess, S., and Thomas, A.: Dynamics of individual development. In Levine, M.D., Carey, W.B., Crocker, A.C., and Gross, R.T., editors. *Developmental Behavioral Pediatrics.* Philadelphia: W.B. Saunders, 1983, pp. 158-175.

born sibling of an affected child is approximately 5% (Behrman, 1987). The need for genetic counseling of the parents of an affected child is apparent, with referral to genetic resources as appropriate.

Cardiovascular Anomalies

Since congenital anomalies, particularly those of the cardiovascular system, pose the greatest mortality threat to infants, the nurse should be familiar with the major signs and symptoms of congenital heart disease. Early recognition and referral facilitate early management and potentially reduce the threat of death. The physical findings in newborns and infants with congenital heart disease include anorexia, cyanosis, delayed development, enlarged heart or liver, dyspnea during feeding, failure to gain weight, heart murmurs, tachycardia (up to 150 to 200 beats per minute at rest), tachypnea (up to 50 to 60 respirations per minute at rest), and recurrent respiratory infections and distress.

Major Organ Systems

Congenital anomalies of other major organ systems may also pose a threat to infant health. (See a basic pediatric nursing text for a review of the major organ system anomalies and their accompanying signs and symptoms.) Although the incidence of these birth defects is less frequent and in some cases not as life threatening as those of the cardiovascular system, the nurse has a responsibility to be knowledgeable of the symptoms when making an assessment. Those most likely to be lethal to the infant in addition to the congenital heart defects are malformations of the brain and spinal conditions involving the combination of several malformations, such as spina bifida and hydrocephalus.

Genetic Disorders

Also included under the diagnosis of birth defects are the genetic diseases. About one fourth of these defects are thought to be genetic in origin. The five types of genetic or inherited disease factors that cause the most illness and death include Down's syndrome, brain and neural tube defects, defects related to ethnic groups (e.g., Tay-Sachs disease, sickle-cell anemia, cystic fibrosis), sex-linked defects (e.g., hemophilia, muscular dystrophy), and metabolic disorders (Behrman, 1987).

External Factors

Birth defects may also result from exposure of the fetus to toxic agents during pregnancy. External factors that increase infant mortality and morbidity include infections, particularly rubella; exposure to radiation and chemicals; and maternal alcohol or drug abuse.

Sudden Infant Death Syndrome

Sudden infant death syndrome (SIDS) is responsible for approximately 8000 deaths per year occurring in infants from ages 1 week to 1 year (Progress Review, 1985). It occurs most often between 2 and 4 months of age and is found to be uncommon before 1 month and after 8 months. SIDS occurs more frequently in males, low birth weight infants, twins, and low socioeconomic groups. It often oc-

curs during normal sleep periods and happens during times of the year when the incidence of upper respiratory illnesses is increased.

Definition

SIDS is the sudden death of any infant or young child, which is unexpected by history and in which a thorough postmortem examination fails to demonstrate an adequate cause of death. Its etiology has eluded identification; multiple theories of causation have evolved over the years. Current theories and epidemiologic factors under review range from nasal obstruction, neurological problems, and respiratory instability to allergic reactions, chronic hypoxia and depressed CO_2 sensitivity. Nurses should be familiar with the theories because they are frequently in a position to provide counseling and answer questions of concerned or grieving clients.

Clinical Presentation of SIDS

The clinical picture presented by the family of a SIDS victim is relatively unremarkable; most infants die at home, during the night while sleeping, without difficulty, and unobserved. Parents often discover their infant lying lifeless in the crib, often in a state of disarray, with a blood-stained fluid in the nose and mouth. Approximately one half have experienced cold symptoms in the week before death (Chow, 1984).

Infants at Risk for SIDS

Currently no reliable screening tool exists for identifying infants at risk for SIDS. However, recent studies have identified a group of infants who appear to be at increased risk. These "near miss" infants have shown a tendency to have episodes of apnea. The use of apnea monitoring for these infants remains controversial. Although at-home monitoring may alert parents to a difficulty that is occurring, it cannot prevent SIDS.

Siblings of infants who have died from SIDS are also at risk. These siblings experience three times a greater incidence of SIDS than siblings whose family history is free of SIDS.

For the family of infants at risk for SIDS, the community health nurse can be a valuable resource, particularly if home apnea monitoring is instituted. Appropriate nursing interventions may include parent teaching about SIDS, monitoring, and CPR; coordinating discharge planning between home and hospital; assisting family to secure appropriate equipment and financial resources; assisting family in preparing home environment; helping family identify changes in lifestyle and how to cope with these; and assisting family to identify support groups and follow-up care (Norris-Berkemeyer and Hutchins, 1986).

Nursing Role

Nursing's role in this perplexing and agonizing experience is to assist the family in coping. The grief reaction is acute, and severe stress is felt by the entire family. The initial reactions are the predictable symptoms and behavior of the grief process: shock, denial, anger, guilt. A sense of emotional numbness may develop in the parents immediately after the initial response, and frequently insomnia, anorexia, fatigue, depression, and preoccupation with the SIDS event occur (Patterson and Pomeroy, 1974). During this time of responding to an unexplained, unexpected loss, the parents and family require tremendous support. The nurse is in a position to provide this through the therapeutic relationship. Interventions need to be made at the time of death as well as after the cause of death has been confirmed (see box below). The family should be contacted at home within 5 to 7 days after the death. During this and subsequent visits the nurse should focus on providing empathetic sup-

port and assisting the family in coping and progressing through the grief process.

Community health nurses should be involved in the implementation of the management plan for parents and siblings of SIDS victims. This involvement requires familiarity with support groups (such as the National Sudden Infant Death Foundation or Council of Guilds for Infant Survival), and current information (available through Sudden Infant Death Syndrome Clearinghouse).

Prematurity

Approximately 6.8% of all live births are newborns weighing less than 5½ lb. (2500 g.). Of these neonates, up to 90% are at increased risk for death during the first year due to birth injury, respiratory distress syndromes, septicemia, and anorexia.

The incidence of morbidity primarily due to hemorrhage, kernicterus, anemia, and infection is much greater for the preterm infant. Factors disposing infants to premature delivery are identified in the box below and should be assessed through history taking by the community health nurse.

In addition, the community health nurse needs to implement early interventions for these high-risk populations such as referral for prenatal care; frequent follow-up on compliance with care management; education regarding diet and health maintenance during pregnancy; and teaching about the specific high risks factors.

Definition of Prematurity

There are several definitions of *prematurity* based on gestation and weight with which the nurse should be familiar. The premature or preterm infant is one born before the end of the thirty-seventh week of gestation, regardless of birth weight. *Low birth weight infants* (less than 2500 g) are classified as follows (Dubowitz el al., 1970):

- Appropriately grown for gestational age (AGA); that is, infants whose rates of intrauterine growth are normal at birth, but who are small because they are born before the end of the thirty-seventh week.
- Small for gestational age (SGA); that is, infants whose

> ## NURSING INTERVENTIONS IN SIDS MANAGEMENT
>
> ### RECOMMENDED MANAGEMENT* AT THE TIME OF SIDS DEATH
>
> - Performance of autopsies on all infants dying suddenly and unexpectedly
> - Prompt notification of the results of that autopsy to the parents
> - Use of the term *sudden infant death syndrome* on the death certificate
> - Follow-up information and counseling for all families provided by a knowledgeable health professional
>
> ### APPROPRIATE MANAGEMENT WITHIN 1 WEEK OF INFANT'S DEATH INCLUDES A HOME VISIT WITH THE FOLLOWING OBJECTIVES FOR CARE:
>
> - Provide emotional support during the grieving period
> - Listen empathetically
> - Provide information on SIDS to the family members as they are generally ready for it
> - Anticipate normal grief reactions, and reassure parents that their reactions are normal
> - Answer all questions asked by parents, and give printed material on SIDS
> - Assist parents in dealing with siblings and relatives
> - Put parents in touch with parent groups and the National Foundation of Sudden Infant Death
> - Support the whole family during the pregnancy and infancy period of a subsequent child
> - Refer parents for psychiatric help if abnormal reactions exist and persist
>
> ### INDICATIONS FOR REFERRAL
>
> - Parent(s) shows no emotion
> - Parent(s) overintellectualizes (e.g., is obsessed with scientific details)
> - Parent(s) persistently denies the infant's death
> - Continuing inability of parent(s) to resume previous responsibilities and level of functioning

*Recommended by National Foundation of Sudden Infant Death (NFSID) from Mile, M., editor: Mental health aspects of SID, Report of a conference sponsored by NFSID and National Institute for Mental Health, Kansas City, July 30, 1975, U.S. Department of Health, Education, and Welfare. Adapted from Chow, M.P., et al.: Handbook of pediatric primary care, ed. 2, New York, 1984, John Wiley & Sons, Inc., p. 1181 and Tackett, J.J., and Hunsberger, M.: Family centered care of children and adolescents, Philadelphia, 1981, W.B. Saunders Co., p. 686.

> ## FACTORS DISPOSING TO PREMATURITY
>
> Chronic hypertensive disease
> Toxemia
> Placenta previa
> Abruptio placentae
> Cervical incompetence
> Low socioeconomic status, including poor nutrition, chronic infection, fatigue, and generally poor personal and environmental hygiene
> Absence of prenatal care
> Multiple pregnancies
> History of previous premature delivery
> Age (highest incidence under age 20)
> Order of birth (highest incidence in first pregnancies)

From Chow, M.P., et al.: Handbook of pediatric primary care, ed. 2, New York, 1984, John Wiley & Sons, Inc., p. 278.

rates of intrauterine growth are slow but who are born at or later than term (38 to 41 weeks).

- Small for gestational age *and* premature; that is, infants whose rate of intrauterine growth is retarded, and who are delivered before 37 weeks.

In general, infants who are born prematurely are SGA, weighing less than 2500 g, although they may be AGA or LGA (large for gestational age).

Nursing Follow-up Care

Follow-up care of premature infants is the primary management. A plan of care is directed toward preventing the health problems associated with immaturity and facilitating the family's coping by providing support and anticipatory guidance to the parents concerning the physical and psychosocial development of the infant. Community health nurses are in a position to implement such a plan of care through home and clinic contacts, while providing the necessary element of continuity of care.

Because of advances in neonatology, many preterm and LBW infants have been saved. However, these infants have an increased incidence and are at risk for developmental delay, neurological, mental, and physical problems (Rice and Feeg, 1985). This predisposition to risk requires the community health nurse to implement early developmental screening, nutritional education and infant stimulation teaching. Development screening should be expanded to include perceptual and psychomotor skills during toddler and preschool years since these problems are often not manifested until then.

The low birth weight or preterm infant requires a special plan for nutrition. Basically these infants require increased calories, protein, vitamins, and minerals for growth. Though able to absorb protein and carbohydrates efficiently, preterm infants absorb fat poorly and readily lose fat-soluble vitamins and calcium through fecal fat loss. Also, iron stores are depleted much earlier than in full-term infants, and stores of vitamin E and folic acid are deficient in the first 3 months of life (AAP Committee on Nutrition, 1985).

Because of these nutritional deficiencies and added requirements, the feeding of a low birth weight infant must be managed very closely. This infant requires approximately 110 to 150 calories/kg/day with vitamins A, C, D, and B group supplementation. Calcium needs to be supplemented as well as iron. Additional vitamin E and folic acid are required in the first 3 months of life.

Hints such as offering small frequent feedings (2 to 3 ounces every 2 to 3 hours), bubbling frequently, resting at signs of tiring and holding the infant's head above stomach level are all appropriate suggestions.

Though a premature infant requires more frequent follow-up visits, the preventive pediatric care does not differ significantly from that of a full-term infant. However, during the follow-up care of a preterm infant or the infant who has experienced complications or prolonged illness of the family of the infant, extra attention in certain areas of physical and developmental assessment is required. Table 21-4 provides an appropriate plan of care for such infants.

Throughout screening and follow-up, the community health nurse should maintain a positive attitude based on

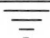

TABLE 21-4

Nursing implications in follow-up care for premature infants

Nursing goal	Nursing implication
Prevent neurological function impairment	Scheduling frequent follow-up visits (initially 1 to 2 times a week, advancing to once a month when a normal pattern of growth is identified)
	Complete physical and neurological assessment at each visit
	Referral as appropriate
Promote physical growth and prevent function impairment	Monitoring of height, weight, and head circumference at each visit
	Nutritional monitoring and education: use of supplemental nutrients and calories to ensure adequate nutrition; suggested techniques for feeding
	Education regarding skin care because of maceration proneness
	Education regarding maintenance of thermal environment
	Education regarding proneness to and avoidance of infections
	Education regarding infant need for rest and gentle handling
	Referral as appropriate, especially early dental assessment and hearing and ophthalmological examinations
Promote maximum development	Routine developmental screening
	Education regarding sensory stimulation
	Promotion of maternal-infant bond and paternal-infant bond
	Promotion of normal newborn experiences and avoidance of overprotection
	Referral as appropriate, especially to community resource support groups

Adapted from Korones, S.B.: High risk newborn infants, ed. 4, St. Louis, 1986, The C.V. Mosby Co.; and Tackett, J.J., and Hunsberger, M.: Family centered care of children and adolescents, Philadelphia, 1981, W.B. Saunders Co.

the knowledge that although potentials for delay and health problems are present, *equally present is the potential for normal outcomes.*

Other Causes of Neonate Morbidity

Although infectious diseases no longer pose the major life threat they once did 20 years ago, they do remain the leading cause of illness and restricted activity for children under 6 years of age in the U.S. Neonates are particularly susceptible to sepsis, a bacterial infection involving the bloodstream and frequently the meninges. Gram-negative bacilli and group β- beta hemolytic streptococci are the most common agents of sepsis in neonates. Sites vulnerable to entry of the infectious agents are the umbilicus, skin, and nasopharynx, and infections may spread rapidly with few signs of symptoms. The neonate is particularly susceptible to these agents and subsequent sepsis for a number of reasons, such as exposure to contaminated equipment and environment, unrecognized infections in other persons, an immature immune system, and the body's inability to carry out effective phagocytosis.

The signs and symptoms of sepsis are subtle and difficult to detect. However, neurological involvement may occur rapidly. Since community health nurses may have the first contact with an infant developing sepsis, they should be alert to its symptoms, which include the following (Chow et al., 1984, Korones, 1986):

Full anterior fontanel that lacks normal pulsations
Hypothermia
Continued lethargy, anorexia
Persistent apneic spells or seizures
Feeding poorly with a weak suck
Persistent diarrhea, vomiting, spitting up
Jaundice and liver enlargement between the fourth and eighth day of life
Petechia, shrill cry, or abdominal distension

The mortality for neonatal sepsis is high, and meningitis is responsible for 60% to 70% of the fatalities. In addition, up to 80% of those who survive sepsis suffer serious neurological complications resulting in brain damage, retardation, and developmental and growth delays.

Nursing Role

The nurse's role is early recognition and assessment. Preventive measures can be implemented by the nurse, aimed at reducing the incidence and spread of the agents of septicemia. Community health nurses can initiate prevention through parental and family education in hygiene techniques. Potential environmental sources of the bacteria can be identified by the community health nurse who can then refer the client for treatment.

Finally, the nurse has a responsibility to provide support to the parents of an infant who develops sepsis. Particular attention to the disruption in the parent-child relationship is needed if hospitalization occurs. The nurse should identify measures that facilitate attachment and parental involvement in the care of the infant. (See Table 21-4 for additional follow-up suggestions.) The community health nurse can be most instrumental in a successful resolution by acting as a client advocate and supporter.

Causes of Infant Morbidity

For the infant 1 month to 1 year of age, infection remains the greatest cause of illness. (This is also true of children up to 6 years of age, although the causative agent for each age group may differ as a result of host susceptibility and development of immunity.) Of greatest significance is the incidence of influenza and pneumonia in infants.

The origin of an infectious disease such as influenza or penumonia may be viral or bacterial. The symptoms gen-

TABLE 21-5

General measures for symptoms of infectious disease

Symptom	Measure
Fever	1. Antipyretic medication 2. Tepid sponge baths 3. Liberal fluid intake 4. Rest and limited activity
Upper respiratory symptoms	1. Liberal fluid intake 2. Cool mist vaporizers 3. Decongestants 4. Warm gargles, saline solution mouth and throat irrigations, cool liquids, and soft foods for sore throat as appropriate to age 5. Petrolatum jelly to protect the skin around the nares 6. Cough preparations generally ineffective and contraindicated in infants and young children
Generalized aching and malaise	1. Rest and limited physical activity 2. Warm baths 3. Body massage 4. Cold compresses for headache 5. Analgesic medication
Anorexia	1. Small, frequent feedings of favorite foods and liquids 2. Relaxed attitude about oral intake; forcing foods and fluids is usually counterproductive
Rash	1. Proper hygiene and bathing to reduce incidence of secondary infection 2. Cool baths, local applications of calamine lotion, and mild anesthetic ointments or systemic antihistamines to relieve pruritus 3. Fingernail care, including frequent cutting and cleaning, to reduce effects of scratching; gloves or mittens may be used at night on younger children 4. Saline mouthwashes if mucous membranes are involved

Adapted from Chow, M.P., et al.: Handbook of pediatric primary care, ed. 2, New York, 1984, John Wiley & Sons, Inc.; and Krugman, S., Ward, R., and Katz, S.L.: Infectious diseases of children, ed. 8, St. Louis, 1986, The C.V. Mosby Co.

erally fall into specific categories such as fever, upper respiratory symptoms, generalized ache and malaise, anorexia, and exanthema. Early recognition and management of symptoms abates their severity and complications (Table 21-5).

Nursing Role

The community health nurse frequently encounters infants and children with infectious diseases. Assisting parents through education in recognition and responsible symptomatic management can prevent further complications. In addition, facilitating client knowledge in the prevention of infectious disease spread is well within the community health nurse's role. Health promotional activities that need to be stressed include adequate nutrition, avoidance of sources of infection or ill persons, use of responsible hygiene measures, and early intervention if symptoms occur.

MAJOR HEALTH PROBLEMS

During the process of physical and emotional maturation, a child passes through many stages. Each presents risks to health and well-being. Nurses should provide anticipatory guidance, and when indicated, assist parents with the management of these problems.

Major health problems during the neonatal period include the phenomenon of jaundice and regulation of body temperature. With infants the health problems of major concern include upper respiratory tract infections, otitis media, allergies, gastrointestinal illnesses, and malnutrition.

Jaundice

Jaundice refers to the yellowish color of the skin and results from the breakdown of red blood cells plus the immaturity of liver enzymes to conjugate and excrete bilirubin. Bilirubin must be conjugated to bind with albumin for excretion. Unbound (indirect) bilirubin cannot be excreted from the body and is subsequently absorbed into the fatty tissue and the brain.

Physiological jaundice (icterus neonatorum) is a normal occurrence between the second and fourth day of life and appears in approximately 50% of all full-term newborns. Bilirubin levels may reach 6 to 10 mg/dl. and resolution generally occurs by the seventh to eighth day. A bilirubin level exceeding 12 mg/dl for the full-term infant is suggestive of more than normal physiology and would be considered hyperbilirubinemia (Behrman, 1987).

Hyperbilirubinemia

Hyperbilirubinemia of the newborn appears in the first week of life but persists rather than resolving. Among the causes may be a more severe form of physiological jaundice, blood group incompatibility (hemolytic disease), or breast-feeding jaundice. The primary cause of the problem is elevated levels of unconjugated bilirubin resulting from deficiency or inactivity of bilirubin glucuronyl transferase, a liver enzyme that conjugates bilirubin. The immediate danger is kernicterus when bilirubin levels exceed 18 to 20 mg/dl. (See a basic pediatric text for a detailed discussion on the causes of hyperbilirubinemia.)

Kernicterus

Kernicterus refers to neurological damage that occurs when unconjugated bilirubin is deposited in brain tissue. The mortality is high, and survivors generally demonstrate signs of central nervous system damage. When serum bilirubin levels reach 18 mg/dl and above, the risk of kernicterus exists (Behrman, 1987). Low birth weight and premature infants are particularly at risk and at lower levels.

Nursing Role

With the advent of early discharge after delivery, the community health nurse in the home or clinic setting will encounter newborns at risk for jaundice. Early recognition and intervention thus become responsibilities that the community health nurse must assume. Observation is the primary tool nurses can use when assessing a neonate for jaundice. Progressive hyperbilirubinemia is accompanied by the appearance of jaundice in a cephalocaudal advancement. The yellow appearance shows first in the head and neck, advances to the trunk and umbilicus, and progresses to the groin, upper thighs, knees, ankles, elbows, and finally to the palms of the hands and soles of the feet. As the yellow appearance progresses downward and outward, the level of bilirubin progresses upward. Management common to all causes of jaundice and hyperbilirubinemia involves adequate hydration and support, education, and counseling of the parents. In some instances phototherapy (placing the infant under fluorescent lights) is indicated. Frequently this therapy occurs in the home. The role of the community health nurse is to teach parents about jaundice, about the proper method for phototherapy and about appropriate safety precautions and to ensure necessary follow-up (Osborn, 1986).

Temperature Control

Temperature control is the result of heat production and heat loss function. In newborns the heat production function is unreliable as are the controls for the rate and amount of heat loss. Since the environment influences the amount of heat loss, regulation and maintenance of the thermal environment are critical to the newborn. By controlling the immediate environment of the newborn, some degree of this thermal imbalance can be offset. The normal infant temperature should be 97.5° to 98.6° rectally. This body temperature can be maintained by keeping a warm room temperature of 74° to 76° and by providing external warmth such as blankets and cloth.

The premature or low birth weight infant requires special attention to thermoregulation. As the weight (body mass) of the baby decreases, the body surface area becomes proportionately greater. In addition, the lesser the amount of subcutaneous fat, the greater the degree of heat loss. For the preterm infant this means a constant effort needs to be made to control body temperature through environmental measures.

Upper Respiratory Tract Infections

Over half of all acute illnesses treated in ambulatory settings include *upper respiratory tract infections* (URIs). Infants and children are particularly susceptible to URIs because of their immunological immaturity; small, easily obstructed airways; underdeveloped accessory muscles; and ineffectual coughing ability (Behrman, 1987).

Nursing Role

Nursing's primary responsibility in URIs is prevention, which includes providing anticipatory guidance in nutrition, rest, and hygiene. In addition, community health nurses should identify infants and children at risk because of numerous URIs, institute preventive measures, and implement close follow-up. Careful assessment is essential and should explore environmental conditions, such as living arrangements, exposure to ill family members, and smoking behaviors of household members. Data retrieved from the assessment determine nursing's management.

Assessment begins with a chronological picture of the present complaint, including data regarding the presence, character, and severity of cough, fever, respiratory difficulty, rhinorrhea, other discharge, pain, and sore throat. The physical assessment should focus on determining the severity and location of the illness.

In addition, measurement of vital signs, particularly the respiratory rate, character, and rhythm, facilitates determination of severity.

Though the management of upper respiratory infections varies according to the severity and location, several general measures can be appropriately instituted. These measures include hydration through generous amounts of fluids, humidification through cool mist or steam vaporizers, and symptomatic relief measures such as bulb syringing for nasal discharge, use of antipyretics for fever reduction, and warm saline gargles for sore throat in older children (Table 21-5).

Otitis Media

Serous otitis media, generally caused by allergy or nasopharyngeal inflammation, is characterized by marked conductive hearing loss persisting for weeks. The fluid produces a "popping" sensation with swallowing and a feeling of fullness. On examination the tympanic membrane is retracted, translucent, and dull. Fluid may be evident behind the drum as may air bubbles. A decrease in drum mobility is a definitive finding (Kaleida and Stool, 1983).

Management is directed toward identification of cause and alleviation of discomfort. The fullness may be alleviated by the Valsalva maneuver (holding nose and blowing) or the use of decongestants, although their efficacy has yet to be proven (Kaleida and Stool, 1983).

Suppurative *otitis media,* a bacterial infection of the middle ear, is a significant complication of URIs in infants and children. Frequently, serous otitis media, an accumulation of fluid in the middle ear, is the sequela of suppurative otitis media.

The common causes of suppurative otitis media vary with age. In infants 6 to 8 weeks of age and younger, gram-negative bacilli and staphylococci are most prevalent. In older infants and children pneumococci, *Haemophilus influenzae,* and *mycoplasma pneumoniae* are common causative organisms. Nasal congestion, irritability, and cough are characteristic. Other associated symptoms may include fever, vomiting, diarrhea, and hearing difficulties. Physical examination reveals outward bulging of the drum with redness and obscured visualization of bony landmarks and light reflex (Kaleida and Stool, 1983).

Management involves the use of antibiotics appropriate to the age and causative organism. Decongestants are frequently used in conjunction with antibiotic therapy. Follow-up for both serous and suppurative otitis media is es-

sential. The status of the middle ear's response to treatment, as well as the hearing response, should be evaluated.

Allergies

Allergies pose a health problem for approximately 20% of children. Though allergies can appear at any age, infants and children at ages 5, 10, and 15 appear to be more susceptible. Over 80% of these allergic children achieve symptom relief after intervention (Bierman and Pearlman, 1980). For this reason nurses must be aware of the origin and symptoms of allergies as well as the appropriate treatment and preventive activities.

Causes

Allergy can be defined as a hypersensitivity to a substance or the environment, which ordinarily causes no response in other persons. When the offending substance (antigen) produces symptoms in an individual, it is designated an allergen. Allergens gain entry into the body through inhalation, ingestion, injection, or direct contact. A list of common allergy-producing substances is outlined in the box on p. 414. The degree of the body's response to the allergen is primarily dependent on the frequency and duration of exposure. Other factors such as state of health, age, and genetic predisposition also affect the allergic response. In addition, variables such as the season, weather, emotional state, and time of day appear to affect the intensity of the response.

Symptoms

The most common allergic manifestations in infancy are atopic dermatitis, gastrointestinal disturbances, and mild rhinorrhea. Foods are the most common allergens, with milk the most frequent offending substance followed by eggs, orange juice, wheat, corn, and beef.

In later childhood environmental substances are the leading cause of allergic conditions with symptoms developing more frequently in those with an infantile allergic history. Symptoms suggestive of allergies in older children include those previously described for infancy and possibly the following (Bierman and Pearlman, 1980):

Tension-fatigue syndrome, including listlessness, irritability, fatigue, facial pallor without anemia, circles of discoloration under the eyes ("allergic shiners")

Recurrent otitis or serous otitis media

Upper respiratory symptoms including:

Allergic salute—itching and rubbing of nose upward, which leads to a crease across the nose just above the tip

Excoriated nares and sometimes epistaxis

Rhinorrhea with seromucoid discharge

Postnasal mucoid discharge leading to a tickling, productive cough

Nasal congestion that causes mouth breathing and pursing of lips

Recurrent laryngitis

Lower respiratory tract problems including allergic bronchitis and bronchial asthma

Skin problems including urticaria and types of dermatitis

Assessment and Management

Assessment of the allergic condition requires a detailed history and complete physical examination. Of primary importance to the assessment is securing a detailed nutrition or diet history as well as information regarding family history, since the probability of allergic problems increases if the family history is positive.

Management of allergies is dependent on the identified allergen source (see box at right). Most frequently, for infants this management requires diet control. Such control in the form of an elimination diet is instituted when sufficient evidence from a history and physical examination warrants removing the suspected substance from the child's diet. The procedure for instituting an elimination diet is given in Appendix J2 (Chow, 1984).

Under circumstances in which environmental allergens are suspected, particularly with the home, desensitization or allergy-proofing measures can be implemented (Appendix J2). Though it is virtually impossible to eliminate all allergens from a child's environment, avoidance of known offending substances and partial relief from exposure can benefit the allergic child (Tackett and Hunsberger, 1981).

Vomiting and Diarrhea

Another health problem of concern during infancy is the *vomiting and diarrhea syndrome.* The etiology of this illness, whether symptoms occur together or singularly, is varied.

When assessing an infant for vomiting and diarrhea it is often necessary to verify the meaning of these terms with parents. Frequently vomiting, which is forceful projectile or nonprojectile retching of gastric contents, is confused with regurgitation, a common benign occurrence in the first year of life involving nonforceful, nonprojectile, effortless expulsion of gastric contents, generally after feeding. Similarly, *diarrhea* is defined as watery, copious bowel movements that are usually green and have a foul odor, but the term is frequently misinterpreted by parents. Assessment of causes should also include viral, diet mismanagement, malabsorption, bacterial and allergic factors.

Management of vomiting and diarrhea is directed toward control of symptoms and prevention of dehydration. *Dehydration* is defined as the percentage of body weight lost as water. For example, a child who is 5% dehydrated has lost 50 ml of water for every kilogram of body weight. Though the majority of children with vomiting and/or diarrhea are less than 5% dehydrated, it is imperative that nurses be knowledgeable of the clinical signs of dehydration, which may include dry mucous membranes, reduction in tear formation, decreased urination, decreased skin turgor, and sunken eyes and fontanel.

Nursing Role

Nursing measures directed toward resolution of vomiting and diarrhea are primarily diet modifications. Clear liquids such as apple juice; flat, diluted ginger ale; Lytren; or Pedialyte are recommended for the first 24 hours. Liquids should be given in small amounts and frequently (1 to 2 oz every 30 to 60 minutes). If fluids are retained or diarrhea does not worsen and/or improves, solids such as rice cereal,

---

COMMON ALLERGY-PRODUCING SUBSTANCES

INHALANTS

Pollen
Mold
House dust
Animal dander
Fabric fiber
Feathers
Dyes
Chemicals

INJECTANTS

Vaccines
Injected drugs
Animal serum
Animal saliva
Animal venom
Insect stings

BACTERIAL INFECTANTS

INGESTANTS

Food
   Cow's milk
   Eggs
   Wheat
   Chocolate
   Cola products
   Fish, pork, chicken, legumes
   Corn
   Citrus fruits, strawberries
Drugs
   Aspirin
   Antibiotics
   Barbiturates
Food additives

CONTACTANTS

Plants
Topical drugs
Resins
Metals
Cosmetics
Dyes
Chemicals

OTHER ENVIRONMENTAL FACTORS

Sunshine
Temperature changes
Air pollution

From Tackett, J.J., and Hunsberger, M.: Family centered care of children and adolescents, Philadelphia, 1981, W.B. Saunders Co., p. 494.

---

applesauce, and bananas can be added to the diet. Generally medications such as sedatives, antiemetics, and antidiarrheals are not recommended for younger children, since they can mask the progression of vomiting and diarrhea. In addition, these medications tend to make children drowsy and in this way decrease fluid intake because of induced sleep.

Nurses must also counsel and educate parents in monitoring of symptoms and their progression as well as assess parental knowledge and compliance with dietary management. Further education in techniques that reduce spread or severity is important, particularly in the home environment. Following the course of illness is essential as referral may be required if symptoms are not successfully abated by the management plan.

Malnutrition

Malnutrition refers to poor or inadequate nutrition. It may result from under or over nutrition and frequently presents as iron deficiency anemia or vitamin deficiencies. An estimated 50% of children age 6 to 24 months are iron deficient, due primarily to poor feeding and eating habits. These nutrition practices are influenced by economic, sociocultural, geographic and educational factors, making nutritional counseling a complex process (Whaley and Wong, 1983). The role of the community health nurse is in the prevention of malnutrition through careful dietary assessment, thorough nutritional education, provision of resources, such as Women, Infant and Childhood (WIC) nutritional program, and periodic follow-up in the home or clinic setting. Early recognition and management of nutritional disturbances is an appropriate nursing responsibility and can be accomplished through dietary screening, instructing parents about iron and vitamin supplementation, meal planning with parents, counseling and educating parents about nutrients, anthropometric evaluation, and close follow-up.

COMMON CONCERNS OR PROBLEMS

A common problem might be defined as a child's behavior, which elicits concern on the part of parents. Frequently parents have behavioral expectations of their children, which may be in regard to some physical or psychosocial aspects of their growth or development. When the infant or child does not demonstrate the expected behaviors, parents often respond in an emotional, anxious, or insecure manner. The child then reacts to the parents' response, creating additional stress in the family situation. For example, the mother of a 1-month-old infant expects the baby to feed every 4 hours and sleep through the night. When the infant wants to eat every 2 hours and is up three times a night, the mother becomes concerned, anxious, and maybe insecure about her mothering abilities. This response subsequently affects her ability to be relaxed and motherly toward her infant, and the infant responds by being more demanding. Table 21-6 outlines common childhood behaviors that normally occur yet may create parental concern.

Many factors contribute to the occurrence of common problems. Significant variables include the following:

Parental expectations of a child's behavior and of their own behavior as parents, which are frequently unrealistic

Lack of parenting experience and knowledge

Emotional impact of becoming a parent

Age, sex, and temperament of the child as it affects the parents and family

Too much concern and emphasis on the part of parents toward common problems

The most frequently identified common concerns or problems of infancy include colic, feeding, sleeping and elimination patterns and behaviors, crying, gas, hiccups, teething, spoiling, weaning, and stranger or separation anxiety. Appendix J5 describes these problems and appropriate anticipatory guidance and management.

SAFETY AND ACCIDENT PREVENTION

Accidents are the most preventable cause of mortality and morbidity in infants and children. During the first year of life accidents are the sixth leading cause of death and become the leading cause after the first year.

Practice of age-appropriate safety measures can sigifi-

TABLE 21-6

Common childhood behaviors

Age (years)	Behaviors
1	Sucks thumb, smears stools, shakes bed, bangs and rocks, and masturbates
2	As above; has temper tantrums, tears books or wallpaper, tears bed apart, removes clothes, runs around, and has many demands before sleep
2½	Above behavior to a lesser degree; stutters and has disruptive aggressive attacks such as hitting and biting
3	Less of the above behaviors
3½	Again an increase in some of the above behaviors; spits, picks nose, bites fingernails, and whines
4	Runs away, kicks, spits, bites nails, grimaces, calls names, boasts, brags, uses silly language, has nightmares and fears, needs to urinate in moments of emotional distress, has "belly" pains and may vomit
5	A decrease in some behaviors, blinks eyes, shakes head, clears throat, and sniffles
5½ to 6	All the above behaviors and increased clumsiness
7	Tries to control behaviors and may have headaches
8	Picks at fingers, cries with fatigue, and makes faces
9	Stamps feet, fiddles, drops and breaks things, picks at self, growls and mutters

From Chow, M.P., et al.: Handbook of pediatric primary care, ed. 2, New York, 1984, John Wiley & Sons, Inc., p. 383.

cantly reduce and prevent most accidents. Nursing in its emphasis on health promotion and supervision can have a significant impact on accident prevention. The counseling and education of parents on the developmental abilities and related safety measures needed to provide an accident-free environment are responsibilities that nursing must meet when delivering well-child care. Environmental assessment tools, such as the Safety Evaluation Program, can be utilized by the community health nurse in evaluating home safety, as well as advocating and referring community safety programs, such as KISS (Kids in Safety Seats). Appendix J6 provides information regarding developmental abilities according to age, implications in terms of incidence of accidents, and appropriate nursing interventions.

TOOLS FOR ASSESSMENT

The nursing process involves the assessment, planning, implementation, and evaluation of the health needs of a client and family. An accurate assessment through data collection is the basis for any further plan of intervention. The tools and techniques used for assessment vary, depending on the child's age. However, basic methods provide nursing with a uniform and reliable approach to assessment of an individual child's health needs, as well as those of his or her family and community.

History

The history and subsequent assessment of the child and his family begin at the moment of contact through observation. This technique of data collection provides information regarding the physical as well as psychosocial, developmental, and interactional growth and development of the child and family. A more formal interview should be directed toward gathering data relative to the child's immediate health status. Traditional information gathered in an initial pediatric health history is reviewed in Appendix A2.

Physical Examination

Data collected from the physical assessment of a child serve as verification for information collected from observation and the history interview. For example, observation may reveal that a 6-year-old is limping; the history may reveal the child is complaining of pain in the right ankle after falling off of a bicycle 1 day earlier. The physical examination verifies these data through findings of edema, bruising, and limited range of motion. Similarly, data collected during a health maintenance visit can verify the observation and history that a child is in good health.

Approaches in conducting a physical examination for a pediatric client are most important and must be adapted to the child's age and developmental level. Suggested approaches and sequence of conducting the physical examination according to age are summarized in Appendix A3.

Health Assessment

Combining the components of history taking and physical assessment with the elements of physical and psychosocial growth and development pertinent to a specific age results in a total health assessment. In pediatrics, health assessments are generally implemented at specific time intervals. In the first 6 years of life, health assessment visits for the normally developing child are generally recommended at the following ages: 2 to 4 weeks, 2, 4, 6, 9 or 12, 15, 18, and 24 months, and annually until 6 years. Outlines for the content of these health visits are included in Appendix A3. Health promotion activities for the specific age groups are discussed later in this chapter.

Recording of the data collected during health assessment visits is as vital as the assessment itself. The documentation of care through recording provides a means for review and evaluation. Consequently, using a tool that facilitates documentation and communication about a child's health status becomes essential to the provision of quality, comprehensive care.

In addition to the history and physical examination, other tools are useful in the monitoring, screening, and evaluation of the growth and development of children and are discussed in the following pages.

Monitoring Physical Growth and Development

Measurement of the child's height, weight, and head circumference is most important in the health assessment process because growth is a major characteristic of childhood. Since atypical patterns of growth are common indicators of pathology, these measurements should be made between five and six times in the first year and annually thereafter. Additionally, these measurements need to be recorded on a growth chart and compared to the norms for the child's age and his or her own previous growth pattern. Appendix K2 illustrates commonly used growth charts.

Accuracy and correct measuring techniques are basic to measurement usefulness as evaluators of growth. Height, as a measure of skeletal and muscular growth, is most accurately measured in the supine position for children until they are 2 to 3 years old (Figure 21-1). The appropriate technique requires two people. The top of the head must touch the headboard perpendicular to the table while the sliding footboard rests against the soles of the feet. Weight, as an indicator of general growth and nutritional status, is

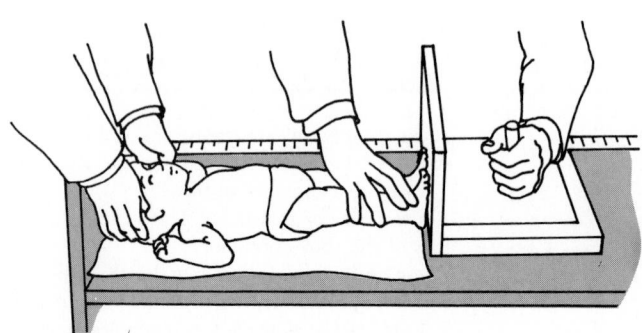

FIGURE 21-1

Measurement of infant height. (From Maternal and Child Health Program: evaluation of body size and physical growth of children, Washington, D.C., 1976, Department of Health, Education, and Welfare.)

measured on an infant scale without clothing (except diaper) for children until they are approximately 2 years of age.

The head circumference is a particularly important measurement, especially in the first year of life when brain growth is most rapid. A nonstretchable measuring tape should be used for the calibration of head size and placed around the largest circumference of the head (around occiput and just above eyebrows). Head circumference should be measured routinely through the first 3 years of life.

Vital Signs

Vital sign measurement is another indicator of health status. Temperature, though not routinely done on health assessment visits, should be measured for every ill child. The choice of thermometer type depends on the child's age, but generally rectal or axillary measurements are done on children under 5 to 6 years and oral temperatures taken after this age.

Pulse readings should be made at every visit whether the child is sick or well. Because an infant's pulse is so rapid, it is best felt in the femoral areas or auscultated in the apical area.

Observation and measurement of the respiratory rate should be done at every encounter. Resting or sleeping respiratory rate measurements are the most reliable. Palpating or auscultating the infant's chest is the most reliable measurement method.

Current recommendations for obtaining blood pressure measurements are to include measurement and recording of blood pressure at the health assessment visit after 3 years of age, unless otherwise indicated. The flush, palpation, or Doppler ultrasound methods are generally used for children under 1 year. For older children, using a cuff that covers two thirds of the upper arm and encircles the arm without a gap is the appropriate method. All blood pressure measurements should be done in the same position, usually seated, and in the same arm, usually the right.

Laboratory Studies

Further means for monitoring physical growth and development include laboratory studies on blood and urine. These studies can be used for (1) monitoring of health status (i.e., hemoglobin, and hematocrit determinations in monitoring anemia); (2) screening for health problems (i.e., Sickledex to identify the presence of sickle-cell trait); or (3) diagnosis of health problems (i.e., Coombs to identify presence of abnormal antigen-antibody levels). In addition, data from laboratory studies may be used for multiple purposes such as diagnosis of a health problem and subsequent monitoring.

Dental Age

Dental age is assessed through knowledge of normal patterns of tooth eruption (see a basic pediatric nursing text). Most humans develop two sets of teeth in a lifetime. By knowing the approximate age of eruption and shedding of teeth, assessment of normal growth for age can be made. In general, an infant's primary (deciduous) teeth begin to erupt around 6 months, and this set is complete by 3 years of age. The primary teeth begin shedding around age 6 and

are replaced by permanent teeth. This replacement process is usually completed by 18 to 25 years of age.

Preventive dental care should be instituted between 1 and 3 years. The community health nurse can facilitate dental health by assessing the family's access to care, referring for care, assessing fluoride content, and teaching brushing and flossing technique.

Screening Tools

See Appendixes A and K for information on additional tools for screening physical growth and development.

Monitoring Psychosocial Development
Developmental Scales

The most useful tools available to nurses are those designed to assess psychosocial and/or developmental skills. Children generally follow similar patterns of development. Subsequently, developmental standards have been established based on studies of the age levels at which the average child masters various motor, language, adaptive, and social behaviors. The Waechter Developmental Guides provide comprehensive summaries of growth and development during infancy and should be a component of the essential knowledge base for nurses involved in pediatric care (Appendix K9).

Purpose of Screening Tests

Developmental and psychosocial screening tests are designed to assess how an individual child is developing compared to the average standard. These tests are a means for determining the need for intervention and perhaps more comprehensive evaluation. Screening tests used most frequently in pediatrics are selected primarily for their ease of administration, economic feasibility, and accuracy and reliability of results. Interpretation of their results requires recognition of the range of normalcy, individual variations, and the variables present in the test situations. Some of the more popular and frequently used screening tests are discussed next.

Overview of Screening Tests

DENVER DEVELOPMENTAL SCREENING TEST. The Denver Developmental Screening test (DDST) was developed to screen children from birth to 6 years for early detection of developmental lags (Appendix K3). It can be used at one time or for periodic screening and assesses personal, social, fine motor, adaptive, language, and gross motor developmental skills and behavior (Frankenburg, et al., 1971).

NEONATAL PERCEPTION INVENTORY. The Neonatal Perception Inventory (NPI; Appendix K1) was developed to determine a new mother's concept of what an average baby's behavior is like and what her assessment is of her own infant's behavior. It is primarily used to identify infants and mothers at risk for developing an unhealthy bond. The NPI is administered in two parts. Part I questionnaire is completed on the first or second day postpartum. Part II questionnaire is administered when the infant is 1 month of age (Broussard and Hartner, 1971).

DEGREE OF BOTHER INVENTORY. The Degree of Bother Inventory is generally used in conjunction with Part II of the NPI (Appendix K1). This inventory questionnaire is administered at 1 month of age and requires the mother to indicate to what degree the listed infant behaviors in her own baby are bothersome or create concern. The purpose of the tool is to identify and rank those behaviors that the mother finds particularly bothersome so that interventions may be initiated. The Degree of Bother Inventory is most useful for first-time mothers as is the NPI (Broussard and Hartner, 1971).

CAREY INFANT TEMPERAMENT SCALE. The Carey Infant Temperament Scale (CITS) is designed to obtain a profile of an infant's temperament. It is appropriate for use in infants 4 and 8 months of age and provides information useful in planning the child's well care and in initiating parental anticipatory guidance. The scale is a questionnaire completed by parents in areas such as feeding, sleep, elimination and play patterns as well as infant response to different stimuli (Carey, 1972).

HOME OBSERVATION FOR MEASUREMENT OF ENVIRONMENT. Home Observation for Measurement of Environment (HOME) is a unique tool using both clinical and home visit observations. It is designed to identify characteristics of the environment of children from birth to 3 years and from 3 to 6 years (Appendix B5). HOME consists of a behavior and interaction inventory each age group. Each inventory scale identifies certain aspects of the quality and quantity of the social, emotional, and cognitive environments available to the child at home. This tool is particularly valuable to the community health nurse as a means of assessing environmental adequacy for development and for initiating interventions (Caldwell, 1976).

Family Assessment Tools

Family-centered care should be the focus of the community health nurse. Although obstacles, such as lack of time, professional and organizational support and knowledge about family assessment, make family centered care difficult, family assessment remains important as the success of nursing interventions is dependent on the family's ability and resources to implement the care. Family assessment is particularly important to pediatrics since children rely on their families for health activities (Speer and Sachs, 1985).

Family assessment tools must be understandable, easily administered and scored, reliable, valid, and appropriate for most families (Speer and Sachs, 1985). Appendix B7 provides an evaluation summary of family assessment tools that the community health nurse may find useful.

IMMUNIZATIONS

Immunity is defined as the body's resistance to the effects of harmful agents. The protection of immunity can be received through active or passive means. (See Chapter 17 for a discussion of active or passive immunity.)

Active artificial immunization is initiated for infants and children to protect them against the once common and dangerous infectious diseases such as measles, mumps, rubella, tetanus, diphtheria, and pertussis. The neonate enjoys a relatively short period (first few weeks to 2 months) of natural passive immunity as a result of placental transfer of maternal antibodies. However, this protection is only against those diseases for which the mother has developed sufficient antibodies, and it is temporary. Young infants then becomes rapidly at risk for infection because of the short-term passive immunity of their own poorly developed and immature immune system. In normal infants the immune system is capable of responding with adequate antibody production by 2 months of age. This is generally the recommended age to begin artificial immunizations.

Active immunization is conferred through two basic types of agents. Antibody production for tetanus and diphtheria is stimulated through the use of a toxoid, which is a bacterial toxin that has been heated or chemically treated to decrease the virulence but not the antibody-producing ability. The use of vaccines, a suspension of attenuated or killed microorganisms, provides an active immunity response for pertussis (a killed bacteria), measles, mumps, rubella, and polio (i.e., Sabin and Salk vaccines, attenuated and killed viruses, respectively), and HBPV (*Haemophilus* b polysaccharide vaccine.) Appendix D2 provides information regarding the basic immunization agents and their administration schedule in pediatrics.

The interval between immunizations is important to the immunity response. After the first injection, antibodies are produced slowly and in small concentrations (primary response). However, the antibody-producing mechanism has been altered in response to this first injection so that subsequent injections with the same antigen are recognized by the body. Once this recognition occurs, antibodies are produced much faster and in higher concentration (secondary response). Because of this secondary response, once an initial immunization series has been started, *it does not need to be restarted if interrupted, regardless of the length of time elapsed.* Once the initial series is completed, boosters are required at the appropriate time intervals to maintain an adequate concentration level of antibodies.

Occasionally, children are encountered who have received no immunizations. The immunization schedule for these children is listed in Table 21-7. However, if compliance with this schedule and follow-up care are doubtful, it is valid to simultaneously administer diphtheria, tetanus, pertussis (DPT) or tetanus, diphtheria (Td) if the child is over 6 years of age, trivalent oral polio virus vaccine (TOPV), measles, mumps and rubella (MMR), and tuberculin test (PPD [Mantoux]).

The HBPV vaccine is administered only once, optimally at 24 months, but up to 5 years. Children under 18 months should not receive the HBPV vaccine. HBPV and DPT vaccines may be given at the same time in different sites.

Contraindications

Contraindications for the administration of immunizations are relatively few. Vaccines should not be administered to children with acute febrile illness or to those who have had severe reactions to the previous dose. Minor illnesses or infections are not contraindications for administration. Specific circumstances for nonadministration of a particular agent are listed in Appendix D2. In addition, the community health nurse needs to be aware of religious and cultural barriers that may prevent immunization. Finally,

TABLE 21-7

Recommended immunization schedules for infants and children not initially immunized at usual recommended times in early infancy

Timing	Preferred schedule	Alternatives* 1	Alternatives* 2	Alternatives* 3	Comments
First visit	DTP† 1, OPV‡ 1, Tuberculin test (PPD)§	MMR,‖ PPD	DTP 1, OPV 1, PPD	DTP 1, OPV 1, MMR, PPD	MMR should be given no younger than 15 months old
1 month after first visit	MMR	DTP 1, OPV 1	MMR, DTP 2	DTP 3	
2 months after first visit	DTP 2, OPV 2	—	DTP 3, OPV 2	DTP 3, OPV 2	—
3 months after first visit	(DTP 3) HBPV**	DTP 2, OPV 2	—	—	In preferred schedule, DTP 3 can be given if OPV 3 is not to be given until 10 to 16 months; HBPV vaccine should be given once, preferably at or after 24 months and up to 5 years. HBPV may be administered with DPT, but not OPV or MMR.
4 months after first visit	DTP 3 (OPV 3)	—	(OPV 3)	(OPV 3)	OPV 3 optional for areas for likely importation of polio (e.g., some southwestern states)
5 months after first visit	—	DTP 3 (OPV 3)	—	—	
10 to 16 months after last dose	DTP 4, OPV 3 or OPV 4	DTP 4, OPV 3 or OPV 4	DTP 4, OPV 3 or OPV 4	DTP 4, OPV 3 or OPV 4	—
Preschool	DTP 5, OPV 4 or OPV 5	DTP 5, OPV 4 or OPV 5	DTP 5, OPV 4 or OPV 5	DTP 5, OPV 4 or OPV 5	Preschool dose not necessary if DTP 4 or 5 given after fourth birthday
14 to 16 years old	Td¶	Td	Td	Td	Repeat every 10 years

Adapted from American Academy of Pediatrics: Report of the Committee on Infectious Diseases, ed. 21, Evanston, Ill., 1986, The AAP, pp. 11. Copyright American Academy of Pediatrics, 1986.
*Alternative 1 can be used in those more than 15 months old if measles is occurring in the community.
 Alternative 2 allows for more rapid DTP immunization.
 Alternative 3 should be reserved for those whose access to medical care is compromised by poor compliance.
†DTP, Diphtheria and tetanus toxoids with pertussis vaccine.
‡OPV, Oral, attenuated poliovirus vaccine contains types 1, 2, and 3.
§Tuberculin test, Mantoux (intradermal PPD) preferred. Frequency of tests depends on local epidemiology. The Committee recommends annual or biennial testing unless local circumstances dictate less frequent or no testing.
‖MMR, Live measles, mumps, and rubella viruses in a combined vaccine.
¶Td, Adult tetanus toxoid (full dose) and diphtheria toxoid (reduced dose) in combination.
NOTE: For all products used, consult manufacturer's brochure for instructions for storage, handling, and administration. Biologics prepared by different manufacturers may vary, and those of the same manufacturer may change from time to time. The package insert should be followed for a specific product.
**Haemophilus b polysaccharide vaccine can be given, if necessary, simultaneously with DTP (at separate sites). The initial three doses of DTP can be given at 1- to 2-month intervals; so, for the child in whom immunization is initiated at 24 months old or older, one visit could be eliminated by giving DTP, OPV, MMR at the first visit; DTP and HBPV at the second visit (1 month later); and DTP and OPV at the third visit (2 months after the first visit). Subsequent DTP and OPV 10 to 16 months after the first visit are still indicated.

those with the following conditions are not routinely immunized and require medical consultation before the agent is administered, especially the live virus vaccines: pregnant women, persons with a generalized malignancy, those on immunosuppressive therapy or with immunodeficiency disease, persons with marked sensitivity to eggs or chicken, or persons who have had recent immune serum globulin or plasma or blood administration, (a wait of 3 months is advised).

Parent Education

An important component of implementing an immunization program is parental preparation and education regarding the program, what responses or reactions to expect, and how to manage these common reactions. Although much discussion has occurred over these issues, parents should be informed of the risks and benefits of each immunizing agent in addition to the common side effects. Appendix D2 discusses potential reactions to specific immunizations and appropriate treatment measures that parents can institute to minimize discomfort.

NUTRITION

One of the most important components of maintaining a child's health is the promotion of good nutrition and dietary habits. The quality and quantity of nutrition influence the growth and development of a child. The nurse's role involves the use of a sound knowledge base to assist parents in providing adequate nutrition for the child.

Basics

Proteins, fats, carbohydrates, vitamins, and minerals are the essential ingredients of a basic diet. These elements must be combined in sufficient quantities to meet the energy or caloric needs of a child, and quantities vary according to age and individual differences. In addition, water requirements must be balanced with the energy produced or the calories metabolized. The distribution of calories and water requirements is summarized in Table 21-8.

The recommended daily allowances (RDAs) are values of levels of intake of essential nutrients considered by the Food and Nutrition Board of the National Academy of Sciences, National Research Council, to be adequate to meet the nutritional needs of almost every person (Table 21-9). The estimates are intended for general use as based on the needs of average individuals expending average amounts of energy. These advisable intakes are generally higher than the actual requirement and represent a safe amount of nutrients.

Factors Influencing Nutrition

As with every aspect of human behavior, nutritional habits that affect nutritional states of health are influenced by a wide variety of variables, which are derived from families as well as the child. Though some habits may be changed, others have to be accepted and accounted for when nursing implements a sound nutrition program. Among the parental factors most influential to food preferences and eating patterns are the ethnic, racial, cultural, and socioeconomic variables. How and what parents eat and their attitude toward nutrition are invariably passed on to their child. The child also brings individual variables to the nutritional situation (i.e., a slow eater, a picky eater, periods of disinterest, development of preferences, presence of food allergy, and alterations in eating patterns during periods of growth).

No one diet is effective for all children or even for one age group. Nurses must accept and be knowledgeable about individual styles, methods, and approaches to child nutrition to assist parents in providing the appropriate nutrients for their child.

Types of Infant Feeding

Supplying essential nutrients to an infant is done primarily through breast- and/or bottle-feeding. The method of feeding is a choice that must be made by parents with guidance and without pressure. The advantages and disadvantages of both methods should be discussed with parents prenatally, and the differences between the basic forms of milk should be reviewed. In addition, parents should also be aware of the need for vitamin and mineral supplementation as well as current recommendations on infant nutrition methods.

With the first choice of whether to breast-feed or bottle-feed, nurses can offer counsel to parents. In addition to providing nutritional facts, nursing must be prepared to instruct, encourage, reassure, and support parents in the method of their choice. For breast-feeding, this means helping the mother establish a successful routine by discussing comfortable positioning, appropriate techniques, feeding frequency, the let-down reflex, care of breasts, and length of feedings. In addition, assessing the mother's feelings about nursing her infant and providing support and encouragement, the presence or absence of paternal and family support, and providing support and encouragement are important to success.

For bottle-feeding, parents require instruction regarding preparation and care of the equipment and formula, positioning of the person feeding as well as the infant and bottle, in addition to the factors of frequency, length, and feelings about the method of feeding. When solids are introduced,

TABLE 21-8

Distribution of calories and water requirements for all age groups

Age	Protein	Fat	Carbohydrate	Total water requirement in 24 hours
Low birth weight infants	10-11%	40-50%	35-45%	200-250
Normal full-term infants	6-8%	30-35%	45-55%	750 at 3 months to 1200 at 12 months
Toddler/Preschooler	10-12%	30-45%	40-50%	1350 at 2 years to 1800 at 4 years
School age child/Adolescent	10-15%	30-45%	35-55%	2000 school age child 2500 adolescent
Adolescent Athletes	10-15%	25-35%	50-60%	2700

nurses need to provide guidance regarding the types, amount, frequency, and progression of foods offered. In addition, nurses must be aware that parents can become overly concerned about their child's eating habits when the child does not meet parental expectations. Overfeeding or underfeeding can ensue. The nurse can prevent such feeding difficulties by being aware of these attitudes and expectations and of parental nutritional knowledge in general. Appendix J5 provides suggestions for anticipatory guidance for common feeding problems.

Currently there is a trend for the new mother to breast-feed her infant. Breast milk is recommended by many health professionals as the preferred method of feeding an infant in the first 6 months of life. Recent studies document the nutritional efficacy and soundness of breast-feeding. However, some supplementation is necessary. For the infant who is solely breast-fed, the following need to be supplemented (Fomon, 1974):

1. Vitamin D. Although breast milk contains adequate amounts of vitamins A and B complex, there is an inadequate amount of vitamin D to meet the 400 IU/day RDA. Additionally, vitamin C in human milk is adequate, provided that the maternal diet contains sufficient vitamin C.
2. Iron supplementation. The normal birth weight infant has sufficient iron stores until 4 to 6 months of age, at which time body stores must be supplied. Breast milk contains adequate amounts of absorbable iron to meet requirements. An infant who is exclusively breast-fed does not require exogenous sources of iron unless breast-feeding is discontinued before 6 months. Use of iron-fortified cereals and formula is recommended in this circumstance.
3. Fluoride. Breast milk contains inadequate amounts of fluoride, and supplementation in combination with other vitamins or alone is recommended.

Milks other than human milk have been used successfully for infant feeding. Commercially prepared formulas are most popular because they are convenient, contain standard ingredients, and are fortified with vitamins and minerals, negating the need for supplements. However, a formula prepared at home with evaporated or condensed milk or use of forms of cow's milk requires supplementation, generally of vitamins A, D, and C, fluoride, and iron (AAP Committee on Nutrition, 1985). Additionally, skim, lowfat, or 2% milk is not recommended for infants under 1 year of age because of insufficient fat and caloric contents.

Advanced-Feeding

Infants receiving breast milk or formula with the appropriate supplementation do not require additional foods before 6 months of age. There are no nutritional, developmental, or psychological advantages to starting infants on solids before this time. However, the trend toward early introduction of solids does exist, and changing this trend does not occur easily. Nurses can make a significant contribution to the nutritional adequacy of infants and children primarily through parental education and support. This requires being up to date on current nutritional findings and also being accepting of parents who for a variety of reasons wish to implement early introduction of solids. Providing parents with sound factual information regarding the best nutrition for their child is the basis for nursing education and ideally for parental decisions.

Development of Feeding Behavior

Feeding behaviors are the outcome of motor development. For example, an infant's ability to swallow solid food is dependent on fine oral motor skills; older infants cannot feed themselves until they have achieved fine and gross motor skills of the upper body. Consequently, from a developmental perspective, infants are not physically able to

TABLE 21-9

Mean heights and weights and recommended energy intake

Category	Age years	Weight kg	Weight lb	Height cm	Height in	Energy needs kcal	Energy needs with range
Infants	½	6	13	60	24	kg × 115	(95-145)
	½-1	9	20	71	28	kg × 105	(80-135)
Children	1-3	13	29	90	35	1300	(900-1800)
	4-6	20	44	112	44	1700	(1300-2300)
	7-10	28	62	132	52	2400	(1650-3300)
Males	11-14	45	99	157	62	2700	(2000-3700)
	15-18	66	145	176	69	2800	(2100-3900)
	10-22	70	154	177	70	2900	(2500-3300)
Females	11-14	46	101	157	62	2200	(1500-3000)
	15-18	55	120	163	64	2100	(1200-3000)
	19-22	55	120	163	64	2100	(1700-2500)
Pregnancy						+300	
Lactation						+500	

From Tackett, J.J., and Hunsberger, M.: Family centered care of children and adolescents, Philadelphia, 1981, W.B. Saunders Co.; as adapted from Food and Nutrition Board, National Research Council: Recommended dietary allowances, ed. 9, Washington, D.C., 1980, National Academy of Sciences.

handle solid food consumption until 5 to 6 months of age. Correlating developmental abilities as they relate to feeding behaviors and subsequent readiness for solid foods may help parents decide when to introduce solids. Table 21-10 provides information regarding the developmental sequence of feeding behaviors.

Nutritional Considerations

Other factors should be considered by parents when making decisions regarding solid food introduction. One such factor is the way calories are distributed in solids versus human milk or formula. Generally solid baby foods are high in carbohydrates, moderate in protein, and low in fat, whereas human milk or formula is high in fat and carbohydrates and lower in protein. When infants are fed solids and also switched to whole, 2%, or low-fat cow's milk, the diet becomes excessively high in protein, sodium, and other solutes. Since the infant cannot excrete these large solutes efficiently unless large amounts of body fluid are used, this type of diet is hazardous for the infant.

Parents should know the diversity of composition and nutritional quality of commercially prepared infant foods. Reading labels carefully and evaluating brands as to their nutritional content are important. Parents also need to know that the cost per unit of calories is considerably higher for commercially prepared foods than for formula. In addition, the incidence of constipation in infants is greater when solid food intake is high, and the introduction of solids too early

TABLE 21-10

Development of feeding skills

Age	Oral and neuromuscular development	Feeding behavior
Birth	Rooting reflex	Turns mouth toward nipple or any object brushing cheek
	Swallowing reflex	Initial swallowing involves the posterior of the tongue; by 9-12 weeks anterior portion is increasingly involved, which facilitates ingestion of semisolid food
	Extrusion reflex	Pushes food out when placed on tongue; strong the first 9 weeks.
	Sucking reflex	By 6-10 weeks recognizes the feeding position and begins mouthing and sucking when placed in this position
3-6 months	Beginning coordination between eyes and body movements	Explores world with eyes, fingers, hands, and mouth; starts reaching for objects at 4 months but overshoots; hands get in the way during feeding
	Learning to reach mouth with hands at 4 months	Finger sucking—by 6 months all objects go into the mouth
		Sucking reflex becomes voluntary, and lateral motions of the jaw begin
	Extrusion reflex present until 4 months	May continue to push out food placed on tongue
	Able to grasp objects voluntarily at 5 months	Grasps objects in mittenlike fashion
6-12 months	Eyes and hands working together	Can approximate lips to rim of cup by 5 months; chewing action begins; by 6 months begins drinking from cup
		Brings hand to mouth; at 7 months able to feed self biscuit
		Bangs cup and objects on table at 7 months
	Sits erect with support at 6 months	
	Sits erect without support at 9 months	
	Development of grasp (finger to thumb opposition)	Holds own bottle at 9-12 months
		Pincer approach to food
		Pokes at food with index finger at 10 months
	Relates to objects at 10 months	Reaches for food and utensils including those beyond reach; pushes plate around with spoon
		Insists on holding spoon not to put in mouth but to return to plate or cup
		Increased desire to feed self
1-3 years	Development of manual dexterity	*15 months*—begins to use spoon but turns it before reaching mouth; may hold cup, likely to tilt cup rather than head, causing spilling
		18 months—eats with spoon, spills frequently, turns spoon in mouth; holds glass with both hands
		2 years—inserts spoon correctly, occasionally with one hand; holds glass; plays with food; distinguishes between food and inedible materials
		2-3 years—self-feeding complete with occasional spilling; uses fork; pours from pitcher; obtains drink of water from faucet

From Scipien, G.M., et al.: Comprehensive pediatric nursing, ed. 2, New York, 1979, McGraw-Hill Book Co., p. 163. Used with permission.

may possibly lead to overfeeding and later overeating. Finally, a greater possibility of food allergy exists for infants when solids are introduced too early as the foreign proteins in foods become antigens because of insufficient IgA production until after the age of 6 months.

Once parents have made the decision to start solid foods, nurses can assist them in developing a program for introducing appropriate foods in sensible amounts and in the best sequence. For example, it is not nutritionally sound to give an infant eggs as the first solid food, primarily because of difficulties in digesting and a high incidence of allergy to the egg protein. Dry cereal fortified with iron is a more appropriate starter food because of the ease of digestion and iron fortification (at a time when newborn iron reserves are low).

Guidelines for feeding infants birth to 1 year are given in Appendix J4. Suggestions on feeding techniques for the low birth weight infant are discussed earlier in this chapter.

Promoting Good Eating Habits

The first 5 years of life are most important in developing sound eating habits in children. Many nursing activities to assist parents in choosing the most nutritionally sound methods of feeding their children have been discussed. However, an additional activity is initiating the diet history.

A diet or nutritional history from parents is one of the most useful tools nurses have. A diet assessment provides information regarding the adequacy of the diet and facilitates identification of areas of parental concern. Such an assessment should take place at every well-child visit, and the data obtained should be used in conjunction with current nutritional information to educate and guide parents in providing a well-balanced diet for their infant or child (Appendix A4).

HEALTH PROMOTION ACTIVITIES

Health is a state each of us wishes to experience, and some take for granted. However, it is not a guaranteed commodity but rather one that must be achieved and maintained. A person must be able to demonstrate behaviors that assist him or her in adapting in a healthy manner to his or her individual life circumstance. Promotion of health is evident in a person when he or she is able to identify and accept realities, adjust to changes in the environment, maintain a wholesome attitude toward self and life, and assume responsibility for managing his or her own health as appropriate for age and development. For the pediatric client, health promotion must involve the family. As primary caretakers, the child's family must also be motivated to assume health promotion responsibilities.

Nursing Role

The role of nursing is to facilitate and support individuals and their families in endeavors for health. Nurses can provide the means and specific activities that promote and maintain individual and family health. This interaction with nursing is especially important for children, who are dependent on others for health. Through objectives that promote health motivation, nurses can assist family members in using their own resources in identifying health needs and assuming responsibility for their own care. Nurses can assist parents in learning and adapting health promotion behaviors that positively affect the health of their children.

Health Assessment Visits

Many of health promotion activities have been discussed throughout this chapter. Of singular importance, however, are the well-child or health maintenance visits. Through these encounters nurses can assess, guide, counsel, and teach parents the basics of child health care.

The specific components of the health assessment visits include (1) gathering of health history information pertinent to the age and needs of the child; (2) collecting physical assessment data pertinent to the history; (3) developing a plan to meet health needs and to promote health in collaboration with parents; (4) implementing the plan of action; and (5) evaluating the plan through follow-up. Of utmost importance to the success of a health assessment and promotion visit is collaboration with the parents or child if old enough. Their involvement throughout the process is essential for compliance and can be achieved by active listening; soliciting parental thoughts, feelings, and opinions; verifying parental knowledge; and promoting parental participation. Appropriate health assessment tools are included in Appendixes A and B.

Group Education and Home Intervention

Group health education is a popular, effective, and time-efficient means of health promotion. Parenting groups often focus on a specific age, developmental stage, or health problem. However, before program development, as discussed in Chapter 11, nurses must assess the learning needs of clients and avoid duplication of current classes or health education resources already available in the community. (See Chapters 10 & 11 for a detailed discussion of program planning for health education.)

Intervention in the home should be based on the health needs of the client and directed toward health promotion. The reasons for initiating a home visit vary. It may be prompted by the birth of a premature infant or may be the result of follow-up needed for a major health problem such as congenital heart disease. Regardless of the originating cause, being in the client's home provides an opportunity for the nurse to assess and teach, using the resources of the client's environment. In addition, observational data gathered while in the client's home provide insights that can greatly influence the overall assessment of the client's health status.

Other Activities

Parental knowledge and understanding of child growth and development are means to ensure child health. To promote this healthy view of children, the development of reading bibliographies for parents is a useful resource. Such readings can focus on a specific age (eg., toddlers) or a specific problem (e.g., the allergic child). These resources can include materials related to parenting approaches or coping with the responsibilities of being a parent. When developing such bibliographies, they should be kept short, be specific to an age or problem, and consist of accurate, pleasant, and easy-to-read material.

Community Resources

Promoting the health of children is largely dependent on the use of available community resources. To identify resources for a specific area or region, nurses should consider the following potential services or interest groups:

Children's services centers or clinics
Well-child clinics
Woman-infant-child programs
Immunization clinics
Communicable disease clinics
Crippled children's services
Child abuse centers or councils
School health programs
Project Grow
Head Start
Parents Anonymous
Youth services bureaus
Crisis or hotlines for parents and/or children
Parent discussion groups
Adult education groups on aspects of parenting (e.g. infant care, coping)
Child development classes
Infant/child stimulation classes
Prepared childbirth and classes or groups on raising children
Local community advocate groups (e.g., single parents, working mothers, nursing mothers)
Day care nurseries

Government sponsored programs have played a major role in child health. Although many maternal-child health programs have suffered or been discontinued as a result of recent federal budged cuts, the following programs have been found to be cost-effective and continue to be funded (Select Committee on Children, Youth and Families, 1986):

Special supplement food program for women, infants and children (WIC)
Prenatal care
Medicaid
Childhood immunizations
Preschool education
Compensatory education
Education for all handicapped children
Youth employment and training

The community health nurse has a responsibility to use these program resources for clients, as well as become knowledgeable and active in legislative processes directed toward child health.

CLINICAL APPLICATION

In the first year of life nursing intervention can greatly affect the health of a child. However, this influence can only be exerted when the nurse puts expert knowledge to use in the clinical setting. For the student in the community health setting this application may take many forms. The primary purpose of all forms is to use knowledge to gain information and insights (assessment) in order to plan and promote the health of an individual child.

This section offers students ways to implement the material presented in this chapter. The suggestions which follow involve direct student participation to enhance learning.

Prenatal Health

Ensuring fetal health is an important first step in pediatric health promotion, which can be accomplished in many ways. Understanding the results of technologies such as sonography, amniocentesis, and fetal monitoring provides valuable data for nurses. For example, amniocentesis results which reveal a Down Syndrome infant should prompt the nurse to seek genetic counseling for the expectant parents. Students in the community health setting may find it useful to observe a genetic counselor's interview with expectant parents and identify relevant information and support given during the session.

Another way to ensure fetal health is to facilitate maternal health, as in prenatal teaching, which focuses on avoidance of alcohol, drugs, and smoking as well as the maternal nutritional requirements during pregnancy. Close monitoring of the mother's health, weight, and emotional state through regularly scheduled prenatal visits is another application for ensuring fetal health through maternal health.

Finally, preparing parents for the birth of their child is an additional way to promote a child's health prenatally. The student may find it useful to observe a prenatal class which offers parents information on early feeding alternatives, infant care such as bathing, diapering, skin and cord care, and use of car safety seats.

Neonatal Health

During the first month of life neonatal health can be monitored through home, office, or clinic visits. During these encounters, physiologic stability can be checked by taking and recording vital signs. Physical growth may be monitored by careful recording of weight and height, and development assessed through questions and observation. Data from the birth history, such as APGAR scoring, gestational age, and physical assessment findings are also useful. For example, a small for gestational age infant with an APGAR score of 8/9 who was discharged in the first 36 hours of life would benefit from a follow-up visit shortly after discharge to assess for the appearance of jaundice and adequacy of feeding.

The student may find it useful to take a prenatal and birth history from the parent of a 1-month-old infant and identify data from the history that does or does not promote health.

Infant Health

Clinical application of health promotion in the remaining 11 months of infancy occurs in the areas of physical growth and health and development of psychosocial and cognitive ability.

Physical growth continues to be monitored in the ways previously described in neonatal health. In addition, factors affecting growth and health are also assessed during health visits. For example, the student may observe nurses taking diet histories to obtain information about nutritional adequacy or assessing the sleep and elimination patterns of an infant. The student may also observe nurses counseling parents about normal newborn patterns and behaviors, feeding methods, and accident prevention methods. This counseling may be done in a one-to-one encounter or a group situation. The student may find it useful to design a class or series of classes for first-time parents on the subject of infant care and health. Content may include the topics previously mentioned with the addition of others such as stimulating infant development, managing minor infectious disease symptoms, taking an infant's temperature, or introducing solid foods.

Illness can be significantly reduced in children through immunization. The student will encounter immunization clinics in the community settings that involve not only the administration of vaccines but also the assessment of an individual child's immunization status and education about vaccine effectiveness and management of side effects. Vision and hearing screenings of infants will also be observed. The student may find it useful to conduct a vision and hearing screen on infants at ages 2, 7, and 12 months comparing the difference of techniques and response. For example, the 2-month-old will quiet when he or she hears a bell and fixate on an object directly in front of him or her, whereas the 11-month-old will turn his or her head toward the sound and see an object approaching from the side.

However, there are some infants and their families who have special needs. The premature infant requires more frequent and closer health encounters. The family of a SIDS victim requires intense, immediate encounters. In the community setting, the student will observe home visits to both of these families, referral to support groups, and frequent follow-up contacts. The student may find it useful to develop a nutritional plan for a preterm infant and compare this infant's nutritional needs, amounts, and frequency to those of a full-term infant to apply nutrition and nursing knowledge.

Developmental Health

Developmental growth and competency must be assessed throughout life. In infancy, the attachment process is important. Nurses in the community setting can facilitate this process in a number of ways: assessment, evaluation, and education. For example, the student may encounter the community health nurse observing a first-time mother in how she holds her infant, if she looks at or talks to the baby, or how she is able to care for the physical needs of the infant. Similarly, the infant is observed for response to his or her mother. Based on this observational assessment, the nurse may teach the mother different ways to hold the baby, encourage her to talk to the baby as she is bathing or diapering, or suggest the use of a front pack for carrying the infant around while keeping close contact. Periodically the nurse will evaluate the mother-infant relationship and offer suggestions for its enhancement. For example, the mother of a 4-month-old could be encouraged to get down

on the floor and play with her infant or spend time rocking and holding the baby before naps. Similarly, the father-infant bond is encouraged through suggestions of paternal involvement in care, such as feeding and bathing, and time for father and infant to be by themselves.

Factors affecting development are also assessed in the community health setting. The student may find it useful to observe a 10-month-old infant and identify characteristics that affect development. Observing for mastery of crawling or temperament characteristics or the amount of contact or support the mother receives from her own mother will help the student recognize the power of these influences on behavior. For example, the health care provider's advice about not starting solid foods too early often ranks last behind grandmother, husband, and friends because the other opinions have more influence with the mother.

Finally, the student will frequently encounter community health nurses doing an overall developmental assessment. Screening tools such as the Denver Developmental Screening Test are most useful in determining adequacy of development progression.

SUMMARY

The promotion of child health provides society with an opportunity to be a well society. The community health nurse has a unique opportunity to work with parents and children to promote positive childhood behaviors that will lead to a healthy adulthood.

Assessing the quality of the atmosphere in which a fetus grows is the first step in ensuring a healthy childhood. At the moment of conception some aspects of wellness are determined. Once conception has occurred, fetal growth becomes dependent on the intrauterine environment. Despite efforts to ensure fetal health through maternal health promotion, fetal difficulties may arise. Fetal assessment and the assessment of the mother's physical and psychosocial environment through the use of current methods and technologies assists the community health nurse in providing interventions that will help families prepare for the baby's first year of life. Prenatal visits help the nurse lay the groundwork for positive influences on the child's health and the parents' adjustment to the child.

Assessment of physical, emotional, and social growth and development and the physical examination are important techniques the nurse can use to evaluate the health of the neonate and infant, predict current and future health problems, and implement early preventive activities to ensure optimal health of the child. Factors that affect growth and development are successful mastery of tasks and milestones of each developmental stage, heredity, temperament, and health and living environment, family, peers, and life experiences.

Although major strides have been made in the past 5 years to improve the safety of life for infants significant problems still exist in infant mortality. The first year of life is the most hazardous period until age 65. The primary threats to infant health and survival are low birth weight, congenital anomalies with associated problems, and sudden infant death syndrome. The community health nurse can assist families to cope with these problems through counseling and teaching.

The major health problems of the neonate include jaundice and regulation of body temperature. With infants the health problems of major concern include upper respiratory tract infections, otitis media, allergies, gastrointestinal illnesses, and malnutrition. Other concerns of this age group include colic, feeding, sleeping, elimination patterns, behaviors, crying, flatus, hiccups, teething, spoiling, weaning, and stranger or separation anxiety. Anticipatory guidance, health teaching, and counseling are appropriate community health nursing interventions that assist families in making the child's first year of life healthy and happy.

≡ KEY CONCEPTS

Children are one third of our population and all of our future. Their health is our foundation.

Human growth and development are orderly, predictable processes that begin with the embryo and continue until death. The phases of growth and development are influenced by many hereditary and environmental influences.

Physical examination of the newborn is one of the most important tools for assessing neonatal health.

A child's growth process includes not only physical development but also emotional and social development.

A *mother* is defined as a biological parent, whereas *mothering* is the means necessary to care for the infant. *Motherliness* is the capacity of the mother to be gratified by the exchange between herself and her infant and to use this gratification for her own growth.

The development of a paternal-infant bond is especially important in today's society.

The quality of the child's living environment also influences his or her growth and development.

The quality of the parent-child relationship has been found to affect the child's development.

The primary threats to infant health and survival are low birth weight (immaturity), congenital anomalies with assoicated problems, and sudden infant death syndrome (SIDS).

For the family of infants at risk for SIDS, the community health nurse can be a valuable resource.

Infectious diseases are still the leading cause of illness and restricted activity for children under age 6 years in the United States.

Major health problems during the neonatal period include jaundice and problems in the regulation of body temperature.

Major health problems of infants are upper respiratory tract infections (URIs), otitis media, allergies, gastrointestinal illnesses, and malnutrition.

Accidents are the most preventable cause of morbidity and mortality in infants and children.

The assessment tools most useful to the nurse are those designed to assess psychosocial and/or developmental skills.

One of the most important components of maintaining a child's health is the promotion of good nutrition and dietary habits. The nurse's role involves encouraging and assisting parents in providing adequate nutrition for their child.

LEARNING ACTIVITIES

1. Develop a plan of immunization for a 2-month-old infant who has never been immunized and a 12-month-old infant who has received one DTP and OPV.

2. Administer the NPI and Degree of Bother Inventory to the mother of a 4-week-old infant. Then develop a plan of anticipatory guidance.

3. Conduct a diet history, and then develop a diet plan for a 4-month-old who is currently being breast-fed.

4. Develop a plan of nursing care for the family and premature infant, the family who has experienced a SIDS death, and the family and allergic infant.

BIBLIOGRAPHY

American Academy of Pediatrics: Report of the Committee on Infectious Diseases, ed. 20, Evanston, Ill., 1986, The Academy.

American Academy of Pediatrics: Committee on Nutrition, Pediatric nutrition handbook, Evanston, Ill., 1985, The Academy.

Apgar, V.: The newborn (Apgar) scoring system, Pediatr. Clin. North Am. 13:645-650, 1966.

Behrman, R.E., and Vaughan, V.C., editors: Nelson textbook of pediatrics, ed. 13, Philadelphia, 1987, W.B. Saunders Co.

Bierman, C.W., and Pearlman, D.C., editors: Allergic diseases of infancy, childhood and adolescense, Philadelphia, 1980, W.B. Saunders Co.

Bowlby, J.: Attachment and loss, vol. 1, Attachment, New York, 1969, Basic Books, Inc., Publishers.

Broussard, E.R., and Hartner, M.S: Further considerations regarding maternal perception of the firstborn. In Hellmuth, J., Jr., editor. Exceptional infant: studies in abnormalities, vol. 2, New York, 1971, Brunner/Mazel, Inc.

Brown, M.S., and Murphy, M.A.: Ambulatory pediatrics for nurses, ed., 2, New York, 1981, McGraw-Hill Book Co.

Caldwell, B.: Home observations for measurement of the environment, Little Rock, 1976, University of Arkansas Center for Child Development and Education.

Carey, W.B.: Clinical application of infant temperament measurements, J. Pediatr. 81:823-828, Oct. 1972.

Chess, S., and Thomas, A.: Dynamics of individual behavioral development. In Levine, M.D., Carey, W.B., Crocker, A.C., and Gross, R.T., editors: Developmental behavioral pediatrics, Philadelophia, 1983, W.B. Saunders Co.

Chow, M.P., et al.: Handbook of pediatric primary care, ed. 2, New York, 1984, John Wiley & Sons, Inc.

Clark, A.L., and Affonso, D.D.: Childbearing: a nursing perspective, ed. 2, Philadelphia, 1979, F.A. Davis Co.

Committee on Infectious Disease, American Academy of Pediatrics: Hemophilus type b polysaccharide vaccine, Pediatrics 76:322-323, August 1985.

DeAngelis, C.: Pediatric primary care, ed. 2, Boston, 1979, Little, Brown & Co.

Dubowitz, L., Dubowitz, V., and Goldberg, C.: Clinical assessment of gestational age in the newborn infant, J. Pediatr. 77:1-10, July 1970.

Dudek, B.: Counseling in sudden infant death syndrome and other childhood deaths, Pediatr. Rev. 7:168-169, Dec. 1985.

Duvall, E.: Marriage and family development, Philadelphia, 1977, J.B. Lippincott Co.

Erikson, E. Childhood and society, New York, 1963, Jeffrey Norton Publishers, Inc.

Food and Nutrition Board, National Research Council: Recommended dietary allowances, ed. 9, Washington, D.C., 1980, National Academy of Sciences.

Frankenburg, W.K., Goldstein, A.D., and Camp, B.W.: The revised Denver Developmental Screening Test: its accuracy as a screening instrument, J. Pediatr. 79:988-995, Dec. 1971.

Kaleida, P.H., and Stool, S.E.: Otitis media with effusion, Pediatr. Rev. 5:108-117, Oct. 1983.

Klaus, M.H., and Kennell, J.H.: Maternal-infant bonding, ed. 2, St. Louis, 1982, The C.V. Mosby Co.

Korones, S.B.: High-risk newborn infants, ed. 4, St. Louis, 1986, The C.V. Mosby Co.

Krugman, S., Ward, R., and Katz, S.L.: Infectious diseases of children, ed. 8, St. Louis, 1985, The C.V. Mosby Co.

Maternal and Child Health Program: Evaluation of body size and physical growth of children, The Maternal and Child Health Program, Washington, D.C., 1976, U.S. Department of Health, Education and Welfare.

Miles, M., editor: Mental health aspects of SIDS. Report of conference sponsored by the National Foundation for Sudden Infant Death and the National Institute of Mental Health, Kansas City, July 30, 1975, U.S. Deparment of Health, Education and Welfare.

Miller, S.J.: Prenatal nursing assessment of the expectant family, Nurse Pract. 11:40-43, May 1986.

Mitchell, K., and Mills, N.N.: Is the sensitive period in parent-child bonding overrated, Ped. Nurs. 9:91-95, Mar-Apr, 1983.

Norris-Berkemeyer, S., and Hutchins, K.A.: Home apnea monitoring, Pediatr. Nurs. 12:259-304, July/Aug. 1986.

Osborn, L.M.: Management of neonatal jaundice, Nurs, Pract. 11:41-46, Apr. 1986.

Progress Review: Pregancy and infant health objectives: Statistical update on the progress highlights of program activities; prepared by Division of Maternal and Child Health Care Delivery and Assistance, Health Resources and Services Administration, June 1985.

Rice, B.R., and Feeg, V.D.: First year developmental outcomes for multiple risk premature infants, Pediatr. Nurs. 11:30-35, Jan./Feb. 1985.

Select Committee on Children, Youth, and Families, 99th Congress, 1st session: Opportunities for success: Cost effectiveness programs for children, Washington, D.C. 1986. U.S. Government Printing Office.

Scipien, G.M., et al.: Comprehensive pediatric nursing, ed. 2, New York, 1979, McGraw-Hill Book Co.

Speer, J.J., and Sachs, B.: Selecting the appropriate family assessment tool, Pediatr. Nurs. 11:349-355, Sept./Oct. 1985.

Suskind, R.M., and Varma, R.N.: Assessment of nutritional status of Children, Pediatr. Rev. 5:195-202, Jan. 1984.

Sutterly, D., and Donnelly, G.: Prespectives in human development: nursing throughout the life cycle, Philadelphia, 1978, J.B. Lippincott Co.

Tackett, J.J., and Hunsberger, M.: Family centered care of children and adolescents, Philadelphia, 1981, W.B. Saunders Co.

Waechter, E.H., and Blake, F.G.: Nursing care of children, ed. 9, Philadelphia, 1976, J.B. Lippincott Co.

Whaley, L.F., and Wong, D.L.: Nursing care of infants and children, ed. 3, St. Louis, 1986, The C.V. Mosby Co.

Weiser, M.A., and Castiglia, P.T.: Assessing early father-infant attachment, MCN 9:104-106, May/Apr. 1984.

Williams, J.: Genetic counseling in pediatric nursing care, Pediatr. Nurs. 12:287-289, July/Aug. 1986.

Nancy Dickenson-Hazard

22

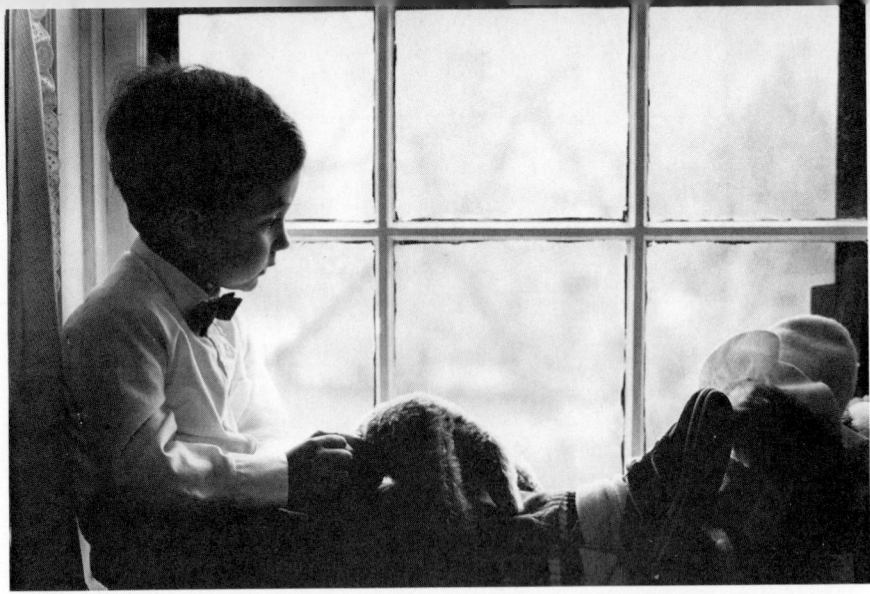

THE SECOND THROUGH SIXTH YEARS OF LIFE

≡ OBJECTIVES

After reading this chapter, the student should be able to:

Identify significant characteristics of physical and psychosocial growth and development in the toddler and the preschooler.

Identify the factors affecting the growth and development of the toddler and the preschooler and discuss the nurse's role in relation to these factors.

Identify the major causes of morbidity and mortality for 1- to 6-year-olds.

Discuss the nurse's role in prevention of the major causes of death and illness in 1- to 6-year-olds.

Identify and discuss appropriate nursing assessment tools specific for 1- to 6-year-olds.

Identify the role of the community health nurse in promoting the health of 1- to 6-year-olds.

≡ KEY TERMS

Erikson's concepts
expansion
expertise
expressive skills
genu valgum

genu varum
integration
Piaget's concepts
play

Preschool Readiness
  Experimental
  Screening Scale
  (PRESS)
preschooler
receptive skills
toddler

Toddlers and preschool children are mobile, curious, and adventuresome. As their developmental abilities expand, so do their environments and life experiences. Through the use of newly acquired physical language and social skills, these children become more adept at mastering and manipulating the world in which they live. The experimentation and learning of these age groups, however, can present obstacles to the child's well-being. The health goal for these children thus becomes the provision of opportunities for maximal growth and development while maintaining a healthy, safe environment. Parents and health care professionals will find a challenge in accomplishing this goal.

This chapter will focus on the assessment, maintenance, and promotion of the health of children in their toddler and preschool years. Significant physical and psychosocial aspects of health will be reviewed as well as the factors that can influence the attainment of the health goal.

PHYSICAL GROWTH AND DEVELOPMENT
The Toddler

The toddler years are the second and third years of life. During this time, physical growth and development rates decelerate from the rapid growth rate of infancy, and by 2 years of age the growth rate has stabilized. A toddler gains approximately 5 pounds (2.6 kg) annually. Birth weight is usually quadrupled by 2½ years. The average toddler gains 5 inches (12.7 cm) in the second year and 3 to 4 inches (7.6 to 10.2 cm) in the third year. A toddler's height at 2 years of age generally represents 50% of eventual adult height (see Appendix K2 for growth measurement averages).

Physiological functioning becomes more competent during the toddler years. The physiological changes of these years are not as dramatic as those of infancy and occur at a slower rate. However, development is continuing throughout all major organ systems.

Skeletal Growth

Skeletal growth is evidenced by the closure of the anterior fontanel by 18 months and the addition of epiphyses to the long bones. The broad-based gait of a toddler is created by a long trunk, short arms and legs, and large head (Fig. 22-1). To compensate for weight distribution, the spine curves anteroposteriorly (lordosis) and legs bow (genu varum). This

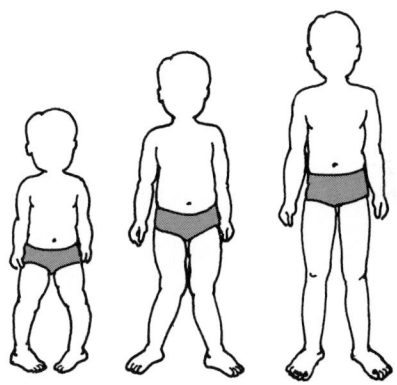

FIGURE 22-1

Progression from bowlegs to profound knockknees to correction. This sequence is perfectly normal and represents the normal pattern of development. (From Bunch, W.H. Reprinted with permission from *Pediatric Nursing*, 5(4), July/August 1979.)

bowlegged appearance generally persists until approximately 18 months of age and is followed by a physiological genu valgum (knock-knee) with protective toeing-in of the foot. See Appendix K6 and accompanying figures, which provide information regarding screening for orthopedic problems. The use of such procedures in a screening clinic situation will be most helpful to community health nurses when assessing young children for potential health problems.

Dental Growth

Dental growth continues with the calcification of first and second bicuspids and second molars. The number of primary teeth by the end of the second year has increased to a complete set of 20.

Preventive dental care should begin as soon as primary teeth erupt. Early care requires parents to wipe the teeth clean daily. By 18 months to 2 years, brushing with a fluoride toothpaste should be done daily. Teaching children to do this activity themselves should also be begun at this age. An initial visit to the dentist should be scheduled by 3 years of age. The use of sealants and fluorides (systemic, topical, or rinses) is very effective in preventing dental decay.

The challenge facing the community health nurse is to

secure access to dental care. Utilizing community-based dental clinics, or private dentists who assess fees on a sliding scale, based on the parents' income, and securing transportation for families are appropriate nursing interventions. Educating families regarding dental health—flossing, brushing and reducing the intake of cavity-causing (cariogenic) foods—is an additional nursing responsibility (Kronmiller and Nirschl, 1985).

Sleeping Patterns

The sleeping patterns of a toddler become more routine and there is often a need for bedtime rituals. The average toddler will sleep 8 to 12 hours a day and by 3 years has usually relinquished the afternoon nap for nighttime sleep only.

Feeding Behaviors

Feeding behaviors of toddlers also change. They are able to express distinct food preferences, and the 2- to 3-year-old is frequently an on-the-run, picky eater. The toddler becomes disinterested in food, the appetite falls, and food jags are common. The development of fine and gross motor skills also influences the ability to eat (see Table 21-10). Nonetheless, the toddler's nutritional requirements of between 1000 and 1500 kcal/day need to be met. Table 21-8 describes the distribution of calories for this age group, which also must be met.

Motor Skills

The toddler years are a time for achieving physical competence in both fine and gross motor skills. Refinement of previous motor skills and mastery of new ones make the toddler a very mobile, busy person. The average toddler should be assessed for motor performance when physical development is evaluated. Appendix K9 describes landmark behaviors and abilities for the toddler and the preschooler.

The Preschooler

The world of the 3- to 6-year-old rapidly expands because of increased physical abilities. Preschool children become active members of a world both in and out of the family unit. Growth patterns for each individual preschooler are fairly well established by the age of 3. During these years, most children increase their weight annually by approximately 5 pounds (2.6 kg). The average height gain is 3 to 4 inches (7.6 to 10.2 cm) in the third year and 2 to 3 inches (5.1 to 7.6 cm) per year until prepubescence.

Physical and physiological growth continues but at a slower pace than before. Some preschoolers grow gradually over the years, whereas others have growth spurts.

Significant Changes

Skeletal growth primarily consists in further bone ossification and epiphysis development. Visible dental growth is minimal until the sixth through eighth years, when primary teeth are lost and replaced by deciduous adult teeth. The lower central incisors are generally lost and replaced first. Musculoskeletal development is aided by central nervous system progression, as evidenced by a more coordinated and adept preschooler.

Visual acuity matures as well. The normally hyperoptic (farsighted) toddler develops into a preschooler with 20/30 vision by 5 or 6 years.

Motor Skills

The fine and gross motor skills of a preschooler also continue development. The clumsiness and oftentimes ineptness of the toddler vanish, and the preschooler becomes a master of physical abilities. The average 3- to 5-year-old needs to be assessed for these skills when physical development is evaluated (Appendix K9).

Feeding Habits

Eating and sleeping habits stabilize over the preschool years. The 3- to 5-year-old usually regains appetite and interest in food. Caloric intake requirement ranges from 90 to 100 kcal/kg/day, and the average daily water requirement is 1½ to 2 ounces per pound (100 to 125 ml/kg). These requirements can be met with a planned, balanced diet focusing on the preschooler's food preferences (Table 21-8).

Sleeping Patterns

The sleeping patterns of a preschooler are generally predictable. Most sleeping time is at night, although occasional daytime naps are not unusual. By 3 years most children have graduated from crib to bed, have developed definite bedtime routines, and display few sleep problems (Table 21-2).

PSYCHOSOCIAL GROWTH AND DEVELOPMENT
The Toddler

During the second through third years of life, a child's personality comes into its own. The individuality of the child becomes more apparent, and psychosocial development is enhanced by improved physical prowess as well as by expanding communicative ability.

Erikson's Concepts

This toddler age period is stage 2 in Erikson's theory of life development. During this time a toddler is charged with the task of developing a sense of autonomy versus one of shame or doubt. This task is partially accomplished through the discovery of the difference between dependence and independence. A toddler is able to make this discrimination if a sense of trust has developed in a significant caretaker. Trusting allows the child to see the separateness of self and the caretaker (usually the mother).

In viewing themselves as separate, toddlers will begin to explore their world. This exploration is facilitated by their physical abilities of walking, climbing, and running. They quickly learn that their own behaviors have an impact on their environment and the people within that world. They are no longer passive contributors to the family, and their newfound ability to effect change in their world facilitates a sense of autonomy and independence.

At the same time a toddler still needs and desires closeness and dependence, especially to significant persons. The exploration and independence are fun and challenging but are also full of unknowns, at times intimidating, at times frightening. Consequently, toddlers must begin to balance behaviors and actions that meet dependence needs with those that meet independence needs.

LEARNING TO BALANCE NEEDS. Achieving this balance is accomplished in a variety of ways. First the toddler learns to tolerate separation from the mother. As children learn more about themselves and their capabilities, they are able to separate from others for longer periods of time. Initially the separation may be merely across the room, but gradually the distance and time of separation increase as the toddler becomes more secure with this independence.

COMMUNICATION SKILLS. The ability to communicate further facilitates achievement of the balance between autonomy and doubt. Language is an important aspect of psychosocial as well as intellectual development, and its development involves comprehension (receptive) as well as speaking (expressive) skills (Lenneberg, 1967). The stages of language development are found in Table 22-1).

Receptive skills. Receptive language skills are known to be achieved earlier than expressive skills, as evidenced by toddlers' early ability to follow simple instructions (Goldberg, 1984). During this time toddlers are absorbing the language of their environment. They are passive participants in the communication process, and their behavioral responses to the language of their world reinforce their sociability, sense of autonomy, and subsequent participation. For example, a toddler responds to mother's request to put the toy in the toybox by doing so. Mother responds with praise, and the toddler feels a sense of pleasure and accomplishment. The act has been an independent one, which increases social acceptability with mother and contributes to wanting to participate in future interactions.

Expressive skills. Expressive language skills make toddlers active participants in the communication process (Goldberg, 1984). Through speech, toddlers expand the scope of

their interactive ability. They can now respond to their environment through verbal and behavioral expression, thereby having a greater impact. For example, imagine the effect the toddler will have if he tells the mother "I did it" after being asked to put the toys away. Both mother and child feel a sense of accomplishment, but the child is now able to verbalize this feeling as well as act it out.

PLAY. The dimension of play becomes an integral part of the toddler's life and serves as a tool to achieve developmental tasks. Play reflects a child's physical, cognitive, and psychosocial development and serves as a medium for the child's orientation to self and the world. Learning is accomplished through play, and play provides the child with a safe, self-controlled means to explore feelings and the environment. In addition, play contributes to a child's development in all spheres: the physical activity of play contributes to coordination; the explorative activity of play contributes to reality orientation; and the experimental activity of play contributes to self-awareness and emotional expression (Caplan, 1973).

Play undergoes development as well, based on the child's abilities and environmental changes and opportunities. The progression of play reflects varying degrees of sociability, from playing alone to playing alongside to playing cooperatively. The younger child spends the most time playing alone or beside another child, whereas the 5-year-old is able to play cooperatively. Types of play have been categorized by Parten (1932) as follows:

Unoccupied behavior: child occupies self with watching whatever happens to be of momentary interest. When nothing exciting is occurring, play is initiated with own body (e.g., sitting, standing, rolling).

Onlooker: child watches others play. May make inquiries or give suggestions but does not interact in play with others.

Solitary independent: child plays alone and independently with toys different from those used by other children who are within speaking distance. Child does not get close but pursues own activity without concern for what others are doing.

Parallel: child plays beside other children, not with them, using similar toys and choosing activities that bring others close.

Associative: child plays with other children in a common activity. Borrowing and lending occur but there is no organization, division of labor, or control by any one child that shapes direction of play.

Cooperative: child plays in a group that is organized for a purpose. Roles and tasks are assigned, activity is organized, and leadership and control are evidenced.

NURSE'S ROLE. Knowledge of the characteristics of play is most useful in assessing the productivity and purpose of play as related to the child's developmental stage. Since play is a child's work, it is important for nurses to be knowledgeable about ways to stimulate play. Concrete, practical suggestions from nurses to parents can promote healthy, productive play. Principles useful in assisting parents to promote play are as follows:

Parents should be taught characteristics and content of play.

TABLE 22-1

Age ranges of language developmental stages

Stages	Age
Cooing stage	0-2 months
Babbling stage	2-6 months
First word, usually imitated	12-18 months
Rapid vocabulary acquisition	18 months-3 years
Open and pivot words	
Telegraphic sentences	
Steady word acquisition	3-5 years
Multiword sentences	
Basic mastery of language by end	
Progressively complex sentences	6-11+ years
Use of pronouns, proper nouns, prepositions	
Basic grammatical mastery by end	

From Tackett, J.J., and Hunsberger, M.: Family centered care of children and adolescents, Philadelphia, 1981, W.B. Saunders Co., p. 151.

Opportunities for play should be provided that are appropriate to the child's age.

The expense of a toy is not necessarily an indicator that it will promote development. Common household items such as plastic cartons provide as much stimulation as an expensive set of stackables.

Parents need to play with their child.

Parents need to be aware of the child's response to play—that is, when to stimulate and when to rest.

Play should be pleasurable.

Toys should be safe, durable, and suitable to the child's developmental abilities.

Toys should promote the child's own creativity and resourcefulness and not be excessive, confusing, or overwhelming.

In addition to adhering to these principles, nurses can assist parents in directing play and selecting toys through suggested readings and provision of information appropriate to child's age and safety needs.

Piaget's Concepts

Children of toddler or preschool age see things only from their point of view. Lifelike qualities are given to inanimate objects, and everything is considered real. They believe they can make things happen just by thinking of them and that the world exists for them alone.

Piaget views this characteristic egocentric thought pattern as the preoperational period of cognitive development. This period, which lasts from 2 to 7 years of age, makes the child appear quite illogical. The child's task is to utilize language and memory and to understand past, present, and future happenings. Specifically, the 2- to 4-year-olds are in stage 1 of this period, or the preconceptual phase. During this time they are able to form mental images that stand for things they cannot see (symbolic thought). Play becomes the primary tool for the development of these images and, coupled with language and imitation, assists children to establish their place in relationship to their environment. Since they are egocentric, much of their play is parallel because they cannot readily focus on what someone else may want. As they become more aware of other influences in their world, children of this age will display more socialized behavior at the end of this period of cognitive development.

NURSE'S ROLE. Assessment of developmental milestones continues to be an important responsibility of nurses. While much of a child's development has occurred, personality formation is ongoing. Fine and gross motor skills have previously been reviewed in this chapter. Knowledge and assessment of social and language skills are also appropriate (see Table 22-1 and Appendix K8).

The Preschooler
Erikson's Concepts

Ages 4 to 8 constitute the third stage of development according to Erikson. During this phase children must learn to develop a sense of initiative versus a sense of guilt as they broaden the scope of their environment. They will come into contact with more peers, more authority figures, and more new life experiences and societal rules. In their eagerness to explore, the preschoolers rush in to accomplish new skills, tasks, and capabilities in the expanded world of home, school, and neighborhood. They begin to initiate themselves and their personalities in a world away from home. They may also have some feelings of guilt for wanting to be dependent and to be close to familiar surroundings and persons. Resolving this conflict and achieving a psychosocial balance requires parental sensitivity in knowing when to comfort and allow dependence and when to encourage independence.

The preschoolers' own developmental progression assists them in resolving this conflict. The comfortable expansion of their social sphere and skills occurs when the 4- to 6-year-old has mastered some degree of self-control. It is at this age that all aspects of psychosocial development begin to have the greatest interaction, because social, emotional, physical, and cognitive development must all come forth in order for the child to be acceptable in social spheres outside the home.

Piaget's Concepts

Cognitive development impacts greatly on this total developmental interaction. According to Piaget, 4- to 6-year-olds begin to move away from egocentricity. At the same time they achieve control over bodily functions and to some degree behavior. In stage 2 of the preoperational period, the preschooler becomes more perceptual and intuitive. Prelogical reasoning appears, and experiences and objects are judged by outside appearances and results. As an example, that father will be angry if father's newly planted flowers are pulled up is deduced by a 4-year-old *before* the act is carried out, thereby demonstrating prelogical reasoning. As for objects being judged by outward appearances, a preschooler will insist that there are more oranges than tangerines when shown an equal number because the oranges are bigger.

Cognition is further enhanced by the child's increasing use of language to express self rather than acting out feelings or desires. This development influences the child's play, which subsequently becomes more social. In sum, as preschoolers move into spheres outside the home, they are equipped to deal with forthcoming experiences because cognition, language, and control have increased while egocentrism and dependence have decreased.

Sociability

With exposure to new life experiences, the preschooler will begin to test out social behaviors for safety and effectiveness. Some of these behaviors will be retained and reused, and others will be adapted for better efficacy. Always the preschooler will continue to develop psychosocially and cognitively, beginning with the foundation acquired in early years and building upward.

A developmental assessment of this age must take into account the basic skills with which the preschooler should be equipped. Fine and gross motor milestones have been previously reviewed. Appropriate social behaviors and language skills are outlined in Appendix K8.

FACTORS AFFECTING GROWTH AND DEVELOPMENT

An overview of pertinent factors that influence the growth and development of children has been discussed in the preceding chapter. These factors continue to be influential in the toddler and preschool years in addition to those discussed below.

Expansion and Expertise

Of singular importance to toddler and preschool children is the expansion of experiences created by their own increasing developmental abilities. A type of feedback mechanism ensues whereby the child is able to do more physically and psychosocially, which expands the manipulative and learning opportunities in the environment. Once new elements in the environment are mastered, the child uses this expertise to practice and expand further to include interactions with people and experiences outside the home. As an example, the toddler, having learned to climb, will push a chair to the countertop to reach a cookie. Once the climbing is mastered in the home, the toddler will then use this skill at the playground, where climbing up the slide will be attempted.

Integration

As the child advances through the preschool years, all the developmental skills will be integrated into the whole personality. Rather than focusing on a specific skill, such as the 2-year-old learning to climb or the 3-year-old mastering language, the child at the end of the preschool years will have incorporated all skill spheres into a repertoire of effective behaviors. Although a distinct individual person exists in the child as an infant, this individual becomes more apparent by the end of the fifth year as a result of this integration process.

Working Mothers

Currently more than 9 million children younger than 6 have mothers who are working outside the home. By 1990 the population of children requiring day care will reach 10.4 million (Hayghe, 1984). The primary motive for mothers working outside the home is monetary need.

Because of this increasing trend toward working mothers, family functioning has changed (e.g., chores and day-to-day parenting must be shared) and many mothers experience conflicting emotions (such as guilt at leaving their children in someone else's care, yet relief at having the additional income). Whatever changes occur because mother works, the child's need for day care remains constant. One half of working families resolve child care needs by arrangements between the parents while the other half choose from arrangements in the community (e.g., day care centers, day care by relatives, or home care by a nonrelative) (Hayghe, 1984).

NURSE'S ROLE The community health nurse can facilitate the family's decision making and adjustment to the mother's return to work and selection of day care at several points in the process. Initially the nurse can assist the parent(s) in identifying the need for a mother to re-turn to work and possible alternatives. For example, part-time work by one spouse may be sufficient to meet financial need, or work in the home by one parent may be an alternative.

Second, once the decision has been made, assisting parents to identify child care alternatives is a responsibility nurses can assume. Care options appropriate to the child's age should be explored with parents (e.g., care in the home, day care centers or homes, nursery school, play schools or groups, kindergarten). To facilitate the choice of child care options, the nurse should advise parents to consider (1) the philosophy, attitude, and emotional tone expressed by the person acting as primary caretaker; (2) the physical environment, its safety, its appeal and diversity, its materials and equipment, and its access or proximity to parents; (3) other participants in the setting, their health, their response to caretaker and environment, and their ages and developmental levels. In addition, it is wise for nurses to counsel parents about the need to visit and observe the care setting before final selection and to periodically evaluate the setting and its effects and influence on the child. Other factors to consider are the licensing and accreditation status of the facility, the amount of parental involvement allowed, the program curriculum if applicable, and the educational qualifications of the administration and staff (Wong, 1986).

Third, the nurse can be instrumental in developing policies at the community level that would positively affect day care. Advocating requirements for up-to-date immunizations for all children and staff, for special care provisions for sick children, and for sanitary codes are appropriate nursing actions. The nurse can also implement interventions such as training day care staff in the prevention of the spread of infectious disease and making recommendations to employers for parental leave from work to care for sick children (Aronson and Gilsdorf, 1986).

Finally, nurses can facilitate parental coping and adjustment to the working-mother family situation. Appropriate nursing intervention would focus on reallocating chores and responsibilities to include all family members; assisting parents to identify feelings (e.g., inadequacy, guilt, anger, resentment, relief, freedom) regarding return to work and the influence these feelings and behaviors have on the child's attitude toward this change; assisting the family to identify stresses created by the change that may produce tension; and assisting all family members in developing adequate coping behaviors.

COMMON CAUSES OF MORBIDITY AND MORTALITY

Since causes and factors are generally studied for the 1- to 5-year-old range, mortality and morbidity will be discussed in terms of both the toddler and the preschooler age groups. Problems relevant to one specific age group will be defined as such.

Mortality

Children over 1 year of age are enjoying better health today than ever before. The death rate for children has fallen to 34.1 per 100,000 population in 1984 versus 330 per 100,000 in 1925. By 1990 this mortality is expected to be reduced further, to 34 per 100,000 (Health, 1986).

The primary cause of death formerly was infectious and communicable disease. Now cases of these once-dreaded diseases (polio, diphtheria, measles, and rubella) are seldom seen. Instead, accidents and injuries have become responsible for the majority of childhood deaths. In descending order of incidence, the most common causes of fatal injuries are motor vehicle accidents, drowning, burns, poisoning, choking, and falls. Motor vehicle accidents are responsible for 50% of all deaths in children ages 1 to 5. Other accidents or injuries are responsible for an additional 20%. No other preventable cause poses such a threat to life as accidents. In addition, the segments of the childhood population most at risk are boys, who demonstrate an annual death rate higher than girls, and blacks, who demonstrate an overall higher mortality rate (Health, 1983).

NURSE'S ROLE. Clearly the goal of nursing should be provision of preventive measures for these major health threats. Using safety measures can prevent most accidents. Appendix J6 provides age-appropriate accident prevention interventions that should be a primary component of every nurse's management plan.

Particular attention needs to be paid to home and auto safety, such as advocating use of seat belts and car seats, referral to a car seat loaner program, and childproofing the home.

Community health nurses have the opportunity to implement education in the home, clinic, and school settings. A reduced number of accident-related deaths and injuries can be realized by the provision of organized education programs from community health nurses.

Morbidity

For children in the toddler and preschool age groups, infections continue to be the most common cause of restricted activity. Although resistance to many causative agents of infectious diseases is developing in children from 1 to 6 years, their exposure and subsequent immunity are by no means complete. The toddler and the preschooler are frequently plagued with upper respiratory infections and secondary complications such as pharyngitis, otitis media, bronchitis, and bronchiolitis. The incidences of influenza and pneumonia as well as allergies can also be high for these age groups. See Chapter 21 for a detailed discussion of these health problems.

NURSE'S ROLE. The role of the nurse clearly is to implement preventive measures. These nursing activities may be directed toward primary prevention (i.e., reducing the incidence of the problem for the child) or secondary prevention (i.e., reducing the incidence of secondary complications). Specific nursing interventions for the health problems mentioned earlier that affect toddlers and preschoolers are discussed in Chapter 21. The reader is referred to that chapter for a review (Appendix J8).

MAJOR HEALTH PROBLEMS

Although the major health problems of infants discussed in Chapter 21 have significant incidence rates in the 2- to 6-year-old, the toddler and preschool groups are also at risk of developing additional illnesses. Of significance are the viral illnesses and exanthems.

Viral Illnesses

Viruses are the most common cause of infectious disease in children. Of particular significance are the incidences of viral hepatitis, influenza, roseola, and varicella. Appendix J7 reviews their presentation and management as well as the features of other common infectious diseases.

Hepatitis

Up to 70,000 cases of viral hepatitis are reported each year in the United States. There are two types of viral hepatitis, type A and type B. Clinical features are compared in Table 22-2. Since children are less likely to demonstrate jaundice and generally have milder symptoms, their symptomatic and supportive care can be managed easily at home with the proper counseling.

Influenza

Influenza is an acute disease of the respiratory tract caused primarily by A, B, and C influenza viruses. Since these viruses have the ability to change (become mutants), epidemics can be anticipated as well as difficulties in implementing an influenza immunization program.

Roseola and Varicella

Roseola is the most common exanthem in infants and young children ages 6 months to 2 years; 95% of the cases of this benign viral illness occur in this age group. Roseola demonstrates a seasonal pattern, with peak incidence in the spring and autumn. Varicella, commonly known as chickenpox, is a highly contagious disease caused by the varicella-zoster virus. Children between 2 and 8 years demonstrate the highest incidence, whereas infants are generally protected in the first few months through maternal passive immunity. Varicella occurs most frequently in the winter and spring months. Appendix J7 reviews the common exanthematous diseases.

Measles, Mumps, Rubella

With the introduction of the measles, mumps and rubella vaccines, the incidences of these once-common childhood illnesses have been reduced significantly. However, unimmunized populations are at risk, with the highest incidence of disease occurring in school-age children. Prevention of these infectious diseases is the primary goal, and education and promotion of immunization are well within the nurse's role. See Chapter 17 and Appendix D for a discussion of immunizations.

Infectious Diseases in Day Care Centers

Epidemics in day care centers are occurring because of the large number of children in day care and because they are of the ages that are most immunologically susceptible. The

TABLE 22-2

Hepatitis A and hepatitis B: comparison of major features

Features	Hepatitis A	Hepatitis B
Synonym	Infectious hepatitis	Serum hepatitis
Incubation period	15-40 days	50-180 days
HB Ag (Australia antigen in blood)	Absent	Present in incubation period
Age group	Usually children and young adults	All age groups
Mode of transmission	Primarily fecal-to-oral route; some parenteral spread (blood products); contaminated water, food, infected shellfish	Primarily parenteral (transfusion of blood or blood products, intravenous drug inoculation); some nonparenteral (body fluids of infected persons)
Season	Fall and winter predominantly but also throughout the year	Any season
Onset	Usually acute	Usually insidious
Fever	Common; precedes jaundice	Less common
Jaundice	Rare in children; more common in adults	Rare in children; more common in adults
Severity	Usually mild	Often severe
Abnormal SGOT	Transient; 1-3 weeks	More prolonged; 1-8 months
Thymol turbidity	Usually elevated	Usually normal
IgM levels	Usually increased	Usually normal
Virus excretion		
Blood	Present during late incubation period and early acute phase	Present during late incubation period and acute phase; may persist for months and years
Feces	Present during late incubation period and acute phase	Probably present but no direct proof
Value of gammaglobulin prophylaxis	Good	Uncertain
Immunity		
Homologous	Present	Present
Heterologous	None	None

From Chow, M.P., et al.: Handbook of pediatric primary care, ed. 2, New York, 1984, John Wiley & Sons, Inc., p. 1079; as adapted from Krugman, S., et al.: Infectious diseases of children, ed. 6, St. Louis, 1977, The C.V. Mosby Co., p. 101.

> ## INTERVENTIONS FOR PREVENTION OF DAY CARE DISEASES
>
> Teach appropriate handwashing technique, emphasizing frequency.
> Instruct in proper disposal of soiled clothes and diapers.
> Instruct in proper cleansing of changing areas.
> Stress staff assignment to small groups that do not cross age groups.
> Encourage proper kitchen cleaning and meal preparation by staff members other than those who change diapers.
> Instruct in toy cleaning.
> Advocate an exclusion policy for febrile or diarrheal children.

primary risk factors for an increased incidence of infectious diseases are day care center size, the presence of diapered children, and the acceptance of drop-in children. The most commonly transmitted diseases are respiratory tract infections, *Haemophilus influenzae* type B disease, hepatitis type A, diarrheal disease, and cytomegalovirus infection (Smith, 1986).

The focus of the community health nurse needs to be on prevention of disease outbreak and spread. Appropriate interventions should be directed toward the day care staff through health education. The community health nurse should pay particular attention to teaching the preventive measures illustrated in the box at left (Smith, 1986).

Child Abuse and Neglect

The epidemic of child abuse is a recently discovered and unfortunate phenomenon. The battered and neglected children in the United States account for many injuries, burns, and accidents, as well emotional problems, brain damage, and even death. Although the actual number of cases of child abuse and neglect is elusive because of difficulties in identification and reporting, estimates range from 200,000 to 4 million a year. At least 4000 children die annually from circumstances associated with abuse or neglect (Chow et al., 1984).

Incidence and Predisposing Factors

Children under three are the most frequent victims and women the most frequent abusers, although men abuse more severely and are involved in sexual assault. All races and socioeconomic groups are involved, but statistics indicate a higher incidence in lower socioeconomic classes (Kempe and Helfer, 1972). Most perpetrators are known to the child victim (Ryan, 1984).

The psychodynamics involved in an abusive situation are characterized by the following factors:

A crisis precipitating the occurrence, preceded by multiple frustrations, problems, and inability to cope

Socially isolated parents and children

A premeditated injury

Parents who were abused as children, who lack support systems, and who display a lack of trust

A child who has been "labeled" as different by the parent, possibly as a result of unplanned pregnancy, illness, or prematurity

Common clinical findings associated with child abuse as given by Chow et al. (1984) are listed in the box below.

NURSE'S ROLE. Prevention is the primary goal in regard to child abuse (Ryan, 1984). Nurses have the responsibility to use their knowledge and skill to identify potentially abusive situations. Risk screening should be implemented prenatally and postnatally and periodically throughout well child care (see Appendix J9). If a family at risk is identified, additional supportive measures need to be implemented in the interest of prevention (see Appendix J9).

Managing a situation of child abuse is difficult and will require a multidisciplinary approach (Fontana and Robinson, 1976). Nurses can be an integral part of this team by offering support to the parents and the child, teaching parents how to nurture and parent, and investigating community services available to the family. Both child and parents will require health care interventions. The goal of management is directed toward the protection of the child, support and rehabilitation of parents, and the return of the child to the home when deemed safe. In addition, it is mandatory that all cases of suspected abuse and neglect in the United States be reported to appropriate authorities.

Although this responsibility is generally the physician's, nurses are also among the professionals who are obligated to report abuse or neglect. Although failure to report suspected cases can result in prosecution, reporters of such cases are immune from court action for civil liability under the Child Abuse Prevention and Treatment Act. Generally, child abuse or neglect is reported to local or state government child protection agencies. Abused children usually are temporarily removed from the home until the family situation restabilizes and the parents have demonstrated a willingness to continue care as well as a positive caring attitude toward their child.

A plan of follow-up is essential to any circumstance of child abuse. Nurses can contribute in this follow-up by assisting parents to deal with the frustrations of parenthood, teaching parenting approaches, providing support and encouragement, and facilitating the identification and use of community resources. Appropriate community services may include the following (Chow et al., 1984):

Crisis hotlines

Parents Anonymous

Single parents' groups

Lay community organizations

Crisis nurseries or child care centers

Day care centers

Parent education groups

Health visitor groups

National Center for Missing and Exploited Children

COMMON CONCERNS AND PROBLEMS

Parents continue to experience concern over common problems as their children grow. This occurrence was discussed in Chapter 21 and Table 21-6 gives an overview of common childhood behaviors.

Specific behavioral habits of toddlers and preschoolers that evoke parental concern may include or involve biting, hitting, masturbation, sleep and eating disturbances, negativism, temper tantrums, toilet training, discipline, and limit setting.

NURSE'S ROLE. Nurses have the responsibilities of educating parents in understanding the normalcy of these behaviors, assisting parents to identify effective coping behaviors when dealing with the behavior of concern, identifying with parents appropriate approaches to handling the child and the behavior, and providing support and reassurance to parents. Appendix J8 provides information pertinent to the nursing assessment and management of the these common problems.

ASSESSMENT TOOLS

The basic tools and techniques of a pediatric assessment, including monitoring physical and psychosocial aspects of health, are discussed in Chapter 23. Additionally, Appendix A3 presents the components of a health assessment, including health promotion activities, which are specific to the toddler and preschool age groups. Variations of these tools and techniques relevant to the toddler or preschool child are discussed in the following section.

COMMON CLINICAL FINDINGS OF CHILD ABUSE

Skin: burns, old scars, ecchymosis, soft tissue swelling, human bites

Fractures: skull, rib, limb, presence of old fractures on x-ray films, epiphyseal separations

Subdural hematomas

Intestinal injuries

Trauma to genitals

Growth retardation

Poor hygiene

Whiplash: shaken infant syndrome, caused by manual shaking of trunk or extremities, resulting in intraocular and intracranial hemorrhage (Caffey, 1974, p. 396)

Abnormal genital findings

Abnormal anal findings

From Chow, M.P., et al.: Handbook of pediatric primary care, ed. 2, New York, 1984, John Wiley & Sons, Inc., p. 1213.

Monitoring Physical Growth and Development

Measurements of a child's height and weight continue to be valuable tools for assessing growth. For children old enough to stand (generally over 3 years), a traditional scale or yardstick may be used (Figure 22-2). The child's heels, shoulder blades, and occiput should touch the wall. Older children can be weighed accurately on an adult-type scale, wearing only underwear. Monitoring growth by plotting measurements on growth charts should also continue (Appendix K2).

Vital Signs

Continued measurement of vital signs provides pertinent health data and should be implemented at each encounter with the child. For older children, reliable pulse measures may be taken in the radial area, and respiratory rate can be counted as they sit, through either auscultation or observation. For blood pressure measurements, the standard sphygmomanometer can be used for children over 3 years. The important point of this technique, which must be remembered, is that a blood pressure cuff should cover two thirds of the upper arm to gain an accurate reading.

Other Indicators of Physical Growth and Development

Additional methods of monitoring physical growth in the young child include assessment of skeletal or bone age and dental age. In addition, laboratory studies may be useful in monitoring healthy growth.

Familiarity with the purpose and interpretation of these specialized tools may be useful to the community health nurse in recognizing the need for such an assessment, in making appropriate referrals, and in developing a nursing management plan (see Chapter 21 for a discussion of dental age and laboratory studies. See a pediatric nursing textbook for a discussion of skeletal age).

Screening Tools

Assessment of a child's vision, hearing, and speech is an essential component of any health assessment. Although it is impossible to test all ages for all the specific aspects of vision, hearing, and speech development, age-appropriate methods for determining general abilities are available and should be used. As the child's ability develops and participation in screening procedures becomes more cooperative, the more complete and accurate the assessment of vision, hearing, and speech will become. For example, an infant can be assessed for an overall ability to see, focus, hear, and utter sound, whereas a preschool or school-age child, because of a higher level of development, can be assessed for visual acuity, visual fields, near and far vision, color vision, hearing acuity, vocabulary, articulation, and syntax. Incorporating the appropriate age-specific screening method of vision, hearing, and speech development is well within the nurse's role. Appendix K5 discusses appropriate vision and hearing screening methods. Table 22-3 reviews age-appropriate development of normal speech sounds.

A useful speech assessment tool is the Denver Articulation Screening Examination (DASE) (Appendix K7). The DASE is a screening tool that requires no special training to administer. It is used to detect speech disorders in children from 2½ to 6 years of age. This word imitation test consists of 22 items complete with pictures. Administration of the test requires the examiner to say the words and have the child repeat them.

Communication Strategies

Communicating effectively with children is a challenge. Use of nonverbal techniques can assist the community health nurse in soliciting information and feelings from children. For the younger child, these strategies may include storytelling, expressing feelings in terms of a third person, play, and drawing. For older children, strategies include such techniques as "three wishes," writing, word associations, and discussing pros and cons (Whaley and Wong, 1985).

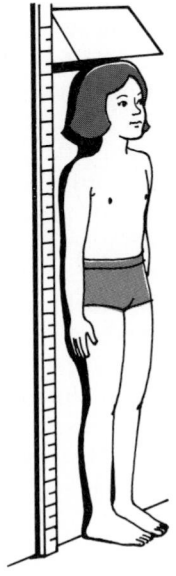

FIGURE 22-2

Measurement of height. Child's heels, shoulder blades, and occiput touch wall. (From Evaluation of body size and physical growth of children, the Maternal and Child Health Program, Washington, D.C., 1976, Department of Health, Education, and Welfare.)

 TABLE 22-3

Development of speech sounds

Age	Sounds
3 to 4 years	Lip sounds—*m, p, b, w, h*
4 to 5 years	Tongue contact sounds—*n, t, d, ng, k, g, y*
5 to 6 years	*f*
6 to 6½ years	(*v, ch, l, sh,* and voiced *th* (as in *thin*)
6½ to 7 years	*z, s, r, th* and voiceless *th* (as in *thin*)

From Brown, M.S., and Murphy, M.A.: Ambulatory pediatrics for nurses, ed. 2, New York, 1981, McGraw-Hill Book Co., p. 295.

Monitoring Psychosocial Development

The need to implement developmental screening and the purpose of such screening are discussed in Chapter 21. The continued monitoring of psychosocial development remains important during the toddler and preschool years. Several of the developmental scales previously discussed can be used in the assessment of children in this age group (e.g., DDST and HOME). In addition to these, tools specific to the toddler and the preschooler are discussed below.

Preschool Readiness Experimental Screening Scale

The Preschool Readiness Experimental Screening Scale (PRESS) is designed to assess the maturational level of children between 4 and 5 years of age. It does not assess intellectual capacity but focuses on knowledge of colors and numbers, ability to draw, comprehension, coordination, and personal-social maturity. This tool is easy to administer and score and provides information indicative of a child's overall readiness to attend kindergarten (Rogers and Rogers, 1972).

Additional Psychological and Intellectual Tests

Many screening tests have been developed with the intent of measuring various psychological and intellectual traits of childhood. Appendix K12 provides a summary of such screening tools that may be useful for the nurse dealing with pediatric clients within the community.

Immunizations

Continuation of the basic immunization schedule implemented in infancy is indicated for the toddler and the preschooler. The reader is referred to the immunization section of Chapter 21 and Appendix D2 for a full discussion of immunizations.

Nutrition

The promotion of nutritionally sound dietary habits remains important during the toddler and preschool years. (See the section on nutrition in Chapter 21 for a review of the basic nutrition principles indicated for children.) Throughout the first year infants will develop significantly in the types and amounts of food they can eat. They will progress from having to be fed to insisting on feeding themselves. As a child progresses through the toddler and preschool years, nutritional status and eating are affected by a decreasing physical growth rate, motor maturity, and cognitive and personality factors. Children learn to feed themselves and demonstrate food preferences and individual eating habits, thereby exerting an influence over their nutritional status. In assisting parents to maintain nutritional adequacy for their toddler or preschooler, the following suggestions can be made:

Offer a balanced diet that meets recommended daily allowances for age (Table 21-8), incorporating food preferences and variety.

Offer food several times a day (i.e., five to six times as opposed to three regular meals).

Limit milk intake to 16 ounces a day to avoid a filling up on milk instead of eating solids as well as milk.

Offer suggested amounts of food as listed in Appendix J4.

Emphasize favorites that are nutritional and are easy to handle.

Continue to avoid nuts, bony fish, and popcorn because of risk of aspiration.

Generally vitamin and iron supplements are not required. However, during periods when appetite and intake decrease, temporary use is appropriate. During such periods, nutritionally sound foods (especially those high in iron and low in sugar) should be offered more frequently.

Diet Assessment

Since toddlers and preschoolers can be unpredictable in regard to the quantity as well as the quality of what they eat, periodic assessment is indicated in determining nutritional adequacy. Appendix A4 illustrates age-appropriate diet histories. Factors specific to these age groups that require consideration in the nurse's assessment and management include the need for (1) increased caloric intake; (2) 10% to 15% protein, 50% carbohydrate, and 35% fat caloric distribution; and (3) increased water intake.

HEALTH PROMOTION ACTIVITIES

The community health nurse can assist families to promote toddler and preschooler well-being in a variety of ways and settings. Many of these activities have been discussed throughout this chapter, but several warrant reemphasis.

Health Assessment

A continuation of an orderly assessment of health is essential during the toddler and preschool years. (Appropriate health assessment tools are included in the appendix section of this book.) The health assessment visit needs to be implemented on a regular basis and should focus on promoting health-oriented behaviors in the parent and child. Parent education and anticipatory guidance from nurses are two means of promoting such behaviors, in addition to emphasis on preventive health measures, particularly safety and accident prevention (see Appendix J6). Also, the nursing management plan for health maintenance activity needs to include the child's participation. For example, even at the age of 2 to 3 years, a child can be taught and encouraged to brush his or her teeth, thereby promoting dental health. Finally, the use of screening tools during the health assessment visit, which are designed to assess physical and psychosocial development, are particularly important in the rapidly changing toddler or preschooler. Age-appropriate tools are discussed earlier in this book and in Appendixes A3 and K8.

Parenting Groups

Parenting groups are an additional way the community health nurse can promote health. Being the parent of a toddler or preschooler can be stressful. Assisting parents to understand and be knowledgeable about their child's developmental phase should be a nursing focus. Courses on parenting techniques are a possible mechanism nurses can use. Table 22-4 illustrates an overview of course content for a group of parents of toddlers.

TABLE 22-4

Content outline for group of parents of toddlers

Session	Topic and content
First	Introduction and getting to know each other Discussion of developmental theories and tasks of age group Review of mastery, investigation, testing, and manipulating
Second	An age of activity: in or out of control Discussion about toddler behaviors: temper tantrums, negativism, jealousy, sibling rivalry, ritualism, separation behaviors, regression
Third	Approaches to toddler behaviors Discussion about limit setting and discipline
Fourth	Changing physically and learning to control body functions Discussion about toilet training, sleeping, eating, and self-comforting behaviors and patterns Discussion about how to handle safety considerations
Fifth	The necessity of play and learning sex role Discussion of learning through play Review of ideas about toys, television, playmates, play groups, and nursery school Discussion of sex role identification and factors influencing this
Sixth	Speech and learning to express self Discussion of timetable, reinforcement, nonverbal activities

Additional health promotion mechanisms appropriate for the toddler or preschool child are discussed in Chapter 21 under this heading.

COMMUNITY RESOURCES

Identification of available community resources is the nurse's responsibility. Groups or services that may be beneficial for parents of toddlers or preschoolers are listed in Chapter 21.

CLINICAL APPLICATION

During the toddler and preschool years, community health nurses continue to implement health promotion activities. Nursing students will observe these interventions in the areas of physical growth and health and developmental competencies.

Physical Growth and Health

Although physical growth slows somewhat during the toddler and preschool years, continued monitoring through height, weight, and vital signs recording is necessary. The community health nurse performs this assessment during annual health maintenance visits, primarily in the clinic setting. By year 3, the monitoring of blood pressure should be added to the nurses activities, using appropriate technique and equipment.

Data obtained from an interval history during the health visit, such as presence or absence of illness, patterns of sleeping and elimination, and development of motor skills, also assist the community health nurse in promoting health. For example, the nurse who discovers that an 18-month-old is pushing chairs over to the counter to climb up will counsel the mother on safekeeping of poisons and medications.

In addition, the community health nurse will assess the dental growth and health of the child 2 through 6. Checking for appropriate tooth shedding and replacement and the presence of dental caries will prompt the community health nurse to educate parents about early dental hygiene or to make dental referrals.

The student may find it useful to collect an interval history from the parent of the toddler-aged child and, based upon the information gathered, develop a teaching plan. For example, if the student finds that the child has a limited source of calcium because he does not like milk, the student can suggest incorporating other foods such as cheese, yogurt, or ice milk into the diet. The student could also offer suggestions about food preparation that would be more appealing to a toddler, such as popsicles made with yogurt and mashed banana or sandwiches cut into different shapes with cookie cutters.

The continued implementation of an immunization schedule and accident prevention counseling can significantly reduce illness in the toddler or preschooler. Students will observe community health nurses assessing the immunization status of 2- to 6-year-olds and implementing clinics in order to administer appropriate vaccines. Since the toddler and the preschool child are among the most accident prone, community health nurses will counsel parents in well child visits, as well as in group settings, on accident prevention issues such as auto restraints, plugging electrical outlets, toy safety, poisonous plants, household products, and medication safety.

Viral illnesses and child abuse and neglect, which are major health problems for the toddler and the preschooler, require nursing intervention. The student may encounter the community health nurse counseling parents in the recognition and treatment of symptoms of viral illnesses. For example, the nurse will teach parents how and when to use normal saline nose drops and humidifiers for upper respiratory congestion; how and when to use antipyretics and tepid sponging for fever reduction; or how and when to use dietary management for diarrhea.

The situation of child abuse or neglect will find the community health nurse acting not only as a primary care provider, but as a liaison and resource person as well. Risk screening for potentially abusive situations will be implemented by community health nurses in home or clinic encounters. For example, the community health nurse will closely follow a single mother who herself has been abused and now finds herself with three young children, no job, and no family support. The nurse will assist this mother in finding employment, support from governmental agencies, and child care in a supportive, caring manner. For the child who has been or is being abused, the nurse will intervene by making referrals for social service and medical care, while providing nursing support and care. The student may find it useful to identify resource agencies and outline the services they provide for child abuse or neglect victims and their families.

Developmental Health
Toddler

During toddlerhood, the child is working to develop a sense of autonomy. The community health nurse will assess the child's behavior for evidence of this competence and offer education that promotes appropriate abilities. For example, the student will observe the the nurse inquiring about the child's language and motor abilities, such as how many words are in the child's vocabulary, whether he or she speaks in phrases or sentences, can run, ride a tricycle, hold a pencil, and so on. On the basis of the information gained, the nurse will make recommendations about ways to promote these skills, such as reading to the child, providing time for outdoor play, and allowing the child to help out with household chores.

Play becomes increasingly important in the toddler and preschool years, and the nurse will offer suggestions (such as those on pp. 431-432) for making play safe and constructive. The student may encounter community-sponsored "Mother's Morning Out" or play group programs for toddler and preschool children that are helpful to the child in learning the sociability of play.

Providing counseling about toilet training is another way the nurse helps parents promote autonomy in their child. Educating parents about appropriate timing and techniques of toilet training will facilitate success. Success for the child means a feeling of accomplishment and independence. The student may find it useful to develop a fact sheet about toilet training that offers suggestions to parents on how to train their toddler.

Cognitively, the toddler is quite egocentric and views the world and its surroundings in relation to self. For this reason, nurses who deal with toddlers are quite concrete and concise in their encounters with them. For example, when a nurse is going to use a stethoscope or otoscope on a toddler, it is helpful if the child can see it used on a doll or his or her mother first, thereby allowing the child to see that the procedure is not harmful.

Preschooler

In the preschool years the child expresses and experiences himself in the home, at school, and with peers. Continued assessment of motor, social, and language skills will be a part of the community health nurse's assessment. Tools such as the DDST, DASE, and PRESS will be utilized by the community health nurse in the assessment. Discussing nursery school and the child's ability to play with peers will be initiated by the nurse. The student will probably observe the nurse offering suggestions about how to select a preschool and what toys and types of play are appropriate for a child of this age. In addition, screening speech ability is an important nursing intervention, since the ability to relate verbally is important to the child's developing social world.

Cognitively, the preschool child is progressing from egocentricity to prelogical thinking. In the clinical situation, the community health nurse demonstrates awareness of this ability by involving the child in what is being done. For example, the nurse might allow the child to examine a doll, performing the activities performed on the child (i.e., nurse listens to child's heart, child listens to doll's heart).

Classes for Parents

Finally, the student will observe the community health nurse offering classes to parents of toddlers and preschoolers. These classes may center around a specific topic, such as toilet training, or may include a variety of topics, such as those outlined in Table 22-4. The student may find it useful to develop a class for parents of preschoolers on how to select a school. This activity would help the student begin to look upon the child as a complex person, who has physical, social, motor, language, and cognitive needs.

SUMMARY

Toddlers and preschool children are mobile, curious, and adventuresome. Erikson and Piaget present theories that help the community health nurse to understand children in these and other age groups as their developmental abilities expand.

The toddler years include ages 1 to 3. This is a period of rapid physical growth and development. The physiological functioning becomes more competent, sleeping patterns become more routine, and feeding behaviors change. These years are marked by achievement of physical competence in both fine and gross motor skills.

Preschoolers, 3- to 6-year-olds, experience expansion of their environment to include experiences in and out of the family unit. Physical growth and development continue but at a slower pace than in the toddler. Eating and sleeping patterns stabilize and become more predictable, and the clumsiness and oftentimes ineptness of the toddler disappear as fine and gross motor skills continue to develop.

Growth and development of the toddler and the preschooler are affected by expansion of life experiences, the integration of the personality, and in many cases, the family's ability to cope when the mother is working. The community health nurse can assist the family in understanding the patterns of growth and development in the toddler and the preschooler and the effect of environmental and life experiences in helping the child to meet growth and developmental milestones.

The major causes of mortality in these age groups are accidents and injuries; infections are responsible for most of the morbidity. Child abuse or neglect is a phenomenon of growing concern in the United States and is becoming a major contributor to morbidity and mortality in toddlers and preschoolers. Prevention is the primary goal of the nurse in regard to accidents, infectious disease, and child abuse.

The basic tools and techniques for assessing health problems of toddlers and preschoolers include monitoring physical growth and psychosocial development. There are many tools available to assist the nurse in identifying problems requiring intervention. Community resources are an integral part of the nurse's techniques for helping assist families to resolve the problems of toddlers and preschoolers.

⩶ KEY CONCEPTS

The toddler years are the second and third years of life. Children 3 to 6 years of age are considered preschoolers.

Physical and physiological growth is slower in toddlers than in infants and continues at a still slower rate during the preschool years.

During the second to fourth years of life a child's personality becomes more apparent and his psychosocial development is enhanced.

The toddler is at stage 2 of Erikson's theory of life development. During this time the toddler has the task of developing a sense of autonomy versus one of shame or doubt.

According to Erikson, ages 4 to 8 constitute the third stage of development. During this stage, the child is developing a sense of initiative versus a sense of guilt.

Piaget views the child's egocentric thought pattern as the preoperational period of cognitive development. According to Piaget, by age 4 to 6 years the child begins to move away from this egocentricity.

The major factors affecting growth and development are expansion and expertise, integration, and the way the family functions when the mother works outside the home.

Major health problems of toddlers and preschoolers include viral illnesses, infectious diseases in day care centers, and child abuse and neglect. Viral illnesses are the most common infectious diseases in children.

The community health nurse can help families promote toddler and preschooler well-being in a variety of ways and settings, including health assessments, physical and psychological screening, diet assessment, and parent groups and parent education.

LEARNING ACTIVITIES

1. Administer the DDST to
   a. An 18-month-old
   b. A 3-year-old
2. Observe a group of toddlers *or* preschool children interacting (at a day care center, a nursery, or a nursery school). Then complete the following, based on your observations of four children:

OBSERVATIONS

Age	Level of play
———————	———————
———————	———————
———————	———————
Fine motor activity	Gross motor activity
———————	———————
———————	———————
———————	———————
Social activity observed	Language observed
———————	———————
———————	———————
———————	———————

BIBLIOGRAPHY

Aronson, S.S., and Gilsdorf, J.R.: Preventive management of infectious diseases in day-care, Pediatrics in Review 7:259-262, Mar. 1986.

Barnard, M.U., et al.: Handbook of comprehensive pediatric nursing, New York, 1981, McGraw-Hill Book Co.

Behrman, R.E., and Vaughan, V.C., editors: Nelson textbook of pediatrics, ed. 12, Philadelphia, 1983, W.B. Saunders Co.

Brown, M.S., and Murphy, M.A.: Ambulatory pediatrics for nurses, ed. 2, New York, 1981, McGraw-Hill Book Co.

Bunch, W.H.: Common deformities of the lower limb, Pediatr. Nurs. 5:18-25, July-Aug. 1979.

Caffey, J.: The whiplash shaken infant: manual shaking by the extremities with whiplash-induced intracranial and intraocular bleedings, linked with residual permanent brain damage and mental retardation, Pediatrics 54:396-403, Oct. 1974.

Caplan, F., and Caplan, T.: The power of play, New York, 1973, Anchor Press.

Chow, M.P., et al.: Handbook of pediatric primary care, ed. 2, New York, 1984, John Wiley & Sons, Inc.

Drumwright, A.F.: Denver Articulation Screening Examination: scoring and interpretation instructions, Denver, 1971, University of Colorado Medical Center.

Fontana, V.J., and Robinson, E.: A multidisciplinary approach to the treatment of child abuse, Pediatrics 57:760-764, May 1976.

Goldberg, R.: Identifying speech and language delays in children, Pediatr. Nurs. 10:252-259, July-Aug. 1984.

Hayghe, H.: Working mothers reach record numbers, 1984 *Monthly Labor Review,* Office of Employment and Unemployment Statistics, U.S. Bureau of Labor Statistics, Washington, D.C., Dec. 1984.

Health: United States and prevention profile, DHHS (PHS) pub. no. 87-1232, Hyattsville, Md., 1986, U.S. Department of Health and Human Services, Public Health Service.

Kempe, C.H., and Helfer, R.: Helping the battered child and his family, Philadelphia, 1972, J.B. Lippincott Co.

Kempe, C.H., and Hopkins, J.: The public health nurse's role in the prevention of child abuse and neglect, Public Health Curr. 15:1-4, May 1975.

Kronmiller, J.E., and Nirsch, R.F.: Preventive dentistry for children, Pediatr. Nurs. 11:446-449, Nov.-Dec. 1985.

Lenneberg, E.H.: Biological foundations of language, New York, 1967, John Wiley & Sons, Inc.

Maier, H.: Three theories of child development, New York, 1969, Harper & Row, Publishers, Inc.

Maternal and Child Health Program: Evaluation of body size and physical growth of children, Washington, D.C., 1976, The Maternal and Child Health Program, Department of Health, Education and Welfare.

Parten, M.: Social participation among preschool children, J. Abnorm. Soc. Psychol. 4:242-245, March 1932.

Rogers, W.B., Jr., and Rogers, R.A.: A new simplified preschool readiness experimental scale (PRESS), Clin. Pediatr. 11:558-562, Oct. 1972.

Ryan, M.T.: Identifying the sexually abused child, Pediatr. Nurs. 10:419-421, Nov.-Dec. 1984.

Scipien, G., et al.: Comprehensive pediatric nursing, ed. 2, New York, 1979, McGraw-Hill Book Co.

Smith, D.P.: Common day care diseases: patterns and prevention, Pediatr. Nurs. 12:175-178, May-June, 1985.

Tackett, J.J., and Hunsberger, M., editors: Family centered care of children and adolescents, Philadelphia, 1972, W.B. Saunders Co.

Whaley, L.F., and Wong, D.L.: Effective communication strategies for pediatric practice, Pediatr. Nurs. 11:429-431, Nov.-Dec. 1985.

Wong, D.L.: Helping parents select day care, Pediatr. Nurs. 12:181-187, May-June 1986.

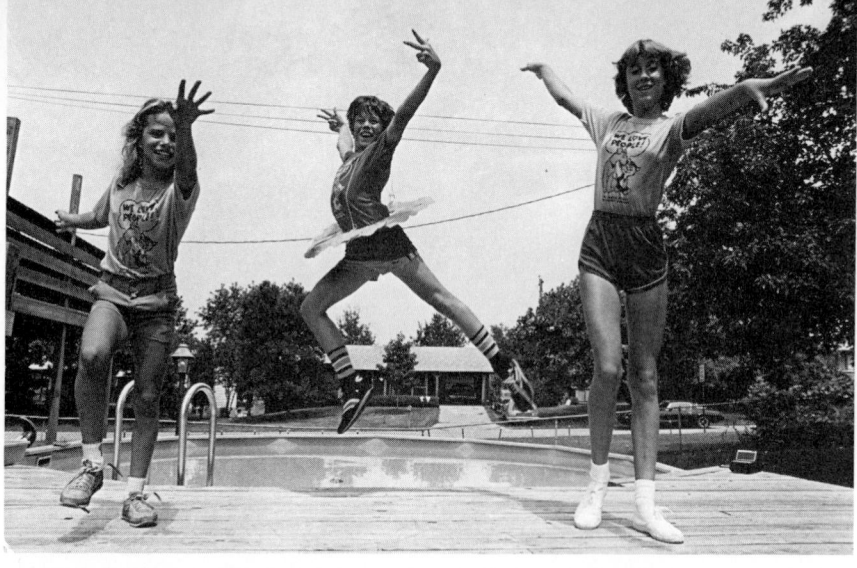

Nancy Dickenson-Hazard

23

SCHOOL-AGE CHILDREN AND ADOLESCENTS

OBJECTIVES

After reading this chapter the student should be able to:

Identify significant physical and psychosocial developmental factors characteristic of school-age and adolescent clients.

Define nursing activities that promote the health of school-age and adolescent clients.

Identify factors that influence the growth, development, and health of school-age children and adolescents.

Discuss assessment tools appropriate for school-age children and adolescents.

Define the role of the community health nurse in the promotion of health for school-age children and adolescents in the home, school, or clinic.

KEY TERMS

acne
adolescence
adolescent mother
amenorrhea
anorexia
bulimia
candida
dyslexia
dysmenorrhea
genital herpes simplex
gonorrhea
hyperactivity
kyphosis
learning disability
lordosis
minimal brain dysfunction
mononucleosis
premenstrual tension (syndrome)
puberty
school phobia
scoliosis
suicide
syphilis
toxic shock syndrome

Both the school-age child and the adolescent live in rapidly expanding worlds. The experiences confronting them are diverse and complex. Although the health of this nation's children and adolescents is better than ever, school-age and adolescent persons are confronted with health problems more complex than those of preceding generations. School and societal influences create many problems for children in these age groups. Nurses in community health settings can educate school-age children and adolescents regarding these problems and the subsequent influence on health. These educational encounters may occur in the school, the clinic, or the home. Through these encounters the community health nurse has an opportunity to assist children and adolescents to learn behaviors that will help them become healthy adults.

This chapter focuses on the health assessment, health maintenance, and health promotion activities germane to the school age child and the adolescent. The physical and psychosocial aspects of health are reviewed, as well as significant factors that can positively or negatively influence health behavior.

PHYSICAL GROWTH AND DEVELOPMENT OF SCHOOL-AGE CHILDREN

The period of life from 6 to 12 years is characterized by steady physical growth, neuromuscular refinement, and rapid expansion of cognitive and social skills. During this phase of life, physical and psychosocial mastery of the expanding environment is the primary task. Developing self-esteem and identifying life-style values are also important during the school-age and adolescent developmental phases. Assisting the school-age child to begin to formulate these characteristics is the basis of anticipatory nursing guidance.

Physical Competence

Physical competence of the school age child is assessed through measurements of physical growth and indicators of normal development—that is, neuromuscular ability, sensory organ development, and tooth shedding and eruption. However, the developmental pace within each of these areas is highly individualized from child to child. The nurse's awareness of the factor of individuality, as well as knowledge of "usual" development, provides the basis of an accurate assessment.

Changes in Height and Weight

Physical growth in the younger school-age child is reflected by an average annual gain of 2 in (5.5 cm) in height and 5.5 lb (2.5 kg) in weight. Boys are generally an average of 1 inch taller and 2 pounds heavier than girls until approximately age 9 to 10. At this time girls begin to grow more rapidly in height and weight, and by age 12, girls are generally 2 pounds heavier and 1 inch taller than boys. The preadolescent growth spurt usually occurs between 9 and 14 years for girls and between 12 and 16 years for boys (Tanner, 1962).

Skeletal Growth

Physiological changes continue through school-age years, which reflect continued maturation and refinement. Skeletal growth in the trunk and extremities is steady, with most of the hand and feet bones present but not complete. Evidence of small and long bone ossification is present. Remodeling of the facial bones is evidenced by visualization of frontal sinuses on x-ray film and a change in eustachian tube positioning to a more downward, anterior direction. As skeletal growth progresses over the school-age years, changes in overall body appearance and posture occur. The stoop shoulder, slightly lordotic posture with a prominent abdomen develops into a more erect posture by the end of this period.

Dental Growth

Dental growth is most prominent during the school-age years. By the tenth year, all primary teeth have been shed and permanent teeth have erupted, with the exception of the second and third molars. The sequence of shedding and eruption is important to proper occlusion, or the alignment of the chewing surface of the maxillary teeth to the mandibular teeth when the jaws are closed.

Patterns of Sleep and Eating

The sleeping and eating patterns of the school-age child are relatively stable. The sleep requirement varies from 8 to 10 hours a night, and the number of meals is usually three plus one or two light snacks. Nutritional needs will increase slightly in terms of quantity rather than quality (see Appendix J4). These patterns are disrupted, however, during the preadolescent and adolescent growth spurt, when caloric and water requirements increase along with appetite.

Sexual Growth

The ages of 10 to 12 are generally considered the prepubertal years. Before this age sexual growth is minimal. However, during the prepubertal period sexual characteristics become visible and maturation begins. A detailed discussion is in the section on adolescent physical growth and development.

Neuromuscular Development

The central nervous system continues to mature slowly. Neuromuscular skills are refined and expanded. Sensory organ development is fine tuned and cognitive skills increase. The school-age child should be able to perform a wide range of physical skills. Appendix K9 presents an overview of all aspects of school-age growth and development on which a nursing assessment should be based.

PHYSICAL GROWTH AND DEVELOPMENT OF ADOLESCENTS

The period of life from 13 to 18 years is characterized by a steady progression of physiological changes. The resultant changes in physical appearance and body function require adolescents to adapt their body image and to adjust to the maturing body. These physical changes, coupled with the emotional, psychological, and social adaptations of adolescence, push the young person to learn to develop coping mechanisms that will be carried throughout life.

Puberty

Puberty refers to the biological stage of development during which physical changes occur that make reproduction possible. Adolescence refers to the psychological maturation of this stage (Tackett and Hunsberger, 1981). Young persons mature at different rates and will complete puberty and adolescence at varying times.

Height and Weight

Physical growth during adolescence is accelerated, with both boys and girls achieving their final mature height by the end of puberty. The majority of this growth occurs over a 2- to 3-year span and begins 2 years earlier for girls than boys. For girls, this growth spurt normally begins at approximately 9½ years, peaks at 12 years, and stops by 14 years. The height spurt for boys begins at approximately 10½ years, peaks at 14 years, and ends at 16 years. Boys will average an 8-inch height gain, while girls average a 3-inch gain during this time (Tanner, 1962). In addition, growth follows a pattern for both sexes. Initially legs lengthen first, followed by widening of thighs, broadening of shoulders, and trunk growth.

Skeletal Growth

As skeletal mass doubles during adolescence, significant gains in weight are noted. In addition, muscle (lean body mass) and fat (nonlean body mass) double. Muscles increase in number of cells and in size for males, whereas only an increase in size is noted in females. Conversely, females average twice as much body fat as males when physical maturation is completed (Behrman, et al., 1987).

Sexual Maturation

Of great significance in the adolescent is the process of sexual maturation that occurs during puberty. Sexual maturation involves the development of primary and secondary sexual characteristics. Primary sex characteristics are those physical and hormonal changes necessary for reproduction. Secondary sex characteristics externally differentiate male from female (Tanner, 1962). The reader is referred to a basic textbook in physiology for a discussion of the hormonal mechanism of puberty.

Girls

Sexual growth is rapid during puberty and follows a specific sequence of events. In girls, puberty occurs in the following sequence (Committee on Adolescence, 1968):

  Initial enlargement of breasts
  Appearance of straight pigmented pubic hair
  Maximum physical growth
  Appearance of kinky pubic hair
  Menstruation
  Growth of axillary hair

  The timing of these sequential phenomena is highly individualized. However, menarche, in general, is occurring earlier with each generation (Daniel, 1977; Kreutner and Hollingsworth, 1978). Presently, adolescent females are beginning to menstruate at an average age of 12 years, with menarche occurring about the time the growth spurt ends. Menstruation generally occurs within 5 years of the beginning of breast development (Tanner, 1962).

Boys

In boys, puberty occurs in the following sequence (Committee on Adolescence, 1968):

  Beginning growth of the testes
  Appearance of straight pigmented pubic hair
  Beginning enlargement of the penis
  Early voice changes
  First nocturnal ejaculation
  Appearance of kinky pubic hair
  Age of maximum growth
  Growth of axillary hair
  Marked voice changes
  Development of facial beard

  The sequence of pubertal events in males follows a timetable as well. Generally the male growth spurt occurs at about the same time as penile growth and about a year after the increase in testicular size. These events usually occur at approximately 14 years of age (Tanner, 1962).

  NURSE'S ROLE. Evaluation of normal sexual development is essential to the assessment of adolescent growth. The nurse must be able to determine the stage of sexual development, evaluate normal progression, identify any abnormalities of development, and educate adolescents in regard to the changes created by their sexual development. Tanner staging is the most widely used assessment tool. It defines sexual development in stages according to sex and developing primary and secondary sex characteristics. See Tanner (1962) or a basic pediatric nursing textbook for a detailed discussion.

PSYCHOSOCIAL DEVELOPMENT OF SCHOOL-AGE CHILDREN
Erikson's Concepts

From the ages of 6 to 12 children expand their social and cognitive spheres. Erikson regards this stage as a period of striving to develop a sense of industry versus a sense of inferiority. To achieve this balance, school-age children direct their energies (industry) toward becoming competent in social and cognitive skills. Physical and cognitive abilities, however, are often lacking, and a sense of inadequacy and inferiority can result (Erikson, 1963). This sense of inferiority is inevitable for most school-age children at some point in this phase of development. However, achieving the positive component of competence generally outweighs the negative aspect of inadequacy, because assets and liabilities are recognized and coping behaviors are developed that do not compromise self-esteem.

During this phase of development a child learns to become a productive member of a peer group. Peers of the same sex become important for judging one's success. Learning to contribute, collaborate, and work cooperatively in relationships toward a common goal becomes a measure of a child's success. In addition, the child works diligently to achieve and improve skills, because success at whatever task is being attempted is desired.

The school-age child who develops confidence in himself and functions well within societal rules will be better equipped to handle the turmoil of adolescence. The nurse can positively influence this adjustment by exploring these feelings with school-age clients and assisting them in developing positive coping behaviors for the pressures of school, home, and friends. For example, the school nurse can hold discussion sessions on how to say no to drugs, sex, and alcohol.

The achievement of these individual and group member competencies occurs gradually over the school-age years. Table 23-1 outlines this progression.

Piaget's Concepts

The thought processes of school-age children undergo significant change over this period of development. Piaget characterizes the cognitive competencies of 6- to 7-year-olds as intuitive. Thinking is based on the immediate unanalyzed relationships between events in the environment and the child's point of view. The child cannot consider wholes or parts simultaneously but focuses only on the whole or the part. A 6- or 7-year-old continues to consider and interpret things and events in relation to self. Consequently, organization and reasoning are not apparent in thought processes or conversation (Maier, 1969).

Between the ages of 8 and 10, cognitive abilities increase in reasoning and realism. According to Piaget, this state of concrete operations allows children to realize their way of thinking is not the only way. They are able to consider more parts of the whole while maintaining a concept of the whole. In addition, 8- to 10-year-olds are able to logically consider a problem or event, arriving at a conclusion or solution. This increased cognitive development allows children to expand their social and intellectual capacity by using the newly acquired abilities to differentiate, categorize, problem solve, conceptualize time and space, and understand causality (Maier, 1969).

PSYCHOSOCIAL DEVELOPMENT OF ADOLESCENTS
Erikson's View of Adolescence

Between the ages of 13 and 20, a person has the task of leaving childhood and becoming an adult. According to Erikson, adolescents must establish their own identity or be caught in confusion regarding their role (Erikson, 1963). As they approach adulthood, teenagers will contend with establishing intimate relationships or remaining socially isolated. Decisions regarding life-style and vocation are most important. Peer and social spheres are expanding, and adult social and cognitive skills need to be developed. In addition, adolescents need to establish an emotional independence from and equilibrium with their families and to adjust to and master their sexuality.

Developmental Tasks

Nine developmental tasks have been defined for adolescents (Havinghurst, 1972). These tasks include (1) accepting one's body and consolidating sex role; (2) expanding peer relationships to include both sexes; (3) gaining emotional independence from family members; (4) achieving economic independence; (5) selecting and preparing for a vocation; (6) developing adult intellectual skills and concepts; (7) becoming socially responsible; (8) preparing for marriage and family responsibilities; and (9) developing realistic values in harmony with the world.

Accomplishing these tasks demands concentrated energy and thought on the part of the teenager. In light of the profound nature of what must be achieved during this period, it is little wonder that the following behaviors and attitudes are characteristic: emphasis on importance of peers, submission and conformity to peer group, preoccupation, ambivalence, idealism, egocentricity, feelings of inferiority, rebelliousness, moodiness, noncommunication, and feelings of insecurity.

Piaget's View of Cognition

In the area of cognition adolescents expand their ability to reason logically at a concrete level and move into the stage of formal operations. According to Piaget, formal thinking involves thinking about thoughts and separating the real from the possible. At this stage, adolescents develop the ability to use abstract logic, examine relationships, construct hypotheses, and, through deductive reasoning, logically test them (Maier, 1969).

These new cognitive abilities allow the adolescent to examine issues and values from differing points of view and to construct individual ideas and values. Thus teenagers can

TABLE 23-1

Social behavior development of the school-age child and the adolescent

Age (years)	Typical behaviors
6	Constant activity; enjoys group activities Spontaneously dramatic Indecisive, explosive behavior; rudeness Strict literal conscience Cheating common; behaves differently at school than at home Eager to learn and help out
7	Cautious in play Self-critical; anxious to do things right Talkative; expressive language Beginning to understand time and money Assumes responsibility; concerned about what is right and wrong Sensitive to feelings of others; concerned about fairness Aware of sexuality; modest
8	Seeks out and initiates group activity Accepts responsibility with greater ease Friendships are tenuous and friendly; segregated by sex Begins to collect items Can recognize individual differences; evaluates own self Relates to past and present (time concepts) Begins to resent authority of parents but needs their support
9	Generally responsible and dependable More reasonable and independent Peer group and conformity as well as hero worship quite important Begins to see parents more realistically (they can be wrong, etc.) Expanding interests; increased ability to plan and to see a project through to completion Self-sufficient and self-critical; strong sense of right and wrong Increased awareness of sexuality and reproduction
10	Cooperative projects and activities dominate; follows and submits to rules Friends of same sex; companions and activities most important Beginning sexual maturation for girls Girls more socially mature than boys Develops distinct hobbies and interests Continues to appraise parents
11-12	Development of "best friends" Feelings of opposition and dislike for opposite sex Characteristic sexual maturation more apparent, especially for girls Increase in physical and intellectual curiosity Group or clubs popular Secretive; demands privacy yet can be unruly, slovenly, and disrespectful Ambivalent feelings regarding parents and independence versus dependence May develop annoying overt behaviors—e.g., hair twirling and nail biting
13-18	Vascillation and ambivalence Family relationships supportive but tumultuous Peer relationships intense but unstable Develops skills in individual and group relationships Increasing involvement with opposite sex Developing independence, self-image Becoming more responsible Discovering reality of world

Modified from Ambulatory pediatrics for nurses, ed. 2, M.S. Brown and M.A. Murphy. Copyright, 1981, McGraw-Hill Book Co. Used with the permission of the McGraw-Hill Book Co.

realistically plan their life events, fully understanding time sequence and the consequences of their actions.

Morality

Moral development also changes during this period of formal thinking. Behaviors now reflect individual conscience and internalized principles rather than acceptance of rules of those in authority. Adolescents now make decisions based on what they perceive as best for them and as the conclusion of introspective thinking. The moral behaviors adolescents display are the result of their own thinking, consciences, and decisions to act (Kohlberg, 1981).

Adolescents struggle during this phase to establish their own identities. The final integration of physical, emotional, and cognitive skills will be evident in the adolescent development and demonstration of social behaviors. Appendix J11 provides an overview of the psychosocial development of the school-age child and the adolescent.

FACTORS INFLUENCING GROWTH AND DEVELOPMENT

As the child continues to grow and develop throughout the school and adolescent years, exposure to a multitude of new factors will influence progression through these stages. As for the earlier years, growth and development are affected by the degree of success or failure a child has had in mastering the tasks of preceding stages. (See Chapters 21 and 22 for an overview of factors affecting growth and development in preceding stages. These factors continue to be influential throughout the life span). However, unlike earlier years, a child is now equipped with more complex cognitive, physical, and social skills, but more complex tasks are faced. In addition, the degree of difficulty a child or adolescent experiences in accomplishing these more complex tasks during these current stages influences overall developmental expression.

Role of Peers

Of singular importance to growth and development is the role of peers. With the exception of family, a child or adolescent's peer group exerts the greatest influence on development (Damon, 1977). It is with and through the peer group that a variety of developmental tasks are accomplished. Peers permit the individual to try out and even fail in new skills, to validate thoughts, feelings, and concepts, and to receive acceptance and support as a unique person. Conversely, a peer group can place demands and pressure on the individual to conform that create feelings of being uncomfortable or even inferior. The balanced effect of this peer influence can be positive at times, negative at others, and almost always lasting.

Role of Family

As the child's world expands outside of the home, the role of family influence changes. Since the child has and is developing individual thoughts and perceptions, parents no longer are viewed as the ultimate, all-knowing authority. The child, and particularly the adolescent, learns that parents are human; they make mistakes and do not have all the answers. Frequently parental values and ideas are questioned and differences and conflicts arise. Despite these confrontations, however, the child still needs parental love and support. Parental guidance, knowledge, and experiences continue to be used by children as resources for verification of their own fast-developing repertoire of behaviors. Parental values, ideas, and expectations become a springboard for adolescents to develop their own. Although adolescents may diverge or digress from parental points of view, the influence remains and eventually affects decisions and behaviors (Sutterley and Donnelly, 1973).

Physical Well-being

The state of health and nutrition will affect a child's ability to grow and develop. Optimal mastery of skills and tasks occurs when physical well-being is optimal. Deficiencies in nutrition and problems with health alter an individual's sense of wellness and perceptions of self. Functioning at a diminished capacity creates difficulties in accomplishing complex tasks. Therefore promotion and maintenance of health and nutrition become important components in the normal developmental progression.

COMMON CAUSES OF MORBIDITY AND MORTALITY
Early Childhood

Although the health of children in the United States is better now than 10 years ago, the slowness of the decline in mortality remains of concern. A major contributor to this slowness is the fact that 50% of all deaths under age 10 occur as a result of accidents (Wegman, 1983). This preventable cause of death requires the attention of health care professionals if the health of children is to continue to improve.

In addition to accidents, children ages 1 to 14 are victims of cancer, birth defects, influenza, and pneumonia (Health, 1983). Although the mortality rates for these are relatively low as compared to accidents, their threat remains. Early recognition of symptoms and preventive measures are largely responsible for minimizing these problems. See Chapters 21 and 22 for detailed discussions of birth defects and respiratory illness.

Screening for cancer through history and physical assessment is an important aspect of the nurse's role. Table 23-2 presents historical data indicative of childhood malignancies, which require immediate referral.

School-Age Health Problems

School-age children face significant health problems, including learning and school difficulties; behavioral disturbances; speech, hearing, and vision problems; and infectious diseases of protozoan and bacterial origin. In addition, children today are rapidly developing risk factors that may eventually lead to adult disease and disability. For example, as many as 40% of children ages 11 to 14 already demonstrate potential characteristics of heart disease, such as overweight, high blood pressure, and high cholesterol levels (Health, 1983).

To enhance healthy growth and development, the health

TABLE 23-2

Historical data for screening for childhood malignancies

	Family history	Review of systems
Leukemia	Relates syndromes or diseases (e.g., Down's syndrome, immune deficiency disease) Carcinogen exposure (e.g., radiation, immunosuppressive drugs)	Signs of anemia: pallor, excessive tiredness, decreased exercise tolerance Bleeding tendencies: excessive bleeding, nosebleeds, petechiae Recurrent infections—local or systemic
Central nervous system disorders	Congenital spine or skull defects Presence of CNS-related disorders (e.g., neurofibromas, tuberous sclerosis)	Signs of CNS dysfunction: headaches; visual problems, e.g., diplopia; nystagmus; decreased acuity; ataxia; vomiting without nausea and on waking; palsies and paresis
Wilms' tumor	Associated congenital anomalies (e.g., hemihypertrophy, hypospadias, cryptorchism, renal masses)	Signs of gastrointestinal dysfunction: abdominal pain, distension or enlargement, diarrhea, anorexia Signs of urinary dysfunction: hematuria General signs: fever, lethargy

Modified from Wolf, W.J., and Bancroft, B.: Early detection of childhood malignancies, Pediatr. Nurs. 5:43-48, Jan.-Feb. 1980.

care professional must be aware of these potential but preventable risks and direct efforts toward their significant reduction, primarily through client education on risk factors, diet, and exercise.

Health in Adolescence and Early Adulthood

As measured by the usual mortality and morbidity indicators, the health of adolescents is relatively good. The death rate for adolescents and young adults is substantially below the rates for other age groups. However, this improvement in the death rate over other groups and over the years has not been sustained. In 1984, adolescent mortality was 96.8 deaths per 100,000, approximately 9 less than the 1960 rate of 106 per 100,000 and quickly approaching the 1990 goal of 92 per 100,000 (Health, 1986; Wegman, 1983).

Violent death and accidents, particularly motor vehicle accidents, account for the majority of deaths in this age group. Three fourths of all deaths are specifically attributable to accidents, homicide, or suicide (Wegman, 1983). The greater risk-taking that occurs in this age group leads to behaviors that are characterized by aggressiveness, errors in judgment, and ambivalence, which more frequently result in death or injury.

Males of this age group are at particular risk. Their death rate is almost three times that of females. Motor vehicle accident deaths are more likely to occur among white youths, whereas homicide is the leading cause of death for young blacks. Although chronic disease is not a leading cause of death, the behaviors and life-styles displayed by this young population may create a later susceptibility.

Adolescents also face other potential threats to health. Substance abuse, pregnancy, and sexually transmissible diseases are among the most common health-related problems for this age group. In 1982 over 75% of all adolescents reported experiences with alcohol and/or drug consumption. 1.2 million American teenage girls report having had at least one pregnancy by age 18, and of 10 million cases of sexually transmitted diseases reported annually, 86% occur in the adolescent group (Health, 1983).

To some extent the presence of these problems represents failure to assist adolescents to secure the help and information they need to solve problems and make decisions. Hence, when dealing with this age group, nurses in the community health setting should center priorities around preventive health and self-care education.

Nursing interventions such as school-based clinics that deal with health issues confronting the adolescent (e.g., substance abuse, violence, suicide, mental illness, sexually transmitted disease, pregnancy, and contraception), that emphasize preventive, on-site counseling, and that provide prompt referral are appropriate and needed and do help the adolescent (Keenan, 1986).

MAJOR HEALTH PROBLEMS OF SCHOOL-AGE CHILDREN AND ADOLESCENTS

Among the major health problems affecting both school-age children and adolescents are accidents and injuries. Since in few other areas of concern can prevention and health education play a major role, nursing's responsibility becomes one of promoting health through prevention.

Accidents
Motor Vehicle Accidents

Motor vehicle accidents are responsible for more than 13% of all childhood deaths ages 1 through 4 and 25% of all deaths for ages 5 through 14. Alcohol consumption has been implicated in many adolescent fatalities, which also accounts for this population having the highest number of motor vehicle accidents (Health, 1986; Wegman, 1983). Prevention of these accidents will require changes in behavior on the part of parents and children. The incorporation of safety education and accident prevention is a necessary component of each health maintenance visit. In addition, educational efforts need to be directed toward and involve the child or adolescent and the parents. Appropriate anticipatory guidance is discussed in Appendix J6.

Of significance to adolescents' involvement in motor vehicle accidents, including those on motorcycles, mopeds, and all-terrain vehicles (ATVs), is their attitude about risk. Excessive speed has been found to be a major factor in almost half the vehicular accidents involving teenagers. Although shoulder and lap belts prevent serious injuries and fatalities in automobiles, more than 70% of adolescents do not use them (Williams, 1976). Moreover, the use of helmet gear for motorcycling is significantly lower for adolescents than for any other population.

Assisting the adolescent to recognize and to try to reduce these risks is a difficult task. However, reinforcement of safety education can be carried out during the health maintenance visit, in collaboration with the school, through driver education classes and through group health education seminars and workshops.

Recreational Accidents

Bicycles, swings, and skateboard injuries account for the most accidental injuries among older children. (See publications from the U.S. Consumer Product Safety Commission for information on toy and play equipment safety and maintenance.) For the preadolescent and the adolescent, injuries from contact sports such as football and basketball are also primary causes of injury. Teaching and reinforcing the need to use and maintain proper recreational and sports equipment as well as safe participation are important factors in implementing safety education. In addition to educating the sports participant, nurses should also include sports personnel and teachers in this safety education. Although emphasis should remain on safety and accident prevention, such programs may also include advice on immediate management (first aid) of the sports injury and appropriate transport of the injured athlete (Smith, 1979).

Health Problems Specific to School-Age Children
School Adjustment

Starting school creates a situation that will require adjustment on the part of the child and parent. No longer are the influences on the child's growth and development limited to the home; both parent and child must now "let go" of some degree of security and comfort to allow the child to develop as an individual (Damon, 1977). Conflict often arises and home becomes a testing ground for new behaviors. Children must learn to cope with new challenges presented by school and peers—for example, learning to be a productive group member, performing and mastering knowledge gained in school, and assimilating the beliefs and values of others. Parents must allow their children to make decisions, accept responsibility, and learn from both positive and negative life experiences. Parents and children will need support and guidance to successfully adjust to the school experience.

NURSE'S ROLE. The implications of nursing's involvement in facilitating parent and child adjustment are numerous. Nurses can promote adjustment to school by assisting individuals to identify potential stresses and by collaborating with parent, child, and teacher to prevent or minimize reactions. Primary areas of intervention include assisting parents to allow the freedom necessary for their child's development, assisting the child to cope with the social and cognitive demands of the school setting, and assisting teachers in dealing with problem or crisis situations involving children and parents. Table 23-3 provides a plan of nursing intervention that facilitates school adjustment.

School Phobia

A problem unique to the school adjustment situation is school phobia, the persistent and abnormal fear of going to school. It occurs across all ethnic and socioeconomic groups, with a slightly higher incidence in girls than in boys. The principal age groups affected are 7- to 9-year-olds and 12- to 14-year-olds. The initial complaints are generally a variety of somatic symptoms and conditions that prevent attendance. Occurrence of these symptoms is greater during the week and rare on weekends, holidays, or vacations. Generally, more illness occurs in the fall, following holidays, and near times when tests or projects are due. The cause of this school anxiety behavior may be related to circumstances at home, at school, or both. Frequently identified factors include pressure to achieve, stressful relationships at school, fear of leaving home, and recent occurrence of a traumatic event associated with death, loss, or abandonment (Brosnan and Fond, 1980).

NURSE'S ROLE. Assessment of the child with suspected school phobia includes a thorough history and physical examination with appropriate diagnostic and laboratory tests to rule out organic causes. Additional assessment tools that may be useful in determining the extent of the problem include the maintenance of a diary by the parent and/or teacher describing the child's daily activities and the administration of intellectual and emotional assessment tests such as the Wechsler Intelligence Scale for Children and the Goodenough-Harris Drawing Test.

The goal of management is to return the child to school. The approach to achieving this goal may involve the immediate return to school, home tutoring for a while, or permission for the child to return voluntarily (Brosnan and Fond, 1980). The choice of approach is based on the individual child and the circumstances that created the fear of school.

Further nursing interventions include supporting the child and family throughout the problem identification and school reentry process; assisting child and family to follow the management plan; assisting the child to develop coping behaviors that will positively affect self-concept and esteem; assisting parents and child to identify other potential support or professional services; and facilitating interaction and relationships between child, parents and school.

Other Health Problems

Several health problems can increase in incidence during the school-age years. Although some of these problems are acute (e.g., bacterial and parasitic infections), others may be ongoing or chronic, reaching an intervention point when the child is older (e.g., dental caries or obesity). Problems

TABLE 23-3

Tasks of children, parents, teachers, and nurses in facilitating school adjustment

Statement of adjustment	Child's tasks	Parents' and teachers' role in facilitating task achievement	Nurse's role in assisting parents, teachers, child
Diffusion into larger world (5 or 6-8 yr)	1. Must adapt to differences in teacher's and parents' disciplinary approach and behavioral expectations.	1. Parents and teacher should communicate their respective expectations for the child to identify extreme differences and to work out compromises that permit the child to meet expectations of each, so that parents and teachers can mutually reinforce their expectations.	1. School nurse can help organize parent-teacher interaction (e.g., preschool roundups; parent-teacher-nurse conferences) or mediate in conflicts. a. During preschool roundup or school physical, learn what child's and parents' expectations for school are.
	2. Must compete with peers for teacher's attention and approval as teacher replaces parent for large portion of day.	2. Teachers should avoid obvious favoritism in classroom, give individual attention and praise to each child, avoid comparisons of achievement.	2. School nurse can offer guidance to teachers and intervene in unhealthy child-teacher relationships. a. During preschool registration or school physical, evaluate parent-child relationship for problems as these often carry over to teacher-child relationships.
	3. Must learn to handle blatant, hurtful honesty and downright rudeness of peers without damage to self-concept.	3. Peer activities and behaviors need close adult supervision.	3. Nurse in well-child facilities or schools can provide this guidance to parents and teachers.
	4. Needs to test out new ideas and behaviors in security of home environment.	4. Parents need to recognize developmental function of "trying on" ideas and behaviors incongruent with family's but set reasonable limits on how much and what type of "trying on" is to be allowed.	4. Nurse in well-child facilities or schools may offer this anticipatory guidance.
Disorganization created by disparities between home and school or peers (8-10 yr)—cont'd	1. Must learn to concentrate on cognitive achievements as the child settles into school life.	1. Parents and teachers need open communication about cognitive tasks that are being focused on at any one time and skills the child finds difficult so that both parties can support mastery of those skills.	1. School nurse observations in classroom will help identify children having difficulty with this task. Investigation of state of health, sensory organ function, and neurological, physical, and emotional function should follow to determine source of problem in achieving task.
	2. Must learn to integrate peer values in a manner that does not deny family values and to transfer family values into larger world in socially acceptable ways.	2. Parents and teachers must understand that just as a child falls while learning to walk, so will falls occur while learning to think. These falls during school age are typically boasting, teasing, fighting, lying, cheating, sassing and whining.	2. School nurses should regularly monitor playground and classroom activities to identify extricated children and then set the task force (parents, teachers, nurses, other pertinent school or health personnel) in motion to uncover source of problem and offer help.

From McElroy, E., and Tackett, J.J.: Growth and development needs of the family with school age children: maintaining wellness. In Tackett, J.J., and Hunsberger, M., editors: Family centered care of children and adolescents, Philadelphia, 1981, W.B. Saunders Co., pp. 1044-1045; as adapted from Laige, J.: The school-aged child and his family. In Hymovich, D., and Barnard, M.: Family health care: developmental and situational crises, New York, 1973, McGraw-Hill Book Co.

TABLE 23-3

Tasks of children, parents, teachers, and nurses in facilitating school adjustment—cont'd

Statement of adjustment	Child's tasks	Parents' and teachers' role in facilitating task achievement	Nurse's role in assisting parents, teachers, child
		2a. Teachers and parents need to develop the art of overlooking minor falls and feel comfortable seeking help for more serious or persistent falls. Children left alone with their peer group often overcome problems with peer assistance rather than adult intervention.	2a. Well-child facility and school nurse should evaluate child's behavior patterns and self-concept at each contact to pick up clues that all is not well in his or her emotional and social relationships. Nurse in clinic or school should offer parental/teacher anticipatory guidance regarding handling of behavior problems.
Disposition of compromise between home and larger world (10-12 yr)	1. Must take increasing responsibility for initiating and carrying out own learning activities at school and home; find internal satisfaction in performance.	1. Family and teacher must acknowledge child's ability to manage responsibility and allocate responsibilities in which child can take pride and feel success.	1. Nurse in any setting in contact with parents and teachers may offer this anticipatory guidance. Nurse may be role model of such interactions in dealings with child.
	2. Must take interest in organized school and peer activities to be accepted as a group member.	2. Parents need to see developmental advantage of child's involvement in organized activities and plan with child how he or she can get to these, financially handle the expenses involved, and still manage home and school responsibilities. Teachers should understand the need for such involvement and appropriate homework reasonably.	2. Same as 1 above. Nurse may help family learn about community activities available to children this age and of financial assistance available through schools, community clubs, churches.
	3. Must become capable of maintaining appropriate personal conduct (control impulses, resist temptation) with little or no adult supervision.	3. Child should be given increasing opportunity to go to school, religious, and peer functions unattended by parents and be praised for reports of good conduct. Digression from appropriate conduct should be dealt with in accordance with the seriousness of digression. Parents need to communicate faith in child's ability to handle self adequately.	3. Same as 1 above.

may be of a physical origin or an emotional-behavioral origin (e.g., enuresis, or involuntary urinary incontinence, and encopresis, or fecal incontinence). The nurse's responsibility is to provide intervention to resolve problems and to reinforce preventive measures that will abate reccurrence. Appendix J10 discusses these health problems and appropriate nursing interventions. (American Academy of Pediatrics, 1982; American Dental Association, 1971; Krugman & Katz, 1985; Behrman, et. al., 1987).

Learning Disabilities

Approximately 10% to 30% of all school-age children experience some degree of learning difficulty in school. The causes are complex, multifaceted, and often unidentifiable. In addition, many types of problems are frequently lumped under the labels of *learning disability* or *minimal brain dysfunction*. Table 23-4 identifies problems associated with learning disabilities, their probable causes, and appropriate intervention (Chow, et al., 1984).

Assessment of a child with learning difficulties involves a comprehensive evaluation involving specialists in language, education, psychology, and medicine. Components of such an assessment are outlined in the above boxed material. A management plan directed toward increasing the child's self-esteem and continuation with education is indicated.

TABLE 23-4

Learning disabilities

Health problem definition	Etiology	Clinical signs	Interventions
MINIMAL BRAIN DYSFUNCTION (MBD)			
Descriptive term for a child of average intelligence who has difficulty learning; a disorder in understanding or using language or adapting behavior	Associated with possible minimal insult to the central nervous system May result from infection, injury, chronic lead poisoning, or the slow maturation of brain function	Normal or above average intelligence May appear as learning, motor coordination, speech, or auditory difficulty, or combination of these Of children affected, 50% demonstrate "soft signs": they have short attention spans and mild speech impairment and are clumsy, impulsive, awkward, talkative, destructive, distractable, hyperactive, and socially immature	Management plan is provided by team and designed for individual child Appropriate nursing interventions may include the following: Administering screening tests Assisting parents to be consistent and to design a workable day-to-day schedule Supporting family when evaluating and venting their feelings Assisting parents to design a schedule that keeps frustrations and obstacles at a minimum Assisting parents to identify ways to positively reinforce desirable behaviors of child Teaching parents to keep directions and tasks simple Assisting parents to work with school, physician, and other therapists to implement plan Assisting family to identify useful community resources
HYPERACTIVITY			
A behavior disorder with characteristic clinical manifestations resulting in non–goal-directed activity in inappropriate amounts	Most common of minimal brain dysfunction disorders, occurring more frequently in boys than girls Appears to involve a delay in the maturation of cerebral inhibitory function Dietary factors may be a contributing factor	Demonstration of characteristic behaviors of increased motor activity, short attention span, poor concentration, emotionally labile, easily distracted, prone to mood swings, and temper outbursts May be accompanied by learning difficulties and "soft" neurological signs	Medical management may include the following: Use of stimulant drugs (Ritalin and Dexedrine), which stimulate release of norepinephrine, thus producing a calming effect Salicylate-free diet that eliminates all artificial colors and flavors as well as salicylates Nursing interventions may include facilitating provision of the following (also see interventions for MBD): Structured external stimuli environment at home and school Special education classes Outlets for family feelings of frustration, inadequacy, guilt, tension, stress Avoidance of labeling child Support and encouragement

NURSE'S ROLE. Nursing activities involve assessment and management of the problem. Participation in the early identification, observation, and data collection is a nursing responsibility, as well as ensuring appropriate referral and follow-up. Coordinating the activities of all disciplines involved in the evaluation and management frequently is the role for nursing. In addition, the nurse can best explain the problem to the parents and child and provide the support and encouragement needed for a successful outcome.

Health Problems Specific to Adolescents
Acne

Acne is a common clinical entity affecting an estimated 90% of boys and 80% of girls. Approximately one third of

TABLE 23-4
Learning disabilities—cont'd

Health problem definition	Etiology	Clinical signs	Interventions
DYSLEXIA			
Inability to read printed symbols or understand oral symbols (materials)	May be primary dyslexia, which is usually familial and may be due to weakness of learning process or immaturity of brain May be developmental dyslexia resulting from cerebral dysfunction About 15% of children have reading skill difficulty and of these 3% are due to primary or developmental dyslexia; developmental dyslexia is more frequent in boys than girls	Demonstrates ability to hear and understand statement but cannot read Usually average or above-average intelligence Demonstrates difficulty distinguishing similar letters (*b* and *d*): may reverse letters when reading (*saw* for *was*); sees letter upside down or mirror image	Measures include the following (also see nursing interventions for MBD and hyperactivity): Early identification thorough screening at health assessment visits Assistance with reading instruction School and family working together Use of repetition and reinforcement Positive, relaxed home and school environment Provision of informal learning at home Games to improve reading and hand-eye coordination Avoidance of negative reinforcement; praise and reassurance for child

---

ASSESSMENT FOR CHILD WITH LEARNING DISABILITY

HISTORY

Complete history with emphasis on the following:
  Parental and child concern and perceptions
  School behaviors and performance
  Family history
  Pregnancy, birth, and infancy history
  Developmental history
  Past medical history

PHYSICAL EXAMINATION

Complete physical assessment with emphasis on the following:
  Neurological examination for "soft" signs (i.e., perceptual or cognitive behaviors that persist beyond normal range)
  Evaluation of fine motor coordination
  Evaluation of sensory skills
  Evaluation of laterality and space orientation
  Evaluation of perceptual-motor function (visual-motor, auditory-motor, gross-motor)

SPECIAL STUDIES AND ASSESSMENTS

  Electroencephalogram
  School readiness screening tests
  Speech/hearing/language screening tests
  Educational/academic evaluation
  Psychological evaluation
  Perceptual motor function screening tests

---

female adolescents experience an increase in papules or pustules in the week preceding menses. Acne is considered a disease of adolescence because of its onset at puberty and increased incidence during the teenage years. Although acne is self-limiting, it is a source of persistent embarrassment, disgust, and stress for the adolescent (Stone, 1982).

PRESENTATION. Acne vulgaris is an inflammatory disease in which sebaceous glands overproduce sebum when stimulated by androgenic hormones. The presentation of this problem is seen as noninflamed comedones and/or inflamed papules, pustules, and nodulocystic lesions. The usual site is the face, but the neck, upper chest, back, and shoulders can be affected. The skin and hair are often oily. The initial assessment and data collection can be facilitated by using a questionnaire that focuses on the pertinent history, hygiene, medical, and social aspects of acne (Stone, 1982). In addition, the data can serve as an initiation point for discussion regarding this sometimes emotional problem. Appendix K11 includes an assessment tool useful in gathering data regarding adolescent acne.

MANAGEMENT. The treatment of acne involves medical management, but client education and counseling are most influential to success. Management generally includes the following measures (Behrman, et. al., 1983):
  Thorough cleansing of the skin two or three times a day using warm water and a mild soap
  Drying and peeling lotions may be used overnight
  Avoid exposure to sun and wind
  Frequent shampooing of the scalp
  Proper diet with added liquids—no diet restrictions are indicated, but should the adolescent feel a certain food aggravates the acne, it should be avoided

Comedone removal by using extractor exerting gentle pressure

When indicated, systemic antibiotics (tetracycline), corticosteroids, injections in lesions, and minor surgery

A multitude of topical medications are available for the treatment of acne. The most effective are benzoyl peroxide and retinoic acid. Preparations do vary in effectiveness, and their recommended use needs to be individualized to the client and the severity of the problem.

EDUCATION. Client education is most important for compliance with and success of therapy. Acne affects young persons at a time when they are struggling to create their own identities and are concerned about body image and peer opinion. The feedback adolescents receive from peers about themselves will influence their self-image and self-esteem. The presence of acne can disrupt receipt of positive peer feedback, affecting the adolescent's self-esteem. The first step in counseling a teenager about acne is to thoroughly explain its cause, its course, and the ways the adolescent can effectively manage and control it (Stone, 1982). The client must understand and be willing to accept responsibility for treatment. The social aspects of acne and the client's feelings about the problem need to be discussed with clients. In addition, clients must be aware of the realistic time frame for outcome and improvement. Acne is a chronic problem, and the nurse must deal with the adolescent's expectations of treatment. Finally, follow-up is essential to the successful treatment of acne. Nurses can provide supportive care and reassurance during this time and help the adolescent with other aspects of management.

Abnormal Spinal Curvatures

Abnormalities of the spinal curvature are most frequently detected during the adolescent growth spurt between the ages of 10 and 15 (Chow et al., 1984). These aberrations are exaggerations of the normal spinal curvature, which may result from organic or structural changes or as the consequence of persistent poor posture. Of particular concern are the incidences of kyphosis, lordosis, and scoliosis, which are illustrated in Figure 23-1.

KYPHOSIS. Kyphosis is an exaggerated convex curve in the thoracic region resulting in a hump or hunchback appearance. Backache and pain generally accompany kyphosis, which may occur as a developmental lesion or secondary to a congenital deformity. Management of kyphosis will require immediate referral. Deformities that are minimal can be treated with Milwaukee braces. However, severe or congenital anomalies need surgical intervention.

LORDOSIS. Lordosis is an exaggerated concave curve in the lumbar region of the spine, resulting in a swayback appearance. A limp and pain are created by lordosis, which is largely caused by failure of hip flexors to stretch and elongate. Referral is indicated and treatment is similar to that for kyphosis.

Nurse's role. Since both kyphosis and lordosis are related to poor posture, nursing actions indicated should focus on assisting adolescents to develop an exercise program and learn proper sitting and standing. To achieve maximal success, a detailed explanation of the problem and its cause should precede development of a program. Incorporating activities of interest to the individual teenager further facilitates compliance and success (Dunn, 1975).

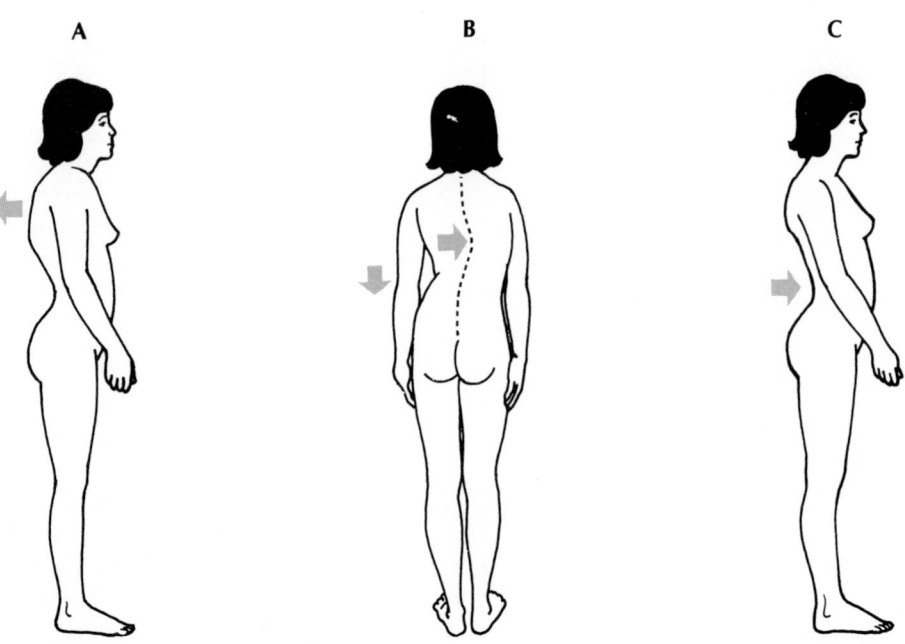

A   B   C

FIGURE 23-1

Skeletal abnormalities of adolescence. **A,** Kyphosis; **B,** scoliosis; and **C,** lordosis. (From Tackett, J.J.: Potential stresses during adolescence: reversible alterations in health status. In Tackett, J.J., and Hunsberger, M., editors: Family centered care of children and adolescents, Philadelphia, 1981, W.B. Saunders Co.

SCOLIOSIS. Scoliosis is an S-shaped lateral curvature of the spine with rotation of vertical bodies. Scoliosis is classified as structural, indicating the curve is less flexible and not completely corrected by postural change, or functional/nonstructural, indicating no specific structural change. Further classification of structural scoliosis includes congenital curves, associated with failure of vertebrae to form or segment; paralytic curves, associated with polio or other neuromuscular disorders; and idiopathic curves, associated with a high familial incidence. Immediate referral is indicated upon recognition of scoliosis. Treatment is aimed toward prevention of increasing deformity and may include use of a Milwaukee brace, traction, and surgery.

Nurse's role. The nurse's role lies in the early recognition of scoliosis and the provision of resources and support during the diagnosis, treatment, and follow-up stages. Early detection and implementation of a plan of care are essential to prevent the secondary complications of lung pathology and future back ailments. Thus screening for scoliosis is a necessary component of health assessment for school-age children and adolescents (Dunn, 1975). Siblings of clients diagnosed with scoliosis particularly need screening because of the potential genetic etiology. Screening procedures are easily implemented in the school setting as well as in special clinics or in the home. The procedure for screening requires complete exposure of back, chest, and hips and is based on observing the child when walking, standing erect, and bending forward (see Appendix K6).

Once problems are identified, nurses can act as advocates and liaisons for children with scoliosis. It is important to support and encourage as well as reassure the child and parents during the time of diagnosis and treatment. Whether the treatment is medical or surgical, child and parents need assistance in coping with the feelings created by the deformity and the ensuing treatment. Self-esteem, body image, and identity are disrupted for the teen. Parents may feel guilty and respond in an overprotective fashion. Both groups develop stress, anger, and worries about leading a normal life in the future. Nurses can facilitate the adjustment necessary to ensure such a normal life.

Each client and family must be dealt with in an individual manner. However, specific areas of intervention are indicated, particularly in the self-care of and adaptation to selected treatment methods. Table 23-5 provides guidelines by which an effective plan of nursing care can be implemented. (Anderson, 1979; Armstrong and Dickenson, 1975).

Menstrual Disorders

Since the hormonal balance of the menstrual cycle is easily disrupted, disturbances in menstruation are common in adolescent girls. The stresses created by adolescence can delay, temporarily halt, or create uncomfortable menstrual cycles (Kreutner and Hollingsworth, 1978). In addition, being different from peers can create embarrassment and anxiety for the teenager experiencing menstrual difficulties. Seeking help for these problems is difficult, and once counsel has been sought, the teenager needs to receive reassurance, information about normal menstrual function, details about

the difficulties she is experiencing, and information regarding the gynecological examination if one is indicated (Wells, 1977).

Menstrual variants frequently encountered in teenage girls are amenorrhea, dysmenorrhea, irregular cycles, and premenstrual tension.

AMENORRHEA. Amenorrhea is a delay in the onset of menses. Primary amenorrhea is a temporary delay in girls over 17 years of age, generally accompanied by delays in other pubertal characteristics. Secondary amenorrhea is a delay between menstrual periods of 12 months or more during the 2 years after the onset of menses, or the absence of three or more periods (Behrman, et al., 1983). Treatment is based on differentiation and identification of causative factors.

Nurse's role. The nurse's primary role in the management of amenorrhea is to provide information regarding the cause and to assist the teenager to identify resources for further treatment and follow-up. A supportive, empathetic approach facilitates acceptance of management.

DYSMENORRHEA. Dysmenorrhea is menses associated with pain. The cause has not been identified definitely, although increased levels of prostaglandins, which stimulate smooth muscle and myometrial contractibility, have been associated with dysmenorrhea. Mental tension and anxiety may also increase the discomforts.

Nurse's role. Most adolescents experience primary dysmenorrhea, and nurses can be most helpful in providing education and counseling in the management phase. Appropriate nursing interventions include the following:

Verification of the client's understanding of the physiology of normal menses

Provision of information regarding causes of discomfort

Provision of support/reassurance regarding discomfort

Development of discomfort alleviation plan: use of analgesics, warmth to lower abdomen, exercises, relaxation techniques

Irregularities in the timing and amount of flow are common in teenagers. Inconsistencies may exist in the length of periods, the time between periods, or the amount of flow. Generally these inconsistencies resolve by the third year after the onset of menses. A familial tendency does exist for these irregularities and should be ruled out by taking the history.

Because the inconsistencies are generally self-limiting, appropriate nursing interventions are similar to those previously discussed. In addition, the nurse needs to explore client feelings and fears regarding the problem.

PREMENSTRUAL TENSION (PREMENSTRUAL SYNDROME). The phenomenon of premenstrual tension has received much attention in the past few years. Although the cause is unknown and therapies remain experimental, it is well known that women may suffer a series of symptoms preceding the onset of menstruation. Once menstruation has begun, these symptoms of headache, abdominal distention, weight gain, changes in mood, irritability, inability to cope, crying spells, lack of energy, and breast discomfort subside. Assisting the adolescent to minimize these symptoms is appropriate nursing action. Counseling the teen to exercise regularly, to wear a well-fitted bra, to follow a nutritious diet avoiding salt and salt-retentive foods, to increase sleep

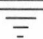

TABLE 23-5

A nursing approach to scoliosis

Areas of intervention	Guidelines
Client knowledge and understanding	Discuss normal anatomy and function of spine
	Define problem as it relates to client and discuss causes of scoliosis
	Discuss potential management methods in relation to how problem will be treated
	Discuss management method for individual client and why chosen and the purpose
	Discuss management course: what will occur, when, how long, how often
	Provide opportunity for questions; second visit may facilitate this
Client self-care	*Devices*
	Discuss application of device to be worn
	Discuss skin care
	Review care and cleaning of device
	Discuss comfortable clothing to wear
	Review appropriate exercise, diet, and safety measures
	Discuss management of activities
	Discuss recognition and prevention of potential problems
	Request return demonstration of appropriate activities
	Casting
	Discuss cast application and drying techniques
	Review care of cast
	Discuss skin care and personal hygiene
	Review safety, diet, and elimination factors
	Discuss impact of immobilization
	Review management of activities
	Discuss recognition and prevention of potential problems, including cast syndrome
	Discuss cast removal, care, and appearance (of skin) after removal
Client psychological well-being	Discuss feelings about management plan (fear, anxiety, lack of control, rejection)
	Discuss impact on body image and self-esteem
	Discuss peer and family acceptance and relationships
	Discuss interaction with general public
	Discuss ways of dressing that disguise cast or device
	Discuss ways to explain cast or device to others
Family support	Discuss preceding client factors with family
	Emphasize self-care activities
	Encourage understanding
	Discuss family feelings, perceptions, and attitudes
	Discuss changes in household routines and physical environment
	Discuss financial responsibilities

and periods of relaxation before onset of period, and to maintain a positive attitude and appearance will assist in reducing symptoms (Lauersen, 1985).

TOXIC SHOCK SYNDROME. Forty-two percent of the individuals with toxic shock syndrome (TSS) are adolescents, and 98% of these cases occur during menstruation (Litt, 1983). TSS is characterized by the rapid, sudden onset of symptoms, progressing from fever, headache, sore throat, nausea, vomiting, diarrhea, and abdominal pain to hypotension, myalia, arthralgia, rash, and desquamation of soles and palms. *Staphylococcus aureus* is the causative agent, and use of superabsorbent tampons is considered a contributing factor.

The role of the nurse is education directed toward prevention of TSS. Adolescent girls (and women in general) should be counseled to use regular tampons, if tampons are used at all, to change the tampons every 3 to 4 hours, to use sanitary pads at night, to wash their hands before insertion, and to use an applicator (Litt, 1983). In addition, general genitourinary hygenic measures should be discussed.

Mononucleosis

Infectious mononucleosis is an acute infectious disease occurring primarily in the 12- to 25-year-old range and caused by the Epstein-Barr virus (EBV). The virus is only mildly contagious; it is primarily transmitted through oropharyngeal secretions and intimate contact such as kissing. The average incubation period is 11 days, and the period of communicability is considered to be during the acute illness.

The initial symptoms of infectious mononucleosis are rather benign. Generally, the client has complaints of headache, malaise, and fatigue. A sore throat occurs by the end of the first week; the tonsils are red, enlarged, and covered with a membrane that peels off in 5 to 7 days. Lymphadenopathy and splenomegaly are common at this stage. Most symptoms subside in 3 weeks, but weakness and fatigue may persist for several weeks (Sapala and Sheldon, 1978).

NURSE'S ROLE. Treatment involves alleviation of symptoms (see Table 21-5). Additional appropriate nursing interventions include the following (Sapala and Sheldon, 1978):

Nutrition counseling that emphasizes high-calorie diet
Bed rest for first 2 weeks with gradual return to activity
Reduced exposure to noninfected persons
No strenuous physical activity if splenomegaly is present
Provision of support and reassurance regarding disease process and confinement

Social Health Problems

Adolescence is a time of discovery of self, of feelings, and of the complexities of society. Complicating these discoveries are enormous pressures from multiple external and internal sources. Teenagers must behaviorally adapt to achieve an equilibrium between these pressures and their sense of self as related to the world. Often adolescents are unable to cope, resulting in health-related problems.

Frequently, adolescent social health problems are related to poor self-esteem and dysfunctional family interactions and communication. Assisting the child early in life to develop a positive view of himself and working with families to develop healthy communication skills constitute primary prevention for social health problems in adolescents. Nursing responsibilities are to assess at-risk clients and families and to implement immediate interventions (Schwartz, 1985).

NURSE'S ROLE. The nurse's role in assisting families and adolescents to adapt to socially related problems includes the following:

Prevention by providing anticipatory guidance
Early problem identification (i.e., case-finding)
Problem intervention through education, resource identification, and referral
Provision of support, nurture, and reassurance

Relevant to prevention and case-finding is the ability to recognize adolescents at risk for social problems. The box below identifies characteristics indicating an at-risk client and family situations that may place normal development in jeopardy. Assessing for the presence of these behaviors or situations facilitates the early recognition of problems, enabling the nurse to seek early intervention for the client.

SUICIDE. Suicide is the second leading cause of death among teenagers. Males have a higher rate (up to four times higher) than females, and it is estimated that the actual suicide rate is probably three times the reported rate (Hart and Prophit, 1979; Health, 1986).

The causative factors for suicide or for attempting to take one's life are not definitive. Among these factors are developmental, social, cultural, psychological, biological, and situational variables. Generally, multiple factors combine to cause adolescents to consider suicide the only solution to their problems (Child et al., 1980; Cohen, 1982).

Most suicidal persons give verbal or behavioral warning, and 80% of those who take their own lives have made previous attempts (Hart et al., 1979). Nurses have a re-

---

CHARACTERISTICS OF ADOLESCENTS AND FAMILIES AT RISK FOR SOCIAL PROBLEMS

ADOLESCENT BEHAVIORS	FAMILY SITUATION
Insecure	Divorce
Poor self-concept or feeling inadequate	Death of one parent
Severe mood changes	Frequent family relocation
School problems	Insufficient parental guidance
Antisocial behavior	Frequent absences of one parent
Substance abuse	Drug or alcohol abuse
Decreased verbal communication	Step-parent
Sleep disturbances	Poor relationships between family members
Prolonged grief reaction following divorce, death, or severing of a romance	Mental illness
Communication problems at home	Economic deprivation
"Loner"	Faulty communication patterns
Friends of questionable reputation	Emotional, physical, or sexual abuse
Premature "growing up"	
Social, emotional, or attention deficits	
Cognitive development disability	
Depression	
Hedonistic philosophy	

Adapted from Bond, L.: Potential stresses during adolescence: managing behavior. In Tackett, J.J., and Hunsberger, M., editors: Family centered care of children and adolescents, Philadelphia, 1981, W.B. Saunders Co., p. 1250; and Schwartz, R.H., et al.: Identifying and coping with a drug using adolescent, Pediatrics in Review 7:133-135, Nov. 1985.

sponsibility to be cognizant of behaviors that are considered danger signs (see following box) and to implement immediate intervention.

Nurse's role. Nursing assessment and intervention, directed toward the depressed or suicidal child, are needed in the community, in the school, and in the ambulatory care setting. Nurses, particularly those in the school and community settings, are potentially the first persons the suicidal adolescent encounters. Frequently a physical complaint is the initial factor precipitating an encounter between the nurse and the adolescent. Masked in the physical complaint is the major problem or concern that is prompting suicidal thoughts. Nurses facilitate the identification of such a troubled teenager by being observant of adolescent behaviors, by encouraging adolescents to discuss their feelings, and by being an available source of support (Child et al., 1980; Hart and Prophit, 1979; Nelms and Brady, 1980).

In addition, family assessment and involvement in nursing interventions are critical. The family's role in exacerbating or alleviating the depressed child's symptoms must be explored through history and interview. Assisting family members to cope with the child's behavior and feelings, helping them solve dysfunctional family relationships, and educating the family to be a support for the child are important nursing tasks.

Community resources are also essential to prevention. Crisis intervention centers and telephone hot lines provide professional help and resource referral. Educational programs directed toward the variables that create problems for adolescents facilitate early identification as well as provide a support group. Such programs should involve adolescents not only in participation but in planning as well (Hart and Prophit, 1980; Nelms and Brady, 1980).

SUBSTANCE ABUSE. The use of alcohol and drugs has been increasing among young adolescents over the past 10 years; 80% of 12- to 16-year-olds report having had a drink, more than half drink at least once a month, and nearly 3% drink daily. Drug use, which was virtually unknown in the 1950s, now represents a major health problem among adolescents. Currently, 60% of adolescents have tried marijuana and 20% have tried harder substances such as cocaine and hallucinogens. Beyond the experimentation phase, adolescents are also increasing the frequency and regularity of use of tobacco, marijuana, and stimulants. Later teens, however, are decreasing their use of alcohol (70% report abstaining) and drugs (89% report abstinence) (Health, 1983).

Cause. The cause of increased substance experimentation and use is not definitive. As with other socially related problems, many factors contribute to this behavioral expression. Among these factors are need for peer acceptance or approval, succumbing to peer pressure, curiosity, availability of substances, poor self-concept, a deteriorated parent-teen relationship, and boredom (Chow, et al., 1984).

Effect. The physical and psychological effects of substance use are highly variable and will differ among individuals. However, chronic use that leads to dependence and addiction can create devastating effects such as change of lifestyle to accommodate drug need, malnutrition, emotional stress, and alienation from family and friends.

Nurse's role. Much substance abuse can be prevented, but assisting adolescents to stop or avoid misuse is not easy. Prevention will require a change in social acceptability as well as individual acceptability (Schonberg, 1978). Strategies for intervention will differ, and nurses have a vital role in these preventive efforts. Appropriate interventions include the following:

Educational programs on substance abuse for adolescents emphasizing their decision-making capabilities

Educational programs for parents in preventing abuse or recognizing early symptoms

Early identification (see box at right) and referral of adolescents with a substance abuse problem

Provision of support and acting as a role model

Assistance for adolescents in identifying stressors in their lives and in developing appropriate coping strategies

Use of youth organizations (such as 4-H and Scouts) and media to reinforce substance abuse education

EATING DISORDERS. *Anorexia nervosa* is a psychosomatic disorder primarily affecting adolescent girls. It frequently begins with a voluntary weight-reduction diet, that is initiated because the client feels overweight, even though weight is within normal range. Weight loss and refusal of food become excessive and are accompanied by denial of any experience of hunger (Boyle et al., 1981; Behrman et al., 1987). Definitive diagnostic criteria include (1) loss of at least 25% of original body weight; (2) delay or cessation of menstruation for at least 3 months; and (3) distorted body image (Bruch, 1965).

Bulimia is defined as recurrent episodes of binge eating frequently followed by self-induced vomiting. It occurs most often in adolescent girls and is characterized by rapid consumption of large amounts of high-calorie, easily digested food in a short time period. Sudden weight loss or dramatic weight fluctuations are common, as are dental erosion, electrolyte imbalance, and menstrual irregularities (Keller, 1986).

Nurse's role. The community health nurse's assessment and intervention in the school, clinic, or home setting are essential to the early recognition and management of the

---

BEHAVIORAL DANGER SIGNS

1. Giving away prized possessions.
2. Becoming increasingly isolated.
3. Recent loss, especially a parent, boyfriend, or girlfriend.
4. Statements such as, "No one cares about me. It would be better for everyone if I were dead." "How many aspirins do you have to take to kill yourself?"
5. A sudden elevation of mood following a depression. This could be misconstrued to mean improvement when actually the teenager may be experiencing a sense of relief that the decision to die has been made.

From Hart, N.A., and Prophit, S.P.: Adolescent suicide, Pediatr. Nurs. 5:22-28, Nov.-Dec. 1979, p. 25.

anorexic and bulimic adolescent. Awareness of behavioral indicators can facilitate the nurse's assessment. Personality characteristics of the adolescent that have been identified as behavioral indicators include obsessive-compulsive traits; setting of perfectionistic standards for self; neat, clean, well-behaved manner; a general immaturity; and difficulty with peer and social relationships (Behrman et al., 1987). Additionally, family dynamics and characteristics and habits require the nurse's assessment (Boyle et al., 1981). Although treatment and management of the anorexic or bulimic adolescent must frequently require hospitalization, the community health nurse is pivotal in facilitating early referral for treatment and in providing continuity of care during hospitalization and follow-up. Nursing activities include (1) liaison contacts with the client, family, and tertiary care management team; (2) provision of support and reassurance; and (3) facilitation of home management and follow-up care by assisting the discharged client and family to maintain normal eating patterns through use of a food journal and education about balancing caloric intake requirements and exercise (Boyle, et al., 1981; Keller, 1986).

Sexual Activity

Sexual experimentation is common during the adolescent years. Recent statistics reveal that one half of the adolescent population is sexually active, that one million teenage pregnancies occur annually, and that an additional 30,000 pregnancies occur in girls under age 15 (Cohen, 1982; CDC, 1981). Peer pressures, physiological and emotional changes, and societal expectations are all contributing factors in early heterosexual relations among adolescents.

HOMOSEXUALITY. Homosexual experimentation may occur as well, particularly in early adolescent years. Boys specifically may pass through a stage of sexual activity with a same-sex counterpart. Early homosexual experiences are not necessarily an indication of later sexual preference but rather are spurred by curiosity and the need to explore. As adolescents satisfy their need to explore various life-styles, they make a sexual preference, generally heterosexual.

The homosexual adolescent encounters unsupporting reactions from family, friends, and society. Nurses can assist the homosexual by being nonjudgmental, educating in ways to reduce exposure to sexually transmitted diseases, and exploring coping mechanisms to deal with family reaction (Rigg, 1982).

SEX EDUCATION. Because adolescents are more sexually active, they and their families need sex education and counseling. Counseling is based on an understanding of the adolescent's need for intimacy and the fact that involvement is a means of fulfilling this need. Society accepts this behavioral expression, even though an adolescent's parent may not. Hence, while prevention of sexual activity is not entirely realistic, educational efforts can be useful tools in assisting the adolescent to make informed decisions. Nurses can provide this education, focusing on (1) the physical and emotional sexuality of adolescents and their options for expression; (2) their attitude regarding sexual activity; (3) their awareness of the potential consequences of sexual activity (e.g., pregnancy, venereal disease, emotional distress); and (4) their available resource or support persons or groups should problems arise.

The nurse can also assist parents to (1) recognize and deal with the present-day realities of increased sexual activity among adolescents; (2) express their feelings about sex positively to their teenagers; (3) handle sex education and discuss sexual issues at home; (4) be a positive role model; and (5) identify support and resources if a problem arises (Chow et al., 1984; Sapala and Strokosch, 1981; Tackett and Hunsberger, 1981).

Two prominent consequences of adolescent sexual activity are sexually transmitted diseases and teenage pregnancy. Both of these health problems have experienced an increased incidence over the past decade, and each poses significant alterations to health.

VENEREAL DISEASE. Sexually transmitted diseases have become the leading type of communicable disease in our nation. Gonorrhea, syphilis, and genital herpes simplex ac-

---

IDENTIFICATION SIGNS FOR ADOLESCENT SUBSTANCE ABUSER

ENVIRONMENTAL	PSYCHOSOCIAL	BIOPHYSICAL
Drug-oriented materials	Falling grades	Bloodshot eyes
Liquor bottles	Change in dress	Slurred speech
Beer cans	Increased aggression	Restlessness
Rolling paper	Change in relationships	Sleepiness
Smoking apparatus	Low frustration tolerance	Erratic appetite
Smoking, alcohol odor	Avoidance of eye contact	Constant sniffles
Syringes	Unaccountable erratic behavior	Clumsiness
Blood spots on clothes	Boasting about drug use	Urinary frequency
Long sleeve shirts	Decreased social participation	Blackouts
Dark glasses		Dilated pupils
		Susceptibility to illness

Adapted from Rice, M.A., and Kibbee, P.E.: Review: identifying the adolescent substance abuser, Matern. Child Nurs. J. 8:139, Mar.-Apr. 1983.

count for an estimated 10 to 12 million cases of venereal disease a year (Health, 1983). Table 23-6 outlines the clinical characteristics and accepted management of these diseases.

Similarly, the transmission of trichomoniasis and *Candida albicans,* most frequently creating vaginal infection, has become a widespread health problem. Trichomoniasis is caused by a protozoan that is generally carried in the vaginal tract; the disease is transmitted by contact with infected perianal discharge, and has a foamy, yellow, foul-smelling discharge as the primary symptom. *Candida* is a normal vaginal fungus, usually kept in balance by normal vaginal flora. The symptoms of infection—itching, and white, cheesy discharge—tend to appear during pregnancy or hormonal or antibiotic therapy, or as a result of factors that alter vaginal pH or flora levels. Microscopic examination or culture is indicated for both conditions. Trichomoniasis is treated with oral medication (Flagyl), and *Candida* infection is treated with an antifungal vaginal preparation.

Nurse's role. Nurses have a vital responsibility in the prevention, identification, and encouragement of prompt treatment of the venereal diseases. Appropriate nursing interventions can be carried out effectively in group or individual counseling sessions, need to be presented in a nonjudgmental manner, and should facilitate adolescent knowledge and understanding about their sexuality. Nursing activities include the following:

   Sex education (written information)
   Venereal disease education (written information)
   Screening of at-risk groups
   Identification and treatment of infected persons and their contacts
   Teaching of preventive practices such as using a condom, washing well after sexual contact, urinating after intercourse, improving personal hygiene, and avoiding contact with persons known to be infected

In addition, school-age children and adolescents need to be made aware of the newest sexually transmitted disease in the United States, acquired immune deficiency syndrome (AIDS). See Chapter 17 for a complete discussion.

Pregnancy

Childbearing during adolescence is a high-risk experience for mother and child. One fifth of the pregnancies in the United States are to teenage girls. Annually 10% of all teenage girls become pregnant, and two thirds of them are unmarried. Eight percent of pregnant adolescents terminate the pregnancy (Health, 1983).

The economic consequences of teenage pregnancy also need to be considered. Less than 18% of teen mothers complete their high school education; therefore the rest have little or no basic training or skills. The incidence of poverty increases as the age of childbearing decreases, a situation that is due in part to this lack of education. Additionally, there is a higher incidence of noncompliance with prenatal care on the part of pregnant adolescents, leading to a higher rate of complications during the prenatal and neonatal periods (Trussell, 1976).

RESPONSE TO PREGNANCY. The teenager responds to the fact of her pregnancy with a wide range of emotion. Initial feelings may include denial, fear, guilt, anger, depression, or happiness. In some instances there may be a motivating factor on the part of the adolescent girl in becoming pregnant. Among the factors contributing to an adolescent's desire to become pregnant are rebellion against parents, viewing pregnancy as a means to leave a stressful home situation or to keep a boyfriend, or unrealistic desires and fantasies about motherhood and having a baby who will love her (Abbott, 1978).

The adolescent father also experiences a wide range of emotion. He may also feel anger, denial, guilt or happiness. Turmoil about his responsibility during and after the pregnancy are common, and frequently he feels left out and shunned.

Frequently the pregnant adolescent is unable to prepare adequately for the pregnancy, labor and delivery, and care of the infant. Because concrete thinking processes are still developing, the realities of the effects of pregnancy are not always understood. In addition, the pregnant teenager still needs association with her peers, and many find this difficult because of the gap pregnancy creates in life-styles. Similarly, because of the pregnancy, relationships with family may become strained at a time when support persons are most needed.

NURSE'S ROLE. The nurse can assist the pregnant teenager in many ways. The initial nursing assessment should focus on identifying the adolescent's feeling about being pregnant; her feelings about options (i.e., termination versus continuation); her support persons and role model; and her short-term goals (e.g., medical care, school continuation, relationships with baby's father, her family, and peers) (Abbott, 1978). A nonjudgmental and supportive attitude is essential during the assessment and management phases. The pregnancy of a teenager affects many people as well as society in general. Handling the implications of the effects of her pregnancy is frequently difficult for the adolescent. Hence the goals of nursing interventions should be short term and directed at definition of the most appropriate way for the individual teenager to handle the pregnancy (Tackett and Hunsberger, 1981). Appropriate nursing activities include the following:

   Providing pregnancy counseling, explaining fully the teenager's choices in regard to termination or continuation
   Assisting the teenager to identify support persons in the family or among friends
   Providing support and encouragement
   Making appropriate referrals for medical care and school placement
   Assisting the teenager to manage her altered life-style
   Providing appropriate health education
   Assisting the family to deal with and provide support to the pregnant teenager and the father
   Assisting the teenage father to identify his role during and after the pregnancy
   Assisting the family, pregnant adolescent, and teenage father to express their feelings about the pregnancy

TABLE 23-6

Characteristics of venereal disease

Venereal disease (pathogen)	Transmission	Incubation	Symptoms	Diagnostic tests	Treatment
Gonorrhea (Neisseria gonorrhoeae)	Direct contact, usually sexual; fomite contact up to 24 hours after fomite contaminated.	2-14 days (average 3-5)	*Early signs:* copious mucopurulent discharge from phagocytosis, vaginal in female and urethral in male. Pharyngeal if oral sex. Pain and frequency of urination from urethritis. 90% of females and 10% of males are asymptomatic. *Other possible signs:* cervicitis, salpingitis, peritonitis, pelvic inflammatory disease, and abscesses of Skene's or Bartholin glands in females. Epididymitis and abscess of prostate glands in males. *Late signs:* arthritis, endocarditis, sterility.	Culture of discharge for gonococcal growth (GC smear) positive. Visualization of discharge in infection on physical exam.	Simultaneous treatment of infected individual and all identified sexual partners with oral (probenecid) or intramuscular (procaine penicillin G, Trobicin) penicillin. The National Institute of Health is currently developing a gonorrheal vaccine. No permanent immunity.
Syphilis (Treponema pallidum)—cont'd	Direct contact, usually sexual, during infective stage. Transfusion.	Primary stage 10-90 days (average 3 weeks)	*Primary*—infectious: chancre (painless, indurated ulcer) that heals spontaneously in 2-3 weeks. Located at site where pathogen entered.	STS reactive. VDRL most common test. STS negative at this stage. Visualization of chancre on physical exam.	*Primary/secondary stages:* 2,400,000 units benzathine penicillin G IM or 4,800,000 units procaine
		6-24 weeks	*Secondary*—very infectious: skin and mucous membrane rash, lymphadenitis, fever, headaches, sore throat that disappears spontaneously. Lasts few months to several years.	STS reactive; becomes nonreactive if treated now.	Penicillin G (half of dose in each buttock) followed by 1,200,000 units of either type penicillin G at 3 days and 6 days after initial dose.
Syphilis (Treponema pallidum)—cont'd		2-4 years	*Early latent*—may be infectious: no physical symptoms.	STS reactive.	*Latent stages:* 3,000,000 units penicillin G given IM (half of dose in each buttock) to be repeated at 7 and 14 days after 1st dose.

From Tackett, J.J.: Potential stresses during adolescence: reversible alterations in health status. In Tackett, J.J., and Hunsberger, M., editors: Family centered care of children and adolescents, Philadelphia, 1981, W.B. Saunders Co., pp. 1294-1295.

Continued.

TABLE 23-6

Characteristics of venereal disease—cont'd

Venereal disease (pathogen)	Transmission	Incubation	Symptoms	Diagnostic tests	Treatment
		After 4 years	*Late latent*—blood infectious: no symptoms.	STS reactive.	VDRL repeated each month for 3 months after treatment completed to establish cure; damage done to body before treatment is not reversible.
			Late active: Gummas in skin, bones, liver, stomach. CNS involvement 10% optic atrophy, deafness. General paresis. Cardiovascular involvement in 80% of cases. Aortic insufficiency or aneurysm. Endarteritis. Insanity.		No immunity is developed.
Genital herpes simplex *(Herpesvirus hominis* [HSV-2])	Direct contact, usually sexual.	3-7 days	*Symptomatic phase:* contagious. Minor itching or extensive rash of genital region followed by a cluster of blisterlike lesions that then rupture and ulcerate; these are pruritic and painful, especially during intercourse. Painful urination, inguinal lymphadenitis and pain, fever, malaise. Symptoms disappear spontaneously after 2-6 weeks. Many cases asymptomatic. *Dormant phase:* symptoms absent but reappear with emotional or physical stress during which person again is infectious; once a person is infected,	Viral culture of lesions. Scraping and staining of ulcer tissue. Antibody blood titer of HVH-2 21 or more days after infection.	Incurable Treatment aimed at pain relief, fostering healing of lesions and preventing other infections: Pain medication. Use of condom during intercourse to prevent spread of HVH-2 or infection with other pathogens. Local application of red dye (0.1% proflavine) followed by light exposure repeated in 18 hours. This shortens course of lesions but is controversial because of increased risk of tumor formation. Acyclovir topically or PO. Cesarean section in all pregnancies if active sores exist at time of birth.

TABLE 23-6

Characteristics of venereal disease—cont'd

Venereal disease (pathogen)	Transmission	Incubation	Symptoms	Diagnostic tests	Treatment
Genital herpes simplex *(Herpesvirus hominis* [HSV-2])—cont'd			virus is harbored for life, though recurrences are less severe and last about 2 weeks. Cervical cancer 8 times more likely in women with HSV-2 virus.		
Chylamydia *(Chlamydia trachomatis)*	Direct contact, usually sexual; also hand to eye.	3-4 days up to 5 weeks	Males: Early: urethritis, gray or clear low-grade discharge Late: epididymitis, inclusion conjunctivitis, sterility Females: Early: vaginal discharge, endocervicitis, urethritis, urinary discomfort, diffuse abdominal pain Late: pelvic inflammatory disease, pain in lower abdomen, fever, chills, salpingitis, endometritis	Tissue culture. Direct specimen identification.	Tetracycline HCl or Doxycline. Abstinence from intercourse until treatment is over. Partner needs to be tested and treated. Follow-up culture after treatment.

CONTINUATION OF PREGNANCY. The adolescent who continues her pregnancy faces a high risk of complications. The incidence of toxemia, prolonged labor, and iron-deficiency anemia are increased for teenage mothers. In addition, teenage mothers give birth to a higher proportion of low-birthweight infants, infants who are retarded, and infants with epilepsy, cerebral palsy, blindness, or deafness. The younger the girl, the greater this risk appears to be for mother and infant (Kreutner et al., 1978). Although some of these risk factors are created by adolescent physical and physiological immaturity, others are attributed to the adolescent psychosocial immaturity resulting in poor compliance with prenatal care and management plans. For this reason the nurse needs to assist the adolescent in understanding the importance of prenatal care and health activities before making a decision about the pregnancy. These health education activities require reinforcement throughout the pregnancy. Information and preparation for labor and delivery and infant care should be introduced into the plan of care later in the pregnancy (Dibble, 1981).

ADOPTION DECISION. The pregnant adolescent who decides

to continue her pregnancy also faces an additional choice: whether to keep the baby or give the infant up for adoption. This decision can be made at any time during the pregnancy, and legally the young mother has 72 hours after delivery before she has to sign adoption papers (Abbott, 1978; Tackett and Hunsberger, 1981). The adolescent who is contemplating adoption needs nursing support and empathy in dealing with the emotions and realities created by giving up a baby for adoption. The family and the baby's father, who has legal rights, may be exerting pressure for one decision or another. Group counseling and interaction with other pregnant teens are often helpful. The final decision belongs to the teenager, and nurses must accept the role of resource people in facilitating the decision.

The Adolescent Mother

The adolescent who decides to keep her infant poses a unique challenge for nurses. The adolescent's adjustment to parenthood relies heavily on being prepared, informed, and supported (Dibble, 1981). Nurses need to be aware that adolescents are continuing to deal with their own developmental tasks in addition to the pregnancy and parenthood. Conflict between her own developmental needs and the pregnancy, and later her infant's needs, is common. The pregnant adolescent frequently discovers she is in a role that requires maturity and decision making but is unable to deal with these responsibilities. Nurses can assist teenage mothers to coordinate their roles and responsibilities as well as to set priorities. Appropriate nursing interventions may include the following:

Assisting teenager and family or father in distributing responsibilities of child care

Assisting teenager to identify and use support persons and groups

Assisting the teenage father to identify his feelings, role, and level of participation in pregnancy, labor, delivery, and care of child

Providing education about infant behavior and physical care

Facilitating use of appropriate health care for teenage mother and infant

Facilitating attachment and bonding

Making referrals as appropriate, identifying appropriate resources (babysitters, living arrangements)

Assisting teenager to identify and meet goals (e.g., return to work or school)

Assisting teenager to use family planning

Facilitating expression of feelings about infant, motherhood, her family, and the infant's father

Acting as an emotional support person and source of reassurance

Birth Control and Sex Education

The adequacy of knowledge and the access to information on sexual behavior and family planning services constitute a major area of concern. Much controversy arises over who should provide information, how much sex education is appropriate, and in what setting it should be given. The decision regarding early sex education generally lies with parents (Bernstein, 1976). They may choose to discuss sex and sexuality with their children or may decide to leave it to the school. Generally, inquiries about sex are best answered by parents. However, parents may feel uncomfortable in discussing sexuality. Nurses can assist parents to work through their feelings of discomfort and provide them with appropriate resources and responses to their children's questions.

NURSE'S ROLE. The nurse's goal is always to promote healthy and informed attitudes regarding sexuality. The opportunity for the community health nurse to plan and present a sex education program can occur in the school or clinic setting. Any age group of children can be the target population. An age-appropriate bibliography of materials on reproduction and sex is often a useful tool for parents and child. The nurse should recommend that both parent and child read the book or pamphlet. Following the reading, a discussion between parent and child should occur so that the child's questions are answered or misconceptions are clarified. Additionally, nurses can assist parents to be pre-

pared for the inevitable inquiries from their child about sexuality. Appendix J12 provides a developmental approach to information on sexuality. When providing parents with information about sex education for their child or in conducting sex education programs, the nurse should observe the following guidelines:

Use the child's curiosity as a guide to the explicitness of the explanation

Avoid inundating the child with information

Explain what the child wants to know in understandable terms

Ask questions of the child that will elicit the child's belief

Convey a positive attitude that reflects comfort with the topic of sex

Avoid belittling or making the child feel foolish

Avoid myths, vague statements, or erroneous information

CONTRACEPTION. Parents and adolescents need to be informed about methods of contraception. Whether this information is sought out by the adolescent or the parent or offered by the nurse, all methods require discussion, emphasizing effectiveness and appropriateness of use for the individual. In addition, the adolescent's knowledge of reproduction needs to be verified and misconceptions and misinformation corrected. An educational tool for methods of contraception is presented in Appendix J13. (See *Contraceptive Technology** for a complete discussion of all methods.)

Follow-up of teenagers using contraceptive methods is imperative. The nurse must assess the teenager's understanding, use, and response as well as the efficacy of the method chosen. Follow-up visits are also a time for the adolescent to voice questions or concerns about contraception and sexuality and to receive support and encouragement.

OTHER COMMON PROBLEMS

Frequently school-age children and adolescents display behaviors of concern to parents or family. Troublesome behaviors are based on expressions of conflict or are a means of testing out a situation, values, or feelings. Their occurrence in most instances is normal. Nurses should encourage parents to continue effective past and current patterns of discipline to facilitate quick passage through this stage.

Of major concern in dealing with the school-age child are cheating, lying, stealing, fighting, scatology, and fears. In the adolescent years concern is created by moodiness, preoccupation with self and body image, rebellion, conformity, inferiority, study habits, and dependent versus independent ambivalence. Appendix J11 defines these problems and discusses appropriate interventions.

Persistence of a minor problem indicates a situation more serious than a developmental deviation. If a child or adolescent repeatedly demonstrates antisocial behavior, a more extensive management plan is indicated, including referral of child and family for counseling. Troublesome behaviors

---

*Published annually by Irvington Publishers, Inc., New York.

may also represent warning signals of deeper difficulties within the family or child even if they are not persistent. For this reason thoughtful assessment is necessary before designating the events or behaviors as normal. The nurse can be instrumental in initiating appropriate guidance whether directed at coping with a normal phase or referring for management of a more complex problem.

ASSESSMENT TOOLS

Once school age or adolescence is reached, the nursing process does not vary significantly from that used for early childhood. Although the basic methods of the nursing process remain the same, variations in tools and techniques are indicated for the older child. These variations occur because the school-age child and the adolescent have the ability to participate more actively in all aspects of health assessment.

The History

The history is a long-term cumulative data base. The amount and type of historical information obtained depend on the purpose of the visit and the expressed concerns of the client and parents. Obtaining a complete health history is essential for a first-time encounter. A summary of health history information appropriate for the school-age child is presented in the box at right. Supplementary information to be obtained for the adolescent in addition to the general history is summarized in the boxed material on p. 466 (Brown and Murphy, 1981; Chow, et al., 1984; Daniel, 1977).

Child as Historian

An added dimension to the interviewing of a school-age child or adolescent is use of the child as the primary informant, or historian. The school-age child can be a reliable historian. The older the child becomes, the greater the degree of detail and accuracy becomes (Gorman, 1980). Focusing on the school-age child and adolescent as the primary informant facilitates the therapeutic relationship by promoting the nurse's trust and confidence in the child's ability. This technique assists children and adolescents in becoming an integral part of their health care and provides an opportunity for expression of concerns or feelings about their own health, growth, and development. If the nurse is concerned about the accuracy of the historical data, particularly in regard to early events, unsure dates, or an identified problem, validation by the parent is indicated. This verification should be done with the child or adolescent's knowledge and is best handled in a separate interview.

Setting for Adolescent Health Visit

Further consideration must also be given to the setting and tone of a healthy assessment visit for the adolescent client. Most adolescents experience some degree of discomfort in coming to a pediatric clinic. The added factor of being accompanied by parents, who possibly wish to discuss issues of concern to them, warrants special consideration. The following measures are useful in facilitating the adolescent health maintenance visit (Daniel, 1977; Marks, 1978):

SUMMARY OF HEALTH HISTORY

1. Identifying information
   Name
   Address
   Phone number
   Clinic number
2. Present concerns
3. Family profile
   Age and health status of family members
   Familial and communicable diseases
   Socioeconomic background
   Support system
4. Child profile
   Past medical history
     Gestation
     Birth history
     Neonatal period
     Immunizations and laboratory tests
     Infectious diseases
     Operations/hospitalizations
     Accidents
     Allergies
     Current medications
     Review of systems
       Head
       Skin
       Eyes, ears, nose, throat
       Dentition
       Heart and lung
       Blood
       Genitourinary
       Skeletal
       Neuromuscular
   Personality
     The child as a person
     Interaction
   Development
     Language
     Fine motor
     Gross motor
   Nutrition
   Sleep
   Elimination
   School
   Past utilization of health care
   Special concerns of the adolescent
   24-hour history

From Chow, M.P., et al.: Handbook of pediatric primary care, ed. 2, New York, 1984, John Wiley & Sons, Inc., p. 7.

Schedule adolescent appointments on days different from baby or younger-child appointments

Provide age-appropriate reading materials in waiting area, which focus on adolescent-related problems

Ask adolescent to complete any previsit history or information forms

Interview the adolescent first and then parents, unless adolescent expresses desire for parent to be present

Explain procedure for present and future visits in detail

SUPPLEMENTARY HEALTH HISTORY DATA PERTINENT TO THE ADOLESCENT

1. Past history
   Use of diethylstilbestrol in mother's pregnancy
2. Social history
   Behavior—as related to school, home, parents, siblings, and peers
   Parent's and adolescent's concerns regarding above behavior
   Smoking, substance usage
3. School history
   Grade, name of school, method of getting to school
   Performance in school
   Favorite, best, most difficult courses
   Attitude about school
   Goals for schoolwork
   Concerns or difficulties related to school
4. Extracurricular activities
   Work
   Social
   Hobbies
   Sports and other activities
5. Peer relationships
   Number of friends
   Relationship with siblings
   Dating activity
   Perception of social self
   Concerns regarding preceding points
6. Sexuality
   Information about sexuality (e.g., physiological)
   Sexual activity
   Knowledge of contraceptive methods
   Knowledge of venereal disease symptoms, prevention, treatment
   Concerns and attitudes regarding sexuality and sexual self
   Worries about body: height, weight, development of sex characteristics, skin problems
7. Review of systems and particular focus on general health as described by client
   Skin: acne
   Dietary history
   HEENT: headaches, squint, hearing difficulty
   Dentition: last dental visit
   Heart: palpations
   Lungs: shortness of breath
   Gastrointestinal: abdominal pain, weight gain or loss
   Genitourinary: discharges, enuresis, dysuria, urinary tract infection
   Musculoskeletal: joint or back pain
   Neurological: emotional stress, fainting, dizzy spells
   Menstruation: age of onset, regularity, frequency, duration, last menstrual period, dysmenorrhea, premenstrual tension, attitude, feelings and beliefs regarding menses

Direct interview to adolescent; be interested in and develop a trusting relationship with adolescent
Reassure adolescent that information shared is confidential (exception being when behavior is dangerous to self or others)
Conduct interview in friendly, concerned manner

When providing health care services to the adolescent, nurses must also be aware of the constitutional rights of minors, including the right to self-consent. All states have legislation pertinent to the aspects of obtaining health care without parental permission. Since state statutes vary, nurses need to be familiar with those within their own jurisdictions. It is important to know the age at which minors can seek health care on their own and the types of health care services that can be offered.

The Physical Examination

The techniques of physical assessment vary little for the school-age child and the adolescent (see Chapter 21). Explaining each portion of the examination is most important for individuals of these age groups, since concern about body functioning, changes, and normalcy is usual (Marks, 1978). Appendix A3 describes approaches to conducting the physical examination for these age groups. In addition, explaining the what and why of the examination technique, including the results of specific parts of the examination, is useful in promoting confidence and trust.

The Health Assessment

A complete health assessment combines the components of health history, physical assessment, and the monitoring of physical and psychosocial growth and development. Based on these data, further activities that promote health can be implemented as needed for the individual child or adolescent. Once the child has reached school age, the frequency of health assessment visits is usually extended to every 2 years, unless the health status of the client warrants more frequent assessment. The general content of these visits is discussed in Appendix A3.

Physical Growth

Monitoring physical growth continues to be a major component of the health maintenance contact. Height and weight measurements need to be taken at these encounters. Similarly, vital sign measurement—heart rate, respiratory rate, and particularly blood pressure—is indicated.

Growth charts continue to be useful tools for recording and monitoring physical measurements (Appendix K2). Since growth spurts occur at varying ages and rates, the monitoring of this upper phase of physical development is essential. Growth charts assist the nurse to identify normal versus atypical growth patterns.

Laboratory Studies

Laboratory studies are a means of monitoring physical health, and selected procedures are indicated for the school-age child and adolescent (Appendix A3). Assessing skeletal and dental age when indicated provides information regarding normal growth patterns (see Chapter 21 for detailed discussion).

Assessment of Sexual Age

An assessment of sex characteristics is important to monitoring the health of older school-age children and adolescents. The tool developed by Tanner is most widely used and recognized. Tanner staging categorizes sexual development according to the appearance of certain physical characteristics (Tanner, 1962). See the section on physical growth and development of the adolescent, found earlier in this chapter, for a detailed discussion.

Screening Procedures

Screening procedures for vision, hearing, and tuberculosis are indicated during health maintenance contacts with school-age children and adolescents. Most frequently, the Snellen alphabet chart is employed for vision screening, an audiogram for hearing screening, and the Mantoux test (intradermal purified protein derivative) for tuberculin screening (see Appendix K5). Additionally, the scoliosis screening previously discussed in this chapter is definitely indicated for clients in this age group. Screening for venereal disease and sickle cell disease as indicated for the individual client is appropriate during health assessment visits (Appendix A3).

Monitoring Psychosocial Development

The psychosocial skills of the school-age child and the adolescent can be monitored in a number of ways. Generally, the therapeutic interview, focusing on aspects of the client's emotional and social development, is conducted during the health maintenance visit (see boxed material on pp. 465 and 466). Knowledge of the development of social behaviors is important to this interview, as are the observations and perceptions of parents and teacher. Data derived from the interview and indicating the need for further assessment prompt the nurse to implement more extensive screening. The tool used for this additional screening is dependent on the area of concern (e.g., family problem, social maturity, intelligence, perceptual ability). The psychosocial tests most commonly used in childhood and adolescence are discussed in Appendix K8. Other tools useful in monitoring psychosocial development are discussed in the following sections.

Family Coping Estimate

The health of a child is largely dependent on the family's health and ability to cope. Comprehensive nursing implies implementing the nursing process for the family as well as the individual client. The Family Coping Index is an assessment tool focusing on the family's need for nursing care, their probable response to care, the plan of care to be given, and evaluation of effectiveness. This tool defines family coping as the ability of the family to be reasonably successful in dealing with problems related to health care (Freeman and Heinrich, 1981).

The Family Coping Estimate consists of a scoring profile, a care plan sheet, and a set of instructions with rationale. Although the tool was designed for use in the community setting, it is versatile and can be used by nurses in other settings as well. A prerequisite to use, however, is the nurse's knowledge of the family's interactions, health attitudes and practices, and living situation (Freeman and Heinrich, 1981).

Home Observation for Measurement of Environment

The Home Observation for Measurement of Environment is another useful assessment tool. This tool was discussed in Chapter 21. See that discussion and Appendix B5 for a review of information.

The School Conference

A major part of the older child's or adolescent's world consists of the time spent at school. Experiences, attitudes, and values encountered at school affect psychosocial development (Damon, 1977). For this reason communication between the nurse and the child's teacher and the school nurse is an essential component in monitoring psychosocial development.

The communication nurses establish with the school can be initiated in several ways: (1) between the nurse in the community and the nurse in the school and/or the child's teacher; (2) between the nurse in the school and the teacher; and (3) between the nurse (in the community and/or the school), the teacher, the parent, and the child.

The dialogue established between nurse, teacher, and child can be focused in the following directions:

A. The adjustment to school (Table 23-3) can be facilitated by:
1. Providing support for teachers and intervening in crisis situations
2. Providing support for parents and offering guidance and a means of participation in child's education and adjustment to school through preschool conferences, parent-teacher-nurse conferences throughout school year, involvement with parent-teacher groups (PTO)
3. Providing support for child and assisting to identify peer group, appropriate after-school activities, and means of coping with new situation of school
B. Preventive health measures can be provided by:
1. Screening for physical and emotional health problems (vision, hearing, and scoliosis screening, conversational conferences about how school is going, etc.)
2. Conducting health education classes geared to specific age group (how to care for teeth, taking care of a cold, sex education, STD education, etc.)
C. Assistance can be offered in managing identified problems, both physical and emotional, such as:
1. Cooperating with a prescribed medication regimen
2. Facilitating a behavior modification plan
3. Facilitating special dietary needs or requirements

The school conference is an essential avenue for health promotion. In order for it to be productive, the nurse must facilitate (1) mutual identification of health goals or problems brought to or created by the setting; (2) collaboration of all parties involved to meet goals or resolve problems; and (3) periodic follow-up to ensure that health is maintained.

Once a child has entered the school system, nursing action can facilitate adjustment to and advancement through the educational process. To do so, the nursing process must expand into many environments: home, school, and peer groups. The nurse must have the knowledge and skill to assess the multiple factors of these environments that influence a child's growth and development. It is the nurse's responsibility, therefore, to intervene, coordinate, and facilitate a positive, healthy outcome for the child.

IMMUNIZATIONS

The process of acquiring immunity continues into the school-age and adolescent years. Boosters are recommended at specific intervals for maintenance of adequate concentrations of antibodies. Between the ages of 4 and 6 years a child should receive a booster of DTP and OPV, and the adolescent should receive a tetanus booster every 10 years (see Appendix D2). Older school-age children and adolescents (particularly females) whose immunity status to rubella is questionable should have a rubella titer (American Academy of Pediatrics, 1986). A rubella titer is the blood determination of the concentration of circulating rubella antibodies. Questionable circumstances of immunity include lack of vaccination, vaccination before 13 months of age, history of disease, or uncertainty of vaccination or disease.

Children who have not received immunizations need to be started on a schedule of primary immunizations. Table 21-7 gives the recommended schedule. As in the case of younger children, the older child or adolescent may experience a mild reaction to immunizations. The treatment primarily includes supportive measures, which are discussed in Appendix D2.

NURSE'S ROLE. Ensuring child and adolescent health through appropriate implementation of the immunization schedule is the nurse's responsibility. Nurses assist parents and children in following the recommended schedule through education and counseling, record maintenance, and referral to apppropriate resources or agencies for receipt of vaccine. Nurses have the further responsibilities of being knowledgeable about state legal requirements for immunizations before school entry and of advising parents and children under their care about the implications of these regulations.

NUTRITION
The School-Age Child

Healthy school-age children are in a period of slow and steady growth, and their nutritional needs are relatively stable. The caloric intake requirement for this age group decreases slightly, as do protein and water requirements. Snacks are most likely to be the primary source of nutrients for the school-age child, and the older the child becomes, the more nutrition is obtained outside the home (Pipes, 1981). Therefore, the continued promotion of good eating habits and nutritious snacks is an essential part of the health maintenance visit. Additionally, implementation of a nutrition education program is indicated for the school setting. The recommended food intake for good nutrition for the school-age and adolescent person is presented in Tables 21-8 and 21-9 and Appendix J4. Foods affecting dental health are presented in Table 23-7.

NURSE'S ROLE. Although the school-age period is generally a time of few nutritional problems, the need for continued nutritional assessment on the part of the nurse is important. The diet history continues to be a useful tool, one that will involve children in their own assessment and potentially their own promotion of sound eating habits (see Appendix A4). The nurse's responsibility is to ensure that previously established healthy eating patterns are maintained and that children with deviant patterns are assisted to recognize them and to change.

The Adolescent

The preadolescent and adolescent years are a time of increased growth that is accompanied by increases in appetite and nutritional requirements (see Tables 21-8 and 21-9). Caloric and protein requirements increase for boys ages 11 to 18. Girls have an increased protein need but a decreased caloric need during the same age span. In addition, the iron needed by the adolescent nearly doubles that needed by adults, and iodine, calcium, niacin, and thiamine requirements increase as well (Pipes, 1984; Torre, 1977).

Adolescent nutritional needs are influenced not only by the physical alterations that are occurring but also by the psychosocial adjustments. Teenagers are generally free to eat when and where they choose. It is a time when eating habits acquired from the family are dropped, snacking outside the home is a major source of nutrition, and fad foods and diets are prominent (Torre, 1977).

The factors of accelerated growth and poor eating habits make the adolescent at risk for poor nutritional health. Adolescents have been found to demonstrate the most unsatisfactory nutritional status of all age groups. Deficiencies in iron, vitamins A and C, calcium, riboflavin, and thiamin are most common.

NURSE'S ROLE. Nursing has a responsibility to intervene and initiate activities that promote improved nutritional status. Such activities include the following:

TABLE 23-7

Foods affecting dental health

Recommended foods	Foods to be avoided
Milk	Foods with added sugar
Cheese	Sticky foods: candy, cake, cook-
Cheese products	ies, pies, ice cream, candied
Salami	popcorn, candy-covered fruit,
Smoked meats	honey-covered foods, dried
Nuts	fruit
Raw fruit and vegetables	Hard candies, breath mints,
Unsweetened fruit juices	cough drops
Vegetable juices	Lemons or acidic fruits that are
Crackers	sucked or eaten
Pretzels	
Corn chips	
Popcorn	
Teething biscuits	

Provision of informational material on good nutrition in group or individual encounters

Diet assessment using a comprehensive diet history or a 24-hour diet diary

Educational activities that focus on:

Effects of fad foods and fad diets

Supplying of "at risk" nutrients and their sources

Provision of a daily food guide (see Table 23-8)

Suggested snacks and "on the run" foods that supply essential nutrients

Relationship of good nutritional habits to healthy appearance

Assessment for signs of nutritional deficiencies (see Table 23-9)

Supplementation
Vitamins

Adequate amounts of vitamins and minerals are necessary for the nutritional health of people of any age. Without these essential nutrients, physical and psychosocial health may be compromised. There is much controversy over the question of whether or not to routinely supplement the diet with vitamins and minerals. Of particular concern is the recent fad of taking megadoses (very large doses) of vitamins and minerals to ensure health.

The decision to supplement a child's or adolescent's diet with vitamins or minerals should be based on (1) the nutritional adequacy of the diet for age and growth requirements as verified by diet assessment and (2) a clinically based nutritional deficiency identified through laboratory studies and physical examination (Chow, et al., 1984).

Fluoride

An adequate fluoride supply is essential for dental health. Fluoride sources include treated drinking water, topical application, and oral tablets and rinses. Nurses should make assessments to verify whether adequate fluoride sources are available and should assist the client to secure a source if current supply is inadequate.

Special Nutritional Situations
Athletic Child

The child or adolescent who is engaged in athletic activities will require additional nursing assessment and intervention. For individuals involved in strenuous activities, at least 2300 to 5000 calories per day is required. Optimal distribution of calories is considered to be 10% to 15% protein, 25% to 35% fat, and 50% to 65% carbohydrate. Increases in vitamins, minerals, and water and salt may be indicated as well (Smith, 1979).

Nurses have the responsibility to be knowledgeable about the potential need for added nutritional supplements of athletic children and to implement appropriate dietary assessment and management to meet these increased needs.

Vegetarian Child

The child or adolescent who follows a vegetarian diet requires special nursing assessment and management. Knowledge of the type of vegetarian diet followed is essential. Generally these types are (1) lactoovovegetarian, a diet of vegetables supplemented by milk, eggs, and cheese; (2) lactovegetarian, a vegetable diet with only milk and cheese added; and (3) pure vegetarian, the diet of a vegan, which excludes all foods of animal origin.

Vegetarian diets can provide the essential nutrients for the growth and development of children. Diets of these types need to be based on sound nutritional principles, and the nurse who is assessing and counseling a vegetarian should be aware of the following points (Williams, 1975):

Protein sources need to be varied to ensure adequate amounts of essential amino acids.

Amino acids in one food can supplement those in another food.

A variety of vitamin C and folacin sources must be included.

A diet that excludes all animal food is deficient in vitamin B_{12}; supplementation is essential if eggs, cheese, and/ or milk are not used.

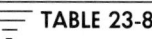

TABLE 23-8

Daily food guide for adolescents

Food group	Servings
Milk and milk products	4
Meats	3
Fruits and vegetables	4
Vitamin A source	1
Vitamin C source	1
Breads and cereals	4

From Tackett, J.J., and Hunsberger, M., editors. Family centered care of children and adolescents, Philadelphia, 1981, W.B. Saunders Co., p. 1244.

TABLE 23-9

Clinical signs indicative of nutritional deficiencies

	Clinical signs
General appearance	Lethargy, excessive or inadequate body fat, muscle wasting
Skin	Dryness, flakiness, scaling, roughness (follicular hyperkeratosis), pallor
Mouth	Angular fissures, redness at corners of mouth (cheilosis); redness, swelling, or atrophic papillae on tongue; red, swollen, or bleeding gums
Teeth	Severe caries
Eyes	Pale conjunctivae
Nails	Spoon-shaped, brittle or ridged
Hair	Dull, easily plucked

From Tackett, J.J., and Hunsberger, M., editors: Family centered care of children and adolescents, Philadelphia, 1981, W.B. Saunders Co., p. 1245.

Adequate iodine can be obtained by using iodized salt. Adequate vitamins and minerals are supplied if protein, vegetables, and fruit are adequate.

NURSE'S ROLE. Sound nutritional counseling includes teaching that a vegetarian diet that includes some animal foods is nutritionally adequate if well planned. Vegans, who observe pure vegetarian diets, require vitamin B_{12} supplementation. Providing sample menus for the vegetarian dieter is often helpful in promoting sound nutritional habits.

HEALTH PROMOTION ACTIVITIES
Health Assessment

Activities implemented by nurses that facilitate health continue throughout the school-age and adolescent years. The health assessment visit, using the health history and physical assessment components that focus on individuals and their potential health risks and stressors, remains a focal point for nursing intervention. Development and implementation of a health plan need to be a collaborative effort involving the child or adolescent, parents, and the school. The specific screening techniques and tools for assessment have been previously discussed. *The most important are screening of hearing, vision, dentition, sex characteristics (Tanner staging), nutrition, and school and social adjustment and screening for scoliosis, tuberculosis, common problems, venereal disease, need for birth control, and learning disabilities.*

Encouraging school-age children and adolescents to assume responsibility for their own health can be an effective health promotion activity (Daniel, 1977). This approach requires close follow-up to ensure that health goals are being met.

The focus of anticipatory guidance is prevention of health problems. See Appendixes A, B, C, D, J, and K for examples of appropriate anticipatory guidance tools. Preventive health counseling should focus on the following aspects:

Nutrition
Safety
School
Peers
Identified or at-risk health problems
Sexuality (including venereal disease and birth control)
Family and sibling relationships
Coping strategies

Group Health Education and Child-Focused Education

Promoting health in the group education setting is an effective technique. The principles for development of health maintenance classes were discussed in Chapter 21 and can be applied to classes focusing on school-age and adolescent persons. An additional technique, which is useful and specific to these age groups, is to solicit participation of the child or adolescent in outlining the content of such courses. As interest evolves, participation can be increased to presentation of material in collaboration with the nurse. In some instances, adolescents may indicate interest in helping with educational classes for younger children. The primary objective, regardless of the technique, is to involve the participants and to encourage self-care responsibilities.

The setting for health education classes varies. However, use of the school setting, where large spans of time are spent, promotes greater participation. In addition, incorporating health education into the school's curriculum is a challenge nurses should undertake. Such health programs could be a required component of the curriculum or be made available during student "free periods." The topics for such programs should be of interest to the participants and focus on a special interest group or an identified problem. In addition to the topics previously discussed under preventive health counseling, potential topics include sex education, participation in sports, taking care of yourself (e.g., focus on dentition, nutrition, or managing a cold), coping as a teenager, the importance of friends, and health risks of smoking.

Parent-Focused Education

Parents, as well as their school-age children and adolescents, are in need of educational programs. Focusing on the topics discussed in the previous section from a parental perspective potentially facilitates more effective parenting skills. For example, classes in how to cope with teenage crises, how to talk to your child about sex, or how to communicate with the teenagers in your family offer parents an opportunity to learn new skills that promote their relationships with their children as well as the children's health. A similar approach can be applied to teachers by offering seminars that focus on problems or concerns they may be experiencing (e.g., how to handle an inattentive child or how to promote a positive relationship with students).

Home Intervention

Home intervention is generally based on an individual's or family's health needs. Certainly intervention at the time of a crisis is indicated. But intervention before a crisis, with the goal of promoting health and preventing a crisis, is a significant contribution nurses can make. Assessing the home situation and environment is the nurse's responsibility. By assisting the family and child to identify problems within the home and by facilitating their resolution, nurses promote individual, family, and community health. A home that maintains health and relies on its resources is engaging in self-care and promoting wellness, both of which are nursing goals.

Additional Activities

Knowledge and understanding facilitate responsible behavior. Nurses are the catalysts who promote these experiences. Many of the activities previously discussed will enhance knowledge and understanding about health. Additional means include making resource material and services available to the child or adolescent and to parents.

Bibliographies directed toward specific concerns, problems, or age groups are useful tools. Printed materials on a diversity of topics are available from governmental agencies, special interest groups, and pharmaceutical companies. Nurses have a responsibility to direct their clients to these resources. Similarly, many community groups provide needed services. A few are listed in Chapter 21. Additional community resources for the school-age child and adolescent include the following:

Mental health hot lines
Drug abuse centers
Planned Parenthood centers
STD clinics
Alcoholics Anonymous
Community recreation centers
Child and youth organizations
Youth athletic clubs

Nurses have the knowledge, skills, and resources to have an impact on the status of child health. The challenge lies in realizing their full potential.

CLINICAL APPLICATION

The school-age and adolescent years present a challenge to the community health nurse when providing health promotion activities. Individuals in these age groups need to be involved in and motivated to make decisions about their current and future health. The community health nurse can promote positive health behaviors through assessment, education, and counseling.

Physical Growth
School-Age Children

In school-age children, physical growth is slow and steady. Monitoring of height, weight, vital signs, and blood pressure continues to be essential to the community health nurse's assessment. Observation of skeletal and dental growth is also valuable to this assessment. The student will encounter the community health nurse making observations about changes in posture and gait as well as the sequence of tooth shedding and eruption.

Promotion of dental health becomes most important during the school-age years. Use the child's cognitive abilities to promote this aspect of health. The student may find it useful to design a health education class for 9- and 10-year-olds on keeping healthy teeth. The use of a tooth model to explain structure is helpful, as well as soliciting the children's involvement in demonstrating good toothbrushing technique. Discussing diet and foods that promote or hinder dental health is also useful.

Adolescents

During adolescence physical growth takes on renewed importance. Monitoring height and weight for the growth spurts of puberty is an important nursing function. Assessment of sexual maturation through Tanner staging observation and recording is a most helpful indicator of physical growth. Facilitating adjustment to these physical and physiological changes is of primary importance. The student may observe the community health nurse using the previously mentioned physical assessment skills in health encounters. The community health nurse will also counsel and educate preadolescents and adolescents about pubertal events. This may include offering a class to a group of girls about menstruation, discussing the physical changes of sexual maturation and their normal sequence, or discussing personal hygiene measures that become necessary with these hormonal changes (need for antiperspirant, skin care, selecting a supportive bra, and so on).

For both school-age and adolescent clients, the community health nurse will continue to monitor immunization and nutritional status. An additional booster for tetanus and diphtheria is indicated for children ages 14 to 16 years. A diet history will provide the nurse with information about nutritional adequacy. Particular attention must be paid to the adolescent's diet as calorie and nutritional requirements increase. The community health nurse will help the adolescent implement a diet plan that incorporates these increased requirements as well as the individual's food preferences.

Psychosocial Health
School-Age Children

During school-age years children are working toward developing a sense of industry, using their expanding cognitive skills of reasoning and realism to achieve this. Being able to differentiate, categorize, solve problems, and conceptualize allows the child to achieve social, cognitive, and physical competencies.

The community health nurse assesses this growth through history taking and observation. By knowing the typical behaviors for a specific age group, the community health nurse can assess the individual child's psychosocial health. For example, knowing that the average 10-year-old can follow rules, participates in cooperative projects, has hobbies or distinct interests, and has a group of special friends would alert the nurse to a child who has few friends, plays alone at recess, does not follow rules, and does not appear to have any special interests. Knowledge of developmental norms can also assist the community health nurse in promoting psychosocial growth. For example, the nurse might encourage a shy child to participate in organized sports, or encourage the parents of a child who is attending a new school to invite schoolmates to play after school. Both of these nursing interventions encourage group and peer activity, which is important for the child's developing social skills.

Adolescents

Adolescents are trying to establish their identities, and at the same time continue to expand concrete and abstract logical abilities. Often these two areas of development collide. For example, most adolescents are aware of the dangers of drinking and driving, yet go along with it because of their need to be a part of the peer group. The role of the nurse is to help adolescents to recognize these inconsistencies and to direct their energies toward positive health behaviors. For example, the community health or school nurse can help students establish a chapter of SADD (Students Against Driving Drunk) or can help them develop a community program that distributes information on safe driving tips at local grocery stores.

The nursing student may further observe the community health nurse motivating and involving adolescents in decisions about health behaviors through education. Knowledge about health facts and risks can help adolescents choose positive health behaviors. The community health nurse will educate and counsel during health visits in the school setting and during home visits. Special adolescent screening and health assessment clinics and special group health education classes in the school or clinic are frequently used by community health nurses. The student will observe community health nurses conducting scoliosis screening in schools, classes on birth control alternatives in the clinic, or health education classes in either setting on skin care, diet, and nutrition.

Additionally, the community health nurse will promote adolescent psychosocial health through education programs for parents of adolescents. These sessions can provide a forum for parents to discuss problems they are encountering—for example—dealing with the influence of peers, the argumentative teenager, and the apparently irresponsible adolescent—or focus on topics of special interest, such as recognizing drug use in the adolescent, communicating with the adolescent, or assisting the adolescent in decision making.

For both adolescent and school-age clients, the community health nurse will take advantage of their increasing cognitive abilities. The student will observe the nurse relying on the school-age child or adolescent as historian, and verifying facts with parents as indicated. In addition, the nurse will explain any physical assessment techniques to clients of these ages and involve them directly in their plans of care. For example, the nurse will explain the Tine test and how to read the results to the 10-year-old client as well as to the parent.

Special Health Problems
Accidents

Accidents continue to pose a major health threat for school-age children and adolescents. Community health nurses will intervene in preventing accidents primarily through education. The student will observe the nurse discussing bicycle and swimming safety tips with school-age children and automobile driving and passenger safety tips with adolescents. In addition, the community health nurse will educate clients of these ages in self-care measures for common health problems—for example, how to take a temperature, what to do for a cold, or how to manage an upset stomach. These educational endeavors are all directed toward the client's level of ability and understanding and toward promoting health behaviors.

Latchkey Children

Another area of concern, particularly for school-age children, is the phenomenon of latchkey children. The student may find it useful to design a program for children who must stay at home by themselves after school and for their parents. Focusing on safety tips is important for such a program. Safety tips include not telling phone callers the child is alone, carrying a house key in a concealed place, calling a parent when the child arrives home, and having a secret hiding place for money and an extra key.

School-age Problems

School-related problems are additional areas of concern for 6- to 12-year-olds. The community health nurse, particularly the nurse in the school setting, is in a position to facilitate school adjustment and minimize school problems through preparation of parent and child for school, early recognition and referral of school problems or learning disabilities, and participation in teacher-parent-child conferences to evaluate the child's progress and performance.

Adolescent Problems

Special adolescent health problems that will require nursing intervention are social and physical in origin. Common health problems such as acne and menstrual disorders can be dealt with during the health encounter or group education session. The student will observe the community health nurse teaching adolescents about skin care or conducting an all-girls session on minimizing premenstrual tension and discomfort. Education about venereal disease, its communicability, and the need for treatment will also be done by the community health or school nurse.

The social problems facing adolescents will be dealt with by the community or school nurse. Educating adolescents about substance abuse, psychosocial problems such as depression, and birth control is an important nursing responsibility. This education occurs in the school, clinic, or individual health encounter. The student will observe the community health nurse assessing the need for such programs, finding out which topics are of interest to the adolescents, designing and implementing an educational program, and encouraging adolescents to be active participants in the program by researching the topic and contributing to the presentation.

Teenage Pregnancy

With the high incidence of teenage pregnancy, the community health nurse is involved with the provision of many services. The student will observe the nurse providing counseling to the pregnant teenager regarding pregnancy continuation or termination. The nurse will act as a referral source for prenatal, postnatal, and social services, and will be directly involved in the delivery of these services. Special prenatal and postnatal clinics for teenagers are planned and implemented by the community health nurse. Close follow-up of the teenage mother in the clinic and at home are also an important nursing function. The student may find it useful to become involved in the implementation of a prenatal clinic for teens. Special attention should be paid to the physical needs of the pregnant teen—for example, increased nutritional needs and state of physical well being—as well as to her psychosocial needs—how or if she will return to school, the father's interaction with her, reactions of family and peers, the decision about whether to keep the infant, and so on.

SUMMARY

Both the school-age child and the adolescent live in rapidly expanding worlds. The period of life from 6 to 12 years is characterized by steady physical growth, neuromuscular refinement, and rapid expansion of cognitive and social skills. Between the ages of 13 and 20, a person leaves childhood and becomes an adult. This period of life is characterized by a steady progression of physiological changes. These changes and the emotional, psychological, and social adaptations to them push the adolescent to learn to develop coping mechanisms that will be carried throughout life.

Growth and development throughout these stages are influenced by the degree of success or failure a child has had in mastering the tasks of preceding stages. Developing self-esteem and identifying life-style values are important accomplishments during the school-age and adolescent developmental phases.

Fifty percent of all deaths of school-age children occur as a result of accidents. Cancer, birth defects, influenza, and pneumonia are other common causes of mortality. The health problems and concerns of school-age children include learning and school difficulties, behavioral disturbances, speech, hearing, and vision problems, and infectious diseases. In addition, children of this age group are rapidly developing risk factors that may eventually lead to adult disease and disabilities.

Three fourths of all deaths among adolescents can be attributed to accidents, homicide, and suicide. Risk-taking behaviors of this age group result in death or injury. Although chronic disease is not a leading cause of death, life-style behaviors at this age may create susceptibility to chronic disease in adulthood. Other threats to adolescent health include substance abuse, pregnancy, sexually transmitted diseases, abnormal spinal curvatures, acne, menstrual disorders, mononucleosis, and eating disorders.

The community health nurse can play a significant role in promoting the health of school-age children and adolescents through physical and health assessment, risk analysis, screening, anticipatory guidance, health teaching, and counseling with children and their parents.

KEY CONCEPTS

Although the health of school-age children and adolescents in the United States is better than ever, these age groups are confronted with health problems more complex than those of previous generations.

Nurses in community health settings can educate school-age children and adolescents regarding health problems and their subsequent influence on future health.

During the preadolescent and adolescent phases of development, physical and social mastery of the expanding environment is the major task.

Helping children develop self-esteem and identify life-style values is the basis of anticipatory guidance.

The physical, emotional, social, and psychological adaptations of adolescence push the young person to learn and develop coping mechanisms that will be carried throughout life.

According to Erikson, between the ages of 6 and 12 a child learns to become a productive member of a peer group.

Piaget characterizes the cognitive competencies of 6- to 7-year olds as intuitive. He states that between the ages of 8 and 10, cognitive abilities increase in reasoning and realism.

Erikson believes that between the ages of 13 and 20, a person has the task of leaving childhood and becoming an adult. Adolescents must establish their own identities or be caught in confusion regarding their roles.

Peers are one of the most important influences on growth and development.

Although the health of children in the United States is better now than 10 years ago, the slowness of the decline in mortality remains a concern. A major contributor to this slow decline is the fact that 50% of all deaths result from accidents.

The significant health problems affecting school-age children are learning and school difficulties; behavioral disturbances; speech, hearing, and vision problems; and infectious diseases.

As many as 40% of children ages 11 to 14 demonstrate potential characteristics of heart disease.

Violent deaths and accidents account for the majority of deaths among adolescents and young adults.

The health assessment visit, using the health history and physical assessment components that focus on individuals and their potential health risks and stressors, remains a focal point for nursing intervention during the preadolescent and adolescent years.

LEARNING ACTIVITIES

1. Develop and implement a program on bicycle safety for 8- to 10-year-olds through the local school.

2. Construct a presentation illustrating the various methods of birth control available to teens.

3. Develop a diet plan for a 12-year-old female who is a competitive gymnast.

4. Develop a nursing care plan for a 16-year-old who has learned she is pregnant.

5. Observe behaviors relating to the first day of school at the local school or bus stop. Note and record the "parting" behaviors of 5- to 6-year-olds and their parents. Return and make the same observation 2 weeks later and compare.

BIBLIOGRAPHY

Abbott, M.: Teens having babies, Pediatr. Nurs. 4:23-27, May-June 1978.

American Academy of Pediatrics: Report of the Committee on Infectious Diseases, ed. 20, Evanston, Ill., 1986, The Academy.

American Dental Association: Your Child's Teeth, Chicago, 1971, The Association.

Anderson, B.: The patient with scoliosis: Carole, a girl treated with bracing, Am. J. Nurs. 79:1592-1598, Sept. 1979.

Behrman, R.E., and Vaughan, V.C., editors: Nelson textbook of pediatrics, ed. 13, Philadelphia, 1987, W.B. Saunders Co.

Bernstein, A.C.: Six stages of understanding how children learn about sex and birth, Psychol. Today 1:31-35, Jan. 1976.

Boyle, M.P., Koff, E., and Guidas, L.J.: Assessment and management of anorexia nervosa, Matern. Child Nurs. J. 6:412-418, Nov.-Dec. 1981.

Brosnan, J., and Fond, K.: School phobia: the student anxiety syndrome, Pediatr. Nurs. 6:9-16, Sept.-Oct. 1980.

Brown, M.S., and Murphy, M.A.: Ambulatory pediatrics for nurses, ed. 1, New York, 1975, McGraw-Hill Book Co.

Bruch, H.: Anorexia nervosa and its differential diagnosis, J. Nerv. Ment. Dis. 141:555-566, Nov. 1965.

Child, A.A., Murphy, C.M., and Rhyne, M.C.: Depression in children: reasons and risks, Pediatr. Nurs. 6:9-15, July-Aug. 1980.

Chow, M.P., et al.: Handbook of pediatric primary care, ed. 2, New York, 1984, John Wiley & Sons, Inc.

Centers for Disease Control: STD fact sheet, ed. 35, DHHS (PHS) pub. no. (CDC) 81-8195, Hyattsville, Md., 1981, U.S. Department of Health and Human Services, Public Health Service.

Cohen, M.I.: Adolescent health: concerns for the eighties, Pediatrics in Review 4:5-7, July 1982.

Committee on Adolescence, Group for the Advancement of Psychiatry: Normal adolescence, New York, 1968, Charles Scribner's Sons.

Damon, W.: The social world of the child, New York, 1977, Jossey Bass, Inc., Publishers.

Daniel, W.A.: Adolescents in health and disease, St. Louis, 1977, The C.V. Mosby Co.

Dibble, J.: ABC for teens-parent education after the baby comes, Pediatr. Nurs. 7:21-25, July-Aug. 1981.

Dunn, B.: Common orthopedic problems of children, Pediatr. Nurs. 1:7-10, Nov.-Dec. 1975.

Erikson, E.: Childhood and society, New York, 1963, W.W. Norton & Co., Inc.

Freeman, R.B., and Heinrich, J.: Community health nursing practice, ed. 2, Philadelphia, 1981, W.B. Saunders Co.

Gorman, G.: The school age child as historian, Pediatr. Nurs. 6:39-41, Jan.-Feb. 1980.

Hart, N.A., and Prophit, S.P.: Adolescent suicide, Pediatr. Nurs. 5:22-28, Nov.-Dec. 1979.

Havinghurst, R.: Developmental tasks and education, New York, 1972, David McKay Co., Inc.

Health: United States and prevention profile, DHHS Pub. No. (PHS) 84-1232, Hyattsville, Md., Dec. 1986, U.S. Department of Health and Human Services, Public Health Service.

Keenan, T.: School based adolescent health care programs, Pediatr. Nurs. 12:365-369, Sept.-Oct. 1986.

Keller, O.L.: Bulimia: primary care approach and intervention, Nurse Pract. 11:42-51, Aug. 1986.

Kreutner, A.K., and Hollingsworth, D.R.: Adolescent obstetrics and gynecology, Chicago, 1978, Year Book Medical Publishers, Inc.

Krugman, S., and Katz, S.L.: Infectious diseases of children, ed. 8, St. Louis, 1985, The C.V. Mosby Co.

Laige, J.: The school aged child and his family. In Hymovich, D., and Barnard, M., editors: Family health care: developmental and situational crises, New York, 1978, McGraw-Hill Book Co.

Lauernsen, N.: Recognition and treatment of menstrual syndrome, Nurse Pract. 10:11-22, March 1985.

Litt, I.: Menstrual problems during adolescence, Pediatrics in Review 4:203-212, Jan. 1983.

Maier, H.: Three theories of child development, New York, 1969, Harper & Row, Publishers, Inc.

Marks, A.: Health screening of the adolescent, Pediatr. Nurs. 4:37-41, July-Aug. 1978.

Meier, J.H.: Development and learning disabilities: evaluation, management and prevention in children, Baltimore, 1976, University Park Press.

Nelms, B.C., and Brady, M.A.: Assessment and intervention: the depressed school-age child, Pediatr. Nurs. 6:15-21, July-Aug. 1980.

Pipes, P.L.: Nutrition in infancy and childhood, ed. 3, St. Louis, 1984, The C.V. Mosby Co.

Rice, M.A., and Kibee, P.E.: Review: identifying the adolescent substance abuser, Matern. Child Nurs. J. 8:139-142, March-April 1983.

Rigg, C.A.: Homosexuality in adolescence, Pediatr. Ann. 11:826-828, 1982.

Rogers, M.: Early identification and intervention with children with learning problems, Pediatr. Nurs. 2:21-26, Jan.-Feb. 1976.

Sapala, S., and Sheldon, S.: Infectious mononucleosis: clinical considerations for practitioners, Pediatr. Nurs. 4:16-27, Nov.-Dec. 1978.

Sapala, S., and Strokosch, G.: Adolescent sexuality: use of a questionnaire for health teaching and counseling, Pediatr. Nurs. 7:33-35, Nov.-Dec. 1981.

Schwartz, R.H., Cohen, P.R., and Bair, G.O.: Identifying and coping with a drug using adolescent, Pediatrics in Review 7:133-135, Nov. 1985.

Smith, N.: Sports medicine, Pediatr. Nurs. 5:39-46, Jan.-Feb. 1979.

Stone, A.C.: Facing up to acne, Pediatr. Nurs. 8:229-239, July-Aug. 1982.

Sutterley, D., and Donnelly, G.: Perspectives in human development: nursing throughout the life cycle, Philadelphia, 1973, J.B. Lippincott Co.

Tackett, J.J., and Hunsberger, M., editors: Family centered care of children and adolescents, Philadelphia, 1981, W.B. Saunders Co.

Tanner, J.M.: Growth at adolescence, Oxford, 1962, Blackwell Scientific Publications, Inc.

Torre, C.T.: Nutritional needs of adolescents, Am. J. Matern. Child Nurs. 2:105-112, March-April 1977.

Trussell, T.J.: Economic consequences of teenage child bearing, Fam. Plann. Perspect. 8:187, 1976.

Wegman, M.E.: Annual summary of vital statistics—1982, Pediatrics 72:755-765, Dec. 1983.

Wells, G.: Reducing the threat of a first pelvic exam, Am. J. Matern. Child Nurs. 2:304-307, Sept.-Oct. 1977.

Williams, A.F.: Observed child restraint uses in automobiles, Am. J. Dis. Child. 130:1311-1317, 1976.

Williams, E.R.: Making vegetarian diets nutritious, Am. J. Nurs. 75:2168-2173, Dec. 1975.

Wolf, W.J., and Bancroft, B.: Early detection of childhood malignancies, Pediatr. Nurs. 5:43-48, Jan.-Feb. 1980.

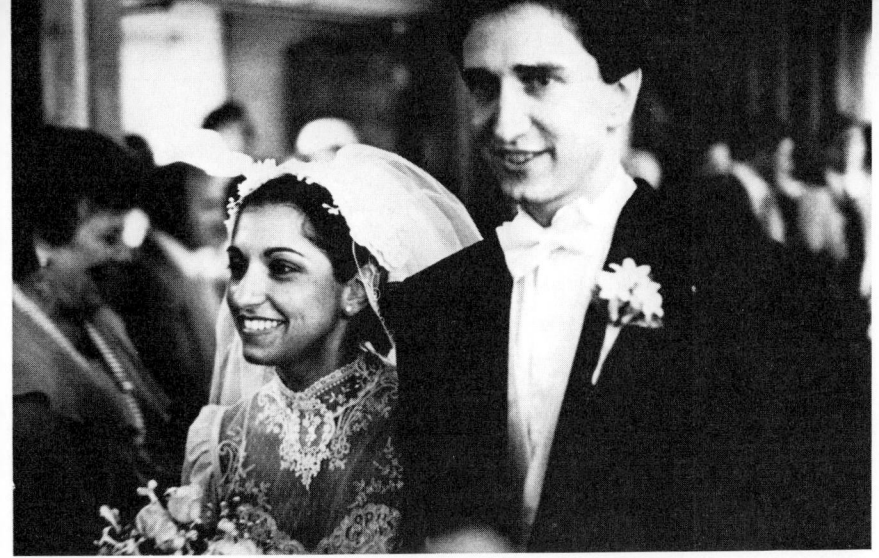

YOUNG AND MIDDLE ADULTS

Patricia Starck

24

OBJECTIVES

After reading this chapter, the student should be able to:

Differentiate the psychosocial tasks of young and middle adults.

Discuss the major health problems of young adults as to causative factors and significant impact on individuals, families, and society.

Discuss the major health problems of middle adults as to risk factors and incidence.

Analyze the role of stress in health and disease as it is related to life-style.

Compare and contrast the terms *impairment, disability,* and *handicap.*

KEY TERMS

aging process

burnout

cancer

dereflection

disability

existential vacuum

handicap

impairment

logotherapy

middlescence

noo-genic neurosis

osteoporosis

periodontitis

personal health profiles

socially naked

Socratic dialogue

The period in life categorized as young and middle adulthood is paradoxically demanding and rewarding. Much is expected of the adult, who must support others on either end of the age continuum. Social role expectations of adults may result in stoicism about or suppression of their own needs, while they take care of the young, cope with the trials and tribulations of adolescent offspring, and take care of elderly parents. Like the middle-income strata of society, the young or middle adult may be considered the backbone of society—being responsible, accountable, and expected to take care of themselves as well as others.

In the health care literature, young and middle adults are a neglected, forgotten group. Other age groups are well-isolated for study and even have identifying labels such as fetus, newborns, infants, toddlers, early childhood, adolescents, preteens, geriatric, and elderly. No such identifying terms exist for adult stages. There are no categories for adults in literature indexes.

Age is used as a criterion for defining adulthood in our society. However, chronological age, maturity, and developmental tasks may vary. For the purposes of this chapter, adults are categorized as young adults (20 to 35 years) and middle adults (36 to 64 years), recognizing that the dividing line is blurred. Indeed, adults may move back and forth between the young adult and the middle adult life-styles when establishing a marriage, home, and family; reentering single life; establishing a second marriage, home, and family; and developing a first and later a second career.

This chapter examines ways community health nurses can assist young and middle adults to meet health needs. Physical development and psychosocial developmental tasks are discussed, including the tasks and responsibilities characteristic of this group and the changes in biological functions and structures along with the concomitant psychosocial changes. Factors influencing progression through this stage of life, including health status, resources in rural and/or urban settings, and life-styles are explored, as are common causes of morbidity and mortality for young and middle adults. The nursing role implied by the major health problems is discussed; discussion includes tools for assessment and strategies for implementation. This chapter also discusses health promotion from physical, psychosocial, and spiritual perspectives. Because a major task for the young and middle adult is career productivity, this chapter dis-

cusses careers and stress in the workplace and considers the special needs of the disabled adult. Exercises to be used by the reader to cope with health needs of this age group are also included.

PSYCHOSOCIAL DEVELOPMENT: TASKS OF ADULTHOOD

Adults progress through successive phases of stabilization and consolidation, followed by change and growth in the pursuit of new goals and in the confrontation of life crises at different stages.

Adulthood is a time of caring for others—children and parents. Caring for children presents challenges that vary with each stage of development of the child. A growing number of single parents face child rearing without partners. These are busy years as the adults keep up with scheduled activities for many family members. The energy drain for adults with such a schedule may adversely affect health.

In addition, adults often encounter the responsibilities of caring for parents. Reversal of the caring role (parent for child) often requires difficult decision making on behalf of a parent's welfare. Deciding on nursing home care versus living alone or with the primary family group may require professional consultation.

The primary burden of income production rests with the young and middle adult. Level of income, which determines living standards, security, and satisfaction, is often considered a measure of success. Adults feel pressure to achieve in a competitive world. During these years, an individual devotes considerable time, often in excess of the traditional 40 hours per week, to economic success.

Adults also feel pressure to fulfill societal responsibilities. Because community progress is dependent on adult leadership, much emphasis is placed on this generation's contribution to posterity.

Developmental Tasks

Common characteristics of the various stages of psychosocial development of adults have been identified by various authors. Table 24-1 compares and contrasts viewpoints by Erikson (1950), Sheehy (1974, 1981), and Diekelmann (1976). In essence, the young adult struggles to achieve intimacy with persons outside the nuclear family while establishing a career, whereas the middle adult concentrates

TABLE 24-1

Developmental tasks for young and middle adults

Stage	Erickson	Sheehy	Diekelmann
Young adult (20 to 35 years)	Intimacy versus isolation *Success:* Intimacy, facing fear of ego loss in situations of self-abandonment such as orgasm, close personal friendships, inspirational experiences *Failure:* Isolation and self-absorption	Stages: a. Pulling up roots (18-22), leaving home b. Trying 20s (23-27), establishing career and mate relationships c. Catch 30 (28-33), reassessing earlier family and/or career decisions d. Rooting and extending (33-35), achieving degree of stability	Tasks: a. Achieving independence from parental controls b. Establishing intimate relationships outside the family c. Establishing a personal set of values d. Developing a sense of personal identity e. Preparing for a career and forming the capacity for intimacy
Middle adult (36-64 years)	Generativity versus stagnation *Success:* Generating an accomplishment—raising a family, writing a book, establishing and guiding the next generation *Failure:* Individual stagnation and interpersonal impoverishment	a. Deadline decade (35-45), recognizing urgency of achieving goals b. Comeback decade (45-55), accepting self and changes in values and life-styles	

on making a contribution to society through work and/or family.

Psychosocial challenges may be complicated by physical changes that begin to occur in adulthood. These changes include graying hair, receding hairlines, changes in fat contours, spinal curvature changes, and skin turgor changes. The effect these changes have varies with each individual. Exercise, nutrition, sleep, rest, play, and mental attitude affect the impact of physical changes.

The community health nurse may encounter individuals who are struggling with psychosocial tasks appropriate to the stages of development or individuals who have failed to achieve normal goals. In either case, frustration impinges on the individual as well as the family system, creating barriers to achieving optimal health.

Middle adults who are single have double demands. They must revert back to the isolation versus intimacy tasks as well as deal with the developmental stage of generativity. Young or middle adults who are married may encounter problems; as Sheehy (1974) pointed out, no two people can possibly coordinate the timing and effect of their developmental crises.

Emotionally healthy adults are able to negotiate psychosocial challenges successfully. Sheehy (1981) identified 10 hallmarks of well-being in the adult.

1. Meaning and direction in life
2. Successful negotiation through transitions
3. Absence of feelings of being cheated or disappointed by life
4. Attainment of several long-term goals
5. Satisfaction with personal growth and development
6. Feelings of mutual love for partner
7. Many friends
8. Cheerful attitude
9. Not sensitive to criticism
10. No major fears

FACTORS INFLUENCING GROWTH AND DEVELOPMENT

Factors that influence growth and development of the adult include health status, a sense of responsibility for self-care, resources in rural and urban settings, and life-style behaviors. A unique factor for the middle adult is the challenge of "middlescence," characterized as a major turning point in life. The consummation of adult growth and development is achieving fulfillment through meaning and purpose in life.

Health

Health for the adult is the balanced state of well-being resulting from the harmonious interaction of body, mind, and spirit. Health care seeks to understand the human condition and to delineate the circumstances of illnesses and the underlying conflicts, hostilities, and griefs (see Chapter 2).

The panorama of health needs for adults includes preventing health disruption, promoting a state of high-level wellness, providing care and/or cure services for illness states, and providing rehabilitation for chronic or disabling conditions. Self-care is a component of adult attempts to maintain or improve health status.

Milio (1981, 1983) described health in terms of freedom—freedom to use one's time in preferred ways, freedom from rigidities and deprivations of medical regimens, and freedom of choice for decisions about the future. Freedom is a mutually sustaining relationship with one's environment. Thus health is much more than the absence of symptoms, problems, or restricted activities. Health is a balance within normal ranges of biological and social parameters. Developmental tasks and ongoing life challenges evoke responses of self-renewal in the healthy individual. As Milio (1983, p. 4) succinctly describes health, it is "continuing success at finding ways to keep time with our biological clocks."

Responsibility: Self-care

Most individuals expect life to provide opportunities to work and play, as well as to find love and meaning in life, and experience joy. Diekelmann (1980) emphasized that people have the conscious power of judgment, decision, and choice to study their own circumstances and to conclude what is best and contributes to overall wellness. Participation is the essential ingredient in self-care or wellness care, and requisite skills include self-centering, self-awareness, or self-reference (Silverman, 1980). These skills allow people to sensitize themselves to others while protecting themselves from the negativity present in the world. Selye (1980) emphasized the need for abilities in learning to gauge innate energies, potential weaknesses and strengths, and, above all, self-discipline and willpower.

Although self-care may be viewed as a modern phenomenon, Johns (1985) pointed out that the passive health consumers are actually the relatively recent phenomenon. Historically, the role of care giving belonged to the family. But with the new industrial age came modern health care technology, which, being foreign to patients, reinforced passive roles and fostered helplessness. These same factors have created a resurgence of self-care as consumers become more involved in and aware of health concerns. Knowledge gained through media coverage and a generalized dissatisfaction with impersonal and costly delivery systems have made self-care a major component of adult health care concerns.

Perhaps the most well-known self-care definition in nursing literature is that by Orem (1985, p. 31), in which self-care is "the production of activities directed to self or to the environment in order to regulate one's functioning in the interest of one's life, integrated functioning and well-being." A broader definition is that of Levin (1981, p. 4) who defines self-care as "a process whereby a lay person can function effectively on his own behalf in health promotion and prevention and in disease detection and treatment at the level of the primary health resource in the health care system." The impact of self-care on the traditional health care delivery system will be significant, with a shift toward patient education as adults become more active in admin-

istering care. Redman (1984) developed a process model for patient education consisting of assessing the need and readiness to learn, setting objectives, teaching, learning, and evaluating and reteaching. The factors influencing self-care are based on what a person believes about health in terms of perceptions of susceptibility, seriousness of the health problem, and advantages and disadvantages of action. This set of perceptions forms a health belief model that is useful in understanding and promoting adherence to a medical treatment regimen. The key point of intervention for the community health nurse is based on understanding, modifying, or enabling factors in the health belief model. Factors such as cultural beliefs and practices, costs, accessibility, and previous experience help to determine the likelihood of behavioral changes. Health teaching involves changing attitudes and values as well as imparting knowledge.

Health risk appraisal as discussed in Chapter 27 is a useful technique in monitoring health states. Though a young adult often takes good health for granted, middle adults become increasingly aware of health hazards and their contributions to these hazards. The health risk appraisal, generating a statement of probability and not a diagnosis, describes a person's chances of becoming ill from or dying from selected diseases. It should not be used as a scare tactic, but rather as a motivator to accentuate the positive aspects of health in the antecedent or subclinical stages of a known preexisting disease.

The most effective means of promoting health and preventing disease is to have a comprehensive understanding of the disease process. Community health nurses must be able to anticipate and predict consequences of poor health practices. For example, community health nurses should be able to predict complications of uncontrolled diabetes, such as a limb amputation, and thus exert preventive measures in the young adult who is presently healthy but has a history of diabetes, and tends to eat foods high in carbohydrates, and has a sedentary life-style. Exercises that demonstrate the predictable flow of pathophysiology from a healthy to a disabled state (Table 24-2) assist in explaining the importance of prevention. As the stage of pathophysiology progresses, risk estimation accelerates for a crippling, permanent state of health.

When healthy adults with particular genetic, dietary, and life-style antecedents become aware of the predictable nature of disease conditions, self-care can be practiced with more vigor. *Personal health profiles* may be useful in health counseling.

Adult health status and opportunities for growth and development are interlinked to environmental influences and resources of the individual, family, and community. A community assessment will identify environmental health stressors as well as services available to the community. Health stressors differ according to community type and industrial focus. For example, the three most dangerous occupations are mining, construction, and farming (Smith, 1986).

Although a wide variety in types of living conditions

exists, one distinction that can be made is rural versus urban settings. Rural is defined by the United States Census Bureau as areas with less than 2500 people and in open country. By this definition, about 27% of the United States population is in a rural area. The criterion for an urban area is the presence of a city with 50,000 or more people (Cordes, 1985).

Health risks and problems have been found to differ according to rural and urban settings. For example, the following conditions are higher among rural dwellers: hypertension, coronary heart disease, stomach and duodenum ulcers, hernias, hypertensive heart disease, gall bladder disease, and emphysema. The incidence of acute conditions is much lower in the nonurban population (Cordes, 1985).

Many of the major health problems of urban dwellers relate to their fast-paced, stressful life-styles. These adults need to learn techniques for assessing risk (described in Chapter 27), receive tools to manage stress, exercise regularly, eat a well-balanced diet, and incorporate leisure and recreational activities in their life-style (see Chapters 28 to 30).

Smith (1986) identified environmental hazards for farm workers and, particularly, migrant workers. Hazardous environmental agents include spore-laden dust and toxic agricultural chemicals that cause pulmonary diseases. Furthermore, infectious agents causing diseases such as rabies, anthrax, Rocky Mountain spotted fever, and tetanus are hazards. Unsanitary conditions in the fields and home, particularly for migrant workers, contribute to tuberculosis, parasitic infections, hepatitis, and typhoid. Allergic reactions to plant foliage and insect bites are also common. Heat-induced illness and exposure to solar radiation are dangerous as well. Because migrant workers do not receive sick pay, they often continue to work when ill. Alcohol and drug abuse and family violence are not uncommon among migrant workers.

Falck (1985) advocated a socioecological model to motivate change for rural health care problems. The model consists of four determinants:

1. Environmental determinants such as transportation and water supply
2. Social role determinants such as community leaders and nurturers
3. Group membership such as family and ethnic group
4. Constitutional determinants such as genetic and biological factors

To be effective, nurses must gain the trust of the clients and structure the care plan according to client priorities. Only then can nurses introduce health improvement ideas that have not been previously valued by the client population. More and more professionals are learning to blend their care with folk practices for greater compliance. That is, if clients engage in certain health rituals that do not harm, nurses can choose to be accepting as long as these individuals also improve other health practices.

Linkage systems between rural and urban areas are the key ingredients in comprehensive, accessible care for rural citizens. Rural areas need adequate emergency services for accidents with farm machinery and for other mishaps. In addition, they need a rapid linkage mechanism with an urban medical center for continued specialized care. When the client returns to the rural area, discharge planning from the urban center must be coordinated.

Personal and Family Life-styles

Life-style, perhaps the greatest influence on health status, involves the practice of health habits and a guiding philosophy of life to promote a positive outlook. Individual and family life-styles vary according to resources, values, traditions, and family members. Like an individual, each family has its particular sources of stressors, and each adopts coping styles in attempts to maintain balance. Further stress within a family is influenced by the roles played by each member and the extent to which the tasks of family living are accomplished.

Changing American life-styles, in which women are now a major part of the workforce, are creating realignment of divisions of labor, roles, and values of the family. What

---

TABLE 24-2

Predictable flow of pathophysiology of diabetes

Stages	Pathophysiology state	Symptoms
I. Antecedent	Genetic predisposition to diabetes Dietary pattern of high carbohydrate intake Smoking Sedentary work and life-style	No symptoms of illness
II. Stress-adaptation	Infection or pregnancy	Glycosuria and hyperglycemia, temporary
III. Beginning pathophysiology	Pancreas unable to meet demands for insulin	Persistent glycosuria and hyperglycemia, diagnosis of diabetes mellitus
IV. Progressive pathophysiology	Vascular plaques; circulatory changes	Numbness in limbs, retarded healing of lower limb lesion
V. Advanced pathophysiology	Occlusion of vessel to limb; necrosis and gangrene	Gangrene, necessitating amputation

health problems will later manifest in today's supermom or superdad? What factors of emerging life-styles will promote health in both men and women? The boxes below and at right contain tools to assist the community health nurse in assessing life-style factors that influence health.

Middlescence

Middlescence is defined as the intermediate stage of life between young adulthood and old age and is marked by physical, psychological, and social changes. The developmental task of middlescence is generativity (see Table 24-1).

The middle years are crossroads in the adult development process, and the transition is as critical as it was in adolescence. Grossman (1979) described this period as a time in the physical trajectory of life when individuals are simultaneously at a peak and yet newly vulnerable. This authenticity crisis occurs between 35 and 45 years of age. Individuals become preoccupied with signs of aging and the inevitability of death, and a last-chance urgency is noted in this period. Sheehy (1974) described

the process as the end of growing up and the beginning of growing old.

The task of middlescence includes moving through a disassembling to a renewal, with less concern for what society expects and attention on redesigning life according to intrinsic needs. Levinson (1978) stated that one of the major tasks for a man in the midlife transition is the acceptance of the feminism in himself. For example, he becomes more sensitive and capable of expressing emotions. In contrast, a woman who has been a caretaker may need to launch a career and actualize traits such as assertion and power, usually identified as masculine traits. Thus both sexes become more comfortable with roles that they previously regarded as sex stereotyped.

Conflicting feelings and states-of-being characterize midlife crises, with people experiencing paradoxical emotions, feeling wise yet confused, seeming to be independent yet dependent. This painful life dilemma is accompanied by anxiety, depression, anger, restlessness, and even physical symptoms.

PERSONAL LIFE-STYLE ASSESSMENT

Directions: Write your response to each of the items, using a maximum of three sentences. Record your answer based on your immediate reaction; do not contemplate items for a lengthy period.

PHYSICAL DIMENSIONS

Describe your habits in a typical week as related to the following activities:

1. Sleep
2. Rest periods
3. Exercise
4. Hair care
5. Dental care
6. Smoking

7. Alcoholic/drug intake
8. Medications
9. Skin care
10. Elimination
11. Sex

12. Foot and nail care
13. Work, job
14. Work, home
15. Diet
16. Medical checkup

How long do you expect to live?

PSYCHOSOCIAL AND/OR SPIRITUAL DIMENSIONS

Describe your habits in a typical week as related to the following activities:

1. Reading for pleasure
2. Reading for intellectual stimulation
3. Meditation
4. Interaction with friends
5. Interaction with family

6. Community activities for pleasure
7. Community activities for service
8. Recreational activities
9. Hobbies
10. Sports

COPING MECHANISMS

How do you handle stress on the job? At home?

What is your personal motto for life? (Eat, drink, and be merry; do unto others as you would have them do unto you, etc.)

What kind of actions by others make you angry? How do you handle the anger?

What goal do you have for this year? How do you plan to meet it?

What goals do you have for the next 5 years? How do you plan to meet them?

Are you satisfied with your present financial status?

What kind of things cause you the greatest anxiety?

How would you describe your relationship with your spouse or most significant other? Your children? Your in-laws and other relatives? Your parents?

What do you consider to be your life task?

On a scale from 1 to 10, how would you rate your present state of health (1-least healthy to 10-most healthy). How does your life-style contribute to or detract from your present state of health?

Sheehy (1974) stated that individuals confront their own deaths through introspection and self-inventory. Additionally, adults in their middle years become aware of the suppressed parts of themselves. They mourn previously abandoned goals and may decide to pursue them with renewed vigor and commitment. They may experience disappointment with their marriage and wish to terminate or restructure it. They confront the reality that their children may have failed to actualize parental aspirations and sadly contemplate the effort that went into those years of raising children. Such disappointments may serve to release inhibitions and cause adoption of a life-style to please oneself, long suppressed for the sake of family convention.

Fulfillment: Meaning, Purpose in Life, and Self-Transcendence

Many adults today suffer from what Frankl* (1959, 1973, 1975) called a society-wide collective neurosis—increasing alcoholism, drug addiction, suicide, and aggression. Adults plunge into meaningless activities to run away from problems and at night are plagued with sleeplessness. Young adults want to be where the action is, experiencing the

---

*Viktor E. Frankl is the founder of the Third School of Viennese Psychiatry—"The Will to Meaning"—after Sigmund Freud's "Will to Pleasure," followed by Alfred Adler's "Will to Power."

illusion of activity through speed. Loved ones are treated only as safety valves for tension reduction. The feeling of emptiness or of having a life with no meaning is widespread among people today. This emptiness, which Frankl called an *existential vacuum,* is created when people feel that life has no purpose, no challenge, and it makes no difference what they do. Such adults feel hopelessly trapped by circumstances beyond their control. This existential vacuum is seen among rich and poor, young and old, the successful and the failures. Business executives try to fill the vacuum with extra work, and students try to fill it with drugs. This new type of neurosis is labeled *noo-genic neurosis,* defined as a mental health problem caused by spiritual (not religious) problems or moral conflicts; a type of mental conflict in which values are not clarified. Such a neurosis is brought about by a conflict of values and emptiness. "Nous" is the human spirit dimension of the individual.

The meaning of life differs for each individual, and according to Frankl, the primary motivation for an individual's behavior is *not* seeking pleasure or power, but searching for meaning and purpose in life. Though we cannot always control the circumstances of life, we can choose the attitude toward our fate. Each adult strives to find meaning in life experiences, and mentally healthy adults seek to lead a purposeful life. From such harmony comes a feeling of fulfillment.

FAMILY LIFE-STYLE ASSESSMENT

Directions: Write your responses to each of the items, using a maximum of three sentences. Record your answer based on your immediate reaction; do not contemplate items for a lengthy period.

PHYSICAL DIMENSIONS

Who in your family do you consider to be the "healthiest" member? The least healthy? How would you rate each family member's health state?

What is your family's pattern as to:

1. Mealtime
2. Sleeping arrangements
3. Family recreation
4. Hygiene, household
5. Dental care
6. Sports, exercises

7. Smoking
8. Alcohol/drugs
9. Medical checkups
10. Work, household chores
11. Work, jobs and schedules
12. Pest control

What hereditary conditions are in your family history?

How long did your parents and grandparents live?

Directions: Contemplate each item as necessary, and record your responses as succinctly as possible.

PSYCHOSOCIAL AND/OR SPIRITUAL DIMENSIONS

Diagram your family constellation (family tree), birth order or position, etc.

What family traditions are most important to your family? Describe a typical Christmas holiday with family.

Name three values that your family holds in high regard to complete the following statement, "One should always . . . (tell the truth, be of service to others, etc.)."

Who fulfills or shares the following roles in your family?

1. Breadwinner
2. Homemaker
3. Peacemaker
4. Counselor

5. Teacher of living skills
6. Caretaker
7. Financial manager
8. Crisis manager

What causes stress within your family system? How does the family cope with stress?

According to Frankl, meaning can be found in three ways:

1. Creative values—a task or mission to complete
2. Experiential values—to experience or know the true, good, and beautiful; to lovingly encounter another human being
3. Attitudinal values—facing one's fate or choosing a positive attitude toward a fate that cannot be changed

Frankl has developed *logotherapy* to assist clients in finding purpose in life and meaning in life experiences. Logotherapy's aim is self-transcendence, or getting outside oneself to help others. Self-transcendence involves focusing on others, as contrasted with self-actualization, or focusing on developing and actualizing potential within oneself. Self-transcendence is commitment to the fulfillment of life's meaning so that the joyous life comes not as a result of direct pursuit but as a by-product.

The community health nurse can use a logotherapeutic approach in working with clients who appear apathetic or otherwise lack the motivation to modify life-style to enhance their state of health. The key to logotherapy is attitude change. The nurse may be innovative in techniques to modify attitudes. Various intellectual exercises, such as analyzing parables, can stimulate discussion that guides the client to a broader view of a fate that cannot be changed. The nursing process may be used as a framework in logotherapy.

1. Assess—determine what is of value to the client and who are the significant others. What are immediate long-term goals? Identify the client's perception of the present state of affairs and the ways in which current health status inhibits or facilitates fulfillment. Assessment also includes comparing verbal and non-verbal behaviors for congruency in values and identifying areas of conflict. Throughout the assessment, analyze the client's abilities and disabilities for feasibility of immediate and long-range goal accomplishment. Isolate restraining and facilitating factors in the environment that influence goal accomplishment.
2. Plan—engage in mutual goal setting that combines realistic abilities with potential growth of abilities. Establish a time frame, methodologies, and criteria for evaluation.
3. Intervene—use innovative strategies to unfreeze attitudes. For example, have the parents of a child diagnosed as having cystic fibrosis discuss the following parable as it relates to their situation.

Two frogs fell into a churn of milk. One said, "I have no chance," and he sank to the bottom and drowned. The other said, "I may not have a chance, but I won't go down without a fight." He splashed around and splashed around until, lo and behold, the milk turned to butter, and he was afloat on top.

4. Evaluate—measure outcomes based on previously established criteria. Make decisions regarding future action. Set new goals and evaluation criteria.

COMMON CAUSES OF MORBIDITY AND MORTALITY IN YOUNG ADULTS

Morbidity and mortality indicators for young adults offer guidance to the community health nurse in planning strategies for this aggregate population. For young adults major threats to health include (1) violent death and injury, involving motor vehicle accidents, suicides, and homicides, (2) alcohol and substance abuse, (3) unwanted pregnancies, and (4) sexually transmissible diseases. The death rate for young men is three times higher than for young women. About 75% of all deaths are caused by accidents, homicides, and suicides; such deaths are often the result of the greater risk-taking characteristic of this age group. Young black adults have a five times greater homicide rate than their white counterparts, with homicide the leading cause of death among black youths; accidents are a close second. Life-styles and behavior patterns that affect health are often established in this period. Health education programs with a community-wide audience should be geared toward avoiding risks and practicing safety precautions. One such program involved television spots regarding the hazards involved in diving into unknown waters, a frequent cause of spinal cord injury.

Motor Vehicle Accidents

Motor vehicle accidents are the leading cause of death in adults 15 to 24 years old. Highest rates are among white men. Death rates per 100,000 population as a result of motor vehicle accidents by sex and race are: white men, 74; black men, 35; white women, 23; and black women, 8. In 1983, 35.0 deaths per 100,000 population in the 15- to 24-year-old age group were the result of motor vehicle accidents, as compared with 22.2 deaths per 100,000 among adults between 25 and 34 years old; 15.4 deaths per 100,000 for adults between 35 and 44 years old; and 14.7 deaths per 100,000 adults between 45 and 54 years old (Health: United States, 1984).

Alcohol use plays a decisive role in accident rates. Although 16 to 24-year-olds account for only 11% of all licensed drivers, they are responsible for 33% of all alcohol-related fatalities (Health: United States, 1984). About one half of fatally injured drivers are found to be intoxicated (100 mg of alcohol per deciliter of blood). Motorcyclists have a seven times greater risk for fatal injury for each mile driven as compared with automobile drivers. Safety precautions such as seat belts, helmets, and enforcement of speed limits should be facilitated to reduce the morbidity and mortality in young adults.

Suicide

In viewing the problem of fulfillment versus emptiness from a community perspective, the incidence of suicide becomes an important indication of mental health. Durkheim, a French sociologist, believed that suicide was a function of social conditions and social forces. Because these circumstances were beyond the control of social scientists or anyone else, suicide was an immutable, unchangeable feature of any society and therefore not always preventable (Durkheim, in

Selkin, 1983). The term *anomie,* literally "without a name," was coined for the type of suicide related to the social change of a sudden and dramatic loss of role. Durkheim (1951, p. 382) predicted that "in a more integrated society with less conflict and more distinctive social roles, suicide rates would decrease." Perhaps the most frequently used measure of anomie is Srole's Anomie Scale. Research by Dodder and Astle (1980) identified two characteristic concepts of anomie: cynicism and valuelessness.

Community health nurses need to be involved with social changes, including public policy, to prevent suicides. A number of current policies and attitudes have been identified by Selkin (1983) as contributing to this health problem, including easy access to handguns and the lack of vocational/educational opportunities.

Statistics of death rates by suicide are given in Table 24-3. In young adults, 12.5 of every 100,000 residents in the United States in the age group 15 to 24 years and 15.5 in the age group 25 to 34 years committed suicide in 1985.

Homicide

Homicide in the United States has a disproportionate impact on young adults, men, and members of ethnic minorities. As can be seen in Table 24-4, the greatest difference is between white and black men.

The overall American homicide rate of 10.2 per 100,000 contrasts sharply with that of France (0.9), Great Britain (1.0), Sweden (1.1), and Japan (1.3). Societal factors thought to influence the high homicide rate are economic deprivation, family breakup, glamorization of violence in the media, and easy access to firearms. Of murders in America, 20% occur among relatives or those with a close relationship and 40% are among acquaintances. Personal disagreements and conflict account for 60% to 80% of homicides, which are more prevalent among the poor, more frequent on weekends and at night, and often associated with alcohol abuse. Men are killed three to five times more often than women, and men are five times as likely to be the offender.

What stressors are contributing to the appalling loss of young American lives? Pressures and frustrations that lead to such violent behaviors are related to life-style and to conflicts experienced in developmental tasks of this generation. For the young adult, striving to establish an identity can be confused by differing role expectations between peer and family groups. Lack of success in educational pursuits and employment goals causes diminished self-esteem and loss of the approval so highly sought by the young adult. Young adults whose task is to establish intimacy find themselves in a culture in which short-term temporary relationships and social mobility are the norms. Lacking the maturity that builds patience and tolerance, young people seek a quick and easy solution (even drastic measures), to bring relief. Drugs and alcohol combined with this immaturity result in reckless behavior that often ends in tragedy. Poverty and crime are related factors.

Alcohol and Substance Abuse

As discussed in Chapter 35, the statistics for alcoholism document the significance of this problem for adults. Alcohol consumption is related to accidents, homicides, suicides, and other disruptive individual and family events. The young adult woman who consumes alcohol during pregnancy risks abnormality in the fetus, resulting in mental retardation and other defects. The community health nurse is likely to be involved with a family who has a child with fetal alcohol syndrome. Alcohol abuse also causes many psychosocial problems in family living. See Chapter 35 for a detailed discussion of alcohol abuse.

There is growing concern about substance abuse, especially in young adults. Marijuana, barbiturates, cocaine, other central nervous system drugs, and heroin are among those abused. Heroin addiction may lead to hepatitis, cardiovascular disease, chromosome damage, diabetes, hepatic cirrhosis, infections, including infection with human im-

---

TABLE 24-3

Suicide death rates, United States, 1985

Ages	Number of deaths per 100,000 resident population
15 to 24 years	12.5
25 to 34 years	15.5
35 to 44 years	15.1
45 to 54 years	16.2
55 to 64 years	17.3
All ages	11.6

TABLE 24-4

Homicide in young adults by race, sex, and age groups*

Age ranges	White (male)	White (female)	Black (male)	Black (female)
15 to 24	11.1	4.3	61.5	14.8
24 to 34	14.1	3.9	96.2	19.3

*Number of deaths per 100,000 resident population for 1984.
From Health: United States, 1984, DHHS Pub. No. 87-1232, Public Health Service, Washington, D.C., Dec. 1986, pp. 114-115, U.S. Government Printing Office.

mune deficiency virus (HIV), and trauma. Treatment should be comprehensive and directed toward meeting total health care needs.

Psychiatric Disorders

Psychiatric disorders are most frequently diagnosed among people with low levels of income, education, and occupation. City residents have a higher incidence of anxiety, mild depression, phobias, self-doubt, and personality disorders, whereas rural residents have a higher incidence of manic depressive disorders. Regardless of the disorder, early professional treatment is advisable.

The community health nurse is often concerned with support care after institutionalization. Aftercare may involve halfway-house residential facilities, a private proprietary home, other innovative group homes, or a return to the family setting. Valenzuela and Hallamore (1979) described a successful "good neighbor network" using natural helpers. Every community has members who are accepted as authorities on helping and healing. They may be called *padrones* in an Italian community, *mavens* in a Jewish community, or *curanderos* in a Mexican community. This folk support system can be linked with the professional care system. This strategy may be essential in an era of legislative cutbacks for human services. The natural, neighborly helping philosophy may also promote community pride.

Cutler and Madore (1980) described an effective approach to mental health services in a rural setting with community-family network therapy. The system is designed to open lines of communication and to strengthen the supportive and adaptive qualities of the client-social network ecosystem. The network consists of family members, nuclear and extended, who relate to the identified problem. Each family member has an assigned advocate who establishes an empathic rapport, intervenes for the family member in group discussion in a supportive manner, and helps facilitate expression of the family member's needs or feelings. The group also has a network organizer, conductor, consultant, and monitor. A network group may contain as many as 30 to 35 people. The group motivation is to create a setting for cooperative, active problem solving. To achieve a balanced perspective from the private, public, and consumer sectors of the community for mental health aftercare services, coordinated planning and cooperation are needed.

Community health nurses play a key role in planning comprehensive health services. Using anticipatory guidance and an approach that emphasizes positive mental health, nurses can provide mental health services that guide family members through stressful times and prepare them for life event changes. Analyzing the community for healthy energy outlets such as recreational opportunities is part of the community assessment. When such resources are lacking, nurses can be instrumental in community planning. On a one-to-one basis, while working with a family in a preexplosive phase, nurses can use the therapeutic approach to help the family members discover some meaning in their circumstances, to see problems as time limited, and to encourage self-transcendence (i.e., getting outside oneself and the im-

mediate problem and focusing on a task to accomplish for others).

Sexually Transmitted Diseases

An additional health problem for 15- to 24-year-olds is sexually transmittable diseases, 75% of which occur in this age group. Syphilis and gonorrhea continue to increase, as do other diseases, including genital herpes and nonspecific urethritis. Each year 75,000 females become sterile as a result of sexually transmitted pelvic inflammatory disease. The incidence of these diseases decreases during the adult years after age 25.

Sexually transmitted diseases are a significant public health problem. Such diseases are caused by bacteria, viruses, protozoa, yeasts, and ectoparasites (Public, 1984). The actual incidence of diseases such as syphilis and gonorrhea is obscured by underreporting, whereas others, such as chlamydia, are not required to be reported.

One of the nation's most prevalent sexually transmitted diseases is chlamydia, which is three times more prevalent than gonorrhea (Centers for Disease Control, 1985). *Chlamydia trachomatis* causes urethritis, epididymitis, proctitis, cervicitis, pelvic inflammatory disease, infant pneumonia, and conjunctivitis. In both sexes, the infection may be asymptomatic. Both men and women can have more than one sexually transmitted disease at the same time. Sexual partners should be treated concurrently.

The most dreaded sexually transmitted disease of all that affects young adults as well as other age groups is acquired immunodeficiency syndrome (AIDS). This disease is discussed fully in Chapter 17. Patient education for safe sex practices may control the rate of spread of this disease.

In addition to physiological problems, the young adult faces many emotional, social, and spiritual stressors that lay the foundation for chronic ill health. Anxiety and pressure from careers and family life interfere with optimum health and plant the seeds for illness later in life.

COMMON CAUSES OF MORBIDITY AND MORTALITY IN MIDDLE ADULTS

Common causes of morbidity and mortality in middle adults are heart disease and strokes, cancer, alcohol and substance abuse, mental health problems, and periodontal disease.

Heart Disease and Strokes

The leading cause of death in middle adults is heart disease, which accounts for over one-third of all deaths and $14.6 billion in personal health costs, and is ranked as first cause in short-stay hospital use (Health: United States, 1984). However, there has been a persistent decline in the mortality rate of about 2% per year since 1968.

The highest mortality rates are among black men and lowest among white women ages 45 to 64 years. Black women have more than twice the mortality rate of white women.

In 1985, heart diseases accounted for 181.7 deaths per 100,000 population, and cerebrovascular accidents, or strokes, accounted for 32.3 deaths per 100,000 population.

Strokes were responsible for $5.1 billion in health costs and ranked as the third leading cause of death in the United States. In 1985, death from strokes occurred most frequently in black men, then in black women, white men and white women. The incidence increases with age (Health: United States, 1986).

Among the major causes of death, stroke has had the most rapid decline over the past 30 years. This decline is thought to be related to improved hypertension control, better diagnosis, improved management, and rehabilitation.

The heart disease problem cannot be analyzed as to a singular cause and effect. Rather, the combination of various predisposing conditions interact to cause disease manifestation in various individuals. Control of risk factors is the most useful strategy in community health nursing practice.

Risk Factors

Thompson (1983) identified heart disease risk factors from epidemiological evidence as being hypercholesterolemia, hypertension, cigarette smoking, type A personality behavior, obesity, lack of voluntary exercise, diabetes mellitus, and family history. Genetic and behavioral characteristics, including diet and metabolic and cellular differences, directly influence the rate of progression of the disease.

Those who smoke cigarettes have twice the rate of heart disease as those who do not. Hazardous substances in cigarettes are nicotine and carbon monoxide; the risk is proportional to the amount of smoke inhaled. Risk is also related to the number of cigarettes smoked. Those who smoke one pack per day are three times more likely to have a heart attack than those who do not smoke.

Hypertension is another risk factor. The World Health Organization classifies blood pressure into the following categories: (1) normal is less than 140/90 mm Hg; (2) borderline is 140/90 to 160/95 mm Hg; and (3) hypertension is 160/95 + mm Hg (O'Connor, 1981). Hypertension, the leading cause of premature disability for industry workers, costs the nation $1.7 billion annually (Lattimore, et al., 1979). About 35 million Americans have hypertension, and those with systolic pressures above 160 are three times as likely to have a stroke as those with systolic pressures under 140. Lowther and Carter (1981) cited factors involved with hypertensive control as compliance with a medication schedule, regular follow-up appointments, sodium-restricted diets, caloric restrictions for weight control, cessation of smoking, and reduction of stress. They found that sending missed-appointment reminder cards significantly increased the client's rescheduling and keeping the next appointment. Community programs can be effective in long-term treatment.

Another risk factor, cholesterol, is associated with heart disease and to a lesser extent with stroke. For the 35- to 44-year-old age group, heart attacks are five times more frequent in individuals whose cholesterol level is above 265 than among those with levels below 220. Low-density lipoproteins (LDL) apparently accelerate cholesterol deposition on vessel walls. High-density lipoproteins (HDL) do not seem to have this effect and may even be protective. Dietary cholesterol is responsible for only 25% to 30% of serum cholesterol. Optimum plasma cholesterol is 200 mg; 250 mg is risky. Exercise and diet modification may increase the HDL:LDL ratio to protect against heart disease.

Individuals with diabetes have an increased risk of cardiovascular disease, with twice as many strokes and heart attacks as the nondiabetic. Women who are diabetic have a risk five times higher than other women for atherosclerotic heart disease.

Primary prevention of heart disease begins in infancy with a diet free from fats, excessive salt, and sugar. Beginning regular exercise at an early age is another preventive measure. Secondary prevention begins at the stage of arterial changes and focuses on arresting and/or retarding atherosclerosis. Tertiary prevention is used with those who already have symptoms of heart disease or actual pathological manifestations.

A valuable resource, the publications of the National Blood Pressure Education Program, are available from the National Blood Pressure Information Center, 120/80 National Institutes of Health, Bethesda, MD 20005.

Cancer

Today more than one American in five dies of *cancer* (American Cancer Society, 1987). The 1985 age-adjusted cancer mortality rate was 195.1 per 100,000 population (Health: United States, 1986). In individuals 35 to 64 years of age, cancer causes more than one third of all deaths. Among the most fatal cancers in adults are those of the lung, intestine, and breast. Experts agree that cancer is not just one disease, but a group of diseases with various rates of occurrence and clinical courses. A carcinogenic agent is defined as a single cancer-inducing substance that triggers a change in behavior of cells, resulting in uncontrolled growth.

Risk Factors

Factors that increase risk for cancer include cigarette smoking, alcohol, certain dietary patterns, radiation, sunlight, occupational hazards, water and air pollutants, heredity, and certain predisposing medical conditions. As noted in Chapter 35, cigarette smoking is the greatest known agent responsible for cancer and cancer deaths; smokers have 10 times the rate of lung cancer as nonsmokers. A combination of other risks with smoking accentuates cancer probability. Alcohol consumers have higher rates of cancer of the esophagus, larynx, oral cavity, and liver. Although no well-established cause-and-effect relationship has linked diet and cancer, food additives may have carcinogenic potential. Roentgenograms should be kept to a minimum to avoid cumulative exposure because low-level radiation, including natural background radiation, affects people. Individuals who spend considerable time outdoors may acquire skin cancer from over-exposure to sunlight. Such cancer, along with premature wrinkling, can be prevented by avoiding sunlight, wearing protective clothing, and using lotions containing paraaminobenzoic acid (PABA).

Data from the National Center for Health Statistics on

occupational diseases indicate that malignant neoplasms of the peritoneum and pleura (mesothelioma) cause more deaths in adult men than other occupational neoplasms. Table 24-5 cites the incidence of deaths for malignant neoplasms for adult males in 1983.

As Table 24-5 shows, the incidence of malignant neoplasms dramatically increases with age. Also, the incidence is higher for black men in every age group except the 15- to 24-year-old group.

Other work-related carcinogens include arsenic, benzene, coal tar, coke-oven emissions, chromium, hematite, nickel, and petroleum distillates.

Industrial carcinogenic agents found in drinking-water supplies include chlordane, aldrin, dieldrin, and benzene. They may become concentrated in fish or shellfish. Air pollution results primarily from automobile exhausts and to a lesser extent from synthetic organic chemicals. Clustering of cancer seems to occur in some families; whether it involves heredity or environmental patterns is not known.

The two most effective strategies for preventing cancer and death from cancer are (1) limiting exposure to carcinogenic agents, and (2) early detection and treatment before a cancer has spread.

For women, breast cancer is the leading cause of cancer-related deaths. The incidence increases with age; women 65 to 74 years old are more than three times as likely to develop breast cancer than 35- to 44-year-old women. Women between 35 and 74 years old account for nearly 75% of deaths from breast cancer; rates are similar for blacks and whites. Other factors are first pregnancies when over 30 years old, nonterm pregnancies before 30 years old, early menarche, late menopause, previous history of benign disease, family history of breast cancer, and certain types of previous cancer. (Health: United States, 1984). Chances for survival improve with early detection and treatment. Thus breast-cancer screening and public education programs are important.

Some authorities believe no significant gains have been made in survival rates since the early 1950s (Kolata, 1985). Although statistics might suggest otherwise, rates look bet-

ter only because of the "lead-time effect" and the "staging effect." The lead-time effect is created because of earlier diagnosis. For example, a cancer patient who would have died in 6 months can now be diagnosed one year earlier, giving the patient 18 months' survival even though nothing has been done to alter the course of the disease. The patient is no better off than before. The staging effect results from early diagnosis and precise determination of spread, causing a milder form of the cancer to be included in stage I. These patients will live longer than others in stage I. Others with metastases (spread of disease to other organs or areas of the body) who previously would have been included in stage I and who now have precise determination of metastases will be placed in stage II. Their absence from the stage I category will further improve that group's rates, and their presence in the stage II category will make that group appear better as well (Kolata, 1985).

The Cancer Client in the Community

Providing care to adults with cancer who are living at home is a challenging opportunity for the community health nurse. Such care includes (1) providing physical care, (2) teaching and counseling, and (3) giving emotional support to the client and family.

Providing physical care may include colostomy care, dressing change, or medication administration. With earlier hospital discharge, more patients are receiving antineoplastic chemotherapy at home. Infusion pumps and venous access lines (peripheral lines, long lines, central lines, and implantable catheters) must be maintained. The nurse must practice safety precautions and teach patient and family to observe those same precautions (Schaffner, 1984).

The major safety precaution is to avoid direct contact with the antineoplastic agent. Family members must be warned not to touch the bag that the medication is in, which is usually kept in the refrigerator. When the nurse prepares the medication, all ceiling, window, and floor heating/cooling units must be turned off to avoid possible aerosol contamination. The work space is lined with a plastic-backed absorbent pad. The nurse puts on polyvinylchloride plastic gloves, a disposable gown with long sleeves and closed cuffs, and protective glasses. (No potentially pregnant nurse should administer chemotherapy.) In the event of a spill, the nurse puts on two pairs of gloves, wipes up the spill with a paper towel, and washes the area thoroughly with water. The company that supplies the medicine also supplies materials for proper disposal. After infusion, all disposable items are put in a red plastic bag that is tied and put into a durable cardboard box, which is lined with a plastic-backed absorbent liner. The box seams are taped shut and the box is placed inside a second red plastic bag, which is then tied and labeled as biohazardous material and later picked up by the supplier. Caution should be exercised so that family members or pets do not disturb the bag.

Periodontal Disease

Diseases of gum tissues are common problems of adults. The initial causative agent is thought to be bacterial plaque, resulting in gingivitis and later periodontitis. Symptoms

---

TABLE 24-5

Deaths among white and black males caused by malignant neoplasms*

Age	White male	Black male
15 to 24	6.7	5.6
25 to 34	12.6	14.7
35 to 44	38.3	70.7
45 to 54	166.7	315.5
55 to 64	499.5	821.6
All ages	158.9	232.2

*Number of deaths per 100,00 resident population.
From Health: United States, 1985, DHHS Pub. No. 86-1232, Hyattsville, Md., Dec. 1985, pp. 53-54, U.S. Department of Health & Human Services, National Center for Health Statistics.

of gingivitis include inflammation, redness, and swelling of gums with a tendency to bleed easily. **Periodontitis** occurs when the supporting bones and ligaments are destroyed, resulting in loose or "drifting" teeth. Periodontitis is the leading cause of loss of teeth after age 35. In the 55- to 64-year-old age group, 30% of adults lose all their natural teeth because of this disease. Proper dental care involves regular brushing and flossing of teeth and regular professional dental care. Antiplaque-forming toothpastes and mouthwashes are now available that can help to prevent or reduce the effects of periodontal disease.

Summary: Morbidity and Mortality

In summary, health for the young and middle adult depends to a significant degree on life-style and health practices, for which the adult must assume responsibility. An individual's risk for disease development can be reduced by compliance with measures known to prevent occurrence and retard progression of disease and maintain a state of good health.

COMMUNITY HEALTH NURSING IMPLICATIONS

The community health nurse uses and integrates knowledge from all clinical specialty areas. Furthermore, the community health nurse has the responsibility for encouraging clients to promote their level of health, change life-styles if necessary, and confront common, inescapable conditions of suffering and death. Several exercises for coping with conflict and stress are given in the appendix.

Promoting Responsibility for Health

A 50-year-old man, a retired military officer, has had essential hypertension for 3 years. He is not employed and spends his days around the house. He has several projects such as repairing a fishing boat, but he paces his day as he likes. His wife is a 38-year-old professional career woman who sometimes is annoyed that he is not working or "making any worthwhile contribution to society." In discussing his health with the nurse, the wife reveals that she suspects that he lies on the sofa all afternoon watching soap operas. He does not get any physical exercise. She puts his medicine in a dish for him every day but is not convinced that he actually takes it. She prepares a healthy lunch for him each day before she leaves for the office but frequently finds evidence that he has eaten salty foods while she is away. He also smokes one pack of cigarettes per day to the annoyance of his wife. She tells the nurse that she is at the end of her rope in trying to take care of his health.

A conference with the client reveals that he feels his wife nags him all the time. He says all he wants is to be left alone. He feels that she treats him like a naughty child and that he deserves to live his life the way he chooses. The nurse also learns that the previous nurse assigned to this case spent considerable time in teaching health to the client and his wife. She found that both comprehended information well, but that the client's attitude was one of indifference.

Who is responsible for the client's health? The thesis of this chapter is that adults are responsible for their own health. The wife in this case has been behaving as if her husband's health is her responsibility. Many who are nurturers, such as mothers, wives, and even nurses, fail to motivate the client to assume self-responsibility. After a discussion with the nurse, the wife had the following conversation with her husband.

> "I realize that I have been nagging you about your diet, exercise, and medications. I also know that you are the one who is responsible for your health, and the choices are yours. From now on I won't constantly hover over you. I'll be glad to do whatever you need to help you carry out your plan." The wife stopped putting out his medicine or preparing his lunch, although she did make certain plenty of nutritious foods were available. Remarkably there was a change in the client's behavior. He purchased two exercise bicycles and began to comply with his diet and medication regimens.

What can the nurse do to promote responsibility for health? Three areas of skills, listed below, are needed.

Communicate an attitude of responsibility for self. Do not say, "You shouldn't eat sweets on a diabetic diet." Such a message presumes a superior-inferior position. It says that the nurse knows what is best, "*I* can tell *you* what *you* should do." It also creates guilt in the client who eats sweets in spite of knowing the dangers. Do say something like, "What do you (or can you) do about your craving for sweets, which would adversely affect your diabetic condition? Are there things you can do to control your desire for sweets?" Stimulate the client to think of chewing sugarless gum, brushing teeth right after meals, or using mouthwash.

Teach health information. Teaching is not telling; giving accurate information does not assure compliance. Client teaching should begin with assessment: it is important to find out what the client already knows so that time and patience are not wasted. To illustrate this point, the following example is given. A nursing student assigned to assist with discharge planning for a client recovering from a myocardial infarction set a priority goal of emphasizing the need for a gradual return to work. The night before the assignment she prepared a simplistic drawing of the heart. She used the diagram to explain to the client how his heart would be affected by overwork. Near the end of her teaching session she said, "By the way, what kind of work do you do?" He replied, "I'm a cardiologist."

After assessment of the knowledge level of the learner, objectives should be set based on mutual goals. Learning activities are designed according to the content and learning style best suited to the client. Evaluation must follow a teaching/learning session. Retention of learned material should not be taken for granted. Reinforcement of the learning is also necessary.

Use positive reinforcement of effective health behaviors. Good health has its own rewards, such as vim, vigor, and vitality. However, the first few days or weeks of losing weight may not bring such a feeling of exhilaration. Nurses must support clients who comply with healthy behaviors, and they also need to accept those who lapse back into unhealthy actions. In the latter case, the nurse can tell the client that it is not unusual to have occasional relapses. Many contracts for health behaviors allow for 1 to 2 free days per week in which jogging, for example, can be omitted. Clients should reward themselves—go to a movie to celebrate a week of adherence to the new diet.

Promoting Changes in Life-style

Life-styles, like personalities, are not easily changed. Personal philosophies about life have a great influence on life-style, as do economic status and peer life-styles. Philosophies about life evolve from parental influence, the educational process, and community activities. Some philosophies may be detrimental to health, such as the hedonistic life-style based on "Eat, drink, and be merry, for tomorrow you may die."

Life-style changes result from reassessing goals, changing values, and making commitments to a new life pattern. These changes can be triggered suddenly through crisis or can blossom from planting a seed and nurturing ideas over a period of time. Significant others are often catalysts in the adoption of new life patterns. Nurses and/or other health professionals can also serve as facilitators of changed attitudes.

When attempting to motivate a client to change his life-style, the circuitous method of communication is often effective. Telling a story about a third party can shed insight on how the client is in the same predicament and can be suggestive of a similar solution that might work. A 19-year-old man injured in an automobile accident while speeding excessively suffered a C7 spinal cord injury. On discharge from the rehabilitation center with instructions to follow a well-defined plan of care, the community health nurse visited him in his home only to discern the following problems:

1. He had been fasting to lose weight.
2. His fluid intake was poor.
3. He decided to drop out of college.
4. He hoped to get married at the end of the year.

While discussing his fasting, the client states that he was getting too big for his clothes, and the wheelchair was feeling tight. In an attempt to get the weight off rapidly, he seemed to discount the risk of protein depletion that could result in skin breakdown and other problems. Although aware of the need for fluids, he said he hated to ask others to get him a drink. He was apathetic about school and yet hung on to the illusion that life would go on as planned when he married his childhood sweetheart. Because he was struggling with the psychosocial task of becoming independent of parental control, the nurse decided against "teaching and preaching scare tactics" but instead told him about a client with similar problems who had made positive plans to resolve them. She gave each the other's telephone number and encouraged them to converse about mutual concerns.

Perhaps the greatest concern for modifying life-styles for the young and middle adult lies in the area of stress level. As discussed in Chapter 30, various relaxation techniques include mediation, progressive relaxation, hypnosis, and biofeedback. Relaxation should be planned and scheduled as a regular part of the day's activities. O'Flynn-Comiskey (1979) emphasized relaxation as a means for increasing efficiency and productivity.

Coping with Conflict and Stress

Stress for the adult often results from speed; the urgency to get many things done in a limited amount of time. Anything and anybody who interferes with this speeding pace causes frustration, conflict, and consequently stress. Community health nurses can help clients assess how they spend time and then evaluate whether other activities would more appropriately meet their personal goals. One way to manage stress is to immunize the body, both physically and emotionally, from stressors that are known and preventable.

Psychosocial immunizations may buffer the adult against stressors to be expected at this time in the life cycle. Anticipatory guidance, helping the adult know what to expect from different phases of life, may be helpful. Often an older friend or mentor eases the way, as is illustrated in the example of a 27-year-old single parent of a 10-year-old boy in fifth grade. Her neighbor has a 15-year-old son who has a motorcycle and wants very much to receive a car by his sixteenth birthday. The friendship between the two women helps the first woman to anticipate what she will face in a few short years as a parent of a teenager. The neighbor also helps by telling the woman parenting techniques she found helpful when her son was 10 years old.

Confronting Suffering and Death

Suffering is a common, natural condition. Frankl (1959) stated that suffering is like gas in a chamber—no matter how much or how little—it fills the whole chamber; suffering is relative. Individuals cannot choose their fates, but they can choose the attitudes they take toward fates that cannot be changed. Suffering can be a growth experience; individuals can learn valuable lessons about life from personal suffering. Those who successfully negotiate developmental tasks grow and evolve from coping with life's challenges. Suffering can have a meaning if it changes the individual; despair is suffering without meaning.

Travelbee (1966) described two types of sufferers from a negative perspective. The *unjustly afflicteds* behave as if they should be exempt from human misfortune and human frailties. Their behavior reflects anger, annoyance, bitterness, rebellion, self-pity, depression, anguish, fear, and/or anxiety. The *punished* focus on their guilt, badness, and punishment for wrongdoing. They exhibit depression, anxiety, and self-pity. They may blame themselves, others, or God.

Frankl (1959) espoused the theory of logotherapy to help clients find meaning and purpose in life. Clients need to find meaning in suffering to cope effectively. Many clients practice hyperreflection, that is, a compulsion to self-observation that creates anticipatory anxiety. Frankl advocated the use of humor as a technique to combat phobias or fears. For example, a client who suffers from hyperhidrosis, or excessive perspiration of the palms, fears a situation that compels handshaking. However, fear precipitates that very symptom. The therapist in this case may encourage the client to try to perspire buckets of sweat the next time he is in this situation—to laugh at himself for even considering taking a bucket with him. Usually the client finds that trying as hard as he can, he is no longer able to produce the state of hyperhidrosis.

Strategies the nurse could use include the following logotherapeutic techniques:

1. *Dereflection*—directing the focus away from the problem and focusing on assets and abilities (e.g., not focusing on paralyzed legs but rather on strong upper arms).
2. *Paradoxical intention*—exaggerating and wishing for the opposite; using humor. (The therapy for hyperhidrosis as just mentioned uses paradoxical intention.)
3. *Socratic dialogue*—engaging in thought-provoking conversation with the client. (An elderly man who has been depressed since his wife's death is asked what would have happened if he had died before his wife. He recounts how unfortunate this would have been, she would have been afraid to live alone and she had no experience managing money. The client is reminded that he has spared his wife this suffering by living past her [Frankl, 1959].)

The nurse's role in coping with death is to be supportive of the family and to assist the client in verbalizing fears and concerns. The nurse can facilitate positive progression through the grieving process as death approaches.

Affecting Health Policy

Milio (1983) suggested that an effective way to approach health policy is to ask two questions. First, what environmental and other changes are needed to measurably improve the health of Americans? Second, what strategies will inspire decisions by organizations and individuals in those new directions? Milio asserted that less-than-healthy life-styles are not a matter of "free" choice but rather the result of opportunities available to people, and that health policies affect those opportunities. Community health nurses have a vital role in developing health policies and must be involved in political activities to ensure implementation.

NUTRITIONAL REQUIREMENTS FOR PROMOTING HEALTH

Adults have normal nutritional needs that may be slightly at variance with other periods of the life cycle. During ill health special nutritional needs may exist. The *aging process* is significantly influenced by nutritional health habits.

Normal Nutritional Needs for Young and Middle Adults

Adults, like children and the elderly, need to be counseled by community health nurses to recognize their nutritional needs and to learn how to eat wisely if poor nutritional habits exist. Several major causes of adult morbidity and mortality are related to diet. Assessment of adult dietary needs, habits, and desires often begins with a determination of nutritional myths and beliefs.

In a survey concerning the level of practical knowledge about nutrition, Poplin (1980) found that the general public holds many misconstrued or erroneous beliefs about nutrition. Some facts that Poplin determined were often misunderstood are listed in the following true statements:

Drinking water is not fattening.

Synthetic vitamins are as effective in the body as natural vitamins.

Nutritionally, honey is no better than white sugar.

Body fat cannot be lost by wearing sauna suits or sweat belts.

Proper weight does not necessarily mean you are getting proper nutrition.

Foods grown with chemical fertilizers are just as nutritious as food grown with natural organic fertilizers.

Neither vinegar nor grapefruit causes the body to burn fat more rapidly.

The young adult, emerging from the adolescent period of high nutritional demand, needs slightly less calcium and protein than before (Diekelmann, 1976). Young adult men need an increase in vitamins C, E, B_6, and B_{12}. Food sources include citrus juices, whole grain products, vegetable oils, leafy vegetables, fish, and cheese. Young women have an increased need for vitamin C and for foods rich in iron, such as organ meats, eggs, fish, poultry, leafy vegetables, and dried fruit. Women need 18 mg of iron daily, as compared with 10 mg needed by men. Signs of anemia include fatigue, low energy level, excess need for sleep, shortness of breath on exertion, and depression. It is safe to say that most young adults should reduce sugar consumption, including sources of hidden sugar. Recommendations for normal adult nutrition include limiting consumption of eggs to three per week and eating foods high in polyunsaturated rather than saturated fats. Care should be taken in consuming foods with perservatives. Foods with nitrates and nitrites—chemicals used to enhance color, flavor, and preservation of meats—may lead to the formation of nitrosamines, a known carcinogenic agent. Such foods include bacon, sausage, lunch meats, smoked fish, and hot dogs. Foods low in cholesterol should be a part of a normal diet. Small-boned fish is an excellent source of calcium. Breakfast is perhaps the most important meal of the day and should not be skipped.

Foods that are high in bulk, whole grain foods, and green vegetables such as broccoli, brussel sprouts, and cabbage may play a role in cancer prevention.

Special Nutritional Needs During Ill Health

One of the most dreaded illnesses of adult life is cardiovascular disease, which has many nutritional implications. For primary prevention of coronary disease, Turner (1980) recommended ingesting half the saturated fats and twice the polyunsaturated fats. This strategy has the effect of reducing total fat by 25%. Most fat is a mixture of three kinds: (1) saturated, which is not essential and is harmful in excess; (2) monosaturated, which is neutral; and (3) polyunsaturated, which is essential and protective. No intake of animal cholesterol is necessary for health, and excessive consumption is harmful. The body manufactures its own sufficient supply for daily requirements. Egg yolks have the highest concentration of cholesterol (250 mg per yolk) followed by dairy fat and meat. Frying can be replaced by other cooking methods. A marbled roast can be cooked a day ahead and refrigerated. The next day the solid fat can be removed before warming. Proteins can also be obtained from mixed sources such as bread, cereals, peas, beans, and lentils. Fish, whether fresh, frozen, or canned, is equally nutritious, as are certain fish oils.

Nutrition for other illnesses depends on the specific diagnosis. However, proper nutrition is necessary to promote recovery from and/or stabilization of a chronic disorder.

Nutritional Influences on the Aging Process for the Middle Adult

Nutrition influences the way people age and may affect the onset or course of degenerative diseases. At this time there is no known diet, food, or food factor that can retard the aging process (Mayer, 1980). A nutritional guideline for the adult is to eat a wide variety of foods, including fresh, raw, or lightly processed foods, which are high in nutrients and provide only enough calories to meet daily energy needs. In addition, adults may need one daily multivitamin/mineral capsule containing levels of nutrients according to the Recommended Daily Allowances.

As the body ages, it replaces some tissue with fat cells. As activity level declines, so should caloric intake. Loss of muscle tissue is another age-related change and may be retarded by adequate intake of high-quality protein. Mayer (1980) recommended 60 to 70 g of protein per day for the adult, the same amount as required in pregnancy. (Protein [50 g] is contained in each of the following: 2 cups of milk or 4 ounces of meat, poultry, or white fish.)

Osteoporosis is a common disorder related to the aging process. Postmenopausal women are susceptible to this condition. In normal bone mineralization, vitamin D and a 1:1 ratio of calcium to phosphorus exist. The typical American diet includes three times as much phosphorus as calcium. Phosphorus is found in meats, soft drinks, and processed foods. To balance the calcium:phosphorus intake, foods that can be added to the diet include leafy dark green vegetables, sesame seeds, and dark molasses. Foods containing the ideal 1:1 ratio are milk and milk products.

WORK-RELATED ISSUES

One of the primary tasks of young and middle adults in engaging in purposeful, productive work. An individual's career, whether domestic or a highly challenging executive position, can affect health negatively or positively. The role of the nurse often involves counseling and referral for counseling regarding job problems or goals for second careers. Job-related problems can be physical, presenting a hazard to health, or psychosocial, creating a feeling of disparity between job and worker. Although Chapter 41 discusses this subject in more detail, this section examines occupational hazards to health, overstress in the workplace, and second careers for young and middle adults.

Occupational Hazards to Health

Occupational hazards to health include musculoskeletal problems, respiratory and circulatory problems, damage to hearing organs, and accidents. Chronic misuse of one's body plus an overload of stressors result in inevitable damage.

An interesting study of 113 mine rescue workers involved examination of the relationship between the workers' perceived health and marital status, use of health services, nonwork physical activity, and absence from work (McKenna et al., 1981). These workers, by definition healthy and fit, averaged approximately 0.5 health problems per worker, and more than 79% of them reported no health problems at all. Of these health problems reported, 40% involved sleep and 25% involved emotional reactions, with the fewest problems in physical mobility (8%) and social isolation (3%). There was a tendency for married respondents and those over 40 years old to perceive more health problems. Those workers who reported little physical exercise outside of work experienced three times as many health problems. The nurse working in an industrial setting may need to study the influence of different variables on absence rates and predict those who are at risk.

Overstress in the Workplace

Stress is the spice of life, but too much of othe wrong kind—overstress—can lead to physical, psychosocial, and/or spiritual problems. The term **burned out** originated from a street expression of the Haight-Ashbury era and referred to hopelessly addicted drug users (Ross, 1980). Such a person experiences an energy drain that cannot be replaced with ordinary measures such as rest or a break in routine. Early signs in persons who are overstressed include the following:

1. Taking the easy way out in decision making or letting others make the decisions
2. Showing only superficial enthusiasm for the job
3. Being too willing to agree with others
4. Being unwilling to take risks
5. Directing anger at oneself and family members
6. Resisting innovations by others
7. Needing alcohol at the end of the day

Ross suggested several ways to prevent burnout.

1. Periodically take an inventory of personal strengths and weaknesses; identifying both stressful and enjoyable conditions; and evaluate family life, health, and personal factors.
2. Learn to manage time more appropriately by planning according to individual rhythms.
3. Keep track of problems and projects, mixing tough tasks with easier ones.
4. Work at cultivating physical and mental health, including regular exercise.
5. Avoid the overload situation by setting decision-making priorities; ration psychic energy needed for coping.

The community health nurse should help clients identify their stressors and find solutions to their occupational problems (Chapter 30).

Second Careers: Becoming a Student Again

Many middle adults and even some young adults struggle with career identity and satisfaction and decide to pursue another career. People often desire to explore new experiences; many yearn for what they wish they had become. This yearning often leads to midlife career changes, many of which require further education (Best, 1978). Baer (1979) described the situation that led up to her decision to make a career change as involving feelings of boredom with routine and dissatisfaction from a lack of challenge in her job. The needs and expectations of adult learners seeking second careers are becoming a major focus of educators as they try to serve this growing population.

Best (1978) described flexible life scheduling as a concept for "recycling people." By being more flexible in the way education, work, and leisure schedules in a person's lifetime are designed, personal dreams and aspirations are more likely to become realities. Present life patterns compress work into the middle years, with little activity for the young or aged. Best suggested alternative lifetime patterns, including cyclic life plans involving working hours that accommodate developmental tasks. For example, during the years of being single or having no children and the later years after raising children; individuals might work longer hours per week (45 to 50) with time-off compensations in vacations and sabbaticals. Individuals in the early child-raising years and old age might work a shorter week (25 to 40 hours) with vacations moderate in length. Leaves of absence in the middle years planned by employers foster health and productivity.

PHYSICALLY DISABLED ADULTS

Approximately 35 million Americans are physically disabled to some degree, making this group the largest minority in the United States, according to Tolentino (1981). Of the 17- to 44-year-old age group, 55% have at least one chronic illness.

Definition of Terms

Several terms are used, often interchangeably, to describe the disability state; various definitions may be found in the literature. For purposes of discussion in this chapter, the following succinct definitions are used:

Impairment: a disturbance in structure or function resulting from anatomical, physiological, and/or psychological abnormalities. For example, a person may have impairment of flexion and extension in the right arm.

Disability: the degree of observable and measurable physical or mental impairment. For example, a person may have a 50% disability of the right arm.

Handicap: the total adjustment to disability necessitated by an impairment or disability that limits or prevents functioning at a normal or usual level. For example, a person may be handicapped in writing, driving a car, and playing tennis because of the disability of the right arm.

People may have a high degree of disability and be minimally handicapped, such as those with quadriplegia who own their own businesses, drive specially equipped vans, and maintain active family roles. Conversely, some clients with little disability may exhibit profound limitations in satisfying life patterns. In either case these clients have

disabilities, but they should not be labeled according to their disabling condition. They are not quadriplegics; they have quadriplegia, just as they have blue eyes or a large frame. They are not cardiacs, diabetics, or any other such label. They are human beings who have impairments that are handicapping to some extent. The nurse's role is to capitalize on the human assets or abilities and minimize and compensate for the disabilities. The nurse should also promote the rehabilitation process for optimal achievement of potential. Rehabilitation is the process by which individuals and/or families strive for the attainment and maintenance of the maximum level of need satisfaction.

A disability may be classified as congenital or acquired, visible or invisible, and stable or progressive. Regardless of the classification or the extent of the disability, individuals are entitled to the rights that anybody has for family, work, social, and sex role responsibilities. They have a right to educational opportunities, health care services, and dignity and respect from others.

Prevention

If a large group of young healthy students were asked to indicate who had a history of diabetes in their families, many would respond positively. Of that group, some may well develop diabetes and eventually have a leg amputated or suffer total blindness. This type of pathological disability is a predictable consequence of chronic illness. Able-bodied people may consider themselves only temporarily so because they are susceptible to disease and/or injury. The importance of prevention and primary health care in the community is that disabling conditions can be minimized and should be approached with vigor. Table 24-6 lists the predictable consequences of certain risk factors that lead to a particular health problem, namely cardiac disability and death. In stage 1, life-style can be modified to promote health and decrease the possibility of impairment.

Impact of Disability

The community health nurse is challenged when assisting a family with a member who has a newly acquired disability. Many rehabilitation agencies discharge clients when they have mastered the physical skills of daily living. Yet total adjustment for the individual and family involves much more. Livneh (1980) described the following 12 stages of adjustment to a disabling condition: shock, anxiety, bargaining, denial, mourning, depression, withdrawal, anger, hostility/aggression, acknowledgment, acceptance, and adjustment. These stages may overlap, and clients may skip or regress to certain stages. The community health nurse may assess the client to be in any stage after discharge from an acute care institution, but often mourning and depression set in after loss of the distracting hustle and bustle of a busy agency. These stages may be evidenced by a slowing of physiological functions such as appetite, sleep, or body movements. The client may express feelings of helplessness, hoplessness, and sadness. Withdrawal is characterized by avoidance of social contacts, increased isolation, sleeping, using fantasy, and a general apathetic attitude. A client who is angry, hostile, or aggressive can be particularly

TABLE 24-6

Predictable consequences of cardiac risk factors

Stage	Conditions	Predictable consequences
1	Risk factors and stress adaptation Dietary pattern—high fat, high carbohydrate, high sodium Sedentary work and leisure Lack of exercise, recreation Heavy smoker	Hypertensive Obesity Arteriosclerotic plaque in vessels
2	Beginning and progressive pathophysiology	Sluggish circulation Decreased oxygenation Shortness of breath Edema
3	Advanced pathophysiology	Death of tissues Dysfunction of heart and lungs Cardiac pulmonale Cardiac crippling Death

enigmatic to his family and the nurse. Fixing blame is often the focus of thoughts and actions. Clients in this stage may be abusive, argumentative, and even violent.

Professionals providing help are no doubt eclectic in approaches used to cope with clients in various stages of adjustment. Logotherapy may be useful in helping the client acknowledge meaning in the suffering experience. As described earlier, Frankl's (1959) logotherapeutic techniques of paradoxical intention and dereflection may be useful. The dereflection technique is illustrated in the following excerpt.

> Milly was injured by a gunshot at age 15 during a domestic quarrel between her parents. The injury left her arms and legs completely paralyzed. She spent her day watching soap operas on television. While responding to the nursing history, Milly expressed surprise when the nurse asked what she did for others. Milly stated that she could not feed herself, bathe herself, write, sew, or even hold a telephone. Using dereflection, deemphasizing the identified problem or deliberately focusing on something other than the problem, the nurse helped Milly to focus on her abilities—a bright mind with retentive and concentration skills, her melodious voice, and lively, expressive eyes. Over the course of nurse/client interaction, Milly learned to type with a mouthstick and wrote letters of comfort to church members who were experiencing sorrow. She began putting her inspirational messages on tape for the church library. Later she volunteered for 4 hours per week of telephone counseling.

The impact of an acquired disability on the individual varies, based on many factors. According to Maslow (1970), all people strive to meet their needs to obtain some degree of satisfaction and fulfillment. The disabled individual is entitled to no less. The Needs Satisfaction Scale found in Appendix A may serve as a useful tool in assessing current need satisfaction level as a basis for planning nursing action.

Family with a Disabled Member

Often health workers focus their entire attention on the individual client and fail to see the needs of the family, particularly the client's caretaker. Disability of one family member can have a significant impact on the entire family. As the costs of institutional care continue to spiral, many families are providing care at home for members with a disability. With these responsibilities, family members become subject to stressors that can affect their health. They may have added roles and expanded or modified patterns and life-styles. The crisis of an injury or the shock of a chronic-illness diagnosis can greatly upset the family equilibrium.

The community health nurse must be cognizant of the impact of the disability on the family system. The beginning point for assessment and planning for family needs is during the initial crisis stage when most clients are hospitalized. Hart (1981) identified the following eight categories of needs of significant others:

1. Feel adequately informed
2. Feel helpful
3. Feel able to cope with responsibilities
4. Receive emotional support
5. Express feelings, positive and negative
6. Feel that the client is getting good care
7. Compare and contrast this with past experiences in coping with crises
8. Explore the future as a result of the client's condition

Family members show grief reactions just as the client does and need to maintain hope and restore balance to family life. Concerns expressed by family members include finances, work, housing, transportation, family activities, sexual activities, social relationships, and coping with the problems (functional and emotional) caused by the disability. Open communication between the disabled person and other family members is crucial to a healthy family pattern. Maintaining contact with extended family through telephone conversations or letter writing is also helpful in providing an emotional support system.

In a study conducted by Davis (1980) several factors were found to be important in a family's decision about home care versus institutional care, including the nature and stage of disability; age and health status of the caretaker; social climate; beliefs about family responsibility, morality, and religion, and the availability, adequacy, and acceptability of the caretaker role. The community health nurse needs to assess the family's patterns for tension management and conflict resolution (e.g., sudden outbursts, passive aggression, and psychosomatic ailments) and to assist the family in using healthy coping techniques. Referral for more intensive professional help may be warranted in some cases. Environmental stimulation and social interaction are necessary for caretakers and family members as well as clients.

The community health nurse should evaluate the client's functional ability and family health, which is complicated by the added responsibilities for a member with a disability. The effects on the major caretaker and others of providing long-term physical and emotional care must be recognized in any nursing care plan for the family. Respite care provides services intermittently to the family or care given to relieve them of the responsibilities associated with caring for a chronically ill or disabled person (Looney, 1987). The long-term effects of unrelieved stress and frustration of needs can cause a breakdown of the caretaker, as demonstrated in the following example.

> Miss A. had never been married, lived with her parents, and assisted with the family business. When her father died, she took on complete responsibilities for providing for herself and her mother. She worked long, hard hours at the store and then assisted her aging mother with the house and yard work. When Mrs. A. had a stroke, her daughter took care of her at home in a devoted manner. As Mrs. A's condition worsened, Miss A. found herself staying up at night yet continuing to put in a full day at the store. Mrs. A became cranky and more demanding. She was incontinent and frequently called for help during the night. Although the doctor urged Miss A. to get help to supplement the daytime nurse, she declined, preferring to take care of her mother herself during the evening and night hours. Friends offered to relieve Miss A. for a weekend and urged her to take a relaxing trip, but she maintained her vigil. One day to the surprise and consternation of relatives, Miss A. lost all control, had her mother placed in a nursing home, and said she never wanted to see her again. At the nursing home Mrs. A. made some degree of progress, and the staff attempted to plan a visit home. However, Miss A. still refused to associate with her mother and in fact had all the locks on the doors changed to ensure that she could not return home. The mother eventually died in the nursing home. The daughter retired from the family business and became a virtual recluse.

Careers for Disabled Adults

Recent legislation has facilitated acceptance of the disabled adult into the work force. The community health nurse can be a source of support because a newly employed disabled adult often faces many barriers, not the least of which are the attitudes of management, fellow workers, and the public.

Technology has enabled many otherwise disqualified individuals to perform satisfactorily in a job (Macleod, 1981). Products of this technology (e.g., the optophone, an electronic sensory aid that translates printed letters into vocal tones) facilitate satisfactory performance by disabled individuals. Several other examples of technology that can be used should be discussed by the community health nurse. The Telesensory Systems' Optacon is a visual to tactile conversion system whereby an optical probe is moved across lines of a text, which converts to letters perceived tactilely and allows a reading rate of about 100 words per minute. Electronic language boards can be controlled by body actions, such as eye movements, and allow for nonverbal communication. Speech prostheses are also available for those with a disability. The Phonic Mirror Handi Voice contains a programmable speech synthesizer in a portable unit. The computer field promises to improve job opportunities for the disabled adult. Financial constraints often limit resourceful devices that would facilitate a self-supporting adult.

Community and National Significance

Disability influences resources and emphasizes needs for services, including inpatient and outpatient services, emergency care services, housing, and transportation. Today's philosophy of mainstreaming, integrating individuals who have disabilities into society rather than isolating them in a protective environment, requires planning; the community health nurse should be actively involved in this planning.

A community may need a variety of modules to provide housing options for its residents. Home as a concept is a central part of our culture, a private, independent, individual place, providing comfort and opportunity for self-expression and intimacy. Falta (1981) described four prototypes of desegregated community housing arrangements.

1. *Group homes* provide independent, semiintegrated lifestyles and are often helpful after leaving a family setting or institution. A home such as a halfway or quarterway house can provide assistance without stifling protection. This type of home may be considered an extended family unit, a home shared with compatible disabled persons and able-bodied helpers in a nonprofit organization. Often this type of facility is created from a typical single-family dwelling or an apartment building. Residents contribute toward room and board, with remaining costs being subsidized by government or private agencies.

2. *Apartment units with in-house staff* are apartment buildings adapted to accommodate disabled clients and/or the elderly, which provide housing with more privacy than group homes. Health care and domestic services for the building complex are provided by in-house staff, and extra security measures are an added feature.

3. *Adapted apartments* onto a private home or within an apartment complex are adapted for a person with a

disability. Needed services can then be provided by family members or agency personnel.

4. *Modified and renovated housing.* The Homebound Program in Alabama provides any person sustaining a spinal cord injury with $1000 to add ramps and otherwise modify the home. Such subsidies to render a home more accessible offer suitable housing at reasonable rates.

The community health nurse should be interested in how well local health services and other aspects of the community take into consideration the needs of individuals who are disabled. For example, do emergency medical technicians receive training on how to handle the needs of a blind person who is injured and may become emotionally hypersensitive? Do restaurants provide braille menus? Do waitresses address family members of a blind person and ask, "What would he like to order?" Are churches accessible to the disabled, or do the churches prefer a ministry to "shut-ins?" Are local government buildings accessible to the disabled?

Rehabilitation following disability is as costly to the nation as providing for special needs such as transportation or housing. However, such services may allow a disabled person and/or the caretaker to return to work. Thus the worker is contributing to the tax base instead of being dependent on government services. Rehabilitation contributes to the economic welfare of the nation and serves to facilitate humanitarianism.

Physical, Psychosocial, and Spiritual Rehabilitation

In a holistic approach to the rehabilitation process, attention must be given to all component parts of human existence. Specialized centers offer a variety of services to meet these needs. Clients are usually discharged from institutions when they master certain physical tasks. The community health nurse monitors treatment plans to maintain physical achievements. Often a client who has learned to work with an artificial limb goes home and hangs it in the closet; hence nurses must constantly encourage physical conditioning. Other nursing care focuses on promoting the health of the nonpathological structures. For example, a client with diabetes who has had one leg amputated for gangrene should be taught to exercise all efforts to keep the other leg healthy.

People with a disability need psychosocial restoration as part of the broad perspective of rehabilitation. The achievement of self-care and mobility does not guarantee reintegration of social functioning. Labi (1980) found that women are slightly more likely than men to decrease their social activity in the home and in hobbies. The findings also indicate that following stroke, social reintegration outside the home is more difficult for women and for those with more education because factors related to body image and feelings of stigma may be more intense. Many disabled persons tend to acquire new friends of lower social status than previously. Dubois (1981) used the term *socially naked* to describe humans who live with little, if any, human contact. The community health nurse must be innovative in individual cases to promote psychosocial restoration. Encouraging self-transcendence helps clients to focus on others. For example, a man who had been injured in a deliberate attempt on his life and left with an ileostomy and spinal cord injury, necessitating the use of a wheel chair, found meaning in volunteering in the recreational program in a nursing home. In meeting needs for others his own psychosocial health improved.

All humans have a spiritual (not synonymous with religious) dimension. The dynamic power of the human spirit can be harnessed to restore the disabled person to satisfaction and fulfillment. Logotherapeutic counseling can assist disabled persons to find meaning in their circumstances and a unique purpose in life, with satisfying roles to fulfill. Life's task becomes finding an answer for the question, "Now that I am in this situation, what will I do with my life?"

CLINICAL APPLICATION

The clinical situation presented here provides an opportunity for the student to apply knowledge gained from this chapter to a typical case involving needs and health problems of young and middle adults. The nursing process is to be used as a framework in making clinical decisions.

> Mrs. Rosa Garcia is a slightly overweight 48-year-old Hispanic woman who comes to the Riverview Community Center diabetic clinic. Her diabetes has been controlled with NPH insulin 30 units for the past 5 years. She explains that recently she has experienced occasional chest tightness and shortness of breath. She is employed as a domestic worker and has noticed symptoms especially after climbing stairs. After a thorough examination by the multidisciplinary team at the center, Mrs. Garcia is placed on nitroglycerine 1/150 gr. p.r.n. for angina. She is referred to the nurse for planning community-based chronic care with emphasis on health maintenance, decreasing cardiovascular risks, and preventing complications of diabetes mellitus.
>
> Other members of the Garcia household include Jose, the husband, a 52-year-old construction worker who is currently unemployed because of the depressed housing market. He has been abusing alcohol in the past three months, which coincides with his length of unemployment. He is depressed, and the nurse suspects his drinking bouts sometimes lead to abusive behavior with his wife and children. The Garcia children are Maria, age 15; Jimenez, age 17, and Anna, age 18. They are all in high school; each has an after-school job making minimum wage.

1. Based upon the information above, what additional assessment data should be collected about the family members and the household during the first home visit?

2. Identify the developmental tasks characteristic of the middle adults in this situation.

3. To analyze the assessment data, an understanding of Hispanic cultural values and life-styles will be necessary. Write a brief paragraph describing common values and traditions of Hispanics who are first generation Mexican-Americans.

> After the first home visit, the nurse identifies several problems within the Garcia household. Mrs. Garcia works 10 hours per day, including housecleaning from 8 AM to 12 PM and managing a laundromat from 12 to 6 PM. In addition, she rises early to prepare breakfast for the family and to make lunches for the children. When she returns in the evening, she prepares dinner and cleans her own house.

Saturdays are usually spent doing the family laundry and baking for the week. Sundays are spent at various church activities. In the past, Sundays were reserved for family outings, but now the children prefer activities with friends their own age. There is evidence that all three children are sexually active, and Mrs. Garcia is worried that Jimenez occasionally experiments with drugs.

Mr. Garcia spends most of his days out of the house, hoping to locate work and drinking. He gets very upset at the suggestion that he is drinking too much. His physical health appears good, but he has not had a thorough physical examination since he started working for the construction company 10 years ago. He is collecting unemployment insurance, but voices shame about it. His parents live in the neighborhood. His father has had a stroke but is doing well at home, cared for by his mother. They are both retired and have a modest, but adequate, income.

1. What factors must be considered in developing a family plan of care?
2. What are the alternatives in modifying Mrs. Garcia's workload and energy expenditure?
3. Develop a 3-month, 6-month, and 12-month plan for the Garcia family that demonstrates gradual change to desired goals.
4. What are the teaching/learning needs of the Garcia family?

One evening, after a particularly stressful day, Mrs. Garcia becomes extremely dyspneic and must be hospitalized. Her complaints of chest tightness and shortness of breath subside with adequate care. Her diabetes is slightly out of control, but with several days of rest and proper diet, it is once more in balance. During the hospitalization, the following family problems are made known to Mrs. Garcia:
Jimenez is addicted to cocaine and has been skipping school for the past 6 weeks.
Maria is pregnant and the father of the baby wants to marry her.
Mr. Garcia has been in an automobile wreck and is arrested for driving under the influence of alcohol.

1. In coordinating discharge planning with the hospital, what priorities should be set for follow-up care?
2. What stress-reducing interventions might be useful as Mrs. Garcia faces domestic problems?
3. How might a logotherapeutic approach to intervening with the family crises be implemented?

Six months after the Garcia family became part of the caseload of the community health nurse, Mrs. Garcia's diabetic and cardiovascular conditions are stabilized. Her work schedule has been reduced to 8 hours per day with no heavy cleaning. Jimenez has entered a residential drug treatment program, where he has developed an interest in the electronics trade. Maria's pregnancy is without complications, and she is conscientious about keeping clinic appointments. She and the baby's father still want to marry but no plans have been made. Anna has entered a nursing program and is progressing satisfactorily. Unfortunately, Mr. Garcia has still not found work, continues to drink, and has recently manifested hypertension.

1. What are the criteria to evaluate the progress, or lack of progress, toward health goals by this family?

2. What are the continued health risks for members of the family?
3. Based on the achievements and/or continued problems for each family member, what are the priorities for future plans?

SUMMARY

The major health problems of young and middle adults are largely the result of life-style behaviors that are influenced by specific developmental tasks. Individuals in this age group have many stressors and pressures from social role expectations to meet not only their own needs, but also the needs of others who are dependent on them. The adult years are fluid, represented by growth and change in the pursuit of new life goals and in coping with various life crises. The responsibilities assumed by adults range from parent to childcare and also include primary burdens of income production.

Physical changes accompany psychosocial changes in adulthood. These changes create various effects in different individuals. However, each person needs to exert a planned effort at maintaining optimum health, including exercise, nutrition, rest, sleep, play, and mental outlook on life. Assuming responsibility for self-care is the adult health task.

The developmental tasks of young adults center around interaction with an intimate other and establishing a career. The middle adult's developmental task involves achieving a significant contribution for future generations and may involve stress in the work-place. Within each age category, special subgroups, such as single adults, require the specialized attention of community health nurses, who attempt to promote health and fulfillment. Morbidity and mortality rates of young and middle adults give direction for the community health nurse. Suicide, homicide, and accidents are serious concerns for young adults. The nurse must assess and analyze pressures and frustrations that lead to such appalling consequences if this major health problem is to be resolved. Positive mental health services are needed in a community so that families can present their problems to professionals and learn to cope with crises. Sexually transmittable diseases are also a major health problem of young adults.

Morbidity and mortality factors for the middle adult include heart disease and stroke, cancer, alcohol and substance abuse, mental health problems, and periodontal diseases. Although singular cause-and-effect factors cannot be demonstrated, various health practices can contribute to disease prevention and health promotion. Avoiding known risk factors is a constructive action. The growing concern for substance abuse can be dealt with in comprehensive health centers. The community health nurse must work in a partner relationship with the adult, who must assume responsibility to reduce risk for disease development and to promote a healthy life-style.

Logotherapy offers an approach for coping with pain, suffering, and illness. Strategies such as dereflection, paradoxical intention, and Socratic dialogue can be useful with the client or family. Such intervention can assist the adult to find meaning and purpose in life experiences.

Self-help groups are beneficial. Groups such as Alcoholics' Anonymous and others are composed of individuals with a common problem who meet regularly to provide support to overcome the problem. These groups apply principles of adult learning and offer peer support. Such groups play a major part in enhancing the quality of life and health in young and middle adults. The nurse must influence (1) health policies, to bring about needed changes in environmental influences on health, and (2) policies on how resources are allocated to health programs.

Assessing the impact of a physical disability on an individual, family, or community is within the realm of the community health nurse. Today's technology has eliminated many barriers to the disabled adult's ability to function in the larger society. As the community health nurse uses this technology and coordinates community resources, attention must be given to what is often the greatest barrier—attitude toward the disabled person.

Health problems of young and middle adults relate to work, family, and community. Though major health hazards are reflected in morbidity and mortality statistics, community health nurses must be cognizant of potential problems from emerging trends of a changing society. Anticipating new health problems depends on analyzing life-styles and values of today's adult population.

KEY CONCEPTS

Like the middle-income segment of society, young and middle adults may be considered the backbone of society.

Young adults are those between the ages of 20 to 35 years; middle adults are those between the ages of 36 to 64 years. However, adults may move forward and backward among the young-adult and middle-adult life-styles.

Adults progress through successive phases of stabilization and consolidation and then change and growth while pursuing new goals and confronting life crises.

Factors that influence growth and development of the adult include health status, a sense of responsibility for self-care, available health resources, and life-style.

Health for the adult is the balanced state of well-being resulting from the harmonious interaction of body, mind, and spirit.

Self-care is defined by Orem (1985, p. 31) as "the production of actions directed to self or to the environment in order to regulate one's functioning in the interests of one's life, integrated functioning and well-being."

Although self-care may be viewed as a modern phenomenon, it is the passive role of health consumers that is a relatively recent phenomenon.

The status of adult health and opportunities for growth and development are interlinked to environmental influences and resources of the individual, family, and community.

The middle years are crossroads in the adult developmental process, and the transition is as critical as it was in adolescence.

For young adults, major health threats include violent death or injury, alcohol and substance abuse, unwanted pregnancies, and sexually transmissible diseases.

Wholly 75% of sexually transmissible diseases occur among young adults age 15 to 24 years.

Motor vehicle accidents are the leading cause of death in young adults age 15 to 24 years.

Common causes of morbidity and mortality in middle adults are heart disease and stroke, cancer, alcohol and substance abuse, mental health problems, and periodontal disease.

Heart disease accounts for over 33% of deaths among middle adults.

The major health problems of young and middle adults are largely the result of life-style behaviors that are influenced by specific developmental tasks.

Approximately 35 million Americans are physically disabled to some degree; 55% of persons age 17 to 44 have at least one chronic illness.

LEARNING ACTIVITIES

1. Conduct an individual assessment on 10 adults. Half of these adults should be between the ages of 20 and 35 years and the remaining 5 between the ages of 36 and 64 years. Compare the psychosocial tasks performed by members of each group as reported on their personal health assessments.

2. Interview at least six single adults. Include males and females in the group and compare the psychosocial tasks mentioned in the interviews to the expected norms.
   a. What similarities exist between the norm and those interviewed?
   b. What differences exist between the norm and those interviewed?
   c. Discuss whether the differences can be attributed to their state of singleness.

3. Design a teaching plan for a middle adult that reflects a maximum level of health promotion.

4. Analyze mortality and morbidity data in your county and rank the order of the 10 most prevalent health problems.

5. Using a community service directory for your county, match available services to the needs identified in the survey of mortality and morbidity data. If gaps are noted, what services would you recommend to overcome this deficit?

6. Consult the most recent annual report of the State Department of Public Health and compare state and national incidence figures for the five leading causes of death in your state versus the nation.

BIBLIOGRAPHY

Anderson, R.: Is the problem of noncompliance all in our heads? Diabetes Educator 11(1):31-34, 1985.

Archer, V.E., et al.: Lung cancer among uranium miners in the United States, Health Phys. 25:351-371, 1973.

Baer, E.: A career change after twenty years, Am. J. Nurs. 79(11):1969-1970, Nov. 1979.

Best, F.: Recycling people: work-sharing through flexible life scheduling. In Cornish, E., editor: 1999 the world of tomorrow, Washington, D.C., 1978, World Future Society.

Bylinski, G.: Science scores a cancer breakthrough, Fortune, 113:16-21, Nov. 1985.

Campbell, A.: The sense of well-being in America: recent patterns and trends, New York, 1981, McGraw-Hill Book Co.

Cancer Facts and Figures, 1987, New York, No. 5008-LE, American Cancer Society.

Centers for Disease Control: Morbidity and Mortality Weekly Report 34(48):722-735, Dec. 6, 1985.

Centers for Disease Control: Chlamydia trachomatis infections: policy guidelines for prevention and control, Morbidity and Mortality Weekly Report Supplement 34:535-745, Aug. 1985.

Colarusso, C.A., and Nemiroff, R.A.: Adult development, New York, 1983, Plenum Publishing Corp.

Cordes, S.M.: Biopsychosocial imperatives from the rural perspective, Soc. Sci. Med. 21:1373-1379, Nov. 1985.

Cutler, D.L., and Madore, E.: Community-family network therapy in a rural setting, Community Ment. Health J. 16:144-155, 1980.

Davis, A.J.: Disability: home care and the caretaking role in family life, J. Adv. Nurs. 5:475-484, Sept. 1980.

DeMoss, C.J.: Giving intravenous chemotherapy at home, Am. J. Nurs. 80:2188-2189, Dec. 1980.

Diekelmann, N.L.: The young adult: the choice is health or illness, Am. J. Nurs. 76:1272-1277, Aug. 1976.

Diekelmann, N.L.: Wellness: approaches and resources, Nurse Pract. 5:41-42, Oct. 1980.

Dodder, R.A., and Astle, D.J.: A methodological analysis of Srole's Nine-item Anomia Scale, Multivariate Behav. Res. 15:329-334, 1980.

Dubois, R.: Celebrations of life, New York, 1981, McGraw-Hill Book Co.

Durkheim, E.: Suicide, Glencoe, Ill., 1951, Free Press.

Eisenberg, M.: The logotherapeutic intergenerational communications group, Int. Forum Logotherapy 2(2):23-25, 1979.

Erikson, E.: Childhood and society, New York, 1950, W.W. Norton & Co., Inc.

Falck, V.T.: A re-evaluation of urban vs rural as ways of life: implications for health educators, Hygie 4:40-44, 1985.

Falta, L.P.: Integration in the community: Canadian housing options for the disabled, Physiother. Can. 33:102-105, March/April 1981.

Francoeur, R.T., and Francoeur, A.K.: The pleasure bond: reversing the antisex ethic. In Cornish, E., editor: 1999 the world of tomorrow, Washington, D.C., 1978, World Future Society.

Frankl, V.: Man's search for meaning, New York, 1959, Simon & Schuster, Inc.

Frankl, V.: The doctor and the soul, New York, 1973, Random House, Inc.

Frankl, V.: The unconscious God, New York, 1975, Simon & Schuster, Inc.

Grossman, R.: Are you dealing with—or denying the mid-life crisis? Fam. Health 11:6-10, Nov./Dec. 1979.

Hart, J.: Spinal cord injury: impact on client's significant others, Rehabil. Nurs. 6:11-15, Jan./Feb. 1981.

Hayne, C.: The body's reaction to noise, Occup. Health Saf. 33:75-83, Feb. 1981.

Health: United States, 1984, DHHS Pub. No. (PHS) 85-1232, Washington, D.C., 1981, Department of Health and Human Services.

Health: United States, 1986, DHHS, Pub. No. 87-1232, Public Health Service, Washington, D.C., 1986, p. 114-115, U.S. Government Printing Office.

Healthy people: the Surgeon General's report on health promotion and disease prevention, DHEW Pub. No. (PHS) 79-55071, Washington, D.C., 1979, Department of Health, Education, and Welfare.

Helander, E.: Training and disabled in the community, World Health Stat. Q. 35:26-29, Jan. 1981.

Johns, J.: Self-care today—in search of an identity, Nurs. Health Care 6(3):153-155, March 1985.

Johnson, J.L., and Norby, P.A.: We can weekend: a program for cancer families, Cancer Nurs. 4:23-28, Feb. 1981.

Karman, J., and Price, J.H.: Community organization for an oral cancer screening program, J. Nurs. Care 13:15-17, Aug. 1980.

Kolata, G.: Is the war on cancer being won? Science, 233:543-544, Aug. 1985.

Labi, M.L.C., et al.: Psychosocial disability in physically restored long-term stroke survivors, Arch. Phys. Med. Rehabil. 61:561-565, Dec. 1980.

Lamb, M.A., and Woods, N.F.: Sexuality and the cancer patient, Cancer Nurs. 4:137-144, April 1981.

Lattimore, S., et al.: Is hypertension a problem in industry? Occup. Health Nurs. 27:19-21, Oct. 1979.

Levin, L.: Self-care: towards fundamental changes in national strategies, Int. J. Health Educ. 24(4):219-228, 1981.

Levinson, D.J., et al.: The seasons of a man's life, New York, 1978, Ballantine Books, Inc.

Livneh, H.: The process of adjustment to disability: feelings, behaviors and counseling strategies, Psychosoc. Rehabil. J. 4:26-35, 1980.

Looney, K.M.: The respite care alternative, J. Gerontol. Nurs. 13(5):18-21, 1987.

Lowther, N.B., and Carter, V.D.: How to increase compliance in hypertensives, Am. J. Nurs. 81(5):963, May 1981.

Macleod, L.: Information processing aids for physically handicapped people, Aust. Nurs. J. 10:46-53, Dec./Jan. 1981.

Maslow, A.H.: Motivation and personality, New York, 1970, Harper & Row, Publishers, Inc.

Mayer, J.: Eating well after 50, Fam. Health 12:52, June 1980.

McGregor, D.: The human side of enterprise: New York, 1960, McGraw-Hill Book Co.

McKenna, S.P., et al.: Mine rescue workers: their perceived health absence from work, Occup. Health Saf. 33:70-74, Feb. 1981.

Milio, N.: Promoting health through public policy, Philadelphia, 1981, F.A. Davis Co.

Milio, N.: Primary care and the public health, Lexington, Mass., 1983, Lexington Books.

Montana, D.E.: Predicting and understanding influenza vaccination behavior: alternatives to the health belief model. Med. Care 24(5):438-453, 1986.

Morbidity and Mortality Weekly Reports: Annual Summary, 1984, U.S. Department of Health and Human Services, Public Health Service 33:91-93, No. 54, March, 1986.

Morris, C.L.: Stress: relaxation therapy in a clinic, Am. J. Nurs. 79(11):1958-1959, Nov. 1979.

N'Kanza, S.: Full participation and equality, World Health 35:3-5, Jan. 1981.

O'Connor, P.: Prevention of coronary heart disease: is there a role for the health visitor, Health Visit. 54:28-30, Jan. 1981.

O'Flynn-Comiskey, A.I.: Stress: the type A individual, Am. J. Nurs. 79(11):1956-1958, Nov. 1979.

Orem, D.: Nursing concepts of practice, New York, 1985, McGraw-Hill Book Co.

Ouchi, W.: Theory Z: how American business can meet the Japanese challenge, Reading, Mass., 1981, Addison-Wesley Publishing Co., Inc.

Poplin, L.E.: Practical knowledge of nutrition in health science, J. Am. Diet. Assoc. 77:576-580, Nov. 1980.

Public health aspects of sexually transmitted diseases, Public Health Rev. 12:131-157, 1984.

Redman, B.: The process of patient teaching in nursing, ed. 5, St. Louis, 1984, The C.V. Mosby Co.

Rix, K.: Alcoholism and the district nurse, Community Outlook, 13:275-276, Sept. 1979.

Ross, A.: Managing executive stress and other related subjects, J. Ambulatory Care Manag. 3:1-10, Nov. 1980.

Schaffner, A.: Safety for chemotherapy at home, Am. J. Nurs. 84(3):346-347, 1984.

Searle, C.: Psychosocial aspects of mammary carcinoma: curationis, S. Afr. J. Nurs. 3:12-15, Sept. 1980.

Selkin, J.: The legacy of Emile Durkheim, Suicide Life Threat. Behav. 13(1):3-14, 1983.

Selye, H.: Stress and holistic medicine, Fam. Community Health 3:85-88, Aug. 1980.

Sheehy, G.: Passages: predictable crises of adult life, New York, 1974, E.P. Dutton.

Sheehy, G.: Pathfinders, New York, 1981, William Morrow & Co., Inc.

Silverman, J.: On the metaphysical aspect of health care: attitudes, values, and other thoughts we use to think, Fam. Community Health 3:93-103, Aug. 1980.

Smith, K.G.: The hazards of migrant farm work: an overview for rural public health nurses, Public Health Nurs. 3(1):48-56, 1986.

Thompson, D.: Dietary advice and heart disease: a nursing dilemma? Int. J. Nurs. Stud. 20(4):245-253, 1983.

Tolentino, A.: 1981: international year of the disabled person, Imprint 28:27, April 1981.

Travelbee, J.: Interpersonal aspects of nursing, Philadelphia, 1966, F.A. Davis Co.

Turner, R.: Diet and primary prevention of coronary disease, Midwife Health Visit. Community Nurse. 16:452, Nov. 1980.

Valenzuela, W.G., and Hallamore, A.G.: The "good neighbor network"—gatekeepers to a rural mental health support system . . . New Hampshire, Psychosoc. Rehabil. J. 3:20-33, 1979.

Volberding, P., and Abrams, D.: Clinical care and research in A.I.D.S., Hastings Center Report 15:16-18, Aug. 1985.

Welch, D.A.: Waiting, worry and the cancer experience, Oncology Nurs. Forum 8:14-18, 1981.

Wilson, J.: Communities re-born, World Health 35:22-25, Jan. 1981.

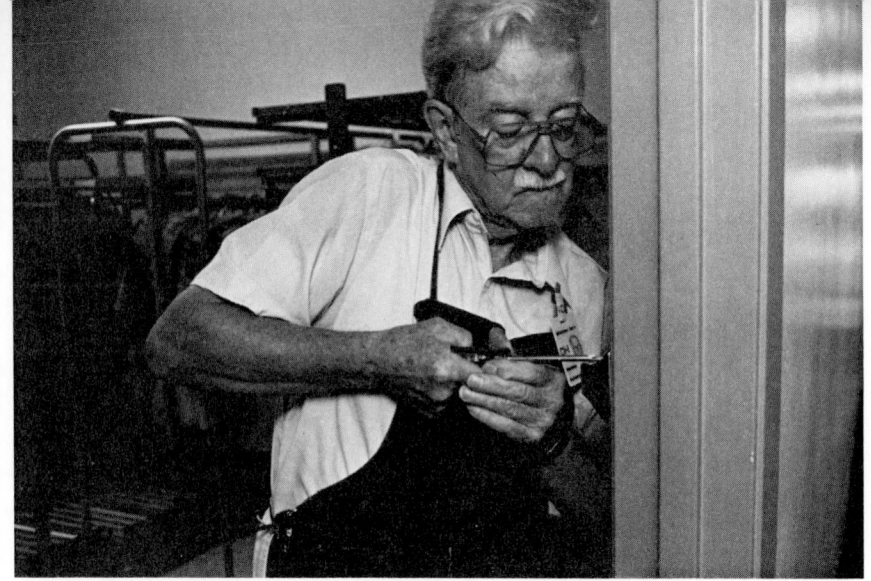

Delois H. Skipwith

THE OLDER ADULT

OBJECTIVES

After reading this chapter, the student should be able to:

List two demographic facts about older adults.

Describe at least two common myths or stereotypes about the older adult.

Identify two of one's personal biases about aging.

Discuss the role of the community health nurse in providing care for older adults who have at least one major health problem.

Describe at least three possible effects of health promotion activities for older adults.

Name at least three community resources and services available for the care of the elderly.

Identify at least three losses that older adults may incur.

List three nursing interventions that could assist the older client to cope with each of the three losses just named.

KEY TERMS

abuse of the elderly
activity theory
Acute brain syndrome
aging network
Alzheimer's disease
autoimmunity theory
Chronic brain syndrome
confusional states
dementia

depression
developmental or
  continuity theory of
  aging
disengagement theory
drug resistance
eight stages of life
life expectancy
psychotropic
respite care

retirement
self-esteem
senility
stress management
substance abuse
time management
wear and tear theory
widowhood

The elderly are the fastest growing population in the United States. Their increased longevity with the accompanying high incidence of chronic disease poses a substantial challenge to the health care system. Technology can keep people alive much longer, yet such care is costly and often uncomfortable. This chapter discusses the following questions: Who are the older adults? What major health problems accompany their increasing longevity? What are appropriate community health–nursing interventions in these situations? What community programs, resources, and legislative support are available to make the older years truly "golden years"?

DEMOGRAPHY

Historically the elderly are described as people who are aged 65 years or older because at age 65 people become eligible to receive *Social Security* benefits. In the early 1900s 1 in every 25 people was aged 65 and over, compared with the 1984 rate of one in every eight people. The 65-years-and-older age group numbered 28 million in 1984. By the year 2010, it is projected that the number of Americans age 65 and over will drastically increase to one in seven. By 2050, one in every five persons will be aged 65 and over (U.S. Senate, 1986). The increasing growth rate of the older population is shown in Table 25-1.

In 1983, the life expectancy at birth was 78.3 years for women and 71.0 years for men. In 1986 the median age of the U.S. population was 31 years; the projected increase for the year 2000 is 36 years, and for the year 2050 is 42 years (U.S. Senate, 1986). Analysis of gender distribution indicates that the 65-years-and-older segment of the population is about two-thirds female (approximately 15.2 million women and 10.2 million men). A breakdown of the older population into smaller age segments illustrates that women outnumber men throughout later life (Table 25-2).

Blacks constitute the largest minority in this country, a total of 28.1 million in 1983. Of this number, 2.3 million are age 65 and older (U.S. Bureau, 1984). Asians and Pacific islanders account for 6% of the 65-years-and-older population, and native Americans and Hispanics account for 4% each (Need for Long-term Care, 1981). Statistics indicate racial and ethnic differences in life expectancy, gender distribution, and median age.

Life expectancy at birth for blacks is less than for whites; however, this gap is narrowing. The 1940 life-expectancy margin of 11 years held by whites over blacks decreased to 5.6 years in 1983. After the age of 80, life expectancy is

TABLE 25-1

Older population growth and projections

Year	Number (in thousands)	Percentage of total population
1900	3084	4.0
1920	4933	4.7
1940	9019	6.8
1960	16,560	9.2
1980	25,544	11.3
1990	31,697	12.7
2000	34,921	13.0
2010	39,195	13.8
2020	51,422	17.3
2030	64,581	21.2
2040	66,988	21.7

Sources: 1900-80: U.S. Bureau of the Census, Decennial Censuses of Population. 1990-2050: U.S. Bureau of the Census, Projections of the Population of the United States by Age, Sex, and Race. 1983 to 2080, Current Population Reports, Series P-25, No. 952, May 1984. Projections are middle series.

TABLE 25-2

Number of men per 100 women in 1984

Age group	Number of men
65-69	81
70-74	72
75-79	63
80-84	53
85-89	43
90-94	36

From the U.S. Bureau of Census: Current population reports, Series P-25, No. 952, estimates, Washington, D.C., 1984, U.S. Government Printing Office.

higher for blacks than for whites. The median age for blacks is 25.8 years as compared with 31.8 years for whites. Black females have gained the largest increase in life expectancy, an increase of 5.5 years for the period from 1970 to 1983. The ratio of black males to black females is 65.5 : 100 (U.S. Bureau, 1984).

The educational level of the elderly population also has improved. The median level of education was 11 years in 1983. By 1990 this figure is expected to increase to 11.9 years for persons 65 years and over. There are differences in education levels between elderly blacks and whites. About 33% of older whites and 66% of older blacks did not attend school beyond the eighth grade (U.S. Senate, 1986).

Although people are living to older ages, Social Security payments and the use of Medicare have benefited the elderly. Only 12.4% of older adults lived below the poverty level in 1984, and the median income for elderly persons was $7349.

Racial and gender differentiations are noted in the economic status of elderly people. Approximately 13% of elderly whites and 39% of elderly blacks live below the poverty level. In 1984 white men aged 65 to 69 had a median income of $12,749, whereas the median income for black and Hispanic men was $7545 and $8778 respectively. Elderly women constitute 64% of the elderly poor. In 1984 elderly women had a median income of $6020 as compared with $10,450 for elderly men (Siegel & Davidson, 1984; U.S. Senate, 1986).

The older adult in America lives in a culture oriented to youth, productivity, and rapid paces. This orientation influences the goods and services produced and marketed, as well as the work, recreation, and rest options available.

A youth-oriented attitude may convey to older adults that they are not respected, valued, or esteemed and that declining health, health problems, and health issues are "natural" or just "old age." Some health problems therefore go undetected, are mislabeled or misdiagnosed, or are ineffectively treated or untreated. There are fewer adequately prepared health care providers for the older segment of the population than for other age groups. Additionally, the allocation of resources—type, amount, and location—may indicate to the older adult that their needs go unmet. Although many demographic and social changes are beginning to alter this youth-oriented attitude, much work is needed to create an attitude recognizing the social worth of all age groups.

Knowledge of the role of the elderly in various cultural, ethnic, and cohort groups is essential to each community health nurse for providing quality care. Across cultures and ethnic groups the roles of the elderly in family relationships and as storers and transmitters of knowledge and information are evident. The black American family esteems its older members for their "adaptation" to many crises and struggles, for their strong religious affiliations and for the life expectancy crossover phenomenon (that is, blacks aged 75 years and older live longer than whites).

In Asian-American families the older adult man may relinquish status and responsibility to his wife and oldest

son. Many older Chinese men live alone by choice and because of cultural beliefs, whereas in Japanese culture the young are expected to respect and care for their elders.*

Mexican-Americans often view health and illness as balance-imbalance between the will of God and their own behavior. Additionally, children are expected to care for the aged, and there is little use of nursing homes (Ebersole and Hess, 1981). Chapter 5 gives additional information on the influence of culture in determining the community health nursing role.

The changes in socialization, social expectations, and lifestyles of each cohort of aged persons determine to some extent what will be paramount needs and issues for the group. Members of the generation who were young during the 1960s and who were characterized as rebellious and concerned with rights and freedom, at age 65 will differ greatly in character, expectations, and social participation from members of the Depression era generation who are now a part of the older population. The cohorts of the 1980s will age with an entirely different set of issues and concerns—influenced by education, consumerism, financial woes of inflation and unemployment, and health consciousness.

MYTHS AND STEREOTYPES

In recent years, aging as a life process has received greater focus and study. The earlier lack of emphasis on this population group perpetuated many myths and stereotypes, the major ones of which are discussed here. It is hoped that, as knowledge expands in this area, the mythography will change. The public often views old people as persons who wear glasses, are hard of hearing, are bald or have grey hair, have wrinkled skin, and are crippled. How many times have such illusions been depicted as typical of old people in dramas, drawings, and other works? The characteristics of older people portrayed on television and the public's conversation and jokes about older people dehumanize and stigmatize this group.

A popular myth is that most older people are institutionalized, yet only about 5% of elderly persons are actually in institutions (U.S. Senate, 1986).

The second most common myth is that the elderly are poor. Although many are poor, the majority of older adults (85%) live above the poverty level (Need for Long-term Care, 1981). However, this figure does not negate the severity of the financial problems stemming from poverty, such as living in older houses in deteriorating neighborhoods, having limited access to transportation, and receiving poor health care.

The myth of the inability of the elderly to learn has serious consequences for the health of elderly persons. Health education opportunities for the elderly are often neglected because providers believe "They can't learn." Yet investigations have shown that older adults are capable of learning, and when learning problems occur, they are gen-

---

*In Japanese culture, children tend to assume responsibility for aging relatives rather than expecting them to live alone and care for themselves.

erally associated with other conditions that interrupt health such as hearing or vision loss. Adjustments are needed in the attitudes of the providers of information, as well as the recipients.

Similar to women, older people have been erroneously characterized as "bad drivers". However, the biggest automobile accident problem for people over 65 years of age is being injured as a pedestrian instead of as the driver of a car causing an accident. Actually, the 15- to 24-year-old group has the highest motor vehicle death rate (Healthy People, 1979).

The perception of older people as "chair rockers" is refuted by Harris' survey (The Myth and Reality of Aging in America, 1975). Harris' study revealed that people 65 years old and older are perceived as spending 42% of their time "sitting and thinking" and 27% of their time "doing nothing," whereas they actually spend only 31% of their time "sitting and thinking" and 15% "just doing nothing." Elder's actual activities include at least 20% of their time gardening, caring for others, walking, participating in organizations and hobbies, and other activities.

Additional myths center on sexuality. Despite the myths, sexual drive and activity are present in old age, with changes in level of sexual activity resulting from physiological causes, sociocultural perspectives or both. However, it is true that health problems and medications may alter sexual activity, as may availability of a mate, stereotypes, privacy, and living arrangements.

DEVELOPMENTAL TASKS AND THEORIES OF AGING

The developmental tasks for old age generally include the following (Burnside, 1979):

1. Adjusting to decreasing health and physical strength
2. Adjusting to retirement and reduced income
3. Adjusting to the death of a spouse
4. Acceptance of one's self as an aging person
5. Maintaining satisfactory living arrangements
6. Realigning relationships with adult children
7. Finding meaning in life

To varying degrees these tasks are incorporated into the theories of aging discussed here. In addition, key tasks and potential problems when they are not met are listed in Table 25-3.

Psychological theories of aging have sought to describe the aging process and to explain behaviors observed during this life phase. Cummings and Henry (1961) formulated the *disengagement theory of aging.* Withdrawal is a key concept in this theory. The disengagement theory postulates that aging people withdraw from customary roles fulfilled during middle years and invest themselves in more introspective, self-focused activities. The protective mechanisms of withdrawal and introspection allow the individual to establish a new balance, permitting adaptation to the numerous changes of aging. Additionally, withdrawal of society from the aged creates a state of mutual withdrawal.

The *activity theory,* at the opposite end of the spectrum, fosters the continuation of activities during middle age as the criterion for successful aging. The active old person who maintains social relationships, is involved in community activities, travels, and has many hobbies and activities is considered the model old person (Havighurst, 1963). Societal expectations and rewards still imply support for this theory of successful aging.

The *developmental or continuity theory of aging* emphasizes a continuation of the individual's unique traits, characteristics, and habits into the later years without much change from earlier age. Interiority, which emphasizes the importance of one's own system of values, introspection, and individuality (Neugarten, 1964), is a key concept in this theory. The developmental or continuity theory represents one balance between the extremes of the disengagement and activity theories.

The work on the *eight stages of life* (Erikson, 1963) provides another perspective for viewing aging. In this theory, timing, sequential order of movement, and accomplishment of certain critical tasks are essential for movement from one life stage to the next. Aging is viewed as the successful resolution of the conflict between the critical tasks of integrity and despair. Positive resolution results in people whose recapitulation of their lives reveals contentment with life and indicates that their relationships have involved a blending of leading and following. The individual suffering from despair regrets that life cannot begin again and be better and that the remaining years are too few.

The *wear and tear* theory of aging emphasizes that aging is a programed process wherein cells are constantly wearing out, affected by harmful stress factors and the accumulation of harmful by-products. Such physiological theories explain

---

 TABLE 25-3

Developmental tasks and potential problems of the elderly

Tasks	Potential problems
Adjusting to decreasing health and physical strength	Hypochondria, anger, anxiety, chronicity, grief, depression, low self-esteem, loss of health
Adjusting to retirement and reduced income	Loss of status, poverty, rejection, low self-esteem
Adjusting to death of a spouse	Loss of spouse, grief, guilt, loneliness, depression
Acceptance of self as an aging person	Rejection, low self-esteem
Maintaining satisfactory living arrangements	Dependency, isolation
Realigning relationships with adult children	Conflict, hostility, rejection, loneliness, isolation
Finding meaning in life	Guilt, despair, suicide

aging as stemming from a breakdown in performance of bodily organs and systems (Steffl, 1984). The autoimmune reaction is the basis of the *autoimmunity theory* of aging (Ebersole & Hess, 1981). With increased age, normal cells within the body are not recognized by the body as its own, and the body sets off a protective mechanism, forming antibodies against the "unknown cells."

Although these theories provide some explanations for the aging process, no one theory completely explains the aging process for all people. However, theories of aging are still important to nursing because they can provide a framework within which practice decisions can be made.

HEALTH PROMOTION

Physical, as well as psychosocial or developmental changes accompany aging. The observed changes represent the cu-

---

NORMAL CHANGES IN AGING

INTEGUMENTARY SYSTEM

Hair and nails: hair thin and gray, receding hairline, thicker nails

Skin: wrinkles, thinning, drier, easily bruised, decreased perspiration, spotty pigmentation

SENSORY SYSTEM

Sight: increased opacity of lens, grayish white corneal ring, less tearing, droopy eyelids, inability to focus on near objects

Hearing: slight decline in hearing (especially for high frequency tones)

Touch: decreased differentiation of cold, heat, and touch sensations

Smell: diminished sense of smell, prominent or protruding nose

Taste: diminished taste bud sensations, less saliva, dry mouth

MUSCULOSKELETAL SYSTEM

Flabby muscles, less energy and more frequent fatigue, slower and shorter gait, less swinging of arms, stooped posture, loss of height, some rubbing of articular cartilage in joints, stiffening of joints, porous and lighter bones

CARDIOVASCULAR-RESPIRATORY SYSTEM

Lessened vital capacity, decreased chest movement, slower pulse, increased systolic and decreased diastolic pressures, poor reaction to increased and sustained demand on heart activity

GASTROINTESTINAL-GENITOURINARY SYSTEM

Decrease motility of gastrointestinal system (organ) function, less secretion of digestive enzymes and acid secretions, slower emptying of stomach, decreased filtering ability of urinary system, polyuria, drier vaginal mucosa, enlarged prostate glands

NERVOUS SYSTEM

Atrophy of brain cells, slower reflexes

---

mulative and lifelong effects of heredity, environment, nutrition, rest, activity, and altered health status. Both men and women experience some changes in hair color and distribution. The thinning epidermis, dehydrated dermis, lessened blood supply, loss of skin elasticity, and reduction and loss of subcutaneous fat culminate in wrinkles. The skin surrounding the eyes is affected by aging. Lines about the lateral canthus of the eyes form shapes resembling crow's feet. The gastrointestinal changes during aging are the result of a reduction in the senses of smell and taste and decreased gastric and intestinal secretion and motility. These changes, in addition to those listed in the box at left represent some of the changes that affect the body. Increased efforts to educate the elderly about normal changes during aging must become a priority nursing intervention.

A life-style of healthy habits during the early years contributes to the well-being of older adults, since the continuation of healthy habits and the addition of age-specific habits improve the quality and quantity of life. Aging can be healthy, and old age is not synonymous with ill health or a pronouncement "to take it easy and retire to the rocking chair." Moderation in exercise, diet, and alcoholic beverage consumption and meaningful activities provide for days of meaningful living. Regular physical checkups, adherence to prescribed treatment regimens, and healthy life-styles must replace expressions such as "medicine won't do any good," "I haven't seen a doctor in so many years, why see a doctor now?" and "I've just got a few years left, so I can eat and do what I please." Discussions of health education topics concerning nutrition, sleep patterns, exercise, older adult development and changes, health care costs and self-care strategies need to be directed to both elderly individuals and groups.

Immunization and nutrition are selected health promotion issues included in this chapter. Other health promotion activities such as exercise are addressed in Chapter 28.

Immunization

Immunization against influenza is a special safeguard for older adults with chronic illnesses and respiratory problems such as emphysema. Pneumonia vaccines also are available. The older adult should discuss the advisability of influenza and pneumonia immunization with his or her private physician in view of the existing controversy about the use of such preventive measures.

Nutrition

As discussed in Chapter 28, a balanced diet including the four food groups is essential to good nutrition. Nutrients such as protein, minerals, calcium, and vitamins must be included in sufficient amounts, which are generally considered the same as for younger people. A diet pattern of three meals per day is just as important during the later years as during the earlier years. Modification of caloric intake is necessary to keep off excess weight, since the physical activity of many older adults declines. Adequate hydration with sufficient amounts of water is good nutritional practice.

Sociological, economic, and biological factors contribute to the eating habits of older persons. Some of these factors are living arrangements, availability of transportation, limited income, dentition, sense of smell and taste, digestion, and myths about nutrition. Some typical statements of older adults are "I don't feel like cooking just for myself. I just eat something light like cereal, soup, and sometimes some vegetables";"I don't like to eat alone";"I don't have an appetite; nothing tastes good." Health status, physical activity, cultural practices, individuality, and physiological changes of aging also must be considered in determining nutritional requirements. Attractive meals, companionship, and good dentition and digestion make mealtimes both healthy and enjoyable.

MAJOR HEALTH PROBLEMS

Although many older adults enjoy good health and freedom of activity, others do not share this distinction. Approximately 80% of the group over age 65 has at least one chronic health problem. Limitation of an activity of daily living is present in half of the elderly population, and 18% of this same group cannot carry on a major activity (Healthy People, 1979). Cardiovascular, arthritic, and visual problems are the three most frequently reported activity-limiting conditions experienced by this age group (Need for Long-term Care, 1981).

The major causes of death in people over age 65 are heart disease, malignant neoplasms, and cerebrovascular diseases (U.S. Bureau, 1984). Other leading causes of death for the elderly are shown in Table 25-4. The following section discusses selected health problems and nursing management of these conditions.

Hypertension

Hypertension is a cardiovascular disease that is a common malady of aging and a major community health problem for elderly and middle-aged adults. In 1981 the rate of hypertension in the 65-years-and-over age category was ap-

proximately 379 per 1000 people, in contrast to a rate of 244 per 1000 for people between 45 and 64 years of age (U.S. Bureau, 1984). Blacks are more often affected by hypertension, as are men. To lower these numbers, risk factors such as smoking, obesity, high salt intake, and lack of exercise must be reduced. Repeated blood pressure readings of 95 mm Hg (diastolic) and 160 mm Hg (systolic) usually indicate hypertension. Prescribed treatment regimens include antihypertensive drugs, optimal weight control, salt restriction, *stress management,* and a balance of rest and exercise. Nursing activities for older adults with hypertension include monitoring blood pressure and weight, giving nutrition and drug education, teaching stress management techniques, and promoting an optimal balance between rest and activity. Blood pressure measurements are important in the secondary prevention of advancement of the illness and of complications. Additionally, routine blood pressure readings establish patients' normal range of blood pressure. Case finding through blood pressure screening is an imporant primary prevention strategy.

In assisting the older adult with hypertension to achieve optimal weight, psychosociocultural factors, life-style, and overall health status must be considered. The community health nurse must assess the client's current life-style and desires so that plans can be made with the client to introduce acceptable changes. A weight reduction diet in conjunction with techniques of self-awareness, motivation, and reward aid the older adult in substituting old eating habits with more health-promoting habits. Food selection and preparation provide the core of nutrition education. For example, canned soups and vegetables, smoked or salted meats, and condiments such as pickles, catsup, and seasoned salts should be avoided. Lemon juice, oregano, thyme, and other spices and herbs may be substituted for salt and fat in the preparation of foods. Older adults must be taught to read labels to determine the financial, as well as the nutritional,

TABLE 25-4
Ten leading causes of death*

Cause	Age			
	55-64	65-74	75-84	85 plus
All causes	1298	2885	6330	15048
Diseases of the heart	469	1156	2801	7342
Malignant neoplasms	440	825	1239	1599
Cerebrovascular diseases	59	194	675	2001
Accidents and adverse effects	37	51	104	256
Chronic obstructive pulmonary disease	42	131	236	278
Pneumonia and influenza	16	48	183	748
Diabetes	26	60	125	212
Suicide	17	17	20	18
Chronic liver disease and cirrhosis	37	40	31	18
Atherosclerosis	5	21	103	563

From National Center for Health Statistics: Advance report of final mortality statistics, 1982, vol. 33, no. 9; Dec. 20, 1984.
*Rates per 100,000 population in specified group.

value of products. It is not enough to explain the prescribed diet to the client. Including the person in the family with the primary responsibility for food selection and preparation and other significant family members along with the client increases compliance with the prescribed diet, food restrictions, and other nutrition teaching. Chapters 28 and 30 discuss stress, exercise, and nutrition further.

Use of the Dietary Modification Activity Guide (see box below) is one strategy the community health nurse can use to assist a client with diet modifications.

Health teaching must also include information about drug and food interactions, as well as interactions among drugs. The replacement of potassium via drugs, food, or both may be necessary for some persons receiving diuretics as treatment for hypertension. For instance, the use of cold remedies by people with hypertension can increase blood pressure. It is essential that hypertensive individuals understand and accept the chronic nature of the illness and the need for lifelong adherence to treatment.

The interrelationship between mind and body is important in hypertension. This interrelationship can be assessed by questions such as the following: What stress or tension have you experienced during the past week (or some other time reference)? Where is the discomfort felt in your body when you are upset? What other things were going on in your life when you started to feel bad and had headaches and dizziness? The total benefits of drugs and dietary management of hypertension cannot be realized without some regard for the individual's stress level. Relaxation techniques, problem-solving skills, and exercise are all strategies for the management of stress. Chapter 30 elaborates further on stress management techniques.

Cancer

Malignant neoplasm, or cancer, is the second most common cause of death in older people in the United States (Healthy People, 1979). Early detection and treatment are still valuable for this age group. Preventive programs for cancer must include cessation of smoking; close vigilance for change in skin moles, altered bowel habits, or nonhealing sores; and regular physical examinations, including pelvic and rectal examinations. Monthly breast self-examinations and annual Pap smears are necessary for older women. Postmenopausal women should establish a consistent time each month for breast self-examination, since there is no menstrual cycle with which to pair the examination. The sociocultural factors affecting this age group must be dealt with so that the goals of regular breast, pelvic, and rectal examinations can become realities. A health history is of immense value, and time must be allocated to focus on data that could provide early detection and diagnosis.

Older adults should be encouraged to become acquainted with their bodies, to attend to physical changes, and to reveal their observations to the health care provider. Often the elderly person's attitude of "It is just old age" and "I don't want to be a bother" creates a barrier to the effective use of the health care system. Correction of misconceptions, emotional support, and quality care during diagnostic and treatment procedures are all activities within the realm of professional nursing.

DIETARY MODIFICATION ACTIVITY GUIDE

1. Ask client to keep a dietary diary for 7 days.
2. Assist the client to compare diary to chart showing recommended dietary pattern.
3. Assist client to modify dietary intake by planning changes to include into next week's meals.
4. Keep dietary diary for 7 days. Follow with steps 2, 3, and 4 as necessary.

FOOD DESCRIPTION	AMOUNT	TIME AND SETTING	MODIFICATIONS
Breakfast			
Grits	½ cup	7:00 AM, kitchen table	
Margarine	4 tb		
Toast	2 slices		
Jelly	2 tb		
Scrambled egg	1		
Coffee	2 cups		
Lunch			
Spinach	½ cup	3:00 PM, kitchen table	
Fried beef patty	1 medium		
Rolls	2		
Margarine	2 tb		
Dinner			
Tea	1 cup	8:00 PM, den	
Dry cereal	¾ cup		
Milk	½ cup		
Sugar	4 tb		

Arthritis

Arthritis is often a devastating disease for the elderly, since it often limits activities and affects comfort and independence. Inflammation, swelling, stiffness, and pain impair mobility and comfort. Approximately 465 per 1000 elderly persons have arthritis, with more women affected than men (U.S. Bureau, 1984). Inflammation and degenerative changes of the joints are usually involved in arthritis. Rheumatoid arthritis generally affects the peripheral joints symmetrically. Symptoms include inflammation, pain, stiffness, swelling, numbness and tingling of the hands and feet, malaise, and weight loss. Treatment generally is medication, combined rest and activity regimens, heat or cold applications, and physical therapy (Luckmann & Sorenson, 1980).

It is important for health care providers to help clients avoid the false hope and expense of arthritis quackery, which offers ineffective and often harmful "cures." Client education should include information on the management of activities, correct body mechanics, and adequate rest. Stress management is also important for controlling the disease process. Persons affected by arthritis may need supportive devices and appliances such as walkers and special chairs, food utensils, and grooming aids. In addition safety measures, such as clear passage-ways to avoid falls, often are needed to avoid injury. As functional dependency and isolation from people increase, human resources and mechanical aids may be needed. The community health nurse can be instrumental in counseling and assisting the client's family to improve open communication, role negotiation, and use of community resources dealing with arthritis.

Sensory Impairments

Sensory impairment in the elderly may involve deficits in any of the five senses: sight, hearing, touch, smell, or taste. Visual impairment in the 65-years-and-over age group occurs in about 137 per 1000 persons. Hearing impairment occurs in 284 per 1000 persons, with more men than women being affected (U.S. Bureau, 1984). Sight and hearing sensory impairments limit the elderly's activities and mobility and creates difficulties in perception and social interaction. Recreational activities, including reading and watching television, also are affected. The older adult who cannot hear has difficulty joining in family conversations and using the telephone. Furthermore, hearing and visual deficits render people more susceptible to victimization by crime because they may not hear or see the attacker.

Major visual problems for the elderly include loss of visual acuity, eyelid disorders, and opacity of the lens. Loss of skin elasticity and diminished muscle tone of the lids can contribute to the occurrence of entropion and ectropion. In entropion, the eye lashes rub against the cornea, causing irritation and discomfort. In ectropion, there is constant tearing and an overflow of tears, which result in dryness and damage to the eye. Additionally, dryness may result from the normal reduction of tear production that occurs in aging. Opacity of the lens, or cataracts, are prevalent in the elderly population. The resulting density of the lens may cause poor vision and a low tolerance for glares (Kahn, 1981).

Presbycusis is a hearing loss that results from aging and is usually moderate in degree for most frequencies; the greatest loss of hearing occurs with high frequency tones. The person may miss sounds within words and thus has difficulty understanding conversations. This condition is caused because high-frequency tones are unclear, not because the volume is too low. Therefore, speech sounds distorted even when comfortably loud (Margolis, Levy, and Sherman, 1981).

Sight problems can cause many problems. For instance, they can impair proper use of medication because the person may be unable to read medication labels. Additionally, many educational materials and health care and insurance claim forms use print that cannot be read by elderly people. The community health nurse must be aware of the older patient's hearing and visual problems when providing health teaching. Strategies such as speaking with clarity and distinction, at a moderate volume and pace, and while facing the audience from a close position are invaluable to successful teaching. A well-lighted, glare-free environment without extraneous noise also enhances sensory perception, as does the use of printed aids with large, well-spaced letters in primary colors. Also, reminding or assisting elderly people to clean their eyeglass lenses is helpful. The community health nurse can help the older person make arrangements for vision and hearing examinations and obtain the necessary prostheses. The nurse must teach the elderly to be cautious of fraudulent advertisement and not to purchase unnecessary aids.

Touch, smell, and taste are other senses that can undergo change in older persons. Decreases in sensory perception necessitate protections against burns (for instance, from heating appliances or bath water) and against exposure to cold temperatures. Increased risk from burns or toxins, such as gas and carbon monoxide, may result from an inability to detect odors. Taste bud changes may affect nutritional habits, requiring a change in food selections and the use of large amounts of seasonings and flavorings to make food tasty. The community health nurse can play a vital role in helping older persons cope with sensory impairments, maximize existing assets, and maintain a safe yet functional environment.

Confusional States

Confusional states include disorientation, memory loss, shortened attention spans, and impaired judgment. Absence of stimulation, toxicity, environmental changes, medications, and metabolic conditions may contribute to varying degrees of confusion. Confusional states are generally classified as reversible or irreversible. Reversible confusion, also referred to as *acute brain syndrome,* occurs rapidly, is limited in duration, and is secondary to a correctable condition. In contrast, irreversible confusion develops slowly and is progressive. *Chronic brain syndrome, dementia,* and *senility* are other terms used to describe irreversible confusion.

Treatment of confusional states consists of a thorough

assessment and diagnosis, correction of underlying causative factors or disease, provision for a protective environment, and activities that reinforce reality. Patience, a caring attitude, calm conversation, and promotion of comfort contribute to the relief of confusional states. Personal hygiene and adequate nutrition and hydration also must be provided. In addition, emotional support helps the family cope with the elderly person's disorientation and confusion. Descriptions of persons who wander into busy streets or forget about food still cooking are familiar reports from families and neighbors. As functions decline, anxiety and frustration increase in both the older adult and his or her family. Confusional states present a challenge to the elderly's adult relations, usually his or her children, who often are involved with careers, family life, and other middle-life tasks or who may, themselves, be elderly. The following case study on confusional states highlights some of the issues presented by this major problem of later life.

> Mrs. Hill, 80 years old, wanders away from the home she shares with her daughter and 10- and 15-year-old grandchildren. She is found by the local police on the expressway. Mrs. Hill is carried to the local hospital for observation and care until her family can be notified.

1. What problems would you identify?
2. What initial plan of care would you develop for Mrs. Hill and her family?
3. What community resources may be helpful to this family?

Alzheimer's Disease

Alzheimer's disease is an irreversible confusional state that is gaining recognition as a major health problem for the elderly (see box below). Approximately 1.5 to 2.5 million older people are affected by this disease (Alzheimer's Dis-

ease, 1984). Obtaining accurate figures is impeded by problems of early recognition and in accurately diagnosing this gradually degenerative disease. Furthermore, difficulties with defining the behaviors and symptoms that constitute the disease compound the problem. The term is sometimes used to refer to the disease and is usually qualified by words such as presenile or senile, depending on when the condition develops. Presenile dementia designates the condition in the young, whereas senile dementia, Alzheimer's type, describes the disease in older people.

Etiological hypotheses such as changes in the cholinergic system, heredity, and the effects of toxins, viruses, and other agents have been formulated and are being investigated by scientists (Alzheimer's Disease, 1984). Although knowledge about the disease is limited, certain symptoms are characteristic, for instance, memory loss and mental deterioration. Hayter (1974) described three stages, or categories, of symptoms (Table 25-5).

Although there is no established cure for Alzheimer's disease, some measures are being studied to manage the progressive, nonreversible processes of this debilitating illness. Medical treatment for Alzheimer's disease includes pharmacological interventions with cholinergic agents (choline, lecithin, or physostigmine); neuropeptides (ACTH and vasopressin analogs); and *psychotropic medications.*

The nursing care treatment goals for individuals with Alzheimer's disease should include maintaining optimal functioning, protection, and safety and fostering human dignity. Assistance with activities of daily living can best be accomplished by a caring person who patiently and firmly instructs, reminds, and assists the person with Alzheimer's disease in eating, dressing, grooming, and toileting. Prais-

---

ALZHEIMER'S DISEASE: RESEARCH PRIORITIES

Research is one strategy for increasing knowledge of Alzheimer's disease. The increased federal support of research from $4 million in 1976 to $25 million in 1983 illustrates the priority that is being given to conquering this devastating illness. Nine areas of research were formulated by the Health and Human Services Departmental Task Force on Alzheimer's Disease:
1. Epidemiology
2. Etiology and pathogenesis
3. Diagnosis
4. Clinical course
5. Treatment
6. Family
7. Systems of care
8. Training of research and clinical personnel
9. Educational materials and information dissemination for professionals and the public

Source: Alzheimer's Disease, Washington, D.C., 1984, U.S. Department of Health and Human Services.

TABLE 25-5

Alzheimer's disease: stages and symptoms

Stage 1 (2 to 4 years)	Stage 2 (several years)	Stage 3 (1 year)
Memory loss	Progressive memory loss	Deterioration of social skills and skills needed for eating, elimination, communication
Time disorientation	Aphasia	Anorexia
Lack of spontaneity	Agnosia	Seizures
Logical thinking exceeds memory ability	Apraxia	Mutism
	Wandering	
	Perseveration	
	Muscular twitching and seizures	
	Confabulations	

Source: Hayter, J. (1974). Patients who have Alzheimer's Disease. *American Journal of Nursing,* 74(8), 1460-1463.

ing the person with Alzheimer's disease for small achievements promotes independence, self-esteem, and dignity. Environments that provide both the least restrictions and the greatest protection and safety should be created and modified as individual needs change. Community health nurses can demonstrate to the primary family caregiver techniques of dressing an adult in garments that are made of easily cared for fabrics and that have simple, easily manipulated openings and few or no detachable objects. Caregivers need frequent encouragement to cope with the frustrations that may arise from repeating the same information and directions.

Respite care and support groups are valuable aids for the client's family. In addition to providing support for family members and functioning as a resource, the community health nurse must continuously be an advocate for the person with Alzheimer's disease. The nurse must ensure that the client's rights are protected, which sometimes requires seeking legal and protective services on the client's behalf. The community health nurse also must be viewed as an advocate for family members. Family support for provision of leisure time, reliefs for anxiety, anger, guilt, and grief, and maintenance of physical and mental health must be promoted by the nurse. The combined efforts of the nurse and the family can prevent mental and physical exhaustion of the family. The economic and emotional impact of Alzheimer's disease on the client's family may require the use of many community resources. Maintaining family stability must be a priority in any plans developed by the community health nurse.

Dental Problems

Many persons aged 65 and over have some, if not all, of their natural teeth; however, the most prevalent dental health problem is tooth loss (Fact Book on Aging, 1978). The loosening of permanent teeth, periodontoclasia, may result from changes in tooth support or periodontal disease. Although normal aging changes must be differentiated from pathological conditions, both can cause serious problems. Diminished salivary secretion and some loss of taste sensation are considered normal changes in aging; however, these complaints still need attention. Complaints of poor dentition, dry mouth, difficult swallowing, taste changes, and sore gums may contribute to changes in eating, chewing, and utimately nutritional status. Problems of constipation, fatigue, loss of appetite, weight loss, and anemia may also occur. Medications affecting oral hygiene include antibiotics, anticonvulsants, phenothiazines, cholinergic blocking agents, and antihistamines.

Dental problems can be reduced by the early establishment of good dental health habits. Regular brushing and flossing, proper nutrition, and regular dental examinations reduce the incidence of dental health problems in the elderly. Vulnerability to oral health problems necessitates continuing oral assessment and care in this age group. Early recognition of problems usually means correction of a minor problem for minimal cost and with minimal discomfort. Oral assessments should include a thorough oral health history and an inspection of the color and condition of lips,

gums, teeth, tongue, and mucosa. Painful swallowing and sore or bleeding gums require further investigation. Caries or loose teeth should be identified and their location and the presence or absence of pain noted. The upper and lower surfaces of the tongue and the floor of the mouth should be inspected, and any abnormal smoothness of the dorsal or upper surface of the tongue should be noted.

The use of mouth wash or a commercial preparation; rinsing with warm tap water; use of lubricants such as lanolin, cocoa butter, or petroleum jelly; drinking increased fluids; and eating frequent, small, nutritionally balanced meals all contribute to correcting some minor oral health problems. The importance of regular dental and physical examinations cannot be overemphasized. People with dentures need to be encouraged to wear and properly care for them. Complaints of malfitting dentures must be investigated, with the necessary adjustments made to ensure proper fit. Areas for oral assessment are summarized in the following list.

    Oral health history
        Health problems
        Medications
        Dentures
        Brushing and flossing practices
        Appetite
        Taste and food preferences
        Painful chewing, swallowing
        Bleeding gums
    Inspection
        Structural components: lips, gums, teeth, tongue, mucosa, palate, pharnyx
        Conditions: odor, dryness-moistness, redness, soreness, color, swelling, bleeding
    Caries
    Loose teeth
    Ulcerations
    Facial grimaces

Encouragement of denture use and praise for appearance are strategies for the successful care of persons with dentures. Oral and dental health are important to digestion, speech, appearance, and body image and therefore must be stressed to older people as worthy of the expenditure of time. Efforts must be made to remove the dental care gap in the health care of the elderly. In addition, problems regarding financing dental care, negative stereotypes and attitudes about receiving dental care, mistrust and fear of the dentist, and access to dental care facilities must be acknowledged, confronted, and resolved.

Drug Use and Abuse

Drug sensitivity, paradoxical reactions, and drug-taking are all factors that contribute to the elderly populations' risk for drug problems. Drug misuse includes overdoses, inadequate doses, and inappropriate drug combinations. Many prescribed drugs are improperly self-administered in amount, frequency, and combination and improperly stored. The cost of medications and the frugality of the elderly combine to encourage the saving of drugs from one occasion to another and the use of previously prescribed drugs after new drugs have been prescribed. It is not uncommon to hear an older adult comment, "My old pill worked better than this new one, so I started to take the old pill again." In addition, the older adult must adjust to changed routines when new medicines with unfamiliar directions are given. Comparing and sharing medicines is another common practice of this age group. The combining of prescribed medicines can be serious, as can the combining or prescribed and nonprescribed over-the-counter (OTC) medicines.

Nursing interventions must include a drug history; directions for safe storage of drugs; cautions about drug-drug and drug-food interactions; and drug information, such as name, purpose, intended benefits, side effects, dosage, and frequency and route of administration. A checkoff system using a date and time calendar and presorting according to medication, dosage, and time of administration are valuable techniques for persons who have difficulty preparing medications or trouble with memory. Presorting strategies include the use of egg cartons or small envelopes, which contain the correct dosage and are labeled with specific administration times. The community health nurse must instruct the older adult in the presorting technique, for example, by saying "Mr. Yates, you are to take the medicine in the envelope marked *1* on Sunday morning at 8:00 AM, envelope *2* on Monday morning at 8:00 AM . . . and I will return on Thursday, the day you take the medicine in envelope *5*." Drugs can be savers or destroyers of life, and community health nurses must help clients capitalize on the life saving aspects.

Substance Abuse

Although *substance abuse,* involving alcohol and other drugs, is present in the older adult population, the exact incidence is difficult to determine because of the life-style of the elderly abuser. The older person who lives alone, drinks to avoid loneliness and boredom, and uses pills for sleep and medications for pain is in an environment that may create substance abuse. Additionally, because the time of many elderly people is unstructured, the daily drinking of alcohol may involve a greater consumption level. The problem of abuse is intensified when coupled with the effects of chronic illnesses. Alcohol abusers include both those persons who begin excessive drinking during old age and long-time alcoholics who have lived into old age. Other abused drugs include sedatives and tranquilizers. As discussed in Chapter 35, treatment approaches in substance abuse generally include monitored detoxification, counseling, stress management, self-help groups, and treatment of any disease stemming from the abuse practices. Community resources such as Alcoholics Anonymous and Al-Anon can be valuable agencies in the total treatment of the older adult. Education of the public continues to be a major task of the community health nurse.

PSYCHOSOCIAL ASPECTS OF AGING
Coping with Retirement

The ability to successfully adjust to *retirement* is affected by such factors as health status, sufficient income, number of situational changes, quality of personal relationships, ability to manage time effectively, flexibility, ability to relinquish the work routine, and anticipation and realistic expectation for retirement. The community health nurse has an important role in assisting to maximize the potential of the retiree. The best preparation for retirement comes years before the event. Good health practices, for instance, begin in utero and continue throughout life. However, circumstances, life-style choice, and other factors sometimes combine to create health problems. In such instances the individual has to learn to adapt to illness. Chronic health problems must be dealt with through life-style adjustments and management of prescribed regimens.

The community health nurse can often provide direction and guidance to the retiree and the family. Professional support for the family is an important nursing role benefiting both the retiree and the family. For instance, the community health nurse may speak to a group of preretirees at a local industry, thus providing them with information about normal expectations and behaviors, *time management,* and other issues often excluded in the customary financial planning programs for preretirees. Education regarding the normal changes of aging, health, retirement, and problems of aging promotes understanding, caring, and positive actions. Two critical aspects of adjustment to retirement relate to how effectively the retiree learns to restructure time and to the quality of personal relationships.

Managing Time

Retirement, formally institutionalized in the United States by the passage of the Social Security Act in 1935, generally occurs at the age of 65 years. At the moment of retirement the worker is confronted with the loss of his or her job, a reduction in income, and the loss of and/or altered relations with co-workers. Time becomes available, and the individual asks, "What will I do with all of this time?"

Time management is crucial for older adults, who generally have a great deal of free time. The day must promise to be a good enough day that an individual is motivated to arise and meet the day's challenges and opportunities. Loneliness is one consequence of inadequate, pleasureless, or absent interpersonal relationships, with many older adults masking loneliness with various complaints such as insomnia, indigestion, muscular aches, and general malaise. Many do not possess leisure-time skills; consequently they feel alienated, lonely, and unhappy with the increased time available in later years. Considering the present life expectancy, a person can anticipate living for several years in retirement. Some realistic plans regarding the pursuit of meaningful activities during retirement must be made. Senior centers offer a social outlet, as well as numerous other services.

Mrs. A, who has to take a taxi to the center, makes the trip on Monday, Wednesday, and Friday to avoid being home alone and thinking and grieving about her deceased husband. Participation in crafts, water exercise, and health education programs have proved to be an effective use of her time. Other people, like Mr. J, Miss T, and Mrs. O, gain purpose and meaningfully use time by volunteering to serve juice, set the table, help in the kitchen, or do the "Thoughts for Living" at the nutrition center. Additionally, they have earned hours as Retired Senior Volunteer Program (RSVP) workers and are publicly recognized for their contribution.

The retired person should plan for ways to satisfy basic needs, to further develop their total person, and to derive happiness from living in addition to planning for fun, entertainment, and leisure. The development of hobbies and interests during earlier years provides a pivotal point for activities during later years. A meaningful activity is one that is congruent with the life-style, interests, resources, and health of the older adult. Health-promoting leisure pursuits for older adults generally include physical fitness activities; visiting in person or via the telephone with relatives and friends; arts and crafts such as painting, sewing and ceramics; viewing television; reading; and travel. New interests should be encouraged by the community health nurse, other health care workers, family, and significant others. Referrals and information about available community activities can be provided by the community health nurse. Many organizations, such as nutrition centers, community schools, and multipurpose senior centers, provide places for older adults to convene for leisure pursuits and to meet other older adults (see Chapter 29).

Realignment of Relationships

Retirees often must reconsider the relationships between themselves and significant others, including spouse, family, and neighbors. Family relationships represent one of the challenges of this age period. The retired person must learn to live with or without his or her spouse. A man who has spent many years working away from home must now spend many hours at home; this requires adjustment. The woman who has been home alone must now become accustomed to having her husband underfoot all day. As families increasingly become characterized by two working adults, it will be interesting to note the adjustment impact on persons who are both retiring at or near the same time and who will have many hours to spend together.

Another aspect of family relationships after retirement is the relationship realignment between aging parents and their adult children. Issues of role reversal, dependency, conflict, guilt, and loss require recognition and resolution.

The community health nurse must consider the parent who has always met the affiliative as well as the physical needs of each household member and who now needs assistance with feeding, bathing, dressing, and mobility and must rely on the adult children to accomplish such daily tasks. Such reversal of "helper-helpee" roles can create a climate of kind caring and love or one of hostile dependency. Many community health nurses hear countless expressions of "when parents grow old they are just like children experiencing second childhood." Such phrases perpetuate a decline in self-esteem, self-worth, and equalitarian relationships.

A second issue, guilt, is highlighted in adult children who feel the pangs of "if only I had 'come sooner,'" made the aging adult move in with us, or realized that the be-

haviors were symptoms of a problem rather than meanness, stubbornness, or cantankerousness." The community health nurse is in a position to assist adult children with their middle-life tasks and crises, as well as to be a resource for helping with the compounding problems of their parents' later-life tasks and crises. In addition, the further compounded effects of the presence and influence of younger children and adolescents must be reconciled. Nursing strategies for providing knowledge about normal developmental needs throughout the life span, communication, conflict resolution, and valuing other people are essential in working with multigenerational families.

Living on a fixed income is another issue of importance to the retiree. Many retirees can expect to receive Social Security benefits and employment-related pensions. An additional segment may have savings or rental or other supplemental income. Thus budget planning and wise shopping can help those on a fixed income. In addition, some supplement their income with part-time work or the exchange of services such as cooking, shopping, childcare, or home cleaning. Other income extenders include food stamps and Supplemental Security Income (SSI) for eligible individuals.

Maintaining Self-Esteem

Self-esteem is critical in the later years of life. One adaptive task associated with later years and aging is to reassess the criteria used to evaluate the self. Ideas used as a basis for self-concept often need to be modified to establish identity and personal worth in roles other than the work role. Planned activities and programs, satisfying interpersonal relationships, good health, quality housing, adequate income, and suitable transportation all contribute to high self-esteem (Schwartz, 1978).

Nursing activities to promote a high level of self-esteem include recognition of achievements; providing positive feedback; granting respect and courtesies; promoting choice, decision making, and control; and encouraging and facilitating interpersonal relationships. An observing community health nurse can comment on certificates, rewards, and pictures that may be visible in the living environment. Encouragement for work or volunteer services that make use of existing knowledge and skills can be valuable; for example, a retired teacher might tutor a group of schoolchildren, another might teach a special hobby to older adults at the multipurpose senior center, a carpenter might assist in building shelves for the display of the center's produced items, and an annual bazaar and sale of crafts might be spearheaded by an older business entrepreneur. Each one can be recognized for at least one desirable trait and thereby feel needed and valued. Additionally, the community health nurse must remember the small yet significant value of addressing older adults with appropriate titles such as Mr., Mrs., Miss, Dr., Rev., and Father. Policy-makers must be made aware of the consequences of various policies on the self-esteem and personhood of elderly adults. Policies can implicitly state that "We care about you," "Old people are of value to this country," and "Minority producers and consumers also have clout."

Coping with Loss and Grief

Loss and grief are common companions of the elderly adult and threaten the maintenance of self-esteem. Loss of roles through retirement, of health from chronic illnesses, and of a spouse are just a few of the losses. *Widowhood* is a problem of later years in addition to other problems; thereby multiplying and making more complex issues that have to be faced. Women are at higher risk for loss of a spouse because women outnumber men and live longer. Married women can expect to live some of their later years in widowhood. Additionally, remarriage following widowhood is less frequent in women because there are fewer older men and older men generally select younger women as spouses.

Loss of a spouse often includes identifiable behaviors. The beginning phase of grief is characterized by a person experiencing shock, disbelief, and denial. Sadness and crying ensue as awareness of the reality of death is experienced. The survivors carry out the ritual of a funeral and other culturally meaningful practices and rites as part of the grieving process. The steps of living alone, relinquishing the lost spouse, and reinvesting oneself in something and/or someone awaits the widow or widower. The nursing activities of providing correct information, a sense of reality, supportive listening, and caring during periods of crying and other emotional releases are essential to healthy grieving. The community health nurse can be a caring individual and provider when the family and friends have returned to their routine activities and the mourner is left alone to deal with problems of loneliness, social isolation, altered finances, changed living arrangements, and a new identity.

Time is important in healing the wound and allowing for successful grieving. Self-help groups, counseling, or both may be beneficial during this phase for assisting the remaining spouse to cope with loss without feeling guilty or losing self-esteem. Present practices of fewer marriages, cohabitation, more divorces, childlessness, geographic mobility, financial instability, and improved educational and health status present special challenges in planning care for future widows or widowers. People must be educated to plan for their later years in life-style choices that are made throughout life. Preparation for widowhood must be of a multifarious nature and must include both financial and psychosocial planning.

Dealing with Depression

Depression is a common health problem of the aged but is often masked by other complaints and problems. Signs to look for when depression is suspected include complaints of sadness, insomnia, anorexia, weight loss, or constipation. Frequently these complaints are undervalued and labeled as normal complaints of old age or as hypochondriasis.

Treatment of the problem must include a thorough history, counseling, and judicious use of medication. Assessment can be made using questions such as the following: Do you awaken during the early morning hours and find yourself unable to return to sleep? Is it hard to "get going" in the morning? Do you feel better as the day progresses? Have your appetite and food intake changed from their usual patterns? Do you have crying spells? Community health

nurses can help older adults adjust to the changes of aging, cope with declining years and health, and view life as meaningful and valuable by aiding in arranging an activity schedule including rest periods, teaching normal expectations of aging and signs of impending health problems, and devising ways of managing financial demands with a fixed income. Nurses as sensitive listeners can be partners for older adults in the life review process. The life review process, including reminiscing and reviewing the past joys, accomplishments, and disappointments, is helpful to the older adult in resolving unresolved conflicts, in bringing order to life, in relinquishing life, and in preparing for death.

After sustaining a major loss, life problems may mount so that some older adults see ending their own life as a viable option, leading to an alarming suicide rate in the elderly. Those over 65 years account for one fourth of the suicides in the United States, with blacks and women committing fewer suicides (Fact Book on Aging, 1978). Thus some of America's most valuable resources are being destroyed by their own hands. Early detection of danger signs and timely interventions can decrease this problem. Cues to the potential for suicide include making a will, giving away possessions and valuables, and planning a funeral. Additionally, subtle and indirect clues include refusing to eat, medication misuse, and noncompliance with health-sustaining treatment regimens. During contacts with older adults, community health nurses should watch for suicide risks, determine lethality, recognize and compliment clients on areas of individual worth and esteem, and encourage meaningful activities and associations.

A sense of purpose, hope, and worth are derived from authentic encounters and experiences with caring people. The community health nurse may determine that the client has been unresponsive to nursing interventions and that additional care is warranted. Referral to a community mental health center, physician, or hospial may be needed. The community health nurse should maintain contact with the referral agency so that the continuity of care may be provided. Additionally, a record of the care rendered by the community health nurse should be sent, with the written permission of the client, to the referral agency to avoid unnecessary delays and duplications.

Abuse of the Elderly

Abuse of the elderly can be physical, psychological, or material abuse, as well as violations of the rights for safety, security, and adequate health care. The classic profile of the elderly victim of abuse is generally an older woman with mental or physical impairments who lives with an adult child or other relative. Abusers are often middle-aged women, related or unrelated caretakers, often experiencing considerable stress. Other contributory factors include economics, interpersonal conflicts, life responsibilities, health, and dependency (Elder Abuse, 1980). Often out of fear, the abused person denies that abusive acts are occurring. The victim's helplessness and resignation to abuse increases as the victim tries to protect self and the caretaker.

Using a family-oriented approach, interventions include counseling for both the abused and the abusers and teaching stress management techniques. In selected instances, placement of the abused adult in a protected setting outside of the home, family vacations as a respite time from the older adult, and sharing of responsibilities among children may be necessary. As described in Chapter 34, family violence continues to be a serious community problem, whether it is violence of child, spouse, or elder. Priorities in the area of prevention must be established if protection of individuals at risk is to become a reality.

Criminal Victimization

Many elderly individuals are the victims of confidence games, fraudulent consumerism, and crimes against person and property. The fear of crime prevents many elderly persons from leaving their homes, thus making them prisoners in their own homes. The frail, sensory-impaired, poor, older woman who lives alone is a prime candidate for criminal victimization. Physical injury often results from the criminal activity. The popularity of confidence games or swindle tactics such as "bank examiner–crooked bank employee" and "pigeon drop–good faith money" continue to be major threats to the security of older adults. The bank examiner–crooked bank employee game consists of a stranger posing as a bank examiner, federal agent, or special police officer telling the older adult the story of trying to catch a crooked bank employee and needing the older person to withdraw a large amount of cash money from the bank to trap the employee. The pigeon drop–good faith money swindle involves a stranger approaching an elderly person with the pretense of having found a large sum of money, which will be shared with the elderly person; however, the elderly person must first withdraw some money from the bank to show good faith. The elderly person may even be given an envelope, allegedly containing the money, and be instructed not to open the envelope, which in actuality contains cut-up paper.

The community health nurse can caution elderly clients about home repair rip-offs, admitting strangers into one's residence, withdrawing large sums of money from the bank on the request of a stranger, flashing or displaying large sums of money, leaving unlocked car or house doors, and walking alone in dimly lighted, deserted areas. Older adults must be assisted to read and understand legal papers and transactions. Evaluation of product use, quality, and safety must be taught to older adults as part of their role as wise consumers. The slogan of "Buyer Beware" can become a household watchword if law enforcement officers, health care providers, businesses, and policymakers join forces to combat the problem of criminal victimization of the elderly.

HEALTH CARE UTILIZATION AND COSTS

Older persons as a group are major users of health services. Persons aged 65 to 74 years average 7.4 physician visits annually. Although the elderly constitute approximately 12% of the population, they are responsible for about 17% of physician visits. Hospital utilization statistics indicate that the 65-to 74-year-old group had an average hospital stay of about 9 days in 1983, whereas persons 75 to 84 years old averaged 10 hospital days. The length of the

hospital stay increases to 11 days for the 85-years-and-older group. Although hospital stays are relatively short, multiple admissions per year are common occurrences within the elderly population (U.S. Senate, 1986).

Soaring health care costs continue to be a problem for all age groups but are of particular concern for the 65-years-and-older age group, whose members each usually have at least one chronic health problem. Health care costs and expenditures for the elderly are approximately a third of the nation's total health care expenditure, yet they only account for 12% of the population. Although the elderly pay for part of their health care costs (25%), public funds such as Medicare and Medicaid are the major sources.

In April 1983, Public Law 98-21 of the Social Security Amendments was signed into law. Title VI of this law stipulates that Medicare reimbursement for hospital inpatient services be on a prospective payment system (Smith, 1985). This payment system, or Diagnostic Related Groups (DRGs), has created a national health care revolution. The DRGs reimbursement approach is based on payment of a predetermined amount for the care of persons who have a medically related diagnosis and treatment and a similar length of hospital stay. Gender and age factors also are considered in the classification of a person into any of the 467 diagnostic groups. In addition to reimbursement for health care, the system also reviews quality assurance and utilization. (Chapter 3 provides further discussion of DRGs.)

Many changes in the health care system have been attributed to DRGs. The most notable is the earlier discharge of clients. Consequently, more formal and informal caregivers are required to provide a variety of services to recovering individuals. The family, when available, has become an even greater partner in health care delivery. However, the increased number of females who are employed outside the home creates a major barrier to providing continuing care at home to elderly persons who have experienced a brief hospitalization, early discharge, or longer recuperation. Furthermore, bureaucratic barriers are encountered if the need for home health care exceeds the provisions as designated by Medicare guidelines and time frames. The needs of the elderly as listed by Auerbach (1986) are for chronic illness monitoring, supportive services, and acute, posthospitalization care. Medicare categorizes this type of care as requiring unskilled nursing except during the immediate postacute phase, which creates many difficulties for elderly people, their families, and home health care agencies. An elderly population that is more ill and that requires more complex care is another variable influencing community health nursing practice and the home health care industry. It is not uncommon for a home health care nurse to be assigned an elderly person who undergoes intravenous therapy and parenteral nutrition and has a respirator. The need for professional nursing services has grown more intense with these health care changes.

HOME HEALTH SERVICES

Many elderly persons require both daily care from a home health care professional and supportive assistance from home health aides. Home health care services coupled with home-maker services prevent or delay institutionalization for older adults who need some assistance with self-care and other activities of daily living and some care for chronic health problems. Agencies providing home health care, home-maker services, or both may be governmental, proprietary, or hospital based and funded. The combined professional–nonprofessional staff may include a nurse, social worker, physician, occupational therapist, and aide. Some states and agencies require some type of training program and certification for home health care aides. Home health care is covered by Medicare for the person meeting a requirement for skilled care. The care is provided by a professional nurse, or home health aide working under the direction of the professional nurse, or both. The aide performs personal hygiene tasks, measures vital signs, and gives technical care. In contrast to the home health care aide, the homemaker aide, whose services are not covered under Medicare, does light housework and cooking. The visiting nurses' association, community health nurses from local public health departments, and nurses from private agencies provide professional nursing services to home-bound persons needing skilled care.

Additional information on home health care can be found in Chapter 42; Chapter 3 contains more information on the economics of health care. Attention to policy issues, problem resolutions, instructions at the time of discharge, and advocacy activities is central to an effective community health care practice. Community health nurses are a vital link in the health care system, they provide care, institute preventive measures, and reduce functional impairment.

ALTERNATIVES TO INSTITUTIONALIZATION

Day-care centers, day hospitals, respite care, and congregate housing are aimed at delaying or preventing institution-alization. Adult day-care centers associated with health care institutions or ambulatory care settings and multipurpose adult day-care centers are two models of adult day care (Emick-Herring, 1983; Koenen, R.E., 1980). Health oriented–day care centers provide health and physical rehabilitation, whereas multipurpose day-care centers provide social activities and interaction. Day-care centers serve the person who has some physical or mental limitation that interferes with totally independent living for 24 hours per day and who needs social, nutritional, or recreational services. Day-care centers also allow the permanent caretaker to use day hours for work or other activities. The day hospital is directed toward providing day-health services to a person who can live at the home during the evening. The respite-care program provides care for the dependent older person while the permanent caretaker has time off for rest, recuperation, recreation, or an emergency. The services may be used for several days to a week; however, the services provide only time-limited care, and their goal is the return of the dependent older person to a refreshed caretaker.

Congregate housing is an alternative-living arrangement that provides shelter and support services to enable the elderly to effectively manage community living. This type of housing arrangement is best suited for the older adult who is independent or semi-independent and has some functional impairment or social deprivation but is otherwise healthy. Congregate housing may include single or multiple units arranged into a community with some commonly shared areas, such as recreational facilities.

The alternatives to institutionalization are not without disadvantages. Problems of eligibility, cost, access, service limitations, and the impact of long-term disability and care on the client and the family exist and are challenges to the health care system. Should chronic care remain in the shadow of acute care, thus receiving only marginal support and importance? Should eligibility guidelines be such that more people are eliminated from services than receive services? Should a family that chooses to keep the older person at home be penalized with lack of assistance or reward? Is the older adult forced into a more dependent role just to obtain minimal help? The political, professional, ethical, and legal ramifications of each answer must be examined as the next decades experience a growing number of persons over 65 years old who will demand more care for and accountability to the older segment of the population.

LONG-TERM CARE IN INSTITUTIONAL SETTINGS

When situations of declining health, depleted physical, financial, and human resources, and increased dependency occur, institutionalization in a long-term care facility may become a necessity. A long-term care facility provides long-term or extended residential, intermediate, or skilled nursing care, medical care, and personal and psychosocial services. The level and type of services offered determine the criteria that must be met to satisfy local, state, and federal requirements. Additionally, federal Medicare and Medicaid guidelines and regulations must be met by participating agencies. Generally guidelines at each level—local, state, and federal—address the type of client; staff qualifications and ratio; environmental regulations; health care; client rights; and food, recreational, and social services. Individual needs and resources dictate which type of facility is most appropriate for the client.

The decision to institutionalize a client is usually a difficult one for the client and the family. The client may experience a sense of helplessness, a loss of control, independence, and love, and an overwhelming feeling of abandonment. Going to a "nursing home" or an "old folk's home" is viewed as a "last resort." Hope often vanishes, for the client knows of no friends or relatives who have recovered in or returned from nursing homes, and thus the client believes he or she is "going there to die." The giving away of possessions and selling of the "home house" indicate that the client is going away, never to return to familiar or loved surroundings. The family has to cope with feelings of conflict, ambivalence, blame, guilt, and helplessness. The community health nurse must support the family, understanding that they have made the best decision for themselves at the present time and under the existing circumstances. The community health nurse can facilitate the expression of feelings by such phrases as the following: "It is usually hard to place a loved one in a nursing home. I wonder what it is like for you?" "Sometimes families have second thoughts about putting a loved one in a nursing home." "I imagine this is a difficult time for you." The family and the older adult must be encouraged to talk *with* each other and not just *to* each other. Listening and hearing become important as the family seeks the best answer.

The community health nurse also must be an advocate for the family, a negotiator between the older adult and other family members, and a resource person. To do this, family contacts should be followed up with visits, telephone calls, or both to determine what actions have been taken by the family and what additional assistance, if any, is needed. During each encounter with the family the community health nurse must remember to apply the concepts of choice, rights, responsibility, and decision making and assist the family in formulating these concepts into a practical solution. The admission of the client to the long-term care facility is not the termination of care to the family. The family needs the nurse during this period of crisis and adjustment. The community health nurse can be the link in the following chain of events: community health nurse↔family↔client↔long-term care facility↔community health nurse↔family↔client↔long-term care facility.

Long-term care facilities cannot be discussed without considering the image of such facilities. Many years ago these facilities were referred to as "nursing homes"; yet neither the staffing pattern nor activities denote very much "nursing" or "home." Perhaps the first effort at changing the image of these facilities is to change the name. A second factor would be to look at staffing and mechanisms for recruiting and retaining capable professional nurses for these facilities. Third, the public needs education about the different types of facilities and how to select the most appropriate facility according to the needs and preference of the individual. The public must also change its values about long-term care facilities so that adequate resources are allocated to correct some of the ills of the long-term care industry. The combined forces of the population growth pattern, prevalence of chronic illnesses, and social forces such as working women, an increasing divorce rate, and a declining birth rate all project a need for vitalization of the long-term care industry and creation of alternative resources.

HOSPICE

A hospice, as discussed in Chapter 42, is a community resource available for the care of the terminally ill. A hospice program has a family orientation and is concerned with the special needs and care of the terminally ill person. The quality of life and decision making for the family and individual are focal points in the delivery of medical, nursing, spiritual, and social care by an interdisciplinary team. Hospice programs may be hospital based or exist as separate entities. Many elderly persons experiencing the later stages of a terminal illness may view this community resource as an answer to the wish to live and die with comfort and dignity and to having the family at one's side. Additional information about hospice care is available in Chapter 42.

LEGISLATION AND COMMUNITY RESOURCES AND PROGRAMS

The legislative and political aspects of aging pervade every other aspect of aging, since most health, social, and economic issues are connected to legislation and programs such as Social Security, Older American's Act, and Medicare. These programs have revamped some of the issues of later life and promise to continue to do so as the nation grapples with balancing the budget, federalism, reductions in social programs, inflation, unemployment, and an increasingly older constituency. Nurses should be informed about the legislative process and legislation and policies that influence health care in general and the elderly population in particular.

During the fourth decade of the nineteenth century when the Social Security Act was passed, population size, employment patterns, and health problems differed. The Social Security Act became law in August 1935 during the administration of Franklin D. Roosevelt. Eligibility for Social Security, a general public retirement pension, is based on previous work history and age. Additionally, there are survivor, disability, and health benefits. The Social Security Act has been amended in several significant ways. Two key amendments, Medicare in 1966 and Supplemental Security Income (SSI) in 1974, have special importance for the elderly. The Supplemental Security Income (SSI) includes a federal supplement to the incomes of adults with inadequate income.

In 1966 Medicare was instituted as a health insurance program for older Americans with hospital and medical insurance provisions. Covered services include hospitalization, skilled nursing, home care, physician's services, and home health care. The services not covered by Medicare are of such magnitude that they are frequently referred to as "Medigap." Many private insurance companies have programs specifically designed to cover this gap.

Medicaid as a health care program for the poor, exclusive of age eligibility, is administered by individual states. These programs, in addition to Social Security benefits, have meant an improved life-style for the poor, including improved health care, food, shelter, and clothing.

The Older American's Act of 1965 and its amendments provide for the establishment of the United States Administration of Aging for program funding, and for training and research. The responsibility for coordinating and planning services for the elderly such as multipurpose senior centers, nutrition centers, employment, and transportation services at a local level is vested in the Area Agency on Aging (AAA). Multipurpose senior centers created by Title V of the Older American's Act provide the locus for a broad spectrum of services for older persons: health, social, legal, educational, and recreational. Title VII of the Older American's Act provides for nutrition programs for the elderly. Nutrition services are offered in congregate settings or are delivered to people at home via Meals on Wheels. In addition to partially meeting individual nutritional requirements, socialization and education needs are met. The Older American's Act Amendments of 1981 provide for a state ombudsman program for long-term care facilities and boarding homes.

AGING NETWORK

The *aging network* includes organizations concerned with advocacy, special populations, and volunteer services by older people. As of 1969 two components of the National Older American Volunteer Program are Retired Senior Volunteer Program and Foster Grandparents Program. Volunteer activities in hospitals, schools, nursing homes, and other settings are provided by members of the Retired Senior Volunteer Program (RSVP). Persons 60 years old and older may volunteer services. These volunteers are provided transportation and meals in connection with their volunteer activities. The Foster Grandparents Program offers an opportunity for older people and children to mutually share, meet needs, and experience gratification across generations. The Gray Panthers, organized by Margaret (Maggie) Kuhn, began as an advocacy group for change and social justice. Now the combined assets and forces of young and old are interested in investigative research, legislative action, monitoring of services to the aged, and organization of training for the Gray Panthers network (Kuhn, 1976). The National Council of Senior Citizens (NCSC) was founded in 1961 out of the need to defeat the American Medical Association's campaign against Medicare, thereby becoming one of the first senior powers (Kleyman, 1974).

Cognizance of and sensitivity to the needs of black Americans and concern about national goals and the necessity for activities to address these needs stimulated Hobart Jackson in the organization of the National Caucus on the Black Aged (NCBA). The NCBA continues to this day as an advocacy group for the improvement of the quality of life for older persons of minority groups (Jackson, 1976). Other organizations concerned about issues involving the aged include the American Association of Retired Persons and the National Retired Teachers Association.

Four White House conferences on aging have been held, one each decade beginning in 1950, to hear concerns and issues of importance to older Americans and to propose plans for national policies on aging for the next decade. The 1981 conference was centered on the theme *The Aging Society: Challenge and Opportunity*. The conference focused on more than 600 recommendations; however, the following recommendations were highlighted: strengthen the Social Security system, prohibit mandatory retirement, increase the availability of home and community-based health care, and emphasize preventive health care. A national policy on aging that emerged from this fourth conference has the following goals (Final Report, 1981):

1. To provide the elderly with the maximum opportunity to live an independent and healthy life and to encourage them to remain in the economic and social mainstream.
2. To provide economic, medical, and social support to the elderly who need help.
3. To encourage serious discussion of the choices we must make as a result of the very large baby boom generation that will become elderly in the 21st century.

The gains have been many, but much work lies ahead. As the constituency of aged persons grows, so do their needs, political power, and demand for participation in the political arena. Nurses can be advocates for the elderly through cooperative efforts with advocacy groups influencing health and social policies. Furthermore, nurses can serve as sources of health information for organizations concerned with the well-being of aged persons.

CLINICAL APPLICATION

This case study and related questions are designed to help the student apply chapter concepts and content to the care of older adults. The use of the nursing process as a framework for care also is presented (see box, p. 516).

◆ ◆ ◆

During your clinical rotation with a local home health care agency you receive the following referral:

Date of Referral: February 15, 1987
Name: Mrs. Rose Lee
Address: 1927 Memory Lane
Age: 70 years
Medicare Number and/or Insurance Provider Number
                000-00-000-0
  Health Information:
  Essential Hypertension since age 35
  Arthritis since age 60
  Discharged from local hospital on February 15, 1987 (hospital stay: 2/10-2/15) where she was treated for uncontrolled hypertension (DRG code: 134.5)
  Prescribed medications include:
    Methyldopa (Aldomet)
      250 mg b.i.d. p.o.
    Hydrochlorothiazide (Hydro Diuril)
      50 mg q.d. p.o.
    Indomethacin (Indocin)
      50 mg t.i.d. p.o.
  Additional therapy:
    Low sodium diet
Reason(s) for Referral:
  Monitoring of blood pressure and medication; health assessment
Physician: Dr. Joe Doe
Referral Source: Social Service Department and local hospital
Date of Agency Receipt of Referral: February 16, 1987
Referral Assigned to: Mary Little

Questions

1. What are priorities for the first visit to Mrs. Lee?
2. What additional data are needed?
3. What special needs must be considered in view of Mrs. Lee's age?
4. Develop a nursing care plan for Mrs. Lee.

APPLICATION OF NURSING PROCESS WITH AN OLDER ADULT IN THE COMMUNITY

ASSESSMENT

Health history

Physical assessment

Observations within each body system that are consistent with normal findings and normal changes in aging

Observations within each body system that deviate from normal findings and normal changes in aging (abnormalities)

Areas for special focus: depends on presenting symptoms, chief complaint, problems

Sensory status: sight, hearing, touch, smell, taste

Limitations of activities

Activities of daily living: feeding, bathing, grooming, dressing, toileting, ambulation

Psychosocial assessment

Living arrangements: housing, physical facilities

Support system: availability of and relationship with family, neighbors, friends, etc.

Finances: income source, amount, date of receipt of income

Community environment: access to transportation, pharmacy, supermarket

Food preparation

Attitudes regarding own health: individual role in management of health problems

Performance of instrumental activities of daily living: shopping, using telephone, preparation of food, cleaning, reading, writing, managing money

Cultural affiliations, beliefs, practices that are relevant to health

Religious affiliations, beliefs, practices that are relevant to health

Emotions and mood: feeling tones; attitudes toward life, self, and others

Educational level: level of reading and comprehension

Mental status: memory, confusion

Hobbies, interests, activities (social, civic, volunteer)

Risk factors to health

Toxins: smoking, pollutants

Optimal weight

Exercise pattern

Dietary habits

Alcohol consumption

Stress

Individual health goals and desires (motivation)

MANAGEMENT PLANS

Optimal balance between rest, activity, and recreation

Optimal nutrition status and weight control

Control of blood pressure within predetermined range

Acceptance and adherence to prescribed treatment regimen

Optimal comfort level

Promotion of optimal functional independence in activities of daily living

INTERVENTIONS

Monitor blood pressure, weight, mobility level, and drug use and response

Provide nutrition and drug education

Assist client with stress management techniques

Arrange a balanced activity-rest-recreation cycle

EVALUATION

Is blood pressure within the predetermined range?

Is weight at the established goal?

Is there a balance between rest, activities, and recreation?

To what degree is there acceptance of and adherence to the prescribed treatment regimen?

SUMMARY

The study of older adults is a study of a growing population with many assets and liabilities. The more than 25 million community-based, high school–educated older Americans are influencing the cultural orientation of this country. This influence is seen in efforts to prevent polarization between generations and to educate the public about and change attitudes toward the elderly, encouraging a perception of the elderly as diverse people who are a national resource and asset. The minority groups—blacks, Hispanics, Native Americans, and Pacific Asians—are obtaining special attention for their unique needs and assets. The myths of older adults as institutionalized, poor, unable to learn, accident prone, passive, and sexless are being replaced with new knowledge, perceptions, and attitudes. The valuing of "oldness" will possibly increase as this nation's population continues to grow old, with members of the great baby boom becoming 65 during the twenty-first century. The theories of aging will again be put to the test as explanations are sought for the aging phenomenon. The disengagement, activity, continuity, or developmental and biological theories will all contribute answers to such questions as the following: Why do people age? How does aging progress? What accelerates and decelerates the process? Is quantity better than quality of life? The developmental task of adjusting to declining health, death, retirement, and changing interpersonal relationships will be researched for its contribution to healthy aging. The major health problems of this population are heart disease, malignancies, and cerebrovascular diseases. Efforts to prevent the development of hypertension are aimed at reduction of risk factors such as smoking, obesity, lack of exercise, and excessive salt intake. Stress management continues to be emphasized for its value in promoting health. Additionally, regular blood pressure screening, diet management, and drug therapy continue to save lives and prevent complications of this major disabler of older adults. Vigilance for changes in the body, regular physical examinations and elimination of smoking will further the decline in the incidence of cancer in older adults.

Health problems such as arthritis, sensory impairments, and confusion limit activity and affect comfort and independence. Decreasing functional dependency is one goal in the improvement of the health of older adults, enabling them to function at their optimal physical, social, and psychological level. The increased years gained through advanced technology will be meaningless unless chronic, disabling conditions are controlled or eliminated and happy healthy years become a normal scenario during later life. Older adults' coping capacity for loss, grief, and depression must be broader so that they do not continue to terminate their lives by their own hands, a practice accounting for approximately one fourth of the suicides in the United States. Prevention, treatment, and rehabilitation must be hallmarks of the care provided within the health care and social systems. Criminal victimization, drug misuse, abuse from relatives and institutional care givers, and social isolation are psychosocial issues affecting the health and quality of life of aged persons. An interdisciplinary approach to solving these problems is necessary to forestall or prevent occurrences of these problems at epidemic levels. Health, social, and political organizations must join forces and form a counterattack on the deadly forces of abuse and victimization.

Health promotion involves adequate nutrition; a balance of exercise, rest, and activity; immunizations against influenza and pneumonia; time management; and optimum self-esteem. These are central to healthy older adults. The years spent dreaming of retirement and "lots of time on hand" have now become a reality for the older population. Are those years going to be the panacea and mecca dreamed or will those years become one horrible nightmare from which relief is sought? The answers begin many years before the magical turning point of age 65.

Community health nurses as care givers must assist older adults to capitalize on their assets and guide them in coping with the process of living with chronic illnesses and disability. A life theme of moderation, variety, and balance contributes to healthy older years. Just as infectious diseases of earlier years were eliminated, the chronic diseases of the present must be conquered to ensure quality of life. The art of decision making, the privilege of choice, and the responsibility of self-discipline are the keys to solving problems of living and aging.

☰ KEY CONCEPTS

The elderly are the fastest growing population in the United States. Their increased longevity with the accompanying high incidence of chronic disease poses a substantial challenge to the health care system. Technology can keep people alive much longer, yet such care is costly and often uncomfortable.

In recent years, aging as a life process has received greater focus and study. The earlier lack of emphasis on this population group perpetuated many myths and stereotypes.

(Erikson, 1963) provides another perspective for viewing aging. In Erikson's theory on the eight stages of life, timing, sequential order of movement, and accomplishment of certain critical tasks are essential for movement from one life stage to the next. Aging is viewed as the successful resolution of the conflict between the critical tasks of integrity and despair.

Physical, as well as psychosocial or developmental changes accompany aging. The observed changes represent the cumulative and lifelong effects of heredity, environment, nutrition, rest, activity, and altered health status.

Although many older adults enjoy good health and freedom of activity, others do not share this distinction. Approximately 80% of the group over age 65 has at least one chronic health problem.

Alzheimer's disease is an irreversible confusional state that is gaining recognition as a major health problem for the elderly. Approximately 1.5 to 2.5 million older people are affected by this disease.

The ability to successfully adjust to retirement is affected by such factors as health status, sufficient income, number of situational changes, quality of personal relationships, ability to manage time effectively, flexibility, ability to relinquish the work routine, and anticipation and realistic expectation for retirement.

Older persons are major users of health services. Persons aged 65 to 74 years average 7.4 physician visits annually. Although the elderly constitute approximately 12% of the population, they are responsible for about 17% of physician visits.

Continued.

LEARNING ACTIVITIES

1. Develop a hypothetical chart that identifies the developmental tasks of the older adult; identify potential problems that might interfere with accomplishing the task.

2. Make a developmental task chart for a client with whom you have been working and enumerate the problems you have observed resulting from inability to satisfactorily master the developmental task(s).

3. Based on the problems with completing developmental tasks identified in the preceding activity, develop a nursing plan of action for at least two of these problems.

4. Interview two elderly people and determine what myths and stereotypes they perceive younger people hold about them.

5. Read your local newspaper to find at least three stories that discuss older adults. Do the stories portray them in a positive or negative way?

The legislative and political aspects of aging pervade every other aspect of aging, since most health, social, and economic issues are connected to legislation and programs such as Social Security, Older American's Act, and Medicare.

The myths of older adults as institutionalized, poor, unable to learn, accident prone, passive, and sexless are being replaced with new knowledge, perceptions, and attitudes. The valuing of "oldness" will possibly increase as this nation's population continues to grow old.

BIBLIOGRAPHY

Alzheimer's Disease, Washington, D.C., 1984, U.S. Department of Health and Human Services.

Auerbach, M.: Changes in home health care delivery, Nursing Outlook 33:290-291, 1986.

Burnside, I.M.: Transition to later life: developmental theories and research. In Burnside, I.M., Ebersol, P., and Monea, H.E., editors: Psychosocial caring through the life span. New York, 1979, McGraw-Hill Book Co.

Cummings, E., and Henry, W.E.: Growing old: the process of disengagement, New York, 1961, Basic Books.

Ebersole, P., and Hess, P.: Toward healthy aging human needs and nursing response, St. Louis, 1981, The C.V. Mosby Co.

Elder abuse, Washington, D.C., 1980, Office of Human Development Services, Department of Health and Human Services.

Emick-Herring, B.C.: Adult day care: support system for disabled elderly and their caregivers, Rehabilitation Nursing 8:29-31, 1983.

Erickson, E.H.: Childhood and society, New York, 1963, W.W. Norton.

Fact book on aging: a profile of America's older population. Washington, D.C., 1978 National Council on Aging.

Facts about older Americans, 1980-1981. Washington, D.C., 1981, Office of Human Development Services.

Final report: the 1981 White House Conference on Aging. Washington, D.C., 1981, Department of Health and Human Services.

Hayter, J.: Patients who have Alzheimer's disease, Am. J. Nurs. 74:1460-1463, 1974.

Havighurst, R.J.: Successful aging. In Williams, R.H., Tibbilts, C., and Donahue, W., editors: Process of aging, vol 1., New York, 1963, Atherton Press.

Health: United States, 1976-77. Washington, D.C., 1977, Public Health Service, Health Resources Administration, National Center for Health Statistics, Department of Health, Education, and Welfare.

Healthy people: Background papers. Washington, D.C., 1979, Public Health Service, Office of the Assistant Secretary for Health and Surgeon General, Department of Health, Education, and Welfare.

Jackson, H.C.: Black advocacy: techniques and trials. In Kerschner, P.A., editor, Advocacy and age, Los Angeles, 1976, The University of Southern California Press.

Kahn, C.: Visual disorders. In Libow, B., and Sherman, F., editors: The core of geriatric medicine, St. Louis, 1981, The C.V. Mosby.

Kleyman, P.: Senior power, San Francisco, 1974, Glide Publications.

Koenen, R.E.: Adult day care: a northwest perspective, J. Gerontol. Nurs. 6:218-221, 1980.

Kuhn, M.E.: What old people want for themselves and others in society. In Kerschner, P.A., editor: advocacy and age, Los Angeles, 1976, The University of Southern California Press.

Luckmann, J., and Sorenson, K.: Medical-surgical nursing, a psychophysiologic approach, ed. 2, Philadelphia, 1980, Saunders.

Margolis, E., Levy, B., and Sherman, F.: Hearing disorders. In Libow, L., and Sherman, F., editors: The core of geriatric medicine, St. Louis, 1981, The C.V. Mosby.

The myth and reality of aging in America, Washington, D.C., 1975, National Council on Aging.

National Center for Health Statistics: Advance report of final mortality statistics, U.S. Public Health Services, Hyattsville, Md., vol. 33, Dec. 20, 1984.

Need for long-term care information and issues, Washington, D.C., 1981, Office of Human Development Services.

Neugarten, B.L.: Personality in middle and late life, New York, 1964, Atherton Press.

Schwartz, A.N.: Counselling the older adults. In O'Brien, B., editor: Aging, today's research and you, Los Angeles, 1978, The University of Southern California Press.

Siegel, H.S., and Davidson, M.: Demographic and socioeconomic aspects of aging in the United States, Washington, D.C., 1984, Current Population Reports, Bureau of the Census, U.S. Department of Commerce.

Smith, C.E.: DRGs: making them work for you. Nurs. '85, 15:34-41, 1985.

Steffl, B.: Theories of aging: biological, psychological, and sociological. In Steffl, B., editor: Handbook of gerontological nursing, New York, 1984, Van Nostrand Reinhold.

U.S. Senate Special Committee on Aging: Trends and projections, Washington, D.C., 1986, The Committee.

U.S. Bureau of the Census: Statistical abstract of the United States, ed. 105, Washington, D.C., 1984, The Bureau.

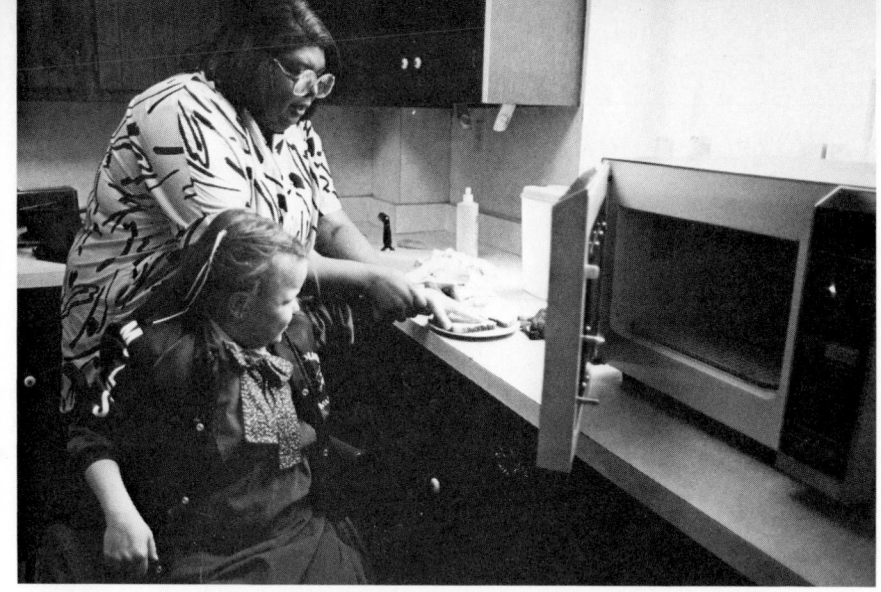

Marcia Kaplan Cowan
Margaret Millsap

26

THE DEVELOPMENTALLY DISABLED POPULATION AS A COMMUNITY HEALTH TARGET

 OBJECTIVES

After reading this chapter, the student should be able to:

Define the term *developmental disability*.

Discuss the recent changes in the definition and their effect on the number of children categorized as developmentally disabled.

List at least five categories of conditions that might cause a child to be developmentally disabled.

Discuss three preventive measures that might reduce the number of children identified in these categories.

Discuss the concept of community-based care for the child who has a developmental disability.

Identify the role of community health nurses in caring for people with developmental disabilities.

Plan a hypothetical program for providing support to families with a member who is developmentally disabled.

KEY TERMS

cerebral palsy

Denver Developmental Screening Test (DDST)

developmental disability

Developmental Profile II

independent living

learning disabilities

mental retardation

Nursing Child Assessment Satellite Training (NCAST) program

retinopathy of prematurity

School Nurse Achievement Program (SNAP)

social isolation

spina bifida

trisomy 21 (Down syndrome)

very low birthweight

Providing care for those who are developmentally disabled is a goal that has been emphasized by the federal government for many years. It is a broad goal that encompasses the work of many people in a variety of professions. Only in the last 26 years have we as a people recognized that all individuals, regardless of condition, have all the rights of other individuals. This implies that all people will be treated with dignity and afforded the opportunity to grow, learn, and enjoy the pleasures of a healthy, rewarding life.

Nurses are in a key role to provide services that have a positive impact on communities. The proper use of their knowledge, skill, and concern can provide the leadership needed to improve the quality of life for this population.

The term *developmental disability* refers to a variety of conditions, mental and physical, that interfere with the ability of an individual to function successfully in society. Public Law (PL) 95-602 (Comprehensive Rehabilitation Service Amendments of 1978) gives the following definition:

A developmental disability is a severe, chronic disability of a person which:
  A. is attributable to a mental or physical impairment or combination of mental and physical impairments;
  B. is manifested before the person attains age twenty two;
  C. is likely to continue indefinitely;
  D. results in substantial limitations in three or more of the following areas of major life activity:
     1. self-care
     2. receptive and expressive language
     3. learning
     4. mobility
     5. self-direction
     6. capacity for independent living
     7. economic sufficiency
  E. reflects the person's need for a combination and sequence of special, interdisciplinary or generic care, treatment, or the services which are of lifelong or extended duration and are individually planned and coordinated.

The current definition has considerably changed the focus of the definition previously used by governmental agencies, which specified conditions such as cerebral palsy, mental retardation, autism, and epilepsy. The definition also expanded the age from 18 to 22. This allows for a longer period of help for this population.

The current definition emphasizes the inability to function in three or more areas of major life activities. The conditions that may interfere with adequate function include environmental deprivation, encompassing sensory and emotional deprivation and biological impairment.

Environmental deprivation may involve intellectual impairment resulting from limited opportunities or stimulation to learn. A number of studies, such as Project Headstart, show the short and long-term benefits of preschool enrichment for environmentally disadvantaged children. The results seem to depend on continued support during school years (Denhoff, 1981).

Biological impairments include genetic, metabolic, neurological, or anatomical defects. A number of coexistent conditions may serve to impair function.

In contrast to the term, *developmental disability, developmental delay* is a broader term referring to a failure to meet developmental landmarks or milestones. Delays do not always indicate a developmental disability. Neither term specifies a diagnosis for the underlying cause of the delay or disability.

Most people who fall within the category of developmental disability are classified as being mentally retarded. A recent definition of mental retardation approved by the American Association on Mental Deficiency has eliminated those previously diagnosed as having borderline intelligence. This definition has thereby reduced the number of mentally retarded individuals and consequently reduced the total number of the developmentally disabled.

A special report on the impact of the change in the definition of developmental disabilities was prepared by the Office of Human Development Services Administration (May 1981). This report states that

There has been a 27% decrease in the estimated total developmental disabilities population, as defined in the 1978 amendments, based on an analysis of the 1980 Developmental Disabilities State Plans. Whereas in FY* 1978 the estimated number of individuals defined as developmentally disabled in the United States was 5,265,846 in FY 1980 the estimated figure was 3,906,913. . . . .Mental retardation in FY 1980 represented 54.8% of those defined as developmentally disabled, compared with 65.5% in FY

*Fiscal year.

1978. During the same time period, the estimated number of individuals considered developmentally disabled with cerebral palsy increased, with epilepsy decreased, and with autism remaining essentially the same. In addition, individuals with other conditions who are now included within the developmentally disabled target population currently account for almost 12% of the population. There continue to be differences in the population considered to be developmentally disabled. Although the total population estimate in the State plans was almost 4 million developmentally disabled individuals, a study utilizing the developmental disabilities definition in conjunction with the 1976 Survey of Income and Education estimated 2.5 million developmentally disabled individuals.

SCOPE OF THE PROBLEM

The problems associated with developmental disabilities are complex, far-reaching, and profound. Despite all the technological and humanistic knowledge abundant today, we do not have the answers to many of these problems. This situation is described by Wallace et al. (1973, p. 931).

> In spite of—and in part because of—advances in medical care, the task of meeting the needs of the handicapped is growing larger, not smaller. Reasons for this include the increasing size of the population, our continued inability to control the incidence of many kinds of disabling conditions, the lengthening survival time of disabled newborn infants (even those with catastrophic disabilities), and the increasing expectations coupled with increasing demands for care.

CAUSES OF DEVELOPMENTAL DISABILITIES

Definitive causes for developmental disabilities are known in only about 25% of the cases. Of this small percentage, the causes are usually categorized as chromosomal aberrations; neural tube defects; central nervous system damage occurring in the perinatal period, including the sequelae of premature birth, teratogens (for example, maternal infection and maternal substance abuse), and neonatal infection; and metabolic disorders.

Trisomy 21 (Down syndrome) is the most commonly found chromosomal abnormality. It is estimated to occur at a rate of 1 to 1.2 per 1000 live births. Maternal age has been demonstrated to be closely related to the incidence of this condition, which increases markedly when the mother is past age 35. However, currently only 20% of the children with trisomy 21 are born to mothers who are older than 35, which is probably the result of the increased availability of genetic screening (Hook, 1982). Some evidence links the father's age to incidence of trisomy 21.

Neural tube defects occur at a rate of 1 to 2 per 1000 live births. This encompasses anomalies ranging from anencephaly to spina bifida occulta. *Spina bifida,* currently the second most common birth defect, usually involves serious physical handicaps and may include mental retardation. In addition, 70% of children with myelomeningocele, the most severe form of spina bifida, also have hydrocephaly, many requiring shunts. Medical complications include serious infections and renal failure and are major causes of morbidity and mortality during infancy and early childhood (Nelson and Crocker, 1983). Early surgical intervention and infant stimulation programs have improved the outlook for these children. However, treatment is expensive, difficult for some families to obtain, and emotionally stressful for the entire family. The constant care, prolonged grief, and financial burden create a tremendous problem for the child and the family.

Most children who have spina bifida are of normal intelligence, but because of severe physical problems, it is most difficult to find suitable educational programs for them. Consequently, many have lower intelligence quotient test scores simply because they lack the opportunity to learn or cannot participate in the educational activities as a result of physical limitations.

Very low birthweight infants (less than 1500 g) are generally considered to be at risk for developmental disabilities. Although advances in neonatal care have improved the survival rate of these infants, recent studies show a 10% to 19% incidence of severe neurological handicap, intellectual handicap, or both (Hack, 1983). Problems encountered include hydrocephaly, cerebral palsy, mental retardation, and sensory impairment, especially involving hearing and vision. It is estimated that 500 to 600 infants are blinded each year by *retinopathy of prematurity* (Phelps, 1981). Alterations in parent-infant interaction that occur as a result of prematurity may also place infants at risk for developmental delay.

Maternal infections during pregnancy that can result in developmental problems include rubella, cytomegalic virus, and toxoplasmosis. Infectious agents, chemicals, drugs, and physical agents can all be considered teratogens. Teratogens are any agents or factors that cause permanent alterations of the fetus in form or function during prenatal development. The extent of damage is determined by the systems developing in the embryo or fetus at the time of exposure. Severe infections during the time of central nervous system development, such as neonatal meningitis, and metabolic disorders, including phenylketonuria and hypothyroidism, can lead to damage during infancy.

Central nervous system damage may result in *cerebral palsy,* which is defined as a disorder of movement and posture. Damage resulting in cerebral palsy may occur prenatally, perinatally, or in childhood. Mental retardation occurs in 50% of affected individuals (Taft & Matthews, 1983).

Some children who have *learning disabilities* may also be classified as developmentally disabled. Since *learning disability* is a poorly defined term, prevalence figures vary widely (from 4% to 20% of the school-age population) (Levine, 1980). Levine notes that the child's performance may be affected in specific areas of neurological function, such as memory, language, selective attention, perception, and motor abilities. Areas of emotional function may also be involved, including social perception and the ability to interact with peers. Learning disabilities include a broad range of problems that may interfere with a child's ability to function normally in society.

PRIMARY PREVENTION
Role of Professionals

If effective, preventive measures must begin with education of the parents before conception. Social behavior, environmental factors, family mores, and moral issues are parts of this complex problem. Technological advances, research, and improved standards of living have contributed to increased infant survival rates and to a longer life span for most people, yet a large number of children continue to have developmental disabilities.

Family planning services, genetic counseling, comprehensive prenatal care, immunizations, decreasing use of drugs and alcohol, and continuing research are all preventive means that need to be used to the fullest extent. It has been predicted that the number of developmentally disabled children could be reduced by one half in the next decade if all the available knowledge was now applied.

"The aim of professionals who deal with handicapped children and their families is to lessen the susceptibility of such children at risk and to increase their sense of mastery and competence" (Waechter, 1975, p. 110). This aim may be reached by recognizing the areas of vulnerability of families through rejection or overprotection of the child. Early assessment of the child and family should help the nurse plan effective intervention. To support the child in the normal development of independence and autonomous living and to increase his or her self-esteem, a complete assessment should be made early in life. This includes (1) a complete physical examination; (2) developmental assessment; (3) psychological testing; (4) evaluation of the quality, quantity, and consistency of environmental support;

and (5) determination of the ego capacities of the parents (Waechter, 1975). Figure 26-1 shows an interdisciplinary team in action.

Nurses play a vital role in preventive measures before conception through family planning and counseling with high risk parents such as teenagers, women over 35, and families known to have histories of developmental disabilities.

Prenatal care that begins early and continues throughout pregnancy has long been recognized as a vital factor in the prevention of problematic pregnancies and births. Included in this care is identification of mothers at risk for having a child with a developmental disability. This list includes women age 35 and older; women who have had a child with a congenital abnormality such as Down's syndrome, spina bifida, or other genetic problems; and those who have a history of drug abuse, alcoholism, infectious diseases, environmental exposure to toxic substances, or premature births.

These families need support from the nurse. They may need information, referral, encouragement, or a combination of these to seek and follow through with services that are provided. Amniocentesis is frequently suggested to these mothers. Both parents need to understand the procedure, its purpose, and its value. Counseling can help them to understand this procedure.

If it is determined that the fetus is at risk for or has an actual developmental disorder, the possibility of aborting the pregnancy presents a difficult decision for most parents. The nurse must be skilled in supporting the parents in the decision they make.

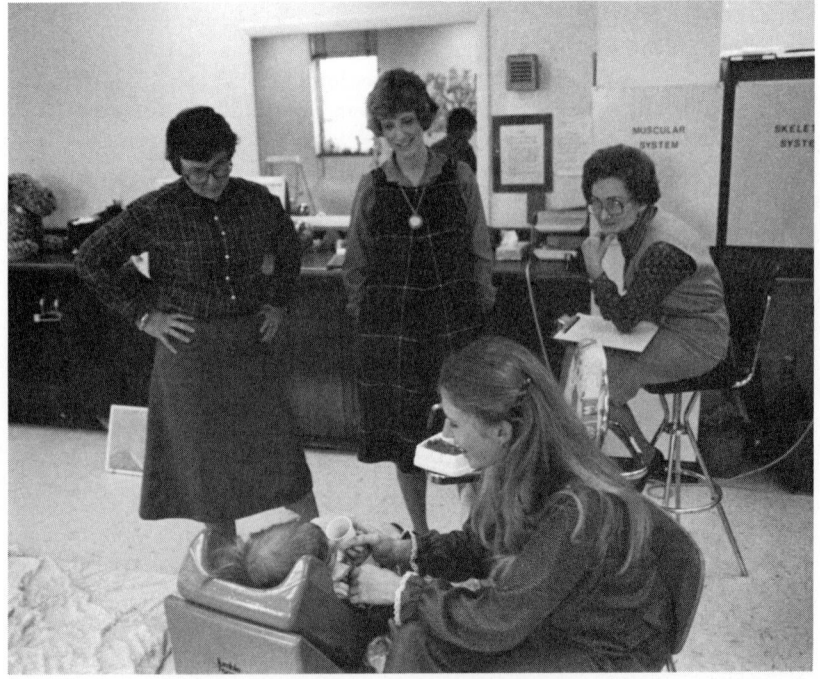

FIGURE 26-1

Interdisciplinary team evaluation.

Prevention of Further Disability: Early Intervention

Early intervention programs are intended to stimulate the development of children who are not progressing at an appropriate rate of motor, cognitive, language, or socio-emotional development. Interventions are ideally aimed at promoting optimal development, prevention of secondary disabilities, and improvement of family function. Programs are based on theories that stimulation strengthens functional connections or enhances the development of new pathways in the central nervous system. Studies of the effectiveness of such programs are plagued with problems related to numbers and outcome criteria; however, these studies generally find improvements in personal and social skills and in family interaction.

Prevention of further disabling conditions is a sound reason for recommending early intervention programs. Although much controversy still exists about the value of early stimulation for the child with a developmental disability, its importance has been recognized by many nurses working with these children and their families. Figure 26-2 depicts an early infant stimulation program.

A 10-month-old child was brought to a university-affiliated program by the mother through a referral from a community health nurse. When examined by the nurse, this child, Amy, could not lift her head, did not attend well to voice commands, and had a weak sucking reflex. The mother was distraught, discouraged, and physically exhausted. She had accepted the physician's diagnosis that Amy had severe brain damage and had been giving the medications as ordered for her child. She had continued to care for her like a newborn infant but expressed the need to know what she could do to help her child.

A team of experts evaluated the child, and a program was designed with the participation of the mother. The program involved some visits to the center for demonstration and reinforcement, but most of the activities prescribed were carried out in the home by the parents. The nurse at the center coordinated the program with the community health nurse, family, and the center.

Progress was slow for Amy, but it did occur. Within 3 months she was lifting and turning her head in response to sound. Moreover, socialization was seen as she began to respond positively to her parents with some eye contact and facial expressions.

Experiences such as this have demonstrated that many of these children can be helped through early stimulation programs. The value to the family is inestimable. This young mother appeared to have a new lease on life as a result of the progress made by her child.

Early and continuous assessment of these children aids in identifying other problems, such as hearing or visual deficits. Recognition and treatment should enhance the learning ability of the child. Physical stimulation helps to prevent contractures and to strengthen the muscular development of the child. Figures 26-3 and 26-4 illustrate the assessment of motor and speech function. Encouraging the parents to keep the child under medical supervision can prevent the development of further physical problems. Nutritional counseling, intellectual stimulation, and up-to-date immunizations are also valuable components of a preventive program for these children.

ROLE OF THE COMMUNITY HEALTH NURSE

The role of the community health nurse in the care of the child with a developmental disability must be built on a sincere concern for the child and his or her family. The child with a problem must first be viewed as an individual worthy of dignity and capable of living for a purpose. The

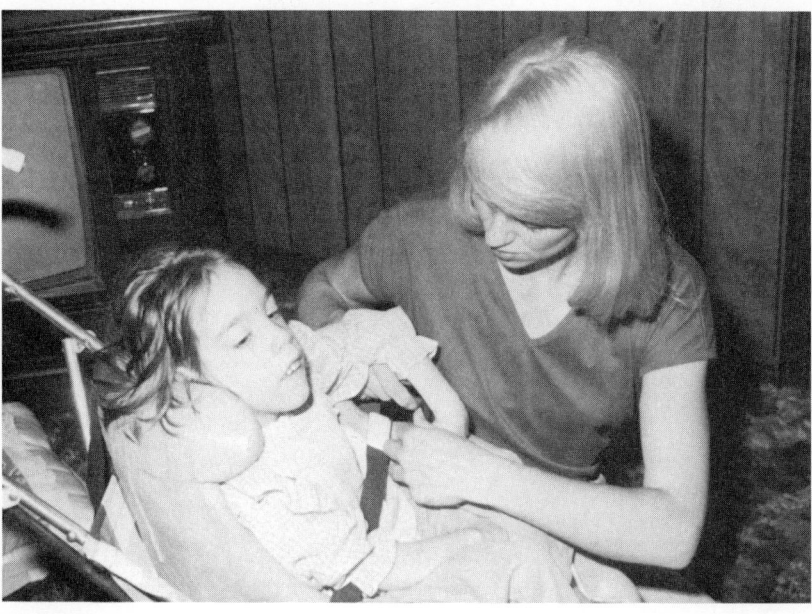

FIGURE 26-2

Early infant stimulation program.

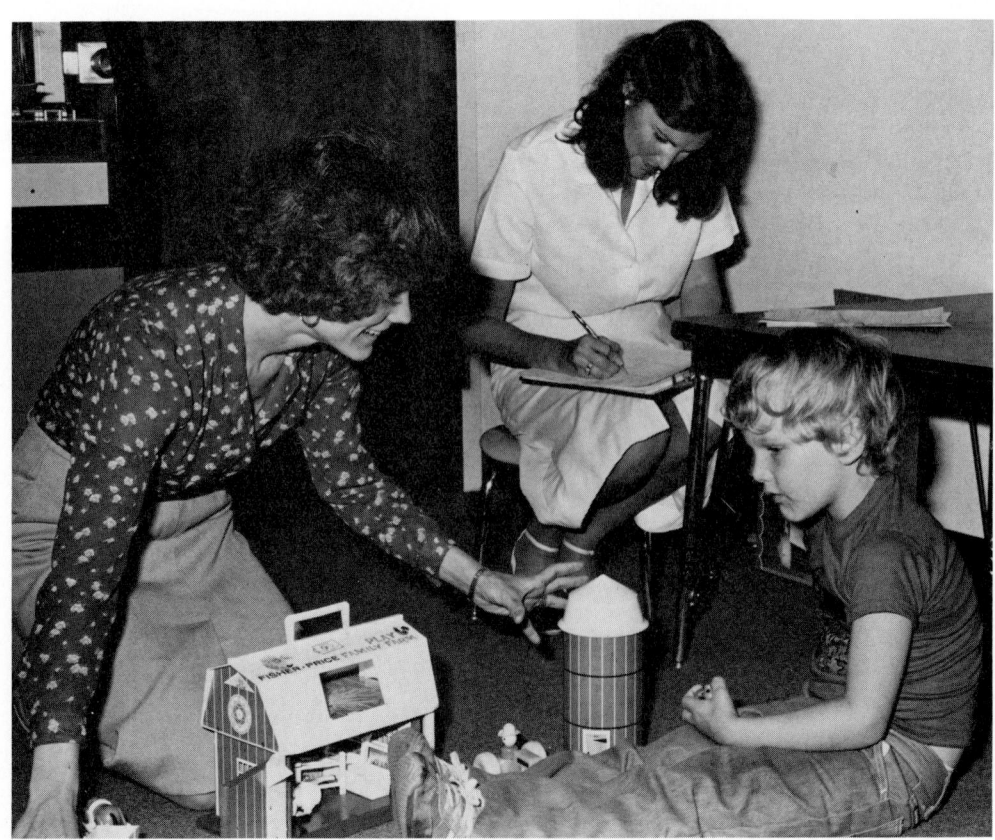

FIGURE 26-3

Assessment of motor function.

attitude of the nurse is reflected in all that is done with, to, and by the nurse. Unless that attitude conveys concern for the child and understanding of the grief and frustration of the family, therapy will be ineffective.

The nurse must help the parents and siblings see the potential in the child and build a program around his or her assets. Dealing with the reaction of the family to the child who has a developmental disability is the first step in working with the child. Sensitivity to this need and acceptance of the family's reaction provide the opportunity to make an adequate assessment of the child and the family.

Ideally, physicians and hospital personnel work more closely with the community nurse so that referral of the child from hospital to home is made early in the child's life. The community health nurse should visit the child and the mother while they are in the hospital. This provides an opportunity for the community health nurse to meet the medical team, nursing staff, and the parents. The community health nurse should have access to all the medical information and the medical plan for the child so that steps for the child's care within the community can be coordinated.

Meeting the mother at this stage is an excellent way to let her know she has an advocate in the community. Understanding the stages of grief helps the nurse to be sup-

FIGURE 26-4

Speech evaluation.

portive rather than intrusive. Plans can be made to visit in the home at a later time. It is essential that a feeling of trust be established between the nurse and the family.

Unfortunately, not all children with developmental disabilities are referred to the community health nurse during the immediate neonatal period. Often the nurse learns from neighbors, the kindergarten teacher, the church, or the clinic that there is a child with a problem in the community.

Developmental Assessment and Health Promotion

Nurses are responsible for pediatric screening and assessments beginning in the immediate neonatal period and continuing throughout childhood. Several conditions that categorize a child as developmentally disabled can be identified at birth, but many do not become apparent until the child is older. Assessments of physical status, development, and behavior are performed by nurses to provide early detection of developmental disabilities and as a part of the ongoing care for disabled children.

Nurses providing care for developmentally disabled children are involved in assessments of growth, maturation, and general well-being to prevent further alterations in health status. Handicapped children are at risk for nutritional deficiencies, alterations in activity and rest patterns, and increased incidence of infections. Regularly scheduled health assessments can provide early recognition and treatment of these problems and the basis for well-child counseling and preventive care. The families of developmentally disabled children have many of the same health promotion and counseling needs as other families; however, these needs often are overlooked because of the emphasis placed on the disability.

Developmental assessments and adaptive behavior judgments are made by observing the child in the home, office, or clinic. One or several tools may be used by the nurse to validate observations. The *Denver Developmental Screening Test (DDST)* is one of the simplest, more economical measures of ability for the child from birth to 6 years. (See Appendix K.) The test can be administered in less than 30 minutes and identifies many of the strengths and weaknesses of the child. Four areas of evaluation included in the DDST are personal/social, fine motor/adaptive, language, and gross motor development. The test may be used repeatedly on an individual child to plot his or her development over a period of time. Instructions for using the test are written on the back of each form.

The DDST must be administered by the examiner to one child at a time. Some items require observation of performance, and others may be reported by the parent. The test yields reliable information that can be most helpful as a screening tool. The DDST may be administered by nonprofessionals with very little training and is relatively inexpensive. It is used effectively to identify developmental delays or for follow-up assessments. The test does not measure intelligence quotient, and those who use the DDST should explain its purpose clearly to the parents to lessen the tension associated with any examination. (See Appendix K for source.)

The *Denver Prescreening Developmental Questionnaire* (PDQ) is a short test designed to identify children who need more testing with the DDST. It is designed for children 3 months to 6 years of age and is a series of questions designed to be answered with a "yes" or "no" by the parent or caretaker. The test requires less than 10 minutes to complete. Referral is recommended for any child with 6 or fewer "yes" answers.(See Appendix K, and use source for DDST.)

The *Developmental Profile II* is another assessment that is based on the responses of the mother or care taker to questions posed by the nurse. This standardized test can be used for measurement of children from birth to preadolescence. The test provides developmental age scores in the following five categories: physical/motor, self-help, social, academic, and communication skills. The test can be administered after a short training period and is relatively inexpensive. The evaluation is made in an interview and can be completed in approximately 30 minutes. Parent responses to the questions can yield valuable information that can be used in developing a program for the child. Referrals for further evaluation or placement into programs for children can be made using this instrument if agreeable to those involved. It is a single test that has been used effectively for a number of years for the purposes of screening and has been a reliable and valid tool. (See Appendix K for source.)

The American Association on Mental Deficiency has two instruments that can be used easily to assess the development of children or adults. Both instruments are called the AAMD Adaptive Behavior Scale. The version of the test first developed is designed to be used by staff members who work with clients in institutions. The later version is called the *Public School Version* and was designed to be used by schoolteachers or school nurses. Either test yields valuable information that can be used to develop appropriate care plans for children or adults. (See Appendix K for source.)

Several guides, such as the Portage Guide, the Washington Guide to Child Development, and the San Juan Development Progression Chart are available to help the nurse develop a program for a child. Sources for these guides are in Appendix K. Each of these guides gives specific steps that parents or teachers can follow to help a child learn a particular skill or advance his or her development. No one guide meets every need, so the nurse must use a repertoire of tools. Most are easy to understand and simple to use. The slow progress that most developmentally disabled children make requires repetition and a great deal of patience on the part of the parents, nurse, or therapist.

Many screening tests have been developed and can be used effectively by nurses and other health workers to plan and give care to children and their families. A useful book by Stangler et al. (1980) provides a comprehensive guide for the selection of tests for evaluating preschool children and developmentally disabled children.

Information acquired from observations, interviews, and test results is used to develop care plans for the child. Often the community health nurse is the health care coordinator for the child and the family. Assessment skills, knowledge of community resources, familiarity with the medical plan, and effective communication abilities are essential assets for such a coordinator.

Family Assessment and Support

Sharing information with the family and including them in the care plan is essential for the plan's successful implementation. The diagnosis of a developmental disability envelops most parents in a paralyzing grief that often lessens their ability to cope. Lacking the medical knowledge to understand the cause, treatment and prognosis, they are frequently frightened, grief stricken, and easily confused.

Parents' Reactions

Parents of developmentally disabled children react to the knowledge of having such a child in a fairly predictive manner, according to Rosen (1955). These stages are:
1. Awareness of a problem
2. Recognition of the basic problem
3. Search for a cause
4. Search for a cure
5. Acceptance of the problem

The time involved in moving from one stage to another varies with each family. *Awareness* may come early in the life of the child, particularly the child with a physical handicap. However, if it is a mental problem, awareness may come as late as the beginning of school. Denial and anger are the dominate emotions as the parent becomes aware.

Recognition of the basic problem, the second stage, helps the parents gain insight and motivates most to *seek a cause,* the third and perhaps most difficult stage in the parents' reactions. Mothers tend to blame themselves, and inability to cope with an unknown cause leads to poor adjustment, which is often manifested in misplaced hostility, anger, or self-pity. Many parents exhaust all their financial, physical, and emotional resources trying to find a reason for the child's problem.

Searching for a cure, the fourth stage, can also lead to family destruction. Hoping that each new drug, therapy, or published bit of research will help their child, many families travel from one physician to another, from city to city, and from school to school only to find little real help. The despair and grief are overwhelming for many. These families need support from the social worker, nurse, or other professionals.

The final stage, *acceptance* of the problem, takes much time. Often it is years before the parents can accept the reality of the child's problem. It is only when they have accepted the problem that they can begin to actively participate in the therapeutic plan of care. Until that time, their grief interferes with their ability to completely understand the information being shared with them. Their participation in the care of the child is essential, and professionals must be aware of the personal struggle the parents face every day as they live and work with the child.

Olshansky (1962) proposed that chronic sorrow is the natural response to a child's disability. He disputed the idea that families move through progressive stages toward a plateau of acceptance of the problem. Instead, he suggested

that families continue to move back and forth between the stages of grief and adjustment. There will be periodic crises that reevoke feelings of intense grief, anger, guilt, hostility, and denial. These periods may coincide with various developmental milestones such as birthdays, the beginning of school, or graduation. Sharing their feelings with other parents and professionals can provide a great deal of support during these periods. When families feel they have adjusted to the situation, they function most smoothly.

Assessment

Complete family assessments are critical for the nurse providing services for developmentally disabled clients and their families. In assessments, particular emphasis should be placed on areas that are unique to families with a disabled family member. Areas that are possibly more problematic for these families include interactions between family members and division of responsibilities. It is also important to compare the family's perceptions of and expectations for the developmentally disabled individual with reality and to assess how each member copes with having a disabled family member. The nurse should assess family functions and the ability of family members to carry on roles within and outside of the family. Support systems should be defined and evaluated for effectiveness. Management of conflicts, stresses, and crises should be described. Each family member's perceptions of the strengths and weaknesses of other family members and of themselves should be obtained.

Intervention

Responding to the needs of families who have children with developmental disabilities begins with recognizing, appreciating, and validating the pain families experience (Tudor, 1981). From the moment the family members learn that they have a "less than perfect" child they need a nurse who is sensitive to their grief.

Planning strategies that support the child and the family should be based more on the development and abilities the child has than on deficiencies. Focusing on the positive qualities of the child first, rather than planning for a developmentally disabled child, is one concept that can be shared with the family.

Recognition by the family that the child does have a problem aids the nurse in assisting the family to set realistic goals. Working with the family in the home affords the nurse the opportunity to appraise the coping ability of the family and to give support and encouragement as needed (Tudor, 1981).

Intervention programs for the child with a developmental disability must be planned cooperatively with the family and other professionals as needs arise. The parents are the first teachers the child knows; they are the caretakers, and the persons who must meet the emotional needs of the child. They must be taught parenting skills that they can accept and practice within the limits of their abilities.

Nurses must identify interventions that assist the child to develop to his or her highest level of health, independence, and growth. It is sometimes difficult for parents to encourage independence in children who have problems.

(Figure 26-5 depicts coordination training activities; in Figure 26-6 a child is being taught activities of daily living.)

These children also need to be accepted by their family and the community as individuals with the same rights and privileges as those with no disabilities. Encouraging the child's capabilities and providing opportunities for enrichment in his or her life through participation in family and community activities can strengthen the child's self-image.

Support Groups

As the child grows, the needs of the child and the parents change. Parents need to be supported by their extended families, friends, and others who have experienced similar problems. Small groups of parents who can identify with other parents of developmentally disabled children and can share their problems and their joys are supportive and rewarding. Voluntary groups such as those sponsored by the Association for Retarded Citizens groups, the Spina Bifida Association, and the Cerebral Palsy Organizations provide a mechanism for communication. As seen in Figure 26-7, parent groups are vital in working with developmentally disabled children. The nurse should encourage the parents to join these groups and share their experiences with others.

Parents are also helped by continued participation in the normal day-to-day activities of the community. They need to be encouraged to find responsible babysitters and respite

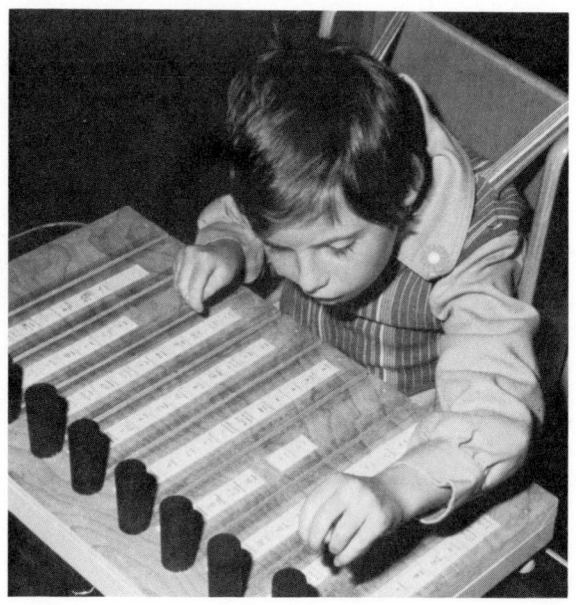

FIGURE 26-5

Coordination training.

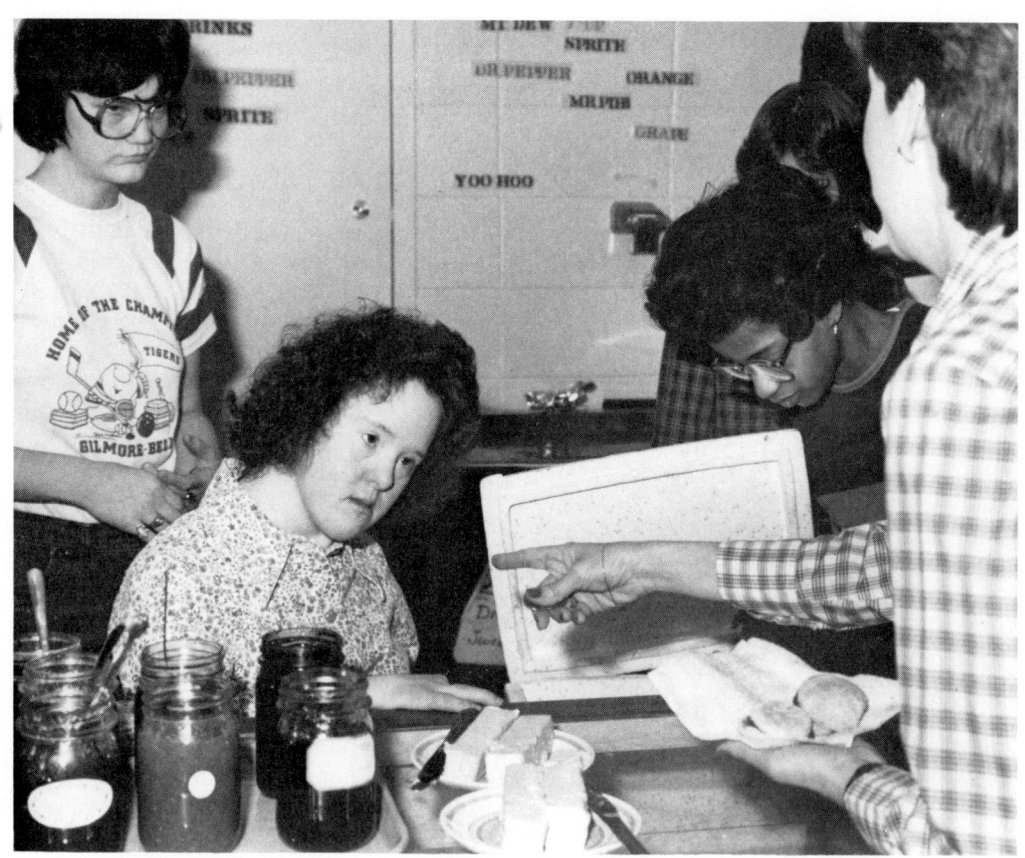

FIGURE 26-6

Activities of daily living laboratory.

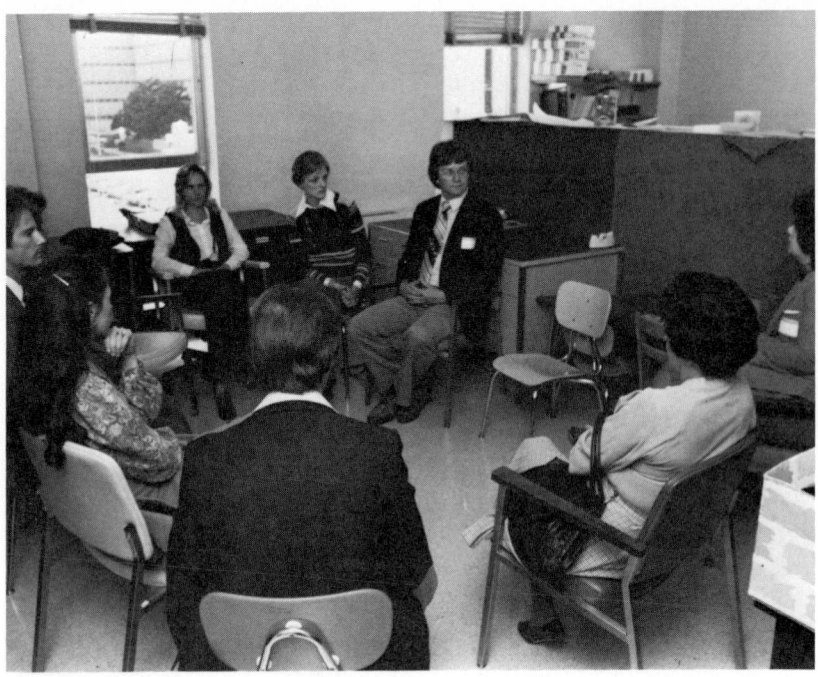

FIGURE 26-7

Parent group.

care services so that they have time to spend with other children, their spouse, and friends.

Adolescence and Adulthood

To provide anticipatory support and guidance, the community health nurse must have an understanding of the needs of developmentally disabled adolescents and adults and their families. Families of older children with disabilities may experience periods of stress during the adolescent years and at the onset of adulthood. These may be times when families receive less support and may have difficulty obtaining needed services. Concerns of parents often involve the adolescent's social, sexual, marital, and vocational possibilities. At this time, the nurse may need to help the family discuss concerns openly and realistically, to offer information they may lack, and to help them find available resources.

Frequently the physical development of the developmentally disabled adolescent is normal. The adolescent must adapt to body changes, often without the full ability to understand the implications of those changes. Information about reproduction and sexuality is needed by both the family and the adolescent. It is important to help the family and the adolescent understand the normality of emergent sexuality and to find appropriate behaviors that are acceptable within the family structure. Family planning referrals may be appropriate. The family and the adolescent should be made aware of the possibility of sexual abuse.

Social isolation often occurs as the adolescent's social and emotional development lags behind peers. Parents are often concerned that the adolescent or young adult is lonely, and these concerns should be addressed.

Plans for the future often include concerns about program needs and living arrangements as adulthood approaches. The trend is to refer disabled adults between the ages of 22 and 30 to institutions. This is probably due to limited services available during the move from school systems to adult service programs (Black et al., 1985).

Current issues concerning the care of adults with developmental disabilities results from three major trends: the increasing number of developmentally disabled adults residing in communities, the increasing advocacy for the rights of developmentally disabled citizens, and the increasing numbers of elderly developmentally disabled adults.

Many of the increased number of developmentally disabled persons remaining in or returning to the community from institutions are residing with family members or in group facilities. Currently the majority of those residing in institutions are severely retarded and have limited self-care and adaptive skills, complex medical problems, or family stressors that interfere with home placement. However, strengthening community services for the individual and the family may allow the trend of home care to continue. Needed services include medical care, sheltered housing, and counseling (Black et al., 1985).

Developmentally disabled adults have the right to marry and have children, and more information is needed about the childrearing abilities of disabled parents. There is insufficient research to predict the possibilities of developmental delay or disability in the offspring of these parents or to suggest the range of supportive services that may be necessary.

Seltzer (1985) estimated that there are as many as

it is the nurse who initiates activities that lead to more and better services for this group of people. Knowledge of the conditions, therapy, and needs of this population should motivate the community health nurse to be active in promoting local, state, and federal legislation for their assistance. Participation in civic and professional groups also provides an avenue for sharing knowledge and concern. Many professionals have little insight into the overwhelming problems faced by individuals who have disabling conditions. Community health nurses have an obligation to demonstrate concern for facilitating continued care for this group.

A well-documented record that follows the child can be a valuable tool in planning for ongoing care. Such a record prevents repetitious evaluations and provides evidence of therapy that assists with the periodic evaluation of the care and progress of the child. Ideally, computerization of records will assist individuals and agencies to maintain accurate records of developmentally disabled persons in our increasingly mobile society.

ABILITIES AND INDEPENDENT LIVING

The goal of care for all the developmentally disabled people in our society is to assist the individual to live a productive life. All are not able to achieve the goal of *independent living,* but many are capable of accomplishing this with help from the community. Figure 26-8 depicts developmentally disabled teenagers practicing sales skills.

In the last 10 years emphasis has been placed on early training, recognition of the rights of all people, and public support for programs that provide services for the developmentally disabled. Ideally, public attitudes can be changed to offer encouragement to disabled people and to support programs that are geared toward helping this population achieve independent living. Many avenues are open today, but all require public support. Figure 26-9 illustrates the development of social skills.

Since the implementation of PL 94-142, these people have an opportunity to be included in the public school system. However, adoption of such a program is expensive and requires a great deal of interpretation to the public and constant surveillance. Yet through these programs, many children and young adults have had opportunities to learn that were never offered to them before this time.

The inclusion of these children in public schools has intensified their need for health supervision. School nurses need additional preparation in the care of developmentally disabled children to help the schools provide this attention.

In addition to academic opportunity, these children are increasingly being taught how to manage activities of daily living. Learning social, self-help, and communication skills requires personnel who have an interest in and an understanding of many disciplines. Often it is the nurse who must learn from a speech therapist, physical therapist, or nutritionist the procedures to be taught to the individual child. In addition, the nurse must teach these techniques to the aides or parents because most school systems cannot support all the specialists that a child might need.

In planning for the child's care at home, his emotional,

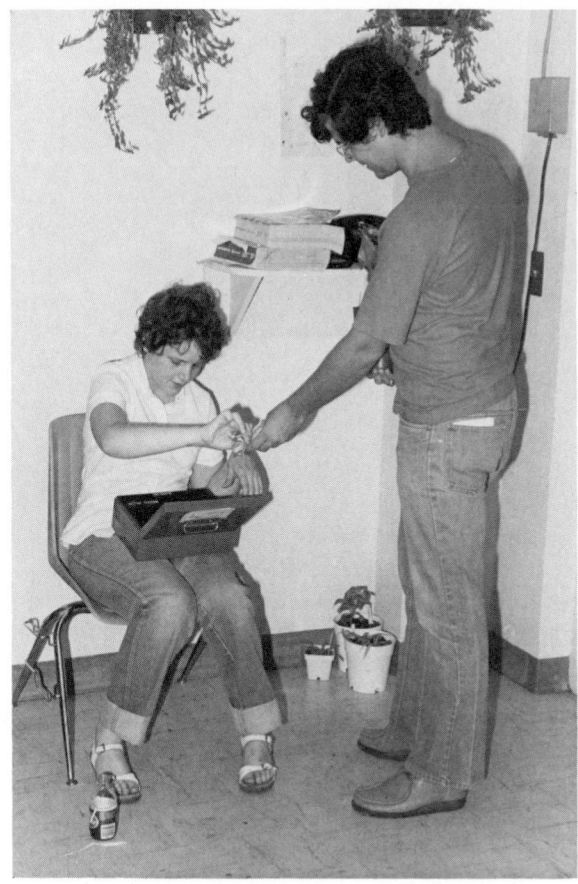

FIGURE 26-8

Teenagers practicing sales skills.

460,000 developmentally disabled adults over the age of 55 in the United States. Unlike most elderly persons, these persons generally do not have children or a spouse to depend on for assistance or support. Addressing the needs of this population can help plan for the anticipated increase in their numbers, resulting from increased survival rates. Providing services will require the coordinated efforts of federal, state, and local agencies.

FOLLOW-UP CARE

With earlier and more comprehensive evaluation of infants and young children, many are receiving better care than a few years ago. It is imperative that children who have been diagnosed as having a developmental disability be assigned to some responsible professional in the community who will maintain contact with the child and document his or her care and program.

It is far more economical for families and professional health providers to develop such plans cooperatively. When this is done, community health nurses are the most logical people in the community to assume the role of coordinator. Their expertise in working with individuals, families, and agencies is usually well-known and accepted in the community. In addition to serving as the coordinator, the nurse also acts as an advocate for the child and the family. Often

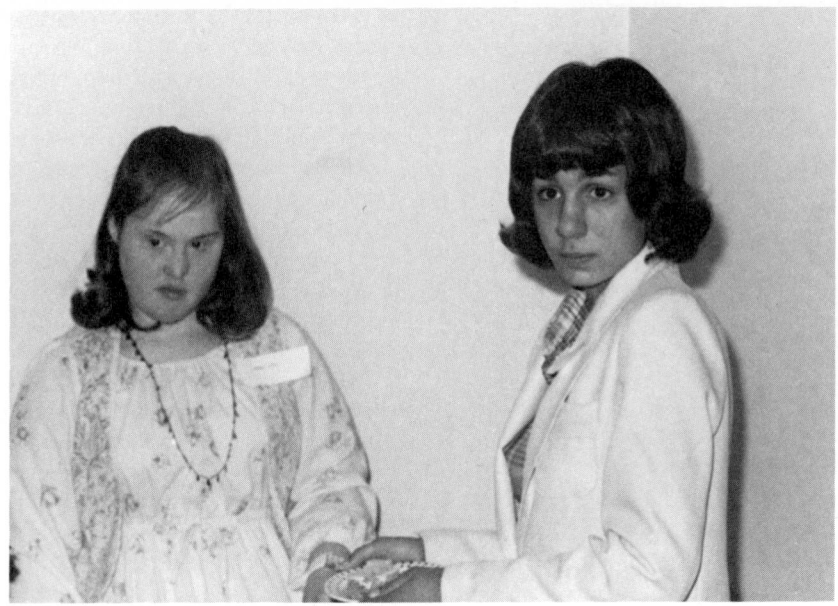

FIGURE 26-9

Development of social skills.

social, and spiritual needs should also be a part of the care program. Again it is the public health nurse who can provide the leadership for such planning. Recognizing the totality of needs of the child and the family is a realistic goal that should be a part of the basic preparation of community health nurses.

THE ROLE OF FEDERAL PROGRAMS

Federal programs for the care of developmentally disabled children were initiated by the legislative mandate of Title V of the Social Security Act. This act required states to identify and provide services to crippled children. Through the years federal programs have been expanded to provide screening and service to many more children. Over 300 categorical programs have been authorized by Congress in recent years (Norris, 1975).

The Social Security Act has been amended many times in the last 25 years to provide services for the developmentally disabled. Title XIX was amended in 1967 to require early and periodic screening, diagnosis, and treatment (EPSDT) of children eligible for Medicaid. These services were designed to provide a program of prevention, early detection, and treatment for our indigent population. This program is financed by federal and state funds and has provided a much needed service. Included in it are the following elements (Norris, 1975, p. 314):

History
Physical growth assessment
Developmental assessment
Physical inspection of unclothed child
Ear, nose, mouth, teeth, and throat inspections
Vision screening
Hearing screening
Screening tests for anemia, sickle-cell anemia, tubercu-

losis, urinary tract problems, and lead-based paint poisoning
Nutritional status
Immunization status with boosters
Other individually determined screenings such as chest x-ray films, throat cultures, pinworm slides, blood pressure, serological tests, drug-dependency screening, and stool specimen tests for parasites, ova, and blood

In 1974 the Office for the Handicapped was created as a result of the Rehabilitation Act of 1973 (93-112). The following are five functions related to the many and varied federally funded programs and are the responsibility of the Office of the Handicapped (Norris, 1975, pp. 315-316):

1. Prepare a long-range projection for the provision of comprehensive services.
2. Continually analyze the operation of the Health and Human Services programs and evaluate their effectiveness.
3. Encourage coordination and cooperative planning among the Health and Human Services' programs.
4. Develop ways to promote the use of research findings and the adoption of exemplary practices.
5. Provide for a central clearinghouse for information and resources available for handicapped persons.

A landmark act was passed by Congress with enactment of the Education for All Handicapped Children Act (94-142) in 1975. This act provides "education for every child, regardless of handicaps, in the least restrictive environment possible." Implementation of this act created both blessings and problems for the state and the children served in the public schools. The focus of Public Law (PL) 94-142 is on the education of the school-age child and not the provision of services for infants and toddlers. However, many states have taken on the responsibility for providing services for infants and toddlers although it is not a federal mandate.

Only a few federal acts have been listed to illustrate the input federal intervention has had on the care of developmentally disabled children and their families. This population needed federal and public support to be able to meet the problems of everyday living.

Nurses and nursing have also benefited from this federal legislation. Nursing skills have been refined and expanded to meet demands in a professional manner. Support through grants to states, schools, scholars, and handicapped individuals has been a great boon to advancing knowledge, concern, and methods of assisting the developmentally disabled population and their families.

These monies have enabled states to fund nursing positions in community health departments, crippled children's services, developmental diagnostic centers, and genetic laboratories. Educational grants have provided the funds needed to update the knowledge and skill of nurses working with this population.

Nurses need opportunities to learn new techniques and add to their knowledge. Nursing skills needed to care for the developmentally disabled are being addressed by a program developed by the School of Nursing at the University of Colorado Health Science Center, where a grant, funded by the Office of the Bureau of Education for the Handicapped, is being used to organize, implement, and evaluate a national educational program for school nurses. This program called the *School Nurse Achievement Program (SNAP),* is a course designed to enable school nurses to deliver health care to children with developmental disabilities during the school day. Since many community health nurses also serve as school nurses, they are invited to participate in these classes. All of these programs should assist the nurse in further developing the expertise needed to plan and implement quality care to developmentally disabled children.

The *Nursing Child Assessment Satellite Training (NCAST) program* developed by Dr. Kathryn Barnard was originally funded by the Department of Health, Education, and Welfare. The NCAST program, which is based on a model of infant-caregiver-environment interaction, can assist community health nurses in early screening, assessment of problems, and intervention techniques. (See Appendix K for information about training.)

Although federal spending for service programs and income supplementation has increased, money for research and training of professionals has declined. In early 1986 enactment of budget-balancing legislation necessitated cutbacks in domestic programs, including mental retardation programs. Continued advances in the prevention of developmental disabilities and the provision of quality services in the least restrictive environment depends on financial support, ongoing research, and preparation of professionals in the field (Braddock, 1986).

THE FUTURE

Plans for the health field must include children and adults who have developmental disabilities. Increasingly they are living in the community and are cared for by their families and local agencies. Support of families through adequate funding for community services, provision of respite care to relieve families from the ongoing burden of constant care, continuation of research into causes and preventive measures, and increased recognition of the rights of this population are concerns that must be addressed by any group that is involved in planning care for the large number of people with developmental disabilities. The community as a whole must not lose sight of the needs of these individuals as they grow from childhood to adulthood and into old age. Far too often in the past, recognition has been given to disabled children, but as they age, less and less attention is given to them. Community health nurses can help add meaning to the life of these individuals and their families.

CLINICAL APPLICATIONS

A referral was made to a public health department from a nearby regional level III neonatal intensive care unit regarding discharge plans for a developmentally delayed infant. The infant, Joel, was born at 27 weeks gestation and remained in intensive care for 7 months. His hospital course was complicated by hyaline membrane disease, bronchopulmonary dysplasia (a chronic lung disorder), and intraventricular hemorrhage. At the time of discharge Joel was receiving neither supplemental oxygen nor medications and was taking all of his feedings orally. There were strong indications of spastic diplegia, and he was diagnosed as having severe retinopathy of prematurity with the expectation of eventual blindness. Family financial resources were extremely limited. Although Medicaid coverage was available for subsequent needs, the family owed over $100,000 to the hospital. Joel's 17-year-old mother, Mary, was unmarried. She planned to complete high school; Joel's grandmother would babysit. Joel's father, who was unemployed, had been active with Mary and her mother in the hospital discharge planning program. The hospital was seeking a home evaluation before discharge.

The nurse planned to evaluate the safety of the home environment and to begin her assessment of the family's understanding of the situation and their concerns. She found that Joel's mother and grandmother were optimistic about the future and delighted to bring him home after such a long hospitalization. They recognized that he would probably suffer motor and visual impairments, yet they wanted to participate in a program to help him develop to his best potential.

The nurse also assessed knowledge of infant care and availability of infant care items. The nurse recommended the purchase of a cool mist humidifier. Since the family had been so involved in providing Joel's daily care in the nursery, they had become skilled in this area and no knowledge deficits were identified.

In planning for early intervention services, several factors were considered. Joel's family expressed a desire for developmental services. Joel's chronic lung disease made him susceptible to complications of respiratory tract infections, making it unwise to expose him to groups of young children. Lack of financial resources limited access to services.

SAMPLE DEVELOPMENTAL PROGRAM FOR JOEL

GOAL	INTERVENTION	TARGET DATE	EVALUATION
Joel will respond to auditory, visual, and tactile stimuli that indicates he is going to be picked up. Caregivers will recognize Joel's cues indicating that he wants to be picked up (holding arms out). Joel will demonstrate decreased extensor tone when lifted from supine.	Before lifting Joel, talk to him about "up," smile at him, and touch him gently. Do not lift him until he indicates a response by cooing, smiling back, or lifting his arms. If he does not give a response, prompt him by guiding his arms forward at the shoulders. When lifting Joel, do not encourage extension; place your hands behind his shoulders and roll him forward, keeping his head and shoulders flexed.	2 weeks	Family consistently demonstrated appropriate lifting technique for Joel. Joel brings his hands forward when signaled that he will be picked up.

Available community resources were center-based, offered no provision for home programs, and primarily served children ages 3 to 6. The neonatal intensive care unit (NICU) follow-up clinic was a multidisciplinary program that could offer periodic evaluations and recommendations for developmental intervention. The health department staff—the nutritionist, physical therapist, and nurse—would be responsible for receiving recommendations from the hospital and follow-up program staff to develop a home program for Joel. Later the community developmental center would serve as the main program.

During the week following Joel's discharge from the hospital, he was seen at the health department by the pediatrician and nurse to establish a baseline health appraisal. The DDST was administered using Joel's corrected age (birth age in weeks minus number of weeks premature). Results showed delays in all areas. Nutritional assessment showed that weight gain was only minimally acceptable but consistent with the growth demonstrated in the hospital. Feeding practices were assessed; Joel continued to take a high calorie formula and rice cereal with a spoon. He tired easily with feedings and was fed small amounts on a frequent schedule. Joel's immunization status was also reviewed. He had received a DPT vaccine in the nursery at 5 months of age but had not been given oral polio vaccine (OPV). Plans were made to establish an immunization schedule for him. Mary and her mother had concerns about his irregular sleeping habits and irritability. The nurse counseled them regarding behavioral and environmental interventions to promote a more organized sleeping pattern. Before the family left the clinic, the nurse checked Joel's position in his carseat and made recommendations about support for correct posture.

The physical therapist and nurse made a home visit in the following week to assess the family's success with interventions begun in the nursery and their readiness to continue the program. Mary and her mother demonstrated the exercises the hospital physical therapist had taught them. They expressed a desire to set goals including: fostering appropriate parenting skills, developing Joel's awareness of sensory stimuli, and facilitating optimal motor functioning. Examples of interventions for promoting development included recognizing Joel's behavior cues (for hunger, sleepiness, overstimulation, boredom), offering auditory and tactile stimulation in addition to visual stimulation, and demonstrating handling techniques that promote appropriate muscle tone (see box above). Joel's mother, father, and grandmother were taught how to incorporate the interventions into Joel's playtimes and daily care. Assessment of the family's coping abilities continued to indicate that the family was adjusting to the complexity of Joel's care and his physical and sensory limitations.

The nurse planned to continue biweekly home visits with the physical therapist to develop further intervention techniques and establish goals in self-help, social and emotional, cognitive, and language skills. Periodic evaluations were performed by the multidisciplinary staff at the follow-up clinic. In collaboration with the physician and nutritionist, the nurse also planned a schedule of health appraisal, nutritional assessments, and family assessments to identify health problems and to guide well-child care.

At Joel's 1 year health assessment (9 ¾ months corrected age), Mary complained of feeling upset about Joel's delays. The nurse encouraged her to discuss her frustrations and pointed out the progress Joel had made. Mary expressed anger and guilt and was unable to handle the constant demands placed on her. She was having difficulty understanding her own feelings, since she usually seemed able to adjust to everything. The nurse supported her in her grief responses and helped her recognize that she was experiencing natural emotions that other parents had also described. The nurse helped her to realize that, although she accepted Joel's limitations, she might have times of intense pain and grief. The nurse recommended that Mary and other family members attend parent–support-group meetings through the community's developmental program.

◆ ◆ ◆

The preceding case study illustrates the role of the community health nurse in providing care for developmentally disabled children and their families. The nurse is often responsible for the coordination of services, the provision of well-child care, the assessment of health status, and the implementation of interventions. The key to the management of care is the involvement of the family in mutual goal setting and the recognition and support of appropriate coping mechanisms of family members. Use of multidisciplinary resources is essential.

SUMMARY

Recognition of the need for community health nurses to become more skilled in meeting the requirements of the developmentally disabled person and his family has led to greater interest in and desire to learn more about this population. Concern and commitment to care can be augmented through the use of specific techniques and the study of problems that have currently become increasingly apparent in communities. With emphasis on care of the developmentally disabled child or adult at home and in the community, nurses must familiarize themselves with the resources available and must plan experiences to enhance their ability to provide professional service for this group. These goals can be accomplished through the cooperative efforts of the service and educational groups found in all the states. Nurses working in harmony with professionals in other fields can help provide a brighter future for our developmentally disabled population and their families.

≡ KEY CONCEPTS

Providing care for those who are developmentally disabled is a goal that has been emphasized by the federal government for many years. It is a broad goal that encompasses the work of many people in a variety of professions.

Nurses are in a key role to provide services that have a positive impact on communities.

Definitive causes for developmental disabilities are known in only about 25% of the cases. Of this small percentage, the causes are usually categorized as chromosomal aberrations; neural tube defects; central nervous system damage occurring in the perinatal period, including the sequelae of premature birth; teratogens (for example, maternal infection and maternal substance abuse); neonatal infection, and metabolic disorders.

If effective, preventive measures must begin with education of the parents before conception.

The role of the community health nurse in the care of the child with a developmental disability must be built on a sincere concern for the child and his or her family. The child with a problem must first be viewed as an individual worthy of dignity and capable of living for a purpose.

Nurses are responsible for pediatric screening and assessments beginning in the immediate neonatal period and continuing throughout childhood.

Complete family assessments are critical for the nurse providing services for developmentally disabled clients and their families.

To provide anticipatory support and guidance, the community health nurse must have an understanding of the needs of developmentally disabled adolescents and adults and their families.

With earlier and more comprehensive evaluation of infants and young children, many are receiving better care than a few years ago.

Federal programs for the care of developmentally disabled children were initiated by the legislative mandate of Title V of the Social Security Act. This act required states to identify and provide services to crippled children. Through the years federal programs have been expanded to provide screening and service to many more children.

LEARNING ACTIVITIES

1. Divide the class into two groups and debate the following issue: Children with developmental disabilities should or should not be mainstreamed into the schools.

2. Make a home visit with a nurse who has a developmentally disabled client and assess how this person's presence (1) affects the family and (2) affects (or alters) the home, and (3) what physical, emotional, and financial costs are involved for the family.

3. Using a telephone book or community resources directory, list and evaluate the services available for developmentally disabled people and their families. Include fees, location, and range of services. What gaps, overlaps, or both exist in your community? What resources are available for (1) prevention, (2) assessment, (3) intervention, and (4) follow-up care?

4. Practice using at least two of the developmental assessment tests described in this chapter.

BIBLIOGRAPHY

American Association on Mental Deficiency: Manual on terminology and classification in mental retardation. Washington, D.C., 1977, The Associaton.

Bernard, K.E., and Erickson, M.L.: Teaching children with developmental problems; a family care approach, ed. 2, 1976, The C.V. Mosby Co.

Better health for our children: a national strategy. Report of the Select Panel for the Promotion of Child Health vols. 1, 2, 3, and 55. DHHS Pub. No. 79-55071, Washington, D.C., 1981, Department of Health and Human Sciences.

Black, M.M. et al.: Individual and family factors associated with risk of institutionalization of mentally retarded adults, Am. J. Ment. Defic. 90:271-276, 1985.

Blackwell, M.W.: Care of the mentally retarded, Boston, 1979, Little, Brown & Co.

Braddock, D.: Federal assistance for mental retardation and developmental disabilities. II. The modern era, Ment. Retard. 24:209-218, 1986.

Brazelton, T.B.: The neonatal behavioral assessment scale, Philadelphia and London, 1973, J.B. Lippincott Co., and William Heinemann Ltd.

Bumbalo, J.A., and Seikel, M.A.: Identifying and serving a multiply handicapped population. Deaf-blind children and their families, Nurs. Clin. North Am. 10(2):341-352, 1975.

Buser, B.N.: The evaluation of school health services, J. Sch. Health. 50:475, 1980.

Caldwell, B.M.: Home observation for measurement of environment (Birth to Three) and (Three to Six), Little Rock, 1970 and 1976, University of Arkansas.

Caldwell, B.M.: Instructors manual inventory for infants. In Home observation for measurement of the environment, Little Rock, 1970, University of Arkansas.

Chinn, P.C., Drew, C.S., and Logan, D.R.: Mental retardation, a life cycle approach, St. Louis, 1975, The C.V. Mosby Co.

Curry, M.F.: Where are we with education of the handicapped: new approaches to screening, J. Sch. Health 51:442, 1981.

Denhoff, E.: Current status of infant stimulation or enrichment programs for children with developmental disabilities, Pediatrics 67:32, 1981.

Erickson, M.L.: Assessment and management of developmental changes in children, St. Louis, 1976, The C.V. Mosby Co.

Fleming, J.W.: Care and management of exceptional children, New York, 1973, Appleton-Century-Crofts.

Groninga, S.: Emotional/behavioral disorders: assessment and management, J. Sch. Health 50:228-229, 1980.

Hack, M. et al.: The very low birthweight infant: the broader spectrum of morbidity during infancy and early childhood, J. Dev. Behav. Pediatr. 4:243-249, 1983.

Haynes, U.: A developmental approach to case finding among infants and children. DHEW, Pub. N. (HSA) 79-5210, Washington, D.C., 1979, U.S. Government Printing Office.

Holmberg, N.J.: Serving the child with MBD and his family, Nurs. Clin. North Am. 10:301-391, 1975.

Hook, E.B.: Epidemiology of down syndrome. In Pueschel, S., and Rynders, J.E., editors: Down syndrome—advances in biomedicine and the behavioral sciences, Cambridge, 1982, The Ware Press.

House of Representatives Conference Committee: Conference report: comprehensive rehabilitation services amendments of 1978, Rep. No. 95-1780, Washington, D.C., 1978, Government Printing Office, pp. 51-52.

Jarvis, L.L.: Community health nursing: keeping the public healthy, ed. 2, Philadelphia, 1985, F.A. Davis Co.

Johnston, R.B., and Magrab, P.R.: Developmental disorder: assessment, treatment, education, Baltimore, 1976, University Park Press.

Levine, M.D.: The child with learning disabilities. In Scheiner, A.P., and Abroms, I.F., editors: The practical management of the developmentally disabled child, St. Louis, 1980, The C.V. Mosby Co.

Phelps, D.L.: Vision loss due to retinopathy of prematurity, Lancet 1:606, 1981.

Miller, L.G.: Towards a greater understanding of parents of the mentally retarded child, J. Pediatr. 733:699-705, 1968.

Nelson, R., and Crocker, A.C.: The child with multiple handicaps. In Levine, M.D. et al., editors: Developmental and behavioral pediatrics, Philadelphia, 1983, W.B. Saunders Co.

Norris, G.J.: National concerns for children with handicaps, Nurs. Clin. North Am. 10:309-317, 1975.

Office of Human Development Services Administration on Developmental Disabilities: Special report on the impact of the change in the definition of developmental disabilities. Washington, D.C., May 1981, Department of Health and Human Services.

Olshansky, S.: Chronic sorrow: a response to having a mentally defective child, Soc. Casework, 43(4):190-193, 1962.

Passo, S.: Symposium on CNS disorders in children. Malformation of the neural tube, Nurs. Clin. North Am. 15:5-21, 1980.

Phelps, D.L.: Vision loss due to retinopathy of prematurity, Lancet 1:606, 1981.

Porter, P.: The role of the independent community nurse practitioner in providing services to the developmentally disabled children and their families, Nurs. Clin. North Am. 15:419-428, 1980.

Robinson T.: Clinics for children with handicaps, J. Sch. Health 52:541-542, 1982.

Rodgers, B.M.: Comprehensive care for the child with a chronic disability, Am. J. Nurs. 79:1106-1108, 1979.

Rose, T.I.: The education of all handicapped children act (PL 94-142): new responsibilities and opportunities for the school nurse, J. Sch. Health 50:30-31, 1980.

Rosen, L.: Selected aspects in the development of the mother's understanding of her mentally retarded child, Am. J. Ment. Defic. 59:522, 1955.

Seltzer, M.M.: Informal supports for aging mentally retarded persons, Am. J. Ment. Defic. 90:259-265, 1985.

Stangler, S.R., Huber, C.J., and Routh, D.K.: Screening growth and development of preschool children: a guide for test selection, New York, 1980, McGraw-Hill Book Co.

Taft, L.T., and Matthews, W.S.: Cerebral palsy. In Levine, M.D. et al., editors: Developmental and behavioral pediatrics, Philadelphia, 1983, W.B. Saunders Co.

Tudor, M: Child development, New York, 1981, McGraw-Hill Book Co.

Waechter, E.H.: Developmental consequences of congenital abnormalities, Nurs. Forum, 14:108-129, 1975.

Wallace, H.M., Gold, E.M., and Lis, E.: Maternal and child practices: problems, resources and methods, Springfield, Ill., 1973, Charles C Thomas Publisher.

Whaley, L.F., and Wong, D.L.: Essentials of pediatric nursing, St. Louis, 1982, The C.V. Mosby Co.

Whaley, L.F., and Wong, D.L.: Nursing care of infants and children, ed. 2, St. Louis, 1983, The C.V. Mosby Co.

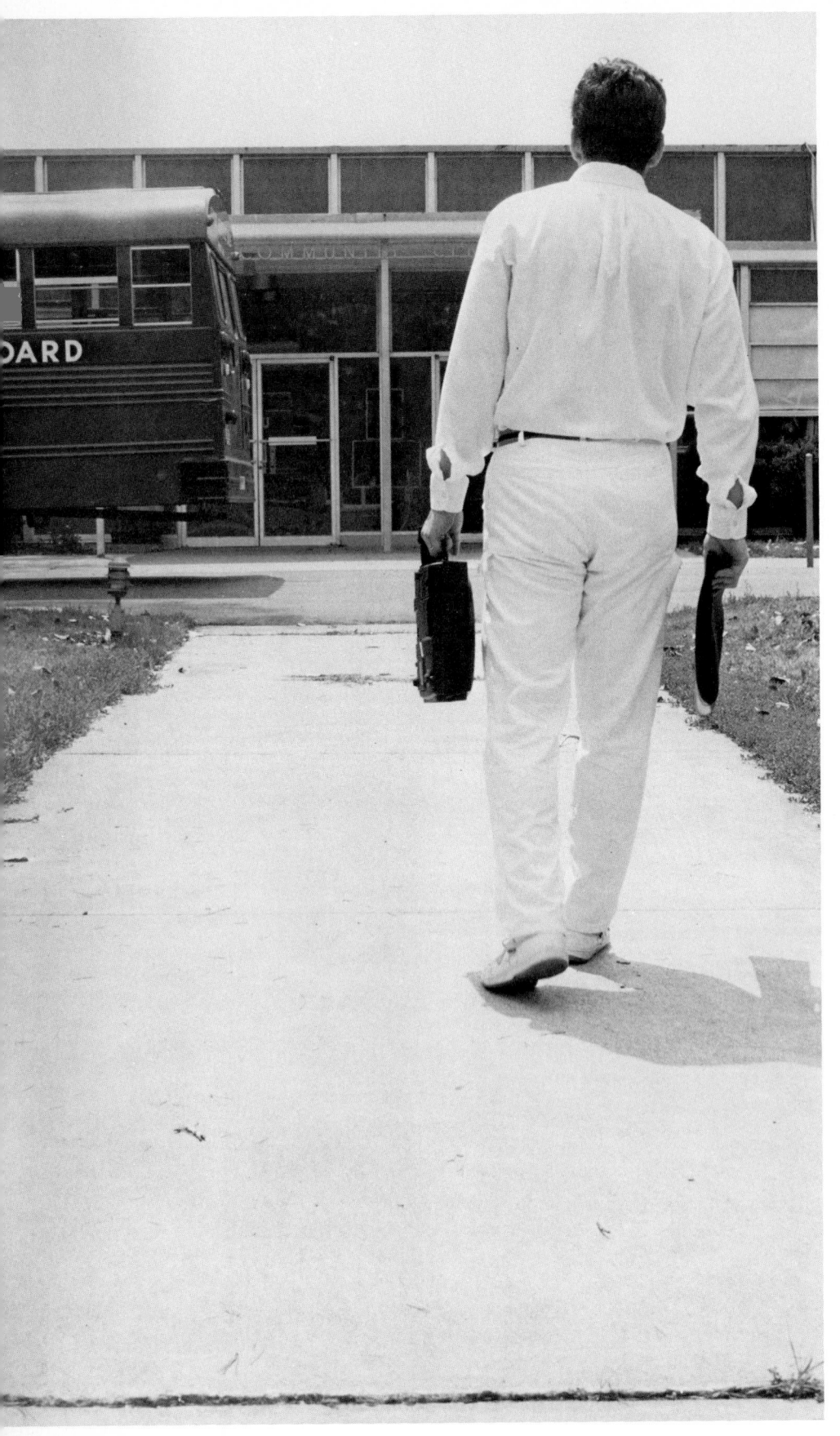

TOOLS
AND TECHNIQUES FOR
HEALTH PROMOTION

It has been estimated that the medical care system affects about 10% of the usual indexes for measuring health. The remaining 90% are determined by factors over which health care providers have little or no direct control, such as life-style and social and physical environmental conditions. The focus of this text is on the processes and practices for promoting health, and the community health nurse is considered an ideal person to personally demonstrate and teach others how to promote health. To be effective, health promotion requires that people cease focusing on how to "fix" themselves and others when they detect physical and/or emotional disequilibrium and instead acknowledge and accept personal responsibility for health. Such a change in emphasis requires that all health care providers shift from a "we will make you well" approach to a "let us work together as partners for better individual, family, and community health."

The chapters in this section document the effectiveness of health promotion and describe specific strategies that community health nurses can practice and teach to clients. The benefits of self-care are described in Chapter 27 followed by chapters that emphasize the way in which nutrition, exercise, recreation, leisure time, stress management, and assertiveness techniques can be incorporated into a plan for personal and client-centered health.

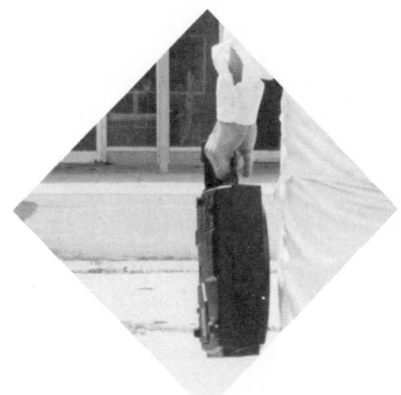

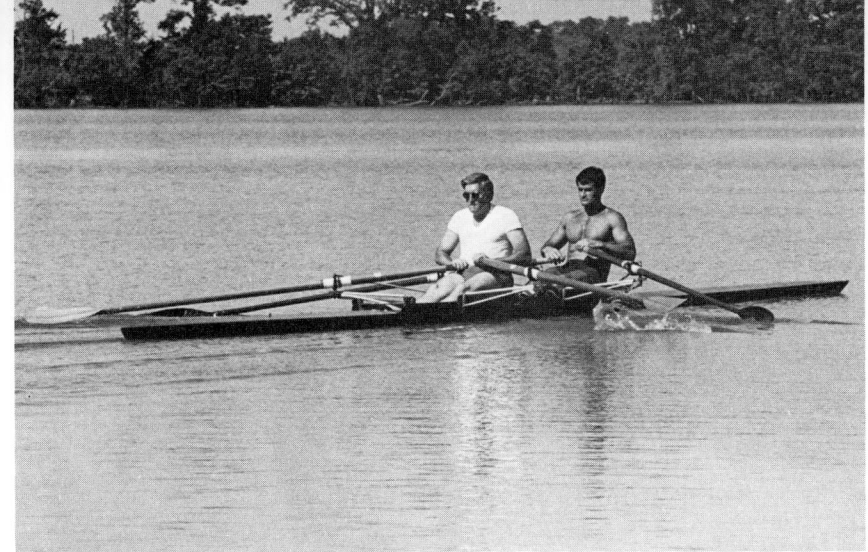

Jean Goeppinger
Karen T. Labuhn

27

SELF-HEALTH CARE THROUGH RISK APPRAISAL AND REDUCTION

⊤ OBJECTIVES

After reading this chapter, the student should be able to:

Identify factors influential in the development and practice of self-health care.

Define self-health care.

Relate self-health care to risk appraisal and reduction.

Compare and contrast methods of appraising individual health risks.

Describe methods of assessing aggregate health risks.

Compare and contrast methods of reducing health risks.

Develop an argument for community health nursing roles in risk appraisal and reduction.

⊤ KEY TERMS

counterconditioning
Framingham Heart Study
Health Hazard Appraisal
health maintenance organizations

health risk appraisal
iatrogenesis
lifetime health monitoring
macrolevel interventions
microlevel interventions
modeling

North Karelia Study
operant conditioning
Pawtucket study
self-health care
self-health management
stimulus control
wellness inventories

A marked resurgence of interest in self-health care is apparent today. Many Americans exercise regularly (even enthusiastically), maintain their weight at recommended levels, and deliberately attempt to manage stress. Some drive at reduced speeds, drink fewer alcoholic beverages than in the past, and no longer smoke. Others jog on country lanes and in city parks, participate in structured physical fitness programs, patronize natural foods stores, garden organically (without the use of pesticides or chemical fertilizers), and engage in a variety of relaxation techniques at home and at work.

Newspaper articles and radio and television programs provide evidence of this growing interest in self-health care as does the rapid proliferation of commerical weight-reduction programs, smoking cessation plans, and health spas. Organizations also have been established to promote self-health care. The San Francisco-based National Center for Health Education, a private institution, was founded in the mid-1970s. About the same time, the health and life insurance industry began supporting the Advisory Committee on Education for Health. The American Hospital Association also instituted its Center for Health Promotion. These organizations have published reviews of literature and programs related to self-health care and have developed recommendations for the insurance and health care industries.

The federal government also has become involved in the self-health care movement. During the past decade, the Office of Health Information and Health Promotion (now the Office of Health Information, Health Promotion, Physical Fitness, and Sports Medicine) was established in the office of the Assistant Secretary for Health, and the Bureau of Health Education (now the Center for Health Promotion and Education) was started in the Centers for Disease Control. In the late 1970s, *Healthy People: The Surgeon General's Report on Health Promotion and Disease Prevention* was published (Healthy People, 1979a). Subsequently, *Promoting Health/Preventing Disease: Objectives for the Nation,* was published (Promoting Health, 1981). The National Heart, Lung, and Blood Institute has sponsored major research projects such as the Multiple Risk Factor Intervention Trial (Neaton et al., 1981) and the Stanford Heart Disease Prevention Program (Maccoby et al., 1977). These studies are described later in the chapter.

Naturally there are critics of self-health care. Critics challenge the self-health care movement on philosophical and political grounds. They argue that (1) social changes, not simply individual changes, are prerequisite to individual health (Kronenfeld, 1979); (2) professional interest in self-health care has overcome the initial orientation toward meeting consumer needs (Fanoroff, 1977; Levin, 1976); (3) the fostering of individual change requires unethical manipulation of human behavior (Warwick and Kelman, 1973); and (4) the focus on self-health care reflects a "blaming-the-victim" attitude (Mitchell, 1982). Other critics question the efficacy and cost effectiveness of self-health care. Breslow (1978b) states that the efficacy of self-health care has not been systematically and convincingly demonstrated; he believes that the movement has been adopted for faddish rather than for scientific reasons. Gori and Richter (1978) and Veatch (1980) also point out that the cost effectiveness of self-health care has not been established.

The debate between the critics and proponents of *self-health care* is important. It suggests that despite the rhetoric of support and recent progress, important questions still remain. The criticisms require careful attention. Health professionals need to be aware of the complexity of the philosophical, political, and practice issues to direct their efforts toward enhancing positive aspects of the self-health care movement. Efforts to address questions of efficacy are of primary importance to the practitioner.

This chapter focuses on *health risk appraisal* and reduction, areas of self-health care in which questions of efficacy are already being addressed. The context within which health risk appraisal and reduction has developed is described, and the scientific basis for risk appraisal and reduction is discussed. A variety of methods for appraising and reducing health risks at the individual and community levels is explained. Finally, suggestions for applications of these methods are given, with specific references to community health nursing practice.

SELF-HEALTH CARE

The concept of people helping themselves in health matters is not new. Very likely the practice of self-health care began

The authors wish to thank Jeanne Allen for her assistance in updating the references.

before recorded history. Early references appear in ancient Greek, Chinese, and Hebrew writings. Americans have been involved since colonial times. Thomas Jefferson, for example, required a medical self-help course for students entering the University of Virginia during the early years of the nineteenth century (Weiss, 1977).

History

References to self-health care in classical literature include mystical and religious elements, as well as pragmatic components. For instance, in Greek literature the goddess Hygeia represented the belief that humans could remain healthy if they lived rationally. Certain activities of daily living, like exercise, were considered essential to the maintenance of health; and tributes to Hygeia were important. Similarly, in biblical times various food laws were promulgated to please Yahweh and ensure health.

With the later development of a scientific and biological orientation toward disease, self-health care was gradually deemphasized. A new focus on treatment and cure displaced the original goals of health protection and illness prevention. This new focus also encouraged a growing dependence on persons with specialized training—health professionals. Despite these changes, the nurturance of health and the provision of care to the ill remained lay functions to a certain extent. Many health-related activities continued to occur within the family environment and were directed or performed by wives and mothers.

Currently self-health care is reemerging as an important factor in health care. In some cases it is competing with, if not supplanting, professional care. For example, some versions of self-health care emphasize lay diagnosis and self-treatment as opposed to professional diagnosis and collaborative management. Other more conservative versions focus on teaching people how to work with their health care providers. In either case, the professional health care system is being dramatically affected. Professional roles are being renegotiated, and the structure of the existing health care system is changing to allow more emphasis on prevention and self-health care. The rapid growth of **health maintenance organizations** (HMOs) and other prepaid medical plans reflects the development of one such self-health care model emphasizing collaboration between consumers and providers.

The revitalization of self-health care in the United States may represent a cyclical recurrence of the more general self-help theme. Americans on the frontier did not have the benefit of expert advice nor were they often close to professional medical help. In the true spirit of Jacksonian democracy, they not only depended on themselves but often scorned advice from outsiders. In health matters, as in other areas, the older, wiser, and more experienced family members were the experts. If these persons were literate and financially secure, they may have consulted the medical encyclopedia on the parlor bookshelf. If they were illiterate and impoverished, they used folk remedies, which were part of the culture's oral tradition. In either case, self-health care retained its original religious links. Early popular self-health care books, such as the *Primitive Physic* by John Wesley

(1747), were recommended regularly at prairie revivals.

The reemerging self-health care movement also has been influenced by the political climate of the past two decades. During the 1960s and 1970s authority in general was challenged. Racial minorities demanded their rights in the 1960s; and women, patients, and the elderly made their demands public in the 1970s. A challenge to the professional health care system, which many believe exemplifies elite rather than democratic control, is illustrated clearly in the ideology of self-health care. Illich, for example, wrote, "The medical establishment has become a major threat to health. The disabling impact of professional control over medicine has reached the proportions of an epidemic" (Illich, 1976a, p. 3).

Illich considers both social and cultural *iatrogenesis* as relevant to self-health care. Iatrogenesis refers to illness acquired in the health care environment, such as an infection contracted during a hospital stay. Social iatrogenesis fosters people becoming "consumers of doubtful nostrums rather than changing the morbid social and political conditions that are the major causes of ill health" (Illich, 1976b, p. 69). Cultural iatrogenesis turns "patients into passive consumers, objects to be repaired, voyeurs of their own treatment . . . It destroys our autonomous ability to cope with our bodies and heal ourselves" (Illich, 1976b, p. 73). Illich chastises American health professionals and society for robbing individuals of their self-health care skills. He warns that politicians and legislators may promote self-health care because of their interest in cost containment rather than a genuine belief in individuals' abilities to preserve health.

Other self-health care advocates believe that modern medicine has been given too much credit for improvements in health. McKinlay and McKinlay (1977) have been articulate and convincing advocates of the position that medical measures have contributed little to the decline in mortality in the United States since the turn of the century. Their secondary analysis of data on mortality from 10 major infectious diseases since 1900 suggests that chemotherapeutic and prophylactic medical measures often were introduced decades after the marked decline in mortality began. McKeown et al., (1975) argue that the main contributors to the decline in mortality seem to have been better standards of living, including improvements in sanitation, personal hygiene, and diet, which led to a more favorable balance in the host-agent-environment relationship.

Conclusions such as these have been drawn for chronic illnesses as well as for communicable diseases. Wildavsky (1977) asserts that the medical system affects only 10% of the variability in health indicators such as infant mortality, disability days, and adult mortality. He attributes the remainder to factors over which physicians lack control, "from individual life-style (smoking, exercise, worry), to social conditions (income, eating habits, physiological inheritance), to the physical environment (air and water quality)" (1977, p. 105).

In the political arena these conclusions first were supported by LaLonde in *A New Perspective on the Health of Canadians* (1974). As the Canadian Minister of National Health and Welfare, LaLonde urged a more comprehensive approach to health care. He identified four major determinants of health: human biology, environment, life-style, and health care (Figure 27-1). LaLonde's ideas influenced policymakers in this country. The three major categories of health risks delineated in the Surgeon General's Report (*Healthy People,* 1979a) were inherited biological factors, the environment, and behavioral factors. These are identical to LaLonde's first three major determinants of health.

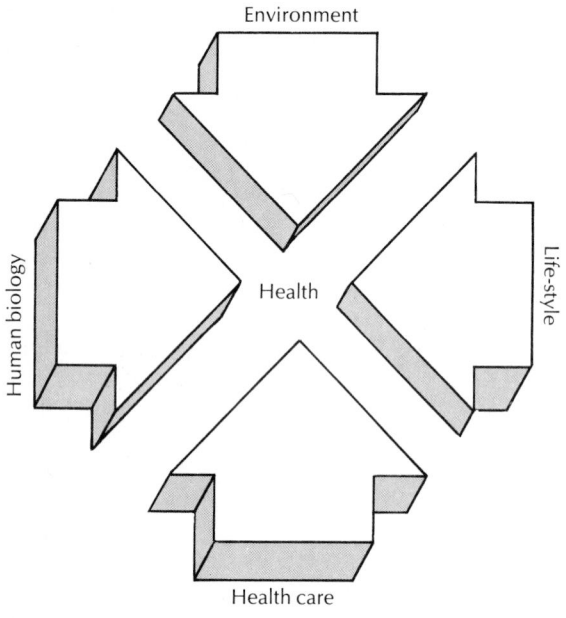

FIGURE 27-1

Determinants of health. (Adapted from Lalonde, M.: A new perspective on the health of Canadians, Ottawa, 1974, Government of Canada.)

Meaning

Despite its renewed popularity, the concept of self-health care lacks a consistent definition. Labels for the concept also vary, from life-style management to self-care, self-health care, and self-health management. Some authors use these terms interchangeably, but others attempt to distinguish among them. Green, a prominent health educator, uses the terms self-care to refer to self-diagnosis, treatment and preventive care and *self-health management* to refer to these self-care activities and the use of professional and educational services (1985).

Lorig (1980) has developed a conceptual paradigm, that is very useful for comparing and evaluating various authors' perspectives on self-health care. The paradigm includes four dimensions: the instigator of care, the target of care, the goal of care, and the type of knowledge on which care is based (Table 27-1). Most commonly the instigators of self-health care are lay persons who carry out health care for themselves. When compliance behaviors are included as a component of self-health care, however, the instigators may be health professionals.

Self-health care may be targeted toward the individual, the community, or the society. Approaches by primary care providers are generally directed toward the individual; they focus on changing health beliefs and behaviors. Self-health care approached from a public health and political perspective emphasizes community responsibility and social change rather than individual reform.

The goal of self-health care refers to the purpose or function of the care. Goals can be directed toward health promotion or toward disease prevention, early detection, and treatment. The goal of risk appraisal and reduction usually involves primary prevention or early detection and treatment of health problems.

TABLE 27-1

A comparison of perspectives on self-health care

Author	Dimension			
	INSTIGATOR OF CARE	TARGET OF CARE	GOAL OF CARE	TYPES OF KNOWLEDGE
Lorig	Usually layperson; professional when compliance included in self-health care	Individual; community; society	Health promotion; disease prevention; disease detection and treatment	Religious-philosophical; scientific-cultural
Levin	Layperson functioning in own behalf as primary resource in health care delivery	Individual	Health promotion; disease prevention; disease detection and treatment	Scientific
Green	Layperson as alternative health care provider	Individual	Self-diagnosis and treatment	Scientific
Orem	Usually layperson; professional if required by self-health care deficits	Individual	Maintenance of life, health, and well-being	Scientific
Goeppinger	Individuals, singly or in groups	Individual; community; society	All activities pertinent to health and illness	Scientific-cultural; religious-philosophical

Interpretations of the final dimension of Lorig's paradigm, the knowledge base of self-health care, have changed over the decades. Whereas early self-health care practices often were based on religious or philosophical tenets, currently self-health care has primarily a scientific base with strong cultural and folk-medicine overtones.

Contemporary literature about self-health care emphasizes varying dimensions of Lorig's paradigm. Levin, a prolific writer on the subject, subsumes self-health care under the professional health care delivery system, bases it on scientific medicine, and targets it toward individual change. He describes the goal of self-health care broadly: "self-health care is a process in which a layperson can function effectively on his or her own behalf in health promotion and decision-making, in disease prevention, detection, and treatment" as "the primary health resource in the health care system" (1977, p. 115).

Green's definition of self-care includes only diagnostic and treatment activities, which formerly were the responsibility of professional health care providers. He excludes basic prevention activities that consumers "may and should take" and that providers have not traditionally controlled (Green, 1977, p. 168). Self-health care from this perspective is a lay alternative to professional health care, is targeted toward the individual, and has a goal of self-diagnosis and treatment but remains based on scientific medicine.

Nurses always have emphasized peoples' natural self-health care capacities. Orem, a contemporary nursing theorist, uses the term *self-care* to describe activities that individuals initiate and perform on their own behalf to maintain life, health, and well-being (Orem, 1971). According to Orem, the nursing profession is essential because individuals are not always self-sufficient. Consequently, though self-health care is a lay responsibility, professional contributions may be required. Like Levin and Green, Orem's focus is on the individual, and the basis of self-health care is scientific.

We agree with Lorig that the conceptualizations of self-health care by Levin, Green, and Orem are too restrictive because of their exclusively scientific basis and focus on the individual only. A more complete definition would include the full range of possibilities, considering all four dimensions of the paradigm. Self-health care then would encompass all "those activities, continuous and episodic, volitional and unintentional, which people can do for themselves, individually or collectively, in a variety of health and illness matters. These activities complement professional health care services" (Goeppinger, 1982, p. 380). They may be directed toward the individual, community, and society and are based on various combinations of scientific, religious, philosophical, and cultural influences. In the following discussion, we consider risk appraisal and reduction in light of this broad perspective of self-health care.

Relation to Risk Appraisal and Reduction

Risk appraisal and reduction is an approach that health professionals can use to help individuals and groups maximize their self-health care. The goal of risk appraisal and reduction is the prevention or early detection of disease. The knowledge base for this approach is the scientific evidence regarding the relationships between risk factors and mortality and the effectiveness of planned interventions in reducing these risks and the mortality that can result.

Since the early 1970s, risk appraisal and reduction have gained popularity among health professionals. This trend has been influenced by the renewed emphasis on health promotion and disease prevention, by epidemiological studies that have provided an empirical data base for making predictions from risk appraisal methods, and by a proliferation of risk appraisal tools for use in clinical practice. The health insurance industry also has recognized the potential of risk reduction for cost containment and has promoted the approach in occupational and health care settings.

Two of the most influential epidemiological studies of health risks have been the *Framingham Heart Study,* initiated in 1949, and the Human Population Laboratory's longitudinal survey of Alameda County, California residents, initiated in the early 1970s. Both of these studies have supported the hypothesis that selected risk factors are directly related to morbidity and mortality.

In the Framingham Heart Study, 5209 adult residents of a small town in Massachusetts agreed to be followed over their lifespans to help researchers identify factors contributing to the development of coronary heart disease and high blood pressure. The subjects received periodic health and life-style assessments, and morbidity and mortality statistics were collected. The longitudinal study was successful in meeting its objectives. Heart disease was found to be more prevalent among persons who had high blood pressure, high cholesterol levels, low levels of exercise, and who smoked. Obesity also was identified as a contributor to high blood pressure and elevated cholesterol levels and thus to heart disease (Haynes, Feinlieb, and Kannel, et al., 1980).

The Alameda County Study was also designed as a prospective study, but it included a probability sample of 6928 subjects, which allows more confident generalizations of the findings than the Framingham study (Breslow, 1972). In this study, a number of social and behavioral factors were studied in relation to mortality. The first 5-year follow-up revealed several self-health care practices inversely related to mortality. These practices included eating three meals daily at regular intervals, eating breakfast, sleeping 7 to 8 hours a night, using alcohol moderately, exercising regularly, not smoking, and maintaining a desirable height-to-weight ratio (Belloc, 1973). Projections of life expectancies for combinations of these health practices also were made. A 45-year-old man who engaged in six or seven of the positive practices could expect to live 11 years longer than a man engaging in fewer than three of the practices. A 45-year-old woman who engaged in six or seven of the practices could expect to live 7 years longer than a woman engaged in fewer than four of the practices. Results from subsequent follow-ups of the sample generally supported these early findings, although some self-health care practices such as dietary habits were no longer found to be significant predictors of mortality. Cigarette smoking, alcohol consumption, physical exercise, hours of sleep, and weight in relation to height continued to predict mortality for white adults (Wiley and Camacho, 1980).

Also in the Alameda County study, social factors were identified as having important influences on health. Berkman (1977) found that the strength of respondent's social networks (such as marriage, contact with close friends and relatives, church membership, and ties with formal and informal groups) was inversely related to mortality. These findings were initially received with a great deal of controversy, but they encouraged the inclusion of social and environmental variables, as well as personal behaviors, in health risk appraisals.

Findings from large scale surveys such as the Framingham and Alameda County studies prompted a number of intervention trials that focused on reducing health risks. Some studies that attempted to evaluate community-based interventions were the Stanford Heart Disease Prevention Program (Maccoby, et al., 1977) the North Karelia Study (Puska, 1978), the Pawtucket Study (Lasater, Abrams, and Artz, et al., 1984), and the Multiple Risk Factor Intervention Trial (Neaton, et al., 1981).

The Stanford study was designed to test the impact of a mass media campaign alone and in combination with face-to-face instruction on three cardiovascular risk factors: cigarette smoking, systolic blood pressure, and serum cholesterol. After 2 years, the investigators found a substantial increase in knowledge about cardiovascular disease and its risk factors and a decrease in risk behaviors in the two experimental communities. A comparable increase in knowledge and decline in risk were not found in the control community. The intervention with the combined mass media and face-to-face instruction was found to be the most effective method of inducing behavioral changes (Maccoby, et al., 1977).

These findings must be accepted with caution. High-risk subjects in the media-only community showed almost no reduction in cardiovascular risks. The lack of a face-to-face instruction-only experimental condition also made it impossible to test the relative efficacy of the two methods (Leventhal, et al., 1980). Finally, the persistence of change after 2 years was not examined. Despite these limitations, the changes found in this study are encouraging.

Tentative positive results likewise were found in the *North Karelia Study* (Puska, 1978). Citizens of North Karelia, a rural area in Finland, experienced extraordinarily high mortality rates from cardiovascular disease in the early 1970s. At this time, more than half of North Karelian men smoked. They ingested large amounts of animal fats and had grossly elevated serum cholesterol levels. In addition, many suffered from untreated hypertension. The government initiated an intervention program at both individual and community levels to assist individuals in modifying their high risk behaviors.

The North Karelia project involved extensive retraining of health professionals; reorganization of public health services; production of low-fat dairy products and low-fat, low-salt sausages; and the development of community health education programs. Follow-up studies demonstrated that

the prevalence of the three major risk factors for cardiovascular disease decreased much more in North Karelia than in a comparison county (Bauer, 1981). Critics of this study point out that changes in behavioral changes have not been adequately linked to changes in morbidity and mortality (Wagner, 1982), but data collection is continuing in an attempt to document these long-range effects.

The *Pawtucket study* is an ongoing ten-year intervention project in a Rhode Island community, that traditionally has had very high rates of cardiovascular disease. As in the North Karelia study, the interventions in Pawtucket are directed toward both individuals and the community. The news media, churches, and numerous social groups have been involved in risk reduction education activities, and the food industry has begun to offer special "Heart Healthy" menus (Lasater, Abrams, and Artz, et al., 1984). The official findings from this study will not be reported until the 1990s, but the study has been publicized widely and has helped to maintain public interest in risk appraisal and reduction strategies.

Unlike the Stanford, North Karelia, and Pawtucket community studies, the Multiple Risk Factor Intervention Trial (MRFIT) was a controlled clinical trial that focused on testing the effectiveness of various counseling techniques in lowering smoking, high cholesterol, and hypertension rates among men at high risk for cardiovascular disease. The study extended from 1972 through 1982 and involved 22 treatment centers and 12,000 patients (Zukel, Oglesby, and Schnaper, 1981). Findings from an early analysis of the data revealed significant differences between the risk factors of counseled patients and the usual-care patients, suggesting that risk reduction counseling in practice settings can be very effective (Neaton, et al., 1981).

These studies, among others, have provided a beginning scientific knowledge base for the implementation of risk appraisal and reduction methods. However, information on the relative effectiveness of specific interventions in reducing risks remains limited. The evidence from intervention studies is insufficient to assess the extent to which reductions in risk produce comparable reductions in morbidity and early mortality. Yet most health professionals agree that we cannot afford to postpone intervention efforts. As Breslow (1978a, p. 456) has stated: "The best we can seek is to avoid action based on imprudent interpretation of available data, and to promote action against risk factors based on prudent interpretations of available data, at the same time, striving for better and more pertinent evidence."

METHODS OF HEALTH RISK APPRAISAL

In *health risk appraisal,* data about health risks experienced by an individual or group are collected and analyzed, and a health-risk profile is generated. Health risk appraisal may be carried out on an individual and community level. A clinical approach is required to establish the presence or absence of risks at the individual level, and epidemiological approaches are used to identify risks at the community level. Both of these approaches are important to community health nurses and are discussed in this chapter (Table 27-2).

Appraising Individual Health Risks

At least three types of individual health risk appraisal tools are common today. These include the Health Hazard Appraisal and its many versions, the Lifetime Health Monitoring Program, and Wellness Appraisals or Inventories. Each type of risk appraisal is rather complex, and only the basic concepts and procedures are described in this chapter. Fuller explanations can be found in the references cited at the end of the chapter. Some examples of risk appraisal tools (the Health Hazard Appraisal, the Lifetime Health Monitoring Program, and the Lifestyle Assessment Questionnaire) are shown in Appendix C.

Health Hazards Appraisal (HHA)

Among the earliest proponents of individual health risk appraisal were two family physicians who called their approach prospective medicine (Robbins and Hall, 1970). Unlike physicians in conventional curative practice, they wanted to deal with an individual's health from the perspective of what was likely to occur, rather than what had already happened. They recognized that most chronic diseases have a predictable sequence and that the characteristic precursors of many diseases can be monitored and controlled. The natural history of one such illness, arteriosclerotic heart disease, is diagrammed in Figure 27-2.

Robbins and Hall (1970) put the concept of prospective medicine into practice by developing a method of profiling risk termed the **Health Hazard Appraisal.** The objectives of the Health Hazard Appraisal are to (1) assess the total risks to a client's health based on knowledge of the client, the natural history of certain diseases, and the major causes of mortality for aggregates of the client's age, sex, and race; (2) initiate life-style changes in the client to avoid disease precursors or to minimize their pathogenic influence; and (3) institute medical treatment as early in the course of disease as possible.

To accomplish these objectives, data are collected by a self-administered questionnaire, basic laboratory tests, and a miniclinical examination. The questionnaire (see Appendix C) elicits information about personal characteristics and behaviors known to predict health status. The laboratory testing is limited to obtaining the serum cholesterol level; and the physical examination consists of height, weight, and blood pressure measurements.

These personal data then are compared with data compiled from the 10 major causes of death for an aggregate of the client's age, sex, and race; the average probability of dying; and the precursors and risk intensities associated with each cause of death. Appraisal and achievable ages are computed. The appraisal age is the health age of the average person in the client's racial, sex, and age aggregate with a similar risk profile. For example, a 20-year-old white woman might have an appraisal age of 15 if she has good health habits and is genetically fortunate. Another 20-year-old white woman might have an appraisal age of 26 if she smokes, fails to use seat belts, and does not perform regular breast examinations. This person's achieveable age, the health age she could achieve by modifying her health hazards, would be considerably lower.

In the decade after Robbins and Hall's initial work, health hazard appraisal instruments proliferated rapidly. At least 12 health risk appraisals are in current use (Doerr and Hutchins, 1981). Some of these are medically focused whereas others include issues related to mental health, social health, and the environment. Two instruments that illustrate these differences are the Health Risk Index (Medical Datamation, 1980) and the Lifestyle Assessment Questionnaire (Hettler, 1978) (see Appendix C).

The Health Risk Index collects data on illnesses; family medical history; and lifestyle factors related to specific diseases, selected physiological areas, and to a lesser extent, emotions and feelings. These data are compared with mortality data. The Lifestyle Assessment Questionnaire includes

---

TABLE 27-2

Health risk appraisal methods

Individual level	Aggregate level
Health hazard appraisal	Epidemiological study; survey with risk appraisal instruments; morbidity and mortality statistics
Lifetime health monitoring program	Vital statistics with demographic data
Wellness inventory	Community Competence Assessment

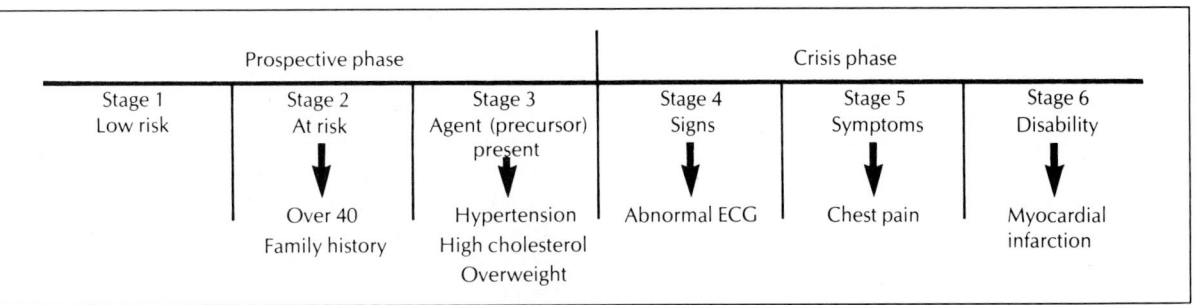

FIGURE 27-2

Natural history of arteriosclerotic heart disease.

(1) a wellness inventory that requests data on personal habits, feelings and emotions, the community, automobile safety, rest and relaxation, and fitness; (2) a life-style assessment with separate sections for personal growth and risk of death; and (3) a medical alert. Only data from the risk of death portion of the life-style assessment are compared with mortality data. Other health hazard appraisal instruments range between these two extremes.

Special versions of health hazard appraisals have been developed for children and adolescents. The Know Your Body program, developed by the American Health Foundation in New York City (Williams, Carter, and Eng, 1980), was designed to identify chronic disease risk factors in school children 11 to 14 years of age. The children receive feedback and health prescriptions in a "health passport". The University of Florida 4-H for Life Appraisal (Moody, et al., 1979) provides teenagers with health risk profiles and educational messages regarding their health behaviors.

Lifetime Health Monitoring Program (LHMP)

Because a substantial portion of physician time is spent in evaluating the health of apparently well people (often considered the "worried well"), Breslow and Somers (1977) proposed a Lifetime Health Monitoring Program (see Appendix C), which is suitable for medical practice settings. Like the Health Hazard Appraisal, it uses clinical and epidemiological data to identify specific needs for health care, but instead of assessing individual health risks, the lifetime health monitoring program provides a detailed list of recommendations for preventive measures appropriate to each of 10 different age groups. An ad hoc advisory committee of the Institute of Medicine drafted these recommendations and developed criteria to guide the choice of procedures for specific age groups (Bauer, 1981).

The overall objective of lifetime health monitoring is to focus routine health evaluations on the specific problems most likely to occur at a given age and, thus, to better prevent these problems. For example, recommendations for women who are 40 to 49 years of age include tests for hypertension and malignancies of the breast, cervix, and gastrointestinal tract, and counseling on changing nutritional needs, physical activity, and the use of cigarettes, alcohol, and drugs (Breslow and Somers, 1977).

In the past several years, *lifetime health monitoring* programs for use in specific settings have been developed. In such cases, the known risk profile of the population under surveillance is used to modify screening recommendations adopted for the general population. Guidotti (1983) describes a lifetime health monitoring program that was developed for managers in an occupational setting. Since the managers were shown (in health surveys) to be heavier smokers and coffee drinkers than other white-collar employees in the company, these behaviors and other psychological stress factors were taken into consideration when developing the monitoring program.

Wellness Inventories

The various wellness inventories are slightly different from the generic Health Hazard Appraisal (Robbins and Hall,

1970) and the Lifetime Health Monitoring Program. They tend to define health risks more broadly and emphasize lay control. The Health Hazard Appraisal is designed to avert disease and premature death; wellness appraisals may encourage disease prevention, but they do so by advocating health enhancement or promotion. "One holds the line, the other moves forward" (Ardell, 1977, p. 56).

Typically, *wellness inventories* are concerned with a wide range of personal self-health care behaviors. For example, Clark's Wellness Assessment (1981) has six categories: eating well, being fit, feeling good, caring for self and/or others, fitting in, and being responsible. Ardell (1977) includes inventories related to self-responsibility, nutritional awareness, physical fitness, stress management, and environmental sensitivity. Travis' Wellness Self-Evaluation (1977) includes a Life Change Index, an Eating Habits Survey, a Wellness Inventory Symptom Checklist, a Medical History, a Purpose in Life Test, Stress Assessments, and a Creativity Index. In contrast with these instruments, the Health Hazard Appraisal assesses only those health behaviors which have clearly documented relationships to disease.

Advantages and Limitations

Risk appraisal instruments are convenient tools that can be used to determine individual health risks. Because these instruments also provide written feedback regarding recommended preventive actions, they support the individual's self-health care efforts. Professionals also receive support and direction in their educational activities. Studies of health risk appraisals in clinical settings indicate that clients who complete the instruments generally are more aware of their health risks (Bartlett, Pegues, and Shaffer, et al., 1983; Schultz, 1984), are more willing to discuss their health behaviors with their physicians (Skinner, Allen, and McIntosh, et al., 1985), and in some cases, initiate suggested changes (Bartlett, Pegues, and Shaffer, et al., 1983; Schultz, 1984). Risk appraisals also are useful for measuring the effectiveness of planned interventions for risk reduction. Completed by individuals at different time periods, they provide feedback about how behavioral changes have influenced health risks and life expectancy.

Despite these advantages, practitioners should be aware of the limitations of risk appraisal instruments. Some of these limitations are inherent in the tools themselves, whereas others relate more to problems in usage. Actual tool limitations include (1) the questionable validity and reliability of some of the instruments, (2) the inconsistency with which different appraisal instruments measure and analyze health characteristics, and (3) a general over-emphasis on life-style factors and lack of attention to other important risks such as environmental hazards and inadequate health care (Bartlett, et al., 1983; Schultz, 1984). Problems primarily are caused by the erroneous assumption that risk appraisal tools alone can effect risk reduction (Frachel, 1984; Schultz, 1984; Wagner, et al., 1982).

Because of the methodological limitations of risk appraisals, practitioners should not rely totally on the instruments to assess individual health risks. If certain risks are not adequately identified, appraisals will give a false sense of security. Most instruments fail to identify important individual and family strengths. Risk appraisal tools are best used to supplement information obtained by a variety of methods. Health risk profiles are a valuable complement to the practitioner's own observational and assessment skills.

Risk appraisal tools, by themselves, should not be expected to stimulate behavior change, or modify health risks. Although they can be effective in increasing individuals' awareness about needed changes, they may or may not sufficiently motivate the individual to take the recommended actions (Bartlett et al., 1983; Schultz, 1984; Skinner et al., 1985). While educational messages may have a great impact on some individuals other persons may deny or avoid the implications (Stryd, 1982).

Even when individuals are motivated by health appraisal feedback, they may not have the behavioral skills necessary to initiate and sustain changes in life-style, especially those behaviors difficult to change, such as smoking habits. Studies show that risk appraisals are most effective when they are followed by a well-planned risk reduction program (Doerr and Hutchins, 1981; Goetz and McTyre, 1981; Schultz, 1984). Some examples of risk reduction methods are discussed later in this chapter.

Appraising Community Health Risks

Health risk appraisals can be used at the community or aggregate level to estimate risks for a number of chronic diseases, accidents, and acts of violence. Three basic approaches to establishing such risks include (1) epidemiological studies, health surveys using risk appraisal instruments, and well established morbidity and mortality statistics; (2) vital statistics showing demographic correlates of health and illness; and (3) *community competence levels* reflecting a community's ability to identify and resolve problems of community life, including those related to health. These approaches have been discussed in Chapter 8 and 13 of the text and are only highlighted here.

The use of mortality data and to a lesser extent, morbidity figures to establish aggregate measures of health risk is the most usual approach. Similarly, the results of health risk appraisals for a given population may be compiled to form a composite picture of risk. This has been done in many occupational settings (Durfee and DeGrassi, 1979; Murphy, 1982; Rodnick, 1982; Smeltzly, 1985) as well as by governmental agencies (Chen and Bill, 1983).

The use of health risk appraisals to assess group risks in occupational settings has become especially popular during the last decade. The risk profiles for the total employee group are used to assess needs for system-wide intervention programs. Individuals completing the risk appraisal instruments generally are given clear and comprehensive feedback and guidance on how to modify their behavioral health risks (Murphy, 1982; Rodnick, 1982; Smeltzly, 1985; Shepard et al., 1982). Unfortunately, the assessment and feedback concerning serious occupational risks, such as exposure to harmful chemicals for environmental conditions, is much less optimal.

An example of health risk appraisal by a governmental agency is Ohio's Health Risk Prevalence Survey, conducted in the early 1980s under funding from the Centers for Disease Control. In this study, a random sample of 607 Ohio residents aged 18 and older were polled by telephone, using random digit dialing techniques. A standardized health risk appraisal instrument was used to collect descriptive statistics on selected risk factors.

Among other findings, the study revealed very high rates of smoking, low use of protective devices such as smoke detectors, and a generally low level of awareness about preventive measures. Goals set as a result of the study include (1) removing economic barriers impeding the installation of smoke detectors in homes, (2) initiating health education at an early age to counter smoking trends, and (3) encouraging more adult self-determination in reducing health risks. (Chen and Bill, 1983).

The use of demographic data that have a documented relationship to health status and illness can also be helpful in estimating health risks at the community level. Dependency ratios, socioeconomic status indexes, race, gender, and education levels can be very valuable pieces of information in identifying community health risks.

The third approach, the use of community competence levels, has been proposed and tested (Goeppinger and Baglioni, 1985) but not widely used. The potential use of this approach is described in Chapter 13. Community competence is a correlate, if not an actual indicator, of the population's health; thus, low levels of community competence should be associated with increased morbidity and mortality risks. Like demographic measures, community competence may be an important contextual variable, occurring at the community process level. The possible use of demographic data and community competence levels to access community health risks needs much further study. Just as critical is the need to develop methods for combining health risk appraisals with high-quality risk reduction programs.

METHODS OF HEALTH RISK REDUCTION

As might be expected, the successful reduction of health risks is even more difficult to achieve than is the adequate appraisal of risks. Broad risk reduction efforts focus on minimizing risks for specific health problems as well as maximizing positive aspects of any of the four determinants of health: human biology, life-style, environment, and health care (Figure 27-3). *Microlevel interventions,* those performed at the individual or small group level, are most feasible in the areas of human biology and life-style. *Macrolevel interventions,* those carried out at the community or societal level, are essential in the areas of environment and health care delivery.

Both microlevel and macrolevel interventions may be required to sustain health risk reduction. Individuals can initiate positive changes in life-style and may even be successful in improving their health care resources, but without corresponding changes at the community or societal levels, these improvements may be very difficult to maintain. Similarly, legislation to control environmental hazards can be implemented, but without cooperation from individuals, these efforts will be ineffective.

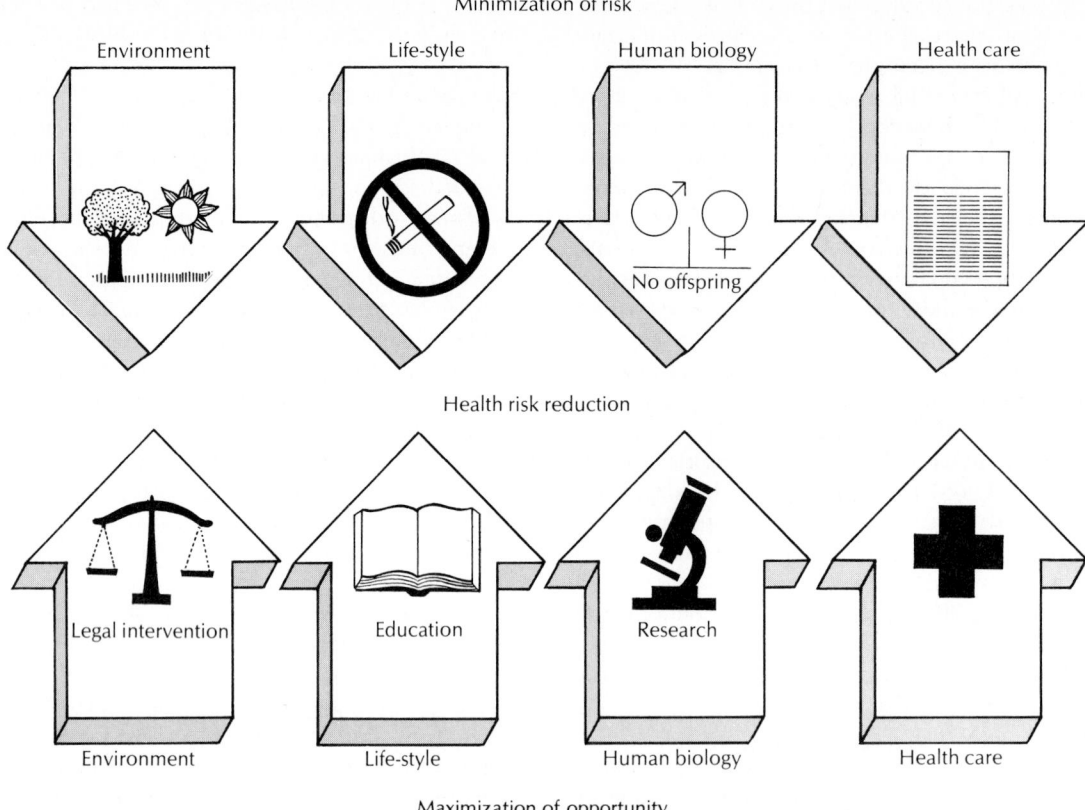

FIGURE 27-3

Aims of health risk reduction.

Microlevel Interventions

Microlevel interventions are the most popular approaches for achieving health risk reduction. Most of these interventions essentially require persons to modify risk behaviors in their individual lifestyles. The philosophical premise is that people "use their own personal interest, knowledge, ingenuity, and resources to achieve risk reduction" (Blum, 1982, p. 23). Other persons, including health professionals, may take supportive roles in the efforts to reduce health risks, but the locus of control for change rests with the individual. Programs directed toward exercise and fitness, nutrition and weight control, smoking cessation, stress management, automobile safety, and other preventive measures are common in health care settings as well as in many educational and occupational settings. Some of the intervention strategies used to modify life-style include individual and group counseling, educational programs and materials, behavior modification, contracting, referral to community resources, self-management, and mass media programs (Schultz 1984).

Pender (1982) has categorized behavior change strategies useful for understanding microlevel interventions as (1) self-confrontation, (2) cognitive restructuring, (3) modeling, (4) operant conditioning, (5) counterconditioning, and (6) stimulus control. Self-confrontation is based on the premise that individuals make changes when they recognize inconsistencies within their own beliefs, values, and behaviors or

between their own behaviors and those of persons whom they emulate. Providing written feedback from health risk appraisals is an example of an attempt to induce behavior change through self-confrontation. The use of nationally known basketball players to communicate health messages about the dangers of drugs through the mass media is another example.

Strategies using cognitive restructuring are attempts to "teach clients to think more rationally and thus gain greater control over their lives and health" (Pender, 1982, p. 215). Rational thinking about obesity and weight loss is reflected in the following statement: "I have difficulty controlling my between-meal snacking." In the same situation, the statement: "I'll never be slender; I've always been chubby," exemplifies irrational thinking. Ellis and Grieger (1977) originally described cognitive restructuring and called their intervention approach "rational emotive therapy." Specific steps for applying cognitive restructuring strategies also have been described by Goldfried and Sobocinski (1975).

Modeling is a common strategy used to help individuals or groups modify their behaviors. The individual desiring to reach a specific goal is provided opportunities to observe the behavior of other persons who have achieved the goal and then practices the desired behavior, identifying with the role models. Modeling is especially helpful when persons are unsure of the behaviors required to reach a specific goal.

The learning of social skills, beginning in early childhood and continuing in adult life, entails much modeling. Alcoholics Anonymous and other self-help groups successfully use modeling (among other strategies) to support their group members. The modeling of both health-protecting and health-promoting behaviors are also "inherent in the professional nurse's role" (Pender, 1982, p. 216).

Some of the most effective self-modification strategies use *operant conditioning,* which is based on the principle that behavior is determined by its consequences. As a result, health-generating behaviors must be identified and rewards provided. Practitioners who use operant conditioning need to be well informed about ways of sensitizing individuals to their health-generating and health-damaging behaviors, the appropriate use of rewards, and the gradual shaping of healthy behaviors. Pender (1982) suggests that the client should control the selection of behaviors to be changed and the rewards to be received. Positive reinforcements are better motivators of behavior change than negative reinforcements. Books that provide information on operant conditioning have been written by LeBow (1977) and Berni and Fordyce (1977).

Counterconditioning, or systematic desensitization, focuses on breaking an undesirable bond between a stimulus and a response. The response represents an irrational or maladaptive response to a specific situation, such as immediately lighting up a cigarette when becoming anxious or angry. The goal of counterconditioning in this example might be to replace the maladaptive response with a relaxation response. Imagery, biofeedback, or progressive relaxation techniques might be used to help promote tension release. These techniques frequently are used in stress management programs.

Stimulus control, the final self-modification strategy identified by Pender, focuses on the antecedents rather than the consequences of behavior. By changing the events that precede behavior, it theoretically is possible to decrease or eliminate undesired behavior and to increase desired outcomes. To use stimulus control successfully, the client must have accurate information about the desirable and undesirable behaviors and must arrange for environmental cues to be encountered in such a way as to promote only the desired behavior.

During a "decision-making phase" in stimulus control, the client determines which health actions will be taken and achieves a "level of readiness" to act. Cues, such as those described in the Health Belief Model discussed in Chapter 10 and the Health Promotion Model (Pender, 1982), then are used to prompt behavior change. Internal cues to action include perceptions and affective states. External cues include interactions with others, media communications, and visual or other stimuli (Pender, 1982). Nurses can assist clients in achieving stimulus control by providing correct information, giving appropriate cues, and helping clients to eliminate any barriers to change.

Microlevel interventions also may be targeted to the area of human biology. The application of new knowledge in genetics is one example in which only individual change would be considered ethically acceptable. Individuals with sickle cell anemia, for instance, might be counseled about the risks to their future offspring, but not proscribed from reproducing.

The effectiveness of any of these strategies varies depending on the targeted behaviors, the client's characteristics, and the intervention setting. Health risk appraisals combined with various educational programs and/or individual and group counseling have been shown to be effective in both clinical settings (Bartlett, et al., 1983; Schultz, 1984) and in occupational settings (Rodnick, 1982; Shepard, et al., 1982). In general, life-style changes that entail the introduction of new habits (such as preventive dental visits, self-breast examinations, and seatbelt use) are more amenable to educational approaches than are changes that require giving up negative habits. The modification of long-term addictive behaviors such as cigarette smoking and drug or alcohol abuse usually requires a combination of education efforts, behavioral modification strategies, and ongoing interpersonal support.

Macrolevel Interventions

Macrolevel interventions, those aimed at the societal level, are less popular than those directed toward individual change, largely because it is easiest to assume that individuals are responsible for their own health risks. Individuals are indeed responsible but only to a limited extent. For example, how can an individual be held solely responsible for reckless driving when overly powerful automobiles continue to be manufactured with government subsidies? Or, how can persons who live in impoverished and volatile neighborhoods take sufficient preventive actions to protect themselves from physical attack?

Obviously, to be effective in reducing health risks, many changes in life-style require concurrent societal level changes. In her book, *Promoting Health Through Public Policy* (1981), Milio points out the realistic limitations of microlevel interventions. She argues for a more ecological focus, in which there is greater emphasis on creating healthy environments for individuals and groups (Milio, 1981).

In areas like the environment, societal change is essential. Only legislation to control environmental hazards from chemical and physical agents will reduce mortality caused by occupationally-induced cancer. The need to earn enough to purchase basic necessities precludes many persons from quitting jobs with well-established health risks. As a result, the risks themselves, and not the individual's exposure to them, must be altered.

Clean air and water, as well as safe jobs, require group action. State legislation mandating the inspection of wells and the laboratory examination of well water is a traditional example of risk-reducing surveillance. Negotiations between the United States and Canada on the pollution of the Great Lakes are a creative example of group action for environmental health at the international level. Recent studies of inner-city violence (Tardiff, Gross, and Messner, 1986) also represent attempts to deal with health problems on the macrolevel.

The current initiatives of antismoking groups to effect smoking bans in businesses and other public places is another example of collective group action directed toward change at both the community and societal levels. Although various individuals and groups have differing opinions concerning the best strategies for meeting their goals, significant progress in implementing anti-smoking policies has occurred. Successes in lobbying against the tobacco industry have been much slower, however, and the goal of a smoke-free society remains elusive.

Multilevel Change

It is clear that effective multidimensional risk reduction involves health-generating changes at both the individual and societal levels. It is equally clear that the community health nurse, acting alone, cannot be very effective in reducing health risks. Change requires the nurse to use multiple intervention strategies, such as individual behavioral contracts, the establishment of coalitions, the use of small interacting groups, cooperation with lay advisors, the mass media, public policy, and legislation (state, federal, and international).

The community health nurse's unique synthesis of clinical and aggregate skills provides a strong knowledge base for applying risk appraisal and reduction methods. At the microlevel, the community health nurse might use health hazard appraisals, wellness inventories, or a lifetime health monitoring program to strengthen her assessment of an individual's health risks. The client then could be counseled regarding his or her individual self-care needs, and interventions collaboratively planned to reduce the health risks. The community health nurse might also seek opportunities for intervening in educational and/or occupational settings. Here health risk appraisals might be used to identify group risks as well as individual risks, and interventions planned to meet these needs.

At the macrolevel, nurses can use data from surveys, compiled statistics, and community assessments to identify the most salient health hazards for a given population. They can work with other health professionals and community leaders in planning system-wide interventions to reduce these hazards. These interventions may involve political and legislative activities as well as education programs. Successful attempts to intervene at the macrolevel will be especially rewarding, since large numbers of persons can benefit from these efforts. Societal-level interventions are more fully discussed in Chapters 6 and 13; in the next section, the nurse's role in individual risk appraisal and reduction is emphasized.

CLINICAL APPLICATION

Sally Jones was a community health nurse employed by a rural county health department in the eastern United States. She had worked in the community for a number of years and was knowledgeable about the demographic and health characteristics of the local population, as well as its resources and leadership patterns. Ms. Jones' typical work week might entail involvement in wellness clinics in the small towns in her district, a number of home visits, visits to two local schools, consultations with lay community leaders, planning with other health professionals, and possible meetings with elected officials to lobby for specific health legislation.

Becoming aware of risk appraisal tools, Ms. Jones recognized their potential usefulness to strengthen her health assessments and intervention efforts. In health clinics and home visits, she began educating her clients about the concept of health risks and used a lifetime health monitoring schedule to advise them about preventive self-health care. She also encouraged her clients to complete health risk appraisals and/or wellness inventories, providing guidance on the selection of instruments that would be most meaningful for the individual's age and overall living situation.

One appraisal completed by Stanley Hess, a 30-year-old truck driver, revealed an appraisal age of 43 years and an achievable age of 25. Mr. Hess was at greater risk than his contemporaries for motor vehicle accidents, arteriosclerotic heart disease, suicide, cirrhosis of the liver, stroke, and cancer of the lungs. He had a sedentary job that kept him apart from his family for long periods, drank 25 to 40 bottles of beer a week, never wore a seatbelt, was hypertensive (blood pressure 200/160), smoked two packs of cigarettes a day when he was "on the road," and drove 198,000 miles annually.

Despite these ominous findings, Mr. Hess was somewhat motivated to improve his health situation. He very much wanted to be a good parent and role model for his two sons, and to please his wife and family. His wife had previously established a trusting relationship with the community health nurse. Both Mr. and Mrs. Hess thus were quite receptive to the nurse's comments when the health appraisal was reviewed.

In planning interventions to reduce this client's health risks, Ms. Jones first assisted him to identify those risks he actually wanted to change and those he considered modifiable. She then worked with him, his wife and family, and his employer in developing a plan that would begin to bring his appraisal age down to the desired achievable age. A behavioral contract between Ms. Jones and Mr. Hess was developed to assist in goal attainment (Pender, 1982; Schultz, 1984). Since several of the client's health risks involved long-term habits, such as smoking and alcohol abuse, referrals to several other community agencies and programs were made to assist with risk reduction. Ms. Jones kept in close contact with Mr. Hess to encourage and support his active involvement in these programs.

Working in the school setting provided Ms. Jones with another opportunity for using health risk appraisals. In one of the parent-teacher organization's meetings, she introduced the idea of risk appraisal. This resulted in a lively discussion concerning health promotion topics. Subsequently, Ms. Jones worked in collaboration with several teachers to plan a program for risk appraisal and reduction in the school.

Because there was interest in testing the effectiveness of risk appraisals and various educational and counseling methods in reducing the students' identified health risks, the nurse helped to design an intervention program to meet these goals. She sought advice from a nurse researcher at a nearby university in designing the experimental program. After the program was initiated, Ms. Jones was contacted by one child's father who expressed interest in developing a similar risk reduction program for the employees in his small industrial plant. He believed that risk reduction would be quite difficult but due to his daughter's enthusiasm, he was willing to give it a try. This contact resulted in collaborative planning between Ms. Jones, an occupational health nurse in the area, an experienced health educator, and the interested employer.

In addition to using health appraisals at the microlevel, Ms. Jones eventually was successful in convincing county health department officials to conduct a prevalence survey in her community to identify aggregate health risks. This, she reasoned, would provide useful data for planning health promotion and disease prevention programs and for documenting the need for increased funding and legislation to support the necessary changes. Plans to seek state funding for the survey were begun. Ms. Jones requested to be actively involved in planning the survey, since she wanted to assure that environmental risks, as well as life-style factors, were adequately assessed. Excited about this new venture, she began considering how she would convince others of the potential impact of macrolevel interventions.

SUMMARY

This chapter presented risk appraisal and reduction as important ways for community health nurses to assist individuals, families, aggregates, and other community groups to improve their self-health care. Past and present self-health care activities were described, and the relationship of self-health care to risk appraisal and reduction was described. Four areas in which self-health care could be targeted were reviewed: human biology, environment, life-style, and health care. The environment and life-style were emphasized as especially important to risk appraisal and reduction because of our growing abilities to successfully modify risks in these areas. A number of methods of appraising individual and aggregate health risks are available for nurses in practice, as are examples of innovative intervention strategies. Both the acknowledged benefits of self-health care, as documented by well-respected longitudinal studies, and criticisms of self-health care were presented. Microlevel and macrolevel interventions were described and compared. In general, it is easier for community health nurses to influence microlevel or individual/small group behavior change than to influence macrolevel or community/societal change although the necessity of intervention at multiple levels was stressed. The chapter concluded with an illustration of how one community health nurse went about appraising and reducing risks at the individual and group levels. Many other possibilities for effecting change exist, including more direct involvement in formulating public health policy.

☰ KEY CONCEPTS

The debate between the critics and proponents of self-health care is important. It suggests that despite the rhetoric of support and recent progress, important questions still remain.

The revitalization of self-health care in the United States may represent a cyclical recurrence of the more general self-help theme.

Risk appraisal and reduction is an approach that health professionals can use to help individuals and groups maximize their self-health care.

In health risk appraisal, data about health risks experienced by an individual or group are collected and analyzed, and a health-risk profile is generated. Health risk appraisal may be carried out on an individual and community level.

At least three types of individual health risk appraisal tools are common today. These include the Health Hazard Appraisal and its many versions, the Lifetime Health Monitoring Program, and wellness appraisals or inventories.

The overall objective of lifetime health monitoring is to focus routine health evaluations on the specific problems most likely to occur at a given age and thus to better prevent these problems.

Health risk appraisals can be used at the community or aggregate level to estimate risks for a number of chronic diseases, accidents, and acts of violence.

LEARNING ACTIVITIES

1. Read any of the current legislative proposals for federal health insurance. Note the position on self-health care taken and/or implied in the legislation and outline the supporting argument. Identify the key factors (religious beliefs, professional attitudes, scientific knowledge, etc.) in the argument.

2. Interview a nurse, client, physician, and businessperson about their views of self-health care. Ascertain their beliefs about each of Lorig's four dimensions of a comprehensive self-health care definition: instigator, target, goal, and knowledge base.

3. Attend a meeting of Weight Watchers, TOPS, Reach for Recovery, or a similar self-help health group. Identify several key themes of the meeting and discuss how they exemplify both self-health care and risk appraisal and reduction.

4. Complete any two of the Health Risk Appraisal forms included in Appendix D. Compare and contrast them on the breadth of health risks covered, the extent to which they require professional involvement, and the ease with which they can be completed.

Continued.

As might be expected, the successful reduction of health risks is even more difficult to achieve than is the adequate appraisal of risks. Broad risk reduction efforts focus on minimizing risks for specific health problems and maximizing positive aspects of any of the four determinants of health: human biology, life-style, environment, and health care.

The community health nurse's unique synthesis of clinical and aggregate skills provides a strong knowledge base for applying risk appraisal and reduction methods.

> 5. Interview a school health nurse, a home health care and/or visiting nurse, or an occupational health nurse about nursing roles in risk appraisal and reduction. If these roles are not now a part of the job description of the nurse you are interviewing, sketch a revised job description that includes such roles.

BIBLIOGRAPHY

Ardell, D.B.: High level wellness: an alternative to doctors, drugs, and disease, Emmaus, Pa., 1977, Rodale Press, Inc.

Bartlett, E.E., Pegues, H.U., Shaffer, C.R., and Crump, W: Health hazard appraisal in a family practice center: an exploratory study, J. Community Health 9:(2):135-144, 1983.

Bauer, K.G.: Improving the chances for health: lifestyle change and health evaluation, San Francisco, 1981, National Center for Health Education.

Becker, M.H., editor: The health belief model and personal health behavior, Thorofare, N.J., 1974, Charles B. Slack, Inc.

Belloc, N.B.: Relationship of health practices and mortality, Prev. Med. 2:67, 1973.

Berkman, L.F.: Psychosocial resources, health, behavior, and mortality; a nine-year follow-up study. Paper presented at the annual meeting of the American Public Health Association, Washington, D.C., Oct. 1977.

Berni, R., and Fordyce, W.E.: Behavior modification and the nursing process, St. Louis, 1977, The C.V. Mosby Co.

Blum, H.J.: Social perspective on risk reduction. In Faber, M.M., and Reinhardt, A.M., editors: Promoting health through risk reduction, New York, Macmillan Publishing Co., Inc., 1982.

Breslow, L.: A quantitative approach to the World Health Organization's definition of health: physical, mental, and social well-being, Int. J. Epidemiol. 1:347, 1972.

Breslow, L.: Prospects for improving health through reducing risk factors, Prev. Med. 7:449, 1978a.

Breslow, L.: Risk factor intervention for health maintenance, Science 200:908, 1978b.

Breslow, L., and Somers, A.R.: The lifetime health monitoring program: a practical approach to preventive medicine, N. Engl. J. Med. 296:601, 1977.

Chen, M.S., and Bill, D.: Statewide survey of risk factor prevalence: the Ohio experience, Public Health Rep. 98:(5):443-448, 1983.

Clark, C.C.: Enhancing wellness: a guide for self-care, New York, 1981, Springer Publishing Co., Inc.

Doerr, B.T., and Hutchins, E.B.: Health risk appraisal: process, problems, and prospects for nursing practice and research, Nurs. Res. 30:299, 1981.

Durfee, J.H., and De Grassi, A.: Health hazard appraisal in the workplace. Proceedings of the fifteenth annual meeting on Prospective Medicine and Health Hazard Appraisal, Bethesda, Md., 1979, Health and Education Resources, p. 71.

Ellis, A., and Grieger, R.: Handbook of rational-emotive therapy, New York, 1977, Springer Publishing Co., Inc.

Faber, M.M., and Reinhardt, A.M.: Promoting health through risk reduction, New York, 1982, Macmillan Publishing Co., Inc.

Fielding, J.E.: Appraising the health of health risk appraisal, Am. J. Public Health 72:337, 1982.

Fonaroff, A.: Issues in self-care: preface, Health Educ. Monogr. 5(2):108, 1977.

Frachel, R.R.: Health hazard appraisal: personal and professional implications, J. Nurs. Educ. 23(6):265-267, 1984.

Goldfried, M.R., and Sobocinski, D.: Effect of irrational beliefs on emotional arousal, J. Consult. Clin. Psychol. 43:504, 1975.

Goeppinger, J., and Baglioni, A.J., Jr.: Community competence: a positive approach to needs assessment, Am. J. Community Psychol. 13:507-523, 1986.

Goeppinger, J.: Self-health care through risk appraisal and reduction: implications for community health nursing. In Stanhope, M., and Lancaster, J., editors: Community health nursing: process and practices for promoting health, St. Louis, 1987, The C.V. Mosby Co.

Goeppinger, J.: Changing health behaviors and outcomes through self-care. In Lancaster, J., and Lancaster, W., editors: Concepts for advanced nursing practice: the nurse as a change agent, St. Louis, 1982, The C.V. Mosby Co.

Goetz, A.A., and McTyre, R.B.: Health risk appraisal: some methodological considerations, Nurs. Res. 30:307, 1981.

Gori, G.B., and Richter, B.J.: Macroeconomics of disease prevention in the United States, Science 200:1124, 1978.

Green, L.W.: Research and development issues in self-care: measuring the decline in medicocentrism, Health Educ. Monogr. 5:161, 1977.

Green, L.W., and Lewis, F.M.: Measurement and evaluation in health education and health promotion, 1985, Mayfield Publishing Co.

Guidotti, T.L.: Adaptation of the lifetime health monitoring concept to defined employee groups not at exceptional risk, J. Occup. Med. 25:731-736, 1983.

Haynes, S.G., Feinleib, M., Kannel, W.B., et al.: The relationship of psychosocial factors to coronary heart disease in the Framingham study, 111. Eight-year incidence of coronary heart disease, Am. J. Epidem. 111:37, 1980.

Healthy people: the Surgeon General's report on health promotion and disease prevention, DHEW Pub. No. (PHS) 79-55071, Washington, D.C., 1979a, Department of Health, Education and Welfare.

Healthy people: the Surgeon General's report on health promotion and disease prevention, Background papers, DHEW Pub. No. (PHS) 79-55071A, Washington, D.C., 1979b, Department of Health, Education and Welfare.

Hettler, B.: Lifestyle assessment questionnaire, Stevens Point, 1978, University of Wisconsin, Stevens Point Foundation.

Illich, I.: Medical nemesis, the expropriation of health, New York, 1976a, Random House, Inc.

Illich, I.: Medicine is a major threat to health, Psychology Today 9:66, 1976b.

Kasl, S.V.: Cardiovascular risk reduction in a community setting: some comments, J. Consult. Clin. Psychol. 48:143, 1980.

Kronenfeld, J.J.: Self care as a panacea for the ills of the health care system: an assessment, Soc. Sci. Med. 13(A):263, 1979.

Kuller, L., Neaton, J., Caggiula, A., and Falvo-Gerard, L.: Primary prevention of heart attacks: the multiple risk factor intervention trial, Am. J. Epidemiol. 112:185, 1980.

LaLonde, M.: A new perspective on the health of Canadians, Ottawa, 1974, Government of Canada.

Lasater, T., Abrams, D., Artz, L., et al: Lay volunteer delivery of a community-based cardiovascular risk factor change program: the Pawtucket Experiment. In Matarayzo, J.D., Miller, N.E., Weiss, S.M., et al., editors: Behavioral health: a handbook of health enhancement and disease prevention, Silver Spring, Md., 1984, John Wiley & Sons, Inc.

LeBow, M.D.: Behavior modification: a significant method in nursing practice, Englewood Cliffs, N.J., 1973, Prentice-Hall, Inc.

Leventhal, H., Safer, M.A., Cleary, P.D., and Gotmann, M.: Cardiovascular risk modification by community-based programs for life-style change: comments on the Stanford study, J. Consult. Clin. Psychol. 48:150, 1980.

Levin, L.S.: Self-care: an international perspective, Soc. Policy 6:70, 1976.

Levin, L.S.: Forces and issues in the revival of interest in self-care: impetus for redirection in health, Health Educ. Monogr. 5:115, 1977.

Lorig, K.: Arthritis self-management: a joint venture. A multiple outcome patient education evaluation, doctoral dissertation, Berkeley, 1980, University of California at Berkeley.

Maccoby, N., Farquhar, J.W., Wood, P.D., and Alexandar, J.: Reducing the risk of cardiovascular disease: effects of a community-based campaign on knowledge and behavior, J. Community Health 3:100, 1977.

McKeown, T., Record, R.G., and Turner, R.D.: An interpretation of the decline in mortality in England and Wales during the twentieth century, Popul. Studies 29:391, 1975.

McKinlay, J.B., and McKinlay, S.M.: The questionable contribution of medical measures to the decline of mortality in the United States in the twentieth century, Milbank Mem. Fund Q. 55:405, 1977.

Medical datamation: health risk index, Bellevue, Ohio, 1980.

Milio, N.: Promoting health through public policy, Philadelphia, 1981, F.A. Davis Co.

Mitchell, J.: Looking after ourselves: an individual responsibility? R. Soc. Health J. 102: 169-173, 1982.

Moody, L., et al.: A computerized health profile model for adolescents. In Proceedings of the fifteenth meeting of the society of prospective medicine. Bethesda, Md., 1979, Society of Prospective Medicine.

Mooney, H., and Rives, N.W.: Measures of community health status for health planning, Health Serv. Res. 2:124-145, 1978.

Multiple risk factors intervention trial group: Statistical design considerations in the NHLI multiple risk factor intervention trial, J. Chronic Dis. 30:261, 1977.

Murphy, D.C.: A realistic method of health hazard appraisal for the occupational health nurse, Occup. Health Nursing 30(1):11-16, 1982.

Neaton, J.D., Kuller, L., Caggiula, A., and Falvo-Gerard, L.: The multiple risk factor intervention trial (MRFIT) VII. A comparison of risk factor changes between the two study groups, Prev. Med. 10:519, 1981.

Orem, D.: Nursing: concepts of practice, New York, 1971, McGraw-Hill Book Co.

Pender, N.J.: Health promotion in nursing practice, 1982, Appleton-Century-Crofts.

Promoting health/preventing disease: objectives for the nation, DHHS Pub. No. (PHS) 0-349-256, Washington, D.C., 1981, Department of Health and Human Services.

Puska, P.: North Karelia project: a community program for the control of cardiovascular disease (abstract), Conference on Prevention, Institute of Medicine, Washington, D.C., Feb., 1978.

Robbins, L.C., and Hall, J.N.: How to practice prospective medicine, Indianapolis, 1970, Methodist Hospital of Indiana.

Rodnick, J.E.: Health behavior changes associated with health hazard appraisal counseling in an occupational setting, Prev. Med. 11(5): 583-594, 1982.

Ryan, W.: Blaming the victim, New York, 1976, Random House, Inc.

Schultz, C.M.: Lifestyle assessment: a tool for practice, Nurs. Clin. North Am. 19(2):271-281, 1984.

Shepard, R.J., Corey, P., and Cox, M.: Health hazard appraisal—the influence of an employee fitness program, Can. J. Public Health, 73(3):183-187, 1982.

Skinner, H.A., Allen, B.A., McIntosh, M.C., and Palmer, W.H.: Lifestyle assessment: just asking makes a difference, Br. Med. J. 290:214-216, 1985.

Smeltzly, J.: Employee health promotion: the Hennepin Wellway program, Am. J. Public Health 75(7):785-786, 1985.

Stryd, A.: Risk appraisal and its effect on lifestyle, Occup. Health Nursing, 11:19-20, 1982.

Tardiff, K., Gross, E., and Messner, S.F.: A study of homicides in Manhattan, 1981, Am. J. Public Health 76(2):139-143, 1986.

Travis, J.W.: Wellness workbook for health professionals, Mill Valley, Calif., 1977, Wellness Resource Center.

Veatch, R.M.: Voluntary risks to health: the ethical issues, JAMA 243:50, 1980.

Wagner, E.H.: The North Karelia project: what it tells us about the prevention of cardiovascular disease, Am. J. Public Health 72:51, 1982.

Wagner, E., Beery, W.L., Schoenbach, V.S., et al: An assessment of health hazard/health risk appraisal, Am. J. Public Health 72:347, 1982.

Wallston, K.A., Wallston, B.S., and De Vellis, R.: Development of the multidimensional health locus of control (MHLC) scales, Health Educ. Monogr. 6(2):160, 1978.

Warwick, D.P., and Kelman, H.C.: Ethical issues in social intervention. In Zaltman, G., editor: Processes and phenomena of social change, New York, 1973, John Wiley & Sons, Inc.

Weiss, D.: Who has been responsible for our health in the past? Paper presented at a workshop of the Kentucky Bureau of Health Services, Lexington, March 22, 1977.

Wesley, J.: Primitive physic: or, an easy and natural method for curing most diseases, London, 1747, Thomas Trye.

Wildavsky, A.: Doing better and feeling worse: the political pathology of health policy, Daedalus 106:105, 1977.

Wiley, J.A., and Camacho, T.C.: Life-style and future health: evidence from the Alameda County study, Prev. Med. 9:1, 1980.

Williams, C.A.: Community health nursing—what is it? Nurs. Outlook 25:250, 1977.

Williams, C.L., Carter, B.J., and Eng. A.: The know your body program: a developmental approach to health education and disease prevention, Prev. Med. 9:371, 1980.

Zukel, W.J., Oglesby, P., and Schnaper, H.W.: The Multiple Risk Factor Intervention Trial (MRFIT), Prev. Med. 10:387-401, 1981.

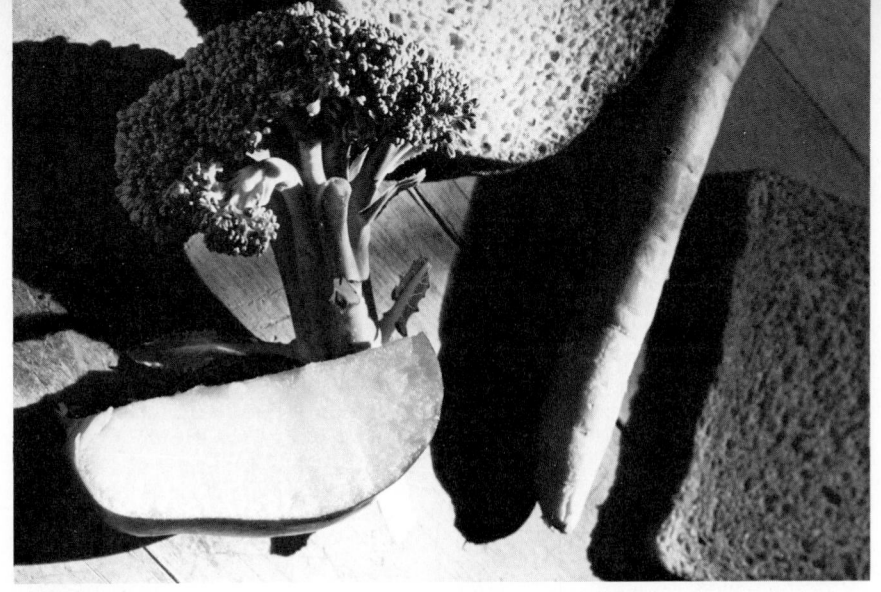

Kathleen Beckman Blomquist

28

PROMOTING HEALTH THROUGH NUTRITION AND EXERCISE

OBJECTIVES

After reading this chapter, the student should be able to:

Identify changes in the dietary habits of Americans that could significantly reduce the incidence of leading disease processes.

Describe factors influencing food selection and consumption.

Discuss the origin and usefulness of the RDAs.

Use dietary guidelines and the nursing process to plan and evaluate diets.

Discuss the reasons nurses should be knowledgeable about nutrition and exercise.

Identify physiological and psychological benefits of exercise.

Explain the factors that must be considered when designing an individual exercise program.

Describe ways in which nurses can promote exercise in the community.

KEY TERMS

aerobic exercise
anticipatory guidance
basic four food groups
cool-down
Dietary Guidelines for Americans
dietary influences

exercise
food exchange system
nutritional assessment
obesity
physical activity
physical fitness

Recommended Dietary Allowances (RDAs)
Special Supplemental Food Program for Women, Infants, and Children (WIC)
target heart rate
warm-up

Hilda and Carl Willow are 60 years old, moderately obese, and mildly hypertensive. Their physician tells them that if they will lose some weight and get some exercise, they might not have to take medication to control their blood pressures. The Willows provide an example of the challenge nurses in the community face in promoting the health of people with chronic diseases induced by sedentary life-styles and inadequate dietary practices. Nurses also play a major role in primary prevention by encouraging people to be more active and eat well.

◆ ◆ ◆

This chapter discusses current trends in nutrition and exercise and the role of nurses in educating community residents about nutrition and exercise. The chapter concludes with the health promotion program planned with Mr. and Mrs. Willow.

PROMOTING HEALTH THROUGH NUTRITION

Nutrition should be an integral component of client care. All people eat to stay alive, and what is eaten affects health from conception through old age. Throughout the world, chronic malnutrition affects physical and mental development. In industrialized societies, diet-related conditions are among the leading causes of disease and death. Many of these (Table 28-1) are the result of nutritional excesses rather than undernutrition. Coronary heart disease is the nation's number one killer and has been linked with excessive intake of saturated fats and cholesterol; high blood pressure has been associated with excessive calories and dietary salt; diabetes mellitus has been associated with excessive calorie intake and obesity; dental caries have been linked to excessive sugar intake; liver disease has been associated with heavy alcohol intake; and obesity is often the result of excessive calorie intake.

Frequent and extended contact with clients in the community affords nurses excellent opportunities to provide information and counseling regarding the role of nutrition in the promotion of health and the prevention of illness. Knowledge and skills related to nutrition will enable the community health nurse to (Nestle, 1985):

This chapter was written by Nannette Worel for the first edition. It has been revised and updated for this edition by Kathleen Blomquist.

1. *Answer questions clients ask about nutrition.* The media bombard people with nutrition information. People are interested and sometimes confused about the relationship of nutrition to health. They expect nurses to be able to answer questions and resolve confusions.
2. *Provide appropriate dietary advice.* Community health nurses should be familiar with basic dietary principles so that they can counsel healthy people, as well as those with disease conditions.
3. *Recommend age-appropriate diets.* Because nutritional requirements change throughout life, knowledge of the special needs of infants and children, adolescents, pregnant and lactating women, and adults of all ages improves the health care of these groups.
4. *Prevent and treat disease.* Diet is an important factor in the etiology and treatment of many disease conditions. Nurses have historically used supportive care

TABLE 28-1

Age-adjusted rates of major causes of death in the U.S. in 1984

Cause of death	Rate per 100,000 people	% of total deaths
1. *Disease of the heart	183.3	33.5
2. *Cancer	133.1	24.3
3. *Stroke (Cerebrovascular diseases and allied conditions)	33.9	6.1
4. Accidents and adverse effects	35.6	6.5
5. COPD and allied conditions	18.0	3.2
6. Suicide	11.6	2.1
7. Pneumonia and influenza	12.2	2.2
8. *Chronic liver disease and cirrhosis	9.8	1.8
9. *Diabetes mellitus	9.9	1.8
10. All others	100.3	18.3

*Conditions associated with overconsumption of energy or nutrients.
Health: United States, 1986; and Prevention Profile, USDHHS, (PHS) 87-1232, Hyattsville, Md., Dec. 1986, U.S. Government Printing Office.

such as nutritional counseling and provision of appropriate food intake in care of healthy and ill clients. Appropriate diets prevent or delay symptoms of disease and support the body in recovery. Anticipatory guidance is an important aspect of care for clients. For example, women planning pregnancy, persons having elective surgery, and middle-aged and aging persons benefit from nutritional guidance.

5. *Identify and appropriately refer malnourished clients.* Dietitians and nutritionists are trained to assess clients' diets and help clients meet their nutritional needs. Appropriate use of their services improves health care services.

6. *Evaluate current research studies.* Controlled studies in clinical nutrition are difficult to design, conduct, and interpret because of the complexity of diets and the varying nutritional requirements of individuals due to age, sex, activity, and physical condition. Three questions might be asked when evaluating nutrition information:

    a. What kind of evidence has been presented relating a specific nutrient to a certain disease process?
    b. What is the quality (strength) of this evidence?
    c. What are the possible risks and benefits of increasing, reducing, and/or eliminating the specific nutrient from the diet?

The answers to these questions assist the nurse in determining the validity of claims made about dietary practices. By combining a background in nutrition principles with this analysis of information, community health nurses can assist clients in understanding the difference between factual and nonsubstantiated nutrition information.

Dietary Factors

What people eat is determined by a variety of factors including biological needs, psychological variables, sociocultural influences, and environmental aspects such as price and availability. Research in the area of nutrition is rapidly producing new information, some of which contradicts old ideas. Politics, economics, and social norms influence the growing, marketing, distributing, and consuming of food products. Figure 28-1 summarizes some factors that influence food selection and ultimately the health of a population. Dietary counseling should be based on an understanding of the biological, psychological, sociocultural, and environmental factors influencing food selection and eating behaviors.

Biological Factors

The human body requires certain nutrients to maintain health. Table 28-2 summarizes the nutrients needed for growth, development, and repair of body structures and maintenance of body processes. Level of activity and stress, age and rate of growth, genetics, and a variety of factors such as hormones, temperature, and taste and smell of food affect intake of food (Nestle, 1985).

Psychological Factors

Both positive emotions, such as enjoyment and tranquility, and negative feelings, like anger and insecurity, often affect the eating behavior of individuals. Food may represent rewards, comfort, and security to clients. Habits, such as skipping breakfast or regular midmorning coffee breaks with pastries, are important factors in determining eating behavior. They require little or no conscious thought and often result in poor dietary practices. Two other important

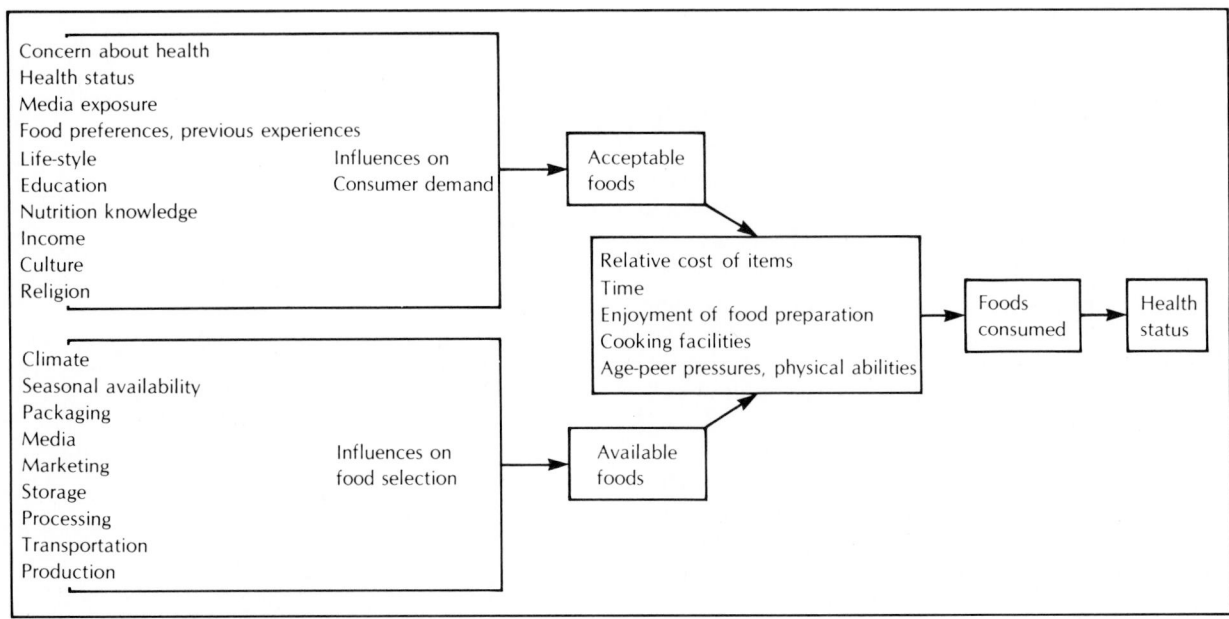

FIGURE 28-1

Factors influencing food selection.

TABLE 28-2
Summary of nutrients for health

| Nutrient | Important sources of nutrient | EXAMPLES OF MAJOR PHYSIOLOGICAL FUNCTIONS | | | Toxicity symptoms |
		Provide energy	Build and maintain body cell	Regulate body processes	Deficiency symptoms
Protein Essential amino acids	Meat, poultry, fish Beans and peas Eggs Cheese Milk	Supplies 4 calories per gram	Constitutes part of the structure of every cell, such as muscle, blood, and bone; supports growth and maintains healthy body cells	Constitutes part of enzymes, some hormones and body fluids, and antibodies that increase resistance to infection	Protein calorie malnutrition	Elevated uric acid and urea in serum
Carbohydrate Fiber Starch Sugar	Cereal Potatoes Beans Corn Bread Sugar	Supplies 4 calories per gram Major source of energy for central nervous system	Supplies energy so protein can be used for growth and maintenance of body cells	Unrefined products supply fiber—complex carbohydrates in fruits, vegetables, and whole grains—for regular elimination	Poor GI function	Flatulence, trace mineral deficiencies
Fat	Shortening, oil Butter, margarine Salad dressing Sausages	Supplies 9 calories per gram	Constitutes part of the structure of every cell Supplies essential fatty acids	Assists in fat utilization Provides and carries fat-soluble vitamins (A, D, E, & K)	Essential fatty acid deficiency	Obesity
Fat soluable vitamins Vitamin A (Retinol)	Liver Carrots, pumpkin Sweet potatoes Greens Butter, margarine		Assists formation and maintenance of skin and mucous membranes that line body cavities and tracts, such as nasal passages and intestinal tract, thus increasing resistance to infection	Functions in visual processes and forms visual purple, thus promoting healthy eye tissues and eye adaptation in dim light	Eye, skin, bone and blood disorders	Toxic at 25-100x recommended dosage
Vitamin D	Exposure to sunlight; fortified milk, fish			Activates calcium and phosphorous	Neuromuscular—cramps, muscle twitching	
Vitamins E and K	Food fats, vegetable oils, nuts, fish			Antioxidants—affect cell aging and immune system; wound healing, modifies blood fats		

Adapted from: Poleman, C.N., and Capra, C.L.: Shakelton's nutrition essentials and diet therapy, ed. 5, Philadelphia, 1984, W.B. Saunders; and Nestle, M.: Nutrition in clinical practice, Greenbrae, CA, 1985, Jones Medical Publications.

Continued.

TABLE 28-2

Summary of nutrients for health—cont'd

Nutrient	Important sources of nutrient	EXAMPLES OF MAJOR PHYSIOLOGICAL FUNCTIONS			Deficiency symptoms	Toxicity symptoms
		Provide energy	Build and maintain body cells	Regulate body processes		
Water soluble vitamins Vitamin C (ascorbic acid)	Broccoli Orange Grapefruit Papaya Mango Strawberries		Forms cementing substances, such as collagen, that hold body cells together, thus strengthening blood vessels, hastening healing of wounds and bones, and increasing resistance to infection	Aids utilization of iron	Skin, blood, digestive, neurologic disorders	Usually nontoxic
Thiamin (B_1)	Lean pork Nuts Fortified cereal products	Aids in utilization of energy		Functions as part of a coenzyme to promote the utilization of carbohydrate Promotes normal appetite Contributes to normal functioning of nervous system	Skin, blood, digestive, neurologic disorders	
Riboflavin (B_2)	Liver Milk Yogurt Cottage cheese	Aids in utilization of energy		Functions as part of a coenzyme in the production of energy within body cells Promotes healthy skin, eyes, and clear vision	Skin, blood, digestive, neurologic disorders	

		Sources	Functions	Deficiency	Toxicity
Niacin (B₆)	Aids in utilization of energy	Liver Meat, poultry, fish Peanuts Fortified cereal products	Functions as part of coenzyme in fat synthesis, tissue respiration, and utilization of carbohydrate Promotes healthy skin, nerves, and digestive tract Aids digestion and fosters normal appetite	Skin, blood, digestive, neurologic disorders	
Minerals Calcium		Milk, yogurt Cheese Sardines and salmon with bones Collard, kale, mustard, and turnip greens	Combines with other minerals within a protein framework to give structure and strength to bones and teeth Assists in blood clotting Functions in normal muscle contraction and relaxation, and normal nerve transmission	Bone loss Osteoporosis Periodontal disease Muscle spasms	Toxic at high dosage
Iron	Aids in utilization of energy	Enriched farina Prune juice Liver Dried beans and peas Red meat	Combines with protein to form hemoglobin, the red substance in blood that carries oxygen to and carbon dioxide from the cells Prevents nutritional anemia and its accompanying fatigue Increases resistance to infection	Anemia, weakness, fatigue	Bronze coloration, liver damage, severe diabetes

factors are self-esteem and knowledge about nutrition. Both have been shown to affect the quality of the diet consumed.

Sociocultural Factors

The cultural and ethnic backgrounds of clients play a major role in food selection and eating behaviors. Many cultural practices have evolved because they are healthful (Wilson, 1985). Recognition of and respect for these food preferences are important for nurses counseling clients in the community. Nurses should gather information about the nutritional value of ethnic foods, tailor recommended changes as much as possible to cultural practices, and encourage major changes only when foods are clearly hazardous to the health of clients. Working with clients of a particular ethnic group for whom a specific diet has been recommended can be quite a challenge for community health nurses. For example, the diet recommended for a client with hypertension who is of Mexican descent is likely to be quite different from that of a hypertensive client of Japanese descent. Attempting to incorporate foods that are low in sodium while staying within cultural limitations necessitates close teamwork between nurse and client.

The number of vegetarians has increased rapidly over the past few years partly in response to information about the relationship of animal fat to cardiovascular disease. Vege-

tarians, especially those who eat no milk products or eggs, may need assistance in planning meals that contain essential amino acids, vitamins, and minerals. Meals will supply essential amino acids if they include legumes (such as soybeans, other beans, or peas) and whole grains, nuts, or seeds. Calcium, iron, zinc, and vitamin B_{12} intake may be deficient, especially for growth and development of children (see Chapters 21-23).

Environmental Factors

Cost, accessibility, convenience, and safety are major factors influencing food selection and eating behavior. With food prices on the rise, consumers attempt to get the most for their money. Unfortunately, foods high in nutritional value, such as fruits and grains, may appear to be more expensive than highly refined sugar products and may require more preparation. Consumers often end up with foods that are easy to prepare but are high in calories, and have minimal nutritional value. By being familiar with cultural limitations and the available resources, nurses can assist clients to select menus that are nutritionally sound. For example, nurses may recommend seasonal fruits and vegetables to minimize cost and maximize nutritional value, or they may recommend that less expensive cuts of meat be purchased and navy beans be used as a source of protein in the diet

---

TABLE 28-3

Food and Nutrition Board, National Academy of Sciences—National Research Council Recommended Daily Dietary Allowances,* Revised 1980

Designed for the maintenance of good nutrition of practically all healthy people in the U.S.A.

	Age (years)	WEIGHT (kg)	WEIGHT (lb)	HEIGHT (cm)	HEIGHT (in)	Protein (g)	FAT-SOLUBLE VITAMINS Vitamin A (µg RE)	Vitamin D (µg)	Vitamin E (mg α-TE)
Infants	0.0-0.5	6	13	60	24	kg × 2.2	420	10	3
	0.5-1.0	9	20	71	28	kg × 2.0	400	10	4
Children	1-3	13	29	90	35	23	400	10	5
	4-6	20	44	112	44	30	500	10	6
	7-10	28	62	132	52	34	700	10	7
Males	11-14	45	99	157	62	45	1000	10	8
	15-18	66	145	176	69	56	1000	10	10
	19-22	70	154	177	70	56	1000	7.5	10
	23-50	70	154	178	70	56	1000	5	10
	51+	70	154	178	70	56	1000	5	10
Females	11-14	46	101	157	62	46	800	10	8
	15-18	55	120	163	64	46	800	10	8
	19-22	55	120	163	64	44	800	7.5	8
	23-50	55	120	163	64	44	800	5	8
	51+	55	120	163	64	44	800	5	8
Pregnant						+30	+200	+5	+2
Lactating						+20	+400	+5	+3

*The allowances are intended to provide for individual variations among most normal persons as they live in the United States under usual environmental stresses. Diets should be based on a variety of common foods in order to provide other nutrients for which human requirements have been less well defined.

of low-income families. Assistance with food preparation ideas is also important when introducing new foods.

Accessibility is a major factor in food selection. Many low-income families have limited mobility and must rely on local merchants for their food choices. Small, local stores tend to be more expensive than supermarkets. Assistance with planning meals over several days and shopping in larger stores may help clients learn to plan more nutritious, less expensive meals.

Convenience plays a large part in food selection. Many women work outside the home, so families are eating more foods that are quickly and easily prepared and are eating out more often. Counseling regarding the nutritional value, deficiencies, and excesses of convenient and "fast-food" menus is an important function of community health nurses.

Safety of food and water is not usually a problem for families in the United States because of the network of inspection services. However, the number of chemicals in use is increasing rapidly, while at the same time the ability to detect potentially harmful substances is improving. Thus, all community residents, especially health professionals, should be alert to the potential for contamination of air, water, and foods. In homes, nurses can teach families about food preparation and storage to ensure intake of food that is not spoiled. For example, the nurse can discuss with the family how to prepare and store lunches taken to school or work.

Recommended Dietary Allowances

Recommended dietary allowances (RDA) are the levels of intake of essential nutrients considered to be adequate to meet the known nutritional needs of practically all healthy persons. Table 28-3 shows the RDA, which is made by a committee of scientists designated by the National Academy of Sciences Food and Nutrition Board. The committee reviews the world's literature on nutrient requirements, paying particular attention to new findings since last RDA publications.

The RDAs are recommendations for the average daily amounts of nutrients that population groups should consume over a period of time. Nutritionists become concerned when someone consistently consumes less than 70% of the RDA for a vitamin, mineral, or protein. It is almost impossible to exceed the RDA limits with foods alone. People who take vitamin and mineral supplements should be aware of possible toxic effects of fat-soluble vitamins (A, D, E, and K) at levels above five times the RDA and some minerals at three times the RDA (Tufts University, 1986).

Since nutrient needs vary by sex and stage of life, the RDAs give recommendations for nutrients by sex and age.

WATER-SOLUBLE VITAMINS							MINERALS					
Vita-min C (mg)	Thia-min (mg)	Ribo-flavin (mg)	Niacin (mg NE)	Vita-min B-6 (mg)	Fola-cin (μg)	Vita-min B-12 (μg)	Cal-cium (mg)	Phos-phorus (mg)	Mag-nesium (mg)	Iron (mg)	Zinc (mg)	Iodine (μg)
35	0.3	0.4	6	0.3	30	0.5	360	240	50	10	3	40
35	0.5	0.6	8	0.6	45	1.5	540	360	70	15	5	50
45	0.7	0.8	9	0.9	100	2.0	800	800	150	15	10	70
45	0.9	1.0	11	1.3	200	2.5	800	800	200	10	10	90
45	1.2	1.4	16	1.6	300	3.0	800	800	250	10	10	120
50	1.4	1.6	18	1.8	400	3.0	1200	1200	350	18	15	150
60	1.4	1.7	18	2.0	400	3.0	1200	1200	400	18	15	150
60	1.5	1.7	19	2.2	400	3.0	800	800	350	10	15	150
60	1.4	1.6	18	2.2	400	3.0	800	800	350	10	15	150
60	1.2	1.4	16	2.2	400	3.0	800	800	350	10	15	150
50	1.1	1.3	15	1.8	400	3.0	1200	1200	300	18	15	150
60	1.1	1.3	14	2.0	400	3.0	1200	1200	300	18	15	150
60	1.1	1.3	14	2.0	400	3.0	800	800	300	18	15	150
60	1.0	1.2	13	2.0	400	3.0	800	800	300	18	15	150
60	1.0	1.2	13	2.0	400	3.0	800	800	300	10	15	150
+20	+0.4	+0.3	+2	+0.6	+400	+1.0	+400	+400	+150	h	+5	+25
+40	+0.5	+0.5	+5	+0.5	+100	+1.0	+400	+400	+150	h	+10	+50

TABLE 28-4

The basic four food groups

Food group	Main nutrients	Daily amounts
Vegetables and fruits		4 or more servings Count as 1 serving: ½ cup vegetable or fruit or a portion such as 1 medium apple, banana, orange, potato, or half a medium grapefruit or melon
	Vitamin A	Include: 1 dark green or deep yellow vegetable or fruit rich in vitamin A, at least every other day
	Vitamin C (ascorbic acid)	1 citrus or other fruit or vegetable rich in vitamin C daily
	Smaller amounts of other vitamins and minerals	Other vegetables and fruits, including potatoes
Bread and cereals	Thiamin Niacin Riboflavin Iron Protein	4 or more servings of whole-grain, enriched, or restored Count as 1 serving: 1 slice bread 1 oz (1 cup) ready-to-eat cereal, flake or puff varieties ½-¾ cup cooked cereal ½-¾ cup cooked pasta (macaroni, spaghetti, noodles) Crackers: 5 saltines, 2 squares graham crackers, and so forth
Meats		
Beef, veal, lamb, pork, poultry, fish, eggs	Protein Iron Thiamin	2 or more servings Count as one serving: 2-3 oz lean, boneless, cooked meat, poultry, or fish
Alternatives: dry beans and peas, nuts, peanut butter	Niacin Riboflavin	2 eggs 1 cup cooked dry beans or peas 4 tbs peanut butter
Milk*		
Milk, cheese, ice cream, or other products made with whole or skimmed milk	Calcium Protein Riboflavin	Children under 9: 2-3 cups Children 9 to 12: 3 or more cups Teenagers: 4 or more cups Adults: 2 or more cups Pregnant women: 3 or more cups Nursing mothers: 4 or more cups (1 cup = 8 oz fluid milk or designated milk equivalent†)

*Milk equivalents: 1 oz cheddar cheese, 2 cups cottage cheese, 1 cup fluid skimmed milk, 1 cup buttermilk, ¼ cup dry skimmed milk powder, 1 cup ice milk, 1⅔ cup ice cream, ½ cup evaporated milk.
Source: U. S. Department of Agriculture.

The USRDAs used for food labeling are a distillation of the 17 separate categories and are based on the highest RDA of that nutrient.

The RDAs are used by federal, state, and local health and welfare agencies for licensing and certification standards for feeding programs for groups, such as day care centers, schools, and nursing homes. They are used to interpret food consumption records, evaluate adequacy of food supplies in meeting nutritional needs, establish guides for public food assistance programs, evaluate new food products developed by industry, establish guidelines for nutritional labeling of foods, and develop nutrition education programs (Poleman and Capra, 1984).

The first RDAs were published in 1943 and have been

revised every 5 years to include new scientific information. The latest edition was to be published at the end of 1985, but the proposed changes were rejected by the National Academy of Sciences Food and Nutrition Board because the committee's suggestions altered the concept of RDA from that of meeting nutritional needs for nearly all healthy people to "protecting practically all healthy persons against nutritional deficiencies." The proposal included significant reductions of RDAs for Vitamins A, C, B_6, manganese, iron, and zinc. Critics feared the changes would pave the way for reductions in federal programs based on the RDAs, such as funding for school lunches and food stamps (Tufts University, 1986). The RDAs will continue to evolve as information becomes available. Current interest is in de-

TABLE 28-5
Dietary Goals for the United States

	PERCENT OF TOTAL CALORIC INTAKE	
	Current diet	Goals
Protein	12	12
Carbohydrates		
Complex carbohydrates and naturally occurring sugars	28	48
Sugars, refined and processed	18	10
Total	46	58
Fat		
Saturated	16	10
Nonunsaturated	19	10
Polyunsaturated	7	10
Total	42	30
Cholesterol mg/day	600	300
Salt g/day	6-18	5

Select Committee on Nutrition and Human Needs, U.S. Senate, Washington, D.C., 1977, U.S. Government Printing Office.

veloping guidelines for fats and carbohydrates, additional minerals, and specific RDAs of all nutrients for the elderly.

Dietary Guidelines

To interpret and apply sound nutrient standards, practical food guides have been developed to assist health care workers with nutrition education. Such tools include the basic four food groups, the food exchange system, and the Dietary Guidelines for Americans.

The United States Department of Agriculture developed the basic four food groups as a guide for planning a well-balanced diet. Although it has its limitations, it provides a practical, general basis for planning meals and evaluating a person's overall food intake. Table 28-4 provides an outline of the basic four food groups.

Another food guide in general use, especially for modified diets such as those for diabetes or weight control, is the food exchange system. There are six food groups in this system: milk, vegetables, fruits, breads and other starches, meats and other protein foods, and fats. These foods are grouped according to their similarity in calories and food values, so measured amounts of foods within the group may be traded off ("exchanged") in meals. This provides an easy way for anyone to learn to balance a meal. Most nutrition texts provide exchange lists.

The first federal statement on the relationship between diet and disease risk factors were the U.S. Dietary Goals. These were developed by the U.S. Senate Select Committee on Nutrition and Human Needs as a general food guide because of concern about chronic health problems, an aging population, and a changing food environment. The specific recommendations of the dietary goals are listed in Table 28-5. The goals propose increases in intake of starches and decreases in intake of fats, sugars, cholesterol, and salt. Because the goals have not been consistently supported by experimental evidence and because they require major changes in food purchases and consumption, they have generated considerable controversy (especially from cattle and dairy farmers). The Dietary Guidelines for Americans are useful statements that support the dietary goals but contain recommendations that are less specific (Nestle, 1985). No guidelines guarantee health or well-being, and people vary widely in their food needs, but these general statements about variety and moderation can lead people to evaluate their food habits and move toward general improvements.

The seven statements that comprise the Dietary Guidelines for Americans and some suggestions for nurses to assist clients to follow the guidelines are described in the following paragraphs. (Williams, 1984; USDA & USDHHS, 1980)

1. Eat a variety of foods. About 40 different nutrients are needed to maintain health and no single food can supply all the essential nutrients in the amounts needed. To ensure variety, teach clients to select foods from all of the major food groups on a daily basis.

2. Maintain ideal weight. Obesity is associated with chronic disorders, such as hypertension, diabetes, and heart disease. What is "ideal" weight must be determined individually, for many factors are involved, such as body composition, body metabolism, genetics, and physical activity. Table 28-6 gives the most recent weight recommendations based on the Metropolitan Life Insurance Company's experience with longevity. Some controversy surrounds these standards (Tufts University, 1987), but they provide starting points for assisting clients to set realistic goals for weight loss, gain, or maintenance. Suggestions on ways to improve eating habits, such as eating slowly, preparing smaller portions, avoiding second helpings, and concentrating on eating rather than reading or TV, may be useful to clients.

3. Avoid too much saturated fat and cholesterol. The American population as a whole consumes a high-fat diet. Some people apparently cannot tolerate fat, and extra fat intake leads to high levels of blood lipids, which are associated with higher risk of heart disease. To assist families to lower fat intake, nurses can suggest the following:

Choose lean meat, fish, poultry, and legumes (such as soybean substances, other beans, and peas) as protein sources.

Trim excess fat off meats.

Use eggs and organ meats (such as liver) in moderation.

Limit intake of butter, cream, hydrogenated margarines, shortenings, coconut oil, and foods made from such products.

Bake, broil, or boil foods rather than fry.

Read labels carefully to determine both amount and types of fat contained in foods.

4. Eat foods with adequate starch and fiber. Complex carbohydrates, such as whole grain cereals and breads, beans, peas, fruits and vegetables, are better fuel sources for energy than are fats and sugars and contain many es-

TABLE 28-6

1983 Metropolitan height and weight tables for men and women according to frame, ages 25-59

Height (in shoes)†		Weight in pounds (in indoor clothing)*		
Feet	Inches	Small frame	Medium frame	Large frame
MEN				
5	2	128-134	131-141	138-150
5	3	130-136	133-143	140-153
5	4	132-138	135-145	142-156
5	5	134-140	137-148	144-160
5	6	136-142	139-151	146-164
5	7	138-145	142-154	149-168
5	8	140-148	145-157	152-172
5	9	142-151	148-160	155-176
5	10	144-154	151-163	158-180
5	11	146-157	154-166	161-184
6	0	149-160	157-170	164-188
6	1	152-164	160-174	168-192
6	2	155-168	164-178	172-197
6	3	158-172	167-182	176-202
6	4	162-176	171-187	181-207
WOMEN				
4	10	102-111	109-121	118-131
4	11	103-113	111-123	120-134
5	0	104-115	113-126	122-137
5	1	106-118	115-129	125-140
5	2	108-121	118-132	128-143
5	3	111-124	121-135	131-147
5	4	114-127	124-138	134-151
5	5	117-130	127-141	137-155
5	6	120-133	130-144	140-159
5	7	123-136	133-147	143-163
5	8	126-139	136-150	146-167
5	9	129-142	139-153	149-170
5	10	132-145	142-156	152-173
5	11	135-148	145-159	155-176
6	0	138-151	148-162	158-179

Source of basic data: *Build Study, 1979,* Society of Actuaries and Association of Life Insurance Medical Directors of America, 1980.
Copyright 1983 Metropolitan Life Insurance Company.
*Indoor clothing weighing 5 pounds for men and 3 pounds for women.
†Shoes with 1-inch heels.

sential nutrients and fiber. Because many processed and refined foods are eaten, the American diet is low in fiber. There is evidence that fiber improves bowel health as well as contributes to better blood sugar control for diabetics.

5. Avoid too much sugar. The major health hazard from eating too much sugar is tooth decay. Americans consume an average of 130 pounds of sugar per person per year, mostly from processed foods. To avoid excessive sugar, nurses can recommend that people:

Use less of all sugars including white, brown, and raw sugars, honey, and syrups.

Eat fewer foods containing sugar, such as candy, soft drinks, ice cream, and cake.

Read food labels for clues to sugar content—if sucrose, glucose, maltose, dextrose, lactose, fructose, or syrup

appears first, the product contains a large amount of sugar.

Select fresh fruits or fruits canned without sugar or in light syrup.

6. Avoid too much sodium. Many processed foods contain extra sodium, and most Americans eat more sodium than needed. People can lower their sodium intake by cooking with small amounts of salt, adding little salt to foods at the table, limiting intake of salty foods, reading labels to determine the amount of sodium in processed foods, and being aware of sodium content in water and medications.

7. If you drink alcohol, do so in moderation. Alcoholic beverages are high in calories and low in other nutrients. Limited food intake may accompany large alcohol intake. Heavy drinking contributes to chronic liver dis-

TABLE 28-7

Clinical signs of nutritional status

Features	Good	Poor
General appearance	Alert, responsive	Listless, apathetic; cachexia
General vitality	Endurance; energetic; sleeps well at night; vigorous	Easily fatigues, no energy, falls asleep, looks tired, apathetic
Weight	Normal for height, age, body build	Overweight or underweight
Skin	Smooth, slightly moist; good color	Rough, dry, scaly, pale, pigmented, irritated; petechiae, bruises
Posture	Erect, arms and legs straight, abdomen in, chest out	Sagging shoulders, sunken chest, humped back
Muscles	Well developed, firm	Flaccid, poor tone; undeveloped, tender
Skeleton	No malformations	Bowlegs, knock-knees, chest deformity at diaphragm, beaded ribs, prominent scapulae
Legs and feet	No tenderness, weakness, or swelling; good color	Edema, tender calves; tingling, weakness
Nervous control	Good attention span for age; does not cry easily; not irritable or restless	Inattentive, irritable
Hair	Shiny, lustrous; healthy scalp	Stringy, dull, brittle, dry, depigmented
Neck glands	No enlargement	Thyroid enlarged
Skin on face and neck	Smooth, slightly moist; good color, reddish pink mucous membranes	Greasy, discolored, scaly
Eyes	Bright, clear; no fatigue circles	Dryness, signs of infection, increased vascularity, glassiness, thickened conjunctivae
Lips	Good color, moist	Dry, scaly, swollen, angular lesions (stomatitis)
Tongue	Good pink color; surface papillae present; no lesions	Papillary atrophy, smooth appearance; swollen, red beefy (glossitis)
Gums	Good pink color; no swelling or bleeding; firm	Marginal redness or swelling; receding, spongy
Teeth	Straight, no crowding; well-shaped jaw; clean, no discoloration	Unfilled cavities, absent teeth, worn surfaces; mottled, malpositioned
Abdomen	Flat	Swollen
Gastrointestinal function	Good appetite and digestion; normal, regular elimination	Anorexia, indigestion, constipation or diarrhea

Adapted from Williams, S.R.: Mowry's Basic Nutrition and Diet Therapy, ed. 7, St. Louis, 1984, The C.V. Mosby Co.

ease and neurological disorders, as well as throat and neck cancer.

Using the Nursing Process to Promote Sound Nutrition

Most meal planning and preparation occur in the home, so community health nurses have many opportunities to provide nutrition education when making home visits. In addition, although physicians, dietitians, nutritionists, and home economists often assist in resolving nutritional problems and related diseases, the responsibility for identification frequently rests with the community health nurse. It is through the nursing process that community health nurses are able to detect and intervene in nutritional difficulties encountered by individuals, families, and groups in the community.

Assessment

Nutritional assessment of an individual or group of people should include biological, psychological, cultural, and en-

vironmental factors. Review of the client's medical history may identify conditions that place the client at risk for malnutrition. Some of these conditions include hypermetabolic states, compromised digestive or absorptive capacity, chronic or acute diseases associated with abnormal nutrient intake or loss, recent major surgery, or a treatment plan with nutritional implications such as chemotherapy or multiple drug therapies (Jensen, Englert, and Dudrick, 1983). Side effects of various medications cause nutritional problems or symptoms of nutritional problems and should be considered when doing physiological assessment. For example, antibiotics may cause stomatitis, nausea, vomiting, gastritis, or diarrhea; and steroids may cause digestive tract disturbances or interfere with protein, lipid, and electrolyte utilization (Poleman and Capra, 1984).

Through a physical examination, nurses can document signs and symptoms of inadequate nutrition. Table 28-7 summarizes clinical signs of nutritional status.

Interviewing clients about their food intake is helpful in obtaining information about patterns of eating, food aver-

> ## KEY QUESTIONS TO ASK DURING NUTRITIONAL ASSESSMENT
>
> How much do you weigh and how tall are you?
>
> What is the most you have ever weighed? When and what circumstances?
>
> Has your weight changed recently? How much? Any idea why?
>
> Do you follow a special diet at home? Type?
>
> Are there any foods you avoid? What and why? (aversions, intolerances, allergies)
>
> Have you recently experienced nausea, vomiting, diarrhea, constipation, chewing or swallowing problems?
>
> Have you experienced any changes in your appetite? in food intake?
>
> Are you taking any vitamins or nutritional supplements? Type?
>
> What is your occupation? Usual activity?
>
> Are you being treated for any disease? taking any medications?
>
> Have you had surgery? When and type?
>
> Recall all the food you have eaten in the past 24 hours.

sions, intolerances, and difficulties in eating or digesting certain foods. Some key questions to ask during nutritional assessment are listed in the box above (Jensen et al., 1983).

During the assessment phase, the nurse may ask the client to keep a food diary of all foods and beverages consumed, the time of day foods are eaten, and environmental and emotional aspects of the eating situation. The diary can be jointly reviewed by the nurse and client, so eating and food selection patterns can be identified and interventions planned.

Any assessment tool that focuses only on the foods eaten and ignores the cultural, environmental, and economic influences on dietary habits does not provide an adequate basis for planning nursing interventions. Information regarding food preferences, preparation time, cost, availability, daily meal patterns, physical limitations, and environmental constraints (such as lack of running water) must be obtained. In addition, the client's relation to the family and community as a whole must be considered in the assessment phase to gain an understanding of all influences on food selection and eating behaviors. For example, before helping a client with hypertension to select a low sodium diet, the nurse would gather information regarding such variables as the major foods eaten, the client's eating patterns (food prepared at home vs. meals eaten out), family support of the dietary changes for one member (how willing other family members are to alter their diets somewhat), and cultural influences (ethnic diet high in sodium).

Planning

The information gathered in the assessment process guides plans for nutrition education. Whether working with individuals, families, or groups, the community health nurse must consider the concerns, interests, and priorities of the potential audience when planning nursing interventions. Clients may have limited food choices because of the cost and availability of foods and confusion over advertising claims.

It is essential in the planning phase of the nursing process to include all individuals who will be affected by the proposed nutritional changes. For example, when assisting an adolescent to plan a weight reduction diet, the nurse would benefit by including family members responsible for selecting, preparing, and financing the food. Inclusion in the planning process generally encourages participation in implementation of the diet.

In the planning phase, additional resource persons, such as nutritionists, physicians, and social workers, are consulted to assist in meeting the identified needs of the clients. Special needs of clients may be met by community nutrition resources or governmental aid programs. For example, families with low-birth-weight infants may be eligible for the Special Supplemental Food Program for Women, Infants, and Children (WIC). Elderly clients confined to their homes may benefit from Meals on Wheels, a local program in which one hot meal is brought to their home daily. Poor families may be able to obtain food stamps to extend their food dollars.

Implementation

The nursing process culminates in the implementation and evaluation of the plan jointly developed by nurses and clients and their families. Involving clients and their families in the planning phase, setting reasonable and achievable goals, and suggesting incorporation of self-rewards into the plans keep clients interested and motivated during implementation of the nursing care plan.

Evaluation

Regardless of the strategies selected for implementation, awareness of how clients and their families are perceiving the benefits of the proposed changes is essential to success. Discussion and feedback about progress is important. Progress can be monitored throughout the plan and corrections made to ensure maximum benefit from the nursing interventions. Evaluation at the conclusion of nursing interventions provides nurses with valuable information about the degree to which objectives and client needs have been met.

To evaluate clients' progress, community health nurses may ask them to keep food diaries for one or more days each week to be reviewed at the meetings. Nurses can use data in the diaries to educate and reinforce clients and their families about a balanced diet.

Weight Control

Obesity is generally defined as being 20% or more overweight. Heredity, interpersonal factors such as family problems, anxiety, unrealistic expectations of self and others, sociocultural factors (e.g., food selection practices), and environmental factors have been identified as probable causes of obesity. Numerous studies have suggested that it is more important to deal with personal, social, and environmental influences rather than biochemical causes of obesity. Because

TABLE 28-8

Health-related physical fitness measures

Measure	Definition	Evaluation
1. Cardiorespiratory endurance	Ability of the circulatory and respiratory systems to supply fuel during sustained physical activity and to eliminate waste products that produce fatigue	Maximum or submaximum oxygen uptake tests on treadmill or cycle ergometer; 12-minute run
2. Muscular endurance	Ability of muscle groups to exert external force for many repetitious or successive exertions	Isokinetic tests; number of repetitions of pull-ups, sit-ups, or lifts of light to moderate weights
3. Muscular strength	The amount of external force that a muscle can exert	Weight lifts by particular muscles or groups of muscles
4. Flexibility	The range of motion available at a joint	Flexometer tests; sit and reach tests
5. Body composition	Relative amounts of muscle, fat, bone, and other vital parts of the body	Underwater weighing; skinfold pinch test

Adapted from Caspersen, C.J., Powell, K.E., and Christenson, G.M.: Physical activity, exercise, and physical fitness: definitions and distinctions for health-related research. Public Health Rep 100:126-131, 1985.

of their holistic approach to care, nurses can be quite effective in assisting obese people to lose weight.

Assessment of individuals desiring weight loss is essential to developing an individualized, effective program. In addition to gathering data regarding current dietary practices and sociocultural influences, nurses should also consider the client's past weight loss program. Persons who derive the greatest benefits from a weight reduction program exhibit adult-onset rather than adolescent-onset obesity, report fewer previous attempts to lose weight, and are more adept at self-reinforcement (Pender, 1987).

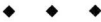

Although controversy exists regarding the value of many nutrients, little doubt remains that nutrition plays a vital role in maintaining health. Attempts are being made to link diseases with dietary practices, and the government has made recommendations regarding the elimination of excesses from the American diet.

The concept of physical fitness and its relation to health promotion and maintenance is also receiving much attention. The next section of this chapter focuses on exercise.

PROMOTING HEALTH THROUGH EXERCISE

Exercise is a means for promoting physiological and psychological health. Community health nurses are in prime positions to observe activity patterns and problems of individuals and groups. By recognizing the potential benefits of exercise and promoting physical fitness, innovative and vitally important nursing interventions can be planned.

The majority of American adults are concerned about their physical fitness and are reasonably convinced that regular exercise is essential to good health. However, only about one third of all adults participate in exercise on a weekly basis, and only 20% exercise at levels recommended for cardiovascular fitness. Recent increases in exercise participation have occurred in well-educated, affluent, young adults. Among Americans over 50 there is limited awareness of the kinds and amounts of activity needed to maintain physical fitness, and there is a widespread belief that exercise may be dangerous (Dishman, Sallis, and Orenstein, 1985; President's Council on Physical Fitness, 1980).

Physical activity is movement produced by skeletal muscles that results in energy expenditure. *Exercise* is a subset of physical activity that is planned, structured, and repetitive and has as its objective the improvement or maintenance of physical fitness (Powell and Paffenbarger, 1985).

Physical fitness is a set of physiological attributes, some of which are health related, that people have or achieve. Being physically fit has been defined as "the ability to carry out daily tasks with vigor and alertness, without undue fatigue, and with ample energy to enjoy leisure time pursuits and to meet unforeseen emergencies" (President's Council on Physical Fitness, 1971). The skill-related components of physical fitness important for performance in particular sports or activities are agility, balance, coordination, speed, power, and reaction time.

The health-related components of physical fitness important for the public's health are cardiorespiratory endurance, flexibility, body composition, muscular endurance, and muscular strength.

Table 28-8 defines each of these components and lists ways they are measured. Levels of physical fitness range from high to low, and the levels of the components may differ greatly. For example, a person may be strong, but not be flexible or not have cardiorespiratory endurance (Caspersen, Powell, and Christenson, 1985).

Effects of Exercise

Exercise has both physiological and psychological effects. Both should be considered during nursing assessment, planning, and evaluation.

TABLE 28-9

Responses of body systems to exercise

System	Responses during exercise	Changes due to conditioning
Muscles and locomotive organs	Increased rate of contraction Increased activity of anaerobic and aerobic energy production systems	Increased strength of bones and ligaments Increased volume and tensile strength of tendons and ligaments Increased thickness, compressibility, and contact area of articular cartilage Increased muscle strength Increased capillary density (number of capillaries per square millimeter of muscle tissue)
Neurological	Increased sympathetic nervous system stimulation, which causes a neural shift toward the muscles and away from the internal organs	Hypertrophy of synapse of nerve fiber with muscle fiber Increased ability for motorneurons to be stimulated frequently Increase in number of fibers contracting at one time
	Increased alertness at beginning of exercise, which may wane as exercise progresses (due to increased brain stimulation at beginning and decrease of circulating carbohydrate for fuel or buildup metabolic waste products as the exercise progresses)	Faster reaction time
Blood	More oxygen is extracted from blood by tissues (up to 3 times)	Increase in total hemoglobin Increase in plasma volume Increased speed of formation of red blood cells
	Blood pH decreases due to formation of lactic acid and carbonic acid Decrease in plasma volume 5% to 10% due to diffusion into interstitial fluid Increase in white blood cell concentration Increase in hematocrit	
Heart	Increase in cardiac output from 5 to 6 L/min to as much as 30 to 40 L/min Increased stroke volume by up to 50% Increased heart rate (up to 5 times) Increased blood flow to the cardiac muscle	Increase in size and weight of heart muscle and chambers, especially the left ventricle due to increased muscle volume Increased maximum stroke volume and resting stroke volume (about 150%) Decrease in heart rate at rest (due to larger stroke volume) Decrease in heart rate at submaximum workloads due to decreased sympathetic stimulation and increased parasympathetic stimulation
Circulation	Increased systolic blood pressure No change in diastolic due to decrease in peripheral resistance Dilation of capillaries of working muscles so circulation increases Increase in pulmonary circulation Increased blood flow to the skin depending on the temperature of the environment Decrease in percent of blood flow to GI tract and abdominal organs Decrease in transit time for blood to make complete cycle from heart back to heart Increased venous return due to increased action of the diaphragm used in increased ventilation	Decrease in blood pressure if hypertensive Increased ability of capillaries to respond to needs of working muscles Some ECG changes at rest, which usually normalize during exercise

Respiratory	Increased ventilation
	  -minute volume increases from 5 to 6 L to as high as 200 L
	  -tidal volume increases from 0.5 L up to 3 L from 12 to 16 up to 50 to 60 breaths/min
	Increased oxygen uptake and carbon dioxide output
		Increase in maximum minute ventilatory volume
		Increase in efficiency and endurance of ventilation muscles
		Increase in tidal volume and decrease in breath rate during exercise
		
		Increase in maximum oxygen uptake

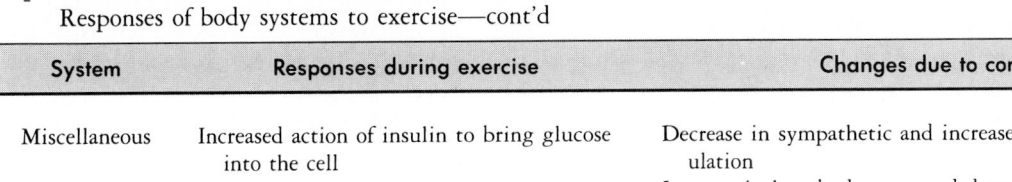

TABLE 28-9

Responses of body systems to exercise—cont'd

System	Responses during exercise	Changes due to conditioning
Miscellaneous	Increased action of insulin to bring glucose into the cell	Decrease in sympathetic and increase in parasympathetic stimulation Increase in lean body mass and decrease in fat if caloric intake is unchanged Increase in fatigue threshold—may be psychological in that person is more willing to exert and has had practice in doing so

Physiological

Nurses have long been aware of the detrimental effects of prolonged bed rest and the resultant lack of exercise. Venous thrombosis, orthostatic hypotension, a progressive increase in heart rate, and a reduction in the strength of skeletal muscles are a few of the problems associated with inactivity. In recent years, much research has been conducted to demonstrate a cause-and-effect relationship between physical inactivity in ambulatory populations and specific disease processes. Although no unequivocal relationships have been demonstrated, physiological responses and benefits to exercise have been determined (Table 28-9). Mounting epidemiological evidence suggests that physical inactivity and lack of exercise are related to the occurence of several diseases that are major causes of death and disability in the United States. The relationship between activity and coronary heart disease has been studied the most extensively, and results suggest that physical activity also contributes to prevention and control of diabetes mellitus, hypertension, and osteoporosis (Siscovick, LaPorte, and Newman, 1985).

Psychological

Claims have been made that exercise produces a variety of psychological benefits. Some of the claims come from anecdotes and self-reports, whereas others have been demonstrated in research studies (Shephard, 1983). The effects may be caused by biochemical changes that result from the activity, by the perceptions of the individual, or a combination of both. Many participants in exercise state they "feel better" when they exercise regularly. Exercise increases arousal, which improves alertness and mood. It improves self-esteem and body image by improving ability to undertake physical and mental work. Regular exercise also tends to relieve depression and anxiety and lessen the frequency of minor medical complaints and industrial absenteeism. Cognitive functioning and psychomotor abilities in children, retarded persons, and geriatric clients are enhanced by exercise. Potential negative psychological effects include mental fatigue and compulsiveness, self-centeredness, and competitiveness, all of which affect work and family life. It is not clear whether exercise causes the negative behavior or if certain personalities are predisposed to abuse exercise as a way of coping with other problems (Dishman, 1985; Taylor, Sallis, and Needle, 1985).

Although the psychological benefits of exercise and phys-

ical fitness have been studied in a variety of settings, no exact mechanisms of action have been discovered. Individual differences in expectations, beliefs, coping patterns, and initial fitness potentially affect benefits received from exercise.

The stimuli for many of the health benefits of exercise are not well defined. Many of the health effects may be related more to physical or mechanical stress placed on the muscles, connective tissue, or skeleton than to increased energy expenditure (Haskell, 1985). Nurses should inform clients of the benefits of increases in activity even at low levels. Success at increasing activity a little improves both physiology and mental status and is likely to promote further activity. Aiming for major changes in exercise may not be as effective as planning small changes.

Fitness Evaluation and Programs

Exercise is a safe activity for most people. Apparently healthy individuals under age 35 can usually begin exercise programs without a physical examination if the exercise program begins and proceeds gradually and as long as the individual is alert to the development of unusual signs or symptoms. Requiring that people consult physicians before beginning any type of program may mean that people do not exercise at all, which is more detrimental to health than beginning without medical approval. The Physical Activity Readiness Questionnaire (British Columbia Department of Health, 1975, cited in American College of Sports Medicine, 1986) may be used to screen people for an exercise program. If a person answers "yes" to any of these questions, he or she should postpone plans for vigorous exercise until given clearance by a physician:

1. Has your doctor ever said you have heart trouble?
2. Do you ever suffer from pains in your chest?
3. Do you often feel faint or have spells of dizziness?
4. Has a doctor ever told you that you have a bone or joint problem, such as arthritis, that has been aggravated by exercise or might be made worse by exercise?
5. Is there a good physical reason not mentioned here why you should not follow an activity program even if you wanted to?
6. Are you over age 65 and not accustomed to vigorous exercise?

Individuals with coronary risk factors, such as history of

high blood pressure; elevated cholesterol; cigarette smoking; abnormal resting ECG; family history of cardiovascular disease prior to age 50; or with pulmonary diseases or metabolic diseases, such as diabetes mellitus, thyroid disorders, renal disease, or liver disease, should be seen by a physician before beginning a program involving vigorous exercise.

Exercise Recommendations

The American College of Sports Medicine (1986) has made the following recommendations for quantity and quality of exercise for developing and maintaining cardiorespiratory fitness and body composition.

TYPE OF ACTIVITY. Activities that improve cardiovascular endurance and functional capacity are recommended. These are activities that use large muscle groups, can be maintained for prolonged periods, and are rhythmical and aerobic in nature, such as walking-hiking, jogging-running, swimming, skating, bicycling, rowing, cross-country skiing, rope skipping, and various endurance game activities (dancing, figure skating, tennis, etc.) if done on a continuous basis over a period of time. Competitive aspects of exercise should be minimized to reduce risk to participants.

INTENSITY. Physical activity should raise heart rate up to 60% to 85% of age-predicted maximum heart rate. A formula for determining the range to which clients should target their heart rates is shown in the box below.

DURATION. Fifteen to sixty minutes of continuous or discontinuous aerobic activity is recommended; aerobic activity for 20 to 30 minutes results in a conditioning effect. Lower intensity activities over longer durations are recommended because of the potential hazards of high intensity activity and because when persons perceive the activity as too intense, they are less likely to perform.

FORMULA FOR DETERMINING TARGET HEART RATE

220 − age = age predicted maximum heart rate
Maximum heart rate × 0.60 = minimum aerobic effect heart rate
Maximum heart rate × 0.75 = target heart rate
Maximum heart rate × 0.85 = maximum safe heart rate

For example, the maximum heart rate for a 45-year-old man is 175; the heart rate for minimal aerobic effect is 105; and the maximum safe heart rate is 149. Target heart rate to be attained during aerobic activity after the initial several weeks of conditioning is 131. An important aspect of planning intensity of exercise is to teach clients how to take their pulses so that they can monitor themselves.

The most difficult problem in designing exercise programs is the prescription of appropriate intensity. This heart rate range is one way of estimating intensity. However, Gaesser and Rich (1984) found that after 18 weeks, middle-aged men who exercised five times per week at 40% of maximum oxygen uptake had just as great aerobic fitness improvement as men who exercised at 80% of maximum oxygen uptake. Their fitness did not increase as rapidly, but they attained the same level at the end of the program.

FREQUENCY. Exercise three to five times per week is recommended for conditioning. Initially a day of rest should follow each day of exercise. Once adaptation is accomplished, a greater conditioning response will be obtained with daily exercise.

RATE OF PROGRESSION. Progression in an exercise program is dependent on an individual's initial fitness level, health status, age, and goals. The initial phase should include stretching, light calisthenics, and low-level aerobic activities after which the participants experience minimal muscle soreness. Discomfort is associated with starting an exercise program without adequate time for physiological adaptation. Program adherence may be reduced if the program is initiated too abruptly. During the improvement phase, intensity is increased to the targeted heart rate level and duration of exercise is increased every 2 to 3 weeks until a satisfactory level of fitness is achieved. During the maintenance phase, workout schedules are maintained and activities may be substituted for variety, but duration and intensity are no longer increased.

Components of a Fitness Program

Any exercise program should include (1) a warm-up period, (2) aerobic exercise, and (3) a cool-down period. The exercise session should gradually progress from a low to a vigorous level of activity and then slowly return to a low activity level.

WARM-UP. The warm-up period lasts 5 to 20 minutes and includes stretching (joint-readiness) exercises, calisthenics and other types of muscle conditioning exercises, and walking or slow jogging. The duration and intensity of each of these activities depends on environmental conditions, the individual's functional capacity and symptomatology, and exercise preferences. For participants who require or prefer greater amounts of muscle strength or endurance, additional calisthenics and exercises using weights may be included. However weight lifting is not recommended for persons with hypertension, arrhythmias, or poor cardiac reserve. Warm-up exercises increase respiration, circulation, and body temperature and gently stretch ligaments and connective tissue to prepare them for more vigorous activity, and decrease the possibility of injury.

AEROBIC EXERCISE. The endurance or aerobic phase of conditioning can be designed to be continuous or discontinuous. It includes aerobic activities involving large muscle groups to produce heart rates of targeted intensity for the desired duration.

COOL-DOWN. The cool-down period includes exercises of diminishing intensities such as slower jogging or walking, stretching, and in some cases, relaxation activities. The cool-down period of 5 to 10 minutes allows body temperature and heart rate to decrease slowly. Blood does not pool in the lower extremities, reducing the potential for dizziness; and metabolites of muscle activity are oxidized, so pain and muscle stiffness are less likely.

Potential Hazards of Exercise

Exercise has many demonstrated benefits, but it also has associated risks. Client education regarding risks of exercise and how to minimize them should be part of a fitness program. Common problems associated with exercise and related nursing interventions are summarized in Table 28-10.

Promoting Fitness of the Community

With the growing public interest in exercise and physical fitness and the strong epidemiological and clinical evidence that supports exercise as a means of disease prevention, community health nurses can become involved in promoting community health through exercise. Programs involve collaboration with other health professionals and leaders in industry, schools, and the community.

Health Professionals

Advice from physicians and nurses is a factor in making life-style changes. As age increases, professional advice becomes more important. Clients want and expect such advice. Health professionals sometimes do not teach clients about exercise benefits because they lack knowledge or they lack confidence that they can help clients change (Powell, Spain, Christenson, and Mollenkemp, 1986). The majority of people have a health care provider who can make an impact on the exercise behavior of clients. Community health nurses can work to increase community residents' and health professionals' awareness of the benefits of fitness and ways to achieve fitness improvements.

Worksite

The worksite is an ideal place to increase physical activity because a large percentage of the population is employed and spends approximately one third of the day at work. Increasing physical activity has economic and performance benefits both for employees and employers (Fielding, 1984). Successful programs have strong leadership, convenient facilities, ongoing recruitment, long-term commitment, a variety of program options from which to select, a system for employee recognition, and involvement of spouses and family (Iverson, Fielding, Crow, and Christenson, 1985). Community health nurses can effectively work with busi-nesses to promote health in the work place. Assessment of employee fitness levels, needs, and desires, as well as the planning, implementation, and evaluation of employee fitness programs are activities that fall within the scope of community health nursing practice.

Schools

The nation's schools underpin the effort to achieve national fitness goals. Programs in schools can provide children with knowledge and the skill base for a lifetime of physical activity. Physical education requirements vary greatly among school districts, and although required in many states, physical education programs are not daily and emphasize team sports, which build skill rather than individual sports, which tend to build aerobic fitness (Iverson et al., 1985). Pressure on schools to emphasize basic academic skills and reduce costs have placed physical education programs in jeopardy. Community health nurses assigned to school districts can be instrumental in promoting exercise in the schools in both formal physical education classes and during free-play recess times.

Community

The largest number and variety of exercise programs are offered by public agencies such as city parks and recreation departments, nonprofit private agencies such as YMCAs and YWCAs, educational institutions, local clubs (skiing, bicycling, running, swimming, tennis, dancing), and for-profit health and fitness clubs. Many communities have a variety of facilities including bike paths; fitness courses; swimming pools; basketball, volleyball, and tennis courts; soccer fields; and open fields for games. Many shopping malls are opening early for walking. Nurses can assess the community to determine gaps in facilities and programs and coordinate efforts to expand exercise options for all age groups.

By enlisting support of community groups and governmental agencies, community health nurses can spearhead

---

TABLE 28-10

Common exercise-related problems and suggested nursing interventions

Problem	Probable causes	Nursing interventions
Nausea and/or vomiting	Delayed gastric emptying secondary to exercise	Encourage client to exercise on an empty stomach
Dehydration	Inadequate fluid intake	Encourage person to drink fluids (preferably water) before, during, and after exercise
Fatigue, lightheadedness	Overexertion	Teach people to exercise at an intensity that they can easily talk and are not breathless; teach people to do body and mind checks every few minutes so they will become aware of symptoms of overexertion and slow down
Orthopedic injuries	Overuse or misuse	Teach people to warm up before vigorous exercise, gradually increase intensity and duration of exercise over several months, rest if muscle or joint discomfort develops. Instruct people in appropriate first aid and follow-up measures
Injury related to heat	Inadequate training Inadequate precautions	Encourage clients to exercise during cool parts of day; lower intensity during hot, humid weather. Teach signs, symptoms and first aid for heat stroke and heat exhaustion

campaigns to educate community residents about the benefits of exercise and how to begin exercise programs. Media campaigns increase awareness about available facilities, the need for additional facilities, and the benefits of exercise. Health fairs can offer fitness assessments (cardiovascular, flexibility, strength) and educational programs related to fitness; neutralize perceived barriers; and portray activity as sociable, enjoyable, and part of a balanced lifestyle (Iverson et al., 1985). Walk-a-thons and bike-a-thons to support worthy causes increase awareness, interest, and sometimes participation in exercise.

The state of Massachusetts offers an example of a community-wide effort toward health promotion and prevention of chronic disease. Information on the benefits of exercise, low-fat and low-salt diets, nonsmoking, blood pressure control, and decreased exposure to toxic substances is disseminated through mass media. Local health program staff are assisted by skilled health professionals in the development of screening and health promotion programs for schools, workplaces, and community gathering places (Havas and Walker, 1986).

Motivation for Exercise

Even the best exercise program will fail if people are not motivated to initiate or follow it. Because community health nurses work closely with individuals and groups over extended periods of time, they can tailor exercise programs to specific needs and motivators. When planning exercise programs, three aspects should be considered: (1) the person and his or her characteristics and social support system; (2) the exercise setting; and (3) the characteristics of the physical activity (Dishman, Sallis, and Orenstein, 1985; Martin and Dubbert, 1985; Shephard, 1985).

Characteristics of People

People who begin and adhere to exercise programs have the following characteristics: they perceive that they lack activity and express a desire for improvement in health, fitness, and/or mental working capacity. They feel they have control over their health and that exercise will affect their health. They perceive they have or can learn the skills needed to exercise successfully and can recover from relapses to inactivity. They have support of significant others and see exercise as a way to socialize and vary routines. Many who exercise have done so sometime in their past. Enjoyment of the activity and feelings of well-being tend to be stronger motivators for participation in exercise than concerns about improvements in health. Persons most likely to drop out are obese and feel less well—just the people who need the activity the most. The challenge for community health nurses is to increase awareness and perceptions of control, teach skills, and gather support for clients to increase their activity levels.

Characteristics of Settings and Programs

Important aspects of the exercise setting are convenient hours and accessible facilities; leaders who individualize the program and offer choices to participants, provide reinforcement, and serve as models; activity partners who expect to have each other's company while exercising; and plans for weather conditions and time constraints. A program that helps people anticipate problems and learn how to deal with them, such as walking in a mall in bad weather or climbing steps for 20 minutes in a hotel when traveling, is more likely to produce adherence.

Activity Characteristics

Activities that are perceived as uncomfortable will not be performed. A program begun with too much intensity will produce dropouts quickly or may produce injuries that prohibit continuation. A person may be unwilling or unable to incorporate structured exercise into his or her weekly routine but might be willing to increase daily activity, such as walking to a nearby store rather than driving, parking in a corner of the parking lot rather than next to the building entrance, climbing stairs rather than riding elevators or escalators, taking a walk during work breaks or meals, or doing yard work rather than delegating it to someone else. Community health nurses can use their creativity to help clients increase activity in ways that are acceptable.

No motivators work in all situations, but the following suggestions can help community health nurses promote exercise (Blomquist, 1981, 1986; Estok and Rudy, 1986; Fixx, 1980):

1. *Involve clients in the planning process.* Clients provide nurses with clues to the types of activities they may enjoy, as well as barriers that may inhibit their participation.
2. *Select activities the people have already mastered.* Clients may become discouraged and quit if they are unable to master a new skill (such as swimming). Also, be alert to clients' desires to learn new skills.
3. *Fit the exercise program into the individual's present life-style.* Programs that require minimal alterations in a person's life-style will meet with less resistance than those demanding greater changes.
4. *Plan the exercise activities at the same time every day or each week to help in establishing a routine.*
5. *Develop realistic, achievable goals.* Clients are likely to participate when a particular goal is in sight. Some clients enjoy plotting their progress on a graph so that achievement is easy to see. Plotting the number of minutes of exercise or the miles walked is one way of determining progress toward goals and offering recognition.
6. *Acknowledge the disadvantages of exercise.* Preparing clients for the daily aggravations of exercise while at the same time expounding on the positive aspects not only protects the nurse's credibility with clients but also helps prevent discouragement with the program.
7. *Encourage and reinforce!* Let the people know that the positive aspects of exercising are readily apparent in their appearance, modification of habits (such as not smoking), or other outward measures.
8. *Teach self-management techniques.* Teaching participants to reinforce themselves may help them maintain enthusiasm. Praising one's self at intervals; relaxation and persuasion techniques such as Lamaze muscle relaxation and breathing, chanting, singing;

consciously planning or looking for something while walking/running; and planning personal rewards for milestones can be encouraged.

9. *Establish rewards.* At the beginning of the week persons may set goals and rewards for themselves if the goal is met. Companies can offer monetary rewards for miles employees walk, run, or swim and well-pay for employees who are neither absent nor tardy for a specified period of time. Facilities can offer T-shirts proclaiming achievements of goals (such as 100 mile clubs). People can make contracts with themselves or with the community health nurse (see Chapters 20 and 38 for more on contracting).

10. *Use exercise time as social time.* Individuals may find it more difficult to stop the program if others are depending on them. Groups, clubs, and teams promote social interaction, cooperation, fun, and variety. Group discussions provide opportunity for comparisons with peers; setting goals; sharing thoughts, feelings and strategies about exercise; and modeling desirable behaviors.

11. *Integrate music into the exercise program.* Music facilitates movement, relieves boredom, and may distract the individual from the repetitive nature of some exercises. People are often amazed at the number of rope jumps or sit-ups they are able to complete during a jazzy song.

12. *Enlist the support of companies and community organizations to provide additional motivations.* Discounts on insurances rates, free group exercise programs, and free clinics in which exercise-related problems can be discussed may be incentives to exercise.

CLINICAL APPLICATIONS

Hilda Willow is a 60-year-old married grandmother with mild hypertension (150/95). She is 5 feet 3 inches tall and weighs 160 pounds. She has no other medical problems. The primary care physician of the health department has referred Mrs. Willow to the community health nurse for guidance in a weight reduction and activity program.

The nurse finds during her assessment that Mrs. Willow is a homemaker who lives with her husband, Carl, who is a butcher in a local supermarket and is also moderately obese and hypertensive. They have three adult children—one in another state and two nearby. They frequently care for their two grandchildren, aged 2 and 4. The Willow home is a small, immaculate bungalow with flower boxes. Mrs. Willow welcomes the nurse and laments that she has been on a diet most of her life but continues to get "a little fatter every year." She is worried about her own and her husband's high blood pressure because her father had several strokes and was an invalid for 2 years before he died.

The nurse and Mrs. Willow discuss the kinds of foods Mrs. Willow eats, how she prepares them, and the milieu of the eating situation. They also discuss Mrs. Willow's activity. The nurse asks Mrs. Willow to keep a food intake and activity log for one week to discuss at the next visit.

The next week Mrs. Willow and the nurse review the diet and exercise log and discover that Mrs. Willow has very little physical activity, eats small amounts almost con-

tinuously during the day, and enjoys foods that are high in fat and salt. Mrs. Willow is quite surprised at these findings and indicates great interest in making changes in both her diet and exercise patterns. She says her husband wants to help and suggests they take walks each evening because it would be good for both of them.

With the baseline data of the diet/activity log, the nurse and Mr. and Mrs. Willow are able to plan and implement a program that helps them both lose weight and control their blood pressure without medication. Components of the program consist of the following (American College of Sports Medicine, 1986; Morgan, 1984; White, 1986).

Assessment

Information was obtained regarding when, where, why, and what cues or stimuli produced eating; what or who were reinforcers for the Willows; and how these reinforcers could be mobilized. They were willing to help each other and their daughter, the mother of the beloved grandchildren, was supportive. Environmental and financial supports and barriers were identified. The Willows have adequate food preparation and storage facilities and live in a clean, safe neighborhood. They have restricted income but are accustomed to watching how money is spent. Both read and write at high school level and have social and vocational skills. Both have a history of dieting with little success but have many health, function, and body image reasons for wanting to lose weight now.

Planning and Contracting

Three major tasks to be accomplished during this phase were (1) making a problem list and setting priorities in terms of easiest to accomplish to more difficult; (2) establishing contracts (weekly initially) that were mutually agreed upon, written, and specific; and (3) discussing the expectations of the Willows and the nurse. The nurse asked the Willows to keep records for self-monitoring. She visited weekly initially to monitor progress and assist with future planning. A typical one-week contract relating to diet called for Mrs. Willow to keep a record of foods eaten and the milieu for the week focusing on eliminating half of the between-meal snacks. According to the terms of the contract the nurse brought information on low-calorie, low-fat cooking methods and food seasonings to replace salt. A contract related to activity called for Mrs. Willow to walk for 15 minutes at a comfortable pace three times in the next week, to record when and where she walked and any thoughts, feelings, or questions she had to discuss with the nurse.

Involvement of the clients in developing plans and contracts is essential. Building of client self-esteem and self-confidence is an important objective of planning and intervention activities. During the process the nurse is teaching clients how to change and monitor their own life-style behaviors.

Intervention

During the intervention phase, the nurse gave the Willows information about nutrition and exercise programs and taught them how to learn new behaviors, how to problem solve, how to cope with relapses, and how to reinforce their healthful behavior. Specific topics included low-calorie cooking, choosing healthful, varied foods incorporating likes and dislikes, tips on stimulus control such as chewing gum or singing while cooking, eating only in the kitchen or dining room, recognizing eating and exercise patterns, and finding patterns that produced a 2-to 3-pound (1 kg) loss of weight per week. Exercise-related subjects were pulse taking and determination of activity to induce conditioning without discomfort, discussion of equipment (shoes, bicycles) relevant to desired activity, safety (weather, night activity, pollution, animals, carrying identification), timing (preferably before meals or at least 1 to 2 hours after meals), control of soreness by watching intensity and doing adequate warm-up and cool-down, companions and competitiveness, fluid intake in hot weather, and ideas for motivation and variety.

Evaluation

A variety of methods of evaluation were used, including nutrition and activity knowledge, activity levels and improvements, weight loss and body dimension changes, blood pressure levels, modifications of eating and activity patterns based on diet/activity logs, and abilities to problem solve and manage relapses.

Nurses helping clients with weight management and exercise programs influence them by modeling health behaviors. Modeling helps nurses bring behaviors to the attention of clients, shows them how to perform more healthy behaviors, and gives examples of the rewards of healthy lifestyles. Besides being a good model, nurses should develop knowledge of nutrition and exercise as well as skills in rapport, patience, flexibility, and awareness of the ways clients can be set up to succeed or fail. Nurses must not consider noncompliance as a reflection on their ability, but rather as an impetus for more creativity and teamwork with clients (White, 1986).

SUMMARY

This chapter has described current trends in promotion of health through nutrition and exercise. Health promotion involves collaboration by clients, nurses, physicians, nutritionists, exercise physiologists, and others. It is often community health nurses who first come into contact with individuals and groups in need of nutritional and exercise guidance. Nurses can play important roles by increasing awareness of benefits of and resources for nutrition and exercise, identifying risk factors, educating and motivating individuals and groups, and interpreting research findings. No diet plan or exercise prescription works for all people at all times, but through the use of the nursing process, nurses can assist people to develop personalized plans for health promotion.

KEY CONCEPTS

In industrialized societies, diet-related conditions are among the leading causes of disease and death. Many of these result from nutritional excesses rather than undernutrition.

Frequent and extended contact with clients in the community affords nurses excellent opportunities to provide information and counseling regarding the role of nutrition and diet in the promotion of health and prevention of illness.

Anticipatory guidance is an important aspect of care for clients.

What people eat is determined by a variety of factors, including biological needs, psychological variables, sociocultural influences, and environmental aspects such as price and availability.

The cultural and ethnic backgrounds of clients play a major role in food selection and eating behaviors. Recognition and respect for these food preferences are important for nurses counseling clients in the community.

Counseling regarding the nutritional value, deficiencies, and excesses of convenient and "fast food" menus is an important function of community health nurses.

Recommended Dietary Allowances (RDAs) are the levels of intake considered adequate to meet the known nutritional needs of practically all healthy persons.

Most meal planning and preparation occur in the home, so community health nurses have many opportunities to provide nutrition education when making home visits.

Through the nursing process community health nurses are able to detect and intervene in nutritional difficulties encountered by individuals, families, and groups in the community.

Nutritional assessment of an individual or group should include biological, psychological, cultural, and environmental factors.

Well-educated, affluent young adults have increased their level of exercise. Americans over 50, however, have limited awareness of the kinds and amounts of activity needed to maintain physical fitness, and there is a widespread belief that exercise may be dangerous.

The skill-related components of physical fitness are agility, balance, coordination, speed, power, and reaction time.

The health-related components of physical fitness are cardiorespiratory endurance, flexibility, body composition, muscular endurance, and muscular strength.

Exercise has both physiological and psychological benefits. Both should be considered during nursing assessment, planning, implementation, and evaluation.

The work site is an ideal place to increase physical activity because a large percentage of the population is employed and spends approximately one third of the day at work.

LEARNING ACTIVITIES

1. Keep a food diary for one week. Record the types and amounts of foods, time, eating situation, and personal thoughts and feelings while eating. Analyze the diary for nutritional adequacy. How does your diet compare with the RDAs for your age and sex, the 4 food groups, and the dietary guidelines for Americans? Where could improvements be made? How will you motivate yourself to eat better?

2. Select two cultures and compare their diets. What similarities can be seen? Identify factors influencing food selection in both cultures. What changes might be recommended to improve nutritional adequacy?

3. Keep an activity log for one week. Analyze your activity and determine how you might get the recommended amount of exercise. Plan an exercise program for yourself and get started!

4. Select an article regarding nutrition or exercise in a current lay publication and analyze the information provided and how it might be understood by people with little background in nutrition or exercise.

6. Design an individualized exercise program for a friend or relative including motivational aspects.

7. Survey local business and industries to discover what health promotion programs are available and how they are used.

BIBLIOGRAPHY

American College of Sports Medicine: Guidelines for exercise testing and prescription, ed. 3, Philadelphia, 1986, Lea & Febiger.

Blomquist, K.B.: Physical fitness programs in industry: applications of social learning theory, Occup. Health Nurs. 29(7):30-33, 1981.

Blomquist, K.B.: Modeling and health behavior: strategies for prevention in the schools, Health Educ. 17(3):8-10, 1986.

Caspersen, C.J., Powell, K.E., and Christenson, G.M.: Physical activity, exercise, and physical fitness: definitions and distinctions for health-related research, Public Health Rep. 100:126-131, 1985.

Dishman, R.K.: Medical psychology in exercise and sport, Med. Clin. North Am. 69:123-143, 1985.

Dishman, R.K., Sallis, J.F., and Orenstein, D.R.: The determinants of physical activity and exercise, Public Health Rep. 100:158-171, 1985.

Estok, P.J., and Rudy, E.B.: Jogging: Cardiovascular benefits and risks, Nurse Pract. 11(5):21-27, 1986.

Fielding, J.E.: Health promotion and disease prevention at the worksite, Ann. Rev. Public Health 5:237-265, 1984.

Fixx, J.: Jim Fixx's second book of running, New York, 1980, Random House.

Gaesser, G.A., and Rich, R.G.: Effects of high- and low-intensity exercise training on aerobic capacity and blood lipids, Med. Sci. Sports Exerc. 16:269-274, 1984.

Haskell, W.L.: Physical activity and health: need to define the required stimulus, Am. J. Cardiol. 55:4D-9D, 1985.

Havas, S., and Walker, B.: Massachusetts' approach to the prevention of heart disease, cancer, and stroke, Public Health Rep. 101:29-39, 1986.

Iverson, D.C., Fielding, J.E., Crow, R.S., and Christenson, G.M.: The promotion of physical activity in the United States population: the status of programs in medical, worksite, community, and school settings, Public Health Rep. 100:212-224, 1985.

Jensen, T.G., Englert, D., and Dudrick, S.J.: Nutritional assessment: a manual for practitioners, Norwalk, CT, 1983, Appleton-Century-Crofts.

Martin, J.E., and Dubbert, P.M.: Adherence to exercise, Exerc. Sport Sci. Rev. 13:137-167, 1985.

Morgan, J.: Behavioral treatment of obesity: the occupational health nurse's role, Occup. Health Nurs. 32:312-314, 1984.

Nestle, M.: Nutrition in clinical practice, Greenbrae, CA, 1985, Jones Medical Publications.

Pender, N.: Health promotion in nursing practice, ed. 2, Norwalk, Conn., 1987, Appleton & Lange.

Poleman, C.M., and Capra, C.L.: Shackelton's nutrition essentials and diet therapy, ed. 5, Philadelphia, 1984, W.B. Saunders.

Powell, K.E., and Paffenbarger, R.S.: Workshop on epidemiologic and public health aspects of physical activity and exercise: a summary, Public Health Rep. 100:118-126, 1985.

Powell, K.E., Spain, K.G., Christenson, G.M., and Mollenkamp, M.P.: The status of the 1990 objectives for physical fitness and exercise, Public Health Rep. 101:15-21, 1986.

President's Council on Physical Fitness and Sports: Physical fitness research digest, Series 1, No. 1. Washington, D.C., 1971.

President's Council on Physical Fitness and Sports: An introduction to physical fitness, DHEW Pub. No. (OS) 79-50068, Washington, D.C., 1980, Government Printing Office.

Shephard, R.J.: Physical activity and the healthy mind, Can. Med. Assoc. J. 128:552-530, 1983.

Shephard, R.J.: Factors influencing the exercise behavior of patients, Sports Med. 2:348-366, 1985.

Siscovick, D.S., LaPorte, R.E., and Newman, J.M.: The disease-specific benefits and risks of physical activity and exercise, Public Health Rep. 100:180-188, 1985.

Taylor, C.B., Sallis, J.F., and Needle, R.: The relation of physical activity and exercise to mental health, Public Health Rep. 100:195-202, 1985.

Tufts University: Your nutrient needs: the facts behind the numbers, Tufts University Diet and Nutrition Letter 4(2, April):3-6, 1986.

U.S. Department of Agriculture, and U.S. Department of Health and Human Services: Nutrition and your health: dietary guidelines for Americans, Home and Garden Bulletin No. 232, 1980.

U.S. Public Health Service: Prevention 84-85, Washington, D.C., 1985, Government Printing Office.

White, J.H.: Behavioral intervention for the obese client, Nurse Pract. 11(1):27-34, 1986.

Williams, S.R.: Mowry's basic nutrition and diet therapy, ed 7, St. Louis, 1984, The C.V. Mosby Co.

Wilson, C.S.: Nutritionally beneficial cultural practices, World Rev. Nutr. Diet. 45:68-96, 1985.

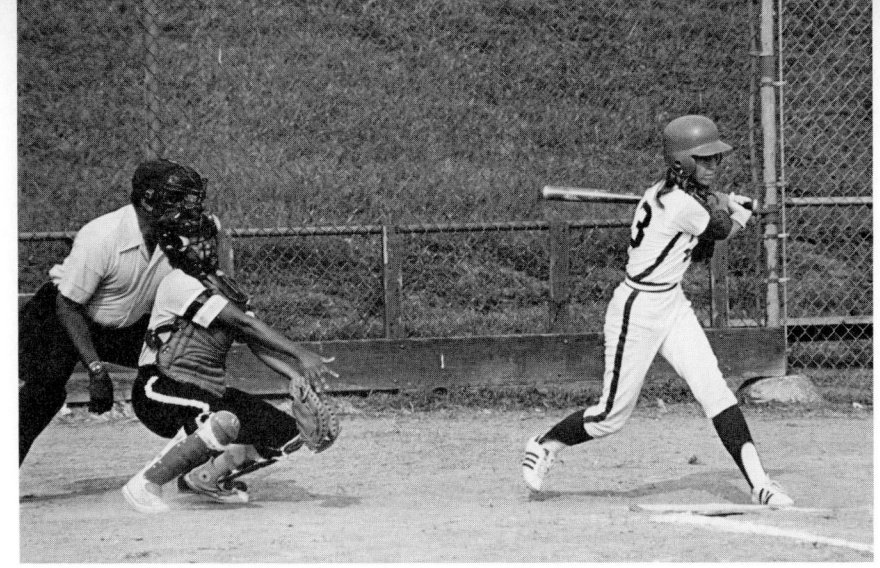

Marjorie Keller

29

LEISURE AND RECREATION

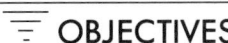

OBJECTIVES

After reading this chapter, the student should be able to:

Recognize the interrelationship between health and use of leisure time and recreational activities and patterns.

Distinguish between the terms *leisure, recreation,* and *play.*

Identify the four dimensions of leisure applicable to the role of the community health nurse.

Describe contemporary societal changes and trends leading to increased leisure time.

Identify and describe concepts and theories relevant to health and leisure/recreation from the biological, psychological, and social sciences.

Analyze leisure/recreational needs of two specific age groups.

Describe and implement a role for the community health nurse in leisure/recreation.

KEY TERMS

biological health
caretakers
catalyst
compensation theory
individual activities
joint activities

leisure
neutrality theory
outreach
parallel activities
play
psychological health

recreation
retirees
social health
spillover theory
triad of work-family-leisure

In recent years the relationship between health and social problems and the ability to use leisure time effectively has been described. However, many Americans are unable to use leisure time in a positive way and participate in meaningful recreational activities. One way to promote the health of our clients is to assist them to learn to use leisure and recreation in a constructive manner. The relationship between health status and the effective use of leisure and recreation is in a developing stage. This chapter discusses relevant leisure/recreation literature and suggests ways in which the community health nurse can apply this information. An assessment inventory, "Personal Inventory Tool" is in Appendix A6. This tool helps people to assess their philosophy, attitude, and practices in relation to leisure and recreation.

LEISURE AND RECREATION: IMPORTANCE FOR COMMUNITY HEALTH NURSES

The field of leisure and recreation is a relatively new discipline. Historically, nurses have included *diversion* for the sick as a nursing function. As nursing care has moved from treating primarily sick people to both caring for sick people and assisting healthy people attain a higher level of health, the use of diversionary activities has been lost. In recent years the roles of recreational therapists, health educators, and fitness experts have expanded. This development emphasizes two issues: first, with recreational therapists gravitating toward institutional settings, what disciplines should be addressing leisure/recreation in the community? and second, should contemporary thinking about leisure and recreation be broader and more inclusive than physical education and physical fitness?

Community health nurses practice in situations in which leisure/recreational needs of individuals and families can be assessed and planning can be initiated to meet needs. With the current emphasis in nursing on health and wellness, community health nurses must look at the deficits present in communities that can be resolved and pay increased attention to the development of leisure skills and increased recreational facilities. Opportunities must be created for people to express themselves creatively without undue constraints.

Berkman and Breslow (1983) demonstrated that leisure and recreational patterns have a direct link to mortality risks. Hence, the community health nurse has a responsibility to help individuals to develop and maintain leisure/recreational habits.

DEFINITIONS
Leisure

Neulinger (1981) describes the term *to leisure:* ". . . to be engaged in an activity performed for its own sake, freely and without pressure or coercion; . . . doing something from which one derives meaning and satisfaction, and which involves one to the very core of one's being." Neulinger introduces the elements of lack of extrinsic control, gratification, and depth of commitment to the traditional concept of leisure time as time away from work or other responsibilities that may or may not be filled with activity. According to Godbey (1985), *leisure* has four dimensions: (1) *time,* which is spent voluntarily in a desired way, (2) *activity,* that which a person does during leisure, including hobbies, sports, watching television, reading, or just relaxing, (3) *state of existence,* a sense of being that incorporates a commitment to the current activity, and (4) *state of mind,* perceived freedom to do as one chooses.

Recreation

Recreation has been defined as "activity indulged in voluntarily for the satisfaction derived from the activity itself and leading to revitalization or re-creation, of mind, body, or spirit" (Goodale and Witt, 1980, p. 25). The phrase "revitalization or re-creation" is an element that separates leisure from recreation.

Recreation is in general how leisure time is used by an individual. Recreation can take a myriad of forms: active or passive participation; alone or with others. One of the most popular recreational activities is sports, as a participant or as a spectator. Hobbies, bicycling, watching television, attending social functions, and travel or camping are well-accepted forms of recreation. A key factor in determining if an activity is recreational is if the activity provides opportunity for revitalization (and meaning) to the person. The essence of recreation is lost if the activity is inflicted or is perceived as a duty or responsibility.

The current emphasis on physical fitness has become confused with ability to recreate. Joining spas and exercise programs with a focus on fitness, albeit the physical and psychological benefits, may be restricting some individuals in recognizing and developing a variety of recreational pursuits. Considering the work-rest-recreation balance the average person has a limited amount of time available for leisure. Should that time be limited to physical fitness?

Furthermore, not all socioeconomic groups participate in fitness programs. Participants are primarily middle- and upper-income white-collar workers and professionals. Blue-collar workers and lower income groups apparently do not feel free to participate or wish to participate or do not have the money to spare.

Play

Ellis (1973, p. 2) defines *play* as "the behavior emitted by an individual not motivated by the end product of the behavior." This definition, according to Ellis, implies that play must be uncontrolled and unplanned. Play activity is generally pleasurable, intrinsically motivated, spontaneous and voluntary, non-productive, and not essential for survival (Garvey, cited in Kalyan-Masih, 1979). Children are expected to play, in fact, permitted and encouraged to play. Adults are discouraged from unproductive and perhaps spontaneous expression of one's self through playfulness.

Kalyan-Masih (1979) summarizes five proposed theories of play: surplus energy, relaxation, preexercise, recapitulation, and psychoanalytic. The first two theories concern the availability and replenishing of energy. Preexercise theory is based on skill development; and recapitulation and psychoanalytic theories reflect the influence of past experiences.

Barnett and Kane (1985) found that children are influenced primarily by parents in their choice of play activities. (Ability to play and the selection of play activities may be encouraged or discouraged by parental interest and concern.) Peers have a positive influence on participation in games and other forms of play for both children and adults.

Play provides an opportunity for children to develop physical coordination and to learn socialization skills, sharing, competing, cooperating, and communicating with others. The ability to form and maintain friendships begins with play in childhood.

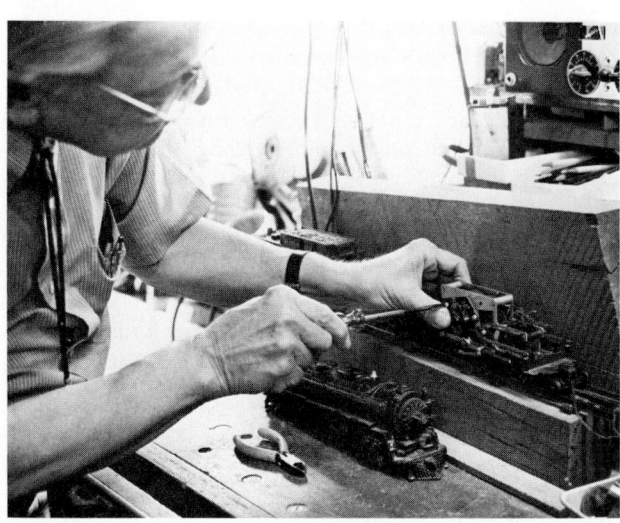

The environment, the family, the peer group, and educational system contribute to shaping play behavior (Barnett and Kane, 1985). The availability of toys can influence imagination in play activities. Toys may be a constraint to developing play behaviors in that they may prescribe the child's activity and minimize the need for creativity. Everyone has observed children playing with an empty carton in the most imaginative ways possible!

SOCIETAL CHANGES CREATING INCREASED LEISURE TIME AND ACTIVITIES

Hayes, Brightwell, and Antozzi (1984, p. 43) suggest that we are living in an "age of leisure rivaled only by the early Greek civilization." In addition, Murphy (1981) reports a number of contemporary societal changes and trends that create increased leisure time and demand for desired activities. These changes and trends are described below.

An actual increase in discretionary time. Employee work hours have become more flexible and in some instances have been reduced in recent years. In addition to reduction in work time, some employers permit flexibility of working hours. Concurrently, the time devoted to care of the home has been lessened by using appliances and convenience foods. The multitude of relatively inexpensive fast-food restaurants has promoted eating outside the home. Furthermore, more individuals are self-employed, unemployed, and retired. Gault (1983) indicates that the potential amount of time for leisure in a year is 4 months. The 4 months are made up of 9 holidays, 52 weekends, and at least 10 vacation days.

A higher level of education. Studies (Murphy, 1981) have demonstrated that levels of education and leisure participation are highly correlated. Higher levels of education generally give rise to broader interests and higher incomes, thereby encouraging and permitting recreational pursuits.

An increasing affluence. Despite inflation, a rising and falling stock market, and high unemployment rates, level of income is increasing although spendable income may be decreasing. The median income for 1983 was reported as $25,757 for whites and $15,887 for blacks and other minorities. Godbey (1985) reports that, according to the U.S. Department of Commerce, over $310 billion is now spent for recreational goods and services yearly. Kraus (1971) identifies nine categories of leisure spending: popular sports, outdoor recreation (e.g., boating, hunting, fishing, camping), travel, commercial entertainment, cultural activities, gambling, television, technological-type activities (e.g., electronic games, ice rinks), and various hobbies.

A changed attitude toward leisure/recreation. With the lessening belief in the traditional American work ethic, which valued hard work and long hours and discounted the value of leisure time, a balance is developing between value of work and value of leisure. Individuals now feel more free to participate in leisure activities. Furthermore, churches are developing recreational activities as part of their spiritual programs. Emphasis is on striving for joy and self-fulfillment, as evidenced by the success of the holistic health movement.

Continued population mobility. Transportation systems, automobiles, and recreational vehicles are easing travel. Tourism has become a major industry. Parks, campgrounds, and amusement complexes provide recreational opportunities for millions of visitors yearly.

Expectations of various groups. There is greater acceptance of ethnic, economic, gender-related, age-related, and handicapped groups in society. Recognition of their needs has created new and expanded opportunities for participation in activities. Various clubs and groups have formed, such as Loners on Wheels, Elderhostels, Special Olympics, and handicapped sports teams.

Despite this trend, single women and single men experience covert discrimination in society. Rural areas, towns, and small cities are usually couple- and family-oriented where leisure and recreation are concerned. The unaccompanied person may be unwelcome at various functions, may be perceived as a threat, and may be considered and treated as an extra or an outsider.

RELATIONSHIP BETWEEN WORK AND LEISURE

The relationship between work and leisure is basic in terms of which has priority and the degree of separation or merging of work and leisure (Godbey, 1985). There are three theories regarding this relationship: spillover, compensatory, and neutrality (Mannell and Iso-Ahola, 1985).

In 1960 Wilansky (Mannell and Iso-Ahola, 1985) suggested in the *spillover theory* that leisure was an extension of work habits, attitudes, and interests. Leisure activities were similar to work activities. For example, many nurses pursue health-related or nursing-related activities during leisure time, such as working at home during nonworking hours or spending vacation days at a meeting or conference. Moreover, friendships may be primarily with other nurses.

Wilansky also suggested that leisure and work may have opposing characteristics; this is termed the *compensatory theory.* For example, the person with the demanding, high-involvement job may choose quiet, relatively isolated leisure activities, or vice versa.

Parker (Mannell and Iso-Ahola, 1985) proposed the *neutrality theory* in 1971 by suggesting that work and leisure may be totally separate and unrelated entities. An example of neutrality is the nurse who skis, hikes, plays cards, or dances.

CULTURE AS A SHAPER OF LEISURE

Beliefs, traditions, and values are major forces influencing the use of leisure time and the selection of recreational activities. Related factors include emphasis on play; centrality of the family; availability of time, activities, facilities, and money; and geographic location (urban or rural), climate and terrain.

Hantrais, Clark, and Samuel (1984) described political policy and attitudes toward the work-leisure relationship from the viewpoint of the work pole thesis, originally set forth by Marx in 1867 in *Das Kapital*. This thesis suggests that in the *triad of work-family-leisure* a powerful and controlling relationship exists between the work setting and the family. "Employers and technocrats are the major agents in structuring the time aspects of work, the family and free time . . . in appropriating blocks of time . . . in generating certain forms of time discipline [directly affecting]

the temporal and spatial patterning of . . . non work life" (p. 302).

Festivals and celebrations also shape leisure. The spacing and manner in which a society celebrates holidays and festivals create leisure patterns and activities. For example, Thanksgiving Day, Halloween, and Valentine's Day have traditional activities associated with them. Celebration of holidays such as Christmas and Hanukkah may differ from society to society. Most states have local festivals that are leisure activities. These festivals may be all-town activities creating opportunities for social contacts and expression of individual abilities and creativity. For instance, in Indiana, about 170 festivals are celebrated yearly, ranging from the Persimmon Festival to the Talbot Street Art Fair to the Covered Bridge Festival.

LEISURE AS A SHAPER OF CULTURE

Leisure activities developed by a population can affect culture. The use of alcohol, drugs, and sexual activity for recreation have a profound influence on life-style and health status. Newspapers, popular periodicals, and relevant statistical reports confirm the effect, not only on the culture but also on the health of individuals and stability of families. A city of about 250,000 was recently reported as having forty-two Alcoholic-Anonymous groups in operation. Another city of about 100,000 in a relatively isolated part of the United States listed twelve treatment sites for drug and alcohol addiction in their telephone directory. Larger metropolitan areas list far more treatment facilities.

The availability and use of money may shape a culture by affecting the type of goods and services that are purchased. For example, boating equipment, home video equipment, and tickets for cultural or sporting events are indicators of priorities set by society. Commercialism and the impact of mass media influence interests, which in turn shape culture.

Sporting events such as baseball, football, and auto racing are particularly influential. The Indianapolis 500 is a major influence for many people during the month of May, creating a sense of excitement and festivity. In contemporary society sports have importance for people of all ages. The availability of televised games provide leisure activities for millions of Americans.

The level of creativity associated with leisure also affects a culture. Amateur plays, off-Broadway presentations, musical offerings, art, crafts, and other creative endeavors serve as mechanisms for conveying cultural beliefs from one generation to another.

LEISURE AND RECREATION CONCEPTS SPECIFIC TO COMMUNITY HEALTH NURSING
Health and Wellness

Leisure and recreation contribute to three major health components of an individual: biological, psychological, and social. Leisure and recreation can have both positive and negative effects on one's health.

Biological Health

The leisure activities most frequently associated with one's *biological health* are athletics, sports participation and ex-

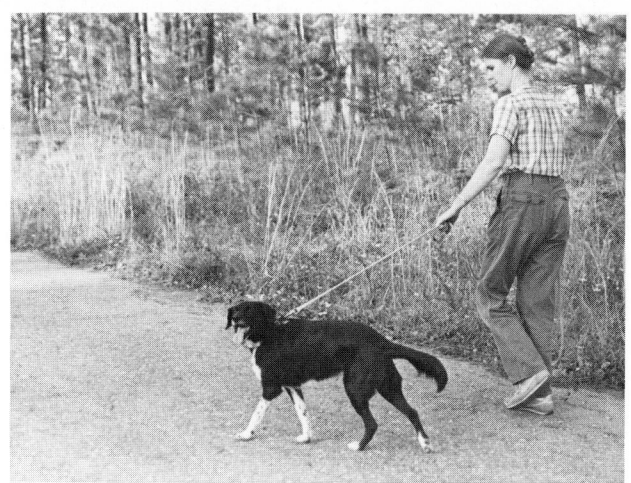

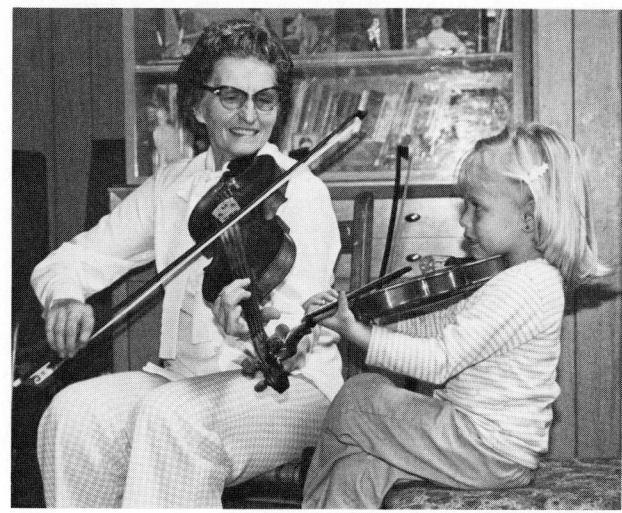

ercise. Muscular and cardiovascular development is an obvious result. The speciality of physical fitness is developing around these factors. Unfortunately, to some extent, physical fitness is being equated with recreation. Recreation is far more encompassing than jogging, aerobics, and other activities leading to physical fitness. There is evidence, however, that much satisfaction can be obtained from jogging. A study by Levenson, Thornby, and Levenson (1985) of 298 joggers in an urban university revealed that the participants jogged for three reasons: emotional and physical benefits, support from others, and potential for increased attractiveness and improved appearance. Obstacles to jogging fell into four categories: lack of information and skill, fear of consequences, geographical or climatic barriers, and attitudinal barriers.

One's eating habits, both nutritional intake and eating practices, are a leisure activity as well as a requirement for good health. Availability of food, the types of restaurants frequented, economic resources, and patterns of eating habits affect the quality of this leisure activity.

Psychological Health

Leisure and recreation can influence *psychological health* because the potential stimulation and development of interests during leisure contribute to the quality of life. It is difficult to separate the interdependent physical and psychological factors; athletics and exercise directly affect emotional status, as does the satisfaction derived from successful completion of a handicraft, reading a good book, or playing music.

Dowd (1984) identified nine functions of leisure that can positively affect mental health. These functions are described in the following paragraphs.

Promotes one's own identification. Leisure activities offer the opportunity to develop an interest, skill, or value unlike one's occupational pursuits.

Provides increased autonomy. Leisure activity can provide the means for establishing independence, self-determination, and self-expression in a society that increasingly values conformity more than individuality.

Provides mastery experiences. Leisure activity can provide opportunity for increasing one's perceived competency.

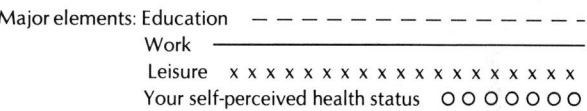

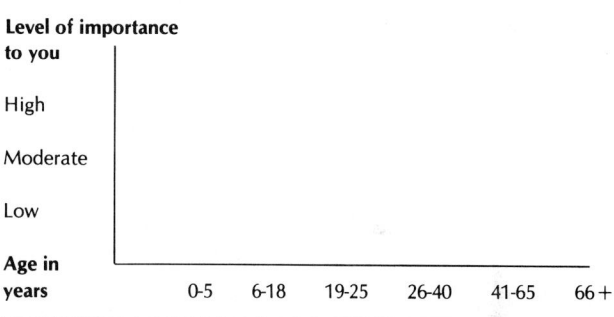

FIGURE 29-1

Analysis of major elements in life-style balance. Plot how you perceive your current life-style balance. Repeat the process by considering how you would prefer your life-style balance. What needs to be changed and what is needed to accomplish the change?

Provides increasing sense of freedom. The opportunity for self-expression is available for internally controlled persons; externally controlled persons may find their niche for self-expression in leisure activities.

Provides spontaneous commitment and involvement. Leisure activities provide opportunities for play and commitment to satisfying activities that are unplanned, unstructured, and just plain fun.

Promotes a sense of community and social network. A sense of belonging can result by establishing a circle of friends and acquaintances. Newcomers to a community are particularly appreciative of efforts by a community to help them fit in and feel welcome.

Promotes balance in life. Three triads involve leisure and recreation as a factor: work-rest-recreation, work-family-leisure, and work-education-leisure. (See Figure 29-1 for a tool to measure three elements in life-style balance, work-education-leisure in relation to one's health.) Although no hard-and-fast rules control these balances, societal norms determine work hours, thereby providing an external control to be considered.

Promotes creativity and self-expression. Through leisure activities, individuals have the chance to develop their own uniqueness, special abilities and interests, with the expectation to moving toward self-actualization.

Provides personal meaning to life. Search for meaning in life is a developmental task of adulthood. Considering approaches compensatory, spillover, and neutrality approaches to leisure discussed previously, leisure activities provide opportunities to pursue interests for satisfaction and meaning in life (p. 580).

Social Health

Social networks are links of personal contacts established by an individual for the purposes of communication, influence, support, understanding, and prestige (Maguire, 1983). Leisure and recreational activities serve as a means for socialization, forming friendships, making acquaintances and contacts, and developing interpersonal skills. These activities can introduce people with similar and diverse backgrounds. Generally a mutual interest is present with each link, such as a hobby; an interest in theater, music, or art; a sport; or membership in a group.

The Alameda County Study (Berkman and Breslow, 1983) included data pertaining to social networks and mortality. In this comprehensive epidemiological study, the review of literature about the relationship of health and social networks was mixed: "data published so far do not show whether the quality of relationship is more significant [in health] than the quantity of contacts, whether intimate ties are more related [to health] than extended ones, or whether cumulative effects [on health] occur with increasing isolation" (p. 121). The study demonstrated that the risk of mortality was lower for people who are married, have contact with close friends and relatives, are members of a church, and are associated with nonchurch groups. The ties of marriage and contact with close friends and relatives were the strongest predictors of low mortality risk.

History-Taking Tools

History-taking questions are presented for use by the community health nurse in Appendix A7. Recognition of preferred types of recreation can guide identification of health teaching needs. Furthermore, responses to the items regarding involvement with other people can suggest (1) counseling needs relative to forming friendships, establishing networks, demonstrating personal growth through independence; (2) opportunity for assessing social networks for categories of acquaintances; and (3) referral or guidance to presently unknown facilities or resources in the community. School or occupational health nurses can use the information gathering in the client history to provide nursing care to children and employees.

Specific Implications for Nursing

Nurses in school and industry can influence attitudes toward exercise and eating habits. School nurses can also assist in the development of life-long leisure and recreational patterns for the children. Nurses can influence administrators and parent-teacher groups in the areas of policy and resource development to broaden the leisure options available to children as well as in attitudes toward accident prevention during recreational activities. School nurses on city-town planning groups can influence the creation and expansion of parks and other recreational resources.

Occupational health nurses are in an ideal position to assist employees and their families to develop and expand their interests and uses of leisure time. Each employee-nurse encounter offers the opportunity to inquire in subtle ways about how leisure time is spent. As the nurse tours a plant, casual but meaningful inquiries can be made about various holiday and vacation plans, how the weekend was spent, interests and participation in groups, and involvement in sports.

Prevention

Although community health nurses are well-informed about disease prevention, the relationship between prevention and leisure and recreation warrants exploration. In the past recreational activity has been perceived as a diversionary activity when an illness or disability is already present. Shamansky and Clausen (1980) in their effort to clarify prevention and its levels, suggest that contemporary nursing practice calls for greater emphasis on primary prevention. The terms *health promotion* and *disease prevention* are used liberally in the mass media, by the public, and by health professionals to describe reduction in the potential for illness. The health practices most frequently identified for change are nutrition, physical fitness, and stress reduction. The selection of appropriate leisure and recreational activities can also contribute to the prevention of physical, emotional, and social problems.

Situations observed by the community health nurse that could be changed with leisure intervention strategies include:

The middle-aged overweight man, apparently content to watch television for hours while eating potato chips and drinking beer

The school-age latch-key child who may lack coping skills for managing alone or is under the influence of adolescents in the neighborhood

The teen-ager who has few interests and social skills and is bored and starved for affection

The elderly woman who sits and looks out of the window; the elderly man who walks to the mailbox five times a day

The youth who has found "friendship" with gangs, drug and alcohol users, crime-prone contemporaries

A mother with little hope and with several children to raise alone

The single man or woman who has sufficient financial resources yet sits home alone night after night, "waiting for something to happen"

These are common situations found in every neighborhood.

The Family as a Unit

Family recreational patterns affect the health of the family as well as each member. Today confusion surrounds the "American family" in terms of composition, roles, group identity, and commitment to the purpose of a family. Chilman (1979 p. 19) states that we are in "a time in which virtually no family can be self-sufficient, a time in which virtually no family is immune from the world situations and resultant ideologies which invade each home in both benign and damaging ways." Not only do community health nurses need to assess internal dynamics of a family, but in contemporary society, the direct and indirect impact of events and conditions nationally and internationally must be considered. The interrelationship between countries cannot be underestimated. Individuals and families from countries in which tensions exist with the United States or which are hostile to the United States may need assistance in meeting leisure and recreational needs in safe, stress-free environments.

In contrast to the commonly observed symptoms of family instability, Stinnett (1979) reports six qualities of strong families: (1) appreciation of each family member, (2) members spend time together, (3) demonstration of good communication patterns, (4) hold commitment for each person's happiness and welfare, (5) hold a high degree of religious orientation, and (6) have the ability to solve problems in times of crises. Furthermore, Otto (1979), in his Family Strength Survey, identifies 36 family strengths for assessment, of which 10 qualities are directly related to leisure and recreation. These qualities are having adequate time together, common interests, mutual support, a good circle of friends, having fun together, a good sense of humor, good food available, encouragement of each other's talents, family traditions and celebrations, freedom to grow as individuals, and fostering creativity in each other. The remaining 25 qualities are generally indirectly related to use of leisure time. Witt and Goodale (1985 p. 227) believe

that satisfying leisure patterns are "important as a means of communication and interaction and as a contributor to individual growth and overall family stability." They conclude that leisure is "an end in itself (by providing fun, enjoyment, and satisfaction) and is a means for achieving a strong, healthy family."

Biological, psychological, and social factors affecting individual and family leisure patterns are affected by developmental stage. Figure 29-2 displays these factors. Furthermore, individual developmental stages influence major group affiliation, leisure and recreational interests, and potential contribution of the community health nurse. These influences are found in Table 29-1.

Orthner (Kando, 1980) suggests that leisure activities fall into three categories: *individual activities, joint activities,* and *parallel activities.* Translated into a family focus, opportunity should be available for members to pursue activities alone, such as a hobby or sport; for considerable interaction, such as playing a game, traveling, picnicing; and for minimal interaction, such as watching television, making a puzzle or gardening.

Witt and Goodale (1985) sought to identify barriers to leisure and recreation at particular family stages based on the age of the youngest child through age 18. The researchers report nine statistically significant barriers parents experience when the children are between the ages of 6 and 18: (1) lack skill in use of resources, (2) lack of knowledge of resources, (3) uncertainty about choice of involvement, (4) lack of companionship, (5) difficulty in planning and decision-making, (6) being ill at ease in social situations, (7) difficulty in carrying out plans, (8) lack of free time, and (9) too many family obligations. Another group of barriers that influence family recreation patterns were lim-

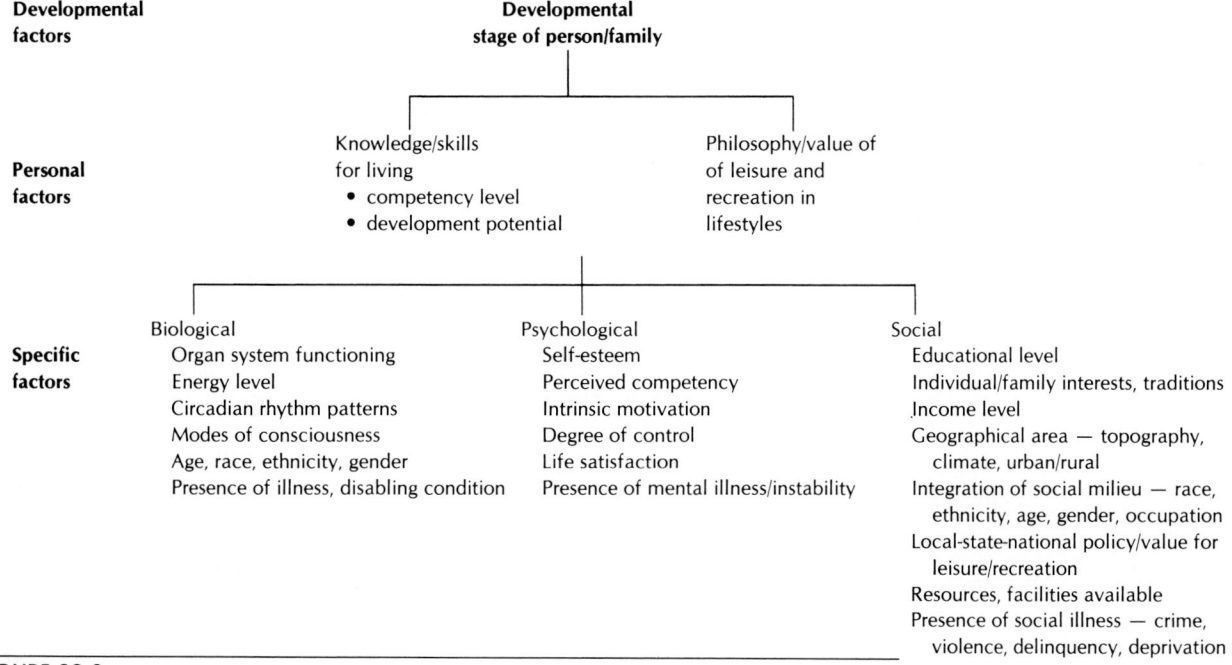

FIGURE 29-2

Personal and family factors affecting leisure patterns.

TABLE 29-1

Implications of individual developmental stage in regard to leisure and recreation

Age	Major group affiliation	Leisure and recreation implications	Contribution of community health nurse
0-1	Family: parents grandparents	Respite for family Socialization with grandparents	Parenting classes; well-baby clinics Pediatrician or family practitioner office
1-4	Family Peers (end of age range)	Play skills Imagination skills Socialization skills Respite for family	Parenting classes Well-child clinics Nursery schools Physicians' offices
4-6	Family Peers	Continue skills above Creating interests and social pattern habits Increased independence Learn give-and-take	Nursery school Kindergarten Special interest groups Information regarding "touch-me-not"
6-12	Family Peers School Church Social groups such as scouts and little league	Increased play skills Increased socialization skills Learn healthy competition Interest in sports as participant and spectator (influenced by region of country) Hobbies Develop special interests, such as music, sewing, hunting, fishing	School health Parent-Teacher organizations Special groups, re development of health habits Information regarding "touch-me-not"

12-15	Peers
	School
	Family
	Church
	Social groups
		Male-female relationships/dating
		Continue socialization skills
		Continue interest in sports, hobbies, special interests
		Joining clubs at school, youth groups at church, in community
		Contemporary music
		Shopping—clothes
		Telephoning
		Visiting friends
		Travel
		Computers
			School health
			  Personal hygiene
			  Sexual development
			  Interpersonal relationships
			  Counseling regarding developing interests, joining groups
			  Problems associated with use of drugs, alcohol, sexual activity
			Speaker at groups regarding developing leisure and recreation interests, nutrition, physical fitness, self-responsibility for health

15-18	(Same as above)	Male-female relationships Proms/parties Automobiles Clothes for girls Sports Travel	(Same as above)
18-21	Work group School faculty Peers Military Family	Social groups, i.e., sororities, fraternities Sports, parties Refining IPR skills, socialization	(Same as above) Occupational health nurse College health nurse Health departments, centers
21-25	Family Peers Work group	Development of family recreational interests Sports, parties, visiting, travel, hobbies	Promotion of family recreational interests Encourage physical activity for fitness Nutrition Self-responsibility for health Child-rearing practices to encourage socialization of children (see ages 0-1, 1-4)
25-35	Family Peers Work group Young people	(Same as above)	(Same as above) (See ages 0-1, 1-4, 4-6, 6-12)

NOTE: Contributions to this chart were made by the community health nursing graduate students, University of Southern Mississippi. After considerable discussion, the age groupings were identified based on observations and personal experiences of the students and faculty member.

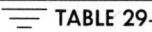

TABLE 29-1

Implications of individual developmental stage in regard to leisure and recreation—cont'd

Age	Major group affiliation	Leisure and recreation implications	Contribution of community health nurse
35-55	Family Peers Work group Young people	Development of personal or spouse's recreational interests Sports (increased spectator role), visiting, travel, hobbies, parties, social clubs	(Same as above) (See ages 4-6, 6-12, 12-15, 15-18, 18-21)
55-65	Peers Family Work group	(Same as above) Eating out	(Same as above) (See ages 21-25, 25-35)
65+	Peers Family	Development of personal or spouse's leisure and recreational interests Sports (spectator role), visiting, travel, hobbies, social clubs	(Same as above) Retirement counseling Respite in caretaking role Interests and activities in declining years, illness Counseling after death of spouse regarding return to activities

itations from the expectations of others on them, too much stress, and lack of motivation.

Aggregates

Williams (in Chapter 15) advocates a community health nursing role that involves primarily groups, or aggregates, as the client. The approach calls for defining group problems and proposing resolutions to those problems at a group level.

Community health nurses have access to groups in a community not generally accessible to recreational therapists, access which offers opportunities for population-focused practice in the use of leisure time and development of recreational activities. A community health nurse can make a significant contribution to community recreation activities as a member of or consultant to the local, county, or state planning groups for recreation. The community health nurse brings knowledge of community strengths and weaknesses, family needs, individual and group health status, and knowledge of normal individual and family developmental stages. Nurses are also aware of special population groups, such as physically or mentally handicapped and disabled people. Other groups in a community that would be responsive to *input* from the community health nurse are schools, industries, and various social agencies and groups, such as Scouts, YMCA/YWCA, Salvation Army, Boy's and Girl's Clubs, and community centers. The Clinical Application section provides a framework using the nursing process for the nurse to use in working with groups.

Two population groups have been selected for particular attention to leisure and recreation needs: adolescents and elderly people. With teenage pregnancy identified as a major community health problem and the projected increase in elderly persons, specific needs of these groups will be considered.

ADOLESCENTS. The characteristics of the adolescent developmental stage have been well documented by Erikson and Havighurst among others. Duvall (1977) has identified tasks of a family with an adolescent. The implications for these tasks in developing and maintaining leisure and recreational interests and activities is being associated with the problem of teenage pregnancy. A community health nurse can influence the health of adolescents and families by applying concepts associated with leisure and recreation, especially prevention, family, and health and wellness.

In the prevention of teenage pregnancy, efforts must be directed at both young women and young men. Although a number of factors influence the sexual habits of adolescents, a crucial question is "what recreational activities are available for them at an affordable cost?" In rural areas the question "what recreational activities are available?" is of particular importance. Recreational activities and facilities are more readily available in urban areas through parks and recreation departments as well as through voluntary agencies. Rural areas may have few activities, thereby inadvertently promoting sexual experimentation as a result of boredom and lack of interesting alternatives. Adolescents need opportunities to develop self-esteem, decision making, and social skills. They may lack goals and have limited hope for the future.

Efforts to prevent teenage pregnancy have focused on birth control measures, thereby minimizing the attention devoted to primary prevention. Questions to be raised include: Are adolescents using sexual activity as a form of entertainment when limited or no recreational activities are available, such as music and dance, sports, special interest groups, and clubs? What opportunities are available for expanding horizons, learning new skills, and developing varied interests? Dumazedier in 1974 (Klieber and Rickards, 1985) identified three purposes of recreation particularly relevant to adolescents: relaxation, stimulation, and self-development.

The community health nursing role can include participation in the development and maintenance of recreational opportunities that provide relaxing and stimulating pastimes for adolescents. Drop-in, community, and multi-service centers afford adolescents easily accessible sites for developing various skills, especially if the centers are located adjacent to schools. School-based clinics can assist adolescents to develop goals directed toward involvement in recreational activities as well as development of self-esteem and decision-making skills. Leisure activities, such as hobbies, sewing, fashion-modeling, artistic skills, dancing, leadership skills, interest in environment and nature, gardening, home decoration, and sports can be a vehicle for enhancing self-esteem and decision-making skills.

The community health nurse can offer regularly scheduled health education and counseling in centers. By direct involvement in the center programs the nurse can become acquainted with the adolescents and use the contacts to identify their recreational interests and potential leadership skills. Adolescents can be given the opportunity to assist in program planning, development, and evaluation. Including active, involved, and interested parents in the program development can be an effective means of promoting stronger parent-child relationships.

The responsibility for instituting primary prevention measures in controlling teenage pregnancy should be part of an expanding role of the community health nurse. All income levels are affected by teenage pregnancies, and with the access a nurse has to groups, opportunities and challenges are many.

ELDERLY PERSONS. Elderly persons are probably the most vulnerable group in society in relation to their leisure and recreation needs. This group is generally retired, has great amounts of leisure time (perhaps too much free time), may be on limited incomes, and is declining in physical and emotional energy. Many elderly persons have transportation problems, or may have personal mobility problems which contribute to lack of companionship. Women are particularly vulnerable (Burrus-Bamell and Bamell, 1985).

Age alone is not a good predictor of potential level of activity. Income, race, gender, and place of residence, such as urban or rural, are better indicators than is age (Burrus-Bamell, and Bamell, 1985). However, the best indicator is educational level, because it is directly related to literacy level. The ability to read and write broadens the available leisure options.

Burrus-Bammel and Bammel report a study by Iso-Ahola in 1980 that activities among the elderly are altered in several ways:

The intensity of the participation;

The site of the activities (tend to be at home);

Companionship available, whether few or many companions, men or women, old or young, close or distant friends;

The reasons for participation;

The time of day for participation

At least two studies have explored the activities preferred by the elderly. Pepper's study in 1976 (Burrus-Bammel and

Bammel, 1985) ranked visiting friends, doing odd jobs at home, group travel, and reading as most popular. In 1979 McAvoy (Burrus-Bammel and Bammel, 1985) found that the elderly most preferred visiting friends, reading, hobbies, gardening, and indoor games. Results showed a mix of isolated versus social activities.

The *outreach function* of the community health nurse is essential in helping the elderly with leisure and recreation. Many individuals must be found and assisted in remaining or being involved in activities. The nurse may serve as a *catalyst* by arranging joint activities, helping promote friendships, church activities, and various groups such as those focused on conservation, hobbies, travel, volunteerism, cultural activities, and fraternal and service activities. An easy, practical entry to meeting unknown elderly is by taking blood pressures. This simple task can be performed almost anywhere and offers the opportunity to "pass the time of day." ("Passing the time of day" reveals much information about an individual frequently not elicited by questionnaires, assessment tools, interviews, and the like.)

Community health nurses providing nursing care in the home must be particularly cognizant of the leisure and recreational needs of family members, particularly *caretakers* (Springer and Brubaker, 1984). Relief of responsibility through respite programs can partially meet the need; however, arrangements should be made for the primary caretakers to have time for themselves each day. The nurses can assist the family and client in understanding this critical need and help with arrangements. A particularly eloquent description of the needs of the caretaker is set forth by Murphy (1984) in her account of caring for her chronically ill mother.

It is also necessary to bring the diversional or even recreational needs of the partially or totally home-bound person to the attention of the caretaker and family. Opportunities must be afforded for fullest use of remaining capabilities, interests, and potential.

In industry, nurses can make a major contribution to meeting leisure and recreation needs of *retirees.* The occupational health nurse can provide impetus to the formation of recreational interests in the years before retirement by encouraging employees to develop appropriate knowledge, skills, and activities. Each contact with an employee provides the opportunity for a few well-chosen words about use of leisure time and retirement. Furthermore, the nurse should participate in planning various employee benefit programs, such as physical fitness centers and preretirement programs.

Many companies are now providing exercise facilities for employees. The key question for the nurse to ask is "how will this program help the employee and family to maintain the exercising pattern when the equipment and stimulus are no longer present?" The resourcefulness and intrinsic motivation of the employee and family must be developed.

Occupational health nurses continue to have responsibility following employee retirement. The interest and activity level of retirees must be maintained, especially when discretionary time increases drastically. Research should be conducted about the relationship between level of leisure/

---

* The author wishes to acknowledge with appreciation the contribution to the section on adolescents by Katherine Ase, R.N., M.S., Marion County Health Department, Indianapolis, Indiana.

recreational activity and health status, particularly as company provided health insurance plans are affected. Faculty in schools of nursing and occupational health nurses might collaborate in such a study.

For additional ideas applicable in nursing, books by Gault (1983), McPherson (1983), Dowd (1984), Wade (1985), and Godbey (1985) are particularly pertinent.

CLINICAL APPLICATION

The following situation focuses on adolescents in a drop-in, community, or multiservice center. A similar strategy is appropriate for urban and rural areas although differences in availability of recreational facilities exists. The role of the community health nurse is suggested using the nursing process as the framework.

Goals for the nursing activity
1. To reduce the frequency of adolescent pregnancies
2. To assist the participants in the center to develop new interests and skills.

Assessment—individual or group
1. Using the tools provided in this chapter, identify attitudes, interests, and existing skills pertaining to leisure and recreation.
2. Observe the participants for potential leadership skills.
3. Apply risk criteria to the participants. Variables to be included are:
   a. Working? how many hours? what is work performed? (Consider the skills used at work relative to transfer to a recreational activity)
   b. Relationship with parents; relationship between parents; single parent family? (Consider the potential for recreational activities including parents)
   c. History of pregnancies in family, particularly of adolescent girls
   d. Urban area? rural area? (Consider the facilities available)
   e. Level of self-esteem; level of social skills; level of decision-making skills; values held
   f. Goal(s) for future; hope for a better future
   g. Leisure and recreational interests, skills, and potential skills

Plan—may be in collaboration with individuals; groups; center staff; volunteers; students in service professions; parents; representatives from the health department, welfare department, park and recreation department or police department

Based on recreational interests and skills elicited, plans may be needed:
   a. For expanding the center program
   b. Planning for other desired facilities in the community
   c. Identifying sites for referrals of individuals to meet needs and interests
   d. For publicity of programs

Implementation—may be in collaboration with persons identified under Plan

Actions include:
   a. Assist individuals to develop interests or skills that "are their very own"
   b. Make referrals to appropriate recreational program, club, other center. To take advantage of the referral, the individual(s) may need to be accompanied to the new site
   c. Assist in development and maintenance of leisure activities and recreational programs
   d. Present needs identified to various groups, such as parent-teacher organizations, business groups, home extension agents, Girl/Boy Scouts, Big Sister and Big Brother groups, Girl's and Boy's clubs, 4-H groups, church groups, women's and men's groups, country clubs, summer camps
   e. Arrange for classes to promote self-esteem, decision-making skills, values clarification, and social skills
   f. Assist with obtaining funding for programs from local government, private donations, and foundations
   g. Visit schools, other community centers, homes of center participants to encourage participation
   h. Assist in developing TV programs, spot announcements, and advertisements regarding recreational opportunities

Evaluation—may be of individuals, groups, or program
   Criteria include:
   a. Decrease in rate of pregnancy
   b. Increase in numbers of adolescents involved in a center; in a program; increased percent of participants maintaining involvement
   c. Observable increase in level of self-esteem, decision-making skills, social skills
   d. Higher grades in school; decreased absenteeism
   e. Increase in referrals between nurses; between nurses and other community centers; between nurses and recreational programs; between nurses and social workers; between nurses and parks and recreational programs
   f. Decrease in police contacts among adolescents for disorderly conduct and other offenses
   g. Increased recognition and participation of community health nurses in leisure and recreation

SUMMARY

Nurses have much to gain through the application of concepts pertaining to leisure and recreation in their practice in community health. The concepts of freedom, locus of control, motivation, health and wellness, disease prevention, and family are especially relevant to understanding the implications of use of leisure and recreation to the growth of a person and strengthening of family life and relationships, and developing community leisure and recreational resources. The developmental stage of individuals and families carries implications for the role of the nurse in identifying and assisting in satisfaction of leisure and recreational needs. Two age groups particularly vulnerable but potentially responsive to the expanding concern are adolescents and elderly persons.

Nurses in schools and industry can play a major role in creating positive attitudes toward leisure and recreation and developing interests and skills. Preretirement and postretirement periods in the work life of employees are particularly amenable to the contribution of the occupational health nurse.

The breadth of knowledge about community needs held by the community health nurse has yet to be fully used in planning recreational facilities and setting policy for a community pertaining to leisure time. The time for the nurse's participation on commissions and planning groups for recreation is here.

☰ KEY CONCEPTS

In recent years the relationship between health and social problems and the ability to use leisure time effectively has been described. However, many Americans are unable to use leisure time effectively and participate in meaningful recreational activities.

Recreation is in general how leisure time is used by an individual.

A key factor in determining if an activity is recreational is if the activity provides opportunity for revitalization and meaning to the person.

The essence of recreation is lost if the activity is inflicted or is perceived as a duty or responsibility.

Play provides an opportunity for children to develop physical coordination and to learn socialization skills, sharing, competing, cooperating, and communicating with others. The ability to form and maintain friendship begins with play in childhood.

The relationship between work and leisure is basic in terms of which has priority and the degree of separation or merging of work and leisure.

Beliefs, traditions, and values are major forces influencing the use of leisure time and the selection of activities.

Leisure activities developed by a population can affect culture.

Leisure and recreation contribute to three major health components of an individual: biological, psychological, and social.

Nurses in school and industry can influence attitudes toward exercise and eating habits. School nurses can also assist in the development of life-long leisure and recreational patterns for the children.

Family recreational patterns affect the health of the family as well as each member.

Community health nurses have access to groups in a community not generally accessible to recreational therapists, access which offers opportunities for population-focused practice in the use of leisure time and development of recreational activities.

Two population groups have been selected for particular attention to leisure and recreation needs: adolescents and elderly people.

The breadth of knowledge about community needs held by the community health nurse has yet to be fully used in planning recreational facilities and setting policy for a community pertaining to leisure time. The time for the nurse's participation on commissions and planning groups for recreation is here.

LEARNING ACTIVITIES

1. Using the Personal Inventory tool (Appendix A6), respond to the questions assessing your and your family's leisure/recreation habits and patterns.

2. Using the Personal Inventory tool, form small groups and analyze the responses of each member using the concepts of social networks, the work-rest-recreation balance.

3. Using the Personal Assessment tool, interview 2 or 3 persons from various age and income groups. Identify commonalities and differences. Analyze the responses from the older interviewees and project how a community health nurse might use the information from the interviews to develop a health education program to assist the younger group.

4. Attend a celebration, such as St. Patrick's Day parade, Mardi Gras event, Christmas season event(s), and write a short paper describing the influences on the health of the participants as a result of the event.

5. Observe in your neighborhood for individuals and families who demonstrate positive uses of leisure time and negative uses of leisure time.

BIBLIOGRAPHY

Barnett, L.A., and Kane, M.J.: Environmental constraints on children's play. In Wade, M.G., editor: Constraints on leisure, Springfield, Ill., 1985, Charles C Thomas, Publisher.

Berkman, L.S., and Breslow, L.: Health and ways of living—the Alameda County study, New York, 1983, Oxford University Press.

Burrus-Bammel, L.L., and Bammel, G.: Leisure and recreation. In Birren, J.E., and Schair, K.W., editors: Handbook of the psychology of aging, ed. 2, New York, 1985, Van Nostrand Reinhold Co., Inc.

Carlley, C., and Peters, F.: Power-load-margin, Indiana University, July, 1981, unpublished manuscript.

Chilman, C.S.: Families defined. In Stinnett, N., Chesser, B., and DeFrain, J., editors: Building family strengths—blueprints for action, Lincoln, Neb., 1979, University of Nebraska Press.

Chubb, M., and Chubb, H.R.: One third of our time? An introduction to recreation behavior and resources, New York, 1981, John Wiley & Sons, Publishers.

Cox, H.: The feast of fools—a theological essay on festivity and fantasy, Cambridge, Mass., 1969, Harvard Press.

Csikszentmihalyi, M.: Beyond boredom and anxiety, San Francisco, 1975, Jossey-Bass Publishers, Inc.

Deci, E.L., and Ryan, R.M.: Intrinsic motivation and self-determination in human behavior, New York, 1985, Plenum Publishing Corp.

Dowd, E.T.: Leisure counseling—concepts and applications, Springfield, Ill., 1984, Charles C Thomas, Publisher.

Dowd, E.T.: Leisure counseling with adults across the life span. In Dowd, E.T., editor: Leisure counseling—concepts and applications, Springfield, Ill., 1984, Charles C Thomas, Publisher.

Duvall, E.R.: Family development, ed. 4, Philadelphia, 1977, J.B. Lippincott Co.

Ellis, M.J.: Why people play, Englewood Cliffs, N.J., 1973, Prentice-Hall, Inc.

Freeman, R.B., and Heinrich, J.: Community health nursing practice, Philadelphia, 1981, W.B. Saunders Co.

Gault, J.: Free time: Making your leisure count, New York, 1983, John Wiley & Sons, Publishers.

Godbey, G.: Leisure in your life—an exploration, ed. 2, State College, Pa., 1985, Venture Publishing.

Goodale, T.L., and Witt, P.A.: Recreation and leisure: issues in an era of change, State College, Pa., 1980, Venture Publicating.

Hantrais, L., Clark, P.A., and Samuel, N.: Time-space dimensions of work, family and leisure in France and Great Britain. Leisure Studies 3:301-317, 1984.

Hayes, G.A., Brightwell, J., and Antozzi, R.K.: Managing stress through leisure awareness, Parks and Recreation, 19:43-47, 69, 1984.

Helvie, C.O.: Community health nursing—theory and process, Philadelphia, 1981, Harper & Row Publishers, Inc.

Information please almanac atlas and yearbook 1986, ed. 39, Boston, 1986, Houghton Mifflin Co.

Jarvis, L.L.: Community health nursing: Keeping the public healthy, ed 2., Philadelphia, 1985, F.A. Davis Co.

Kalyan-Masih, V.: Play: Implications for building family strengths, in Stinnett, N., Chesser, B., DeFrain, J. (eds.), Building family strengths—blueprints for action, Lincoln, Neb., 1979, Univ. of Neb. Press.

Kando, T.M.: Leisure and popular culture in transition, ed. 2, St. Louis, 1980, The C.V. Mosby Co.

Kaplan, M.: Leisure in America, New York, 1960, John Wiley & Sons, Publishers.

Klieber, D.A., and Dirken, G.R.: Intrapersonal constraints to leisure. In Wade, M.G., editor: Constraints to leisure, Springfield,Ill., 1985, Charles C Thomas, Publisher.

Kraus, R.: Recreation and leisure in modern society, New York, 1971, Appleton-Century-Crofts.

Levenson, P.M., Thornby, J.I., and Levenson, A.J.: Dimensions, benefits, and barriers to jogging perceived by joggers and nonjoggers. Health Values 9:6, 1985.

Maguire, L.: Understanding social networks, Beverly Hills, 1983, Sage Publications.

Mannell, R.C., and Iso-Ahola, S.E.: Work constraints on leisure: A social psychological analysis. In Wade, M.G., editor: Constraints on leisure, Springfield, Ill., 1985, Charles C Thomas, Publisher.

Maxey, W. Personal communication, 1986.

Mead, M.: The pattern of leisure in contemporary American culture. In Larrabee, E., and Meyersohn, R., editors: Mass leisure, Glencoe, Ill., 1958, The Free Press.

Murphy, D.: Wheels within wheels, New York, 1984, Viking Penguin Inc.

Murphy, J.F.: Concepts of leisure, ed. 2, Englewood Cliffs, N.J., 1981, Prentice-Hall, Inc.

McClusky, H.Y.: The course in the adult life span. In Hallenbeck, W.C., editor: Psychology of adults, Washington, D.C., 1963, Adult Education Association.

McDowell, C.F.: Leisure: consciousness, well-being, and counseling. In Dowd, E.T., editor: Leisure counseling—concepts and applications, Springfield, Ill., 1984, Charles C Thomas, Publisher.

McPherson, B.D.: Aging as a social process—an introduction to individual and population aging, Toronto, 1983, Butterworths.

Neulinger, J.: The psychology of leisure, ed. 2, Springfield, Ill., 1981, Charles C Thomas, Publisher.

Otto, H.: Developing human and family potential. In Stinnett, N., Chesser, B., and DeFrain, J., editors: Building family strengths—blueprints for action, Lincoln, Neb., 1979, University of Nebraska Press.

Pearse, I.H.: The quality of life—the Peckham approach to human ethology, Edinburgh, Scotland, 1979, Columbia University Press.

Pearse, I.H., and Crocker, L.H.: The Peckham experiment—a study in the living structure of society, London, 1947, George Allen & Unwin, Ltd.

Pearse, I.H., and Williamson, G.S.: The case for action, ed. 4, Trowbridge, England, 1982, Pioneer Health Centre Ltd.

Peiper, J.: Leisure: The basis of culture, New York, 1952, New American Library.

Rotter, J.B.: Generalized expectancies for internal versus external control of reinforcement, Psychol. Monogr. 80:1, 1966.

Shamansky, S.L., and Clausen, C.L.: Levels of prevention: examination of the concept, Nurs. Outlook 27:2, 1980.

Springer, D., and Brubaker, T.H.: Family caregivers and dependent elderly—minimizing stress and maximizing independence, Beverly Hills, 1984, Sage Publications.

Stallibrass, A.: Child development and education—the contribution of the Peckham experiment, Nutr. Health vol. 1, 1982.

Stevenson, J.S.: Construction of a scale to measure load, power, and margin in life, Nurs. Res. 31:4, 1982.

Stinnett, N.: In search of strong families. In Stinnet, N., Chesser, B., and DeFrain, J., editors: Building family strengths—blueprints for action, Lincoln, Neb., 1979, University of Nebraska Press.

Wade, M.G.: Constraints on leisure, Springfield, Ill., 1985, Charles C Thomas, Publisher.

Witt, P.A., Ellis, G., and Niles, S.H.: Leisure counseling with special populations. In Dowd, E.T., ed.; Leisure counseling—concepts and applications, Springfield, Ill., 1984, Charles C. Thomas, Publishers.

Witt, P.A., and Goodale, T.L.: Barriers to leisure across family stages. In Wade, M.G., ed.: Constraints on leisure, Springfield, Ill., 1985, Charles C. Thomas, Publishers.

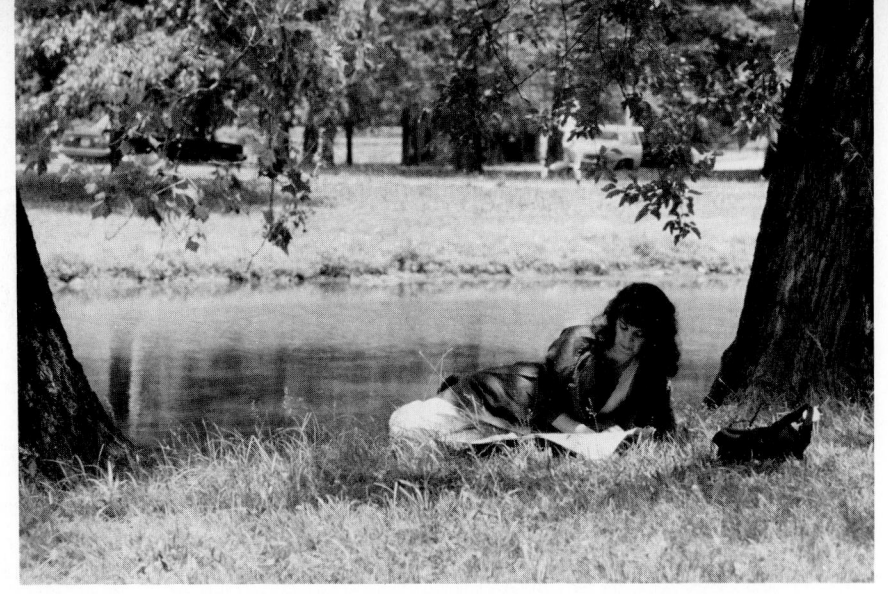

EFFECTIVE STRESS MANAGEMENT

Jeanette Lancaster

30

≡ OBJECTIVES

After reading this chapter, the student should be able to:

Define stress.

Describe the bodily response to stress.

Discuss how change can cause stress.

Discuss burnout as a common response to stress.

Identify three common physical stressors in many communities.

Describe at least three psychosocial-cultural stressors.

Identify five alternatives for managing stress.

Select at least one alternative for managing stress and practice it regularly.

≡ KEY TERMS

adaptation

adrenocorticotropic hormone

autonomic nervous system

biofeedback

burnout

creative imagery

crisis

distress

eustress

general adaptation syndrome

homeostasis

meditation

perception

progressive relaxation

Schedule of Recent Events

Social Readjustment Rating Scale

somatotropin

stress

stressor

Stress and its effects on health and well-being are areas of concern for many health care providers. The concept of *stress* dates to such pioneers as Bernard and Cannon who in the early 1900s described stress as a biophysical process (Sutterly, 1986). Selye, well known for his extensive work in stress research, proposed the theory of the *general adaptation syndrome* (GAS), which viewed stress as resulting from an outside force acting on the organism. During the 1950s, Selye proposed that stress resulted from the "nonspecific response of the body to any demand" (Selye, 1978, p. 1). In the broadest sense, stress is viewed as resulting from either physical or psychosocial forces that require the organism to alter existing modes of coping. Stress places a demand on the organism to change in order to cope with physical or psychosocial demands.

Since stress is ever present and influences the ability to cope, adapt, and lead a productive life, the nature of stress, stressors, the stress response, levels of stress, and sources of stress (for example, life change events and occupation) have implications for community health nursing. Community health nurses must understand the effect that stress has on them and be able to deal effectively with it to be a role model and teacher of clients.

RELATIONSHIP OF STRESS TO HEALTH STATUS

Stress is related directly or indirectly to many emotional and physical illnesses including coronary heart disease, anxiety states, ulcerative colitis, cancer, and sleep disorders (Woolfolk and Lehrer, 1984). Since personal life-styles and environmental conditions are also related to many of the major health problems people are increasingly encouraged to assume responsibility for their own health and to preserve health rather than to rely on the health care system to repair them once health is disrupted. The goal of health promotion is to assist people to be as healthy as they can.

NATURE OF STRESS

According to Selye, (1974) the demands causing stress for a person can take a variety of forms, each requiring adaptation and readjustment. Selye (1965) perceived all people as being constantly under stress, with each *stressor,* whether pleasant or unpleasant, having the ability to cause wear and tear on the body.

Hartl (1979, p. 91) defined stress as "that emotional and physical experience which results from a requirement to change from the condition of the moment to any other condition." This definition emphasizes the relation between change and stress. Stress is increased when people are faced with personal, social, and environmental changes; these changes can be perceived as being either positive or negative. The key is that each change experience requires new coping abilities and often novel forms of adaptation.

Similarly, Lazarus, Cohen, and Falkman found stress to be dependent on the person's appraisal of a situation as neutral, benign, or stressful. Stress develops from a person's appraisal that the demands exceed one's ability to cope (Clarke, 1984). *Perception* or appraisal of a given situation is crucial to determining the potential for stress. Consider the varying experiences of a group of college students at a large amusement park. Many of the rides and attractions are mild, funny, and essentially nonthreatening. However, the roller coaster may arouse a variety of feelings in the students. The majority of the group may feel exhilarated over the promise of a fast, thrilling ride; whereas the "silent minority" is anxious and perhaps would prefer to avoid this ride. Because of peer pressure and the desire to be part of the group, some of the frightened members ride the roller coaster although they are afraid. Despite the varying anticipation of the ride, each of the students would have a similar bodily experience. Bounding over the loops and curves, whether finding this fun or frightening, leads to a characteristic bodily reaction.

Perception also includes the cumulative effects of stressors. Often a person responds in what seems to be a disproportionate manner to a minor stressor. The observer does not know about the multiple stressors already at work in the person's life. For example, a man may go into a blind rage when his car stalls on a busy street. What would not be apparent to others is that the problem with the car is "the last straw." The man had been fired on Friday, his wife was hospitalized on Saturday, and he was on his way to the unemployment office.

Factors Influencing Stress

The Chinese word for *crisis* is a combination of two symbols—one representing danger and the other opportunity. Whether a situation is a threat or a challenge is largely dependent on perception. Selye (1975) pointed out the difference between adequate stimulation and overload when he described people as being racehorses or turtles. A racehorse would be driven to distraction on a quiet beach, whereas a turtle would have considerable difficulty trying to live the life of a racehorse.

The way in which people experience stress depends to a large extent on predictability (the degree to which people can anticipate the occurrence of an event), social context (the psychosocial setting or factors present in the environment), and control (the degree to which one can alter a situation or event). The effects of stress are less disruptive if the onset is expected or preceded by some warning. The social context of a stressor influences the reaction. It is easier to tolerate loud music if it is your own rather than if it is coming from someone else's apartment. The running and yelling of small children are generally better tolerated by their parents in their own homes than in a crowded restaurant or a friend's house. In addition, the degree of perceived control influences how a situation is interpreted. For example, listening to loud music in your own automobile may be less stressful than if the music were playing in a public building where your presence was required. In your automobile you could turn the volume down, whereas in the building you might not be able to leave or adjust the volume.

In the last 20 years, attention has focused on the influence change exerts on health status. In 1967, Holmes and Rahe began publishing research on the relationship between major life changes and alterations in health. Their scale, *The Social Readjustment Rating Scale* (SRRS) assigns numbers to specific life changes. The greater the number of life changes experienced by a person during a specified period of time, the greater the risk of developing a stress-related illness. The SRRS, which has been more recently called the *Schedule of Recent Events* (SRE), has received its share of criticism because of its simplicity of viewing the cumulative effect of positive or negative life events as cause of stress-related illness (Custer, 1985). Rahe (1978) was one of the first to acknowledge the simplistic nature of the tool. He cautioned that, "there are several intervening steps which exist between subjects' recent life change experiences and their subsequent near future illness symptoms and reports" (Rahe, 1978, p. 12). According to Custer (1985) demographic factors, coping ability, social support, focus of control, and desirability of events are often viewed as influential in affecting health outcomes.

How stress is experienced also depends on the person's ability to cope with life events. Coping has become the emphasis of stress research in the 1980s. Some researchers believe that "positive health outcomes are more a product of effective coping rather than simply a consequence of the presence or absence of stress" (Sutterly, 1986, p. 38). Research on coping is complex because one cannot effectively study coping styles without considering the total situation; that is, the interactions that are occurring, the quality of the support system, and the person's perception and general emotional state.

Coping with stressful events also depends on the meaning a person assigns to the event. What is stressful for one person may be energizing for another. For example, deadlines, writing papers, and public speaking affect people in different ways. Each person's response to stress is different because of the interplay of such factors as genetics, organ vulnerability, general state of health, fitness, sociocultural background, and previous experience with stress.

Additionally, not all stress is bad. Stress-related problems occur when the degree of stress remains high for a prolonged period of time. Stress is especially useful in times of danger when people need to mobilize physical and emotional forces for their own defense. In tolerable levels, stress is a motivator; it keeps people moving toward goal accomplishment and prevents boredom and feelings of uselessness. Selye (1974) described a positive form of stress as being *"eustress."* The "eu" means good or positive, as in euphoria. This form of stress results from an optimistic orientation toward life events coupled with the ability to regulate one's life and alter attitudes to view stress positively rather than negatively (Petosa, 1985).

STRESS RESPONSE

Stress theory is based on the concepts of *adaptation* and *homeostasis.* People strive to adapt to their stressors to maintain some semblance of balance. Stressors elicit a response from a person's entire body, including psychological and physiological components. Based on his definition of stress cited earlier, Selye (1978) identified the general adaptation syndrome (GAS). In this syndrome, physiological responses in the nervous and endocrine systems alert people to the occurrence of either *distress* or eustress. These sensations produce a wide range of feelings, varying from joy to fear, and serve as an alerting mechanism so that individuals can summon their resources to fight stress. The physiological changes brought about by stress are nonspecific and affect the entire organism.

The stress involved in the bodily reaction to a stressor occurs as the body attempts to normalize once it has been disrupted from its previous state of homeostasis. When humans are in distress too long or intensively, the GAS becomes decreasingly effective and makes a person vulnerable to mental or physical health disruption. The bodily response to stress has three phases:

1. *Alarm reaction:* physiological indications of alertness during which defense mechanisms are mobilized.
2. *State of resistance:* a state in which the individual resists the alarm and fights back to normal.
3. *Stage of exhaustion:* a point when stress is sustained, and adaptation energy is depleted.

To minimize the effect of stress, interventions should prevent a person from ever reaching exhaustion. People need to be keenly aware of internal and external stress-producing events and recognize their personal signs of stress accumulation. Essentially, stress is a response of the bodily and perceptual systems to a stressor, and the potential causative agent comes from either internal or external sources.

The bodily reaction to stress typically includes increases in the following:

1. Metabolism (oxygen consumption)
2. Blood pressure
3. Heart rate
4. Rate of breathing
5. Amount of blood pumped by the heart
6. Amount of blood pumped to the skeletal muscles

During a stress response the hypothalamus is stimulated, which in turn stimulates the *autonomic nervous system* (ANS) and the anterior pituitary gland. Stimulation of the ANS causes the heart to speed up, the digestive systems to slow down, and epinephrine and norepinephrine to be released. When the anterior pituitary gland is stimulated, it releases *adrenocorticotropic hormone* (ACTH), which subsequently stimulates the cortex of the adrenal glands and causes the release of steroids or anti-inflammatory hormones. A second hormone, *somatotropin* (STH), is also released from the anterior pituitary gland and stimulates the growth of the body as a whole and increases the activity of proinflammatory corticoids (Selye, 1978).

When the sympathetic portion of the ANS is activated, a "fight-or-flight" reaction is manifest in the accelerated heart rate, increased respiration, and redistribution of blood from peripheral areas of the body into the head and trunk. Each stressor activates the sequence just described, thereby enabling the body to fight or take flight.

The autonomic response occurs quickly and lasts only a short time; the endocrine response initiates more slowly and lasts longer. Setting off this response many times over a long period has a wear-and-tear effect on the body; eventually it lowers resistance to diseases. The hormones flowing through the system, along with the accompanying tensions, also have a psychological effect. Over a period of time, the chain reaction of the stress response can cause depression; irritability; nervousness; apathy; sleep difficulties; and changes in smoking, eating, and drinking habits, etc.

This reaction to stress originally evolved to help humans escape from predators. Once safe, escapees were able to proceed with their normal routines when the physical effect wore off. Today we have the same physiological response to stress, but the kinds of stressors we encounter are different.

STRESS IDENTIFICATION

Stress cannot and should not be avoided; the secret lies in successful management of stress. All machines wear out with excessive use, and the human body is no exception. Selye (1978, p. 405) stated that the critical first step in managing stress is "to know thyself." Everyone is familiar with the sensation of being keyed up from nervous tension. It has been noted that this feeling has a physiochemical basis and that people respond in unique ways to stressors. It is often difficult to learn to "tune down" or decelerate the pace of life. Simple rest is no panacea for managing stress for everyone. Successful stress management judiciously balances activity and rest to meet the individual's unique requirements.

Although each person reacts in a unique way to stress, there are several commonly observed physical, behavioral, and emotional indicators of increased stress, as depicted in the following box. As noted earlier, a key part of stress diagnosis includes determining one's own way of responding to stressors. Each person demonstrates some of the indicators listed in the box below.

A key part of stress diagnosis includes determining if perceptions are accurate. Occasionally, the anxiety present during a stressful time diminishes the ability to accurately perceive reality. Thus, it is important to disengage from a stressful situation long enough to make certain that what is perceived is really happening. For example, passing remarks of co-workers or supervisors may be perceived negatively if people are tired and feeling worthless. Once it is determined that perceptions are accurate, the next phase of

---

INDICATORS OF STRESS

PHYSICAL

1. Elevated blood pressure
2. Increased muscle tension (neck, shoulders, back)
3. Elevated pulse and/or increased respiration
4. "Sweaty" palms
5. Cold hands and feet
6. Slumped posture
7. Tension headache
8. Upset stomach
9. Higher pitched voice
10. Change in appetite
11. Urinary frequency
12. Restlessness
13. Difficulty in falling asleep or waking up; frequent awakening
14. Dry mouth and throat

BEHAVIORAL

1. Decreased productivity and quality of job performance
2. Tendency to make mistakes; poor judgment
3. Forgetfulness and blocking
4. Diminished attention to detail
5. Preoccupation, daydreaming, or "spacing out"
6. Inability to concentrate on tasks
7. Reduced creativity
8. Increased use of alcohol and/or drugs
9. Increased smoking
10. Increased absenteeism and illness
11. Lethargy
12. Loss of interest
13. Accident proneness

EMOTIONAL

1. Emotional outbursts and crying
2. Irritability
3. Depression
4. Withdrawal
5. Hostile and assaultive behavior
6. Tendency to blame others
7. Anxiousness
8. Feeling of worthlessness
9. Suspiciousness

stress identification deals with targeting the stress source, and the following list of questions can be asked:

1. Is the stress work-related?
2. Is something going on in my personal life that is worrisome and unfavorable?
3. Is the stress a combination of demands made on me at home and at work?
4. Do I set unrealistic goals and standards for myself that make me anxious?
5. Do I resist change because it threatens me?
6. Do I feel anxious most of the time?

Appendix C includes Health Style, a test used for determining the level of health risks present due to one's lifestyle.

STRESSORS

Stressors are defined as internal or external environmental stimuli that trigger physiological and psychological coping mechanisms. Some stressors are positive, whereas others elicit a negative response. Similarly, what serves as a negative stressor for one person may be energizing for another.

Robinson, Bridgewater, Molla, et al. (1982) differentiated the nature of stressors into three categories: bio-physiological, psychosocial and sociotechnical. Examples of causative factors in each of these stress categories include:

1. *biophysiological:* lack of exercise, poor nutrition, trauma, bacteria
2. *psychosocial:* low self-esteem, faulty interpersonal relationships, developmental crisis
3. *sociotechnical:* mass media, industrialization, pollution, changing economic conditions

Similarly, Sutterly (1979) classified stressors into two categories: biophysical-technical and psychosocial-chemical. These categories form the basis for the following discussion.

Biophysical-Chemical Stressors

As seen in Figure 30-1 a variety of biophysical-chemical stressors can elicit the stress response. However, the response does not necessarily result from a cause-and-effect situation. For this reason nurses must carefully monitor individual responses to stress and note what provokes the stress response and in what ways stress is manifested.

The substances many people use to combat stress actually are stressors themselves. For example, coffee, cigarettes, and alcoholic beverages are often used to promote relaxation; yet these substances actually are toxic to the body and act

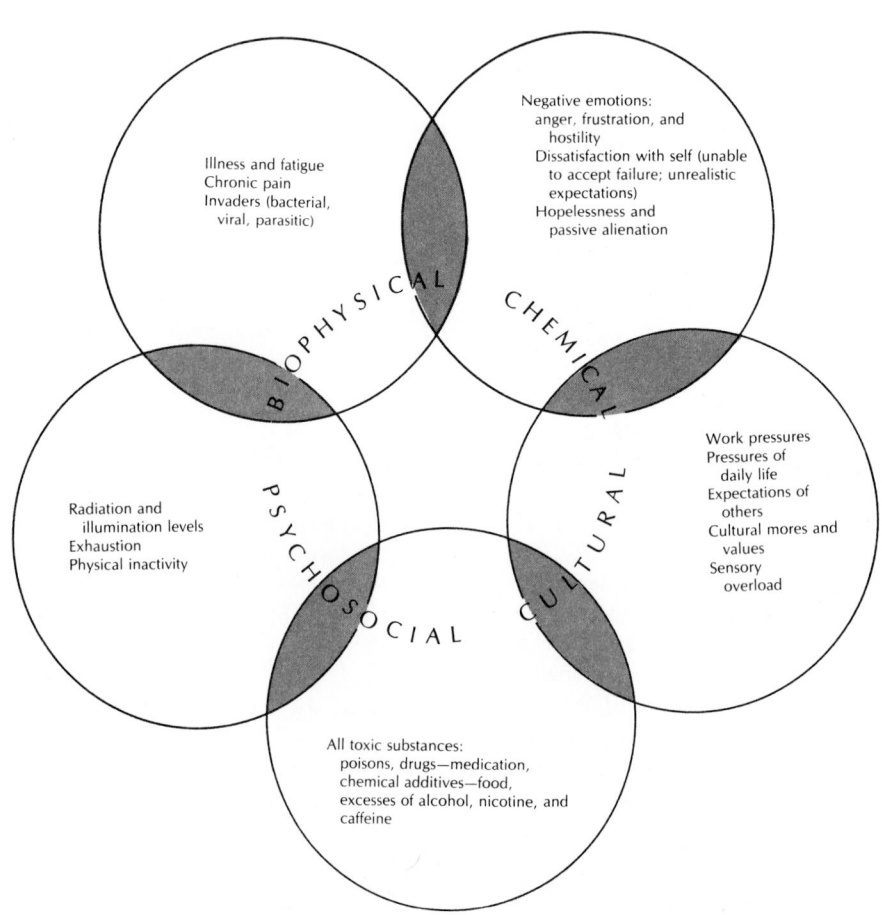

FIGURE 30-1

Multiple sources of stress: biophysical-chemical and psychosocial-cultural stressors. (Reprinted from Sutterly, D.C.: Stress and health: a survey of self-regulation modalities, Top. Clin. Nurs. 1:1-20, April, 1979. By permission of Aspen Systems Corp., © 1979.)

as stressors. Similarly, overeating stresses biophysical-chemical adaptation, especially if the food taken in is composed of excessive amounts of refined carbohydrates, salt, fats, and animal protein. Foods that Americans consume without awareness of the potential for generating stress include sugar, salt, caffeine, alcohol, nicotine, and food additives. When combined with the effects of air pollution, insecticides, and other toxins, the cumulative impact of these substances is considerable.

Physical sources of stress that are often overlooked or taken for granted include any form of trauma, accidents, weather changes, poor light, noise, physical work or living conditions, infectious agents, or inactivity. It is estimated that remaining in bed for a week generates as much stress as having a broken leg. Community health nurses should continuously estimate the cumulative stress effect on clients. For example, a bedridden person recovering from the physical stress of a stroke is more affected by an upper respiratory infection than is a relatively active, physically fit person. It is important to help clients learn what stressors are present in their lives and how to remove the optional ones and learn effective ways to cope with inevitable ones.

Living conditions affect stress. Crowded living conditions provide limited privacy. Under such conditions tempers tend to flare as people feel overstimulated by the presence of others.

Noise is another physical source of stress present in most communities. Excessive noise is considered irritating, and in recent years accumulated data have indicated that it also influences people's behavior. Thus, what may be pleasant to one person is often irritating to others. Consider the variable reactions of teenagers and their parents to a loud stereo. For one group this noise is thrilling, whereas to the other it is often deafening. Unpredictable noises tend to be more disruptive than steady repetitive sounds. Also, workers continuously exposed to high intensity noises show an increased incidence of nervous complaints, nausea, instability, argumentativeness, sexual impotence, mood changes, and anxiety (Cohen, 1981).

Climate has historically been associated with emotions. For example, happiness is equated with sunny weather and sadness with clouds. Extremes of temperature also seem to inhibit efficiency, and tempers seem to flare in exceedingly hot weather. With the advent of air conditioning and central heating, people have grown accustomed to expecting predictable weather and find themselves stressed when temperatures reach record highs and lows; thus, clients may need to be counseled about preparation for inclement weather conditions. Do they know where they can go to find relief when it is exceptionally hot or cold? Is it helpful to have canned foods ready if they become unable to get to the store?

Psychosocial-Cultural Stressors

As noted, a considerable amount of today's stress is brought about by the rapidly changing social environment, increasing technology, economic constraints, accelerated pace of living, and increased mobility. Many stressors arise at home and work. Conflicting values among family members may cause strains and tension. Also, work situations often serve as stressors by causing people to feel overwhelmed with either the quantity or quality of work expected. People seem to cope better in work situations in which they are regarded as valuable, contributing members of the group rather than when their only value seems to revolve around the amount of output they produce. Psychosocial-cultural stressors can arise from one of three general causes: societal, situational, and personal.

Societal Stressors

Some examples of societal causes of stress have already been identified. The range of societal stressors is vast and may differ from one community to another. It should also be noted that stressors have an interactive effect. One or two isolated stressors may not tax the coping ability of an individual or community. However, multiple stressors or the combination of a few highly emotional stressors can greatly affect stability. A community might effectively cope with encroaching forest fires by team effort and personal assistance to one another. However, if an escaped convict begins burglarizing homes and businesses concurrent with the threat of fire the community's coping ability may be severely taxed.

Other societal stressors include economic fluctuations, changing social values and attitudes (e.g., male-female roles and relationships and attitudes toward sexuality), increasing threat of violence, availability of illicit and prescription drugs, and pornography.

Situational Stressors

Examples of situational causes of stress include varying aspects of the work situation, such as too much or too little structure and unclear communication or lines of authority. French and Caplan (1980) observed that people experience more stress at work when they are not given adequate information to do their jobs and remain unclear about what is expected. This lack of clarity about role expectations is called role ambiguity. In contrast, role conflict occurs when information is contradictory or when there are substantive differences and disagreements among workers. Likewise, role overload increases stress and generally decreases productivity. Two general categories of role overload include: qualitative and quantitative. Qualitative role overload is seen when people do not know how to do what is expected of them or do not have access to the information, skill, and resources necessary for task completion. In contrast, quantitative role overload occurs when there is simply too much to do in too short a time.

Other work-associated causes of stress include conflicts across organizational boundaries where each group may hold different goals and expectations. New situations and settings which involve adapting to a new set of rules and expectations, are usually more stressful than familiar settings and situations. Additionally, responsibility for people rather than things tends to be more stressful because of the potential for interruptions from human needs requiring attention (Pope, 1982).

Major sources of situational stressors facing workers have been reported by Schwartz (1980, p. 100):

1. Work overload or stagnation
2. Extreme ambiguity or rigidity
3. Extreme role conflict or too little conflict
4. Extreme amounts of responsibility
5. Cutthroat and negative competition or no competition at all
6. Constant change and daily variability
7. Ongoing contact with "stress carriers" or people who cause others to experience stress because of their unreasonable goals, expectations, or ways of speaking or responding to others.
8. The corporation (for its own survival) discouraging individuality and clearly rewarding deference of one's own goals to that of the group.

Although these stressors are observed in many work situations, some groups have unique stressors. Nursing is a stressful profession because of factors such as poor communication; politics within the organization; conflicting demands for time and attention; lack of knowledge of what is expected; underuse of skills; changes in the organization; lack of participation in making decisions; limited job progress or career advancement; relations with other nurses, supervisors, subordinates, physicians, families, and clients; role overload; and responsibility without authority (Ivancevich and Matteson, 1980).

Changes in a person's life also prompt a stress response, especially if there is an accumulation of changes. Relocation is a situational stressor that affects many individuals. When people move from one city to another, they disrupt established support networks. New support systems must be developed in an unfamiliar place. Simply getting to school, work, or the grocery store is initially difficult in a new place.

Throughout history periods of social unrest and rapid change have tended to precipitate depression. Some groups are at higher risk for depression under these conditions than others. The following factors seem important in the onset of stress-related depression (Jacobson, 1980, p. 12).

1. Discrete life events and ongoing stressors (including their meaning to the person)
2. Being unmarried (especially if previously married)
3. Being female
4. Belonging to the lowest socioeconomic group
5. Age (youth or elderly)
6. Family history of affective illness
7. Premorbid personality characteristics as described by the dominant other

Labeling and prejudice comprise a situational stressor that is often present yet at times difficult to define. People tend to be appraised by others according to a wide range of characteristics such as race, sex, age, income, appearance, family status, and other personal qualities. Many groups, including women, children, the aged, mentally ill people, minorities, and poor people are often discriminated against just for being themselves.

Economic conditions constitute an increasing source of stress for people in many parts of the world. Specifically, inflation has an insidious effect on the health of communities. Instead of experiencing an obvious change in income, people often realize slowly that their buying power has slowly eroded and that their standard of living is decreasing rather than increasing. The American dream of working hard and making life better has disappeared for many. Only about 20% of Americans are socioeconomically mobile, with 15% moving up, and the remaining 5% moving downward (Johnson, 1979).

Personal Stressors

Personal causes of stress include low self-esteem, a need for perfection, a need to control others, or a need to be dominated and controlled by others. For many people irrational beliefs constitute stressful situations.

People often have unrealistic personal expectations for themselves, others, and the environment. People often expect to be perfect; they then experience considerable anguish when they fail to meet this expectation. Clients must be reminded that no one is perfect; everyone makes mistakes. The goal is to learn from mistakes and not repeat the same ones.

People also tend to have unrealistic expectations of others. For example, a middle-aged widowed woman may expect that her 30-year-old married son will always do as she says and expects. She may consider it reasonable to call him two or three times a week and to ask him to come over and fix something. Because of his own busy schedule and family demands, he may not always be able to comply with his mother's wishes, causing her to feel rejected. A nursing goal could be to help the mother have more realistic expectations of her son as well as develop additional support networks.

Other people have unrealistic expectations of the environment. For example, some expect that raises and promotions will automatically occur. Although this may be possible in some situations, effort, initiative, and productivity are usually essential to ensure promotions.

STRESS MANAGEMENT TECHNIQUES

According to Donnelly (1980a), there are two ways of dealing with stress: reactive and active. Reactive techniques are based on the belief that stress is inevitable and that all people can do is sit back and wait for "it" to happen. This view is similar to the flight response to stress. Behaving in a reactive way, people simply take what comes along. For example, they work late when the poor planning of others causes extra work. They blame themselves for all that goes wrong at home, school, or work. When self-blame and overconscientiousness fail, the reactive person may lash out at others in an irrational or aggressive manner or may resort to consuming drugs or alcohol, overeating, smoking, or oversleeping as an escape. The reactive pattern can lead to chronic fatigue, irritability, depression, feelings of inadequacy, and finally stress-related diseases such as colitis or hypertension.

The alternative to dealing with stress in a reactive manner is to gain control and assume an active role in fighting stressors. The ability to actively fight stressors, however, does not depend only on one's willingness to assume personal responsibility. Complex, interrelated factors such as past experiences in assuming personal responsibility; cultural variables, which may or may not sanction certain behaviors; and the availability of support systems also play a part. People are more likely to continue stress-reducing behaviors such as managing diet and regularly participating in exercise if friends or family members either actively encourage them or join with them in the effort.

Some of the generally accepted methods for managing stress appeal more to some cultural and socioeconomic groups than others. People with limited educational backgrounds and restricted incomes may not adapt to or have access to techniques such as biofeedback, progressive relaxation, yoga, or so forth. Also, Woolfolk and Lehrer (1984) caution that some techniques for managing stress alleviate symptoms but fail to influence the actual problem. As Sutterly (1986, p. 41) points out "Practicing stress management techniques in lieu of a direct change in life-style can be counterproductive, such as teaching relaxation skills to abused wives." Figure 30-2 depicts several general ways to regulate stress. Finally, although many stress management techniques appear simple, their success depends on the skill of both the teacher and the client. Nurses should not attempt to teach skills unless they are thoroughly grounded

in the technique. Similarly, clients are not likely to learn and effectively use techniques they do not like and support. The techniques selected must be ones with which the teacher is proficient and the client is receptive.

Clarke (1984) classified methods for coping with stress into three types: direct, indirect, and palliative. The first two methods reflect an active technique and the third is reactive. Specifically, direct coping involves the individual in some action to alleviate the demand made by the stressor such as preparing for an examination by carefully studying relevant information. Indirect coping does not alter the situation but alters one's reaction to it. Examples of indirect coping including changing the bodily experience when confronted by a stressor by learning techniques such as relaxation, biofeedback, or hypnosis. In contrast, palliative coping includes temporary relief measures such as using alcohol, drugs, cigarettes, or the use of defense mechanisms including denial or rationalization.

The following are four general ways for intervening in stress:

1. Alter exposure to stress by establishing priorities and setting limits (Sutterly, 1986).
2. Alter the environment so that it is less stressful.

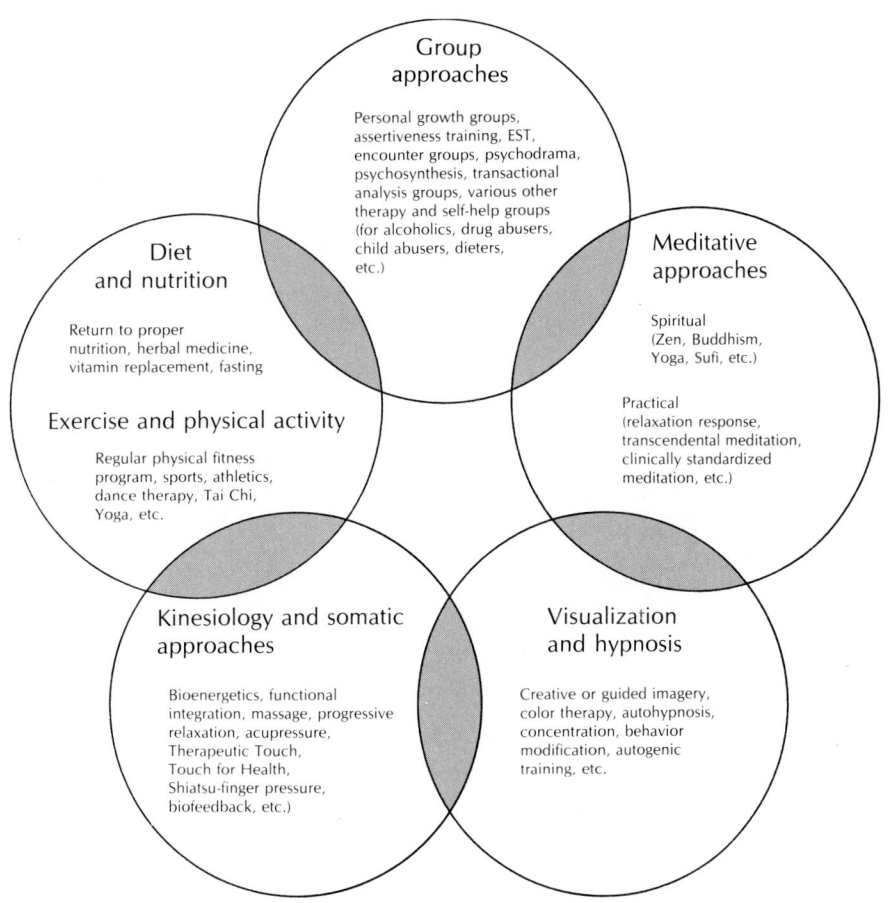

FIGURE 30-2

Various approaches used in self-regulation of stress. (Reprinted from Sutterly, D.C.: Stress and health: a survey of self-regulation modalities, Top. Clin. Nurs., 1:1-20, April, 1979. Used with permission of Aspen Systems Corp., © 1979.)

3. Change one's own beliefs and/or behavior so that situations are perceived differently and are subsequently responded to in a different manner.
4. Learn to lower physiological arousal to stress by countering the long-range effects.

There are many ways to manage stress, and people have preferences in the method they find most successful. Also, certain techniques require more skill and resources than others. A variety of techniques are discussed to equip the community health nurse with many choices for developing personal stress management programs with clients. Some general principles of stress management are presented in the box below followed by specific and detailed techniques.

To determine the most appropriate mode of intervention for stress reduction it is important to apply the nursing process. The assessment phase for determination of individual stress include questions such as the following:

1. What specific demands is the person experiencing?
2. What are perceived as stressors?
3. How has the person previously coped with stressful situations?
5. What support systems have assisted in the past?
6. Is the discomfort proportional to the event?
7. What are the person's current resources, limitations and level of motivation?

The stress reduction plan is unique for each client depending on the level and nature of stress, the person's interest and motivation to be actively involved in reducing stress, and the comfort in practicing skills on a regular basis. As is discussed in the section on meditation, certain personal and environmental characteristics must be present to ensure the potential for success.

Various avenues are available for implementation of a stress reduction plan including diet, exercise, recreational activities, changing attitudes, relaxation, creative imagery, biofeedback, hypnosis, and acupressure. Chapters 28 and 29 describe in detail the benefits of diet, exercise, and recreation on health promotion. Chapter 31 discusses assertiveness as a tool for promoting health. The skill management techniques discussed here deal with cognitive and interpersonal tools for the personal management of stress.

Changing Attitudes

Changing attitudes is an essential part of stress management. It is important to handle stressors as they occur and to deal directly with feelings to avoid bottling up thoughts or emotions. It is also important to find something to substitute for worrying thoughts and to chase them away. Nothing erases unpleasant thoughts more effectively than conscious efforts to focus on positive things. Adams (1980) describes a process for shifting attitudes to more effectively deal with feelings:

1. Notice the feeling or sensation by being consciously aware that something is occurring.
2. Give the feeling a label such as anger or happiness.
3. Decide whether or not the feeling or cluster of feelings is appropriate to the present situation being perceived in the environment.
4. Give expression to feelings in a way that is safe, will get what is wanted or needed, and will do no harm to another. That is, it is much more appropriate to talk with people about being angry than to hit them.

Creating and Using Support Networks

One of the best ways of coping with stress is by seeking support from members of a reliable and caring work, family, or social group. Everyone needs someone to trust and with whom stress-producing situations can be discussed in depth without fear of rejection or retaliation. Talking with one or more members of a trusted support network provides opportunities for testing reality, obtaining feedback from someone whose opinion is valued, working through feelings, and constructively planning future actions.

Seashore (1980) described a support network as a resource pool which one can draw on selectively to provide support and strength. People need several options in their resource pool so they do not consistently draw on the same one and also so that the responsibility for choosing how to deal with the situation remains with the person and is not delegated to the support system. Clients should be guided in identifying the support networks currently available. Who are the members of their support network? How many people can they call on in a crisis or a stressful situation?

The purpose of support groups is to assist members in growing and developing through support from people who understand (often because they have lived through a similar circumstance) and who care about one another. Usually, a

---

STRESS MANAGEMENT TIPS

1. Get to know your body so that you can recognize the first signs of stress. (Have clients recall their last stressful situation and describe their physiological reaction).
2. Learn to relax. Deep breathing is a natural relaxant.
3. Practice simple relaxing exercises.
4. Exercise. Take a brisk walk, run, play tennis, or dance to stimulate blood flow.
5. Learn to smile and laugh and to balance work and recreation. (Ask clients to recall the last time they had fun; what were they doing, and how did they feel?)
6. Learn to worry effectively by doing something about it. (Instruct people to talk out their worries with someone they trust and respect.)
7. Learn to accept things and people. Some situations are beyond your control. (Instruct people to change their attitudes about a situation or to develop a stress-reduction plan.)
8. Take one thing at a time. A sure way to become overwhelmed is to find yourself in the middle of a dozen projects.
9. Give in once in a while, and try to avoid getting angry. Once you are angry, you are conquered because the ability to think clearly and rationally is diminished in the face of anger.

common bond holds the members of a support group together. In many support groups there are no agendas for the meeting, but rather the mission is to support, encourage, and at times challenge one another. Seashore listed the following four functions of a support group (1980, p. 157):

1. *Reestablish competence:* In times of high stress people often devalue their ability and fail to recognize their own strengths.
2. *Maintain high performance:* In good times when excessive stress is not present, support groups help members "keep their batteries charged."
3. *Gain new competencies:* Some members of the group may be better able to challenge, teach, or motivate others.
4. *Achieve selected objectives:* Group membership can help in the clarification, formulation, and refinement of short-term and long-term objectives.

Group members can help validate the effectiveness of poor selection of a coping mechanism and assist members in learning and practicing new responses. Often people think that they have behaved so badly that no one else could possibly understand, much less accept them.

Community health nurses have for many years recognized the value of group sessions in helping clients deal with problems. Successful group experiences have included people with alcohol and/or drug dependencies, those with problems of obesity, individuals with major chronic illnesses, those suffering the loss of a child or spouse, and victims and/or perpetrators of human abuse. Historically, groups have been a significant avenue for health maintenance and promotion. Stress management groups offer a rich potential for clients and nurses. These groups can be oriented toward discussions, activities, or a combination of both. Group membership is a natural and desirable social phenomenon. People are born into a group and throughout life, either consciously or unconsciously, attempt to find their place in the group. Groups can have a healing effect by providing opportunities for self-understanding and acceptance (Donnelly, 1980b).

Support systems are useful in helping people reestablish their competence by assisting during times of high stress as well as serving as sources of strength and encouragement during ordinary situations. In using support systems, clients need to rely on them sparingly so that they are not "worn out" by giving such assistance. To maintain a support system it is useful to keep in contact in times of homeostasis as well as when under stress.

Relaxation

Although relaxing is a universal human ability, this activity tends to be cast aside in the busy hustle and bustle of life. For many people, relaxing is viewed as a waste of time rather than an opportunity for unwinding and passively dealing with the stresses of life.

Community health nurses are in an ideal position to teach relaxation techniques; before teaching them, however, they should learn and practice the techniques themselves to gain comfort in this ability. Several brief relaxation exercises are

included in the box below to provide variety in practice sessions.

Relaxation exercises are simply "journeys into self," which provide a mechanism for unwinding. The primary purpose of relaxation is to relieve muscle tension and induce a quieting response whereby the body can rebuild needed energy resources. Nurses can assist clients through teaching and role modeling to control autonomic functions by altering their state of consciousness to assume a mental state of relaxation. One form of relaxation, progressive relaxation, is discussed in some detail.

Progressive Relaxation

Progressive relaxation provides a way of reducing stress by altering the relation between muscle and psychological tension. Jacobson (1974) did extensive research on mind/muscle interaction and postulated that anxiety and relaxation are mutually exclusive. This technique was developed as a method of combating tension and anxiety by instructing clients to systematically tense and relax muscle groups. The goal of progressive relaxation is not to eliminate all stress but to allow people to monitor and control their stress levels.

Progressive relaxation, a rudimentary form of biofeedback, is based on the person's ability to differentiate tension from relaxation and to feel the difference as each of 14 major muscle groups is consecutively tensed and then immediately relaxed. The procedure follows a systematic format moving from the feet to the head (see box on p. 600). This form of relaxation is within the scope of nursing practice and has been successful in treating clients with borderline hypertension, headaches, insomnia, and anxiety.

Specific assessment areas before instituting progressive relaxation include, in addition to a history, a determination

---

RELAXATION EXERCISES

BRIEF RELAXATION SHOULD BE A PART OF EVERY DAY
EXERCISE 1

1. Take 5 minutes, three times a day.
2. Sit comfortably and close your eyes.
3. Concentrate on bringing to mind a picture of the most peaceful setting you have experienced.
4. With each breath say to yourself, "Relax, relax."
5. With practice you can let your thoughts and problems float away for a few minutes.

EXERCISE 2

1. Sit in a comfortable position.
2. Close your eyes.
3. Inhale a deep breath through your nose—hold—exhale through your mouth. Repeat five times.
4. Breathe normally.
5. Concentrate on breathing. Each time you exhale, say the word "one" silently to yourself. Breathe in, breathe out, with "one."
6. Open your eyes.
7. Sit quietly for 1 minute.

PROGRESSIVE RELAXATION: MODIFIED APPROACH FOR COMMUNITY HEALTH NURSING PRACTICE

This activity simply involves relaxing one step at a time, as follows:
1. Sit or lie in a comfortable position.
2. Close your eyes.
3. Concentrate on breathing easily.
4. Once your body feels calm, instruct all bones and muscles of the lower body to relax in the following order:
    a. Feet   d. Knees
    b. Ankles   e. Upper legs
    c. Lower legs   f. Hips
5. Shift attention to the upper parts of your body, instructing all bones and muscles to relax in the following order:
    a. Hands   e. Upper arms
    b. Wrists   f. Neck
    c. Lower arms   g. Shoulders
    d. Elbows

By this time, your arms and legs should feel heavy and unmovable. However, if you become uncomfortable, shift your position. Then continue with step 6.

6. Spend some time concentrating on relaxing the main part of your body, instructing each organ and all muscles to be relaxed.
7. Relax your head muscles in the following order:
    a. Jaws   b. Face   c. Scalp
8. With the relaxation process complete, spend a few minutes focusing on (but not altering) your breathing, which probably has become quite shallow.
9. Gradually increase your breathing to "get the blood flowing again." To prevent dizziness, take one or two relatively deep breaths before standing up.

---

that the stressful situation should be treated in this manner rather than with medication. It must also be determined if any contraindications exist relative to the relaxation of certain muscle groups. For some types of low back pain, strengthening rather than relaxing certain muscle groups is preferred (Richter and Sloan, 1979). The planning and implementation phases are consistent with all other forms of relaxation. In the evaluation phase of the nursing process, it is necessary to carefully observe any factors that may have compromised the effectiveness of this technique.

Bernstein and Borkovec (1973) defined the following common problems relative to progressive relaxation: (1) muscle cramps, (2) movement, (3) laughter or talking, (4) other noise, (5) intrusive thoughts, (6) sleep, (7) coughing and sneezing, (8) inability to relax certain muscle groups, (9) strange or unfamiliar feelings, (10) losing control, (11) internal arousal, (12) failure to follow instructions, and (13) problems with practicing and avoiding certain words and phrases. Many of these problems and the suggested solutions also apply to other stress reduction techniques.

In progressive relaxation cramps may occur in the neck, calves, feet, or any other muscle group held especially tense. These cramps can often be avoided by suggesting that the client reduce the tension and hold these muscles tense for a shorter period of time. The affected muscles can be gradually tensed and relaxed to reduce the level of strain on them. If cramps do occur, the client should manipulate (move or rub) the affected muscle, wait a few minutes before going on, and then continue. When progressive relaxation is practiced in a group, clients may move around excessively during the exercise, and this may be disruptive to others attempting to maintain their concentration. If comfort is a problem, the client may need some assistance in finding a

desirable position. Also, it is not uncommon for participants to either laugh or talk during the early sessions because of anxiety and fear of embarrassment. Some of the muscle-tensing exercises, especially those involving facial muscles, cause participants to look "funny." They may laugh at one another or at themselves as they feel their faces assume strange positions. It is usually helpful if the nurse performs the exercises along with the client to promote a feeling of comfort and acceptance in the session.

The ideal site for beginning progressive relaxation training is a quiet, soundproof room. Since such rooms are not always readily accessible, the best alternative is to find a quiet room that is free from distractions, especially sudden interruptions. Clocks, music, telephones, people talking, horns blowing, etc. often go unnoticed during an active day; but they are highly distracting during relaxation.

In addition to external intrusive noises, some people are disturbed by their own intrusive thoughts. One approach for dealing with this is for the nurse to increase the dialogue or assist the client in selecting a new set of relaxing thoughts. For example, the person may want to build in some pleasant imagery such as thinking of being on a raft in a calm sea with the blue sky above and the clouds gently moving.

Clients should not be encouraged to go to sleep during the relaxation exercise; the word *sleep* is avoided in giving instructions in favor of a suggestion such as being "relaxed and awake." Any words or phrases that produce tension should be avoided; thus the client's reactions to the choice of words used should be noted. If people do fall asleep, they should be gently awakened and the tempo speeded up slightly to see if that helps.

Some people have difficulty tensing certain muscle

groups and may need assistance in developing an alternative tensing pattern. Others have difficulty following instructions either because they were not listening carefully or they simply forgot what was said. Some people benefit from keeping their eyes open during early sessions so that they can model after the nurse, and this also may decrease their fear of the unknown (Richter and Sloan, 1979).

Other clients have strange or unfamiliar feelings during progressive relaxation such as a floating sensation. If this occurs, they may want to look away and become reoriented to their surroundings. Some people feel uncomfortable when they become relaxed because of their loss of control of the situation. If this occurs, it may be helpful to spend more time discussing the situation, introducing the steps slowly, and after the session focusing on the positive experiences that occurred. Others may feel externally relaxed at the end of a session but "uptight" inside. They need to know that internal responses are involuntarily controlled, whereas the peripheral relaxation is controlled voluntarily. Practice increases the degree of internal relaxation.

It is not uncommon for heavy smokers to have episodes of coughing, and people with colds or allergies may begin sneezing. It may be helpful to encourage less deep breathing to diminish stimulation of coughing and sneezing. Some clients have difficulty establishing a schedule for practicing, and they may need assistance with time budgeting. The following approach, meditation, is often used in combination with progressive relaxation. Additionally, progressive relaxation can be included in the creative imagery approach to reinforce the process.

Meditation

Meditation can produce an inhibition of the sympathetic nervous system, thus reducing the effects of chronic stress by producing a state of hypometabolism (Sutterly, 1979). The physiological responses observed in meditation are opposite those seen in the "fight-or-flight" syndrome. One of the most widely used forms of meditation is that devised by Benson (1975). While studying the physiological results of meditation at the Harvard University laboratory, Benson demonstrated that meditation brought about reduced oxygen consumption and blood lactate levels. He was able to identify the basic elements of meditation, which he labeled the *relaxation response.*

Meditation requires (1) a quiet setting with few distractions, (2) a mental device or *mantra* such as a word or sound to be repeated mentally with each exhalation to help avoid distracting thoughts from invading the tranquility, (3) a passive attitude that allows the meditation experience to occur, and (4) a comfortable position that does not induce sleep.

Bates (1979) suggested the following instructions for the meditation process:

1. Sit quietly in a comfortable position with eyes closed.
2. Using progressive relaxation, deeply relax all muscles beginning with the feet and moving to the face.
3. Breathe through the nose being consciously aware of the breathing pattern. While exhaling, mentally say the word *one.*

4. Continue the breathing process of step 3 for 10 to 20 minutes, but do not set an alarm; instead open your eyes to check the time. When finished, sit for several minutes with eyes closed first and then with them open.

The value of meditation as a tool for relaxation in nursing is that it can easily and successfully be used and taught to clients in a variety of clinical settings. Modifications of this response, which are applicable to community health nursing, can incorporate relaxation tapes or a personally developed schedule of steps. For example, one way to learn the relaxation process is to take five minutes three times a day and sit comfortably with the eyes closed and concentrate on a peaceful picture or mental image. For some people, visions of the water such as a lake or the ocean are restful, whereas other people may choose the mountains or some other unique sight. With each breath, say the word *relax.* At first this exercise may seem unnatural, but it serves to divert the mind from the problems at hand and in essence provides a "psychological coffee break" or time out from ordinarily experienced stressors. Other mental devices include repeating the word *one* or the phrase *I am relaxed.* To practice relaxation techniques it is necessary to (1) find a comfortable place to sit; (2) place the feet flat on the floor generally with hands in lap; (3) close the eyes; and (4) breathe steadily and with purpose for about five minutes while taking particular notice of the parts of the body that feel tense and willing them to relax.

Creative Imagery

Creative imagery has gained considerable attention as a way to involve people in creating a milieu for their own healing processes to occur. The concept behind creative imagery is that "the body is equipped to heal itself from every manner of disorder, and that under most circumstances the body requires no special instructions to accomplish this feat" (Achterberg and Lawlis, 1982, pp. 55-56). Mental images or internal representations of events or places use the senses to mentally and consciously alter bodily functioning (Achterberg and Lawlis, 1980). The concept of creative imagery involves any or all five of the senses, including visual, auditory, olfactory, tactile, and kinesthetic (end organs lie in the muscles, joints, and tendons; and this sense is stimulated by bodily tension). Although this concept is often used in attaining and maintaining health, its usefulness applies also to psychotherapy and spiritual care.

Creative imagery is particularly well suited to incorporation in the community health nursing role, since contact with clients often is long term allowing for the development of trust. Heidt (1982) described the use of creative imagery in conjunction with therapeutic touch and found it to aid in the formation of close relationships with clients in a shorter than usual time; it allowed them a nonthreatening means of expressing their feelings about being sick; and it encouraged clients' beliefs about their own abilities to heal. Using tape recordings to facilitate relaxation and the imagery process, clients were asked to draw a picture of their perception of their disease or discomfort and the treatment for it.

Visualization exercises help to demonstrate the relation between the mind and the body. The mind can focus on a peaceful and tranquil imaginary scene, and the body tends to respond by becoming more relaxed. Clients can be assisted to relax by suggesting that they visualize the one place they would like to be. They should become specific and thorough in the visualization to encourage active participation in the process. For example, a client might find the seashore relaxing. First, the nurse asks the client to imagine sitting beside the sea listening to the many sounds. Next, the client asks questions such as what kinds of sounds are most prominent at the sea and how do I feel as I sit, listen, and look at the calm, gently moving blue sea.

The research by Simonton, Simonton, and Creighton (1978) demonstrated the use of visualization in treating cancer. They combined visualization with other methods of cancer treatment, including radiation and chemotherapy to provide patients with a mechanism for fighting rather than being consumed by the cancer. The patients are taught to visualize their concern in an attempt to combat the disease. "For many cancer patients, the body has become the enemy. It has betrayed them by getting sick and threatening their lives. They feel alienated from it and mistrust its ability to combat their disease" (Simonton et al. 1978, p. 125). These researchers devised a cancer treatment program based on the assumption that relaxation helps to reduce fear, which can itself become overwhelming. They combined the progressive relaxation technique developed by Jacobson with mental imagery. They recommended that patients practice this program three times a day for 10 to 15 minutes each time. Several principles form the foundation for the relaxation and mental imagery program developed by these researchers. By forming an image of a desired event, people can make a personal statement of what they want to occur. By repeating the statement, clients come to expect that the desired event will occur, and they begin acting in ways consistent with the achievement of the desired outcome.

Similarly, a hypertensive person could use the creative imagery process to see the problem as being little muscles in the walls of blood vessels that clamp down under stress so that greater force is required to carry the blood to its destination. The next step would be to suggest that they visualize their medication relaxing these little muscles in the blood vessels so that the heart pumps smoothly, evenly, and with minimum resistance.

These same approaches can be used in dealing with arthritis. Clients can be instructed to picture their joints as being irritated and having many small granules on the surface. Next they are urged to see their white blood cells coming in, cleaning up the debris (including the little granules), and smoothing over the joint surfaces. Finally they visualize themselves as being active and free of joint pain.

Relaxation and mental imagery are useful, since these processes can decrease fear by allowing people to have some responsibility for and control of themselves. These processes can also bring about an attitude change moving from despair and often despondency to anticipation and the will to live. Also, physical changes can occur that enhance the immune system, and it can be a basic method for stress reduction.

Biofeedback

The basic principles of biofeedback are (1) monitoring a physiological index that is sensitive to stress, (2) feeding the information back to the person involved, and (3) using the information as a guide in attempting to alter the physiological state (Donnelly, 1980c). Biofeedback provides immediate confirmation of personal control of oneself. Various stress reactions have been effectively controlled with biofeedback, including excessive anxiety, phobias, tension, headaches, insomnia, essential hypertension, bruxism (teeth grinding), colitis, ulcer, or menstrual distress. Kolkmeier (1982) reported on the use of biofeedback to teach hypertensive clients to normalize their blood pressure with minimum medication. At the Biofeedback Laboratory at the Dallas Diagnostic Association, clients are taught what causes elevated blood pressure and what they can do to alter the situation. They also are counseled by a dietitian about salt restriction and weight reduction. Group support is provided to encourage compliance with the therapeutic regimen.

Through *biofeedback* electronic sensors can make people aware of normally unconscious processes. Alpha brain waves, muscle tension, and skin temperature are often used to provide people with an immediate interpretation of their bodily reaction. One popular way to use biofeedback is by using an electromyograph, a machine designed to gauge the state of muscle tension by detecting electrical signals through the skin. Through biofeedback, people learn to reduce increasing tension as a sign of stress.

Several simple procedures, which do not require any machinery, may be used to detect how people are responding to stress. It is commmon practice for nurses to monitor clients' reactions by noting changes in breathing, heart rate, and blood pressure. Clients can easily be taught to monitor pulse as a gauge to their emotions. The first step is to establish a baseline resting pulse. This can be done by having the person sit quietly for 5 minutes and then recording the pulse. The next step is to practice any desired type of meditation or relaxation for at least 5 minutes and record the pulse. The pulse rate should decrease; however, this does not always occur, since for some people the resting pulse is already rather low (Donnelly, 1980c).

Another simple and inexpensive type of biofeedback evaluates temperature of the extremities. Clients can be taught to use a sensitive thermometer for measuring skin temperature of the fingers while repeating the relaxation sequence described for pulse regulation. It is important to tape the thermometer firmly to the finger to obtain an accurate reading.

Another variation of temperature monitoring includes the warming of hands via biofeedback. Before warming the hands, the person's palmar skin temperature of the index finger should be measured using a standard thermometer. Readings below 85°F indicate distress. Once the temperature is recorded, the person can be taught to raise it by a variety of relaxation techniques, including sitting or lying in a comfortable position with shoulders relaxed and attention focused on slow, even breathing. The next step in warming the hands includes concentrating on and repeating the autogenic phrase, "My arms and hands are heavy and warm." As relaxation occurs, the hands begin to warm, and they may tingle as the temperature rises. Temperature should be recorded before and after each session to motivate and encourage participants.

If the person's blood pressure is elevated considerably, medication is initially used to bring it under control before entry into the biofeedback program. Clients are aided in identifying their personal sources of stress, what physiological changes they typically experience in response to stress, and what changes can be made either in their lifestyles or in their responses to the stressor (See Kolkmeier [1982] for a more detailed description of this program). The main benefit is that through a reasonably simple, painless method, clients can be taught to control hypertension while simultaneously reducing their reliance on drugs.

Hypnosis

Hypnosis has been used extensively in health care often in conjunction with other treatments. Successes with hypnosis have been reported to reduce a client's fear of surgery or dental procedures and to reduce the anxiety of childbirth.

Nurses wishing to use hypnosis in their practice should become trained in this skill before practicing with clients. To stimulate interest in hypnosis as a stress-reducing effort a brief description is presented. This technique has in recent years been recognized as a medium for reducing or eliminating pain as well as managing stress.

Six basic components to hypnosis are pretalk, induction, utilization, awakening, posttalk, and assessment. The basic technique can be practiced in 10 to 15 minutes in an unconditioned client who has not previously been hypnotized (Daley and Greenspun, 1979).

During the first stage, pretalk, clients are not told that they will be hypnotized, but rather the hypnotherapist simply explains the process, emphasizing the need for cooperation to achieve maximum relaxation. The subjects are informed they will enter a subconscious state similar to that of being partially awake.

The induction phase usually follows a technique similar to progressive relaxation in which clients sit or lie in a comfortable position with their feet uncrossed, teeth unclenched, and all restrictive clothing loosened. The room should be free from noise. Next, clients are directed to close their eyes, breathe deeply three times, and concentrate on relaxing each part of the body starting with the crown of the skull.

Once relaxation ensues, utilization can begin when clients are ready to receive positive reinforcement. The therapist suggests that the clients will be peaceful, tranquil, calm, and comfortable and that at a specified signal that can be given anytime in the future they will return immediately to their present level of relaxation. An example of a signal given under hypnosis might be, "at any time when I point to your forehead and say the words deep sleep, you will immediately return to this level of relaxation" (Daley and Greenspun, 1979, p. 63). This posthypnotic suggestion eliminates the need for lengthy subsequent inductions.

Awakening is usually a simple process that begins once the beneficial suggestions are given. The therapist might say that at the count of five the client will awake, feel calm, and be in a peaceful frame of mind. Awakening is done slowly so that clients do not experience untoward reactions such as headache, nausea, or vomiting.

The fifth stage, posttalk, begins once clients have reoriented themselves to their setting, without rushing. During this phase, clients are especially susceptible and receptive, and goals should be set and agreed on, giving as much positive reinforcement as possible.

The last step, assessment, deals with the clients' further needs for lessons in relaxation, and should take place 3 or 4 days after the hypnosis. Once clients learn to relax by hypnosis, a program of self-management can be developed.

Acupressure

Another form of stress reduction, acupressure, reduces tension by "reestablishing the harmony and balance of the flow of electromagnetic energy" (Sutterly, 1979, p. 12). In this process, like acupuncture, selected metabolic and circulatory processes can be stimulated by finger pressure on certain points on the body. The value of this technique lies in its use for self-regulation of chronic pain and tension. Several self-help books have been written to teach people this technique (Chan, 1974; Kurland, 1977; Thie, 1973; Warren, 1976). The book by neurologist and psychiatrist Kurland is particularly useful, since it describes the use of acupressure in eliminating tension headaches.

Therapeutic Touch

Therapeutic touch is a nursing method pioneered by Dolores Kreiger (1975) and used by many nurses to aid healing in their clients. This approach uses "the meditative state to enter the energy field of the client and to passively visualize or free the flow of energy from practitioner to recipient with the intent to support or promote healing" (Sutterly, 1979, p. 13). Clients are helped to achieve self-healing by drawing on the energy flow of the practitioner. Also, practitioners trained in therapeutic touch can assess bodily areas out of harmony in a client by alterations and sensations in their own energy flow as they touch the client.

BURNOUT: INEFFECTIVE COPING WITH STRESS

The term *burnout* was coined by psychologist Herbert Freudenberger in 1975 to describe a reaction to excessive job-related stress (Bunch, 1983). It may also be observed in individuals who suffer major losses, such as a job or a close family member, within a short time span. Burnout may also be observed in persons experiencing chronic illness. Whatever the cause, the person experiencing burnout is unable to respond successfully to stress.

Both internal and external stressors contribute to burnout. Inadequate leadership, poor working conditions, long hours, heavy workloads, lack of control over work, and bureaucratic decisions are examples of external stressors. Internal stressors include the need for autonomy, respect, recognition, feelings of competence, and involvement in meaningful activities (Bunch, 1983).

The physiological concomitants of burnout include cardiac irregularities and electrolyte imbalance (hypokalemia), which may result in decreased cardiac output and the subsequent symptoms of irregular pulse, hypotension, dependent edema, decreasing kidney function with alteration in urinary output, mental confusion or forgetfulness, weakness, or even cardiac arrest. Additional physical symptoms include fatigue, gastrointestinal problems, persistent colds, back pain, weight loss or gain, loss of appetite, susceptibility to infections, headaches, insomnia, dyspnea, or angina.

Some or many of these physical signs are generally accompanied by several behavioral symptoms including irritability, rigid thinking and general resistance to new ideas or any threat of change, finding fault easily with other people, and often displaying a generally negative and cynical attitude. Other behavioral indicators of burnout are absenteeism, tardiness, decreasing accuracy in work assignments, and a tendency to "take problems home." The person approaching burnout becomes increasingly exhausted physically and emotionally and, in general, begins to show lack of respect, empathy, or warmth for others. For nurses these signs of burnout are often followed by decisions to leave the profession, go into administration, or use drugs or alcohol to cope with the stress.

Burnout, as a stress reaction in response to work or organizational pressures, is comon among human service workers who spend considerable time and energy helping others. An unfortunate aspect of burnout is that the people who suffer from it tend to be those the organization values most highly. Victims of burnout typically are high achievers who thrive on accomplishments.

Three categories of events have been found to be instrumental in precipitating burnout among health care workers.

1. Environmental deficits, such as not enough supplies or equipment, poor physical layout of the institution, and a shortage of staff.
2. Professional relationships characterized by ineffective communication or personality conflicts.
3. Relationships with clients and families in which the nurse identifies with the client and feels guilty that the best possible care is not being given.

Strangely enough, increased knowledge can precipitate burnout. For example, as health care technology has improved, greater knowledge is available on preventing and treating diseases. People know what they could or should do; yet lack of time, energy, commitment, or resources interfere with their taking the necessary actions. A failure to act leads to stress, especially if lack of action brings about untoward results. For example, a home health care nurse, Ms. Smith, was visiting an elderly client to change her indwelling catheter. Ms. Smith had one sterile catheter kit with her. She considered stopping by the office to get an extra catheter just in case she contaminated the first one. However, she was running late and decided to risk having only one catheter with her by convincing herself that she was quite skilled at changing catheters and rarely had any difficulties. As luck would have it, Ms. Smith dropped the sterile catheter just as she was about to insert it. Not only

did she drop the catheter on the floor, but because of her tight schedule and feeling of pressure to complete her work on time, Ms. Smith picked up the contaminated catheter and used it. The following week Ms. Smith visited this lady and saw signs indicating a urinary tract infection; she felt depressed, guilty, and overwhelmed by her inability to effectively manage her time and use good judgment. If Ms. Smith continued to have many days like the one described, she would be a likely candidate for burnout.

Coping with burnout includes basically the same stress management techniques as those discussed in the text. The core of these efforts begins with self-awareness to recognize accumulating stress, followed by a carefully developed intervention plan with exercise, recreation, open communication, group or individual support, outside interests and resources, and a recognition that burnout is not a function of "bad" people but rather of "bad" situations that need to be modified. The box below lists two approaches for self-management of burnout, prevention and intervention.

COPING WITH A COMMUNITY STRESSOR

This chapter has dealt with stress assessment and management on an individual level. However, the importance and complexity of community stressors should not be underestimated. The dynamic factors in contemporary society are increasing community levels of stress. As discussed under biophysical-chemical stressors, factors such as crowding, excessive noise, and climate influence the community's level of stress. Other community stressors include, but are not limited to, high crime rates, chemical and other pollution, natural and man-made disasters, poverty and homelessness, economic down-turns as evidenced in company closings and lay-offs, or the decision to close a local school.

SELF-MANAGEMENT FOR BURNOUT PREVENTION AND INTERVENTION

1. Know yourself; pay attention to your feelings to see what sets off negative feelings.
2. Delegate whenever possible; do not try to do everything for yourself and others.
3. Recognize that burnout is a function of poor situations and work to change them.
4. Plan a variety of self-care activities to increase resistance to stress.
5. Vary the amount and type of client contact so you are not consistently caring for the same kind of people. Staff members working in tense clinical situations may plan regular, brief "time-outs" to mobilize their personal resources.
6. Keep work and home separate. Leave feelings and problems in the proper place.
7. Form a peer support group to discuss reactions and feelings about work.
8. Negotiate roles and responsibilities to do what you feel competent to do.
9. Regularly show appreciation to others; positive expressions can become contagious!

Far more research has been conducted on how individuals cope with the stressors of daily life than on how people cope with community stressors. Bachrach and Zautra (1985, p. 127) define community stressors as "problems that affect a large number of people in a given area (which) . . . cannot be readily resolved by the individual alone and thus require collective action." Stressors such as these may be acute or chronic and originate either within or outside the community.

Swift (1980) has developed the following equation to examine the relationship between at risk populations and environmental variables that lead to increased incidence of emotional or behavioral dysfunction.

$$\text{mental illness (incidence)} = \frac{\text{stress} + \text{physical vulnerabilities}}{\text{social supports} + \text{coping skills} + \text{self-esteem}}$$

The equation can be applied either to individuals or to populations. From a community perspective, mental illness would result from stress interacting with the strengths and weaknesses of the population at risk. To reduce the incidence you must decrease the size of the numerator (stress, physical vulnerabilities, or both) or increase the value of the denominator (social support, coping skills, and self-esteem). Attempts to increase the value of the numerator have been more prevalent than those to decrease the size or value of the numerator. Efforts to reduce environmental stressors assume "the stressor is known, the technology exists to control it, and the political and economic power is available to accomplish the task" (Swift, 1980, p. 10).

Some community stressors for which known interventions exist include reducing the consumption by children of lead-based paint, selected nutritional deficiencies, and communicable childhood diseases. Nevertheless, barriers exist to achieving complete eradication of these problems. Some paint manufacturers may resist legislation prohibiting production of lead-based paints, fearing loss of profits. Deficient diets may require more than the provision of nutritious foods in schools. Parents may oppose inoculations because of religious beliefs.

Areas in which community health nurses could participate in planning with community groups to decrease stress and physical vulnerabilities might include:

1. *Building project:* In the Bachrach and Zautra (1985) study, for example, residents with a strong sense of community involvement and a belief that their efforts could be effective worked to prohibit the construction of a hazardous waste facility in their rural community. When residents feel threatened by the construction of facilities such as airports, shopping areas, highways, chemical disposal facilities, and so on, community health nurses could assist with cohesive group development so that residents can work constructively to oppose the project.

2. *Programs for special populations:* Community awareness and organized neighborhood protection programs can reduce crime toward vulnerable groups such as children, the elderly, and shopkeepers who run small businesses with few employees present at any given time.

3. *Legislation:* Laws affecting social practices such as legal drinking age, use of seatbelts, and possession of firearms can decrease community stress and vulnerability.

4. *Regulations:* Regulatory bodies can be urged by community pressure to enforce building and fire safety codes, investigate accidents in a timely fashion and increase support for educational and social programs.

The role of the community health nurse in stress reduction extends to individuals, groups, and communities. Although the challenge is complex, the rewards for successful stress management are great.

CLINICAL APPLICATIONS

Students and practicing nurses must become proficient with the strategies for stress management outlined in this chapter and integrate them into their own lives before they can teach them to clients and co-workers. As Webster (1985, p. 713) so aptly states "Nurses spend a large amount of time giving to and taking care of others. Unfortunately, some nurses do not take good care of themselves." To effectively teach stress management techniques nurses must serve as role models for healthy life-styles.

The first step in implementing stress management strategies is to complete a self-appraisal of one's fit between self and the environment. This assessment may be completed individually or in a small group. Questions to be answered include What do I mean when I say I am experiencing stress? What is the source of my stress? and What strategies are available to me for coping with stress?

In assessing stress, people are encouraged to brainstorm in order to elicit all possible answers. It may be helpful to differentiate the stress into mild and strong groups and to decide if the stress elicits thoughts, feelings, or actions. Next, determine whether the source is internal or external. The third major assessment task is to determine if the coping strategies used to deal with each type of stress are adaptive or maladaptive (Woolfe, 1984). If the strategies typically used for coping with certain stressors are maladaptive, explore alternative strategies such as those described in the chapter. Hamilton (1984) succinctly discussed 15 ways to relieve stress. Not all of these will apply to each reader at any one time, but all apply at one time or another.

1. Choose carefully among alternatives, weighing the pros and cons of each trying to avoid indecision.
2. Plan your future by deciding what you really want to be.
3. Manage your time effectively.
4. Pace yourself; don't try to do too much at once.
5. If you decide to do something, commit yourself fully to the effort.
6. Say no when you mean no.
7. Learn to argue successfully.
8. Master the art of flight or find time to be alone each day.
9. Share your feelings with others.
10. Listen with your feelings to others.

11. Improve your environment to make it a more pleasant place.
12. Find opportunity in problems.
13. Surrender to the inevitable or don't waste time and energy trying to change what can't be changed.
14. Accept the unknowable.
15. Encourage yourself.

The goal of these 15 suggestions is to help relieve stress. When stress is minimized people think more clearly; plan more effectively; make better use of their memory; feel better about themselves; and have a more positive attitude toward self, life, and others.

SUMMARY

Stress is a frequent and generally personal experience that can cause considerable mental and physical wear and tear. The positive aspects of stress can be maximized so that they can be used to motivate and energize people. The magnitude of the stress response to changes in life events and expectations can be minimized by a variety of stress management techniques such as relaxation, creative imagery, hypnosis, use of support networks, exercise, and diet.

People respond to stress differently based on their own needs and resources for adapting to changing life events. Stress is manifested in a variety of ways: physically, behaviorally, and emotionally. Each person tends to develop a unique way of handling stress. Some bottle up their feelings and turn the stress response into physical ailments such as ulcers and heart attacks; whereas other people handle stress by screaming, crying, or instituting constructive stress-reduction strategies. It is unrealistic to hope for or anticipate a "stress-free" world. There will always be stress; the key element is learning to use rather than be used and abused by it. Community health nurses can play a vital role in teaching stress-reduction techniques. Perhaps the most effective way to teach clients how to manage stress is to practice this skill and demonstrate it through formal instruction as well as through role modeling.

All life situations are potential sources of stress; however, work is a major stressor for many people. Several problem areas within work settings have been mentioned to alert nurses to the potential for stress-management skills in occupational settings. A major portion of the chapter dealt with the techniques for managing stress including, group discussion, changing attitudes, relaxation (particularly progressive relaxation), meditation, creative imagery, hypnosis, acupressure, and creating and using support networks. The task now is to learn, practice, and teach these skills.

To assist community health nurses in recognizing the magnitude of stress in society and also to teach ways of managing this phenomenon, various contemporary stressors were identified. For example, in any community, biophysical-chemical and psychosocial-cultural stressors are present. It is the task of the nurse to assess the particular community to determine specifically what stressors are present; what populations are most affected (at risk); what resources are currently available for assisting clients to deal more effectively with stress; and finally what actions can be taken by nurses to institute new programs, assist in reducing community stress, and teach clients more effective responses. Although this chapter has focused on ways to work with individuals and families in reducing stress, it in no way discounts the vital role of community health nurses in serving as catalysts in working with the entire community to alleviate those stressors that can be altered or eliminated. Other chapters have dealt with the nurse's role in responding to the community as client and in dealing with crises.

KEY CONCEPTS

Stress and its effects on health and well-being are areas of concern for many health care providers.

Because stress is ever present and influences the ability to cope, adapt, and lead a productive life, the nature of stress, stressors, the stress response, levels of stress, and sources of stress (for example, life change events and occupation) have implications for community health nursing.

Stress is related directly or indirectly to many emotional and physical illnesses, including coronary heart disease, anxiety states, ulcerative colitis, cancer, and sleep disorders.

The way in which people experience stress depends to a large extent on predictability (the degree to which people can anticipate the occurrence of an event), social context (the psychosocial setting or factors present in the environment), and control (the degree to which one can alter a situation or event).

In tolerable levels, stress is a motivator; it keeps people moving toward goal accomplishment and prevents boredom and feelings of uselessness. Selye (1974) described a positive form of stress as being "eustress."

Stress theory is based on the concepts of adaptation and homeostasis.

Although each person reacts in a unique way to stress, there are several commonly observed physical, behavioral, and emotional indicators of increased stress.

Stressors are defined as internal or external environmental stimuli that trigger physiological and psychological coping mechanisms.

Changing attitudes is an essential part of stress management.

One of the best ways of coping with stress is by seeking support from members of a reliable and caring work, family or social group.

Progressive relaxation provides a way of reducing stress by altering the relation between muscle and psychological tension.

The term *burnout* was coined by psychologist Herbert Freudenberger in 1975 to describe a reaction to excessive job-related stress. Both internal and external stressors contribute to burnout.

The role of the community health nurse in stress reduction extends to individuals, groups, and communities. Although the challenge is complex, the rewards for successful stress management are great.

LEARNING ACTIVITIES

1. Interview three people, other than nursing students and faculty, to elicit their definition of stress. Then ask them to identify the five most significant stressors in their lives. Contract to work with at least one person to develop an actual stress management plan.

2. Drive through your community and identify possible stressors during a 15-minute tour. Be aware of biophysical-chemical and psychosocial-cultural stressors.

3. Make a chart and administer it to yourself and two other people, asking them to complete the following questions: How do I have fun alone (with and without spending money)? How do I have fun with someone else (with and without spending money)?

BIBLIOGRAPHY

Achterberg, J., and Lawlis, F.: Bridges of the body-mind; behavioral approaches to health care, Champaign, Ill., 1980, Institute for Personality and Ability Testing.

Achterberg, J., and Lawlis, F.: Imagery and health intervention, Top. Clin. Nurs. 3:55-60, 1982.

Adams, J.D.: Understanding and managing stress: a workbood in changing life styles, San Diego, Calif., 1980, University Associates.

Bachrach, K.M., and Zautra, A.J.: Coping with a community stressor: the threat of a hazardous waste facility, J. Health Soc. Behav. 26(2):127-141, 1985.

Bates, C.: Stress and health, health values: achieving high-level wellness, 3:136-143, 1979.

Benson, H.: The relaxation response, New York, 1975, William Morrow & Co., Inc.

Bernstein, D.S., and Borkovec, T.D.: Progressive relaxation training, Champaign, Ill., 1973, Research Press.

Bunch, D.: Are you ready to explode? Burnout may make you feel that way, AAR Times 7:21-24, 1983.

Chan, P.: Finger acupressure, Los Angeles, 1974, Price/Stern/Sloan Publishers, Inc.

Clarke, M.: Stress and coping: constructs for nursing, J. Adv. Nurs. 9:3-13, 1984.

Cohen, S.: Sound effects on behavior, Psychology Today, 15:38-46, 1981.

Custer, M.: Stress, life events, and the epidemiology of wellness, J. Comm. Health Nurs. 2(4)215-222, 1985.

Daley, T.J., and Greenspun, E.L.: Stress management through hypnosis, Top. Clin. Nurs. 1:59-65, 1979.

Donnelly, G.F.: Why you just can't take it anymore! . . . coping, RN 43:34-37, 1980a.

Donnelly, G.F.: Remember . . . you're not in this alone! . . . how group methods can help you cope . . . and how to pick a group that's right for you, RN 43:3033, 1980b.

Donnelly, G.F.: How do I know I'm on the right track? . . . simple new biofeedback gadgets can help you chart your course to deep relaxation, RN 43:44-46, 1980c.

French, J.R.P., and Caplan, R.D.: Organizational stress and individual strain. In Adams, J.D., editor: Understanding and managing stress, LaJolla, Calif., 1980, University Associates.

Hamilton, J.M.: Effective ways to relieve stress, Nurs. Life 4:24-27, 1984.

Hartl, D.E.: Stress management and the nurse, Adv. Nurs. Sci. 1:91-100, 1979.

Heidt, T.: Patients tell their stories, paper presented at the second annual Conference on Imaging and Fantasy Process, Chicago, November 1979. In Achterberg, J., and Lawlis, G.F.: Imagery and health intervention, Adv. Nurs. Sci. 3(4):55-60, 1982.

Holmes, T.H., and Rahe, R.H.: The social readjustment rating scale, J. Psychosom. Res. 11:213-218, 1967.

Ivancevich, J.M., and Matteson, M.T.: Nurses and stress: time to examine the potential problem, Super. Nurse 11:17-22, 1980.

Ivancevich, J.M., Matteson, M.T., and Preston, C.: Occupational stress, type A behavior, and physical well-being, Acad. Management J. 25(2):373-391, 1982.

Jacobson, A.: Melancholy in the twentieth century: causes and prevention, J. Psychiatr. Nurs. 18:11-21, 1980.

Jacobson, E.: Progressive relaxation: a physiological and clinical investigation of muscular states and their significance in psychology and medical practice, ed. 3, Chicago, 1974, University of Chicago Press.

Johnson, C.L.: The American family during inflationary times, Psychiatric Opinion, 16:13-16, 1979.

Johnson, J.W.: More about stress and some management techniques, J. School Health 51:36-42, 1981.

Kolkmeier, L.: Biofeedback-relaxation therapy for hypertension, Adv. Nurs. Sci. 3:69-73, 1982.

Kreiger, D.: Therapeutic touch: the imprimatur of nursing, Am. J. Nurs. 75(5):784-778, 1975.

Kurland, H.D.: Quick headache relief without drugs, New York, 1977, Ballantine Books.

Lazarus, R.S., Cohen, J.B., and Falkman, S.: Psychological stress and adaptation: some unresolved issues. In Selye, H., editor: Guide to stress research, New York, 1980, Van Nostrand Reinhold Co.

Moss, V.: Beating the stress connection: self-hypnosis. AORN J. 41:720-722, 1985.

Petosa, R.: Eustress and mental health promotion, Health Values, 93:7, 1985,

Pope, R.: Identifying organizational stressors: the nurse's role, Occup. Health Nurs. 30:34-36, 1982.

Rahe, R.H.: Life change and illness studies: past history and future directions, J. Human Stress 4:3-16, 1978.

Richter, J.M., and Sloan, R.: Stress: a relaxation response, Am. J. Nurs. 79:1960-1964, 1979.

Robinson, K.M., Bridgewater, S.C., Molla, P.M., and Wather, C.A.: Concepts of stress for nursing, Issues in Mental Nursing 4:167-176, 1982.

Schwartz, G.E.: Stress management in occupational settings, Public Health Rep. 95:99-108, 1980.

Seashore, C.: Developing and using personal support systems. In Adams, J.D.: Understanding and managing stress, LaJolla, Calif., 1980, University Associates.

Selye, H.: The stress syndrome, Am. J. Nurs. 65:97-99, 1965.

Selye, H.: Stress without distress, Philadelphia, 1974, J.B. Lippincott Co.

Selye, H.: The stress of life, ed. revised, New York, 1978, McGraw-Hill Book Co.

Simonton, C.O., Simonton, S., and Creighton, J.: Getting well again: a step by step self help guide to overcoming cancer for patients and their families, Los Angeles, 1978, J.P. Tarcher, Inc. (Distributed by St. Martin's Press, Inc., New York.)

Sutterly, D.C.: Stress and health: a survey of self-regulation modalities, Top. Clin. Nurs. 1:1-20, 1979.

Sutterly, D.C.: Stress management: grazing the clinical turf, Holistic Nursing Practice 1:36-53, 1986.

Swift, C.: Task force report: National Council of Community Mental Health Centers Task Force on Environmental Assessment, Community Ment. Health J. 18:7-14, 1980.

Thie, J.: Touch for health, Marina Del Ray, Calif., 1973, De Vorss and Co., Publishers.

Warren, F.: Freedom from pain through acupressure, New York, 1976, Frederick Fell Publishers, Inc.

Webster, J.A.: The wellness model: feeling good about you. AORN J. 41:713-718, 1985.

Woolfe, R.: Coping with stress: a workshop framework. Br. J. Guidance Counselling, 12(2):141-153, 1984.

Woolfolk, R., and Lehrer, P.: Clinical stress reduction: an overview. In Woolfolk, R., and Lehrer, P.: Principles and practice of stress management, New York, 1984, Guilford Press.

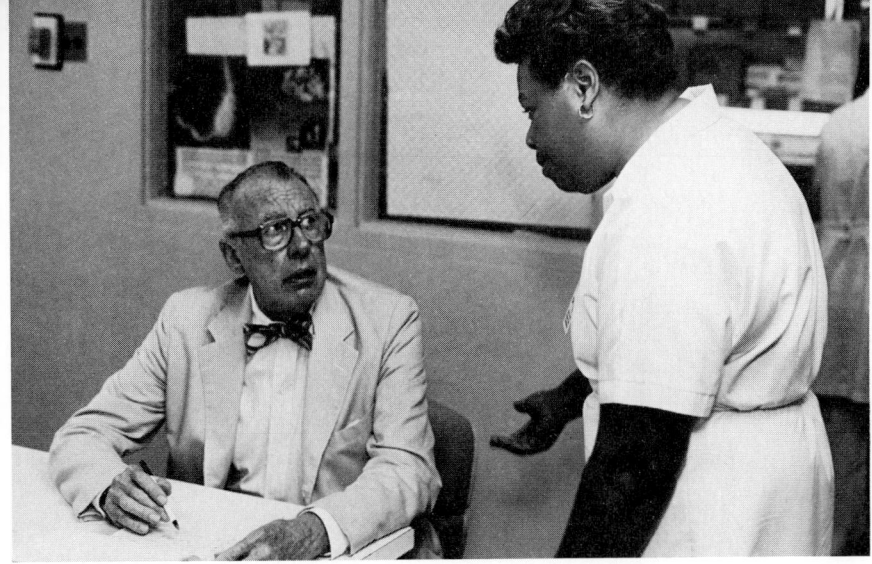

ASSERTIVENESS

Paula Pointer
Jeanette Lancaster

31

OBJECTIVES

After reading this chapter, the student should be able to:

Describe how a person's self-concept affects behavior.

Discuss the process of socialization into the nursing role.

Differentiate nonassertive, assertive, and aggressive behavior.

State the basic rights of all people as advocated in an assertive philosophy.

Discuss the nonverbal components of assertive behavior.

Describe three ways of dealing with manipulation which reflect an assertiveness view of behavior.

Differentiate between constructive and destructive conflict.

Explain the three stages of confrontation.

Define negotiation.

Describe four potential reactions of others to assertive behavior in nursing practice.

KEY TERMS

active listening
aggressive behavior
assertive behavior
assertiveness
conflict
confrontation
criticism

flattery
fogging
guilt
insecurity
manipulation
negative assertion
negative inquiry

negotiation
nonassertive behavior
power
role prescriptions
role strain
self-concept
sense of obligation
socialization

This chapter and others in this section are included to emphasize that the practice of health promotion is a part of community health nursing. Assertiveness, like stress management, is a skill that nurses can teach to their clients and use to promote their own health.

Assertive people reflect confidence in their interpersonal relationships and are able to express feelings and emotions honestly and spontaneously, and they are respected by others for these qualities (Jenkins, 1982). Assertive behavior is learned behavior; *assertiveness* means standing up for one's own rights without violating the rights of others. Assertive techniques help people meet their own needs while respecting the needs of others.

This chapter discusses assertiveness by reviewing theories of the self, exploring basic assumptions of assertive behavior, and discussing techniques for evaluating personal actions and making informed choices about one's actions. The final section discusses conflict as a part of human interaction and describes the use of confrontation and negotiation as assertive techniques for dealing with conflict.

SELF-CONCEPT AS A BASIS FOR BEHAVIOR

A person's attitude and self-concept continuously affect behavior. People hold attitudes reflecting what they think and feel about themselves, which are acquired throughout life and are influenced by the way others respond to them. These attitudes form an abstraction known as the *self-concept* and are represented by the symbol *me*. The terms *self-esteem* and *self-concept* are used interchangeably in this discussion.

Early Theories on the Origins of Self-Esteem

Cooley (1902, p. 152) described the "looking-glass" self in which an individual imagines the reactions of others to this image and is satisfied or ashamed as a result.

For example, nurses who were obese as children often continue to think of themselves in this way even though as adults they have attained through diet control and exercise an average physique. Imagining that others see them as overweight, the nurses feel unattractive and ashamed of their appearance.

William James (1890), one of the early theorists about the concept of self, believed that aspirations and values have an essential role in determining whether people regard themselves favorably. When achievement approximates aspirations in a valued area, high self-esteem develops; low self-esteem results from a discrepancy between aspirations and achievement.

Similarly, Mead (1934) elaborated on James' social self by addressing the process by which people become compatible and integrated members of their social group. In this process, people internalize the ideas and attitudes expressed by the key figures in their lives through observing their actions and attitudes and often unknowingly adopting them as their own. Mead's formulations led to the notion that self-esteem largely derives from the reflected appraisals of others.

Current Theories on the Origins of Self-Esteem

Horney (1950), focusing on the interpersonal processes influential in the development of self-esteem, postulated that feelings of helplessness and isolation constitute key determinants of self-esteem and sources of "basic anxiety." According to Horney, anxiety occurs in situations characterized by domination, indifference, lack of respect, disparagement, and lack of admiration and warmth, as well as in situations of isolation and discrimination.

In many families, parents dominate children, fail to acknowledge their accomplishments, and find fault rather than praise for their actions. If they earn a B, the parents question why it was not an A. These children grow up questioning their competency. Their lack of faith in their abilities and diminished self-regard generate considerable anxiety in adulthood as they frequently question whether they are adequate and as capable as others. In a later section, methods for dealing with such anxieties are discussed, since nurses are by no means immune to feelings of low self-esteem.

Sullivan (1953) accepted Mead's interpretation of the social origins of personality and emphasized the interpersonal relationships influencing self-esteem. According to Sullivan, other people play a significant role in the development of self-esteem for each person.

Based on a review of many early views of self-esteem, Coopersmith (1967) described four major factors contributing to the development of self-esteem. First, stating that the most significant factor in the enhancement of self-esteem was respectful, accepting, and concerned treatment from significant others, Coopersmith concluded that people develop their self-esteem in accordance with how others view and value them. Second, a history of previous successes, position, and status contribute to self-esteem. Third, a person's values and aspirations influence the interpretation and modification of experiences; thus the degree of felt success influences status in the community. Success and status achievements for one person may seem totally insignificant to another. Fourth, a person's manner of responding to devaluation also affects self-esteem; some people defend themselves against negative responses more effectively than others.

Branden (1969) said that no other value judgment is more important to people than their self-estimates, since self-esteem has a profound effect on thinking processes, emotions, desires, values, and goals. Combs (1965) extended Branden's emphasis on the significance of self-esteem to say that what people believe about themselves affects every aspect of functioning. Clinard's (1971) synthesis of the concept of self states that when interpreting events around them, people sort out the meaning of an occurrence in terms of their individual self-perceptions.

SOCIALIZATION AND SOCIAL ROLES

Social behavior must be acquired; it is not present at birth but rather develops through socialization with others. Almost all behavior results from social interaction and is modified in response to the demands and expectations of others (Clinard, 1971). People acquire social roles linked to status and position and with a set of role prescriptions that influence actions. In addition, each person plays a number of roles, depending on age, sex, social class, occupation, and birth order in the family. Although considerable socialization occurs in childhood, it continues into later life as people encounter new situations.

Social behavior develops not only as people actually respond to one another but also in accordance with their perceptions of the responses of others. For example, people respond to one another in different ways when they perceive the reaction of the others to be anger rather than joy. A frown can represent anger in some people, while others frown when in deep contemplation.

Socialization, then, represents the learning of roles and refers to the "process by which the individual acquires the skills, knowledge, attitudes, values, and motives necessary for performance of social roles" (Sewell, 1963, p. 163). According to Clinard (1971, p. 176), "the required behaviors (habits, beliefs, attitudes and motives) are an individual's prescribed roles; the requirements themselves are the role prescriptions." Interactions as well as specific positions affect *role prescriptions,* or the script that occupants of a position enact. In addition, because of the complexity of life situations, some people play more roles than others. Hence, *role strain* results from situations requiring complex role demands and the fulfillment of multiple roles. Whether or not a new role or a change in self takes place depends on several factors, including the following:

1. Whether the proposed new role enhances the person's self-perception or fulfills a basic need
2. Whether the new role is compatible with the person's other roles
3. How clearly defined the new role expectation is
4. Whether a transitional procedure is available in the acquisition of the new role

How Roles are Learned

Never static, roles are constantly changing as a result of maturation processes, external stressors, and unique life situations. The earliest lessons about roles occur in families when children are taught the expected ways to behave in social situations. The next significant form of intentional role instruction occurs in schools when children are rapidly and clearly apprised of the expected behaviors. At this point, children learn that others hold expectations about what their actions should be.

Behavior that is rewarded is repeated, and both boys and girls are rewarded for sex-specific behaviors. In childhood, girls have a greater range of behaviors available to them in that they can be both feminine and tomboyish without causing consternation. In contrast, society expects young boys to rapidly develop masculine behaviors and avoid any sign of femininity.

Stereotypes also affect the roles members of different groups hold. The communications media typically portray women as consumers and housewives, often depicted as nurturing, emotionally unstable, weak, intuitive, inconsistent, dependent, passive, sensitive, and interpersonally oriented creatures (Dean, 1982, p. 251). In contrast, the media characterize men as aggressive, independent, competitive, task-oriented, stoic, analytical, rational, self-disciplined, objective, and confident. The traits attributed to men tend to be more highly valued by society. These stereotypes influence behavior because roles do not exist in isolation, but rather role behavior results from interactions in which one individual (or group) responds to the behavior of another.

Society specifies behaviors for people in specific roles. According to Biddle (1979, p. 5), the most common notion in role theory associates roles with social positions or an "identity that designates a commonly recognized set of persons." The terms *nurse, physician, mother, sister,* and *brother* all refer to recognized sets of people. Members of a given social position exhibit a common role because of expectations attached to that role.

SOCIALIZATION IN THE NURSING ROLE

It has been said that female nurses are "twice socialized"; first into their roles as women in a paternalistic society and then into their roles as wives or mothers in the hospital or health care agency family (Milauskas, 1985). A thorough treatment of the historical process of socialization of nurses is not presented here, but selected aspects of this socialization are discussed to emphasize the importance of assertiveness in nursing practice.

Several unique features in nurse-physician relationships

have influenced the socialization of nurses. Historically, nurses have been expected to be subservient to physicians. Deference to the physician developed from a variety of factors, including the following: physicians tended to be older when they began their practice than were nurses; physicians initially came from a higher socioeconomic class than nurses; society recognized physicians as experts who cured them and therefore were willing to reward them with money and admiration.

Faculty in schools of nursing have, in the past, reinforced the idea that nurses were subservient to physicians. Nursing schools have not traditionally encouraged students to question persons in authority in the health care system. Kalisch and Kalisch (1977) noted that nursing schools have not traditionally generated bold and fearless thinkers. In some instances the creative, questioning student with the highly stimulated mind has been labeled a "troublemaker." Fortunately, this tendency has changed and students are expected to have inquiring minds, to question faculty, and to seek new and better ways to practice nursing.

Certainly, there have always been assertive nurses who defied efforts to be socialized into a passive role. Often these were the most respected nurses in an agency; they dared to stand up for the profession and their beliefs. In recent years the need for nurses to become vigorous proponents of quality care has increased, and assertiveness has been viewed as an easily applied tool to stimulate advocacy for clients and the profession of nursing.

ASSERTIVE STYLE OF BEHAVIOR

There is a common misconception that being assertive means being "pushy." In fact, *assertive behavior* is defined as "standing up for personal rights and expressing thoughts, feelings, and beliefs in direct, honest and appropriate ways which do not violate another person's rights" (Lange and Jakubowski, 1976, p. 7). Basically, assertive communication declares to the world, "This is how I perceive and interpret the situation; this is what I see, think, and feel." Assertive behavior develops most readily when a person has a healthy self-esteem and projects confidence and assurance. Assertive behavior at its best takes into account the rights and needs of all persons involved in the interaction. An assertive community health nurse might say to a client, "I can't schedule a routine visit on Tuesday—I can come on Monday or Wednesday."

Contrasting Styles

In contrast to being assertive, nurses' behavior may be either nonassertive or aggressive. Nonassertive actions generally deny the self by failing to express thoughts, beliefs, and emotions honestly. The nonassertive style implies, "My thoughts and feelings don't count. I am not as important as you. Take advantage of me. I aim to please others and avoid conflict." Nonassertive people often let others make choices for them. By forfeiting their rights to make their own choices and decisions, nonassertive people elicit responses of disgust or pity from those whom they seek to please. For example, because of an inability to say "no" a nurse may schedule so many home visits that she is frazzled at the end of the day, thereby doing a disservice to herself and her clients. *Nonassertive behavior* does not help nurses develop nor maintain good relationships with patients, physicians, or colleagues.

Aggressive behavior, in contrast to nonassertiveness, occurs when people infringe on the rights of others while standing up for their own rights. Aggressiveness implies "My thoughts and feelings are more important than yours. You have no right to be different from me. I plan to dominate and win even if you lose in the process." While *aggressive behavior* may help people meet short-term goals or have their way temporarily through intimidation, it generally prevents the development of good relationships. The intent of aggressiveness is to dominate: "aggression is a hostile, insensitive, and socially inappropriate attack that demeans, coerces and humiliates others" (Jenkins, 1982, p. 52).

Assertive Rights

Assertiveness purports that people have basic interpersonal rights. Specifically, people have a basic right to be respected as unique persons of worth and to express who they are in ways judged to be appropriate. Each one has the right to express thoughts, feelings, opinions, doubts, and preferences without feeling guilty as well as the right to decide how best to use resources—time, property, and one's body—to help meet personal goals. Responsibility to be fair and reasonable and to accept the consequences of one's behavior accompanies these rights. The responsibilities to the profession and to the team influence the behavior of nurses.

Recognizing Choices

Assertive behavior creates an atmosphere of openness in which people can engage in mutual goal setting and action toward reaching their goals while recognizing the uniqueness, strengths, and limitations of others. A key element in developing skills of assertive behavior is the recognition of the choices available to participants in every situation. Often, nurses limit themselves when they fail to recognize their ever present range of choices. Assertiveness training helps participants recognize, evaluate, and act on their choices. An assertive philosophy recognizes that although circumstances and the behavior of others may be beyond nurses' control, they can control their own responses.

On occasion, people may choose not to be assertive. Choosing to remain silent is not the same as remaining silent because of anxiety or failure to see other choices. People may choose not to be assertive when the other person would profit from learning and practicing assertiveness. Nurturing nurses may want to do more than is best for the client. People benefit from doing for themselves; however, nurses often do for clients what they could do for themselves with instruction and practice. There may also be situations when the perceived penalty for being assertive may outweigh the benefits gained. For instance, an opinion may be withheld when it is unnecessary or when it may distract persons or a team from moving toward common goals. This risk must be estimated and taken into account. In reality, people choose daily which opinions, ideas, and feelings to assert and which to refrain from asserting. The sense of actively making choices gives nurses a sense of being in control, an important component of self-esteem.

Self-Assessment

Where can nurses begin? Assertiveness starts wherever people are in their personal development through a program of small, systematic, gradually learned, and practiced steps. The first step includes a personal assessment. Self-assessment may be done individually or in a group or class where the interaction serves as a catalyst for each nurse. Research reported by McIntyre, Jeffrey, and McIntyre (1984) points to the validity of a group approach to assertiveness training with professional nurses. Involvement with peers offers support and a sense of "fun" to the learning process.

Increasing self-awareness usually accompanies assertiveness. As people become aware of how their thoughts, emotions, and intentions influence their behavior as well as how others respond to their behavior, they become better able to modify behavior and more effective in interpersonal relationships. Just because assertiveness can be simply described in a sentence does not mean it is a simple process! It takes persistence and patience to develop new, more satisfying ways of behaving—persistence in the practice of the skills and patience with oneself in a slow, but rewarding process of growth. Just as patterns of behaving in a certain way do not develop overnight, major shifts from either nonassertiveness or aggressiveness to assertiveness will not occur instantly. Furthermore, setbacks do occur. Remember, though, each assertive action is a step forward in promoting health by exercising the full range of rights and privileges. As nurses learn to be assertive, they can teach these behaviors to others including clients, families, students, and colleagues.

Assertiveness is really a style of living and interacting in the broadest sense. For purposes of learning, the style may be characterized as having a number of facets or aspects that can be discussed separately though each facet is only part of the person's style.

SKILLS FOR BEING ASSERTIVE
Nonverbal Components of Assertive Behavior

Body language communicates more than words about self-image and confidence, as Figure 31-1 illustrates. As the old saying goes, "A picture is worth a thousand words." Thus the picture or image nurses present conveys a great deal about both the individual nurse and the profession. Assertive nurses convey with their entire bodies through erect posture and with feet firmly on the ground, "I am a person of value, worth paying attention to." Level, steady eye contact also communicates willingness and readiness to see and be seen and inspires self-confidence as well as the confidence of patients and professional colleagues. Eyes cast downward often accompany nonassertive behavior and communicate insecurity.

Appropriate voice tone and loudness, facial expressions, and hand gestures emphasize an assertive message. For example, a whispered message with eyes downcast conveys different information about the nurse than a message delivered in a clear, carefully modulated tone of voice with the nurse looking directly into the eyes of the listener. A nurse's view of self and others is communicated by the total person—body language as well as the way of speaking the chosen words. Behavior that says to others "I have a right to take up space in the world" increases the individual nurse's self-esteem and invites others to believe and affirm the person's worthiness. Assertive behavior actually stimulates assertive behavior in others and teaches others the necessity for fair, professional treatment.

Speaking Clearly

The core of assertive behavior is taking responsibility for self. Nurses, like other people, acknowledge self-responsibility primarily by using "I" messages—"I think," "I feel," "I want" rather than the commonly used "You should" or

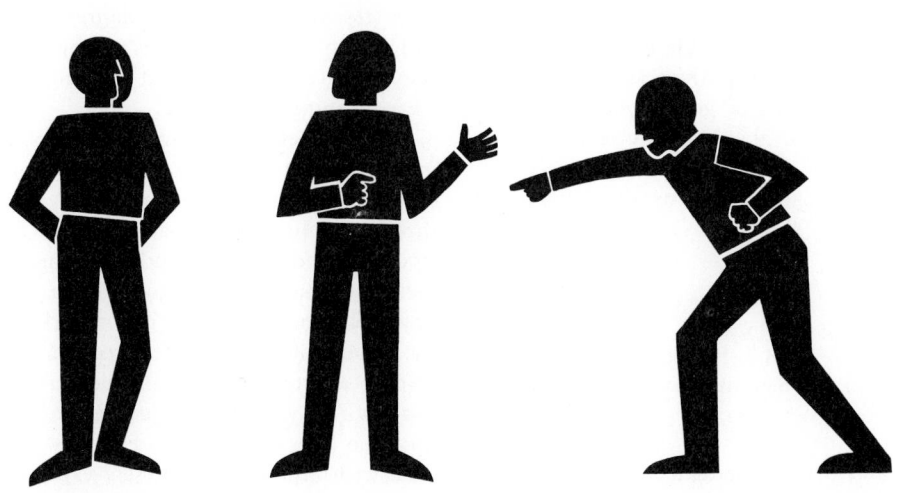

FIGURE 31-1

Body language makes a difference.

"You did." The use of "I" messages minimizes the likelihood that the other person will feel defensive and simultaneously creates an atmosphere of trust. For example, people respond more positively to "I want you to turn in a neat, typed paper" rather than "You always turn in messy, hand-written and hard to read papers." Such messages do not eliminate conflict, which is always possible when people interact. However, the messages foster problem-solving and give the listener an opportunity to know the speaker through self-disclosure. What people disclose of themselves gives others information about their self-image, values, and goals; they reveal who they are and what makes them tick. Self-disclosure is always risky, for others may not like what one reveals, but the potential reward is affection and respect from others. Action always involves risk; the alternative is to be passive and safe.

Steady, nonhesitant speech has the best chance of communicating confidence. Elimination of "uhs" and "ahs" is a step toward assertive speaking. Good eye contact, voice of appropriate loudness, suitable hand and arm gestures, and erect but relaxed posture constitute assertive speaking. When speaking, nurses should make their messages complete and specific and should include all the information the other person needs to understand the message.

> *Incomplete message*
> Nurse: "Your recovery depends on proper eating."
> Patient to herself: "I wonder if that means I have to give up chocolate bars?"
> *More complete message*
> Nurse: "If you are to recover, your diet should contain foods from each of the four groups listed on this page and a limited amount of refined sugar."

Similarly, the verbal and nonverbal aspects of the message must be congruent to avoid the confusion that typically results from mixed messages. When the voice says one thing and the body another, most people hear the nonverbal message. Gentle words accompanied by rough and hurtful handling convey a message of anger or apathy or both.

A facet of clear speech is behavior description that leaves no doubt about what is being discussed. Describing behavior means reporting specific, observable actions of others without placing a value judgment on them as good or bad and without making accusations or generalizations about the other's motives, attitudes, or personality traits. Such objective descriptions enable participants to hear what is being said with the least chance of the listener's becoming defensive.

> *Examples of behavior description*
> Supervisor to nurse: "Mrs. Brown, you have been late to work three times in the last 2 weeks."
> Administrator to nurse: "Mary, I've noticed that you haven't said anything in staff meeting today and you look unhappy."

After a behavior description, a statement of feeling can be added, using "I" messages that are honest and direct without carrying the threat of judgment.

> *Examples of statements of feeling*
> Supervisor to nurse: "When you are late, Mrs. Brown, I'm frustrated because I have the responsibility for seeing that every job is covered. I like your work and wonder what we can do about the situation."
> Administrator to nurse: "I'm afraid the proposal we just discussed doesn't suit you and that you are hesitant to say so. I would like to have your opinion before we reach a final decision."

In both examples, the speaker assumes a problem-solving attitude and invites a collaborative effort for mutual benefit. The message is honest, clear, and nondefensive. Such messages make no value judgments or inferences about the nurse as a person or about other unrelated characteristics of the person. Clear, direct, descriptive messages should also be given to clients. For example, in the following material it is much more supportive of health promotion to discuss lack of compliance with a systematic diet by using the first approach rather than the second.

> Nurse: "Mr. Brown, I am concerned that your blood sugar is high and you have been eating quite a few sweets. Can we reexamine your diet plan and determine how you can reduce sugar and still be satisfied?"
> Nurse: "Mr. Brown, you received an hour and a half of instruction last week about excluding refined sugar from your diet. Don't you want to try to help yourself?"

Note the use of "I" messages in the first example as well as the focus on mutual problem solving. This markedly contrasts with the accusing nature of the second example in which the blame is placed on the client for not adhering to prior nutrition counseling.

Active Listening

Although volumes have been written on the art of listening, many people need to improve this skill. Assertive behavior recognizes the needs and rights of all participants in an interaction; *active listening* is the key to discovering the other person's needs and values.

Communicating the desire to hear and understand is the first step in listening. That desire is communicated largely through body language, such as by facing the speaker, establishing eye contact, and showing with the whole body that listening is the goal.

One can let another know the message is heard by paraphrasing what was said and by affirming the speaker's feelings before making comments. Frequently nurses fail to hear what clients say because they are busy with their own thoughts and needs, including lining up their arguments, before carefully listening to the message. When Mrs. Smith says, "The new medicine is not working," a response such as "You're feeling discouraged that you aren't getting better" affirms her as a valuable person and sets the stage for her to say, "Well, I guess it will take more time." A brusque "It's too soon to tell" may be true but does not deal with Mrs. Smith's present experience.

Active listening lets clients know in a concrete way that you value them and truly want to understand them. Assertive nurses express themselves directly and try to understand their client's needs and desires. Cuming (1982) stated that an important interpersonal skill that gets others to help you meet your goals is projecting the attitude "I'm okay, You're okay." The "I'm okay" attitude is projected largely by "I" messages with appropriate nonverbal action while the "you're okay" message is sent largely through listening, responding with empathy, and drawing others out. One of the goals nurses have in community health settings is enlisting patients' participation in their own health. Listening and building trust are ways to accomplish this end.

Nurses may think that because they are busy and often feel harried and overworked, they don't have time for such amenities. The actual time used in active listening is minimal compared with the value to the client. Actually time may be saved in the long run by hearing the message before responding. Frequently we answer what seems to be the question asked or the concern expressed only to learn later that we were 90 degrees off target. The client may not have been worried about the surgery when she said, "I guess the operation will take a long time," but rather she may have been worried about who would stay with her retarded son if she had to remain in the hospital more than 2 or 3 days.

In taking instructions from a physician or supervisor, the time spent in clarifying and understanding is well spent if the job is done with more competence and understanding. Nurses often think that asking clarifying questions indicates inadequacy or is insulting to the one giving the instructions. Not so! All people are so influenced by their own interpretations of what they hear that they should not assume they understand. This truth is reflected in the epigram, "I know you believe you understand what you think I said but I'm not sure you realize that what you heard is not what I meant."

Dealing with Manipulation

According to Phelps and Austin (1975), *manipulation* is the conscious or unconscious use of indirect and dishonest means to achieve a desired goal. All nurses need attitudes and techniques that allow them to protect themselves from being "used" by others.

Saying "No"

Nurses have the right to set priorities on the use of their time and energy in order to meet their goals. To be able to say "yes" to the priorities, they must say "no" to other things. This presents a dilemma to a profession that has traditionally been "at your service" and to each professional nurse who wants to please everyone (whether consciously or unconsciously). If nurses try to say "yes" to every possibility or request they become fatigued and overstressed and feel inadequate for the high-priority activities in their life and work. Hence, nurses must be vigilant in the use of their time and energy and direct these resources toward accomplishing their goals.

Learning to say "no" is the primary tool to use against manipulation. No one wants to feel or be manipulated.

Nurses do not want to be manipulated by other staff members, physicians, clients, friends, spouses, or children. Likewise, clients do not want to feel used by people in their personal life or by health care providers. However, the way "no" is said is of prime importance. "I" messages delivered firmly and kindly make one's position clear without offending the other person.

"I won't be able to get to that today. I'll be glad to do it tomorrow." Or "Today I was planning to make visits in the community. Is this job more important? If I do your work today, my community visits will have to be delayed. Which takes priority?" In the latter example the nurse adopts a problem-solving stance and invites negotiation toward resolving conflicting demands on time.

Generally the person making the request will stop asking when the "no" is decisively spoken. Hesitant, vague responses say to the asker, "Persuade me." In some situations the most assertive response to a request is to say, "I'll have to check my schedule and let you know if I have some time to do that" or "I'll need to think about that and let you know." Such actions give the nurse time to gather her thoughts carefully and decide on a response without feeling pressured or threatened by the presence of the person making the request. Few requests cannot be delayed a few minutes or even longer if schedules and other factors need to be checked. Nurses often fail to exercise the option of "I'll check and let you know in 10 minutes (tomorrow)." Such reluctance reflects lack of respect for one's rights and privileges as a person of worth. Likewise, clients should be afforded time to consider the alternatives and make careful and thoughtful choices.

Negotiating compromises is an assertive skill worth cultivating. It is appropriate to compromise except when one's integrity is at stake. If a visiting nurse is asked to make a home visit every day and determines that twice a week would be sufficient for the patient's needs, the answer to the original request may be "no" but a workable compromise will be offered. Negotiation as an assertive skill is discussed in depth in a later section.

In the case of a request to obtain drugs or perform a service not within one's professional scope, no compromise should be offered because the nurse's integrity would become an issue. Refusal of such a request might provoke a response of anger and create temporary distance in the relationship, but in the long run the nurse's self-esteem will be increased by such an action. Furthermore, on occasion nurses would be legally jeopardizing their role by not saying "no." To provide services not within the realm of either nursing or appropriate health care is, of course, inadvisable. For example, just because a physician orders an excessive dosage of medication for a home health care client does not mean that the nurse should give it. To do so would make the nurse legally liable for this erroneous action should complications arise.

Manipulative Ploys

It is particularly distressing to feel manipulated and perceive that you have no power to do anything about it. In their efforts to meet personal goals many people use other people's time, talent, and energy. However, such actions cannot happen without one's own participation in the manipulation—good news indeed! So the question becomes: How can nurses protect themselves from manipulation in their professional roles as well as in their personal lives?

The first step, as always, begins with self-awareness about what promotes or allows manipulation to take place. What are the vulnerable areas that a manipulator can touch to get what is desired? Most people, including nurses, respond to various ploys outlined by Chenevert (1978), and several are discussed in the following paragraphs.

FLATTERY. How many people are unresponsive to *flattery*? Each person has one or more areas vulnerable to "buttering-up" efforts. An assertive nurse certainly wants to be able to accept a genuine compliment graciously and yet resist the urge to comply with a request from a flatterer simply because that person's regard is highly valued. Therefore, one must learn to differentiate between flattery and an honest and sincerely delivered compliment. For example, two nurses at a home health care agency have equal client loads yet Ms. Jones seems to be more efficient than Ms. Smith. On a rainy Friday when Ms. Smith is running late in getting started with her home visits, she is overheard saying to Ms. Jones, "You know your new hairstyle really looks great. You look younger and more excited about life these days," Ms. Jones replies, "Thanks, I appreciate your opinion; that makes my day." (Pause.) "By the way," says Ms. Smith, "would you mind visiting Mr. Hall for me? I'll just never finish by four if I have to drive to his home. Anyway, he has always liked you better." Manipulators exploit the human desire to be needed and often feign helplessness to get what they want. Female nurses may be more inclined toward this kind of behavior because of their socialization, but men are certainly not immune to it.

ASSUMING RESPONSIBILITY. Nurses need to resist the urge to rush in and "rescue" the situation when the other person is capable of assuming personal responsibility. For example, if a client is trying to decide how to manage the details of her recovery, she may ask the nurse, "What do you think I should do?" Responsible action may include assisting the client to consider alternatives and solve her own problem. Nurses should not assume the decision-making role for clients. Taking over may stem from an innate desire to be helpful to other people; however, every person has strengths that outnumber weaknesses, and often the way to be most helpful is to help others stand on their own feet. It generally is a disservice to do for others what they can be taught to do for themselves. Such behavior actually deprives the recipient of independence and personal integrity by conveying "I really don't think you can do. . . ."

SENSE OF OBLIGATION. A *sense of obligation* or duty may make nurses vunerable to manipulation. Women, particularly in American culture, have been taught to feel responsible for the welfare and happiness of others. Mutual, freely accepted obligations go with any relationship, professional or personal, and nurses must not allow themselves to get out of balance in this area.

INSECURITY. *Insecurity* occasionally makes people suscep-tible to manipulation. Those who know you can play on your particular fears to get agreement on any number of things. Nurses should become aware of their individual fears so they can protect themselves against those who would use fears maliciously. Common fears include fear of being replaced (the nurse may agree to all sorts of extra tasks), fear that love or approval will be withdrawn (the nurse may comply with unreasonable demands), fear of what people will think (nurses may hesitate to take risks that are in their interest), or fear of offending someone (nurses may hesitate to express their opinion even when it is needed).

GUILT. Skilled manipulators use *guilt* as one of their primary weapons. Feelings of guilt persuade nurses to do things they would not consider or choose otherwise. Guilt feelings, easily evoked in many nurses, make assertiveness difficult. For example, in the previous encounter between the nurses, Ms. Smith could have played on her colleague's feeling of guilt by continuing with "If you won't help me by visiting Mr. Hill, I probably will have to skip his bed bath and that sure would be a step backward in all the hard work we have done to prevent him from getting a decubitus ulcer." A nurse, troubled by dysfunctional guilt, may benefit from rethinking the ideas that underline these feelings, which will be discussed in the later section, "Why are nurses not more assertive?"

CRITICISM. *Criticism* is the weapon that manipulators use with more success than all others. When one is criticized, all those old feelings of inadequacy surface from childhood. Even a mature, professional nurse who has accepted that being human also means being imperfect must relearn this lesson from time to time. However, when one's self-esteem is high, criticism can be evaluated and used for personal and professional growth and development.

Most people respond to criticism in two characteristic ways—either by denial or defense. Both responses are generally accompanied by anxiety, which blocks evaluation of the criticism. As Smith (1975) said, people need to develop skills that can minimize the typical emotional response of anxiety to criticism. They need coping behaviors to enable them to feel comfortable when they are reminded of some truth about themselves which is interpreted, explicitly or implicitly, as wrongdoing in another person's value system. Furthermore, nurses need coping skills to help them feel comfortable with their errors that may have been inefficient, wasteful, awkward, or stupid but have nothing to do with right or wrong.

According to Smith (1975), a change in external verbal behavior in the face of criticism allows for internal changes, for example, less anxiety and more assertive behavior. To facilitate such changes, Smith suggested several techniques that may be used to protect oneself from criticism.

TECHNIQUES FOR PROTECTING AGAINST CRITICISM

Constructive criticism can be useful and encourage growth; manipulative criticism can render people vulnerable. Several techniques for dealing with criticism are described below. These techniques serve to interrupt a pattern of criticism; they do not necessarily facilitate open discussion, but they can defuse a potentially negative situation by terminating the criticism.

Fogging refers to the technique of agreeing with truth, agreeing in principle, or agreeing with the odds. It is called "fogging" because the person criticized reacts much like a fog bank—without reaction. A nurse might use such a response with a patient who complaints chronically. When the patient says, "You are late getting here again. You certainly took your sweet time," the nurse might respond, "You are right. I might have gotten here earlier" (agreeing with truth). If the patient then responds, "It seems like nurses should get to the patient as soon as possible," the nurse's fogging response might be, "It certainly does seem the nurse should be there when the patient is sick" (agreeing in principle). If the patient then says, "I guess I could have died and no one would have known it," the nurse might respond, "I suppose that is possible" (agreeing with the odds).

Lange and Jakubowski (1976) question the use of fogging because it is not straight communication and could be manipulative if carried to extremes. They prefer a more direct assertion in the face of criticism. While their comment is worth considering, fogging does have a place in developing a repertoire of assertive skills. Fogging is useful in situations where the criticism has been discussed repeatedly or where one just does not want to "get into it" at that time. In no case should fogging be used to prevent listening to criticism offered. For example, if an instructor or supervisor is criticizing behaviors involved in carrying out nursing actions, fogging is not usually applicable. Instructors and supervisors want to discuss, rather than avoid, the issue.

Negative assertion is a more active assertive skill described by Smith (1975). Negative assertion openly admits negative things about oneself, acknowledging that perfection is not one's goal. This technique helps change verbal behavior and modify the belief that guilt is automatically associated with making a mistake. If your supervisor says, "You did not handle that situation in a very professional manner," and you recognize the truth of the criticism, you might respond, "You're right, I was rather awkward." Professional nurses want to do what they can to rectify errors after admitting them. The skill of negative inquiry discussed in the next paragraph offers a way of discovering how the mistake can be corrected or avoided in the future.

Negative inquiry is the most assertive skill available to cope with criticism, according to Smith (1975). In essence, it involves prompting more information about statements of wrongdoing in an unemotional, low-key manner. The criticizer can then state what is wanted through the help of the questions asked by the criticized person. In the example just given where the first response was negative assertion, the next response (negative inquiry) might be "What do you think I might do next time that would be more professional?" Nurses must be careful not to become sarcastic as they ask the question because verbal aggression may trigger an aggressive response. Often the tone of voice may give an aggressive ring to a response such as the example just given. The same words spoken angrily would carry a different message than if spoken with sincerity and honesty.

In professional relationships the use of negative inquiry can let the supervisor know a nurse wants to do a good job and will listen to suggestions about how to improve performance. This technique also indicates that one does not crumple under criticism but rather listens and uses the information for professional development. Negative inquiry can also be a way of soliciting regular, constructive feedback that will help improve the handling of the job.

> Supervisor: "I have been concerned, Mrs. Brown, about the way you have been doing your job lately."
> Nurse: "What have your concerns been?"
> Supervisor: "I understand you have been giving the insulin injection to your diabetic patients when they come for their clinic appointments."
> Nurse: "What would be a better way for me to handle that?"
> Supervisor: "It would be more helpful to ask them to demonstrate their self-injection practices so that you can evaluate their skill and accuracy with these techniques."

Through negative inquiry the person who is criticized can learn what the specific behavior in question means to the critic and what is really wanted in the situation. Using criticism for growth is one more assertive skill to help nurses do a good job and feel good about themselves.

Assertive behavior therapy and education historically have focused on the "standing up" behaviors that help people protect their rights and prevent manipulation by others. An often neglected, though crucial, aspect of being assertive is the ability or capacity to behave in ways that build relationships and that help in approaching and getting closer to others, sometimes called "soft" assertions. Many people have great difficulty expressing affection, tenderness, appreciation, and caring. Nurses, as caring professionals, can augment their competence through verbal and nonverbal expressions of warmth and compassion.

SKILLS FOR BUILDING RELATIONSHIPS
Compliments

Giving and receiving compliments presents problems for many. To offer a compliment puts one at risk of rejection or even ridicule. For example, if you say, "You did a good job today with that client," and the response is "It was really nothing. Anyone could have done better," you might become discouraged and hesitate to voice your approval next time.

The person who receives a compliment by down-grading the giver reduces the possibility of future compliments and fails to acknowledge the giver. Both parties to the interaction probably feel vaguely uneasy and discouraged. Everyone needs reinforcement from others and each of us needs to learn to accept that reinforcement in an assertive manner.

"Thank you" is the only necessary reply to a compliment. That response acknowledges the giver and allows the receiver to accept the compliment and be warmed by it. Of course, you may add to the "thank you" a phrase such as "I appreciate your saying that," "It feels good to know you liked that," or "I'm glad I did the job well, I've worked hard at it."

Making Conversation

Making conversation is the starting point for every relationship. Without the basic skills used in conversation people become isolated from others, personally and professionally. The first step is to speak up! Say something. The discussion in the earlier section, Speaking Clearly, applies here.

Everything that is said discloses something of the speaker and can be a conversation starter. Generally the more you disclose of yourself, the more you will receive of the other. A warning—too much too soon can frighten the listener. Few people want instant intimacy in the beginning of a relationship. The amount of self-disclosure sets the limits of intimacy and lets the other person know what is acceptable to discuss.

Every disclosure is information for the other person to use in developing the conversation. Listening for the free information, that is, information given not in response to a direct question, gives possible subjects for further discussion. The listener then has choices about which information to respond to.

> Patient: I really wish my children could be here while I'm in the hospital, but they all live so far away and they're so busy. My son on the farm lives especially far away; it's about time for the harvest, so he couldn't possibly come. And all the grandchildren have to be taken care of."

What shall the nurse respond to when there is so much information given freely? Some possible responses might be: "Tell me more about your family." "I wonder if you're feeling a bit neglected since they aren't here?" "You want your grandchildren to come first even though you'd like your children here. How many grandchildren do you have?" "Where do your children live?" Or you might respond "So one of your children is a farmer. I grew up on a farm and I know timing is important for the harvesting." This latter response gives information about the nurse which establishes a common interest.

Developing a Support Network

The development of the social skills of conversation helps nurses develop a support system—a network of relationships that builds self-esteem, provides camaraderie and companionship, and thereby nurtures the professional care giver. All people need a resource group whose presence in their lives can help them both to *be* and to *become*. A special pleasure is provided by friends—those trusted people with whom mutual give and take is experienced. As Francis Bacon said, "Friendship redoubleth joys and cutteth griefs in halves."

A functional support network may include relationships other than traditional friends. An older, more experienced nurse may become a mentor or a guide through the professional labyrinth. A mentor gives support and feedback while fledgling nurses develop professional identity and learn to trust their own judgment. More experienced professionals provide role models whom a novice can admire, respect, and emulate. Frequently, a professor, supervisor, or more experienced colleague fills this role. Asserting one's needs

and asking for guidance may help in locating a mentor. Some supervisors are unable to serve as mentors because they are threatened by the competence of those they supervise while others are uncaring about the professional development of colleagues.

There may also be support people who challenge nurses to grow, who believe in their talent, and who offer encouragement as they grow and develop. Common interests also provide the base of some relationships—a colleague with whom racquetball or a passion for mystery novels is shared. Some occasions call for a confidante who willingly offers a listening ear without judgment, who holds the mirror so oneself can be seen, and who encourages the next step in growth.

A common thread in all the different kinds of relationships nurses might have is the sense of strength that comes from the relationships. All people need others who enhance their lives through support, affirmation, sense of humor, and even challenge and caring confrontation. Nurses feel more able to cope after encounters with such people. These encounters serve as buffers between the nurse and the relationships and situations that threaten one's self-esteem and sense of competence. Bergman (1985) cites the need for nurses to reward each other for assertive behavior as well as for teachers to reward students and for nurses to reward patients and clients. Herman (1978) says it is essential for nurses to have good emotional support and honest feedback, to be available for one another, and share the successes as well as the stresses.

WHY ARE NURSES NOT MORE ASSERTIVE?

The traditionally female nursing profession has defined itself in terms of the feminine cultural stereotype—passive and dependent. This belief system blocks individual nurses and the profession as a whole. The belief of nurses (both male and female) that they are to play a secondary, subservient role retards the development of assertive behavior patterns. Early conditioning into sex roles is difficult to transcend; however, it must be done if nurses intend to take their proper place on the health care team.

Fear

Fear blocks effective functioning for many nurses. Fear of rejection and fear of inadequacy retard many nurses' ability to be actively involved in decision making in their practice. These fears may contribute to a self-defeating cycle when they inhibit assertive behavior. Nonassertive behavior is often followed by a decrease in self-esteem and an increase in anxiety. The pattern is dysfunctional to a professional nurse; it may be altered by learning more effective assertive behavior.

Anxiety

Anxiety blocks the development of assertive behavior. Because nurses deal with high-stress situations, they must learn to monitor and reduce their anxiety in both present and long-term situations.

Chapter 30 discusses ways nurses can deal with their own anxiety and also teach clients to manage stress and anxiety.

One anxiety-reducing method is progressive relaxation, a deep-muscle relaxation method developed by Jacobson (1974) and based on the tensing and relaxing of specific muscle groups. It can be used to develop awareness of early signs of tension so measures can be taken to relax (see Chapter 30 for a description of the specific process). The more nurses can be aware of their own early anxiety responses, the more they can take charge of combating them through relaxation.

Creative imagery, another relaxation method discussed in detail in Chapter 30, focuses on releasing tensions through deep breathing and imagery, using mental scenes of pleasant places, and visualizing words such as "calm" or "relax."

Lack of clarity about the role of nurses has created confusion and anxiety in the minds of nurses, clients, and other health providers. The image of nursing must be redefined if the profession is to grow in scope of practice. A more definite assertive image—or belief about nursing as a profession—can help nurses and the public develop a more realistic view.

Belief System

The development of a positive belief system is one element in the process of becoming more assertive. Nurses must believe that "assertion, rather than manipulation, submission, or hostility enriches life and ultimately leads to more satisfying personal relationships with people" (Lange and Jakubowski, 1976, p. 55). Assertive styles of interaction that grow out of rational thinking patterns enhance professional relationships. Fortunately, nurses can identify irrational thinking patterns that underlie ineffectual behavior and can substitute more productive thought processes through conscious rethinking of their perceptions of a situation.

Ellis (1977) has made a persuasive case that faulty behavior is caused by irrational beliefs. Based on the belief that "men's minds are disturbed not by events, but by their interpretation of events," he developed a system of exploring and challenging beliefs so one can develop a rational belief system that leads to effective behavior. Believing one is "dumb," "inadequate," or "only a nurse" can block expressions of positive thoughts and feelings. Such self-labeling, says Burns (1980) leads to procrastination and lethargy. Being assertive with yourself in facing your negative thoughts (cognitive distortions) can open the door to more realistic and effective ways of dealing with the world and other people.

Lack of Assertiveness Skills

Lack of appropriate skill is probably the largest block to assertive behavior. Early conditioning, sex role stereotyping, peer pressure, and low self-esteem are among the factors that inhibit the development of adequate skills of interaction and assertiveness. Nurses can learn needed skills by taking classes for that purpose, by reading, and by practicing. Proficiency in any skill develops through practice. A planned program of small steps developed in a group or on your own can set the stage for the persistent practice that

reaps such great rewards for nurses. The support of a network will augment a program of personal and professional growth. As they begin to take small steps, many feel more confident immediately, and the confidence then encourages taking the next step. Success indeed builds on success.

HANDLING CONFLICT ASSERTIVELY

In any organization in which nurses are likely to work, conflict is inevitable; conflict is a normal occurrence when people work together. However, conflict is often viewed as a disruptive force that should be avoided whenever possible. In applying assertive skills and standing up for personal rights, conflict should not be ignored. It must be recognized, understood, and resolved. One way to do so is by using negotiation skills. Before exploring the strategy of negotiation, the nature of conflict needs to be briefly reviewed.

Conflict can be either constructive or destructive. When used solely for personal gain or to work out hidden angers or when directed toward the demise of another person, it is a destructive force. However, conflict is a clue that something is amiss and thus should generate the need for open communication and problem solving.

Conflict arises for a variety of reasons. One reason may be that each participant in a situation does not have the same information. One missing fact may completely alter the perception of a situation; thus clear communication, as previously mentioned, is one way to minimize conflict.

Another source of conflict lies in incompatible goals among participants. When new ideas or plans are to be implemented, it is important to have participants carefully describe their own goals for the project. This process is complex because people tend to be guarded about some goals. When the level of trust is low or when competitiveness is particularly keen, people may be unwilling to share their own goals openly for fear of weakening their position relative to that of their opponent. Such people are said to have a "hidden agenda."

Whether conflict enhances the functioning of the involved parties, leads to a stalemate, or causes major hostilities within the group depends on how it is handled. Constructive handling of conflict leads to individual and group growth. Should a conflict arise in a work group as to the best method for handling a client situation, a variety of alternatives exist. The following are four common responses to conflict. First, some members could persuasively convince the others that only one approach would work. Second, people may withdraw from the discussion if their point of view is not accepted. Third, members can become aggressive and may personally attack one another's point of view. Fourth, participants could engage in a thorough discussion of all possible alternatives and collectively arrive at a solution.

The advantages of handling conflict via active group discussion include:

1. When participants present their points of view, everyone has the opportunity to gain a broader view of the problem.
2. When open discussion takes place, participants have

more alternatives to consider. People generate more alternatives when they disagree than when they agree.

3. Lively discussion encourages active participation and discourages apathy and withdrawal (Fisher, 1985).

Conflict resolution can occur when participants do not feel threatened by different views and when there is a commitment to open handling of the issue. Stepsis (1974) purports that conflict resolution strategies can be categorized as avoidance, defusing (or cooling down), and confrontation. Although each strategy has both positive and negative features, confrontation seems most consistent with assertiveness skills.

Confrontation, assertiveness, and negotiation use many of the same principles for guiding behavior. Prerequisites for confrontation useful for promoting an environment of assertiveness or negotiation include the following (Thurkettle and Jones, 1978, p. 40):

1. Willingness and ability of participants to accurately identify the issue
2. Open communication, including astute, active listening
3. Focusing on the issues, not the people involved
4. Mutual responsibility for the communication outcome

Confrontation

Smoyak (1974, p. 1632) describes *confrontation* as a "concept, a process, and a technique" with application in nursing practice. Confrontation, like assertiveness, is not "telling the other person off" but rather is a problem-solving strategy for conflict resolution. Confrontation skills, which are briefly discussed here, are quite compatible with the negotiation process described later.

Confrontation is essentially a three-stage process: assessment, direct confrontation, and resettlement. The first step, assessment, can be carried out by asking the questions in the box below. As can be seen from these questions, assessment includes *who* is involved, *what* is the issue or problem, *what* are possible consequences, and *how* is the discussion going to be handled. Confrontation is a direct approach, like assertiveness, which deals only with the identified problem. Side issues are not drawn in nor is attention

directed toward the participant's personal attributes. In confrontation all participants are apprised of the need for an open discussion about the conflict. Preplanning as to issues, participants, time, and place are part of the assessment process.

The second step, implementation or direct confrontation, is composed of basic skills of communication. Key points include sticking to the facts, handling only one subject at a time, and avoiding any interruption of other speakers. No matter how much a person may want to clarify, defend, explain, and so on, it is essential to listen carefully to what the other party has to say. People have the innate tendency to begin defending their behavior before they have heard the speaker's entire message. Once each participant has presented the issues, it is helpful to have each repeat what was heard. This form of feedback provides immediate clarification of any misperception or lack of understanding.

The last stage in confrontation, resettlement, includes agreeing that a problem exists and jointly devising a strategy for resolution. Until this point, only one participant may have perceived that a problem existed. Now it is time to take specific steps to resolve the problem.

> Three students have been assigned to a work group in community health nursing. Their task is to assess a rural community near the university and establish nursing diagnoses and action plans for the community. In the first meeting the students divide the areas to be assessed and agree to meet in two weeks with their information.
>
> During their second meeting, one of the group members, Sue, explains that she has had the flu and has not collected her community data. She assures her group that if they can give her a week's extension she will come well prepared to their next meeting. However, at the next meeting, Sue explains that her car broke down and she was unable to gather much information. She requests another week's extension. What should the other two members do? If they give Sue another extension are they adhering to principles of assertive behavior? Should they confront Sue now or hope she will mobilize her energies and do her part?

During the past week the other two group members had spent time assessing this situation and had decided that a problem exists. Since they have previously been in Sue's class, they know she tends to procrastinate. Thus when they raised questions such as those in the box at left, they decided that Sue's inability to meet her acknowledged obligations was the problem. They are becoming anxious about the outcome of their project and simultaneously getting angry with Sue. They believe that the potential cost to them of Sue's behavior may be an unfinished project on the due date. They decide to confront Sue by explaining that either she will have to negotiate with them for a series of deadlines that she can meet or withdraw from the group and allow them to finish the project without her. The latter option will mean that Sue will have to discuss this situation with their instructor and request a new assignment.

Negotiation

Another strategy that uses principles of communication, conflict resolution, and assertiveness is negotiation. Ways (1979, p. 87) defines *negotiation* as "a process in which two

---

ASSESSMENT QUESTIONS TO BE RAISED WHEN ANTICIPATING AND PLANNING FOR CONFRONTATION

1. What is the problem?
2. What (who) seems to be causing the problem?
3. How is it affecting me? others?
4. How and what kind of power is involved?
5. What kind of changes can be expected as a result of confrontation?
6. What are the potential consequences of a confrontation (positive and negative)?
7. What might be the cost of raising the issue?
8. What might be the cost of ignoring the issue?
9. Who is involved in the situation?

or more parties, who have both common interests and conflicting interests, put forth and discuss explicit proposals concerning specific terms of a possible agreement." Similarly, Cohen (1980, p. 27) describes negotiation as an attempt by two parties to satisfy their mutual needs and involves time, information, and power. According to Cohen, *time* means that most people wait until the deadline is fast approaching before they commence to negotiate. *Information* means learning as much as possible about the situation and participants before the process starts. *Power* is somewhat more complex and is the ability to use resources to achieve goals and influence people and events. Power is influenced by perception; people who believe they have power convey this notion by their actions, posture, and voice tone. Cohen described nine types of power used in negotiations, and these are defined in the box below.

The power component of negotiation is illustrated in the dilemma of a group of students.

The student group was unable to meet the deadline for a group project because an important piece of information was not received from a publishing company in time for them to complete the project on schedule. They believe their request for an extension is legitimate, since they have been conscientious in their efforts; however, their instructor likes work turned in on schedule. The students realize they must negotiate a new deadline and, based on Cohen's power principles, plan their strategy.

First, they carefully organize their position to clearly state their request to their instructor, realizing that a positive anticipatory attitude is necessary. When they approach the instructor, they do so by setting up an appointment, selecting a spokesperson to begin the discussion, and assuming total responsibility for the delay. They present the facts regarding the needed extension, carefully sticking to the issue and posing an alternative deadline without becoming aggressive.

The instructor listens to their recommendation and agrees that situations beyond the students' control led to the delay. The students request a two-week extension which means that their project will be turned in during exam week. The instructor agrees with the concept of an extension but says that receiving the project during the week of final exams will create a personal burden. They brainstorm as to alternative sources of data collection for securing the missing information and agree on a 10-day extension.

In this example of negotiation both the students and the instructor were winners; the students received their much-needed extension and the faculty member arranged to receive the paper before the onslaught of final examination grading. This example illustrates several of Cohen's additional principles of negotiation. First, it points out that negotiation does not need to be a win-lose situation in which one party does all the giving and the other party receives the concession made. Cohen (1980, p. 119) describes a *win-lose* strategy as the "Soviet style" of negotiation, which is most effectively used when there is no continuing relationship between parties, when neither will feel remorse afterward, and when the victim is unaware of the strategy being used. These characteristics do not apply to most ongoing student-faculty interactions, since both parties may feel remorse (Cohen, 1980). Also, students are not generally in a powerful bargaining position because they cannot reward or punish faculty. However, students can gain power in several ways, as illustrated earlier.

A more useful form of negotiation is called *win-win*, in which participants negotiate for mutual interest. As mentioned in the case of the students-instructor negotiation for turning in the paper, win-win forms of negotiation are positive for all participants. The key components of this approach are building trust, gaining commitment, and managing opposition (Cohen, 1980). In this approach participants avoid embarrassing one another in public, and each tries to remain calm and stick to the issues.

As mentioned, negotiation includes time, power, and information. In considering information, one must be aware that negotiation is a process not an event. Before beginning to negotiate participants should gather all relevant information so as not to appear confused and poorly prepared. Throughout the process it is essential to practice active listening to hear clearly what the opponent is really saying.

CLINICAL APPLICATION

Behaving assertively is the basis of an effective interpersonal style; thus it is impossible to separate being an assertive nurse from being a professional, competent, proficient nurse. Being assertive means relating well to oneself through discipline, goal setting, and taking care of oneself. It means relating well to physicians, supervisors, and peers by being reliable, trustworthy, creative, and professional. And it means relating effectively to clients through competent nursing practice and modeling behaviors that enable them to be actively involved in their own treatment.

Assertiveness promotes openness and honesty in all relationships and builds self-esteem in nurses, physicians, and clients. Interactions between people who feel good about themselves have the best chance of being based in reality and offering a win-win outcome.

People are seen by others largely through their behavior.

TYPES OF POWER USEFUL IN NEGOTIATION

1. Power of "knowledge of needs"—what are the verbalized versus the real, yet unstated needs?
2. Power of investment—settlement often follows a substantial investment of time, energy, and money in the process of negotiation.
3. Power of rewarding or punishing—to what extent can the participants help or hinder each other?
4. Power of identification—people will identify with you if you convey knowledge, warmth, and empathy.
5. Power of morality—doing what is right.
6. Power of precedent—"we have always done it this way."
7. Power of persistence—stick to the issue.
8. Power of persuasive capacity—if you are going to persuade me, I have to know what you are saying and it must be overwhelming so that I cannot dispute it.
9. Power of attitude—keep a positive attitude with your emotions under control.

From Cohen, H.: You can negotiate anything. Secaucus, N.J., 1980, Lyle Stuart, Inc.

To develop the repertoire of behaviors called "assertive" allows people to feel good, build relationships, do competent work, solve problems, and live relatively stress-free lives.

Nurses use assertiveness skills in their own lives and teach clients to use these skills. Patients often demonstrate either passive or aggressive behavior in contrast to the positive expression of needs, desires, thoughts, and feelings reflected in assertiveness.

However, once community health nurses learn and become skilled in assertive techniques, it is important to remember that not everyone is going to be pleased with this behavior in nurses or clients. Not all assertive efforts are warmly and enthusiastically received. Assertive behavior can be disruptive to a relationship or environment, since it tends to affect the status quo. Virtually all change meets with some degree of resistance; people whose usual patterns are upset by new assertive actions may seek revenge. Before looking at some typical reactions to the demonstration of assertive behavior, it is useful to discuss the concept of *resistance.*

According to New and Couillard (1981, pp. 17-18), people resist change for one of five reasons:

1. Threatened self-interest in which their perception of personal costs outweigh their anticipated personal benefits
2. Inaccurate perceptions where they do not understand the nature and/or implications of the change
3. Objective disagreement in which the person does not think the change will benefit the organization
4. Psychological reaction that occurs when people perceive that their personal freedom is being threatened
5. Low tolerance for change in which the person understands the change but is emotionally unable to make the transition from the old behavior or situation to the new one

All of these five forms of resistance seem to stem from fear. When one member of a family, social, or work group become more assertive, those influenced by this change wonder how they will be affected. Thus, when changing one's own behavior or teaching others to modify their behavior, it is important to assess who may be affected by these changes. What is their usual or likely reaction to any alterations? Anticipating resistance increases alertness to possible reactions and provides for early resolution of such conflicts.

Alberti and Emmons (1980) describe the most common reactions to assertiveness as being backbiting, aggression, psychosomatic reactions, and revenge. *Backbiting* occurs when someone is displeased with another's behavior; however, rather than approaching the actor directly, the person makes comments to others such as "What's wrong with her these days?" or "Wonder who he thinks he is, anyway?" One must be careful not to respond to backbiting in like fashion but instead ignore these remarks.

Aggressive reactions to assertive behavior are usually verbal. Consider the reaction if a physician ordered a dosage of medication four times the recommended amount. You are a home health care nurse, and the client is in your caseload. Rather than give the incorrect medication, which could have serious effects on the client, you assert yourself by calling the physician and asking him to double-check the order. He immediately yells into the telephone, "No fiesty nurse is going to tell me what to do." He slams down the telephone. Instead of visiting the client you return to the office to consult with your supervisor. As might be expected, the physician has already called your supervisor *and* the director of the agency. Although you know your position was both medically and ethically correct, you begin to wonder if it was really worth all the aggravation. However, you also realize that had you given an excessive dosage of medication and had it caused the patient to have serious effects you would have been liable for your actions. Of course, this is an extreme situation, but it illustrates that nurses must not back down because of a harangue caused by actions when they are doing what is correct and necessary.

Donnelly (1979b, p. 31) describes *psychosomatic responses* to assertiveness as the "weeping willow reaction." Often when one demonstrates new behaviors, others will accuse the person of giving them a headache or a backache or will indirectly complain (weep) that they are not treated fairly, that their workload gives them a headache or their back aches from lifting so many people or things without any help. Nurses do not like to think that they caused someone else to get sick. Remember, one never causes anyone else to feel a certain way. People are in charge of their responses to the behavior of others.

A final response to assertiveness is to *seek revenge.* Such reactions may be seen as public taunts about one's behavior or direct or veiled threats to retaliate. Such behavior may be demoralizing and painful, especially if people other than the two directly concerned become involved. In some cases the revenge can have serious consequences including the loss of a job or damage to one's credibility. Thus in choosing when to be assertive it is important to evaluate the potential consequences rationally.

In some instances assertiveness may influence job mobility in either a positive or negative direction. Some supervisors and administrators do not want people who can think for themselves, who behave in ways they consciously choose, and who are accountable for their actions. When supervisors are threatened by perceived competence of subordinates or when they prefer an autocratic style, assertive subordinates are usually not valued. In contrast, many administrators believe that the best run organizations are those in which co-workers are bright, assertive, skillful, and decisive decision makers. Hence, the individual nurse must critically assess the work situation and decide if the fit is a compatible one.

The emphasis on the potential negative consequences of assertiveness is not intended to belittle the positive outcomes. Many benefits of assertive behavior have been previously mentioned. However, it is important to summarize the potential positive effects on the nurse, the setting, and the client. When nurses use assertiveness, they essentially stand up for their personal rights while simultaneously respecting the rights of others. Such behavior leads to increased feelings of self-worth and personal confidence. Essentially this message is incorporated into the person's self-perception: "I am a valuable person who is entitled to say what I think and feel in a way nondetrimental to others."

Clear, assertive messages not only enrich the nurse's self-view but also stimulate positive feelings among others. To be honest with another person (family, colleague, client) conveys respect for that person's worth by saying "I value you enough to be open and honest in my communications with you." Such behavior tends to keep communication patterns clear and to minimize misunderstanding and inaccurate perceptions. Being assertive with people allows them to take responsibility for their own behavior.

In dealing with clients, there are times when the nurse may choose to refrain from being assertive *for* clients in order to teach them to be assertive. This was the case in the following example.

Mrs. Brown was being treated by Dr. Smith for hypertension. His primary approach was medication, and he had provided no specific instruction relative to diet and nutrition. When Jane, the community health nurse, made her regular visit to Mrs. Brown, who was recovering from a stroke, they discussed the implications of hypertension. Mrs. Brown told Jane that her neighbor who is also hypertensive was not taking much medication but did go to the health department every week for a nutrition and exercise class. In the past 2 months her neighbor lost 4 pounds and declared that she never felt better. Mrs. Brown wanted to attend the class too but feared that Dr. Smith wouldn't write a referral. She asked Jane to call her physician and explain the value of this program.

Jane, however, knows that Dr. Smith thinks such classes are foolish and there is nothing a nurse could teach his patients that he has not already shared with them. What should she do? Should she use assertive skills in this instance for patient advocacy?*

The most useful nursing approach at this juncture would be to teach Mrs. Brown to be assertive in this specific situation. This could be done by role-playing whereby Mrs. Brown and Jane alternate enacting the potential responses of both Dr. Smith and Mrs. Brown. Since Dr. Smith's first response may be negative, Mrs. Brown can practice using "I" messages to express clearly her desires along with a version of "broken record" where the main point is made

---

*Advocacy refers to "speaking in another's behalf" (Donnelly, 1979a, p. 49). The community health nurse as a client advocate is described in detail in Chapter 33. This chapter defines only one time in which advocacy is not recommended. In contrast, assertive behavior refers to an attitude of self-responsibility. Thus using assertive principles to speak for others violates the basic intent unless they are unable to speak for themselves.

over and over in a low-key manner. If Dr. Smith perceives that this class is really important to Mrs. Brown, he may agree.

Essentially the nurse wanted to foster Mrs. Brown's independence so she could translate the learning from this situation to other similar ones. Thus one should avoid doing for people what they can do for themselves and should reinforce independent actions. Clients may not be aware that they have rights and are entitled to be part of the decision-making process relating to their health and lives.

SUMMARY

A health promotion goal is to attain and maintain the highest possible level of human functioning. Community health nurses can enrich their own functioning and adaptation to their various environments as well as teach clients to do likewise by learning and practicing the skills of assertive behavior. This technique, often confused with aggressiveness, refers to clear, straight-forward communication of one's needs, goals, and rights. Assertive behavior avoids using or taking advantage of others as well as being used by others. This form of communicating, behaving, and even standing, walking, and dressing conveys self-confidence and comfort with oneself as a person of value.

An assertive stance opposes the traditional female, and especially nursing, stance of subservience and deference to others. Because nurses assume responsibility for most of the health care given in all segments of the health care system, a passive posture is not in the best interests of either nurses or clients. Nurses must model and teach others to stand up for what they believe, to be clear and honest in their messages, and to learn to practice negotiation and conflict resolution so that there are no losers, only winners, in the health care system.

Specific skills are needed to be assertive. Nurses can learn communication techniques such as fogging, negative assertion, and negative inquiry to help them respond more constructively to criticism. In addition, an assertive approach includes social skills such as giving and receiving compliments, making conversation, and developing and relying on a support network.

Attainment of an assertive style may be blocked by several things. Anxiety, fear, an irrational belief system, and lack of skill have been discussed as impediments to nurses' increased assertiveness. Many of the examples cited have directly applied to nursing practice skills so nurses could identify with them and practice the skills described. The goal has been twofold: to teach community health nurses assertive skills and to offer the potential that these skills can be taught to clients.

≡ KEY CONCEPTS

Assertiveness, like stress management, is a skill that nurses can teach to their clients and use to promote their own health.

Assertive people reflect confidence in their interpersonal relationships and are able to express feelings and emotions honestly and spontaneously, and they are respected by others for these qualities.

Social behavior must be acquired; it is not present at birth but rather develops through socialization with others. Almost all behavior results from social interaction and is modified in response to the demands and expectations of others.

It has been said that female nurses are "twice socialized"; first into their role as women in a paternalistic society and then into their roles as wife or mother in the hospital or health care agency family.

There is a common misconception that being assertive means being "pushy." In fact, assertive behavior is defined as "standing up for personal rights and expressing thoughts, feelings, and beliefs in direct, honest and appropriate ways which do not violate another person's rights."

Aggressive behavior, in contrast to nonassertiveness, occurs when people infringe on the rights of others while standing up for their own rights.

Assertive behavior creates an atmosphere of openness in which people can engage in mutual goal-setting and action toward reaching their goals while recognizing the uniqueness, strengths, and limitations of others.

Appropriate voice tone and loudness, facial expressions, and hand gestures emphasize an assertive message.

The core of assertive behavior is taking responsibility for self.

Constructive criticism can be useful and encourage growth; manipulative criticism can render people vulnerable.

The development of the social skills of conversation helps nurses develop a support system—a network of relationships that builds self-esteem, provides camaraderie and companionship, and thereby nurtures the professional care giver.

Fear blocks effective functioning for many nurses. Fear of rejection and fear of inadequacy retard many nurses' ability to be actively involved in decision making in their practice.

In applying assertive skills and standing up for personal rights, conflict should not be ignored. It must be recognized, understood, and resolved.

LEARNING ACTIVITIES

1. Select a person you know well and assess how (specifically) that person's self-concept affects behavior. Take specific examples of behavior and relate it to your perception of the person's self view.

2. Think back to your first contact with the nursing role and trace the pattern of socialization that has taken place. Identify the positive and negative aspects of your socialization into nursing. What would you change about your socialization if you could redo the past?

3. Interview someone who has been a practicing nurse for at least 15 years. The focus of the interview is to be a discussion of that person's perception of his or her socialization process into nursing. How does that person's pattern of socialization differ from yours? What commonalities exist?

4. Interview at least three high school students to determine their perception of nursing as a career and what type of people (from among their classmates) they think will and should enter nursing school.

5. For 1 week observe the behavior of people with whom you come in contact. Keep a log of the instances in which you or someone you observed used either an assertive, aggressive, or nonassertive form of behavior. If the behavior was either of the latter two, redesign the interaction so the person behaves in an assertive way.

BIBLIOGRAPHY

Alberti, R.E., and Emmons, M.L.: Your perfect right, San Luis Obispo, Calif., 1980, Impact Publishers, Inc.

Bergman, P.E.: The use of assertiveness training in the clinical environment, J. Nurs. Ed. 24(3):33-35, 1984.

Biddle, B.J.: Role theory: expectations, identities and behaviors, New York, 1979, Academic Press, Inc.

Branden, N.: The psychology of self-esteem, San Francisco, 1969, W.H. Freeman & Co.

Burns, D.D.: Feeling good, the new mood therapy, New York, 1980, Signet.

Chenevert, M.: Special techniques in assertiveness training for women in the health care professions, St. Louis, 1978, The C.V. Mosby Co.

Clinard, M.B.: Sociology of deviant behavior, New York, 1971, Holt, Rinehart & Winston, Inc.

Cohen, H.: You can negotiate anything, Secaucus, N.J., 1980, Lyle Stuart, Inc.

Combs, A.W.: The professional education of teachers, Boston, 1965, Allyn & Bacon, Inc.

Cooley, C.H.: Human nature and the social order, New York, 1902, Charles Scribner's Sons.

Coopersmith, S.: The antecedents of self-esteem, San Francisco, 1967, W.H. Freeman & Company.

Cuming, P.: Getting others to help you meet your goals, Nurs. Life 2:65-72, May/June 1982.

Dean, P.G.: Toward androgyny. In Muff, J., editor: Socialization, sexism and stereotyping, St. Louis, 1982, The C.V. Mosby Co., pp. 248-254.

Donnelly, G.F.: When it's best not to assert, RN 10:49-51, Sept. 1979a.

Donnelly, G.F.: When assertiveness exacts a price, RN 10:29-31, Oct. 1979b.

Ellis, A.: How to live with and without anger, New York, 1977, Reader's Digest Press.

Fisher, D.W.: Group conflict may promote positive solutions, Ethicon 22(2):16-17, 1985.

Herman, S.: Becoming assertive: a guide for nurses, New York, 1978, D. Van Nostrand Co.

Horney, K.: Neurosis and human growth, New York, 1950, W.W. Norton & Co., Inc.

Jacobson, E.: Progressive relaxation, ed. 3, Chicago, 1974, University of Chicago Press.

James, W.: Principles of psychology, 2 vols., New York, 1890, Holt, Rinehart & Winston, Inc.

Jenkins, L.M.: The concept of assertion: from theory to practice, Issues Mental Health Nurs. 4(1):51-63, Jan. 1982.

Kalisch, B.J., and Kalisch, P.A.: An analysis of the sources of physician-nurse conflict, J. Nurs. Admin. 7:51-57, Jan. 1977.

Lange, J., and Jakubowski, P.: Responsible assertive behavior, cognitive behavioral procedures for trainers, Champaign, Ill., 1976, Research Press.

McIntyre, T.J., Jeffrey, D.B., and McIntyre, S.L.: Assertion training: the effectiveness of a comprehensive cognitive-behavioral treatment package with professional nurses, Behav. Res. Ther. 22(3):311-318, 1984.

Mead, G.: Mind, self & society, Chicago, 1934, University of Chicago Press.

Mereness, D.: Your self-image and your practice, Am. J. Nurs. 66:96-100, Jan. 1966.

Milauskas, J.: Will nursing assert itself? Nurs. Admin. Q. 9(3):1-15, 1985.

New, J.R., and Couillard, N.A.: Guidelines for introducing change, J. Nurs. Admin. 11:17-21, March 1981.

Phelps, S., and Austin, N.: The assertive woman, San Luis Obispo, Calif., 1975, Impact Publishers, Inc.

Rawnsely, M.M.: The six A's of assertiveness, J. Cont. Ed. Nurs. 11:15-18, Jan.-Feb. 1980.

Sewell, W.H.: Some recent developments in socialization theory and research, The Annals 349:163-181, 1963.

Smith, M.J.: When I say no I feel guilty, New York, 1975, The Dial Press.

Smoyak, S.A.: The confrontation process, Am. J. Nurs. 74:1632-1635, 1974.

Stepsis, J.: Conflict resolution strategies. In Jones, J.E., and Pfeiffer, J.W.: The 1974 annual handbook for group facilitators, LaJolla, Calif., 1974, University Associates, p. 139.

Sullivan, H.W.: The interpersonal theory of psychiatry, New York, 1953, W.W. Norton & Co., Inc.

Thurkettle, M.A., and Jones, S.L.: Conflict as a systems process: theory and management, J. Nurs. Admin. 8:39-43, Jan. 1978.

Ways, M.: The virtues, dangers and limits of negotiation, Fortune 99:86-90, Jan. 15, 1979.

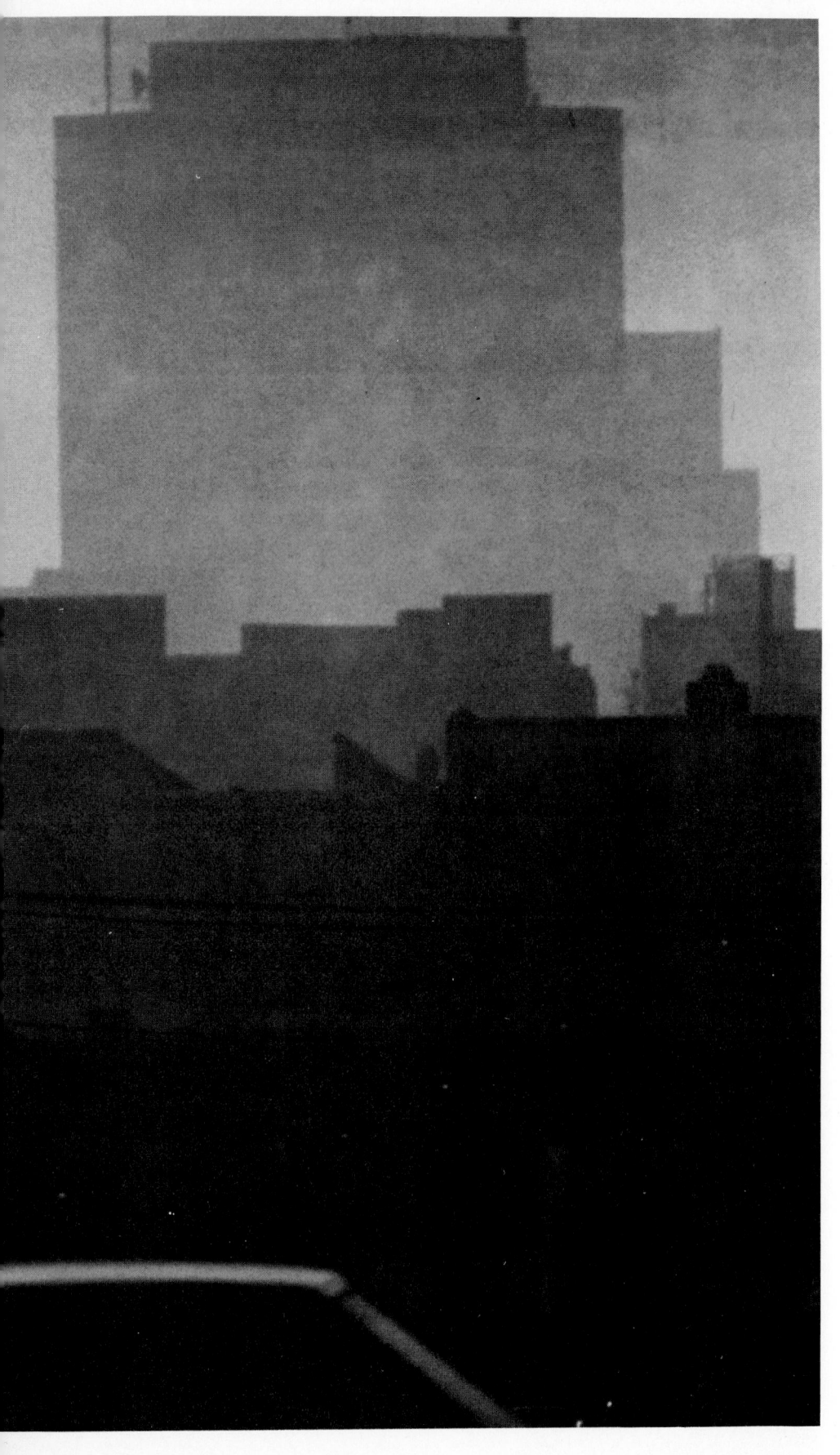

INTERVENTIONS
FOR MAJOR COMMUNITY HEALTH PROBLEMS

Communities continue to experience an alarming rate of violence and mental illness. Declining federal support for health programs has greatly influenced the effectiveness of treatment programs for dealing with crises, violence, and mental health needs. Primary prevention is the desired way to maintain community mental health, yet efforts directed toward this aim are not supported at the fiscal level necessary to enrich communities. Problems related to unemployment, crowding, poverty, lack of education, and ineffective family role modeling continue to challenge the stability of communities. Chapters 32 to 34 describe the incidence, characteristics, and strategies for intervening in selected community mental health problems, crises, and abusive patterns.

Chapter 35 documents the significant problem substance abuse is for all population groups. Strategies for intervening in this increasing, yet preventable, health hazard are also reviewed.

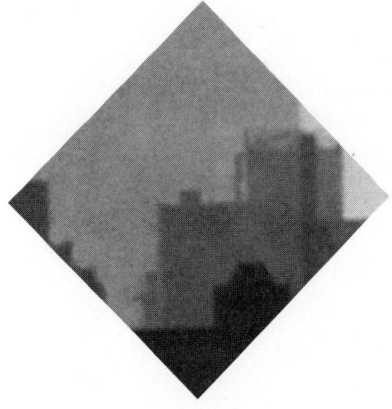

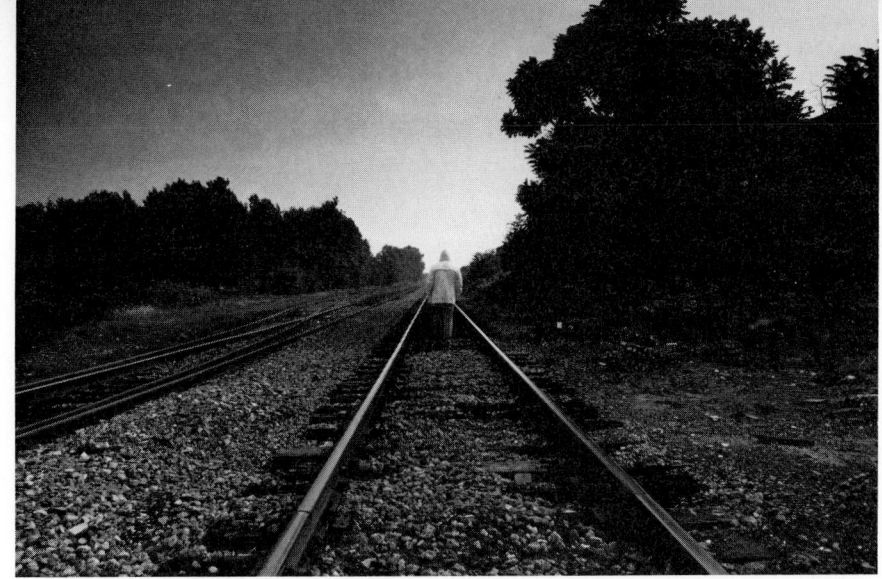

Jeanette Lancaster
David Kerschner

32

COMMUNITY MENTAL HEALTH: PROBLEM IDENTIFICATION, PREVENTION, AND INTERVENTION

☰ OBJECTIVES

After reading this chapter, the student should be able to:

Identify client information necessary for the management of psychotropic drug regimens.

Identify psychotropic drugs and the psychiatric disorder that they are commonly used to treat.

Identify the common side effects that may be associated with psychotropic drugs.

Briefly summarize the development of community mental health as a system of care.

Discuss the impact of *Action for Mental Health*.

Discuss legislation leading to the establishment and continuation of community mental health centers.

Explain primary, secondary, and tertiary prevention in relation to mental health.

Identify factors in the community that may decrease host resistance to the maintenance of mental health.

Identify how a variety of social changes in American society have influenced mental health.

Evaluate deinstitutionalization as a viable mechanism for caring for chronically ill psychiatric patients.

☰ KEY TERMS

affective disorders
catchment area
continuity of care program
deinstitutionalization
homelessness
least restrictive alternative

markets
market segmentation
mental deficiency
mental health
mental illness
monoamine oxidase inhibitors

National Institute for Mental Health (NIMH)
new mental health paradigm
psychotropic medications
public health paradigm
schizophrenia
tardive dyskinesia

Persons with mental health problems and needs frequently are clients of community health nurses. These problems are often complex and result from the interaction of many factors, including heredity, family relationships, living conditions, and social and economic constraints. Because people suffering from psychological maladies often remain in or return to the community following treatment, community health nurses must be able to assess the presence of mental health problems and plan and implement interventions within the confines of the resources available in the community. To do this, it is necessary to understand how mental health services are typically organized, including the history of their development. Other sections of this chapter discuss current challenges to the maintenance of mental health, creation of a preventive framework, major risk factors working against maintenance of mental health, major mental health problems, and selected methods of intervention. Particular attention is given to medication management of mentally ill persons in the community.

CONCEPTS OF MENTAL HEALTH AND ILLNESS

Mental health and *mental illness* represent an area filled with unknowns. Definitions of mental health vary considerably, and the cause of most forms of mental illness remains elusive or highly debatable. Because no universally accepted definition of mental health exists, program planning in community health for this population group is complex. Definitions of mental health range from the absence of mental disease to the attainment of one's maximal capabilities.

Concepts of mental health and illness have changed dramatically in the last five centuries. In the fifteenth century the mentally ill were considered to be "possessed," and witch-hunting and exorcism of demons were ways in which communities responded to this health disruption (Wilner et al., 1978). A book published in 1489 entitled *Malleus Maleficarum (Hammer Against Witches)* contained instructions for identifying a witch. This book served as a guide for "handling" mentally afflicted people for nearly 300 years; many of the criteria used in 1489 to detect witches are symptoms currently associated with mental illness (Wilner et al., 1978).

Following the era of demon possession it was next thought that disease resulted from organic defect or injury. If no lesion was found, people demonstrating aberrant behavior were considered immoral or criminal, and suitable punishment was leveled against them.

In recent times efforts have been directed toward differentiating mental health from illness. Anthropologists, however, point out that what seems like illness in one culture may be viewed as acceptable behavior in another. Chapter 5 describes social and cultural aspects of community health nursing. Considering social, cultural, and individual differences affecting and evidenced in people, it can be seen that mental health is always relative—to time, place, and situation (Taylor, 1982). However, several characteristics of mental health are generally accepted: the ability to cope with maturational and situational stressors, to cope with reality, to love and be loved in return, to accept oneself, and to think and act independently (Taylor, 1982). Marmor and Pumpian-Mindlin (1950, p. 30) defined mental health as "that state in the interrelationships of the individual and his environment in which the personality structure is relatively stable, and the environmental stresses are within its absorptive capacity."

Like mental health, mental illness is usually determined in terms of an individual's relationship to the environment. According to Taylor (1982, p. 115) "Mental illness is a complex problem that is thought to be a unique response involving an individual's personality as it interacts with his environment at a time when he is particularly vulnerable to stress."

The breadth of these definitions allows their adaptation to specific situations. The maintenance of mental health, viewed from a community health perspective, is a complex process whereby people attain at least a moderate degree of adaptation to the environment and are able to function in everyday activities and cope with daily stressors. Illness ensues when the person is unable to maintain a state of equilibrium with the environment and thereby becomes incapable of acceptable performance of daily activities. The next section briefly traces the development of community mental health as a system of care and significant changes in the concept of mental health. Historical antecedents serve as determinants of many of today's beliefs and forms of care in community mental health.

DEVELOPMENT OF COMMUNITY MENTAL HEALTH AS A SYSTEM OF CARE

The methods of treating mental illness have changed dramatically in the past century. Community mental health, as a treatment philosophy, was mandated by the Community Mental Health Centers Act of 1963 and is discussed in detail in a later section of this chapter.

Community mental health, a treatment approach implemented through comprehensive community mental health centers, is considered the fourth revolutionary development in the field of psychiatry. The first revolution occurred in 1793 when Pinel removed the chains from mentally ill patients confined in Bicêtre, a hospital outside Paris. The second revolution was ushered in with the inception of Freudian psychoanalytic treatment about 100 years after the work of Pinel. The advent of psychotropic drugs commenced the third revolution and in many ways made it possible to treat mentally ill persons from a community mental health approach.

The basic philosophy underlying community mental health is that behavior is determined by two sets of variables: the person and the situation. This philosophy is consistent with public health thinking. To implement this philosophy, community mental health requires a different orientation from the medical model that prevailed in psychiatry for many years. Treatment is more encompassing than merely removing an emotionally disturbed person from the stressful setting, making the necessary psychological repairs, and returning the person to the same setting. Community mental health focuses on helping the individual, the family, and also the community to interact in more adaptive ways so that mental health is maintained.

Humanitarian Reforms in Mental Health

Before 1840 people deemed to be mentally ill were sent to jails, asylums, or county homes. These forms of shelter and removal of the afflicted person from society protected the afflicted people from being harmed and from harming others and provided them with food and shelter. Treatment was unheard of for the mentally ill person. Mental illness was viewed as an incurable affliction, and the only logical goal seemed to be to remove the sick person from the community so that no harm would come to anyone. During this era a few private hospitals were available for patients who could afford this luxury.

Benjamin Rush, often called the "father of American psychiatry," led the movement for humane treatment of mentally ill people. Although instrumental in introducing a humanitarian way of thinking into psychiatry, he continued to use remedies such as blood-letting, purgatives, and a torturelike device known as the "tranquilizer."

The work begun by Rush was carried on enthusiastically by a former schoolteacher, Dorothea Dix, who in 1841 appointed herself inspector of institutions for the mentally ill. Traveling the land, she crusaded for enlightened treatment for patients. Dix insisted that each state should assume the financial and caretaking responsibility for its own residents. Her exhaustive efforts on behalf of mental health

led to the establishment of 32 mental hospitals in the United States. At this time most of the hospitals were built in rural areas both for the patients to benefit from fresh air and also to keep them isolated from the mainstream, since they were feared by others.

As the population of the United States grew, the number of hospitals did also, until 1900. At this time the completion of new hospitals virtually came to a halt, which meant that existing facilities soon became overcrowded and deplorable conditions became the standard. The care of mentally ill people in the United States continued to deteriorate until Adolf Meyer took up the crusade that had been carried on by Dix. Meyer, the first person to describe and campaign for community mental health, proposed that a clinic for the mentally ill be established in communities so that certain population groups could be studied and treated. The mental health movement received a major impetus in 1908 from the publication of Clifford Beers' book *A Mind That Found Itself*. In this book Beers graphically recounted his experiences as a psychiatric patient and urged reform and public education for mental health (Hanlon and Pickett, 1984). He is credited with the establishment of the Connecticut Society for Mental Hygiene, whose purpose was to combat ignorance about the cause and nature of mental illness. In 1909 the National Committee for Mental Hygiene was organized. This organization was a forerunner of the National Association for Mental Health.

In the following decade, 19 state mental hygiene societies and 16 societies in other nations were organized. The International Congress for Mental Hygiene was established in 1922, and in 1930 the first International Mental Hygiene Congress was held in Washington, D.C. (Hanlon and Pickett, 1984).

Governmental Involvement in Mental Health

The federal government first became involved in the financing of mental health services with the 1935 passage of the Social Security Act. This shift in responsibility from the state to the federal government grew out of the notion during the depression that if local communities could not care for their ill people, then the government should undertake this responsibility. The impact of World War II on community mental health was unprecedented: 875,000 draftees of 15 million, or almost 6%, were rejected from military service because of existing mental illness (Snow and Newton, 1976). The end of the war witnessed a significant increase in the government's role for the mentally ill; in 1946 Congress enacted the National Mental Health Act, making grants available to states to develop programs outside of state hospitals. This legislation sought to apply a community health approach to the treatment of mentally ill people; in reality, individual psychotherapy based on a medical model was the primary mode of treatment used (Ramshorn, 1971). The act did establish the *National Institute of Mental Health (NIMH)* in 1949 and designated it as the agency responsible for mental health in the United States. Also during the 1940s, two important types of treatment facilities came into existence: outpatient clinics and psychiatric units in general hospitals.

The next major piece of legislation to affect mental health was the creation in 1955 of the Joint Commission on Mental Illness and Health (Snow and Newton, 1976). This commission consisted of representatives of 36 organizations and agencies chosen by NIMH. Five years after its inception, the Joint Commission submitted its report to Congress. This historical document, *Action for Mental Health,* was published in 1961 as a 338-page report emphasizing the need for better training of personnel, providing early and intensive treatment for the acutely ill, and carrying out research activities. The report also recommended the development of additional facilities, including units in general hospitals and clinics and programs for aftercare, rehabilitation, and mental health education (Joint Commission, 1961).

Following the publication of this report, President John F. Kennedy appointed a cabinet-level committee to review the report and make recommendations regarding the need for federal action. Based on this report, in 1963, Kennedy made the first presidential address on behalf of the mentally ill and called for a "bold new approach" to maintain and return patients to their local community. These actions culminated in the community mental health centers concept (Rubin, 1971).

Legislation for Community Mental Health

Community mental health centers became a reality on October 31, 1963, when Congress enacted Public Law 88-164, the Mental Retardation Facilities and Community Mental Health Centers Construction Act of 1963, authorizing federal matching funds of $150 million over a 3-year period to be used by states in construction centers. This act sought to provide comprehensive mental health services to all residents in a specific area known as a *catchment area.* Each catchment area was to consist of 75,000 to 200,000 people. Besides providing five essential services to qualify for funding, centers were encouraged to implement five additional services. Both the essential and supplementary services are listed in the box above.

The original legislation envisioned that funding would be provided to centers to enable them to get started, at which time federal funds would decrease as state and local funds increased. This plan did not work in many areas, since state and local funds rarely increased sufficiently to take over much of the federal portion. To keep the centers operational, Congress extended Public Law 89-105 (the 1964 legislation to establish the "seed money" concept of financing centers based on a declining formula of federal support over a 51-month period) nine times. In 1975 Congress overrode a presidential veto to pass the Community Mental Health Centers Amendments of 1975 (PL 94-63). These amendments provided a more stable source of funding for centers, made available distress grants, and extended the funding cycle to a maximum of 12 years. The amendments also provided grants for specialty areas, including child care, aging, court screening, care for discharged mentally ill people, transitional services, and substance abuse. Actually the 1975 amendments legally defined the com-

---

ESSENTIAL AND SUPPLEMENTARY SERVICES OF COMMUNITY MENTAL HEALTH CENTERS AS SPECIFIED IN FEDERAL LEGISLATION

ESSENTIAL SERVICES

Inpatient care for patients requiring short-term hospitalization

Partial hospitalization including day and night care

Outpatient treatment

Emergency services on a 24-hour basis

Consultation and education for members of the community

SUPPLEMENTARY SERVICES

Diagnostic services including the making of treatment recommendations

Rehabilitation services and vocational counseling

Precare and aftercare

Training for all kinds of personnel

Research and evaluation

From Landsberg, G., and Hammer, R.: Community Ment. Health J. 13:63-70, 1977.

---

ponents of a community mental health center's services and documented those that must be provided. These amendments have been severely criticized because of their lack of flexibility and limited responsiveness to the unique needs of individual communities (Citizens Guide, 1977). For example, each center was required to offer the same essential and supplemental services regardless of the unique needs of the population within the catchment area. The needs of an aging population would be different from those of families with young or adolescent children.

The 1977 report of the President's Commission on Mental Health recommended strengthening the community mental health system and again extended funding. The 117 recommendations of the report were divided into eight sections: community support systems, service delivery, financing, personnel, patient's rights, research, prevention, and public understanding. The main thrust of the recommendations was to establish a new federal grant program for community mental health services where they were inadequate and to increase the flexibility of communities in planning a comprehensive network of services. In general the report called for many of the same priority areas as mentioned in the original legislation of the 1960s (President's Commission, 1978).

Following publication of the President's Commission on Mental Health report, legislation passed in 1980 emphasized the need for communities to be flexible in planning services to meet their unique needs. This legislation gave states greater authority over mental health funds, allowed flexible and innovative program planning and development, and emphasized prevention, as well as the development of new approaches to meet the mental health needs of priority populations. Communities became eligible to plan according to their needs and were not restricted to federally mandated services. Linkages were also supported among agencies to promote coordination and reduce duplication (Nation's Health, 1981).

In the 1980s there have been continual cuts in mental health funding. With the onset of federal block grants in the early 1980s, lump sums of money were awarded to states; agencies within each state were forced to compete for a portion of the funds. Mental health programs do not have a history of success in capturing funds from block grants.

Criticism of Community Mental Health Centers

Despite over two decades of federal and local funding, few centers have met the dreams of their architects to provide comprehensive, accessible mental health services at the local level. The community mental health movement has been plagued with requirements and stipulations for funding that have largely ignored the unique needs of the communities being served. Centers often fail to define program boundaries and priorities. Frequently they are accused of trying to be all things to all people, regardless of program priorities, personnel, and other resources. The legislation mandated services with no consideration to community characteristics or needs. Despite an initial intent to apply public health principles to mental health, few centers assessed the needs of their communities and planned accordingly. Specific additional criticisms include:

1. The concept of catchment area is often rigid and fails to take into account unique community differences (e.g., an area in Wyoming with a population of between 75,000 and 200,000 would be much different from the same area encompassing that population in a large city such as New York or Los Angeles).
2. Originally centers were managed by health care providers inexperienced in areas of business such as marketing, finance, accounting, and labor relations.
3. Centers were often seen as places for the poor or chronically ill to receive care.
4. The inability to develop a comprehensive community mental health system led to a "revolving door" syndrome.
5. Community resources were not always well coordinated.

Benefits of Community Mental Health Centers

In recent years the benefits of community mental health centers have increased, and the criticisms have decreased. As federal funds diminished, many centers developed successful marketing strategies to promote their programs and also secured increased funding sources through linkages with insurance companies, federal reimbursement, grants, and community support. Centers have altered the image of mental illness by reducing the mystery associated with emotional illness. They have also successfully provided services to a variety of age groups, ranging from children to the elderly. Many centers developed effective prevention programs to strengthen community residents' ability to cope with stress and provide forms of secondary and tertiary interventions.

Successful centers have developed strong community linkages and focused on local needs rather than solely on federal guidelines. The Committee on Psychiatry and Community of the Group for the Advancement of Psychiatry lists 13 ingredients of successful centers:

1. Consistent and adequate funding
2. Assignment of top priority to the needs of the most seriously ill
3. Accessibility of services
4. Availability of a full range of treatment and rehabilitation measures for individual patient needs
5. Responsiveness to expressed local needs
6. Effective interagency collaboration
7. Maximal use of existing community resources and development of new services to meet documented gaps
8. Active involvement of psychiatrists as caregivers and planners
9. Use of well-trained professionals
10. Internal harmony among the staff
11. Pursuit of staff development and "antiburnout" strategies
12. Encouragement of active participation of the private psychiatric sector in patient care
13. Objective assessment of needs and well-designed program evaluation

The 1980s have been more prosperous times for many Americans, but threats other than economic have prevailed. Violence against people and property increased in the 1980s, causing Americans to question the safety of their cities and neighborhoods; families continued to break up at an alarming rate, and social institutions such as schools and churches came under public scrutiny and attack. A variety of social conditions influence the maintenance of mental health: inflation and unemployment, the increasing number of women who work (thereby changing roles within the family for both men and women), and an increasing tendency to use drugs or alcohol to cope with life stresses. A framework for prevention is described in preparation for a detailed description of major mental health stressors, high-risk groups, and nursing implications.

FRAMEWORK FOR MENTAL ILLNESS PREVENTION

Leavell and Clark (1965) described levels of prevention in 1953 when they identified the approaches to preventive medicine as primary, secondary, and tertiary. In the 1960s psychiatrist Gerald Caplan described levels of prevention specific to psychiatry. Caplan (1974) defined primary prevention as efforts directed toward reducing the incidence of mental disorders in a community; secondary prevention referred to decreasing the duration of disorders; and tertiary prevention referred to reducing the level of impairment.

Bloom (1979) described intervention to prevent mental disorders according to prevalence and incidence figures. The first type of intervention is designed to reduce the number of persons with the disorder in a given population (prevalence). Primary prevention attempts to reduce the onset of new cases by reducing incidence through programs aimed at either an entire population group or only at persons at risk. Techniques for mental illness control focusing on early

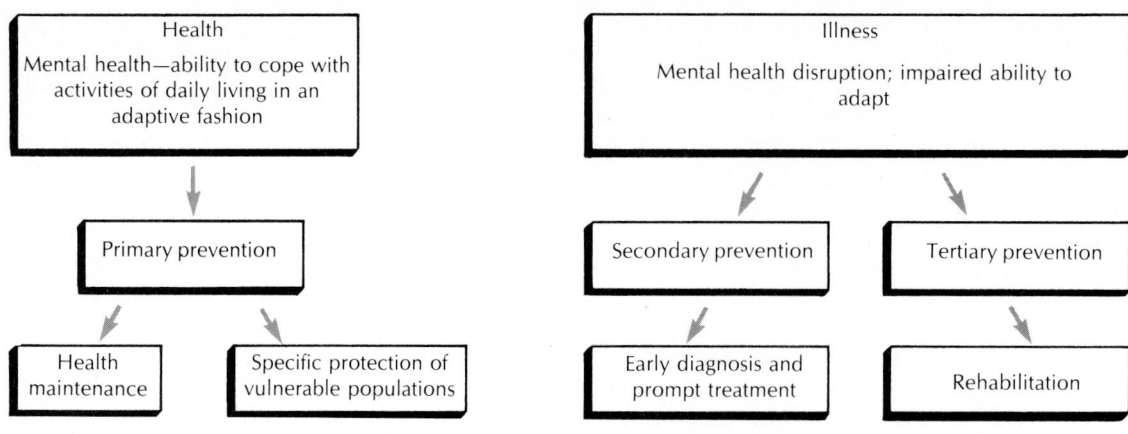

Figure 32-1

Mental health–mental illness continuum.

case finding and prompt treatment are secondary prevention. Tertiary prevention is unrelated to incidence and may actually increase the prevalence as it increases life expectancy for people with chronic illness. Figure 32-1 depicts the mental health–mental illness continuum and includes levels of prevention.

The *public health paradigm* for disease prevention is based on Leavell and Clark's model (1965), which describes the interaction between host (affected person), agent (stimulus causing disease), and environment as the period of prepathogenesis. Pathogenesis extends from the person's first contact with the disease-producing stimuli to the actual change in functioning. The combination of prepathogenesis and pathogenesis makes up the natural history of the disease. Based on this tracing of disease development, specific interventions can be established. This approach holds that each disorder has a necessary and identifiable precondition.

Although this classic public health paradigm explains many forms of mental illness, an approach developed by Bloom (1979) offers more promise for community health nursing. The basis for the *new mental health paradigm* is that stressful life events affect mental health, especially the mental health of vulnerable people. This new approach does not begin by searching for the cause of each disorder but rather " . . . preventive intervention programs can be organized around facilitating the mastery or reducing the incidence of particular stressful life events without undue regard for the prior specification of which forms of disability might be prevented" (Bloom, 1979, p. 183). The steps of this paradigm can be summarized as follows:

1. Identify a stressful life event that seems to have undesirable consequences for health and develop methods to identify people at risk.
2. Study the consequences of the event and develop intervention approaches.
3. Implement and evaluate the success of intervention.

The most effective primary prevention approach requires a union of public health and mental health concepts. Such a model blends the classic public health triad of host, agent, and environment with the paradigm developed by Bloom.

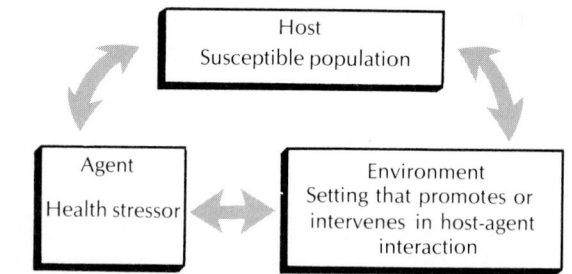

Figure 32-2

Epidemiological triad.

Figure 32-2 demonstrates this combined model. The nursing goal in relation to this triad is to help people (hosts) strike a balance between factors that might disrupt mental health (agents) and the available supports (environment). Both Chapters 8 and 17 provide additional ways of looking at this triad.

Factors such as crowding, poverty, inflation, racism, mobility, family disintegration, type of occupation, and level or threat of crime and violence potentially decrease host resistance to mental health disruption. In contrast, timely and effective physical and psychological care and support, police protection, social and family support networks, and educational opportunities increase resistance on a community level. On a personal or small group basis, mental health education, anticipatory guidance, crisis intervention, counseling, and support groups decrease host susceptibility. Community health nurses are in key positions to identify individual family and group needs, conflicts, and stressors.

Additional factors deserve consideration in establishing a framework for examining mental health. First, it is unlikely that all mental illness will ever be prevented. Unlike the relationship between vitamin C and scurvy, predisposing factors for mental illness are difficult to pinpoint. Second, how people respond to life events depends on the interaction of inherited characteristics, previous experience, perception, and environment. It is also important to recognize that prevention deals with both high-risk groups and high-risk situations.

MAJOR RISK FACTORS WORKING AGAINST MENTAL HEALTH

Changes in social situations carry an increased risk for some people because of their coping ability, the nature and quantity of stressors, and the amount and availability of support networks. Further, because of the complex, interactive nature of factors leading to mental illness, it is impossible to precisely assign events to a particular risk category. This section describes several physiological and psychosocial factors influential in mental health status. The adage "all people are created equal" is not true. Some are born with physical and psychological handicaps, and the odds in life seem stacked against them. The choices discussed in this section are not meant to be inclusive; rather, they set forth examples of risk factors often seen in community health.

Severe Mental Deficiency

Severe *mental deficiency,* different from mental illness, is often defined as an IQ less than 50. This disorder occurs in all socioeconomic groups and frequently results from structural or biochemical abnormalities of the developing brain. Many causes of severe mental deficiency are the result of prenatal insults, which are often genetic or chromosomal in origin. The financial and emotional costs associated with these deficiencies are high, and in many cases documented forms of prevention are known. Some of the examples cited in this chapter have known preventive measures. Chapter 26 presents detailed information about developmental disabilities. This chapter highlights selected forms of mental deficiency not covered in detail in Chapter 26.

Metabolic Abnormalities

Screening often prevents severe mental deficiency caused by metabolic abnormalities. Early detection and prompt treatment minimize brain disruption. These disorders include phenylketonuria (PKU), galactosemia, and congenital hypothyroidism. Screening of newborns indicates that PKU occurs in approximately 1 in 11,500 live births, galactosemia in 1 in 40,000 to 60,000, and congenital hypothyroidism in 1 in 3500. Untreated, each disorder can produce a severely defective child, yet effective dietary or medication treatment enables these children to develop at a normal or nearly normal rate (Eisenberg and Parron, 1979).

Noxious Substances

In addition to population screening and intervention in metabolic disorders, other high risk situations for severe mental deficiency occur when pregnant women are exposed to noxious substances either in the environment or through direct consumption. For example, exposure to radiation, environmental pollutants, and certain medications produces detrimental effects on a developing fetus. Pregnant women should be advised to take as few medications as possible during the first trimester and to avoid drinking alcoholic beverages and smoking cigarettes.

Consumption of more than 3 ounces of absolute *alcohol* (about six drinks/day) has been shown to result in a defined abnormality known as the fetal alcohol syndrome. Fetal alcohol syndrome occurs in about 2 per 1000 live births. Alcohol use during pregnancy is considered the third leading cause of mental retardation in the United States. As few as two drinks per day has been associated with lower infant birth weight (Women's Health, 1985). These infants also often suffer behavioral, craniofacial, skeletal, neurological, cardiac, or genital abnormalities. Chapter 35 presents more detailed information about the hazardous effects of substance abuse.

Lead poisoning also contributes to severe mental retardation, cerebral palsy, convulsive seizures, blindness, and death. Even low doses of lead can cause impaired cognitive, verbal, perceptual, and motor skills. Screening for the presence of lead, especially in paint, is a major community health nursing role. Lead exists in many forms in the environment; it is highly toxic when inhaled or when eaten in flaking paint. Children are particularly susceptible to lead poisoning.

Developmental Attrition

Developmental attrition, or children's cumulative loss of intellectual and emotional potential, results from many sources, including unwanted pregnancies, complications of pregnancy and parturition, malnutrition, infection, insufficient cognitive stimulation, inadequate emotional support, poor schooling, and racial or class discrimination. The last trimester of pregnancy and the first 2 years of life are susceptible times for the effects of malnutrition and infection (Richmond and Filner, 1979).

Learning disorders may result from the fetal and neonatal deficiencies described earlier. Although the etiology of learning disorders is complex and often involves a variety of factors, several patterns are noted. For example, pregnancy-related factors include a "maternal malnutrition, or toxemia, during pregnancy, difficult labor or delivery producing anoxia and prematurity" (Richmond and Filner, 1979, p. 322). Similarly, childhood-related factors, such as head injury, fever, meningitis, encephalitis, lead poisoning, drug intoxication, and severe nutritional deficits, can cause learning disorders. Just as with lead poisoning and malnutrition, prevention is essential.

Nursing Implications for Mental Deficiencies

The implications for nursing are numerous, since many types of mental deficiency are preventable. Special target areas include health education to inform the public of risk factors, careful assessment to detect potential high-risk individuals and groups, early identification, treatment, and follow-up. Specific interventions are directed toward the following:

1. Preparation for parenthood through education in the schools and community
2. Availability of family planning services and screening of high-risk pregnancies
3. Prenatal care throughout the pregnancy, beginning in the first trimester

4. Optimal nutrition during pregnancy and the developmental stages of childhood and adolescence
5. Prevention and treatment of congenital abnormalities and inborn errors of metabolism and early detection and treatment of developmental disabilities

Schizophrenia

Although the etiology of *schizophrenia,* a psychotic disorder characterized by disturbances of thought, mood, and behavior, remains unclear, there is an increasing·correlation with a genetic predisposition. It is often thought schizophrenia may be the result of ineffective parenting and faulty family communication instead of, or as well as, heredity. In spite of the relatively low incidence of schizophrenia, the impact of this disease is significant because of its often chronic nature and early age of onset, usually in the teenage or young adult years.

Studies of children born to schizophrenic parents have indicated some differences between those who do and those who do not develop the disorder. Those who later become schizophrenic are more likely to have experienced vulnerability in infancy, such as early separation from the mother or being born when the mother was in an acute stage of the disease. Poor school performance, low peer acceptance, and disruptive behavior tend to characterize the children of depressed or schizophrenic mothers (Tableman, 1981).

Genetic counseling is not effective as a prevention measure in schizophrenia, since the adult-onset disorder usually follows the age at which the first child is born, and childhood schizophrenia is less common than adult-onset schizophrenia. Measures currently being used for schizophrenic families include day-care services, after-school enrichment programs, homemaker services, and supportive social service efforts during episodes of acute illness. Although these efforts do not prevent schizophrenia, they can relieve stress and potentially prevent additional mental health problems.

Tableman (1981) reported on enrichment projects for children of schizophrenic parents that supplement regular day-care programs. The aim of the supplemental services is to assist children with motor development, self-care, receptive language development, cognitive development, graphic and prereading skills, social behavior, and speech.

Schizophrenics are often hospitalized during acute episodes. However, many schizophrenic individuals are poorly managed once they leave the hospital because the concept of deinstitutionalization, discussed in the following section, has not been adequately implemented across the nation.

Deinstitutionalization

Providing nursing care to families with a chronically ill member is a complex process. Of the chronic psychiatric illnesses, schizophrenia is the most frequently seen in the community. In recent years *deinstitutionalization* affected the services provided by community health nurses. Deinstitutionalization sought to move long-term psychiatric patients out of the warehouse atmosphere of large, public hospitals and back to their communities. However, many communities failed to plan in advance of this trend and

were unable to provide coordinated and comprehensive services; instead patients were "dumped" onto the community with no systematic plan for aftercare.

Statistically, psychiatric deinstitutionalization seems to have been a success. In 1955 there were approximately 559,000 patients in state and county mental hospitals compared with 138,000 in 1983. Of the more than 400,000 patients who left state hospitals, only a minority found a "supportive therapeutic haven" in the community; that is, money simply did not follow the patients (Friedman, 1983, p. 89).

The aim during the early days of deinstitutionalization was to provide patients with the least possible restrictions and to ensure them of as much liberty and freedom as possible. The concept of *least restrictive alternative (LRA)* has merit; however, community resources were often unavailable to meet the needs of the chronically mentally ill. The fact was often overlooked that some of the characteristics of the syndrome referred to as "institutionalism," such as lack of initiative, apathy, withdrawal, and submissiveness to authority, may be attributed to the schizophrenic process not merely to the length of hospitalization. The need of chronic mentally ill patients for structure, medical care, and a social network was seemingly forgotten in the rush to remove them from the "shackles of hospitalization."

Where have the chronically mentally ill gone? Many went to nursing homes, group homes, apartments, to live with their families, or to live on the streets. Increasingly, these patients turn to the emergency rooms of urban hospitals whenever anything goes wrong (Friedman, 1983). In a recent study of families of schizophrenic patients who returned home after deinstitutionalization, the consensus was that the families experienced a diminished quality of life and had increased concerns about their own physical, social, and emotional well-being (Seymour and Dawson, 1986). In studying the quality of life of a primary care provider before and after discharge of a schizophrenic family member, Seymour and Dawson (1986) found that threats to personal safety, including freedom from actual or threatened physical, social, or emotional abuse, constituted the greatest concern. The older the caregiver, the greater was the negative impact on quality of life. The longer the hospitalization, the more negative was the effect on the caregiver's quality of life when the schizophrenic person returned home.

Not surprisingly, the family environment in which schizophrenics live can influence the course of their illness. For this reason, families need guidance and support in learning to respond effectively to discharged patients. What is typically needed with discharged psychiatric patients is aggressive case management whereby clients are linked with basic resources, provided support during crises, monitored closely, and supervised by someone who can serve as an advocate as the client attempts to deal with a complex social and health care system.

Three groups of mentally ill people have been particularly affected by deinstitutionalization: the young chronically ill, the elderly, and the mentally retarded. The young adult chronic patient is typically between the ages of 18 and 35 and is sufficiently psychiatrically and socially impaired to make them continual or recurring clients of the mental health system. These individuals constitute the first generation of mental patients who have had to cope with the tasks and stresses of community living throughout their lives. These young adults do not typically view themselves as patients and are particularly vulnerable to alcohol, marijuana, and other mind-altering drugs. Viewing themselves as "just like everybody else," they take refuge from the pain of difference and the despair of failure by acting out, being aggressive, taking drugs, staying in bed, or blaming parents, therapists, landlords, police, or the health care system for their inability to cope (Pepper et al., 1981).

Deinstitutionalization has displaced many mentally ill elderly people from the only home they have known. Additionally, the shortage of affordable housing, the revitalization of urban areas, and poverty have affected the elderly. Because there typically is a shortage of affordable housing, older people often must live in cheap hotels, boarding homes, "family care" facilities, or the streets or parks. In New York City between 1970 and 1982, 110,000 single-room occupancy hotel units were lost; the consequence of urban redevelopment is the "involuntary removal, uprooting, and dislocating of neighborhood's original residents, now grown old" (Boondas, 1985, p. 4). Poverty among the elderly is widespread. With low incomes and often limited or no family support, elderly people must often choose whether to buy food or pay the rent.

As mentally retarded individuals make the transition from institution to the community, they often display emotional disorders ranging from transient behavioral disturbances to psychoses. The number of residents in public institutions for the mentally retarded in the United States has declined from 193,000 in 1967 to 115,000 in 1985 (Hodgins and Monfils, 1985). These "dual-diagnosis" patients offer special challenges to nurses in that many of the syndromes of mental retardation are accompanied by allied medical needs, such as congenital cardiac defects, intestinal obstructions, or obesity. Many are nonverbal; others demonstrate low self-esteem, primitive defense mechanisms, and diminished coping ability. Most require consistent structure in their daily lives.

Continuity of Care Program

Davies (1981) describes a *continuity of care program* that incorporates a full range of services designed to help chronically ill psychiatric patients return and remain in the community following hospitalization. The components of this program have implications for community health nurses, who are often in key positions for implementation. The program begins during hospitalization, with the selection of a primary clinician who coordinates care and community services following discharge. The specific services include a continuum of care designed to meet individual needs, allowing easy access to and reentry into the community, and crisis intervention. Three major service categories are provided: direct, community network, and case management.

Direct services include individual, group, and/or family counseling, as well as assessment of basic skills. If essential community survival skills are absent, a teaching plan is developed to overcome this deficit. Outreach services in the form of home visits and telephone calls comprise the direct service component. The *community network* component works with community residents and other health care providers to increase awareness of mental health needs and discuss better ways to integrate former psychiatric patients back into the community. *Case management* includes coordination of services for maintaining the person in the community and flexibility so the plan of treatment is modified as the person's needs and abilities change. Community health nurses can become active participants in such a program by first serving as client advocates, then as coordinators of care.

A continuity of care program for chronic psychiatric patients would include at least five major components: (1) community acceptance, (2) client advocacy, (3) individual supervision, (4) client education, and (5) group supervision. For a continuity of care program to be successful, community residents must accept the presence of discharged psychiatric patients in their midst. Residents often fear these patients and believe their presence will decrease property values or bring harm to community members.

Community acceptance can be fostered by open dialogue, public education programs, and support from local radio, television, or newspapers. Mental health volunteers, such as representatives from the local mental health association, can speak to community groups to convey the message that the majority of chronically ill psychiatric patients are withdrawn rather than violent, and they need acceptance, support, and encouragement.

Client advocacy is especially useful for discharged persons. In an organized continuity of care program, one person, typically a community health nurse, makes regular visits to clients to determine their needs relative to obtaining community services. These clients often have difficulty being sufficiently assertive to get through the "red tape" of some agencies and secure information or services.

Home visits provide *individual supervision* and typically emphasize medication maintenance, discussed in detail later in this chapter. In addition to monitoring medication usage, nurses observe the client's appearance, nutritional status, level of cleanliness (both of person and environment), and clarity of thought processes.

Client education is essential for many discharged psychiatric patients who must relearn basic living skills. These skills are appropriately taught before discharge, but if community health nurses note clients who are unable to perform services for themselves, such as cooking, cleaning, shopping, or paying bills, then a referral to the mental health center or a community program is indicated. Client education is essential to aid clients in relearning previously known skills that may have been forgotten during a lengthy hospitalization.

Many clients benefit from *group supervision* where they can share feelings and experiences with understanding peers and staff. Some groups are nondirective, and members discuss any topic of interest; others focus on a specific topic and are led by a member or outside resource person.

Homelessness

Homelessness is increasingly becoming a community health problem. The homeless are a large, diverse, and vulnerable group. Economic problems, unemployment, urban renewal, fire, and eviction contribute to the problem of homelessness. Discharged psychiatric patients are particularly vulnerable to becoming homeless because many have limited resources and restricted abilities to earn an income. Baxter and Hopper (1981, p. 6) define homeless persons as " . . . those whose primary nighttime residence is either in the publicly or privately owned shelters or in the streets, in doorways, train stations and bus terminals, public plazas and parks, subways, abandoned buildings, loading docks. . . ." No age group is immune from becoming homeless. Young women with children can be found living in the streets, as can the elderly.

The homeless are vulnerable to a variety of physical health problems, including:

1. Maintenance of body temperature
2. Exacerbation of chronic illness
3. Exposure to pollutants
4. Incomplete or delayed resolution of acute health problems
5. Constant mobility (foot and leg problems, sleep deprivation)
6. Infectious diseases (Sebastian, 1985)

Constant mobility creates a unique set of problems, including foot and leg blisters, ulcerations, and fatigue. Many of the homeless suffer from chronic sleep deprivation. As can be imagined, it is difficult to find satisfactory places to sleep on the street. Many of the homeless must defend their territory, including their sleeping place, from other street people.

The mental health problems of the homeless are exacerbated by their inability to take medications at scheduled intervals and to be present for counseling appointments and their frequent lack of funds to get medications refilled. Loneliness, depression, and low self-esteem are among the problems faced by the homeless.

To address the problem of the homeless mentally ill in America, the American Psychiatric Association Task Force called for the establishment of a comprehensive and integrated system of care with designated responsibilities, accountability, and adequate fiscal resources. Some of the Task Force's recommendations included:

1. Basic needs such as food, shelter, and clothing must be provided.
2. Adequate numbers of supervised community housing programs must be established.
3. Adequate, comprehensive, and accessible psychiatric and rehabilitative services must be available.
4. General medical assessment and care must be available.
5. Crisis services must be available and accessible.
6. A system of responsibility for chronically mentally ill living in the community must be established.

7. Legal and administrative procedures must be changed to ensure continuing community care.
8. Adequate numbers of professionals and paraprofessionals must be trained for community care of the chronically ill (Lamb, 1984).

The community health nurse may be one of the few individuals in a community with the ability to recognize, evaluate, and coordinate follow-up care for the homeless mentally ill.

Affective Disorders

Affective disorders comprise one of the most common psychiatric syndromes and are essentially of three types: depressive disorder; manic disorder; and bipolar affective disorder, in which episodes of manic and depressive behavior alternate. As with the schizophrenias, the etiology of affective disorders is not clearly understood but does seem to result from multiple factors, including genetic predisposition, stressful life events, high risk for stress based on personality characteristics, and either inherited or acquired biological abnormalities (President's Commission, 1978). Affective disorders are the number one mental health problem in the United States. It is estimated that 25% of the population experiences depression requiring professional care at some point in their lives (Pelletier and Cousins, 1984). Although more men successfully commit suicide, twice as many women attempt suicide. Married women have higher rates of depression than single, widowed, or divorced women and all categories of men. Marriage seems to have a protective effect for men and a detrimental effect for women. After the age of 65 men seem to become more depressed, and the rate of depression becomes nearly equal for men and women. The increase in depression is attributed to the effect of environmental stress and role adjustment after retirement.

All depressive disorders include mood disturbances characterized by blue, sad, hopeless feelings, irritability, and despair. Sleep may be disrupted by inability to fall asleep, middle of the night or early morning awakening, or hypersomnia. Eating habits may change and be accompanied by either weight gain or loss. Other symptoms include fatigue, lack of interest, feelings of self-reproach, guilt, hopelessness, helplessness, or anger.

Recent studies reviewed by Pelletier and Cousins (1984) indicate that depression is more serious than previously believed; recovery may take several months, and relapse occurs in many instances. Treatment typically includes psychotherapy, medication, and/or electroconvulsive therapy. Medications most useful in treating depression (described later in this chapter) include tricyclic agents, monoamine oxidase inhibitors, and antidepressants. Lithium carbonate is being used with manic depressive cycles and recently has been found effective with serious recurring depression.

Community health nurses must be aware that certain medical illnesses, such as hypothyroidism, anemias, cancer of the pancreas, and some neurological difficulties, can cause or mimic depression. Depression can also be a side effect of medications such as reserpine and propranolol (Pelletier and Cousins, 1984).

Although genetic factors seem to partially explain depressive predisposition, especially when manic episodes are also present, there does appear to be considerable environmental influence. It is well established that early parenting behaviors contribute to level of self-esteem, personal belief system, and feelings of security and trust of others. Currently, a number of social influences contribute to depression. As mentioned previously, economic conditions can precipitate depression and feelings of inadequacy. The media present the American life-syle as happy, carefree, and always smiling and purchasing things, yet many people are confronted with a variety of unpleasant and often painful life stressors that dispute this image.

The primary prevention of depression is directed toward building adaptive strengths and coping resources in people, especially those at high risk. Thus addressing broad social issues and initiating programs are indicated as primary preventive measures for depression. People need to learn more effective ways to cope with life events before a crisis to self-esteem and personal worth develops. In addition, attention should be devoted to high stress periods, such as the early childrearing years when parents' worth and competency may be threatened when children do not conform to social expectations. For example, not all children are healthy, normal, attractive, intelligent, and well-mannered regardless of parental behaviors. Parents can become involved in educational programs for parenting or support groups to help them cope with family responsibilities more effectively.

Community health nurses see clients at risk for depression in a variety of settings, including clinics, the home, the workplace, and schools. Group education, as well as individual counseling, can be carried out by community health nurses for people at risk for depression. For example, classes in stress management, parenting, assertiveness, and coping with crises can decrease the tendency to become depressed by enriching self-esteem and teaching skills needed for successful coping.

PSYCHOSOCIAL FACTORS INCREASING THE RISK OF MENTAL ILLNESS

Psychosocial factors increasing the risk of mental health disruption refer to the accumulation of psychological, social, economic, and cultural forces affecting adaptation. People do not respond to one stimulus at a time but react to the cumulative impact of variables in their lives. Of particular interest is the effect of life events on the maintenance of psychcosocial stability. As Hamburg and Killilea (1979, p. 257) point out, "Life change events of predictable and unpredictable nature are an inevitable aspect of human experience. These events may produce life stress that exceeds an individual's coping ability." Changes in life events are inevitable; it is the rapidity at which they occur, the significance they hold for those involved, and each person's coping ability that determine their influence. In general, factors that influence whether life events are viewed as disruptive to psychological equilibrium include the following (Hamburg and Killilea, 1979):

1. A person's biological and psychological characteristics
2. The social and environmental context of the life event
3. Individual coping ability
4. The rate and number of changes occurring at a given time

Holmes and Rahe (1976) devised a social adjustment rating scale in which numbers are assigned to the effect of predictable life events. Examples of life events having either a negative or positive effect included marriage, moving to a new home, assuming a mortgage, death of a spouse, divorce, or a minor traffic violation. Each change event had a different numerical outcome, depending on the way the researchers determined its effect on their study sample. In addition, the outcome of each event depended on both the perception of the people involved and their ability to cope with the change. For people with limited competence in handling change, even minor life events such as receiving a traffic ticket can be disruptive, whereas more adaptive people may seem barely affected by what appear to observers to be major life disruptions. Four broad approaches for dealing with stressful circumstances include the following (Hamburg and Killilea, 1979):

1. Containing distress within limits that are personally tolerable
2. Maintaining self-esteem
3. Preserving interpersonal relationships and a sense of belonging to a valued group
4. Meeting the conditions and demands of the new situation and simultaneously preparing for the future

Various interventions and coping strategies are available for dealing with change. The strategy chosen depends on the developmental and family history of the person, the specific circumstances surrounding the event, (including the number of stressors at any one time), and the nature of the available support system.

Before discussing specific community mental health nursing interventions, two mental health stressors—divorce and two-career families—that are increasing both in number and impact on family stability are discussed. By no means are these stressors meant to represent an inclusive list but rather they are two common life events in typical communities that are not ordinarily addressed in community health nursing literature.

Divorce as a Life Change Stressor

In recent years the divorce rate has increased dramatically, confronting individuals and families with new and often multiple problems. The divorce and annulment rate per 100 population was 5.3 in 1981 compared with 2.5 in 1965 (National Data Book, 1985), with the median duration of the marriage being 7.0 years and the median age of divorce for first marriages of males being 31.5 versus 29.2 years for females.

The first year after a divorce is often considererd the most difficult period. In an 18-month study of 49 once-married and newly separated men and women, Caldwell, Bloom, and Hodges (1983) found that women were most often the initiators of the separation and during the early months of the separation were most likely to see the benefits of their decision. Both groups reported a high incidence of psychological symptoms before separation. Over time women experienced greater support from their social network than men. Also, younger women who held nontraditional sex role attitudes seemed to adjust better than their older, more traditional counterparts.

The community health nursing role is that of supporting all members of families going through a divorce as each attempts to reestablish psychological stability. Before looking at each member's possible reactions, it is useful to note several key components and reactions to the experience. For all involved, divorce is both a disorganizing and reorganizing process that may take several years to resolve. Divorce is both a maturational and a situational life crisis, and like other life crises, the potential for growth and personal development exists, although considerable support and understanding may be needed. At this time, all involved need acceptance and nonjudgmental understanding. People going through or adapting to a divorce often behave in ways that seem contrary to societal expectations; it is essential to accept the person while recognizing that the observed behavior is an effort to cope with a threat to stability.

For example, divorced women often feel worthless, helpless, or physically unattractive. Many have only known a role as someone's wife; when a divorce occurs, they may temporarily lose their sense of identity. The challenge facing these women is to find meaning and purpose in their own life experiences, such as through work or school. Children both help and hinder the process of divorce adjustment. They help in that the pattern of life goes on much the same as before, since children's needs remain constant or become intensified by the experience. Meals must be prepared, carpools driven, and schedules met. On the other hand, children deplete energy reserves when one parent has major responsibility for meeting their needs. Frequently mothers retain custody of children. Wilk (1979), reporting on a study of single divorced mothers who attended a Planned Parenthood Center, found through interviews that these women, when asked to describe themselves, used terms such as "lost," "flighty," "lonely," "floating," and "trying to make it through one day at a time." Compounding these feelings of loneliness, the women felt considerable pressure from the greater parenting responsibilites than from that experienced in two-parent families. In many instances a major concern stemmed from not having someone to talk with about their problems. Those interviewed requested that a group be formed to help them deal with problems related to parenting, community resources, housing, transportation, and child care.

Men, too, experience pain and disruption to their lives when a divorce occurs. Regardless of the events and feelings surrounding a divorce, there is a threat to stability and a necessity for learning new ways to adapt. Both men and women seek validation of their worth from members of the opposite sex. Also, in most divorces men leave their familiar home and often miss the furniture and treasured items they were accustomed to seeing and using. Barhopping, staying out all night at singles parties, buying fancy clothes and cars, and spending hours on the telephone reflect efforts to cope with feelings of alienation, loneliness, and rootlessness. No matter how stressful and strained a marriage is, it does represent a familiar way of life; being single requires an entirely different set of behaviors.

Individual and/or group counseling helps people cope with the feelings, fears, and need to develop new personal resources. Such sessions, for both children and adults, assist the involved parties to disengage from their past relationships with a minimum of pain and destructive feelings. Many of the feelings surrounding a divorce are similar to the grief over the death of a loved one. People need to express and deal with feelings of denial, anger, depression, acceptance, and resolution in an unbiased environment. Although family and friends are immensely needed, they are rarely unbiased in their views, which limits their ability to assist in the resolution of feelings.

The children of divorcing parents comprise a special concern for community health nurses, both because of the numbers involved and because of the disruption and stress attendant on family disruption (Tableman, 1981). The research of Kelly and Wallerstein (1977) indicates that all children initially react to family disruption with aberrant behavior, and all profit from support during this stress period. Some children experience continuing problems, and community health nurses need to assess whether children's reactions are within normal ranges or if more extensive counseling is indicated. In general, children's reactions vary according to the child's age, sex, developmental stage, and amount of conflict surrounding the event. Table 32-1 provides information about age-specific reactions to divorce.

Children often are delayed in their progress in working through their feelings of loss because they become immobilized in denial by maintaining the fantasy that their divorced parents will someday reconcile and they will live "happily ever after." Moreover, Kelly and Wallerstein (1977) found that stresses and/or resources in the environment, including parental interactions and the availability of the noncustodial parent, influenced coping ability. Based on their research, they developed a "divorce-specific" assessment guide, which is modified and shown in Table 32-1. This guide provides critical information for nurses working with families who are involved in a divorce by identifying typical behaviors that occur at each stage of growth and development.

Over time the characteristics of a child's response to divorce depends on the parents' reaction to the experience and their ability to recognize and provide support for the child's needs. Frequently parents are so caught up in dealing with their own feelings related to the divorce that they have limited resources available to share with their children. Lack of parental nurturance is particularly detrimental to preschool children who under normal circumstances have substantial dependency needs. According to Tableman (1981), preschool girls are particularly vulnerable to the decreased parental attention, especially from the mother, that may occur during a divorce. Typically during the later preschool years children form identities with the same sex parent. Lack of time and attention at this developmental stage disrupts this process.

Children are also at risk for mental health disruption when they are caught in the middle of parental conflict.

TABLE 32-1

Age-specific reactions to divorce

Observed behavior	Nursing intervention
EARLY PRESCHOOL (2½-3½ YEARS)	
Acute regression, heightened aggression and irritability, fearfulness, separation anxiety, bewilderment, acute sadness, tearfulness	Provide guidance to the custodial parent, who serves as the child's best support person Teach communication skills to parents so they can assist the child to interpret the meaning of divorce Help parent look at alternatives for intervening in the child's regressive behavior
LATER PRESCHOOL (3½-6 YEARS)	
Fear, excessive worrying, heightened anxiety, whininess, restlessness, moodiness, general irritability, and symptomatic behaviors, including phobias, sleep disturbances, compulsive eating, aggressiveness, and temper tantrums Difficulty understanding what is happening Frequently asking where the absent parent is Increasing use of fantasy to substitute for absent parent Some experience considerable feelings of guilt and self-blame	Help parent become increasingly consistent and predictable about visitation, discipline, and support Provide support and encouragement to parents and babysitter (when appropriate) concerning child's need for reassurance that he is loved and will be cared for
EARLY LATENCY (6-9 YEARS)	
Behavioral changes in school Obvious pain, suffering, and fear Often immobilized by the divorce Less able to use denial than are younger children, yet open confrontation with reality is painful Nearly insatiable need to maintain contact with both parents Frequent outbursts of anger Feelings of deprivation; focused on fantasies of getting new toys, clothes, or pets Feelings of responsibility	Open discussions may be too threatening but these children can talk about how "other kids react to . . ." Help parents support the child's need for contact with them; for assurance that he is loved and that anger is all right Respect the child's need for the defenses of denial or repression; let children verbalize on *their* timetable Use "divorce monologue" to discuss common reactions of many children; this lets the child know that his reactions are all right and does not force him to talk before he is ready
LATER LATENCY (9-12 YEARS)	
Behavioral changes in school Torn in loyalty between parents Considerable worrying Have the ability to express their feelings and can also channel them into organized activities Child's superego controls may be threatened as external controls are decreased or become inconsistent because of parental stress Have an increased need to discuss the divorce experience with someone outside the family, but they feel very loyal to at least one parent and often have trouble talking about that parent At first may appear poised and calm about family situation as they actively try to make order of their lives Anger well organized and object directed (expressed outwardly and also as demandingness; a dictatorial attitude)	Encourage the child to talk with both parents about fears and worries, hurts and anger Support children as they express pain and anger; help them channel these feelings into socially accepted outlets Help parents become increasingly consistent and firm in their approach to the children Listen, listen, listen
ADOLESCENCE (12-18 YEARS)	
Intense feelings of pain (anger, sadness, sense of loss and betrayal) Strong feelings of shame and embarrassment Concern about their future as a marital partner Concern about adequacy as a sexual partner in their current dating or future married life Often unrealistic concern about finances Shortened disengagement from and shift in perceptions of parents Accelerated individuation of parents Heightened awareness of parents as sexual objects Loyalty conflicts Strategic withdrawal as a defense against pain	Provide an opportunity for open discussion of feelings, including helping adolescents plan ways to express their feelings directly and constructively Discuss feelings of shame, embarrassment, and fear of the future Use communication strategies such as role-playing or psychodrama to help adolescents learn new ways to deal with feelings Practice improved, honest, and open communication patterns

Based on data from Wallerstein, J.S., and Kelly, J.B.: Am. J. Orthopsychiatry, 47:4-22, Jan. 1977.

Frequently there are legal contests over custody, visitation rights, amount of child support, and decisions about who gets which of the joint possessions. For children caught in the middle of parental hostilities and battles, resolution of the divorce trauma is difficult; rather than coping with a single crisis, their emotions are kept in a turmoil through an ongoing experience. Children from divorced families tend to be overrepresented in the caseloads of psychiatric facilities. Common presenting symptoms are depression, aggressive outbursts, and behavioral problems in school (Kalter, 1977; Shanok and Lewis, 1977).

Divorce is considered by many to be the most potentially serious mental health disrupter of the next decade. When a divorce occurs, each family member is confronted with the task of resisting mental health disruption and yet responding to multiple changes and demands for new roles. Divorce frequently is both a disorganizing and a reorganizing process for all people involved. Counseling, support, and guidance can be provided to each person to reinforce host resistance by strengthening coping ability.

Two-Career Families

Few married people today grew up in a two-career family with both parents working outside the home.

Although women have in the past helped with farming or with the family business, only since World War II have women comprised a significant portion of the work force. Also, women, as they become better educated, are pursuing careers demanding of time, attention, and energy. Both men and women are taking jobs that do not end at five o'clock; problems and challenges of the workplace are felt at home as people carry projects and problems home with them. It is not surprising that the reorganization of the family that always exists when a wife enters the labor force can lead to marital disagreements and a decline in marital satisfaction (Booth, et. al, 1984).

In a study of family stress in dual-earner families, Sund and Ostwald (1985) found in a sample of 92 dual-earner families with children under 6 years of age a moderate level of stress when compared with national stress level norms for families in the preschool stage of development. The stress levels were categorized as being either high, moderate, or low. Factors that seemed to mediate stress included the age of the parents, age of the children, family income, and satisfaction with income.

Also, job-related travel has increased in the last 10 years for both men and women, leading to additional responsibilities for the parent who remains at home. If one spouse travels considerably more than the other, there may be feelings of resentment or the common ground for discussion of work events may be altered. The one who stays at home may feel put-upon when the spouse is perceived as having so much fun. In contrast, travel is tiring, often hectic, and usually not as exciting as it seems to observers. Hence, the traveling spouse may come home tired and irritable and desire peace and quiet, which may conflict with the expectations of other family members.

Men may feel threatened by highly successful and visible women. The traditional family prototype has been for husbands to gain recognition for their achievements outside the home and for wives to be supportive of the husband's career and provide a family environment that enriches the entire family. As women gain recognition and acclaim for their career accomplishments, even the most enlightened men may feel twinges of envy and discomfort. There have been few role models for women to turn to in regard to learning how to be a participant in a successful two-career family. Thus men may need as much, if not more, support as women do in adapting to contemporary family life-styles. Opportunities to discuss what being a man in today's society is like can be helpful, such as in support groups led by a knowledgeable nurse. Many communities have begun such groups by using vounteer professionals who provide services to various agencies and community programs.

GOALS OF COMMUNITY MENTAL HEALTH NURSING

Goals of community mental health nursing are multifaceted and are only summarized here. The first goal deals with primary prevention and seeks to prevent the occurrence of mental disorders by strengthening individual, family, and group coping abilities.

The second goal, consistent with secondary prevention, aims to detect early signs of mental health disruption so that prompt counseling, treatment, and referral can be provided. In clinics, schools, home health care, and the work place, community health nurses detect early signs of increased levels of anxiety, decreased ability to cope with stress, and failure to perceive self, the environment, and/or reality accurately. Finding cases in mental health, as in all other areas of community health nursing, is a major goal.

In terms of tertiary prevention, community health nurses play vital roles in monitoring the progress of discharged persons, especially their medication regimen, coordination of care, use of advocacy, and response to referral.

An additional goal that cuts across all levels of prevention is coordination among agencies serving mental health clients. Frequently, support, encouragement, and interpretation of agency resources help clients become more comfortable with the facilities they must visit and the often multiple types of care they must seek.

Many nursing interventions have been integrated throughout the chapter. However, because the effectiveness of any plan for nursing intervention is based on careful and systematic assessment, a model for community assessment that has particular application to meeting community mental health needs is discussed.

Community Mental Health Needs Assessment

To effectively assess the mental health needs of community residents, the assessment should focus on the special needs and wants of the population rather than on the nurse's (or other health care provider's) perception of client needs. Two marketing tools can be employed in a community assessment: *market segmentation* and target marketing. A community is made up of multiple heterogeneous groups known as *markets*. To effectively develop community programs, the total population needs to be subdivided into smaller, more homogeneous groups. Once markets are segmented, interventions can be developed to meet the unique needs of the group chosen for attention.

Three conditions influence market segmentation: measurability, accessibility, and substantiality. Measurability refers to the degree to which information exists or is available about specific characteristics of consumers. Many characteristics, such as values, attitudes, and beliefs, are not easy to measure. Accessibility means that the information does exist and is relatively easy to locate. Some information, while of great potential value, is difficult and often costly to obtain. Substantiality refers to the degree to which market segments are large enough to warrant subdividing for separate programs.

There is no one way to divide a community into segments. Common approaches include segmenting according to demographic variables such as age, sex, income, education, occupation, race, and religion. Markets can also be segmented according to such groupings as stage of the family life cycle or psychographic variables such as activities, values, interests, attitudes, opinions, and life-styles. Another method is to segment according to identified mental health problems or to target "at-risk" groups such as families under stress, victims of violence, or discharged psychiatric patients.

Once the community has been segmented, the following information should be obtained. A geographic area should be defined to limit the size of the market. The size and location of the target market need to be considered; strategies differ when markets are small in their geographic area or densely as opposed to sparsely populated.

Once the needs of the community have been assessed, look at the available resources. Information should be gathered concerning what services already exist in the traditional mental health area, as well as resources such as schoolteachers, clergy, halfway houses, nursing homes, and so on.

A final input is an identification of community attitudes toward mental health. The approach depends largely on the attitudinal information gathered from the groups and individuals working with clients, such as private practitioners, staff and administrators in public and private hospitals, social workers, clergymen, and power groups in the community who may control resources and may or may not sanction certain services. The box on p. 644 summarizes a community assessment tool that is easily used in determining the mental health needs of a community.

Supervision of Patients Receiving Psychotropic Medications

A major goal for community health nurses in assisting the mentally ill is to supervise their taking of *psychotropic medications.* The nurse must know the client's medication regimen, the purpose for which the medication is being used, and the potential side effects and complications of the medication. In addition to routine monitoring, testing should be done periodically when clients are taking these medications to avoid serious side effects associated with long-term use. Testing often includes complete blood cultures,

hepatic function studies, blood sugar tests, and ophthalmic testing. The box below lists data to be gathered in assessing medication management.

Table 32-2 lists the common uses of and side effects from antidepressants, antipsychotics, antianxiety agents, and manic and extrapyramidal symptom agents.

The antidepressants known as *monoamine oxidase inhibitors* (MAOIs) need careful monitoring because these drugs have dangerous side effects when certain foods are eaten. Some of the effects of MAOIs can be dangerous or even fatal. Paradoxical hypertension can occur when certain foods rich in amines (such as tryramine) or in amino acids (such as tryosine) are ingested. The pressor amines are normally inactivated by MAO but because MAO is inhibited, they can produce hypertension and intracranial bleeding. Foods that contain these amines include liver, aged cheeses, yogurt, alcoholic beverages, excess caffeine and chocolate, and foods that have been aged, pickled, or smoked. These foods should be avoided for at least 2 to 3 weeks after discontinuation of drug therapy because of continued MAO inhibition. Jaundice and leukopenia are also known side effects of MAOIs. Because of these possible complications, use of MAOIs is usually reserved for hospitalized patients. Suicidal tendencies also occur more often near the end of the depressive cycle; thus clients warrant close attention at this time.

Alcohol potentiates the effect of antianxiety agents and

DATA BASE FOR MEDICATION MANAGEMENT

Psychiatric/medical diagnosis
Vital signs
    Blood pressure
    Pulse
Medication history
    Present medications
        Routine and PRN medications
        Name of the medication
        Prescribed dosage
        Frequency of administration
        How long the individual has been taking the medication
    Past medications (especially those that caused the individual problems)
        Name of the medication
        How long the individual was taking the medication
        Any side effects from the medication
    Over-the-counter medications frequently taken
        Sleep aids
        Laxatives
    Leftover medications that the individual may take occasionally
Past medical history
    Liver disease
    Glaucoma
    Kidney disease
    Visual problems
    Alcohol or drug abuse
Mental status examination

COMMUNITY ASSESSMENT TOOL

MARKET ANALYSIS

Environmental analysis describes major trends or developments with respect to demography, economy, technology, government, and culture affecting the community.

Demographic developments will affect the ultimate size of the community and its needs. The main demographic factors are size of the population, its age distribution, trends in the birth and death rate, and its geographic distribution.

What major demographic developments and trends pose opportunities or threats for this community?

What actions have been taken in response to these developments?

What effect will the forecasted trends have on the community?

Economic developments have a strong effect on the demand for products and services and the cost of providing them.

What major developments and trends in income, prices, savings, and credit have an impact on the community?

What actions have been taken in response to these developments and trends?

Technological developments have a great significance for possible new products and services and cost savings.

What major changes are occurring in product technology?

What major changes are occurring in service technology?

What major changes are occurring in process technology?

Governmental developments are difficult to predict but can have a profound effect on the community.

What new legislation could affect this community?

What laws are being proposed that may affect this community?

What federal, state, and local agency actions should be watched?

What actions has the community taken in response to these developments?

Social-cultural developments have an effect on values and life-styles in the community.

What changes are occurring in life-styles and values that might affect this community?

What actions have been taken in response to these developments?

Market definition defines the characteristics of the community's major mental health care markets.

Who are the primary (actual and potential) markets for mental health care in this community?

Market segmentation divides a market into groups of people who have relatively similar needs. *Bases* for segmenting include:

Geographic
Demographic
Psychographic (life-style)
Service usage

Benefits sought
High-risk groups
Readiness or predisposition to respond

What are the major market segments in this community?

What are the characteristics of each market segment?

Criteria for segments:

Substantiality—must be large enough to justify effort

Measurability—information can be obtained

Accessibility—groups can be reached

What is the present size of each market segment?

What is the expected size of each market segment?

Needs assessment identifies needs unique to each segment.

What is the present state of needs of each market segment?

What is the expected state of needs of each market segment?

Satisfaction assessment identifies level of needs satisfaction within each market segment.

How satisfied are the needs of each market segment?

Identifying target markets focuses on unsatisfied or undersatisfied needs.

Which market segments have needs requiring attention?

On which market segments are our resources best directed?

RESOURCE ANALYSIS

Competitor identification enumerates the community's major competitive professional resources.

Forms of competition include generic, service form, and enterprise professional resources.

Generic: other broad service categories that might satisfy the same need

Service form: specific versions of the service that may be competitive

Enterprise: specific organizations that are competitive purveyors of the same services

Who are the community's major competitive professional resources?

How are these competitive professional resources defined? Generic, service form, or enterprise?

What types of competitors?

How many in each category?

What trends can be foreseen in the competitive environment?

Attitude and image analysis profiles the attitudes and images held by various constituencies within the community.

What are the attitudes of those professionals who work with mental health clients?

What are the attitudes and images of special interest groups regarding community mental health issues?

What are the attitudes and images of clients regarding community mental health issues?

What are the attitudes and images of nonclients regarding community mental health issues?

From Lancaster, J., and Lancaster, W.: The psychiatric nurse's role in community mental health. In Stuart, G.W., and Sundeen, S.J.: *Principles and practice of psychiatric nursing,* ed. 3, St. Louis, 1987, The C.V. Mosby Co.

TABLE 32-2

Psychotropic drugs: action and side effects

Name	Action	Side effects
Antipsychotics	To control acute and chronic psychotic conditions (schizophrenia, mania, paranoid symptoms, agitated psychotic depression)	Unpleasant behavioral effects (feelings of lassitude, fatigue, depression, atropine psychosis) Postural hypertension Extrapyramidal symptoms Pigmentation of the skin and eyes
Antidepressants	To control the following symptoms: Appetite disturbances Lowered mood Difficulty in thinking Inability to concentrate or make decisions Loss of interest in work, recreation, or activity Somatic complaints (headaches, sleep disturbances, insomnia, or hyposomnia, decreased sexual drive) Psychomotor retardation or agitation Suicidal ideation	Hypotension, restlessness, visual disturbances, dry mouth, urinary retention, rashes, liver damage
Antianxiety agents	To control symptoms associated with psychosomatic conditions, as well as insomnia, anxiety, nausea and hyperbilirubinemia, chronic cholestasis, acute seizure disorders, and muscle spasms	Acute poisoning, respiratory failure, chronic barbiturate poisoning (slowness of thought, depression, incoherent speech, failing memory, rash, weight loss, GI upset, anemia, ataxia, tremors)
Antimanic agents	Management of the manic phase of bipolar disorders (manic-depressive illness)	Metallic taste in the mouth Fine tremor of the hand Nausea Polydipsia Diarrhea or loose stools Muscular weakness or fatigue Faulty coordination Dizziness Slurred speech Blurred vision Edema of the face, hands, feet, or abdominal wall
Extrapyramidal symptom agents	Used to control the extrapyramidal symptom side effects of antipsychotic drugs such as akathisia, acute dystonia, or tardive dyskinesia	Cardiovascular system Tachycardia, paradoxical hypertension, bradycardia, transient hypotension Central nervous system Disorientation, nervousness, weakness, irritability, headache, hallucination, euphoria, delusions Ear, eye, nose, throat Blurred vision, mydriasis, increased intraocular pressure, dilated pupils, photophobia, difficulty in swallowing Gastrointestinal system Dry mouth, nausea, vomiting, constipation, sore mouth and tongue Genitourinary system Urinary hesitancy/retention Skin Rash

may lead to injury or accidental overdose. People need to be informed of the addictive potential of chronic excessive use, as well as the symptoms associated with abrupt withdrawal.

Special precautions need to be included in the management of clients taking the antimanic drug lithium. This drug has a narrow therapeutic index, which means that the body cannot tolerate accumulation of lithium salt in the bloodstream. Blood levels of lithium need to be monitored regularly.

The *tardive dyskinesia,* or involuntary, repetitive movements of the muscles of the face, limbs, and trunk, associated with long-term antipsychotic agents is not alleviated by antiparkinsonism agents and may be worsened by them (Krupp and Chatton, 1982). Community health nurses should educate clients taking antipsychotic drugs to watch for symptoms of tardive dyskinesia. Symptoms include involuntary movements of the face, mouth, jaw, and tongue; puffing of the cheeks; eye blinking; and abnormal movements of the extremities. A detailed summary of the side effects of psychotropic drugs is found in Appendix D.

CLINICAL APPLICATION

Mrs. Brown, during a routine home visit to two elderly clients, learned that their 52-year-old son was posing serious problems for the couple. Both Mr. and Mrs. Ables are in their late 70s. They each have several chronic illnesses but are able to maintain their independence because the nurse visits once a week to regulate Mrs. Ables' insulin and assist her with diet supervision and foot care. They also have a cleaning lady who comes twice a week to clean their small home and purchase their groceries.

The Ables have a married daughter who lives in the same city and stops by at least two times a week to visit and assist them with errands, paying their bills, keeping appointments with health care providers, and general management of their affairs. Their only son, Tom, has a long history of manic-depressive illness. For many years he and his wife lived in another state. Tom was able to maintain a job, although he periodically needed brief hospitalizations to regulate his lithium dosage.

Two years ago, Tom's wife died as a result of an automobile accident. Since that time Tom has had frequent hospitalizations and has lost his job. Six months before the nurse's visit, Tom had hitchhiked to the city where his parents live. He often came to their house in a state of acute agitation and disarray. Frequently he appeared malnourished yet refused their constant offers of food. Mr. and Mrs. Ables realized that their son needed medical care, yet they were unable to persuade him to seek such care. He would at times listen to his sister, but of late he had refused to follow her suggestion and visit the community mental health center.

On learning of this situation, Mrs. Brown realized that the Ables' son had a negative effect on the well-being of the elderly couple. They were increasingly anxious and seemed less able to manage their lives. The nurse suggested that the Ables contact their daughter and see if she could arrange for Tom to be present the following week when the nurse visited.

During Mrs. Brown's next visit, both Tom and his sister were present. The nurse observed Tom was much less active than he had been described as being in the recent past. In fact, the nurse assessed that Tom's illness had swung into the depressed stage, as judged by his slowness of movement and speech, downcast eyes, weight loss, and reported difficulties in sleeping. The nurse explained to Tom that he needed to have his medication regulated to control the mood swings caused by his illness. As it turned out, Tom had not been taking his lithium. In fact, it had been 5 months since he had run out of his medication. With considerable encouragement from Mrs. Brown and the Ables' daughter, Tom agreed to be taken to the mental health center. The counselor who assessed Tom determined that he needed to be hospitalized so that his physical and mental health could be completely assessed and his medication regulated.

Although Tom was not a client of the community health nurse, his well-being was affecting his parents. Without infringing on Tom's rights, the nurse was able to persuade him to voluntarily seek treatment.

SUMMARY

The pressures and stresses of the twentieth century are taking their toll on the mental health of the population. People are increasingly succumbing to stress-related illnesses, thereby impairing their ability to cope and adapt to changing life events. In the early 1960s tremendous financial resources were channeled into the development of community mental health centers, yet critics contend that these centers have not fulfilled their original promises. Instead of being truly community oriented, the mental health system is accused of being a "revolving door" where clients are treated briefly in the hospital then released to the community, often without adequate advance preparation. Some communities have been able to develop comprehensive programs to adequately meet the needs of the returning psychiatric client; however, this has by no means been a universal realization. In too many instances, clients are returned to the community only to be housed in inadequate boarding or nursing homes. Critics contend that the only thing that has changed over the years in regard to community-based treatment for psychiatric clients has been "who pays the bill." The implications for community health nursing are evident: Who, more than community health nurses, has access and visibility in the community? Who can better serve as a client advocate to help the chronically ill navigate a complex social and health care system? For many, the tasks of locating health care facilities and arranging transportation are overwhelming responsibilities. Advocacy, caring, and coordination are imperative challenges for the community health nurse.

Like the chronically ill psychiatric client, those who are coping with numerous and often taxing life struggles need the attention of the community health nurses. Families are changing, and the ability to adapt to new roles is not as easy as it might seem at first glance. Mutual support groups are a special kind of assistance that can be provided in communities to help people obtain primary mental health services before any disruption in the ability to cope effectively. Just talking about life pressures with a group of similar and concerned people is often a major source of relief.

Considerable problem solving can also be provided in support groups as people share with one another what has helped them. Nurses can be instrumental in serving as catalysts or leaders of such groups.

≡ KEY CONCEPTS

Persons with mental health problems and needs frequently are clients of the community health nurse.

The definitions of mental health vary considerably, and the concepts of mental health and mental illness have changed dramatically in the last five centuries.

The maintenance of mental health, viewed from a community health perspective, is a complex process whereby people attain at least a moderate degree of adaptation to the environment and are able to cope with daily stressors and function in everyday activities.

Despite more than two decades of federal and local funding, few mental health centers have achieved their original goals of providing accessible, comprehensive mental health services at the local level.

In recent years the benefits of community mental health centers have increased, and the criticisms have decreased.

The most effective primary prevention approach requires a union of public health and mental health concepts.

In recent years the deinstitutionalization of chronic psychiatric patients has dramatically altered the services provided by community health nurses.

Homelessness is increasingly becoming a community health concern.

Psychosocial factors that increase the risk of mental health disruption are psychological, social, economic, and cultural forces affecting adaptation. Among the most significant mental health stressors are divorce and the two-career family.

An effective assessment of community mental health needs should focus on the special needs and wants of the population rather than on the health care provider's perception of client needs.

In addition to the goals of primary, secondary, and tertiary prevention of mental illness, major goals of community health nurses in assisting the mentally ill include careful, systematic assessment of community mental health needs and supervision of mentally ill patients in their taking of psychotropic medications.

LEARNING ACTIVITIES

1. Obtain from at least two different clients all information necessary to assess the clients' medication regimens.

2. By reading your local newspaper, observing happenings in your community, listening to the radio, and watching television, determine what potential threats to mental health exist in your community.

3. Using a community resources guide, determine what resources are available in your community for chronically mentally ill clients and their families.

4. Interview a career woman with young children and one with teenagers concerning their perceptions of the stressors in their lives.

5. Interview a parent who has been divorced and a child from a divorced family concerning their perceptions of the stressors they experience.

6. Interview a parent and a child from what you judge to be a typical family in your community to determine their perceptions of their stressors.

7. Evaluate the preceding three sets of interviews for consistency, contrasts in types, and amount of stress.

BIBLIOGRAPHY

Baxter, E., and Hopper, K.: Private lives/public spaces: homeless adults on the streets of New York City, New York, 1981, Community Service Corporation.

Bloom, B.L.: Prevention of mental disorders: recent advances in theory and practice, Comm. Ment. Health J. 15(3):179-191, 1979.

Boondas, J.: The despair of the homeless aged, J. Gerontol. Nurs. 11(4):9-13, 1985.

Booth, A., Johnson, D., and White, L.: Women, outside employment, and marital instability, Am. J. Sociol. 90(3):567, 1984.

Caldwell, R.A., Bloom, B.L., and Hodges, W.F.: Sex differences in separation and divorce, Iss. Ment. Health Nurs. 5:103-120, 1983.

Caplan, G.: Support systems and community mental health, New York, 1974, Behavioral Publications.

Citizens guide to the Community Mental Health Centers Amendment of 1975, Washington, D.C., 1977, U.S. Government Printing Office.

Davies, M.A.: Continuing care unit: a model of services for chronic psychiatric patients, J. Psychiatr. Nurs. 19:42-45, Feb. 1981.

Eisenberg, L., and Parron, D.: Strategies for the prevention of mental disorders. In Healthy people: the surgeon general's report on health promotion and disease prevention: background papers, Washington, D.C., 1979, U.S. Government Printing Office.

Friedman, E.: The light that failed, Hospitals 57(16):88-94, Aug. 1983.

Hamburg, B., and Killilea, M.: Relation of social support, stress, illness, and use of health services. In Healthy people: the surgeon general's report on health promotion and disease prevention: background papers, Washington, D.C. 1979, U.S. Government Printing Office.

Hanlon, J., and Pickett, G.: Public health administration and practice, ed. 8, St. Louis, 1984, The C.V. Mosby Co.

Harris, E.: Psychotropic drugs: lithium, Am. J. Nurs. 81(7):1310-1315, July 1981.

Harris, E.: Antipsychotic medications, Am. J. Nurs. 81(7):1316-1323, July 1981.

Harris, E.: Extrapyramidal side effects of anti-psychotic medications, Am. J. Nurs. 81(7): 1324-1328, July 1981.

Harris, E.: Sedative-hypnotic drugs, Am. J. Nurs. 81(7):1329-1334, July 1981.

Harris, E.: Somatic treatment. In Lancaster, J., editor: Adult psychiatric nursing, New York, 1984, Medical Examination Publishing Co.

Healthy people: The surgeon general's report on health promotion and disease prevention, DHEW Pub. No. (PHS) 79-55071, Washington, D.C., 1979, U.S. Government Printing Office.

Hecht, A.: A guide to the proper use of tranquilizers, FDA Consumer Guide 19:9-11, Dec. 1985/Jan. 1986.

Hodgins, P.M., and Monfils, M.J.: Nursing care and treatment of the retarded mentally ill. J. Psychosocial Nurs. 23:31-33, 1985.

Holmes, T., and Rahe, R.: The social readjustment rating scale, J. Psychosom. Res. 11(2):213-218, 1976.

Joint Commission on Mental Illness and Health: Action for mental health, New York, 1961, Basic Books, Inc., Publishers.

Kalter, N.: Children of divorce in an outpatient psychiatric population, Am. J. Orthopsychiatry 47:40-51, Jan. 1977.

Kelly, J.B., and Wallerstein, J.S.: Brief interventions with children in divorcing families, Am. J. Orthopsychiatry 47:23-39, Jan. 1977.

Kelly, J.B., and Wallerstein, J.S.: Divorce counseling: a community service for families in the midst of divorce, Am. J. Orthopsychiatry 47:4-22, Jan. 1979.

Krupp, M., and Chatton, M.: Current medical diagnosis and treatment, Los Altos, Calif. 1982, Lange Medical Publications.

Lamb, H.R.: Deinstitutionalization and the homeless mentally ill, Hosp. Commun. Psychiatry 35:899, 1984.

Lancaster, J.: Community mental health nursing: an ecological perspective, St. Louis, 1980, The C.V. Mosby Co.

Lancaster, J., and Lancaster, W.: The psychiatric nurse's role in community mental health. In Stuart, G., and Sundeen, S., editors: Principles and practices of psychiatric nursing, ed. 3, St. Louis, 1987, The C.V. Mosby Co.

Landsberg, G., and Hammer, R.: Possible programmatic consequences of community mental health center funding arrangements: illustrations based on inpatient utilization data, Commun. Ment. Health J. 13:63-70, 1977.

Leavell, J., and Clark, E.: Preventive medicine for the doctor in this community: an epidemiological approach, New York, 1965, McGraw-Hill Book Co.

Marmor, J., and Pumpian-Mindlin, E.: Toward an integrated conception of mental disorders, J. Nerv. Ment. Dis. 3:19-29, Jan. 1950.

National Data Book: Guide to sources: Statistical abstract of the United States, 1985, 105th ed., U.S. Department of Commerce, Washington, D.C., Bureau of the Census.

Nation's Health, Washington, D.C., 1981, U.S. Government Printing Office.

Newton, M., and Godbey, K.: How you can improve the effectiveness of psychotropic drug therapy, Nursing '78 8(7):46-55, 1978.

Oulette, E., et al.: Adverse effects on offspring of maternal alcohol abuse during pregnancy, N. Engl. J. Med. 297:538-540, 1977.

Pelletier, L., and Cousins, A.: Depression update, J. Emerg. Nurs. 10(6):315-318, Nov./Dec. 1984.

Pepper, B., Kirshner, M.C., and Ryglewicz, H.: The young adult chronic patient: overview of a population, Hosp. Commun. Psychiatr. 32(7):1463-1469, 1981.

President's Commission on Mental Health: Report of the task panel on the nature and scope of the problem, vol. 2, Appendix, Washington, D.C., 1978, U.S. Government Printing Office.

Ramshorn, M.: The major thrust in American psychiatry: past, present and future, Perspect. Psychiatr. Care 9(4):144-154, 1974.

Richmond, J., and Filner, B.: Infant and child health needs and strategies. In Healthy people: the surgeon general's report on health promotion and disease prevention: background papers, Washington, D.C. 1979, U.S. Government Printing Office.

Rubin, J.: The community mental health movement in the United States circa 1979, Am. J. Psychoanal. 31(1):68-79, 1971.

Sebastian, J.: Homelessness: a state of vulnerability. Fam. Comm. Health 8:11-24, 1985.

Seymour, R.J., and Dawson, N.J.: The schizophrenic at home, J. Psycholsocial Nurs. 26(1):28-30, 1986.

Shanok, S., and Lewis, D.: Juvenile courts versus child guidance referral: psychological and parental factors, Am. J. Psychiatry 134(10): 1130-1133, 1977.

Snow, D., and Newton, P.: Task, social structure and social process in the community mental health center movement, Am. Psychol. 31(8):582-594, 1976.

Sund, K., and Ostwald, S.K.: Dual-earner families' stress levels and personal life-style related variables, Nurs. Res. 34(6):357-361, Nov./Dec. 1985.

Tableman, M.: Overview of programs to prevent mental health problems of children, Public Health Rep. 96(1):38-44, 1981.

Taylor, C.: Mereness' essentials of psychiatric nursing, ed. 11, St. Louis, 1982, The C.V. Mosby Co.

Wilk, J.: Assessing single parent needs, J. Psychiatr. Nurs. 116(6):21-22, 1979.

Wilner, D.M., Walkley, R.P., and O'Neill, E.J.: Introduction to public health, ed. 7, New York, 1978, Macmillan Publishing Co., Inc.

Women's health: report of the Public Health Service Task Force on Women's Health Issues, Public Health Reports 100(1):73-106, 1985.

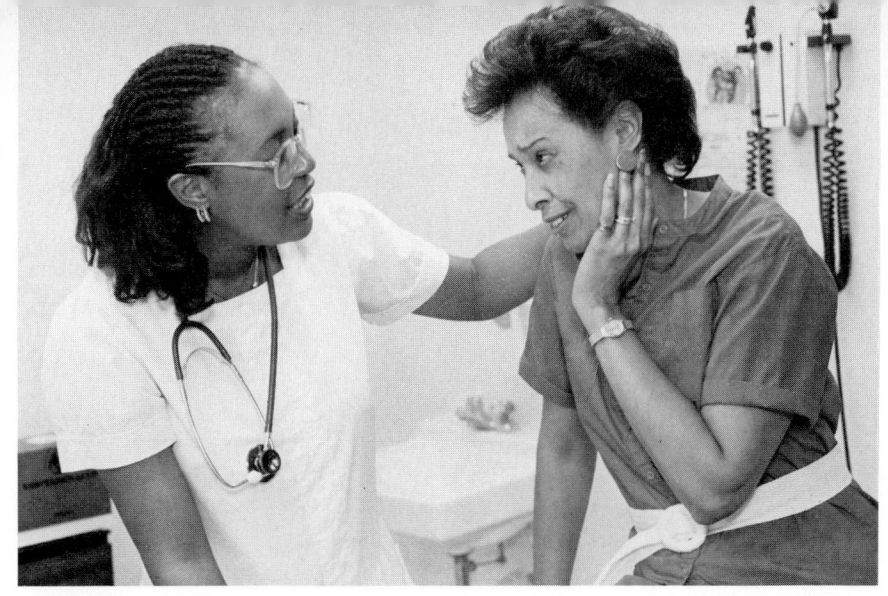

INTERVENING IN CRISIS

Phyllis Graves

33

☰ OBJECTIVES

After reading this chapter, the student should be able to:

Recognize the characteristics of crisis.

Describe the levels of function and tension in each of the four phases of crisis.

Contrast maturational crisis and situational crisis.

Give two examples of anticipatory guidance activities to prevent the occurrence of specific maturational crises.

Discuss two possible roles of community health nurses in (1) primary prevention, (2) secondary prevention, and (3) tertiary prevention of crisis.

Identify the focus of crisis intervention and the roles of the nurse and client.

☰ KEY TERMS

community resources

crisis

crisis intervention

crisis phases

disequilibrium

family life cycle

maturational crisis

primary crisis
  prevention

secondary crisis
  prevention

tertiary crisis prevention

Crisis is a term commonly used in our society for instances in which circumstances are suddenly altered. Headlines may reveal that a city has no more funds and is in crisis or that an unexpected interruption of an energy source and thus a crisis has occurred. Although anticipated and unanticipated events are not in themselves crises, they may predispose individuals, families, and communities to crises. The nature and characteristics of crises are distinctive and set apart from other changes in circumstances. In addition, crises progress through a series of identified phases, each with its own possibilities for intervention.

Crisis intervention techniques can be used by health professionals, nonhealth professionals, and volunteers trained to assist individuals or groups in crisis. Crisis intervention helps clients resolve situations so that the state after the crisis reflects an improvement over the state before the crisis. Responsible community health nurses know about facilities available for crisis prevention and intervention, and they know how clients may gain entry to those resources.

This chapter considers the nature, characteristics, and phases of crisis and the types of crises that individuals, families, and communities experience. An overview of crisis intervention is presented, and the concepts of primary, secondary, and tertiary prevention as they relate to the crisis are discussed. A case is used to illustrate how community health nurses can use the nursing process in crisis intervention. Community resources for crisis are considered in the last section of the chapter.

NATURE OF CRISIS

An essential property of crisis is the potential for promoting growth. Crises present challenges and call for new responses (Rapoport, 1965). Assisting those in crisis to achieve growth is an inherent role for community health nurses.

Caplan (1964), a leader in the development of crisis theory, described *crisis* as an "upset," or disequilibrium in a steady state, occurring when usual problem-solving strategies are ineffective. Typically, a problem situation causes a change in equilibrium, whereby the effected person initiates a previously successful problem-solving or coping strategy to reinstitute a state of balance. Because of the magnitude of the crisis, the person's usual problem-solving strategies are often ineffective, leading to an intense level of disequilibrium. New strategies for problem solving must

then be initiated to alleviate the disruption; the effectiveness of the new strategies leads to one of three potential outcomes. First, effective strategies often lead to psychological growth and a better state of functioning than existed before the crisis. Crises provide opportunities for people to learn new coping mechanisms that can later be applied to other situations. In the second potential outcome, the person returns to the level of functioning before the crisis, with no appreciable gain or loss in functioning. In the third outcome, a loss occurs in that the person reaches a less favorable state than previously existed. When the new strategies are ineffective or the problem continues or intensifies over time, the risk of major psychological disorganization increases.*

As with individuals, when families and communities experience problems that are not solved by usual coping strategies, a crisis occurs. The upset of the steady state of a family or community also offers the possibility for growth and improved function and the danger of major disorganization. Whether the crisis occurs to an individual, family, or community, the situation is one in which a problem is not solved by usual coping strategies, disequilibrium exists, and there is opportunity for growth through the development of new coping strategies.

CHARACTERISTICS OF CRISIS

People in crisis feel helpless and often desire assistance in relieving their misery. The duration of the state of disequilibrium, the individual's perception of the event and problems, and the functioning pattern of the individual (each of which is discussed in the following paragraphs) are characteristic of crises. In addition, cognitive processes may be altered, subjective feelings are usually present, and physiological symptoms occur in many people.

The degree of disequilibrium is related to the duration of the crisis; most crises tend to be temporary and self-limiting and last between 4 and 6 weeks. Thus individuals in crisis are in disequilibrium that cannot be tolerated in-

---

*These possibilities are reflected in the Chinese characters used for the word *crisis* (Aguilera and Messick, 1982). The characters mean danger and opportunity. In a crisis, previous coping strategies are not effective in solving the problem, and there is opportunity for growth through developing new ways of coping.

definitely, and a successful or unsuccessful resolution is reached within a relatively short period of time. For the community health nurse this means that intervention must be prompt and concentrated in a brief time span.

To the individual in crisis the event and accompanying problems are perceived as having serious consequences, but whether or not an event and its problems lead to crisis depends on the perception and coping abilities of the individual. For example, if a person loses his job after being with a company for 20 years and has no experience with unemployment, he may experience a crisis. However, for a high school student who works only for additional spending money, job loss is much less likely to be followed by crisis.

The pattern of functioning is also a feature of those in a state of crisis (Caplan, 1964). In crisis, a decrease in the level of function and associated disorganization occurs; in the disequilibrium state of crisis even routine tasks may not be effectively completed. Recognition of this impairment of functioning level is exemplified by the custom in many communities of taking food to the homes of families who have experienced events such as death, accident, or serious illness. Families in crisis are not expected to function at the same level as others.

Both the increased need for assistance and the increased receptivity to interventions are important considerations for nurses working with those in crisis. Christensen and Harding (1985) illustrated these facets of crisis. A family receiving hospice care refused to allow the nurse to demonstrate a bed bath until the client's first episode of incontinence. For this family the incontinence was the event which precipitated a crisis. At this point the family quickly learned the skills demonstrated by the nurse that allowed them to cope with similar events.

Lindemann's (1979) work with the victims of the Coconut Grove fire is a classic study of individuals in a crisis and provides an understanding of psychological and physiological responses. Further, he was a pioneer in developing interventions that promote growth through successful resolution. Fire engulfed a Boston nightclub on November 28, 1942, while the Harvard-Yale football game was being celebrated. The magnitude of the fire was tremendous, and the death toll reached 491; only 39 people in the nightclub survived. Responding to a request for psychiatric assistance, Lindemann worked with the burn victims, their relatives, and the relatives of those who died. Physical and psychological reactions were noted. Frequent physical responses included sighing respiration, exhaustion, lack of strength, and altered gastrointestinal patterns. For example, usual activities such as walking resulted in a feeling of exhaustion. However, even with the exhaustion, there were feelings of restlessness and the need for activity. Routine tasks were sought and carried out with much effort. Psychological responses in the crisis of acute grief included guilt, hostility, and preoccupation with the image of the deceased.

Although Lindemann found that reactions to the crisis usually closely followed the precipitating event, there were instances of delayed responses. An individual's need to deal with an important problem was a factor in the later grief response. One example involved an adolescent girl who was burned and whose parents were killed in the Coconut Grove fire. Two younger siblings were her chief concern during her hospitalization and resettlement time. Only after more than 2 months did she show depression, frequent crying, and other symptoms of grief.

A more recent crisis situation occurred when within one day, three girls were raped in a New Jersey suburb (Underwood and Fiedler, 1983). Adults and children became apprehensive. The Community Mental Health Center initiated a multi-focus program to cope with the crisis of rape. Meetings for parents, which focused on communicating with children of various ages, correcting misinformation, and reinforcing the amount of control children possess, were begun. Police, the county prosecutor, counselors from the local women's crisis center, and mental health professionals participated in presenting a filmstrip, videotapes, and written materials to the community, and preparing a coloring book for children. Ensuring that the effort occurred quickly after the assault and involving a variety of agencies contributed to the success of the intervention.

The problems resulting in crisis stem from events of loss, threat of loss, or overwhelming challenge (Spradley, 1981). However, undesirable events, such as the death or serious illness of a significant other, are not the only events that may precipitate crises. Desirable events, such as an important new job, may produce problems for a person who lacks effective coping strategies. The problems that could arise following a much desired promotion include establishing relations with new peers and former coworkers, changes in family life-style, and changes in social obligations. Associated problems are inevitable once a significant event has occurred, and in the absence of adequate coping strategies crisis can result.

Another feature of crisis is "cognitive uncertainty" (Spradley, 1981), which means the individual in crisis cannot predict the outcome of the situation. This uncertainty increases the tension experienced by the person in crisis, who experiences many emotions; feelings of helplessness and ineffectuality are characteristic (Caplan, 1964). In addition, depending on the situation, feelings of anxiety, guilt, fear, or shame can occur. For instance, if a child is severely injured while playing, the parents may feel guilty and think that if they had been more attentive, the accident could have been prevented.

Physiological symptoms are often present in individuals in crisis; these responses to crisis vary from person to person and depend on the individual's response to stressors. Sleep disturbances, gastrointestinal symptoms, muscle tension, shortness of breath, irritability, need for routine activity, and exhaustion are among the possible manifestations. For example, a widow whose husband had died 2 days before said that the night he died she had been able to sleep only intermittently, and at 4 AM she had begun cleaning the kitchen.

PHASES OF CRISIS

The progression of an individual through a crisis is described by Caplan (1964) as occurring in four phases (Figure 33-1). In phase 1 a problem is encountered and an initial rise

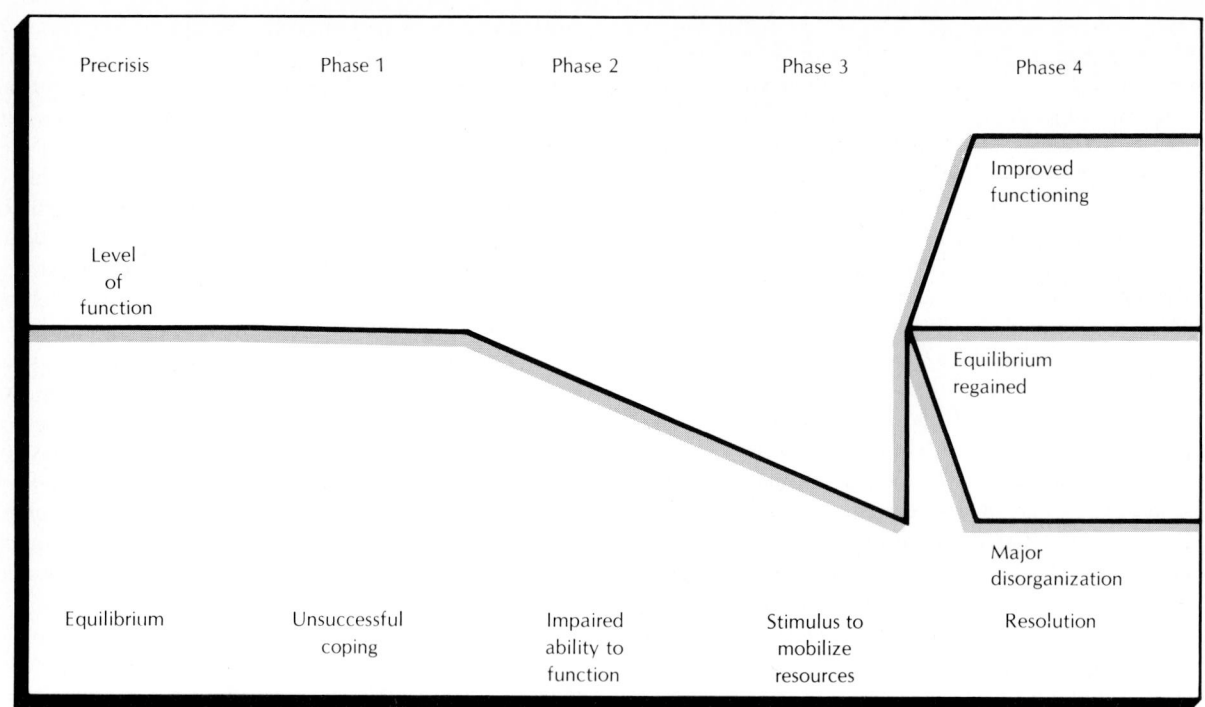

FIGURE 33-1

Phases of crises.

in tension occurs, which causes the person to recall coping strategies that have been successful in the past. When past strategies do not solve the problem and it remains, phase 2 occurs, with a further rise in tension. In phase 2 disequilibrium is evident with the appearance of characteristic psychological and physiological crisis responses; the person's ability to function is impaired. Phase 3, with another rise in tension, stimulates the individual to mobilize resources. Activities in phase 3 can include becoming aware of previously overlooked aspects of the problem, redefining the problem, setting aside irrelevant aspects, and developing new problem-solving mechanisms. If the stategies used in phase 3 are successful, the problem will be resolved and the individual will either return to the previous state of equilibrium or move to an improved level of functioning. If the strategies of phase 3 are not successful, phase 4 follows. With continuation of the problem, lack of success in resolution, and increased tension, a breaking point is reached, and major disorganization results.

TYPES OF CRISIS

Crisis may be categorized as maturational or situational. Also, maturational and situational events may occur concurrently and result in crisis. *Maturational*, or developmental, crises occur during natural transitions in the developmental process. Coping successfully with a maturational transition leads to the next developmental level. The popularity of articles and books that address predictable changes in individuals' lives demonstrates a public awareness of and concern about transition periods. Entering school for the first time, marrying, and retiring are examples of

events that can lead to maturational crises. *Situational*, or accidental, crises follow unanticipated sudden events over which no control can be exerted. Divorce, death, illness, and natural disasters are examples of events that can lead to situational crises.

INDIVIDUALS AND CRISIS

Throughout life, individuals are faced with transition when moving from one stage of development to the next. Because the transitions can be anticipated, measures can be taken to lessen their impact. For example, discussion groups for young teenagers can ease the transition into adolescence. Programs before retirement can help an individual cope with the problems of old age. Developmental psychologists such as Erikson (1950) have identified normal major states of transition in humans (see box at right).

Maturational Crises

As with all crises, maturational crises hold the possibility for growth and the danger of stagnation or regression. For example, adolescents confront issues such as dating, sexual activity, and career choice. Young adults face establishing their own households, securing jobs, and possibly having children. (Problems across the life span are considered in Part Four.)

Situational Crises

Unlike maturational crises, situational crises affecting individuals are frequently sudden and unexpected. Thus anticipatory guidance is not possible, but prompt contact and early intervention can assist the individual to cope with a

NORMAL STATES OF TRANSITION

Infancy to toddler
Toddler to preschool
Preschool to school age
School age to adolescence
Adolescence to adult
Adult to middle age
Middle age to old age

From Erikson, E.: Childhood and society, New York, 1950, W.W. Norton & Co., Inc.

situational crisis. Centers for battered women, laryngectomy self-help groups, and rape crisis centers are examples of organizations developed to assist individuals in coping with specific events that can lead to situational crises.

Some events that lead to situational crises occur precipitously, whereas others have some lead-in time, which can be used to avert or lessen their impact. For example, relocation of an elderly person may cause disequilibrium and subsequent situational crisis (Rosswurm, 1983). The relocation may be moving from one home to another, from one institution to another, within an institution, or from a home to an institution or the reverse. Community health nurses have several opportunities to work with the elderly who are being relocated. Encouraging the older person to discuss the meaning the move has to him and his thoughts and feelings can assist in promoting a realistic perspective of the situation. In addition, several visits to the new residence before the move will not only orient the older person to new surroundings, but also allow him to actively participate in planning the move. Bringing familiar furniture and treasured belongings to the new residence can also ease the transition. Together the community health nurse, elderly person, family, and if an institution is involved, staff can discuss strategies for coping with the move and the new situation. These measures would allow the elderly person to gain a realistic perspective, participate in the planning, and have the support of family and health care providers.

Maturational-Situational Crises

If an unexpected, hazardous event occurs during transition from one maturational state to another, an individual who normally could complete the necessary developmental task may experience crisis (Moynihan and Hayes, 1982). If coping mechanisms are depleted in dealing with the situational event, the developmental task will not be achieved. On the other hand, if coping mechanisms are insufficient or if the coping mechanisms are devoted to the maturational task, it is not possible to adequately cope with the situational event. For example, if a young man who is engaged and just beginning to establish his career is suddenly partially paralyzed because of an accident, he has experienced events that could lead to a combined maturational-situational crisis. Not only is he developmentally in the process of establishing a career and achieving intimacy, but now he must

also cope with the changes made necessary by his paralysis. Strategies for coping with both the maturational and situational events are necessary.

FAMILIES AND CRISIS
Maturational Crisis

Family life is a dynamic cycle requiring readjustments as one phase is completed and another begun. Typically, periods of relative calm are followed by more intense activity at family-life transition times. As with individuals, families may face either maturational or situational crises. Like individuals, families progress through developmental stages, with each presenting a unique set of circumstances and requiring new coping strategies. For successful progression through the developmental stages, all family members must cope with the new situations. Each developmental stage requires members to relinquish some roles previously held and to assume new roles.

Duvall and Miller (1985) developed an eight-stage family life cycle based on a variety of family patterns, age and school placement of the oldest child, and family function and status before children were born and after children left home. The following list provide general guidelines; however, stages may be altered depending on the age and past experience of the couple getting married.

Stage 1—married couples—includes establishing a residence, allocating responsibilities, developing effective ways of settling differences, and learning how to live together on a daily basis. If there are children from a previous marriage of either or both partners, additional negotiations take place to form a blended family.

Stage 2—childbearing families—begins with the birth of the first child and requires the parents to assume new roles and relationships. Parents must learn to effectively meet the needs of a totally dependent person. The way parents previously spent their time, money, and energy may change dramatically. Challenges to new parents are many and include developing parenting skills and reestablishing a good marriage relationship.

Stage 3—families with preschool children—occurs when the first child is between 2½ and 6 years of age. One or more additional children may be born during this time. Demands on the parents include providing adequate space and equipment for the expanding family. The roles of the parents and each child change as subsequent children enter the family.

Stage 4—families with schoolchildren—begins when the oldest child goes to school. During the school years, as children gain independence and establish relationships outside the home, the roles of parents and siblings change again. Parents must often work through situations in which they are no longer the whole world to their children. Teachers, church workers, club leaders, coaches, and others become increasingly important to the children. At this stage of family development, marriage problems, especially those concerned with child rearing and expression of affection, may be more serious than at previous times since the birth of the first child.

Stage 5—families with teenagers—involves children in adolescence experiencing rapid physiological and psychosocial changes and brings a distinct set of problems to the family. As adolescents cope with sexuality and development of autonomy and social skills, parents must set limits that protect the adolescent while simultaneously allowing the freedom necessary to successfully complete developmental tasks.

Stage 6—families launching young adults—occurs from the time the first child leaves home until the last child leaves. During this period, when the family is shrinking to the original pair, parents may become in-laws and grandparents. The major task of this stage is reorganizing the family while meeting the goal of continuity. Children need the freedom to lead their lives, and parents need to encourage their efforts.

Stage 7—families with middle-aged parents—extends from the time the last child leaves home until the retirement or death of the husband or wife. This stage is often longer than any previous stage of family development. With the children gone, the husband and wife must establish a new relationship. If parents devoted little attention to their relationship as a couple while rearing their children, they may be relative strangers to one another when the children begin to leave home. An additional stressor during both stage 6 and 7 is that created by aging parents. Whereas in earlier years the older generation provided for and nurtured the younger generation, problems of aging (described in Chapter 28) may reverse these roles, thereby necessitating new coping strategies by both generations.

The extent to which the developmental tasks of stage 6 were met largely determines the nature and quality of stage 7. If parents adjusted to their children's departure and either continued to or learned to occupy themselves, this "empty nest" stage can be a time of freedom of choice and exercise of creativity. Adults often travel and engage in hobbies and career pursuits that were neglected during the busy child-rearing years.

Stage 8—families with aging family members—is the final stage of family development. This stage begins with retirement and ends with the death of both spouses. Adjusting to retirement, usually with a decrease in income, and deteriorating health are problems which many couples in this stage face. In addition, housing that probably met the needs of a family with children may not meet the needs of the elderly couple. Maintaining emotional, sexual, and marital relationships are also important to the elderly couple. Elderly couples vary greatly in their need for assistance. Some remain vigorous and active maintaining a household and pursuing many interests, whereas others become frail and require assistance with activities of daily living. All need safe surroundings and life-styles, continuing contact with family, and finding meaning in life.

The stages of family development are predictable, and nursing intervention in the form of anticipatory guidance can help families cope with the inherent problems of each stage. Programs designed to promote growth through the family developmental process include premarital conferences, which are often sponsored by churches, classes on preparation for parenthood, parenting groups, and classes that focus on living in the empty nest and preparing for retirement. If a family successfully progresses through the developmental stages, the individual family members and the family as a whole benefit from growth.

Situational Crises

Situational crises affecting families can occur in any of the developmental stages. Stressful, unanticipated events that may precipitate a family crisis include the birth of a premature infant, the death of a family member, a diagnosis of serious illness, and relocation. A crisis ensues when family resources are insufficient for effective coping. Although anticipatory guidance is not always possible for family situational crises, resources are available to assist families confronted with stressful situations. People who have experienced a particular event often band together to form an organization of support for others facing the same situation. Organizations for families of retarded children, hyperactive children, cancer victims, and children lost as a result of sudden infant death syndrome have been useful as crisis intervention strategies.

Not all families who encounter a stressor event experience crisis and some families are more prone to crisis than others. Whether or not crisis occurs depends on the nature of the event, the family's perception of the event, and the family's coping resources (Hill, 1965). If a family defines an event as threatening and impossible to overcome, crisis is more likely than if an event is seen as a challenge to be met. Families in which there is effective communication, coalition formation, and the ability to work together toward a goal have internal resources that aid them in averting crises (Hall and Weaver, 1974). Nurses can assist families to cope by using interventions such as objective clarification of events, promotion of the development of internal family resources, and referral to community resources.

Events such as unemployment and natural disaster create situations that hold the potential for crisis. In recent years sudden unemployment has been experienced by many; often thousands in one community. Not only the worker, but also all family members and family-unit functioning are affected (Voydanoff, 1983). The unemployed person loses, in addition to income, the role associated with a job and relationships with an employer and coworkers. In addition, roles at home change as the unemployed husband is expected to assume responsibility for household chores or the unemployed wife is expected to resume household chores from which she had been relieved by working. Adolescent children may be required to alter educational plans and obtain part-time work.

Families affected by natural disasters such as floods or tornadoes face many adjustments. Relocation at the time of warning or after the disaster places the family in a shelter or unfamiliar residence. This is especially difficult if the family includes an infant or an elderly or disabled member. Loss of belongings accumulated over a lifetime occurs when a home is destroyed. In addition, insurance may be insufficient to replace the home and furnishings lost. Community resources and friends that are usually available for support will themselves be attempting to cope with the aftermath of the disaster.

An organized effort to aid families at risk of situational crises occurred in Israel during the Yom Kippur War in 1973 (Caplan, 1976). Caplan, an expert in crisis intervention, worked in Israel at the time and implemented methods of intervention for families of soldiers killed in the war.

The first method Caplan used was to ensure that families were linked to significant others who could provide emotional support and assistance. This began by bringing family members together in one location to inform them of the death. External support was simultaneously provided by friends, neighbors, and members of religious congregations. Nurses in the community and other health care providers monitored the status of bereaved families to identify those who needed additional attention. For most families, no additional crisis intervention was required.

Five other methods served as guides for families needing further assistance. The second method called for limiting further aid to only those families truly needing help. This meant that careful assessment was required to determine families at greatest risk for disequilibrium from the effects of the war.

The third method dealt with avoiding psychiatric labels for families struggling to cope with their loss. Families were treated and referred to as normal people under stress rather than dysfunctional families or people to whom a label connoting an illness was assigned.

The fourth crisis intervention method addressed the need to use professional and nonprofessional volunteers who were members of the community to act as interveners. By being community members they could understand the nature of the crisis and convey sincere empathy; they were easily accessible and usually knowledgeable about resources and services available. Community health nurses were among the health professionals who provided crisis intervention.

The fifth method involved establishing mutual self-help groups and support networks. By joining other families who had experienced the same loss, energy could be mobilized to cope and group support gained.

The last method dealt with providing assistance to the supporters. People helping others to cope with crises often feel drained of their energy. Unless the supporters receive some nurturance, they are prime candidates for burnout or high stress reactions. Expert consultation was made available to community health nurses and others working with bereaved families in crisis.

Situational and maturational crises can occur in families, and they may happen simultaneously. For example, job loss at the time a family's first child is born would require adaptation to a developmental and situational event. Both types of crises require involvement of all family members and additional strategies to cope successfully.

COMMUNITIES AND CRISIS
Maturational Crises

Communities are also at risk for both maturational and situational crises through tasks such as growth, expansion, and retrenchment. Growth early in the life of a community often takes place when people in the region move to a concentrated area. As growth in a community occurs, there is a need for formal governmental structure and services to meet such basic needs of citizens as health care, education, safe water supply, sewage disposal, utilities, public safety, fire protection, and transportation. Unless problems resulting from growth are successfully solved, stagnation or loss of population will result. The West is dotted with ghost towns that did not cope with developmental events.

During expansion there is diversification and continued growth. A community originally established on one or two economic bases, such as manufacturing or agriculture, expands and becomes a center for a variety of activities such as education, medical care, trade, and industry. The diversification brings people of different cultural backgrounds, talents, and experiences into the community. While expanding, there is a further need for basic services and a need for the blending of the newcomers into the life of the community. During successful expansion, basic needs are met and the community is richer for the contributions of the newcomers. Crisis can arise when any basic need is not met or when there is conflict among the various segments of the population.

With retrenchment, loss of population and therefore loss of economic support for basic needs occur. Loss of population can result from movement to suburbs and/or loss of economic bases, such as industries closing. Individuals who are elderly, poor, or have few job skills are less likely to leave a community. If the needs of those remaining in a community are not met, crisis can result.

Young people predominate in growing communities, thus maternal and child services are especially needed. These services include facilities for prenatal care, well-child care, disabled children, appropriate day-care, and school health. As communities and their populations mature, there is greater need for chronic illness services and programs for the elderly.

Anticipatory preparation to avoid crisis in the growth and expansion stages of a community can include forecasting the population growth and planning and providing facilities to accommodate that growth. In retrenchment, financial support must be found to provide basic services. One example of a revenue source for such communities is a local tax on all income earned within the community. In this way people who are employed in the community but choose to live outside the area contribute to meeting the needs of the community. Communities in retrenchment as a result of the loss of an economic base often begin aggressive programs to attract new businesses and industry to the area.

By being active members of boards and committees charged with the responsibility for planning and providing basic services, community health nurses make health needs known and play a part in developing coping strategies to prevent a maturational crisis in the community. Political activity by nurses through election to public office or support of candidates for public office can also influence the development of a community.

Situational Crises

Situational crises in a community can result from events such as natural disasters or the sudden influx of a large number of refugees. When these unexpected events lead to crisis, resources beyond the community are needed to successfully resolve the situation.

Intervention in situational crises in communities includes mobilization of local disaster plans and assistance from governmental and voluntary agencies. Community health nurses are involved in maintaining the health of citizens affected by disaster. In shelters, they work to assist parents to care for their children under adverse conditions, to meet the needs of the chronically ill so that complications do not occur, and generally to either provide support or identify support systems to prevent individual and family crises. As part of the health department, the Red Cross, or voluntary organizations, community health nurses work at all levels, from making policy to rendering direct service in a community crisis.

CRISIS INTERVENTION

Because crisis is a temporary state of upset, the aim of intervention is to promptly assist the individual, family, or community to resolve the situation so that growth with an improved level of function is achieved when equilibrium is regained. In crisis intervention, clients are not viewed as harboring pathologic conditions but as needing to acquire support and coping mechanisms to resolve a specific situation. The summary of crisis intervenntion that follows is based on the work of several authors (Aguilera and Messick, 1982; Caplan, 1964; Hoff, 1978; Schwenk and Bittle, 1979).

Crisis intervention is a short-term method focused on solving immediate problems. The usual length of a crisis with or without intervention is 4 to 6 weeks. To be effective in preventing disorganization, intervention must take place while disequilibrium is present. Unlike psychotherapeutic techniques such as psychoanalysis, which are long term and focus on the past, crisis intervention is short term, includes one to six contacts, and focuses on the present.

Crisis intervention can be used by health professionals, nonhealth professionals, and volunteers after special training. Nurses, physicians, psychologists, and social workers are among the health professionals who use crisis intervention. Many nonhealth professionals in the course of their work are confronted with crisis situations and are able to intervene. Police, clergy, and teachers are among the nonhealth professionals who typically use crisis intervention. Trained volunteers in rape crisis centers, drug abuse facil-

ities, and self-help groups for people who have experienced a traumatic event such as a mastectomy or the birth of a disabled child use crisis intervention skills.

Because of their educational backgrounds, acceptance by clients, and frequent encounters with individuals and families in crisis, community health nurses can be an integral part of a community's crisis intervention efforts. They may provide crisis intervention to individuals, families, and groups; participate on crisis intervention teams; and serve on communities that manage crisis programs.

To provide specific crisis intervention services, crisis teams may be formed. The composition of the team depends on the purpose of the service and the resources available. A crisis team at a drug abuse facility could consist of a psychiatrist, nurse, social worker, and rehabilitated drug abuser. Members of a team bring their own unique backgrounds plus crisis intervention expertise. For any one client, leadership of the team is assumed by the member who can best assist the client in resolving the crisis. As discussed earlier in the chapter, present crisis intervention techniques are based on the work of Caplan (1964), Hill (1949), Lindemann (1979), and other pioneers in the field. For example, after working with the Coconut Grove fire victims, Cobb and Lindemann (1979) described a three-phase model for crisis intervention. Objective presentation and clarification of the event occur in phase 1. In phase 2 the care giver assists the person in crisis to work through the problems resulting from the stressor event. Phase 3 deals with readjustment, with the care giver assisting the individual to plan for the future.

Community health nurses and other health professionals (with training) function as crisis intervention therapists. In crisis intervention, assessment of the client and the problem is the first step during the initial contact. Information is gathered on the following: (1) precipitating event, (2) resulting problem(s), (3) onset of the crisis, (4) impact of the crisis on the life of the client, (5) impact of the crisis on the life of significant others, (6) previous coping strategies, (7) strengths of the client, (8) individuals in the client's life who can provide support, and (9) risk of homicide or suicide.

Assessment of the client in crisis reveals a characteristic composite (Brownell, 1984). The individual has experienced a distressing event followed by ineffective attempts to cope. The client perceives the event as significant and his attempts to cope with the event as ineffectual, and he feels helpless and anxious. The stressor event and its meaning to the client and the family are explored. The resultant problems, attempts to deal with them, and coping mechanisms used in the past are reviewed. In addition, strengths of the client and external supports are identified.

To assess potential for suicide or homicide, direct and specific questions are asked (Aguilera and Messick, 1982). Are you considering suicide? Are you planning to kill someone else? If so, how and when? The more specific the plan and the more lethal the method, the greater the risk of suicide (Dixon, 1979). Clients at risk of harming themselves or others are not candidates for crisis intervention and should be referred for psychiatric evaluation and possible hospitalization.

With candidates for crisis intervention, information obtained during assessment is organized and presented to the client so that the relation between the event, problems, and crisis is evident. This organized summary of information allows for client validation and serves as a therapeutic technique for a person who does not recognize the relation among the components of the crisis. To plan the intervention the problem must be broken into manageable parts.

The intervention techniques used in crisis are varied and include listening actively with concern, helping the client express feelings, exploring new ways of coping, helping the person find and use supports, and assisting him to gradually accept reality. Immediate goals are set, workable plans of action are explored, and specific actions are chosen with the client. The client leaves the session with certain tasks to perform. In crisis intervention the therapist is an active and direct participant. For example, the therapist may contact community agencies that require referral from a health professional. However, the resolution of the crisis rests with the client. In crisis intervention the assessment remains focused on the crisis situation. As in other community health nursing interactions, the client is an active participant in planning, intervention, and evaluation.

In the first contact it is important to maintain focus on the crisis. The therapist and client should be aware that crisis intervention lasts only a few weeks at most. For some clients one contact provides the assistance necessary for resolution of the problem. In future contacts, progress in using new coping methods and meeting goals is reviewed, and the therapist provides reinforcement for client successes. Other aspects of the crisis problem, in manageable parts, are explored, and ways of coping are considered. Throughout crisis intervention individuals and/or groups who can provide support are identified and mobilized. The length and frequency of client contacts with the therapist depend on the nature of the crisis, but usually range from one to six contacts.

In the last interview a summary of new strategies attempted—successful and unsuccessful—and progress made reinforces the gains of the client. To help the individual maintain the achieved level of function, realistic plans for the future are discussed. The client who achieves resolution of a crisis at an improved level of function has experienced growth and gained coping mechanisms that can prevent a crisis in the future.

The familiarity of the crisis process to the community health nurse lies in its parallelism to the nursing process of assessment, nursing diagnosis, planning, intervention, and evaluation. Steps in crisis intervention as they occur in the initial nursing process are shown in the accompanying box.

Crisis intervention may be provided in individual, family, or group settings, with the choice depending on the need of the client and the availability of services. One example of group intervention following a community disaster with crisis potential is the efforts of a Washington, D.C. area Health Maintenance Organization (HMO) after a Hanafi Muslim sect seized and held hostages for more than 1½ days (Sank, 1979). Mental health professionals from the HMO offered the released hostages eight group sessions that began 4 days after the ordeal. During the group sessions former hostages discussed their perceptions of the event, their feelings while being held hostage, resultant problems they were having since their release, and methods of coping with those problems. The aims of the intervention were to provide support for the ex-hostages and to assist them in developing the coping skills necessary to deal with problems resulting from the traumatic event.

Three aspects of crisis add to the possibility of favorable resolution through crisis intervention (Caplan, 1964). First, the crisis outcome is determined most often by internal and external factors during the course of the crisis, not by the client's past experiences or the nature of the event leading to crisis. Crisis intervention using techniques such as developing new ways of coping and mobilizing support can provide internal and external factors that tilt the resolution in favor of a successful outcome. Second, the client in crisis has an increased desire for help. Therefore the client in crisis is more likely to seek and accept crisis intervention. Third, clients in crisis are more likely to be influenced by others than they are in periods of equilibrium. Because of these aspects of crisis, therapists skilled in crisis intervention have a unique opportunity to influence crisis outcome.

PRIMARY, SECONDARY, AND TERTIARY CRISIS PREVENTION

Primary prevention aims to avert crises in stressful maturational and situational circumstances. Primary prevention

---

THE FIVE STEPS OF CRISIS INTERVENTION

ASSESS

Clarify precipitating event
Explore meaning of event to the client
Identify problems
Identify present and past coping strategies
Identify resources

DIAGNOSE

Clearly define the problems
Label the problems

PLAN

Separate problems into manageable parts
Explore alternative coping methods
Set goals
Define specific tasks to meet goals

INTERVENE

Formulate an objective statement of the situation
Carry out tasks to meet goals
Mobilize resources

EVALUATE

Appraise progress toward goals
Evaluate the success of coping methods used
Reinforce the progress made

for maturational crisis is based on the knowledge of the problems accompanying transitions across the life span. Community health nurses working with individuals and families can provide anticipatory guidance for individual and family developmental transitions. Settings such as prenatal classes, parenting groups, and adolescent discussion groups also present the opportunity to discuss transition problems and helpful coping mechanisms. By sitting on community boards, participating in civic and voluntary organizations, and speaking at public functions, community health nurses contribute to the primary prevention of developmental crises in communities.

To prevent crisis following a stressful situation, prompt action is needed. The group sessions for ex-hostages are one example of an effort to provide primary prevention for a group who experienced a traumatic event. A situational event for which some communities provide primary intervention is rape. Comprehensive rape crisis intervention considers care of the victim from the time of the assault through courtroom appearances testifying against the assailant (McCombie, 1980). Community health nurses encounter many individuals and families at risk of situational crisis and have the opportunity to use primary prevention methods, either by providing direct assistance or by making referrals. Individuals who have experienced loss of meaningful relationships through death or disease, birth of a high-risk infant, or loss of income are among those who may benefit from primary prevention of crisis.

Secondary prevention entails finding cases early to prevent sequelae. Early identification of those in crisis and prompt institution of crisis intervention can promote a favorable outcome. Because a crisis has a limited duration, intervention must not be delayed. The client in crisis needs an appointment today, not next week. If referral to an agency is needed, the nurse should be certain the agency is aware that the client is in crisis and is not to be deferred.

Tertiary prevention consists of rehabilitation when resolution of a crisis has resulted in a level of function that is lower than the level before crisis, accompanied by major disorganization. To assist clients whose resolution of crisis is not successful, referral to mental health specialists is needed. Whereas the goal of primary prevention is to avert crisis and the goal of secondary prevention is to successfully resolve the crisis, the goal of tertiary prevention is to return the client to his former or a higher level of function following an unsuccessfully resolved crisis.

Community Resources

Crisis resources available in a community depend on the size of the community, crisis needs, and the interest and expertise present. The community health nurse in a rural community may be the only health care professional available but need not be the only resource. Other professionals, such as ministers and cooperative extension agents or home economists employed by the agricultural component of a state university, may provide primary and secondary prevention. For example, the cooperative extension agent works on a daily basis with homemakers and has an educational background that includes knowledge of individual and fam-

ily development. Parenting classes and groups to discuss transitions in family life are examples of activities aimed at primary prevention of crisis and may be conducted by cooperative extension agencies. In organizing crisis resources in a rural community, the community health nurse should consider the roles that could be played by both professionals and volunteers.

In larger communities, resources for crisis include both official and voluntary agencies. Among official agencies, the health department and mental health center may offer programs of primary and secondary prevention for individuals and families. In health departments, community health nurses participate in assessing needs for crisis services, diagnosing specific areas for intervention, planning, intervening, and evaluating actions. Tertiary prevention is offered by mental health centers and private psychiatric facilities for clients in whom crisis resolution resulted in a decreased level of function accompanied by disorganization.

Voluntary agencies in a community are concerned with a wide variety of conditions including infertility, drug abuse, birth defects, mental retardation, hyperactivity, cancer, kidney disease, child abuse, battered women, and rape. Services provided by these agencies range from distributing information to sponsoring support groups to offering crisis intervention. In some communities, traditional agencies are expanding their scope of services to include crisis assistance. For example, some Young Women's Christian Associations (YWCAs) offer help to battered women. Religious institutions may also offer programs of primary prevention and, less often, secondary prevention of crisis. Community health nurses have opportunities to support voluntary crisis efforts through joining the membership, serving as consultants, accepting board membership, and providing direct services through the agency.

Minimally, community health nurses provide primary prevention services and have knowledge of the resources for secondary and tertiary crisis prevention. For effective referral to a community resource, the community health nurse must know the specific services of the agency, eligibility requirements for clients, and the procedures for obtaining services. If the community health nurse does not provide crisis intervention, a prompt and appropriate referral of clients in crisis is needed.

CLINICAL APPLICATION

The following example illustrates secondary crisis intervention by a community health nurse with a client in crisis. A summary of the nursing process used in this situation is described after the example.

Susan Jones, a community health nurse employed by a county health department, had been given several new clients. Among them was Betty Steward, a 23-year-old unmarried mother of a 4-year-old girl; Betty was expecting her second child. A review of Betty's record revealed that she was in her thirty-ninth week of pregnancy and had missed her clinic visit the previous week; a home visit was planned. On arriving at the home, Susan was greeted by a young woman with uncombed hair and a rumpled housecoat; she was obviously not pregnant. Betty said she had delivered twin boys 3 days ago, and she and her sons had arrived home earlier in the day. Betty's daughter, Karen, was at home and eager to show her brothers to the nurse. Susan's examinations of Betty and the infants revealed no physical problems. As Susan talked with Betty, she noted Betty's slow movements and sad expression. Susan told Betty she appeared to be sad and asked if there was a problem. Betty began to cry and said that throughout the pregnancy she had planned to give the infant up for adoption, but when the twins were born, she thought they were "special" and changed her mind. Now she was uncertain of her decision and felt overwhelmed.

Although Betty's only income had been child support from Karen's father, Betty felt that Karen needed her at home during the preschool years and was unemployed at the time of the pregnancy. However, Betty looked forward to the time when Karen would enter school. Betty would get a job, and their situation could improve. Keeping the infants meant loss of a goal to Betty. In addition, she expressed concern about her ability to provide for the infants. Not expecting to keep the infants, no care items were available; the only formula was the take-home package from the hospital, and little food was in the house. Repeatedly Betty said she needed to decide whether or not to keep the twins. Susan inquired about individuals in Betty's life who had helped when she had decisions to make in the past. Betty said she had neither family nor friends with whom she could discuss the situation about the twins. However, Betty's minister was a person she trusted and who had been of help previously.

The plan developed by Susan and Betty was for Betty to contact her minister and meet with him and for Susan to contact a community agency to arrange for emergency formula, supplies for the infants, and food for Betty and Karen. If Betty's decision was to keep the infants, further plans would be made on the next visit. They agreed that Susan would return in 2 days, and if Betty needed her before then, she would call.

On Susan's next visit Betty was smiling and said that after talking with her minister she had made a final decision and would keep the twins. Her biggest problem was how she would provide for them because she did not want to leave them to work. Susan informed Betty about Aid to Families with Dependent Children and told her how to go about contacting the social worker. Susan was to call the social worker so that he would expect Betty's call, and Betty would arrange for an appointment. The next visit was scheduled for 1 week later.

By the next visit Betty had seen the social worker, interim assistance was arranged, and she would soon receive regular benefits. Betty's concern now was providing a suitable environment for the children. When asked what kind of place she would like, she referred to a clean place that did not have roaches and mice, which were her main objections to the present house. They discussed options for the problem, and the action planned was for Betty to contact the landlord and request that he have the pests exterminated. Because Betty had little experience taking assertive action with someone she considered an authority figure, they role-played the contact with the landlord. The next visit was scheduled for 3 weeks.

At the next visit Betty, neatly dressed, met Susan at the door and began to tell her about the telephone call to the landlord. She related that she had been firm in her request for extermination services, and, as a result, the landlord agreed. She proudly showed Susan the twins and her cleaner house. Susan commended Betty for the progress she had made and spoke of her recent achievements. Although life with her daughter and the infants was not without problems, Betty was successfully coping with the situation. As a result of her contact with her minister, members of the congregation had come to visit, and Betty talked of her plans to participate in church activities. With the present situation resolved, routine health care plans for the family were agreed on, and Betty was to contact Susan if assistance was needed in the future.

The steps in the nursing process—assessment, nursing diagnosis, planning, intervention, and evaluation—are reviewed here as carried out in the previous example. The first step in the nursing process is assessment, and Susan began assessment of the Steward family by checking the biophysical status of the mother and infants. Assessment of the emotional status revealed problems subsequent to the birth of twins. Further assessment revealed lack of coping strategies and loss of a life goal, leading to a diagnosis of crisis. There was no evidence that Betty was suicidal or would have harmed another. Using crisis intervention, the remainder of the first visit focused on the problems associated with the crisis. Assessment included identification of individuals who could be a support, and this revealed Betty's minister.

Plans were developed jointly by Susan and Betty with priorities established so that problems of greatest importance were dealt with first. Consistent with crisis intervention, problems were considered in manageable parts. Implementation of the plans involved active participation by the nurse and client and allowed Betty to develop new coping skills. The role-playing to prepare Betty for the contact with the landlord is an example. In the last contact, Betty's successful efforts and achievements were reviewed and reinforced, and plans for the future were discussed.

Throughout the crisis period, reassessment, client participation in planning, intervention, and evaluation occurred. The last visit reviewed progress and future plans. In this case study the client successfully resolved the problems resulting from the birth of the twins and developed new coping strategies.

SUMMARY

Crisis is an upset in a steady state, a disequilibrium, resulting from problems that follow an event of significance to the client and for which coping skills are inadequate. With crisis there is both the opportunity for growth and the achievement of a higher level of psychological functioning if successful resolution occurs, and the danger of a decreased level of psychological function and disorganization if resolution is not successful. The disequilibrium of crisis cannot be long endured; with or without intervention a new state of equilibrium is reached in 4 to 6 weeks.

The individual in crisis perceives the event, which may be desirable or undesirable, as having serious consequences. The person also perceives a state of upset, an uncertainty of outcome, and feelings of helplessness and ineffectuality.

Physiological manifestations of crisis are varied and depend on the individual's response to stressful situations.

As defined by Schwenk and Bittle (1979), the four phases of crisis are characterized by changes in tension and function levels. As the crisis progresses, the individual experiences increased tension and decreased function levels.

Maturational and situational crises can affect individuals, families, and communities and are not mutually exclusive; a situational crisis may develop concurrently with a maturational crisis. Because transitions in individual, family, and community life are predictable, anticipatory guidance to provide effective coping skills is possible for situations having the potential for maturational crisis. When a sudden and unexpected event occurs, intervention quickly following the traumatic event can provide coping mechanisms sufficient for prevention of a situational crisis.

Crisis intervention is a short-term treatment modality by which clients in crisis are assisted in developing coping mechanisms and are provided support to resolve the situation so that the client reaches equilibrium at an improved level of psychological function after the crisis. With training, techniques of crisis intervention are suitable for use by health professionals, nonhealth professionals, and volunteers. In crisis intervention the focus and orientation remain on the present situation. The steps of the crisis process are essentially those of the nursing process—assessment, diagnosis, planning, intervention, and evaluation. Throughout crisis intervention the client and therapist play active roles. The client deals with the crisis problems in manageable parts, and progress made is reinforced.

The concepts of primary, secondary, and tertiary prevention are useful in organizing crisis services in a community. With primary prevention, efforts are directed at averting the occurrence of crisis. Secondary prevention entails finding cases early and instituting crisis intervention promptly. If crisis resolution is unsuccessful, tertiary prevention with rehabilitation by mental health specialists is necessary.

By working with official and voluntary agencies, community health nurses can participate in assessment, diagnosis, planning, intervention, and evaluation of crisis services for individuals, families, and communities. Community health nurses may provide direct intervention for clients in crisis or may refer them to resources best able to meet their needs.

⩲ KEY CONCEPTS

An essential property of crisis is the potential for promoting growth. Crises present challenges and call for new responses. Assisting those in crisis to achieve growth is an inherent role for community health nurses.

People in crisis feel helpless and often desire assistance in relieving their misery. The duration of the state of disequilibrium, the individual's perception of the event and problems, and the functioning pattern of the individual are characteristic of crises.

Crises may be categorized as maturational or situational. Maturational, or developmental, crises occur during natural transitions in the developmental process.

Unlike maturational crises, situational crises affecting individuals are frequently sudden and unexpected.

The stages of family development are predictable, and nursing intervention in the form of anticipatory guidance can help families cope with the inherent problems of each stage.

Because crisis is a temporary state of upset, the aim of intervention is to promptly assist the individual, family, or community to resolve the situation so that growth with an improved level of function is achieved when equilibrium is regained.

Crisis intervention can be used by health professionals, nonhealth professionals, and volunteers after special training.

Primary prevention aims to avert crises in stressful maturational and situational circumstances. Secondary prevention entails finding cases early to prevent sequelae. Tertiary prevention consists of rehabilitation when resolution of a crisis has resulted in a level of function that is lower than the level before crisis, accompanied by major disorganization.

Crisis resources available in a community depend on the size of the community, crisis needs, and the interest and expertise present.

By working with official and voluntary agencies, community health nurses can participate in assessment, diagnosis, planning, intervention, and evaluation of crisis services for individuals, families, and communities. Community health nurses may provide direct intervention for clients in crisis or may refer them to resources best able to meet their needs.

LEARNING ACTIVITIES

1. Identify either a real or a fictional account of a crisis situation. Novels, movies, or television programs may provide the situation. For the individual in crisis, describe perceptions of the crisis event and problem, level of function, feelings expressed, somatic symptoms, and length of disequilibrium.

2. Using the crisis situation in number 1, describe the behaviors of the individual in crisis during the phases of crisis.

3. From your clinical experience, select a family and identify the stage of family development and of individual development for each member.

4. In your community, identify two programs that either offer anticipatory guidance for maturational crises or could offer such anticipatory guidance.

5. Identify programs in your community that offer primary, secondary, and tertiary prevention of individual, family, or community crises. For each type of prevention, discuss the ways in which nurses participate or could participate in the assessment, planning, intervention, and evaluation efforts of the programs.

6. Using a newspaper account of an event that could lead to a situational crisis for a family or community, describe how you as a community health nurse could use the nursing process and principles of crisis intervention to provide primary prevention.

BIBLIOGRAPHY

Aguilera, D., and Messick, J.: Crisis intervention theory and methodology, ed. 4, St. Louis, 1982, The C.V. Mosby Co.

Brownell, M.J.: The concept of crisis: its utility for nursing, A.N.S. 6:10, 1984.

Caplan, G.: Principles of preventive psychiatry, New York, 1964, Basic Books, Inc., Publishers.

Caplan, G.: Organization of support systems for civilian populations. In Caplan, G., and Killilea, M., editors: Support systems and mutual help: multidisciplinary explorations, New York, 1976, Grune & Stratton, Inc.

Christensen, S., and Harding, M.: Integrating theories of crisis intervention into hospice home care teaching, Nurs. Clin. North Am. 20:499, 1985.

Cobb, S., and Lindemann, E.: Neuropsychiatric observations after the Coconut Grove fire. In Lindemann, E.: Beyond grief, New York, 1979, Jason Aronson.

Dixon, S.: Working with people in crisis, St. Louis, 1979, The C.V. Mosby Co.

Duvall, E.M., and Miller, B.C.: Marriage and family development, ed. 6, New York, 1985, Harper & Row, Publishers, Inc.

Erikson, E.: Childhood and society, New York, 1950, W.W. Norton & Co.

Hall, J., and Weaver, B., editors: Nursing of families in crisis, Philadelphia, 1974, J.B. Lippincott Co.

Hill, R.: Families under stress, Westport, Conn., 1949, Greenwood Press, Publishers.

Hill, R.: Generic features of families under stress. In Parad, H.: Crisis intervention: se-

lected readings, New York, 1965, Family Service Association of America.

Hoff, L.A.: People in crisis understanding and helping, Menlo Park, Calif., 1978, Addison-Wesley Publishing Co.

Lindemann, E.: Symptomatology and management of acute grief. In Lindemann, E.: Beyond grief, New York, 1979, Jason Aronson.

McCombie, S., editor: The rape crisis intervention handbook, New York, 1980, Plenum Press.

Moynihan, M.M., and Hayes, E.R.: Combined developmental-situational events: a theoretical model for nursing practice and research. In Infante, M.S.: Crisis theory: a framework for nursing practice, Reston, VA, 1982, Reston Publishing Co., Inc.

Rapoport, L.: The state of crisis: some theoretical consideration. In Parad, H.: Crisis intervention: selected readings, New York, 1965, Family Service Association of America.

Rosswurm, M.A.: Relocation and the elderly, J. Gerontol. Nurs. 9(12):632, 1983.

Sank, L.I.: Psychology in action: community disasters, Am. Psychol. 34:334, 1979.

Schwenk, T.L., and Bittle, S.P.: Applicability of crisis intervention in family practice, J. Fam. Pract. 8:1151, 1979.

Spradley, B.W.: Community health nursing: concepts and practice, Boston, 1981, Little, Brown, & Co.

Underwood, M.M., and Fiedler, N.: The crisis of rape: a community response, Community Ment. Health J. 19:227-230, 1983.

Voydanoff, P.: Unemployment: family strategies for adaption. In Figley, C.R., and Cubbin, H.I., editors: Stress and the family, vol. 2, New York, 1983, Brunner/Mazel, Inc.

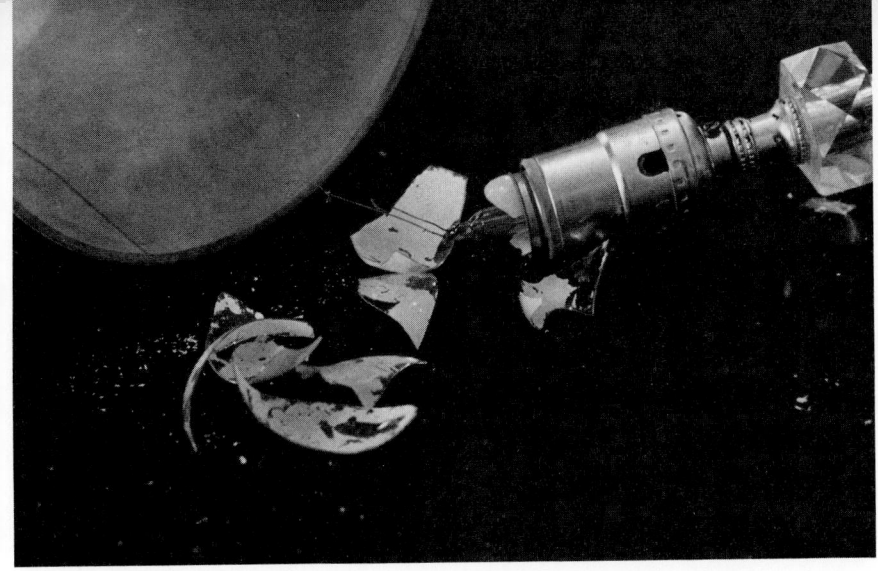

Jeanette Lancaster
David Kerschner

34

VIOLENCE AND HUMAN ABUSE

≡ OBJECTIVES

After reading this chapter, the student should be able to:

Discuss the scope of the problem of violence in American communities.

Describe at least three factors existing in most communities that influence violence and human abuse.

Identify at least three types of common community facilities that can help mitigate violence.

Evaluate a family's vulnerability to violence from an unwanted intruder.

Identify typically noticed indicators of child abuse.

Define four general types of child abuse: neglect, physical abuse, emotional abuse, and sexual abuse.

Describe the three-phase cycle often seen in instances of spouse abuse.

Discuss abuse of the elderly as a growing community health problem.

Evaluate the role that can be assumed with rape victims by community health nurses.

Analyze the six subroles described by Scharer as being applicable to work with abusive parents. Can these subroles be used in all abusive situations?

≡ KEY TERMS

battered child syndrome

crises

developmental
    disabilities

elder abuse

emotional abuse

helplessness

hostility

incest

physical abuse

powerlessness

primary prevention

secondary prevention

sense of cohesiveness

sense of confusion

sexual abuse

spouse abuse

subroles

survivors

tension building

therapeutic intervention

The most powerful obstacle to culture, according to Freud (1955) is the human innate, independent, and instinctual tendency toward aggression. Other scholars have argued that aggression and violence are not innate, but rather are learned behaviors. However, violence seems to be ever present in our society. Headlines in newspapers report political kidnappings, terrorist attacks, and senseless killings. Television news displays in vivid color the capture of a rape suspect, victims of a family shooting, and battles among Third World countries. People continue to harm and kill others as well as themselves.

Underlying most violence toward oneself or others is a deep-seated sense of hostility, which the affected individual may or may not recognize. Hostility tends to be a motivating force and is exhibited in impulses, urges, and tendencies to behave in ways that lead to injury or destruction of either animate or inanimate objects (Saul, 1971). *Hostility* includes active aggression, anger, and hatred as well as passive gestures such as gossip, neglect, and the withholding of affection and fair treatment. Particularly in our fast-paced society, people may have either harbored more hostility or used fewer constructive channels for venting pent-up feelings.

All people, to some degree, are pulled by two opposing forces: to be acceptable to self and society and to exhibit strong asocial and antisocial tendencies (Saul, 1971). To understand community violence, one must recognize the presence of these opposing forces. Each person has an innate ability to lash out and harm or destroy self or others. The crucial factor in dealing effectively with violence and abuse lies in what causes some people to unleash these forces while others keep their hostility and aggression in check.

It is important to realize that violence is a community health nursing concern. The Surgeon General's Workshop on Violence and Public Health Report (1986) points out that medical, nursing, psychology, and social service professionals have been slow in developing a response to violence that is integral to their daily professional lives. As a result, we are not sure if the estimated 4 million victims of violence annually will receive the best care possible. This chapter examines violence as a community problem and how the community health nurse can help individuals, families, and the community cope with and reduce violence and human abuse.

SCOPE OF THE PROBLEM

Violence and human abuse are not new phenomena but are increasingly becoming public health concerns. Communities around the country are voicing anger and fear about rising crime and violence rates.

Crime in the previous decade and a half has undergone dramatic changes. In the period from 1971 to 1979 violent crimes (homicide, forcible rape, robbery, and aggravated assault) and property crimes (burglary, larceny-theft, motor vehicle theft, and arson) increased 60% and 54%, respectively (Uniform Crime Reports, 1980). Crime in the period from 1980 to 1984 appeared to take a downward turn in most categories. Murder was down 19%, robbery decreased by 14%, larceny-theft dropped 12%, and burglary declined 25%. There was an increase of 1% in forcible rape and an increase of 2% in aggravated assault during this same period (Uniform Crime Reports, 1984).

Some criminologists suggest that this decline in crime rates marks the beginning of a long-term decline. The reason, they argue, is the aging of the post–World War II baby-boom generation, maturing from its crime-prone years. In addition, federal officials attribute the declining rates to a national hard line on crime that has led to tougher sentences (Time, 1984). Despite this recent decrease, the overall crime rate continues to be higher in 1984 than it was 25 years ago. Table 34-1 shows the daily rates for crimes, as estimated in the Uniform Crime Reports for 1984.

Violence against family members is more difficult to measure, since many crimes of this nature go unreported. However, the extent of this community health problem should not be underestimated. About 50%, or more, of killings occur between people who know one another (Allen, 1981), and about 30% occur within the family (Newman, 1979). Domestic disputes account for more than half of all police night calls and often result in violent encounters with the police as they answer these calls (Allen, 1981). Detection of family violence and abuse can be particularly difficult because of the nature of the problem, guilt, and the possibility of punishment. Community health nurses, like social workers, are in key positions to detect and intervene in community and family violence, since they have access to clients in a wide variety of settings, including the home.

FACTORS INFLUENCING SOCIAL AND COMMUNITY VIOLENCE

Numerous variables within a community can support or minimize violence. Changing social conditions, multiple demands on people, economic conditions, and the institutions that make up a given society or community influence the level of violence and human abuse. To understand key factors that affect people so that they inflict abuse on themselves and/or others, selected contemporary social conditions are reviewed.

Work

The American way of life reinforces competition for goods and services as an essential and valued aspect of free enterprise. People are expected to be productive, contributing, and self-sufficient. The American work ethic dates to the Industrial Revolution, when arduous child and adult labor was expected. People are expected to work hard to enjoy the "good life." However, in inflationary times when unemployment is high, willing people are not always able to find sufficient work to maintain a satisfactory standard of living.

Work as an institution cannot be relied on to meet basic human needs. Jobs can be repetitive, boring, and nearly lacking in stimulation. Also, even in jobs with the potential for stimulation, supervisors and other forms of organizational control may discourage creativity and reward conformity and "following the rules." In many work settings people try to get ahead regardless of the cost to others. Adults often go home feeling physically and psychologically drained. They may have worked at a back-breaking pace all day only to be yelled at by the boss for what seemed like a trivial oversight. It is hard to separate feelings generated at work from the home environment. A father arrives home tired, angry, and generally feeling inadequate because of a series of reprimands. Soon after he sits down, his 4-year-old son runs through the house pretending to fly a wooden airplane. After about three loud trips past his father, who keeps shouting for the child to be quiet and go outside,

the airplane hits the father in the head. This provides a fertile setting for striking out in frustration and anger.

In addition, in times of economic constraints people are often afraid to give up even those jobs that are frustrating or boring or create great stress; at such times any job seems better than none. People feel trapped; their family needs necessitate that they keep the hated job, which often engenders resentment toward those who are dependent on them, such as children, unemployed spouses, older relatives, and handicapped or sick family members.

Unemployment often precipitates abusive outbursts. The inability to secure or maintain a job may lead to feelings of inadequacy, guilt, boredom, dissatisfaction, and frustration.

A recent study has shown that a wife's employment increases marital instability, especially if her job entails working more than 40 hours per week (Booth, 1984). The wife's entering the labor force almost always leads to a change in the family structure in ways to which most men and women are not accustomed. These changes in structure can cause feelings of resentment, failure, and anger, which may ultimately lead to acts of violence.

Education

In recent years schools have assumed many responsibilities traditionally assigned to the family. Schools teach sexual development, discipline children, and often serve as holding stations for children who have no other place to go. Large classes often mean that teachers spend more time and energy monitoring and disciplining children than challenging and stimulating them to learn. In large classes isolation is often the primary method of dealing with children who do not conform to norms of expected behavior. The nonconforming child is simply removed from the classroom because time does not permit concerted efforts toward helping the child learn alternative ways of behavior.

Ironically, children are often punished for hitting or biting other children by being spanked. Such punishment only reinforces the child's tendency to strike out at others because adults are seen as directing the forbidden action toward the child.

Prince (1981) contends that five basic human needs—stimulation, power, intimacy, interdependence, and "anger outlets"—could be provided by major social institutions but in most cases are not. She believes that the educational system, especially in urban areas, fails to meet these needs largely because of a lack of financial resources. Schools, according to Prince, are often lonely, boring places where the expression of anger is discouraged by the threat of punishment and where children gain feelings of self-esteem from achievement on tests.

Media

Television, movies, newspapers, and magazines portray happy, fun-loving people. Television parades in front of 6 million eyes, in brilliant living color, all the wonders money can provide. Yet for many Americans the hope of buying many of the nonessentials seems unrealistic. Such polarization between what is available and what is possible provides

TABLE 34-1

Incidence of selected crimes: 1984

Crime	Incidence of one crime	Actual number crimes in 1984
Murder	Every 23 minutes	18,600
Forcible rape	Every 6 minutes	84,233
Robbery	Every 58 seconds	
Aggravated assault	Every 48 seconds	
Burglary	Every 8 seconds	
Larceny-theft	Every 4 seconds	
Motor vehicle theft	Every 28 seconds	

From Uniform crime reports for the United States, Washington, D.C., 1985, Federal Bureau of Investigation, U.S. Department of Justice.

fertile ground for the development of abusive patterns. Frustration, unfilled dreams, and unmet wishes are often handled through hurting someone who is limited in the ability to fight back.

The media cater to children by presenting products intended to stimulate their curiosity and desire to purchase. Parents subsequently may get angry when their children frequently request the foods, toys, and clothes they see on television, in magazines, or in newspapers or hear advertised on the radio.

Not only do the media tantalize children and adults with the vast array of possible items to buy and things to do, but they often portray the world as a violent place. Hitting, kicking, stabbing, and shooting are seen daily as ways to handle anger, frustration, and so forth. By the age of 18 the average child has seen 18,000 murders and countless acts of nonfatal violence on television (Roesch, 1984). Often in these acts of violence the good guys conquer the bad ones. Thus violence is often seen as being justified when the perpetrator views the cause to be worthy.

Organized Religion

Three of the human needs cited by Prince (1981) are often provided by the church—stimulation, a sense of worth or power, and some degree of closeness and intimacy. Interestingly, throughout history a seemingly contradictory relationship has existed between abuse and religion. For example, many religious groups uphold the philosophy of "spare the rod, spoil the child." Also, some faiths uphold victimization of people with their disapproval of divorce. Families may stay together, although at emotional or physical war with one another, because of religious commitments (Prince, 1981).

Although controversial, the role of guilt as a form of victimization needs to be considered. Although every society has its own rules and sanctions for what is acceptable, rigid guidelines complete with predictions of dire spiritual consequences can produce guilt and lower self-esteem. The dividing line seems to be between those religious bodies that offer guidelines and encouragement for behavior and those that exercise their beliefs to keep members "in line" (Bruhn and Fuentes, 1981).

Population: Density and Characteristics

A community's population, size, location, and surroundings can influence the potential for violence. High-population-density communities with a *sense of cohesiveness* may have a lower crime rate than areas of similar size that lack social and cultural groups to support unity among members. Bonds formed among church groups, clubs, and professional organizations may promote harmony rather than violence among members. Such groups allow members an opportunity to talk about stressors rather than to respond through violence. For example, residents of public housing projects often form neighborhood associations to deal with situations common to many or all residents. Tension can often be released in a productive way through projects carried out by the association.

Some high-population-density areas experience a community feeling of *powerlessness* and *helplessness* rather than one of cohesiveness. Fear and apathy may cause community residents to withdraw from social contact. Withdrawal can foster crime, since everyone assumes someone else will report suspicious behavior and all fear reprisals for such reports.

Youth often attempt to deal with feelings of powerlessness and helplessness by forming gangs. In many cities these gangs have been highly destructive, as adolescents and young adults have attempted to deal with their feelings by turning to crime against people and property to release frustration.

Other high-population-density areas may be characterized by a *sense of confusion,* resulting in disintegration and disorganization. These areas often have transient populations whose members have limited physical or emotional investment in the community. Lack of community concern allows crime and violence to go unchecked and may become a norm for the area. Also, as crime increases, residents who are able to move and who desire a safer way of life will leave the area. This often reduces the capability for increasing community integration, since the residents who leave a disintegrating neighborhood are often the most capable members of the population.

The potential for violence tends to increase among highly heterogeneous populations. Differences in age, socioeconomic status, ethnicity, religion, or other cultural characteristics may lead to system stress and disrupt community stability. Highly divergent groups may neither accept nor understand one another. They may not communicate effectively, and many such groups become hostile and antagonistic toward one another. Isolation or hostile attacks can occur, thereby increasing tension and decreasing the potential for community cohesiveness and integration. Each group may see the other as different and not belonging. The alienated group may become the focal point for the other's frustrations, anger, and fears.

Community Facilities

As discussed in Chapter 13, communities differ in the resources and facilities they provide to residents. Some are far more desirable as places to live, work, and raise families. With regard to the potential for crime and violence in a community, recreational facilities, such as playgounds, parks, swimming pools, movie theaters, tennis courts, and other areas for exercise and play, provide socially acceptable outlets for a variety of feelings, including aggression.

Spectator sports, organized by the community, such as football or hockey, also allow members of the community to vicariously express feelings of anger and frustration. However, viewing sports can often encourage a sense of violence as participants hit or shove one another or take balls or other items from participants against whom they are competing. Educational institutions such as schools and libraries also provide places and resources for constructive use of time. Religious institutions can provide spiritual and social support as well as aid in forming a sense of community unity.

While the absence of such facilities can increase the likelihood of violence, their presence alone does not prevent violence or crime. These facilities are adjuncts and resources to be used by residents for pleasure, personal enrichment, and group development. Chapter 13 provides information about community health assessment.

◆　◆　◆

Familiarity with factors contributing to a community's violence or potential for violence enables community health nurses to recognize them and intervene accordingly. When factors are discovered that need correction or improvement, it is the nurse's role to work with the citizens and agencies of the community to correct or improve these deficits.

VIOLENCE AGAINST INDIVIDUALS OR ONESELF

The potential for violence against individuals (e.g., murder, robbery, rape, and assault) or oneself (e.g., suicide) is directly related to the level of violence in the community. Persons living in areas with high rates of crime and violence are more likely to become victims than those in more peaceful areas. Identification and correction of factors affecting the rates of community violence (violence against individuals) is one way of reducing violence against the family.

First, persons can take measures to reduce their vulnerability to violence by improving the physical security of their homes and learning personal defense measures. Community health nurses can encourage people to keep windows and doors locked, trim shrubs around their homes, and keep lights on during high crime periods. Many neighborhoods organize crime watch programs and post signs to the effect, as well as signs indicating that certain homes will assist children who need help; these homes are identified by the sign of a hand, usually posted in a window. Other neighbors informally agree to monitor one another's property and safety. Also, many law enforcement agencies evaluate homes for security and teach individual or neighborhood safety programs. Individuals install home security systems, participate in personal defense programs such as judo or karate, and purchase firearms for their protection. The method of protection chosen should be carefully evaluated and meet the family's needs and abilities. Personal defense methods and owning firearms can be dangerous without proper instruction.

Homicide

Almost 17% of the homicides in the United States occur within families; half of these occur between spouses (Crime, 1983). These figures are misleading in that they exclude couples who are not married but are living together or who are either divorced or estranged lovers. Homicide is the eleventh leading cause of death in the United States (Rosenberg and Mercy, 1985). For minority men and women age 15 to 34 years, homicide is the number one cause of death. Approximately 1000 women are killed by their spouses annually in the United States, and a similar number of wives kill their husbands. This latter fact is misleading in that self-defense is involved approximately seven times

more often when women kill men than vice versa (Campbell, 1986).

Rape

Currently rape is one of the most underreported yet fastest-growing forms of human abuse in the United States. The rate of occurrence of this crime is rising annually.

Since many rapes are not reported because of fear of retaliation or stigma, or because of a feeling of guilt about having somehow provoked the attack, the actual incidence is many times higher than reported.

For reported rapes, cities constitute higher-risk areas than rural settings, and the hours between 8 PM and 2 AM, on weekends, and during the summer are the most critical times. In about one half of the rapes the victim and the offender meet on the street, while in the remaining attacks the rapist either gains entry to the victim's home or somehow entices or forces the victim to accompany him.

Primary, secondary, and tertiary preventions are needed. Primary prevention refers to averting the occurrence of rape; secondary prevention involves early treatment to prevent complications; and tertiary prevention is aimed at stopping the progression of the results of the initial health problem.

Primary prevention of rape includes providing information about the dangers involved in going places with strangers, avoiding high-risk locations, and safeguarding one's home against possible entry. Primary prevention of rape, as in other forms of human abuse, requires a broad-based community focus for educating both the community as a whole and key groups such as police, health care providers, educators, and social workers. Public awareness is directed toward increasing knowledge about rape, raising questions about beliefs and attitudes about victims, and discussing and developing intervention alternatives.

Secondary prevention for rape victims begins with an understanding of the commonly accepted dynamics. Rape is generally more an aggressive than a sexual activity. The underlying issues are more often hostility, power, or control than sexual desire, with the defining issue being lack of consent of the victim. The danger that accompanies rape is keen; often, resisting victims are hit, kicked, or stabbed. Although the act of rape is sexual, it is the violence that traumatizes the victim because of the fear for her life, helplessness, lack of control, vulnerability, and the experience of being the living target for someone's wrath.

People react to rape differently, depending on their personality, past experiences and background, and support received after the trauma. Some victims cry, shout, or discuss the experience, while others withdraw and fear discussing the attack. During the immediate as well as the follow-up stages, victims need to talk about what happened and to express their feelings and fears in a nonjudgmental atmosphere. No matter what people think or feel, they are entitled to these views. Therefore nonjudgmental listening is an essential nursing measure.

In any psychological trauma the right to privacy and confidentiality is of the utmost importance. Victims should not be expected to answer questions in an area where others can hear them. Nurses are responsible for providing continuous care once the victim enters the health care system, including monitoring the actions of other workers who may be less sensitive to the psychological needs of the victim (Dietz, 1978).

Since rape is a situational crisis for which advance preparation is rarely possible, nursing efforts are directed toward helping victims maximize their ability to cope with the stress and disruption of their lives caused by the attack. Counseling focuses on the crisis and the concomitant fears, feelings, and issues involved. The goal is to help the victim use problem-solving skills to develop ways to regroup personal forces. Counseling includes assessing the appropriateness of the reaction to the event. Is the person distorting reality? Is the anxiety level so high that it interferes with coping and problem solving? How much has this crisis affected the person's daily life?

The next major area to assess is the nature, availability, and quality of the victim's support system. It is important to determine if family and friends are part of the support network or whether they hold the victim somehow responsible for the crisis. Whom has the victim told about the experience? The victim of rape may need assistance in talking with and asking for support from family and friends because of fear of rejection, anxiety, or guilt.

Five key areas that are crucial nursing interventions include the following:

1. Avoid viewing the woman as a victim and begin to think of her as a client. In a crime such as rape people often have difficulty moving out of a victim role and seeing themselves as coping, capable people. The crime has been committed; the person must reorganize personal resources and learn new ways of adapting.

2. Help the individual confront the reality of the crisis and deal with the attendant feelings. The emotional wound, just like a cut or burn, cannot heal until it has been cleaned. The emotions must be opened up, cleaned out, and treated.

3. Assist the person to confront the crisis one step at a time. Problem solving, reorganizing emotional resources, and planning new coping strategies take time and should be attacked one at a time.

4. Help the person gain an understanding of the crisis. Often people who experience a situational crisis will ask "Why me?" Such questions may indicate a cause-and-effect kind of reasoning whereby the person keeps saying "If only I had (not) done _____, this would not have happened." If the woman used poor judgment before the rape, such as leaving a bar with a stranger or walking down a dark street, help her examine alternative behavior for the future, while reinforcing the fact that her behavior did not justify the violence brought against her.

5. Examine alternative actions for coping with current situations. One residual effect of situational crises is to reduce the victim's ability to deal with daily occurrences and problems. When this happens, these people need to turn to their sources of support and

evaluate alternatives while mobilizing their resources and relearning previous coping abilities.

Secondary prevention often continues into *tertiary prevention,* when rape victims are helped to deal with the crisis of rape so their lives are not emotionally scarred for the future. Just as during secondary prevention, victims must be reminded that they may have delayed reactions to the rape. They need to recognize that they are not "falling apart" emotionally but rather that their phobias, nightmares, or increased motor activity (reflected in moving, taking trips, or frequently changing telephone numbers) are reactions to a crisis. Many rape victims need follow-up mental health services to help them cope with the long-term effects of the crisis. They may be hesitant to ask for help or to follow through on these services, so community health nurses must not only make appropriate referrals but also take the initiative in calling the victim to check on her and remind her of appointments. Rape victims need support, encouragement, and acceptance from those with whom they come in contact.

Suicide

Suicide can be viewed in much the same way as homicide with relation to the abuse-prone individual. *Suicide* can be a means of escape not only for the abused family member but also for the abuser.

Suicide is the tenth leading cause of death in the United States, with approximately 11.6 suicides per 100,000 people. The incidence of suicide increases with age, reaching a high of 40 per 100,000 among persons over 75 years old. Suicide attempts are most common in teens and college students (Hanlon and Pickett, 1984).

Among teenagers the incidence is alarming. The American Academy of Pediatrics reported that according to the National Institute of Mental Health, more than 6,000 teenagers killed themselves in 1984. This figure means that every 90 minutes a teen commits suicide and that every day 1000 more will attempt it (Oliphant, 1986).

Suicide is observed three times more frequently among males than among females, although females attempt suicide more often. Suicide is four times more frequent among whites than among blacks. Affluent and educated people have higher rates of suicide than do the economically and educationally disadvantaged (Hanlon and Pickett, 1984). Laborers, teachers, clergymen, and miners have low rates, in contrast to entertainers, artists, businessmen, professionals such as dentists, lawyers, and physicians, and people in the military. Suicide rates for military people are highest in times of peace.

A group often overlooked is family members and/or friends of suicide victims. *Survivors* often feel angry toward the dead person yet frequently turn the anger inward; likewise, survivors frequently question their own liability for the death. The impact of suicide can affect family, friends, co-workers and the community. Survivors may have difficulty dealing with their feelings toward the dead person, they may have difficulty concentrating, and they may limit their social activities, since it is often difficult for both survivors and their friends to talk about the suicide, yet the topic looms like an overhanging cloud on social contacts. When a person commits suicide, the event causes many other people to confront their own mortality.

Community health nurses often encounter survivors of suicide victims and should be able to implement appropriate interventions. Intervention deals with helping survivors cope with the trauma of the loss and may include referral to a counselor so the family can handle the acute symptoms of grief. Intervention may also include referral to support groups, informing the community of the needs of these individuals, and serving as a catalyst in establishing support groups for survivors if none is available in the community (Praeger and Bernhardt, 1985).

The leading factors associated with suicide attempts are listed by Hanlon and Pickett (1984) as broken homes or frequent moves during childhood, marital disharmony, emotional immaturity, cruelty to children, and jealousy bordering on the pathological. One can clearly see how the abuse-prone family could have one or more of these factors present in their lives.

Exposure to the violence of war may also contribute to the causes of suicide. A study of veterans who were in military service during the Vietnam War found that veterans were 65% and 49% more likely to die from suicide and motor-vehicle accidents, respectively, than nonveterans (Hearst, et. al, 1986).

FAMILY VIOLENCE AND ABUSE

Society has traditionally considered the family one of the most powerful examples of social unity. The family unit in society shapes and is shaped by all the forces surrounding it. In the past, many of the behaviors and actions sanctioned within the family were severely punished by society if they occurred elsewhere. Roman law gave fathers the power of life and death over their sons. For centuries female offspring were considered parental property to be sold or forced into marriage. Once married, women became the property of their husbands.

No member of the family is guaranteed immunity from abuse and neglect. Spouse abuse, child abuse, abuse of the elderly family member, serious violence among siblings, and mutual abuse by members all occur. Although these examples are not inclusive, they demonstrate the scope of family violence. Roesch (1984) points out recent research that indicates that as many as 16 million Americans are assaulted each year by members of their own families.

Recognizing the battered child or spouse in the emergency room is painfully simple after the fact. Unfortunately, by the time medical care is sought, serious physical and emotional damage may have been done. Community health nurses are in a key position to predict and deal with abusive tendencies. By understanding factors contributing to the development of abusive behaviors, the nurse can identify abuse-prone families.

Families differ in their degree of effectiveness as a system. Effective families are able to promote the growth and development of members while maintaining cohesion as an identifiable system (Taylor, 1982). An effective family is not necessarily free from problems but rather has developed a structure and method of functioning that allow it to deal with problems as they arise. Learning to be a responsible family member does not come naturally to all people. Most people receive minimal, if any, preparation for parenthood. They therefore repeat the patterns learned in their own family. In many instances, patterns of family interaction are passed from one generation to another, leading to ineffective family members who are unable to handle stress, frustration, and anger constructively. Family stress may be manifested by the entire system, with overt tension and hostility among members, or may be directed primarily toward one member.

Development of Abusive Patterns

Several factors characterize people who become involved in family violence, including the way in which individual members were raised, the unique characteristics of members, and/or a crisis.

Of all the factors that characterize the background of abusers, the most predictably present is previous exposure to some form of violence. Past episodes of family violence are almost universal in the history of abusers. As children, abusers were often beaten themselves or witnessed the beating of siblings or a parent. Children raised in this fashion may abhor the use of violence, but they have had no experience with other models of family relationships.

Abused children learn early which behaviors lead to abuse and which do not. Typically they relate to their parents in either of the following two ways or in a combination of the two. Compliance is one pattern whereby the child learns what the parent expects and behaves accordingly. This type of child begins at an early age to take care of the parents, such as by bringing them coffee, cigarettes, and so on (Scharer, 1979). Other children learn that they only get attention when they are being noncompliant, so they provoke abuse to avoid being totally ignored. They seem to feel that any attention is better than no attention.

The abuse need not be violent to cause dysfunction. Even gentle physical punishment as a child can lead to the development of family violence in later years. Negative inferences can be drawn from such violence even though it is gentle. A child may learn to associate love with violence inasmuch as parents are usually the first to hit a child, and the child can come to believe that those who love him also are those who hit him. The moral rightness of hitting other family members may be established when physical punishment is used to train children. The child may learn that physical force is justified when something is really important (Roesch, 1984). This type of experience only prepares children to use violence with their own children.

People who become abusers may also learn parenting skills from dysfunctional role models. Their parents may have set unrealistic goals, and when the children failed to perform accordingly, they were criticized, demeaned, and punished and affection was often withheld. The children were told how to act, what to do, and how to feel, thereby discouraging the development of autonomy, problem-solving skills, and creativity (Scharer, 1979). Children raised in this fashion grow up feeling unloved and worthless and may want a child of their own so that they will feel assured of someone's love.

To protect themselves from feelings of worthlessness and fear of rejection, these children form a protective shell and increasingly grow hostile and distrustful of others. The behavior of potential abusers reflects a low tolerance for frustration, emotional instability, and the onset of aggressive feelings with minimal provocation. Because of their emotional insecurity, they often depend on a child or spouse for meeting their needs so that they may be valued and feel secure. When their needs are not met by others, they become overly critical. Critical, resentful behavior and unrealistic expectations of others leads to a vicious cycle. The more critical these people become, the more they are rejected and alienated from others.

Abuse-prone people are emotionally labile, often adopting behaviors that reflect a belief that nothing in life is stable or permanent. Aggression is their primary mode of responding to others, since they only know one way of dealing with internalized resentment, fear, and anger. Lacking personal acceptance, abuse-prone people are suspicious of others and question overtures of kindness as well as authority. Almost predictably, abuse-prone people marry one another, and neither partner knows how to relate in a mature fashion to the spouse. Many abusers were socially isolated because of family mobility. Abusive parents often feel guilty for being unable to cope smoothly with the needs of a developmentally disabled child, and they deal with their feelings of guilt, frustration, embarrassment, or helplessness with violence.

A perceived or actual crisis typically precedes an abusive episode. Abuse-prone people generally are not adept at problem solving; even a small crisis can seem overwhelming. Since crisis reinforces feelings of inadequacy and low self-esteem, it is often the number of events occurring in a short time that precipitates abusive patterns. Factors such as unemployment, strains in the marriage, or an unplanned pregnancy may set off violence.

Mobility also constitutes a precipitating stimulus, since frequent moves disrupt social support systems and tend to isolate people, at least briefly. For the abuse-prone family the difficulty of mobility is keen in that they do not readily seek out new relationships, which means that they only have the family to turn to for support. Resources may be unfamiliar to them because of the location, name, or inaccessibility of the resources. They are alone in a new place and cannot find resources, yet they hesitate to ask for help.

Crowded living conditions may precipitate abuse. The presence of numerous people in a small space tends to heighten tensions and to reduce the possibility of any privacy. Tempers flare because of the constant stimulation from others.

Many factors may precipitate a violent or abusive episode. Community health nurses may be able to predict a potential abusive episode and refer the person to a social or health care agency. The accompanying box summarizes behavioral indicators of potentially abusive parents. Many of these characteristics pertain to all aspects of family abuse, specific types of which are discussed below.

Child Abuse

A recent national survey projected that nearly 1.5 million children and adolescents are subjected to abusive physical violence each year (Gelles, 1985). This is probably a conservative figure, since only the most severe cases are reported. Child maltreatment is not new; it can be traced to ritualistic infanticide among early tribes and is documented in the Bible, the writings of Charles Dickens, and in history texts (Misener, 1986). Child maltreatment was rarely discussed in medical literature until Henry Kempe et al. published their classic article in 1962, which coined the term *battered child syndrome.*

Kempe and his associates (1962) have been highly successful in generating public and professional concern over child maltreatment. The 1973 Congressional hearings on child maltreatment led to the passage in 1974 of the Child Abuse Prevention and Treatment Act (Misener, 1986). One provision of the act requires states to enact mandatory reporting legislation in order to be eligible for grant funds. Although all 50 states have enacted laws to mandate reporting of child maltreatment, underreporting continues to exist because of the lack of consistent definitions of what constitutes abuse and a reluctance on the part of health care providers to get involved in family matters.

The presence of child abuse signifies ineffective family functioning. Abusive parents who recognize their problem

---

BEHAVIORAL INDICATORS OF POTENTIALLY ABUSIVE PARENTS

The following characteristics, while not inclusive or definitive indicators of abuse, do constitute warning signs in couples expecting a child that abuse may be present or may occur at some future time.

1. Denial of the reality of the pregnancy, as evidenced by a refusal to talk about the impending birth or to think of a name for the child
2. An obvious concern or fear that the baby will not meet some predetermined standard: sex, hair color, temperament, or resemblance to family members
3. Failure to follow through on the desire for or seeking of an abortion
4. An initial decision to place the child for adoption and a change of mind
5. Rejection of the mother by the father of the baby
6. Family beset by stress and numerous crises, so that the birth of a child may be the "straw that broke the camel's back"
7. Initial and unresolved negative feelings about having a child
8. Lack of support for the new parents
9. Isolation from friends, neighbors, or family
10. Parental evidence of poor impulse control or fear of losing control
11. Contradictory history
12. Appearance of detachment
13. Appearance of misusing drugs or alcohol
14. Shopping for hospitals or health care providers
15. Unrealistic expectations of the child

are often reluctant to seek assistance because of the stigma attached to being considered a child abuser. Child abuse ranges from violent, physical attacks, resulting in severe injury, to passive neglect, resulting in insidious malnutrition or other problems. It is not limited to physical maltreatment but includes emotional abuse such as yelling at or continually demeaning and criticizing the child.

Children are frequent victims of abuse because they are small and relatively powerless in the family hierarchy. In many families only one child is subjected to abuse. Parents may identify with this particular child and be particularly critical of that child's behavior, or the child may have certain qualities, such as looking like a relative, being handicapped, or being particularly bright and capable, that provoke the parent.

The box at left depicts behavioral indicators of potentially abusive parents. These indicators do not show the pain and often poor emotional stability of the parents. As described in the previous section on family patterns supportive of violence, abusive parents are typically emotionally impoverished people with many unmet needs and poor impulse control (Taylor, 1982).

It is essential that community health nurses recognize the physical and behavioral indicators of abuse and neglect. The box below summarizes indicators of physical abuse, physical neglect, sexual abuse, and emotional maltreatment. The sections that follow describe additional characteristics of child abuse.

FACTORS THAT MAY INDICATE PRESENCE OR POTENTIAL FOR ABUSE

The following characteristics, while not inclusive of all possible behaviors leading to abusive patterns, serve as cues that abuse may be present or could occur at some future time.

Abuse should be investigated when a child:

1. Has an unexplained injury
   a. Skin: burns, old or recent scars, ecchymosis, soft-tissue swelling, human bites
   b. Fractures: recent or ones that have healed
   c. Subdural hematomas
   d. Trauma to genitals
   e. Whiplash (caused by shaking small children)
2. Seems dehydrated or malnourished without obvious cause
3. Is given inappropriate food or drugs (alcohol, tobacco, medication prescribed for someone else, foods not appropriate for the child's age)
4. Shows evidence of general poor care: poor hygiene, dirty clothes, unkempt hair, dirty nails
5. Is unusually fearful of nurse and others
6. Is considered to be a "bad" child
7. Is not dressed appropriately for the season or weather conditions
8. Reports or shows evidence of sexual abuse
9. Has injuries not mentioned in history
10. Seems to need to take care of the parent and speak for the parent

---

Child neglect in general can be divided into two categories: physical and emotional. Physical neglect is defined as failure to provide adequate food, proper clothing, shelter, hygiene, or necesssary medical care (Leaman, 1979). The child is not valued to the extent that even basic requirements for successful adaptation are met. In contrast, emotional neglect is the omission of basic nurturing, acceptance, and caring essential for healthy personal development. These children are largely ignored or in many cases treated as nonpersons. Such neglect usually affects the development of self-esteem in that it is difficult for a neglected child to feel a great deal of self-worth because no one ever seems to care. Neglect is much more difficult to assess and evaluate than abuse because it is more subtle and may go unnoticed. Astute observations of children, their homes, and the way in which they relate to their care givers can provide clues of neglect.

Physical abuse refers to one or more episodes of extreme disciplining or displaced aggression or frustration, often resulting in serious physical damage to the internal organs, bones, central nervous system, or sense organs. This form of abuse is most often seen in episodes of beating, burning, kicking, branding, or shaking the child.

Emotional abuse includes extreme debasement of a child's feelings so that the child feels inadequate, inept, uncared for, and worthless. Examples are constant criticism and ridiculing directed toward a child, who ultimately may believe himself to be a "bad" person. Victims of emotional abuse learn to hold in their feelings to avoid incurring additional scorn. Repressing feelings can lead to symptoms of hyperactivity, withdrawal, overeating, psychosomatic dermatological problems, vague and often difficult-to-pinpoint complaints, stuttering, truancy, or general hostility and aggression toward others or themselves.

Sexual abuse ranges from fondling to rape. A particularly destructive form of sexual abuse, incest, deserves attention because of the nature and magnitude of the problem. Incest is not limited to "backwoods" people but occurs in all races, religious groups, and socioeconomic classes. Incest is receiving greater attention because of mandatory reporting laws, yet all too often its incidence remains a family secret.

Because of hesitancy to report sexual abuse the actual incidence is unknown. It is estimated that approximately one of every four girls is molested sexually during childhood or adolescence (Brunngraber, 1986). In about one third of the cases of sexual abuse, the perpetrator is related to the victim (Finkelhor, 1979). Although reporting systems are improving, it is estimated that one girl in 100 is abused sexually by her father (Brunngraber, 1986). Many cases of parental incest go unreported because the victim fears punishment, abandonment, rejection, or family disruption if she acknowledges the problem.

Because nurses, particularly community health nurses, are often involved in helping women deal with the aftermath of incest, it is essential to understand the typical patterns as well as the long-term implications.

The daughter involved in paternal incest is approximately 11 years old at the onset and is often the oldest or only daughter. The father seldom uses physical force but more likely relies on threats, bribes, intimidation, or misrepresentation of moral standards or exploits the daughter's need for human affection (Brunngraber, 1986).

The immediate effects of incest can include guilt, depression, learning difficulties, sexual promiscuity, running away, somatic complaints, fear of sexuality, disturbed object relations, isolation from the family, and various emotional sequelae such as anxiety, restlessness, truancy, and gastrointestinal symptoms.

No clear picture can be drawn as to the long-term effects of incest in that researchers have found markedly different response patterns. Brunngraber (1986) defines "long-term" as more than 6 months after termination of the incest. In reviewing extensive research on the long-term effects of incest, she noted that findings ranged from minimal emotional damage to promiscuity, illegitimate pregnancies, homosexual tendencies, drug and alcohol abuse, and fear of forming close and trusting relationships.

In her own retrospective study of 21 female victims of incest, Brunngraber found that both the immediate and the long-range effects of incest were diverse in type, nature, and severity. She noted that the type of assistance provided to victims both during the time of the incestuous experience and afterwards influenced the reaction. Nurses must be aware of the incidence, signs and symptoms, and psychological and physical trauma of incest.

Spouse Abuse

Spouse abuse is an increasing social problem requiring the attention of nurses and other health care professionals. Only recently has this phenomenon been openly talked about; in the past, spouse abuse was often considered a family secret. *Spouse abuse* is defined as any physical attack by one marital partner against another, ranging from a slap to homicide. Although spouse abuse usually refers to instances in which husbands behave in a violent way toward wives, it must be remembered that wives do abuse husbands. Wives emotionally and physically strike out at their husbands and leave scars on the mind and body that are difficult to heal. Although this discussion focuses on battered women, a more common occurrence than battered husbands, many of the dynamics apply to either situation.

Spouse abuse is not only a physical act but also is seen in emotional abuse. Emotional abuse takes many forms, but it is often manifest as the overly critical attitude of a spouse: the marital partner, seemingly, does nothing right. Criticism is demeaning and tends to lower the self-esteem of the one who is criticized. Emotional abuse occurs also when a person is hampered in accomplishments in accordance with innate potential by the limits and restrictions of another. For example, spouses often demand that the marital partner not do something, like go to school or secure a job; a husband may fear that his wife will intellectually or socially surpass him if she gets a college education or finds a satisfactory job. Likewise, a wife may limit her husband's potential by complaining when the husband is away from home on business trips or pursuing a degree.

Battered women often have bruises, lacerations, and broken bones. A swollen face, reddened hands, and bruises and cuts on the legs are key signs. Frequently the injuries are carefully inflicted on parts of the body that can easily be disguised by concealing clothing, such as the abdomen, upper thigh, and back. As in families with a history of child abuse, a large portion of spouse abuse victims and victimizers have a violent family history. Interviews with battered women indicate that batterers come from all socioeconomic levels and professions. Batterers are typically described as moody, angry, impulsive, tense, suspicious, and resentful (Weingourt, 1979).

Many battered women have low self-esteem and a general sense of worthlessness. They often remain in a fear-filled marriage for reasons such as an innate cultural or religious belief that it is the woman's role to make the marriage a success. To admit that they are battered is to admit failure as a wife. Other women use the rationalization of "'oh-but-he-needs-me,' how can I desert him?" (Weingourt, 1979). The woman thus sees herself as worthy only when she is taking care of a dependent, needy man. The sicker he gets, the more he needs her; hence her basic human worth is validated by remaining in this pathological marriage.

In a study of 150 battered women, Roy (1977) documented the seven highest-priority factors that kept the women in their marriages. In order of importance these reasons were (1) hope that the husband would reform, (2) feelings of no place to go, (3) fear of reprisals from the husband, (4) children making it difficult to find an alternative place to live, (5) financial problems because of unemployment and lack of money, (6) fear of living alone, and (7) belief that divorce is a shameful state.

Women often experience animosity from parents, friends, neighbors, the police, and health care providers when they openly acknowledge that they cannot keep their own house in order. To avoid society's reaction to being battered, women may hide injuries by staying at home until bruises and scratches heal or by wearing concealing clothing. Because of unpredictable reactions, battered women may hesitate to discuss how their injuries occurred.

Spouse abuse can also lead to violent solutions. Very often the murder of a spouse is the final act in a long history of physical and psychological assaults. A California study in a state prison found that 28 of the 30 women imprisoned for killing their mates had been victims of spouse abuse, (Jordan, 1985). It was also pointed out by Jordan that in a study by the Kansas City Police Department of spouse killings, the police had been called to the home at least once in the two previous years in 90% of the cases.

It is important to recognize that spouse abuse often accompanies child abuse (Hendrix, 1981). Van Stolk (1976) contends that many women are beaten along with their children or are beaten when they try to shield their children from injuries. Beating a pregnant woman may reflect the man's desire to terminate the pregnancy and thereby relieve him of the impending burden of another dependent. Some batterers are emotionally disturbed and unable to recognize the consequences of their actions. This lack of awareness may result from mental illness or the influence of drugs or alcohol.

Prince (1981) described a three-phase cycle often present in spouse abuse. During the first phase, *tension building,* the victim tries to calm the abuser by being compliant, nurturing, and generally nonoffensive. Despite the presence of compliant behavior, *battering* may ensue, motivated by rage as the abuser punishes the woman for "misbehavior." Severe injury or death can occur during this second phase. During the third phase, however, the batterer is *apologetic* and contrite, even attempting to convince the victim that the out-of-control episode will not be repeated. Often victims are misled by this behavior, especially since they are trying to convince themselves that "things will work out and we'll live happily ever after." The hopes and dreams of the past for a happy, loving relationship tend to overshadow the reality of recent behavior and reinforce the continuation of the relationship.

It is important to understand this cyclical pattern so as to curb the impatience felt toward women who are reluctant or unwilling to remove themselves from such a harmful situation. If abuse is suspected, the person should be asked directly about such a possibility. Because of shame and fear, women are hesitant to volunteer such information, but they often feel relieved to discuss their fears and life realities. Women are often defensive and apologetic about their spouse's behavior. A listening, nonjudgmental approach is useful in encouraging a description of past events and planning for the future.

Victims of abuse are often reluctant to leave the familiar, abusive situations because they do not envision themselves as having options. although they may keenly fear for their safety, at least their present life-style is familiar. In providing care for these women, community health nurses should help them identify and set priorities for their alternatives. Individual or marriage counseling may help some, while others must leave the abusive situation and begin a new life. It is not uncommon for women to simply refuse to do anything besides worry about the future. When this occurs, the most useful preventive effort is to assist the woman to plan ahead by considering what the quickest escape route is if violence erupts. Where could she go? Who could she call? The most critical step is for the woman to regain some mastery over her life. She must plan ways to take care of herself in the event that the battering recurs. These plans must include income, shelter, legal aid, and child care.

Abuse of the Elderly

Abuse of the elderly seems to be more prevalent than reported cases would indicate. Abuse of the elderly includes neglect as well as physical or psychological assault. The elderly are neglected and abused when others fail to provide adequate food, clothing, shelter, and physical care and to meet physiological and safety needs.

Roughness in handling elderly people can lead to bruises and bleeding into tissue because of the fragility of their skin and vascular systems. It is often difficult to determine if the injuries of the elderly result from abuse, falls, or other natural causes. Careful assessment both through observation and discussion assists in determining the cause of injuries. Other ways in which the elderly are physically abused occur when caretakers impose unrealistic toileting demands, as well as when the special needs and previous patterns of the elderly person are ignored.

The elderly are also abused with regard to nutrition. They may be given food that they cannot chew or swallow or that is contraindicated because of dietary restrictions. Care givers may overlook food preferences or social or cultural beliefs and patterns about food. Elderly people may become undernourished if they can neither prepare their own food nor eat that prepared for them.

Care givers occasionally give elderly people medication to induce confusion or drowsiness so they will be less troublesome, need less care, or allow others to gain control of their financial and personal resources. Once medicated, the elderly have few ways to act in their own behalf.

The most common form of psychological abuse is rejection or simply ignoring elderly people, conveying that they are worthless and useless to others. On incorporating these feelings into their self-view the elderly regress and become increasingly dependent on others, who tend to resent the imposition and demands on their time and life-styles. The pattern becomes cyclical: the more regressed the person becomes, the greater the dependence, and so on. Furthermore, the elderly people's past accomplishments and present abilities are not consistently acknowledged, causing them to feel less capable than they may actually be.

Care givers abuse elderly people for a variety of reasons. The elderly family member may impose a physical, emotional, or financial burden on the care giver, leading to frustration and resentment. The abuser may be reversing earlier family patterns, whereby the abuser was previously abused by the elderly person (Elder Abuse, 1980).

A subgroup particularly vulnerable to abuse are the confused and frail elderly. There are large numbers of frail elderly people, many with serious physical or mental impairments, who live in the community and are cared for by their families. Living with and providing care to a confused elderly person is a difficult, round-the-clock task, which often exhausts family members. Family stress increases as members simply must work harder to meet their prior responsibilities as well as the needs of the elderly person.

Signs to look for when abuse of the elderly is suspected are listed in the box below.

SIGNS TO LOOK FOR WHEN ABUSE OF THE ELDERLY IS SUSPECTED

Unexplained or repeated injury
Fear of the care giver
Untreated sores or other skin injuries, such as decubitus ulcers, excoriated perineum, burns
Overall poor care (e.g., unclean, given inappropriate food)
Withdrawal and passivity
Periods of time when elderly person is unsupervised
Failure to seek appropriate medical care
Contractures resulting from immobility or restraint
Unwillingness or inability of care giver to meet elderly person's needs
Improper home repair
Unsafe home situation (e.g., poor heating, ventilation, dangerous clutter (Ferguson and Beck, 1983; and Phillips, 1983)

Elderly people need to retain as much autonomy and decision-making ability as possible. Community health nurses have multiple avenues for detecting abuse among the elderly and have skills and responsibility for finding cases, giving treatment, or making referral. Many families caring for elderly members exhaust their resources and coping ability. Community health nurses can assist in finding new sources of support and aid. Block and Sinnott (1979) identified the following resources for easing stressors of both caretakers and elderly people: (1) home-related services such as home aides, medical and/or nursing care, meal delivery service, home repair, and home visits; (2) monetary assistance; (3) day-care and respite day-care centers; (4) transportation services; (5) counseling and other mental health services; and (6) educational programs focusing on the care of the aged.

Abuse of Developmentally Disabled People

Many of the same aspects of child abuse apply to abuse of developmentally disabled people. The term *developmental disabilities* refers to a variety of mental and physical impairments that interfere with an individual's ability to function in an acceptable manner in society because of limitations in the ability to care for oneself, learn, speak, or accomplish other self-care. Several unique characteristics cause this group to be at a high risk for abusive treatment. For example, developmentally disabled people tend to require more attention and supervision than their normal counterparts, which may increase care-giver frustration because of the seemingly never-ending needs and demands. Parents may perceive themselves as trapped with responsibility and feel resentment, anger, and guilt toward their developmentally disabled children.

In addition, these children often fail to live up to the hopes and expectations of their parents. With normal children, parental self-esteem tends to increase because of the accomplishments of the children. Children with developmental delays may not enhance parental status and esteem because their achievements are limited and not comparable to those of normal children.

Infants who begin life by being premature or having mental or physical deficits are especially vulnerable to abuse by both parents and care givers (Sandgrund et al., 1974). These children are viewed as sickly, demanding, and in general "problem children." Their care is expensive in both energy and time; because of the differences from other children, parents tend to worry about their ability to provide adequate care. Also, these children are often less responsive or respond negatively to attention provided, causing care givers to feel insecure in their abilities. As parents become insecure and frustrated and feel inept in eliciting the normal responses of smiling, cooing, and so on, they may be tempted either to ignore the child or to strike out physically. Interventions by community health nurses working with families with a developmentally disabled member are similar to the interventions described in the following section. Community services to assist families in dealing with the stress and crisis associated with a child's handicap and referral to agencies able to assist with education and child

care are key ingredients of nursing action. Families may need to learn how to seek outside diversions to provide them strength to cope with their life situations. Homemaker services, day care, or sitters may be realistic aids for many of these families. Chapter 26 presents additional information about this group.

COMMUNITY HEALTH NURSING INTERVENTION
Primary Prevention

Primary prevention of human abuse can occur when the problem can be predicted. Presently, we are unable to predict with certainty when abuse will occur. However, earlier sections of the chapter have described a variety of factors that tend to influence the onset and support the continuation of abusive patterns. Additionally, lists of early signs of abuse are included. Community health nurses are in an excellent position to identify potential victims of abuse, since these nurses see clients in a wide variety of settings, including homes, schools, work, and clinics.

Factors to include in an assessment of an individual or family's potential for violence are categorized by Logan and Dawkins (1986, p. 743) as illustrated in the algorithm in Figure 34-1.

Essentially, the primary prevention of abuse includes strengthening individuals and families so they can cope more effectively with multiple life stressors and demands and reducing the destructive elements in the community that support and encourage the use of human violence. Nurses in their work with schools, community groups, employees, day care centers, and other community institutions can foster healthy developmental patterns and identify signs of potential abuse.

Prevention of psychosocial problems cannot easily be documented; however, many clinicians believe that providing support and psychological enrichment to at-risk individuals and families prevents the onset of health disruption. For example, community health nurses have varied opportunities to strengthen and even teach parenting abilities. Parenting skills do not come naturally to all people. Basic skills such as diapering, feeding, quieting, and even holding and rocking a baby can be the focus of a class or home or clinic visit. Parents also need to learn acceptable and workable ways to discipline children so that limits are maintained without breaking the child's spirit or causing physical harm.

Mutual support groups are valuable for new parents, families with special children, or abused people themselves. Such groups have variable formats and can provide information, support, and encouragement. Nurses can help begin such groups or can actually serve as group leaders. Chapter 14 describes the role of the community health nurse in working with community groups.

Secondary Prevention

When prevention of abuse has not been possible, community health nurses can initiate preventive measures to reduce or terminate further abuse. It is helpful to review Chapter 33 and to recognize that both developmental and situational *crises* present opportunities for abusive situations to develop. The occurrence of violence represents a family

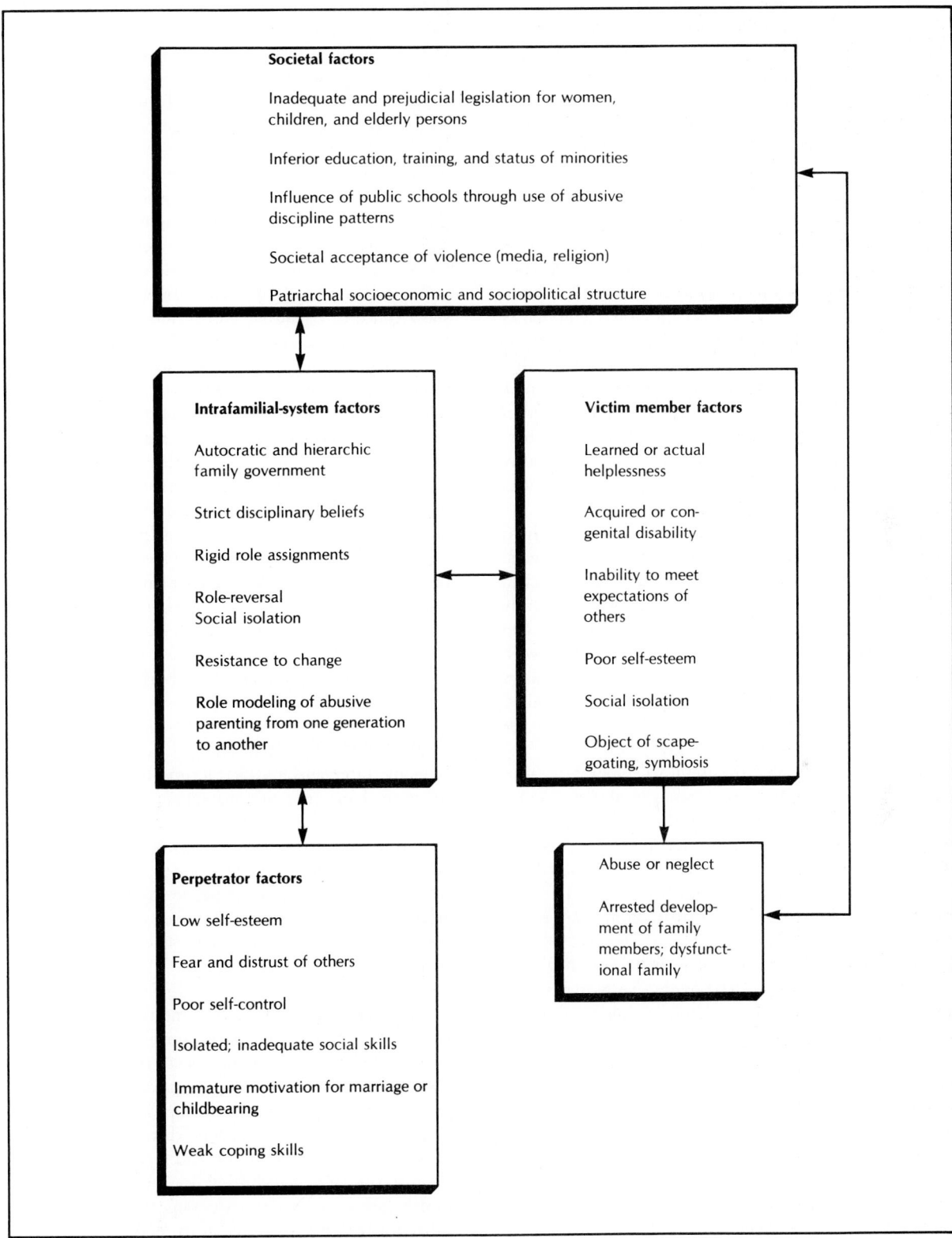

FIGURE 34-1

Factors to include when assessing an individual or family's potential for violence.

crisis and should be handled using the strategies presented in Chapter 33.

Effective *communication* with abusive families is important. Typically, these families are not eager to discuss their problems. Many members of such families are embarrassed to be involved in an abusive situation either as the victim or as the abuser, or as a passive observer who has been unable to terminate the abusive pattern. Often considerable guilt is involved. Effective communication must be preceded by an attitude of acceptance. It is often difficult for nurses to value the worth of an individual who willfully abuses another. The behavior, not the person, must be condemned. Nursing intervention is directed toward helping participants discuss the problem, seek alternatives for dealing with the tension that led to the abusive situation, or seek placement of the injured person either temporarily or permanently. Family members must trust the nurse in order to allow themselves to be helped in dealing with a situation as sensitive and fraught with emotion as human abuse. The nurse must radiate caring, acceptance, understanding, compassion, and a nonjudgmental attitude. These expectations are by no means easy to uphold; every nurse has her own feelings and beliefs about human treatment of others.

In addition, community health nurses bring to client encounters their own past experiences, attitudes, and values. As a child or young adult the nurse may have been a victim of abuse or may have had classmates, friends, or family members who were abused. The emotional investment and sheer drain of energy required for effectively working with abusers and victims of abuse cannot be disregarded. Abusers present difficult clinical challenges because of their reluctance to seek help or to remain actively involved in the helping process.

Preventive measures are most useful when potential abusers recognize their tendency to be abusive and seek help. For children, in addition to the general measures described, there is often a need for 24-hour child protection services or care givers, where parents can take the child until the acute family or individual crisis has been resolved. Telephone crisis lines can be used to provide immediate emergency assistance to families.

The nurse must also be able to identify "red-flag" antisocial behaviors that might lead to abusive patterns. According to Klingbeil (1986), high-risk categories of behavior include the following:
1. Psychiatric diagnosis such as depression
2. Pattern of substance abuse
3. Loss and grief after death of a loved one
4. Isolation
5. Lack of support system
6. Homelessness
7. Previous history of assaultive or suicidal behavior
8. Chronic unemployment
9. Presence or use of weapons, previous arrests
10. History of runaways
11. Single-car auto accidents
12. Psychosomatic complaints

Tertiary Prevention

Tertiary prevention includes a wide range of services with primary emphasis on therapeutic intervention and referral. Community health nurses should know about available community resources for abuse victims. Most larger cities have community resource directories available for a nominal fee. If no such directory is available, then a group of nurses can work together to compile information on what services are available for various clients' needs, who the contact person is, who will be served, and if a fee is charged.

Questions to be raised regarding services for abused people include the following: Are temporary shelters available, and if so, what population do they serve? What emergency funds, transportation, and legal aid are available? How do police and courts respond to abuse and violence? Do they show concern, empathy, and a sincere wish to help, or is the attitude accusatory, punitive, and judgmental?

If attitudes and resources are inadequate, what are the nursing implications? For example, it is often helpful to work with local radio and television stations and newspapers to provide information about the nature and extent of human abuse as a community health problem and also to acquaint people with available services and resources. Frequently people fail to seek services early in an abusive situation because they simply do not know what is available to them. Ideally a program or planned emphasis for abused people begins with a needs assessment to identify potential clients and to determine how to effectively serve this group. Not only can community health nurses serve as catalysts for getting programs started and as a major source of public education, but they often treat both the abused and the abusers.

Protective Measures

Nursing interventions for victims of abuse assist clients either to change the circumstances that have previously led to abuse or to remove themselves from the abusive environment. Protection of victims of abuse is a primary goal of any intervention. As mentioned, not only the abused person but also the abuser needs to be protected. Paying attention to only the abused person reinforces the abusive person's feelings of hopelessness, lack of trust, and belief that no one really cares.

Protective measures are called forth especially when child abuse occurs. All states have some type of child abuse reporting law. In most states the nurse suspecting a child has been abused must report the case to the authorities. Deliberate failure to report abuse cases may result in further injury or death for the child and criminal punishment for the nurse. The community health nurse needs to check local and state laws governing the definition and reporting of child abuse. Despite the fact that child abuse must be reported, some health care providers are reluctant to accept the responsibility for making the decision to report it.

Physicians and nurses often hesitate to report a suspected battered child even though they know not to do so is illegal. All state statutes provide protection from civil suit for anyone making or participating in the reporting of child abuse

(Cazalas, 1978). The child's protection must be the first concern of health care providers once any emergency medical concerns have been treated. Only through proper notification of authorities can the child's protection be assured. Once the child's health and safety are provided for, measures can be started to help the family members deal with their abusive behavior.

Therapeutic Intervention

Therapeutic intervention requires a longer period of time than other types of intervention. It involves dealing with the psychological damage caused by being abusive and having been abused. Dealing with the guilt of abusing a child and developing new resources for coping with crisis are not easy tasks. Referral to community mental health or social work services is necessary and may even be required by the authorities.

The community health nurse can meet the families' therapeutic needs in a variety of ways. Besides referral to appropriate community agencies, nurses can act as role models for the family. During clinic and home visits nurses can demonstrate constructive adult-child interactions. Nurses often teach mothers child care skills such as proper feeding, calming a fretful child, effective discipline, and constructive communication. Nurses not only give parents information about how to feed a child, but should go a step farther and demonstrate this skill. Parents are often frustrated when they try to feed an infant or young child who spits back most of the food. The nurse can calmly show how to offer small amounts of food, use finger foods where appropriate, and remain calm when all efforts at feeding are met with rebellion.

When nurses see families in any setting, they can demonstrate good communication skills and discipline by teaching both parents and children in a calm, respectful, and informative manner. Also, if children behave in undesirable ways, such as handling equipment destructively, the nurse can model appropriate discipline by removing the equipment from the child and redirecting the child's attention to areas or items more suitable for play. Parents watch and listen to what nurses say and do. Talking about children in their presence should be avoided; parents and children should be shown positive types of communication.

Role modeling can be used with abuse victims of all ages. When providing nursing care to abused spouses or to the elderly, nurses can demonstrate communication skills, conflict resolution, and skill training. For example, adult children often become abusive toward their parents when they become frustrated and taxed in their abilities to care for the elderly person. Nurses, during home visits, can demonstrate ways to physically and psychologically care for family members. For example, some elderly people resist having baths, having their clothes changed, taking medications, eating, or exercising. The nurse can work with care givers to help them develop approaches that will be acceptable to the individual elderly person. No standard set of approaches applies to all people. Assessment, creativity, and critical thinking help the nurse, family, and client together devise ways of meeting client and family needs without causing undue stress and frustration.

Tools for Working with Abusive Persons

Scharer (1979) applies six subroles of nursing originally described by Peplau (1952) as tools for working with abusive persons. These subroles apply to abusive situations regardless of the age of the victim. Abusers often fear they will be condemned for their actions, so it is often difficult to make and maintain contact with abusive families. Although community health nurses convey an attitude of caring and concern for them, families may doubt the sincerity of this concern. They may avoid being home at the scheduled visit time out of fear of the consequences of the visit or an inability to believe that anyone really wants to help them. If the victim is a child, parents may fear that the nurse will try to remove the child.

The *subroles* are as follows: mother-surrogate, managerial, technical, teacher, counselor, and socializing. These subroles do not necessarily occur in a sequential or hierarchical order. More than one subrole may occur simultaneously, or they may occur in random order. For example, the sixth subrole, socializing, may be the first one incorporated in the nurse-client interaction.

Mother-surrogate, the first subrole, is used in developing the nurse-client relationship and continues to some degree throughout the duration of the relationship. To convince the family that the nurse really wants to help them, the initial focus should be on the needs of the abusers. By responding first to their difficulties and conflicts, nurses convey an understanding, nonjudgmental attitude. Generally abusers do not want to hurt their victims, and when abuse is discovered, they often feel ashamed of their actions. When nurses convey willingness to listen to the fears, conflicts, and pain of the abuser, a trusting relationship often develops. This interaction may represent the first time someone has devoted time, concern, and energy to listening to the abuser's fears and concerns. Frequently abusers strike out in times of intense frustration. They lose control of their own actions and are later appalled by what they have done.

As a mother-surrogate the nurse teaches basic parenting or adult-to-adult interaction and care-giving skills. Often both abusers and victims need assistance in locating community resources where they can learn skills such as shopping, budgeting, meal preparation, and ways to manage stress, be assertive, or seek a job.

Care givers, especially those caring for children, handicapped people, or the elderly, may need to learn age-appropriate expectations. It is unreasonable to expect a 14-month-old to have moral judgment and be able to differentiate between what is right and wrong. Children at this age do not deliberately annoy care givers by breaking delicate pieces of china. Nor do they set out to spill things; toddlers and young children simply do not always have fine motor coordination. Likewise, a person with poor sphincter control does not willingly soil clothes or bedding. Care givers must learn to deal with their frustrations when soiling occurs and take appropriate preventive measures, such as using thick underwear or bed padding.

Additionally, families do not always know how to have fun. Nurses can assess how much recreation and opportunities for tension release are integrated into the family's lifestyle. Through community assessment the nurse will know what resources and facilities are available and how much they cost. Families may need counseling about the value of recreation and play in reducing tension and appropriately channelling aggressive impulses.

In the *managerial subrole* the nurse organizes and coordinates activities with the family. Examples include helping the family to schedule and arrange clinic appointments, transportation, and babysitters; to find job training programs; to explore career choices and opportunities and pursue them; or to establish linkages with neighbors or social agencies. Nurses should avoid doing for families what they can do for themselves because this can call forth old memories of dependence and lack of autonomy. Doing for other people what they are capable of doing for themselves is not growth producing. Families and community health nurses should jointly plan ways to increase the family's responsibility for their own well-being.

The use of the *technical subrole* depends on family needs and abilities. For example, if abuse has caused injuries, the nurse may need to teach basic skills such as dressing changes, cast care, or vital sign monitoring. Although this role is usually minimal, the nurse does assess the family's care-giving and personal care skills. If a handicapped or elderly person was abused when the care giver tried to provide physical care, the care giver may not have the technical competence to perform necessary skills. In such an instance the nurse should teach the skill and provide an opportunity for the care giver to practice it with supervision and feedback as to the accuracy of the performance.

The *teacher subrole,* like the technical, also includes many traditional nursing actions, such as role modeling, anticipatory guidance, and health education. It is important not to overwork this role, since abusers are often told what they should do. Giving advice should be avoided, since this may undermine the person's ability to be responsible and make informed choices while living with the consequences of the decisions. The teacher subrole includes careful listening to problems and concerns, helping people clarify their needs, and helping to examine possible solutions and alternatives for action (Scharer, 1979).

For example, if a mother were unable to discipline her son without resorting to abuse, the nurse could listen carefully to the mother's recounting of an incident in which discipline failed. Together they could examine the past situation and determine what other actions the mother could have tried. If the 2-year-old broke a favorite vase and the mother spanked the child, finding that her rage increased as the spanking continued, the nurse and mother might consider other forms of discipline. Restricting the environment so the child does not come into contact with valuable items would be an alternative to spanking. The mother might send the child to a quiet place for 10 minutes instead of spanking him, or breakable items might be eliminated from the environment until the child has better impulse control.

The *counselor subrole* comes into play once a trusting relationship has been established. In this subrole the nurse helps abusers explore feelings and look at alternative ways of coping. For example, if adults are involved in marital conflicts, the nurse helps them explore feelings, decide what is expected from one another, identify how the spouse's behavior differs from that expected, describe previous responses to one another, and determine less destructive ways to respond.

Socializing is the sixth and final subrole. It is evidenced by focusing on abusers as people, such as by providing them with opportunities to talk about their interests or what they have been doing that has been enjoyable. Abusers may be inept at social skills; they may profit from opportunities to practice socializing in a safe environment. This does not mean that nurses merely chat with clients, but after determination that a client or family lacks social skills, the nurse systematically engages the client in such interaction. This stage of the nurse-client relationship may occur quite early and increase comfort and trust among participants.

Role of Health Departments

Health departments in most areas of the United States are not strong enough or influential enough, or do not have enough money to provide programs directed at anti-violence interventions by themselves. The community health nurse can act as a focus to bring together many community agencies and groups to work with their health departments in dealing with violence.

What can the role of the health department and community groups be? Foege (1986) describes five roles. First, they could help to get violence into the mainstream of public health. Public health could provide a consistuency for anti-violence activities. Second, health departments and community groups could be involved in problem definition. Third, they could be involved in the education of politicians and others who can produce change, the education of children through the development of appropriate curricula, and the education of the public by providing information to the media. Fourth, health departments could develop intervention strategies and evaluate their impact. Fifth, health departments and community groups must work to keep this interest from being a fad.

The community health nurse can contribute substantially to meeting these roles by becoming the catalyst to bring together the health department and community groups.

◆ ◆ ◆

Intervention in human abuse requires a multidisciplinary and coordinated team approach, since many facets of human existence are involved. Often the nurse serves as the coordinator of the team and ensures that appropriate disciplines are included in the plan of care.

CLINICAL APPLICATON

Mrs. Smith, a 75-year-old bedridden woman, consistently became rude and combative when her daughter attempted to bathe and change her clothes each morning. During a home visit, the daughter told the nurse, Mrs. Jones, that she had gotten so frustrated with her mother on the previous morning that she had hit her. The daughter felt terrible about her behavior but also knew that her mother's incontinence made it essential that Mrs. Smith be kept clean; her clothes had to be changed every day for her own safety and physical well-being.

Mrs. Jones, in taking Mrs. Smith's vital signs and examining her skin turgor, engaged Mrs. Smith in a conversation in which she learned that Mrs. Smith felt stiff and seemed to have more joint pain from her arthritis in the mornings. By late afternoon, her joints were more flexible and less painful. Nurse, daughter, and client discussed their options and decided that the daughter would only wash her mother's anal area in the morning and put clean pads under her if indicated. Total hygienic care would be done in the late afternoon. The nurse was able to demonstrate to the daughter alternative ways of moving, turning, and washing her mother so as to minimize the strain on the arthritic joints and also incorporate some effective exercise into the bath. They also decided that two mornings a week a home health aide would be employed to stay with Mrs. Smith while her daughter did the family shopping and errands and participated in selected community activities in which she had previously been involved and received considerable personal gratification for her contributions.

Nursing assessment and intervention relied on several of the nursing subroles mentioned earlier. The mother-surrogate subrole was used when the nurse listened carefully to the pain and anguish the daughter had felt when she hit her mother. The nurse conveyed a nonjudgmental attitude and helped the daughter and mother explore ways both their needs could be more effectively met. The managerial subrole was used to plan for relying on an outsider to come into the home periodically to give the daughter a break from the constant role of caretaker. The nurse used the technical subrole to teach bathing and exercise techniques and the teacher subrole to role model and demonstrate these techniques. The counselor subrole was employed through the inclusion of the client in the planning of her care. By careful assessment, listening, and problem solving, early intervention served to reduce the possibility of further abuse and to provide the daughter with some relief from feelings of pressure, guilt, and conflict.

SUMMARY

The potential for human abuse and neglect is acquired over many years and stems from a multitude of factors, including societal influences, family history, behavioral characteristics of both the abuser and the abused, and a number of specific precipitating events. Community violence is also influenced by many factors, such as unemployment, dysfunctional community interactions, and lack of cultural activities. Increasing attention is being focused on these age-old problems as varying groups seek to establish a safe environment to live and work in. Women, children, and the elderly are no longer content to be considered the property of others. All people have rights, including being able to live without abuse directed toward them. Because of the stigma attached to the occurrence of human violence, there have historically been poor reporting mechanisms, yet the occurrence seems significant and also increasing in the face of rapidly changing events and social conditions.

Community health nurses must play a key role in prevention, early detection, and prompt intervention. Helping people learn parenting skills as well as ways to care for their elderly relatives are only two examples of prevention. It is erroneous to assume that everyone knows about the normal childhood milestones or the changes that typically occur with aging. Prevention of abuse and violence is the most critical task for community health nurses.

⬒ KEY CONCEPTS

Violence and human abuse are not new phenomena, but they have increasingly become community health concerns.

Communities throughout the United States are voicing anger and frustration about the increasing levels of violence.

The community health nurse is in a position to evaluate and intervene in incidents of community and family violence; to intervene effectively, the community health nurse must understand the dynamics of violence and human abuse.

Factors influencing social and community violence include changing social conditions, economic conditions, population density, community facilities, and institutions within a community, such as organized religion, education, the mass communication media, and work.

The potential for violence against individuals or against oneself is directly related to the level of violence in the community. Identification and correction of factors affecting the level of violence in the community constitute one way of reducing violence against family members and other individuals.

Violence and abuse of family members can happen to any family member: spouse, elderly person, child, or developmentally disabled person.

People who abuse family members are often persons who were themselves abused and who react poorly to real or perceived crises. Other factors that characterize the abuser are the way the person was raised and the unique character of that person.

Child abuse can be physical, emotional, or sexual. Incest is a common and particularly destructive form of child abuse.

Spouse abuse can be physical or emotional. It can lead to violent reprisal by the victimized spouse against the abusive spouse.

Community health nurses are in an excellent position to identify potential victims of family abuse because they see clients in a variety of settings, such as schools, businesses, homes, and clinics. Treatment of family abuse includes primary, secondary, and tertiary prevention and therapeutic intervention.

LEARNING ACTIVITIES

1. For 1 week keep a log or diary related to violence.
   a. Make a note of each time you feel as though you are losing your temper. Consider what it might take to cause you to react in a violent way.
   b. Think back; when was the last time you had a violent outburst? What precipitated it? What were your thoughts? What were your feelings? How might you have handled the situation or those feelings without reacting in a violent way?
   c. During this same week make note of the episodes of violent behaviors you observe. For example, do parents hit children in the supermarket? What seems to precipitate such outbursts? What alternatives might exist for reacting in a less violent way?

2. If you learned after a careful assessment of your community that family violence is a significant community health problem, what plan of action might you take to intervene? Remember that the goal is to promote health; outline a plan of action with objectives, time table, implementation strategies, and evaluation plan for intervening in family violence in your community.

3. Complete a partial community assessment to determine the actual incidence and types of violence in your community.

4. What resources are available in your community for victims of violence? Interview a person who works in an agency that seeks to aid victims of violence. What is the role of the agency? Do its services seem adequate? Who is eligible? Is there a waiting list? What is the fee scale?

BIBLIOGRAPHY

Allen, J.: Violence in the family. Fam. Community Health 4(2):19-33, 1981.

Block, M., and Sinnott, J., editors: The battered elderly syndrome: an exploratory study, College Park, Md., 1979, University of Maryland Press.

Booth, A., Johnson, D., and White, L.: Women, outside employment, and marital instability, Am. J. Sociology 90(3):567-583, 1984.

Bruhn, J., and Fuentes, R.: Child Abuse: a societal paradox, 1981. (Unpublished data.)

Brunngraber, B.S.: Father-daughter incest: immediate and long-term effects of sexual abuse, ANS 8:1-14, July 1986.

Campbell, J.: Nursing assessment for risk of homicide with battered women, ANS 8(4):36-51, 1986.

Cazalas, M.: Nursing and the law, Germantown, Md., 1978, Aspens Systems Corp.

Crime in the United States, 1983. Washington D.C., 1984, U.S. Department of Justice.

Dietz, P.: Social factors in rapist behavior. In Roda, R., editor: Clinical aspects of the rapist, New York, 1978, Grune & Stratton, Inc.

Elder abuse, Washington, D.C., 1980, National Clearing House on Aging.

Ferguson, D. and Beck, C.: H.A.L.F.—A tool to assess elder abuse within the family, Geriatric Nursing vol. 4. Sep/Oct 1983, p. 301-304.

Finkelhor, D.: Sexually victimized children, New York, 1979, Free Press.

Foege, W.: Violence and public health. In Surgeon General's workshop on violence and public health report DHHS pub. no. HRS-D-MC 86-1, Washington, D.C., 1986, Health Resources and Services Administration, U.S. Public Health Service, U.S. Department of Health and Human Services.

Freud, S.: Civilization and its discontents. In Strachey, J., editor: The complete psychological works of Sigmund Freud, London, 1955, Hogarth Press, Ltd.

Gelles, J., and Cornell, C.: Intimate violence in families, Beverly Hills, Calif., 1985, Sage Publications.

Hanlon, J., and Pickett, G.: Public health: administration and practice, ed. 8, St. Louis, 1984, The C.V. Mosby Co.

Health: United States, 1985, DHHS pub. no. (PHS) 86-1232, Hyattsville, Md., December 1985, U.S. Department of Health and Human Services, U.S. Public Health Service, National Center for Health Statistics.

Hearst, N., Newman, T., and Hulley, S.: Delayed effects of the military draft on mortality, N. Engl. J. Med. March 6, 10:620-624, 1986.

Helfer, R., and Kempe, C.: Child abuse and neglect: the family and community, Cambridge, Mass., 1976, Harvard University Press.

Hendrix, M.: Home is where the hell is, Fam. Community Health 4(2)53-59, 1981.

Jones, C.: The fate of abused children. In Franklin, A., editor: The challenge of child abuse, New York, 1977, Academic Press, Inc.

Jordan, N.: Till murder us do part, Psychology Today 19:7, July 1985.

Kempe, C.H., et al.: The battered child syndrome, JAMA 181:17-24, 1962.

Kinard, E.: Mental health needs of abused children, Child Welfare 59(8):451-462, 1980.

Klingbeil, K.: Interpersonal violence: a comprehensive model in a hospital setting—from policy to program. In Surgeon General's workshop on violence and public health report, DHHS pub. no. HRS-D-MC 86-1, Washington, D.C., 1986, Health Resources and Services Administration, U.S. Public Health Service, U.S. Department of Health and Human Services.

Leaman, J.: Recognizing the abused child, Nursing, '79 9(2):65-67, 1979.

Logan, B.B., and Dawkins, C.E.: Family-centered nursing in the community, Menlo Park, Calif., 1986, Addison-Wesley Publishing Co.

Misener, T.R.: Toward a nursing definition of child maltreatment using seriousness vignettes, ANS 8(4):1-14, July 1986.

National Center for Child Abuse and Neglect: Study findings: National Study of Incidence and Severity of Child Abuse and Neglect, U.S. Department of Health and Human Services pub. no. 81-30323, Washington, D.C., 1981, U.S. Government Printing Office.

National Data Book: guide to sources. Statistical abstract of the United States, ed. 105, Washington, D.C., 1986, U.S. Department of Commerce, Bureau of the Census.

Newman, G.: Understanding violence, New York, 1979, J.B. Lippincott Co.

Oliphant, C., editor: Health scene, Pendleton Community Hospital, Pendleton, Ore., Winter 1986.

Phillips, L.R.: Elder abuse—what is it? Who says so? Geriatric Nursing vol. 4. May/June 1983 p. 167-170.

Peplau, H.: Interpersonal relations in nursing, New York, 1952, G.P. Putnam's Sons.

Praeger, S.G., and Bernhardt, G.R.: Survivors of suicide: a community in need, Family and Community Health 8(3): 62-72, Nov. 1985.

Prince, J.: A systems approach to spouse abuse. In Lancaster, J.: Community mental health nursing: an ecological perspective, St. Louis, 1980, The C.V. Mosby Co.

Roesch, R.: Violent families, Parent 59:74, Sept., 1984.

Rosenberg, M.L., and Mercy, J.S.: Homicide and assaultive violence. In Violence as a Public Health Problem, Atlanta, 1985, U.S. Public Health Service, pp. H1-H47.

Roy, M.: A current survey of 150 cases. In Roy, M., editor: Battered women, New York, 1977, Van Nostrand Reinhold Co.

Sandgrund, A., Gaines, R., and Green, A.: Child abuse and mental retardation: a problem of cause and effect, Am. J. Ment. Defic. 79(3):327-330, 1974.

Saul, L.J.: Emotional Maturity, Philadelphia, 1971, J.B. Lippincott Co., pp. 124-141.

Scharer, K.: Nursing therapy with abusive and neglectful families, J. Psychiatr. Nurs. 17(9): 12-21, 1979.

Surgeon General's workshop on violence and public health report, DHHS pub. no. HRS-D-MC 86-1, Washington, D.C., 1986, Health Resources and Services Administration, U.S. Public Health Service, U.S. Department of Health and Human Services.

Taylor, C.: Mereness' essentials of psychiatric nursing, ed. 12. St. Louis, 1986, The C.V. Mosby Co.

Time, p. 64, April 30, 1984.

Uniform crime reports for the United States, Washington, D.C., 1980, Federal Bureau of Investigation, U.S. Department of Justice.

Uniform crime reports for the United States, Washington, D.C., 1984, Federal Bureau of Investigation, U.S. Department of Justice.

Van Stolk, M.: Beaten women, beaten children, Child. Today 5(2):9-12, 1976.

Weingourt, R.: Battered women: the grieving process, J. Psychiatr. Nurs.17(4):40-47, 1979.

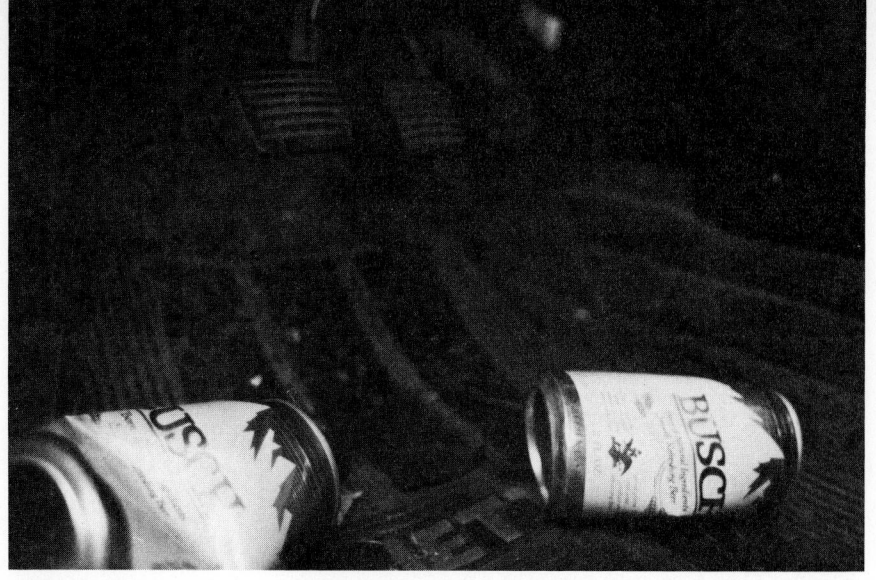

Jeanette Lancaster

35

SUBSTANCE ABUSE

OBJECTIVES

After reading this chapter, the student should be able to:

Identify two attitudes often held by people regarding substance abuse.

List four areas of assessment that might be included in early detection of substance abuse.

Discuss the scope of the alcohol abuse problem.

Describe the physiological effect of excessive alcohol consumption.

List the signs of withdrawal from alcohol.

Identify at least three groups at high risk for alcohol abuse.

Discuss at least three drug-alcohol reactions.

Discuss at least three substances other than alcohol which are often abused.

Identify both short- and long-term effects of smoking on health.

Analyze three smoking cessation programs as to their potential effectiveness.

KEY TERMS

Alcoholics Anonymous
alcoholism
aversive techniques
benzodiazepines
chemical dependency
cocaine
denial
detoxification

fetal alcohol syndrome
freebasing
heroin
mainstream smoke
marijuana
methadone
phenytoin
projection

rationalization
regression
self-control strategies
sidestream smoke
smokeless tobacco
substance abuse
stress
tolerance

Heavy tobacco, alcohol, and drug use has been linked to numerous forms of morbidity and mortality and present serious social and economic problems. Because community health nurses promote the health of individuals, families, and communities, *substance abuse,* or the use of chemicals having undesirable effects, is a major problem for community health nurses to address. In one way or another substance abuse affects all ages, races, sexes, and segments of society.

◆   ◆   ◆

This chapter examines ways to minimize health disruptions attributed to substance abuse. The first section discusses the scope of the problem. Following sections describe the abuse of alcohol, drugs, and cigarettes and tobacco-related products. Each section describes groups at greatest risk for becoming involved in abuse, behavioral and physiological implications of abuse, and avenues of intervention.

SUBSTANCE ABUSE IN MODERN SOCIETY

The necessity for community health nurses to become actively involved in the prevention and cessation of substance abuse is particularly evident when one considers the consequences of substance abuse. Heavy tobacco, alcohol, and drug use has been associated with low birth weight and congenital abnormalities in the children of users; accidents, homicides, and suicides; chronic diseases, such as cardiovascular diseases, cancer, and lung disease; violence and family disruption.

Attitudes and Social Conditions Influencing Substance Abuse

Historically, confusion has existed as to whether substance abuse is a health care or criminal justice problem. Abusers have often been viewed as weak, misguided, irresponsible people who should try harder to help themselves (Green, 1984).

If community health nurses are to help chemically dependent people, it is essential to recognize them as individuals with health problems who cannot always clearly ask for help. Substance abuse, because of its addictive nature and its effects on both physiological and psychological functioning, is a complex phenomenon. Treatment and rehabilitation are possible, and substance abusers can be pro-

ductive members of society. Goals should be realistic, mutually established, and implemented gradually, with continuous support and reinforcement for positive steps taken.

Attitudes toward substance abuse are influenced by the way society categorizes "good" and "bad" drugs. Good drugs are those prescribed by a health care provider, yet this makes them no less addictive and problematic. Americans have come to rely heavily on legal drugs to relieve (or mask) fear, tension, and physical or emotional pain. We have sanctioned the "path of least resistance." Rather than learn to cope with stress, hurt, and so forth, people take pills to blot out feelings.

Social conditions, such as the fast pace of life, competition at school or in the workplace, the search for excellence, and the urgency to accumulate material possessions, influence the use of chemical substances. Also the communications media often presents a positive view of consumption of pain relievers and substances to make people feel better, to cope better, and to live a happier life. The problem is complex; the cost is great. Community health nurses must play a role in promoting health by minimizing substance abuse. To do so, it is necessary to understand selected abusive patterns. Alienation from family and friends often occurs. The dependent person may go to great lengths to assure a supply of the drug, including securing it from a variety of sources to avoid embarrassment and detection. Substitute chemicals may be used; meals tend to be neglected, as does grooming.

During the advanced stages, severe physical problems or psychological symptoms occur. Drug usage becomes continuous, and afflicted individuals become increasingly dependent on others to organize and manage their lives.

Chemical Dependency Syndrome

Various components make up *chemical dependency,* including psychological, social, medical, economic, and legal aspects. Generally, more males than females are involved; the greatest incidence is among young and middle-aged adults. Exposure, availability, and price are key determinants in the rates and distribution of chemical dependency. The various drugs used can lead to similar problems, including unemployment, bankruptcy, family disruption, neglect of children, and traumatic injury or death. Use of some chemicals, because they are highly addictive, expensive, or run the risk of being contaminated, have significant consequences.

Westermeyer (1976) divided the clinical course of chemical dependency into three stages; early (problematic heavy use); middle (chronic dependence and addiction); and advanced. During the early stage, greater doses are taken and the drug assumes an increasingly important role in the person's life. The person thinks more and more about the drug and structures activities to maximize drug benefit. Problems often encountered during this phase include traumatic injury (from falls, fights, accidents) or legal problems (from assaults, child abuse, and automobile accidents).

During the middle phase, as the dosage is increased, the cost of acquiring the drug rises, and longer periods of intoxication ensue. The drug is required to prevent the onset of withdrawal. People close to the chemically dependent person notice personality changes during periods of drug use as compared to periods of sobriety. Family- and job-related problems are frequent at this time because of the lack of predictability of behavior when using the drug.

Effective health promotion and intervention begin with an understanding of the psychological dynamics of both the chemically dependent person and the family. Typically, chemically dependent people have many negative feelings toward themselves. While on the exterior they may appear either hostile, aggressive, and blaming of others, or charming and gracious, inside they are likely to feel fear, hurt, pain, guilt, or shame. To withstand these negative self-feelings, spontaneous defenses often arise and develop with no conscious recognition on the person's part. The major defenses seen in chemical dependency include the following:

1. *Denial:* the inability or unwillingness to acknowledge that a problem exists.
2. *Regression:* the spontaneous forgetting of shameful and painful memories.
3. *Rationalization:* the intellectual process of making irrational behavior seem rational.
4. *Projection:* the unconscious unloading of personally unacceptable thoughts, feelings, and attitudes about self onto others.

These defenses cause chemically dependent people to be out of touch with the severity of their symptoms in that they forget, explain away, and blame others for their problems.

Families play a crucial role in chemical dependency. Frequently they deny the problem and minimize in their own minds the degree to which the family member abuses drugs or alcohol. The family often assumes a protective function, trying to hide the problem from others. They make excuses for absences or tardiness to work, school, or social activities and support rationalizations about the use of chemicals. Every time they say that the chemically dependent person has "the flu," they reinforce the wall of self-deception.

The process of chemical dependency becomes a self-perpetuating cycle. As more chemicals are used, the dependent person often blames family members for troubles, instilling guilt and feelings of inadequacy in the family. To prove their own worth, then, the family continues to protect the dependent member by apologizing, making excuses, and doing for the abuser what the individual is often capable of doing himself.

As the process progresses, and if intervention has not occurred, the family may move to the middle stage as defined by Westermeyer (1976), where they monitor the dependent person's intake of chemicals, hide or throw away the supply, and plead with the dependent person to quit. However, typically the more the family attempts to control substance use, the more the dependent person uses chemicals, and the more inadequate the family feels.

During the advanced stage, families often compensate for their low self-worth by blaming the dependent member for all their troubles. The family's attempts to control and manipulate the chemical dependency actually support the abuse and perpetuate the cycle. To reverse this process the family must gain some insight into how the disease affects them and the dependent person as well as what they are doing to perpetuate the cycle.

Community health nurses are often in a key position to detect the early onset of chemical dependency and to guide clients and families to appropriate referral sources such as a mental health center, private practitioner, or hospital clinic. Through home visits, clinic appointments, and various screening activities, nurses can detect the presence of chemical dependency. The next section examines the type of preventive efforts that hold the greatest potential.

Prevention

The most effective way to handle chemical dependency is to prevent its onset. Since chemical dependency results from a variety of social, psychological, cultural, and physiological factors, prevention involves a multidisciplinary approach. Research indicates that junior and senior high school students are the most vulnerable population for becoming involved in substance abuse. Well-designed prevention programs for youth in these age groups offer the greatest hope for preventing substance abuse.

Durell and Bukoski (1984) reviewed primary prevention strategies and evaluated three as having minimal success and two as having far greater potential. Strategies with limited success are:

1. Media campaigns
2. Drug information in the schools
3. Humanistic education in the schools designed to intervene in the risk factors associated with substance abuse

The two strategies found to offer promise were:

1. Creating a nondrug use climate in the community by simultaneously emphasizing the adverse effects of drugs, reducing the presence of factors motivating drug use, and offsetting pro-drug media messages.
2. Strengthening positive peer pressure to help young people refuse drugs.

Early Detection

If prevention is not accomplished, the next phase is early detection. The identification of substance abuse requires both sensitivity and inquisitiveness on the part of the nurse and the ability to recognize signs and associated risks. In eliciting data about substance abuse, it often helps to start with questions about use of caffeine and cigarettes, then move to discussion of use of prescription drugs and alcoholic beverages, and end by asking about past and present use of illicit drugs. Chychula (1984) developed a useful addiction assessment tool.

Later sections of the chapter provide detailed information about specific substances; several signs and associated risks of drug dependence are outlined here.

Diet is often associated with drug dependence for several reasons. Opiates such as morphine or codeine serve as appetite suppressants, as do psychostimulants or amphetamines, including Benzedrine, pesoxyephedrine and methamphetamine (Desoxyn). Alcohol-dependent people consume many nonnutritious calories in their beverages. Additionally, drug dependence is expensive, and chemicals rather than food may receive priority for limited funds. Chemically dependent people also tend to transfer their behavior from one item to another. For example, on giving up cigarettes, ex-smokers may overeat or drink to excess to compensate for unmet needs. Thus, people who abuse substances should be carefully monitored as they attempt to cease one habit, lest they transfer the needs to another one.

Many severely drug-dependent people neglect their appearance and hygiene as they increasingly focus their attention on the chemicals they tend to use. Particular health risks from these tendencies include skin disorders, dental caries, and gum disease. Living conditions often suffer, thereby predisposing people to additional diseases associated with filth and pest infestation. The box at right lists general behavior characteristics of substance abusers.

Sleep deprivation and disturbances are associated with use of barbiturates and other hypnotic agents. Although one of the clinical uses of these substances is to induce sleep, chronic use leads to sleep impairments. To achieve the desired effect, the drug-dependent person may increase the dosage, thereby leading to a vicious cycle. Sleep deprivation then leads to an entirely new set of symptoms, including feelings of depersonalization or memory and concentration disturbances, with severe deprivation leading to a psychotic state.

Pain suppression is associated with narcotic addiction, and central nervous system depressants with analgesic properties. Many diseases go unnoticed because pain is not experienced; some reach an irreversible state, when earlier detection and treatment could have effected relief.

Biorhythms tend to be interrupted by chemical dependency and affect many complex functions, including secretion of hormones, production of enzymes, metabolism of food and drugs, and usual levels of activity (Westermeyer, 1976). In addition, the life-style associated with drug dependence and acquisition (crime) often increases stress.

The drug-dependent person often experiences various types of physical pathology, including skin, musculoskeletal, respiratory, cardiovascular, blood and lymphatic, gastrointestinal, genitourinary, and central nervous system disorders. Many body systems are at risk from substance abuse, with specific systems at greater risk depending on the substance being used.

As discussed in Chapter 17, users of intravenous drugs

GENERAL BEHAVIOR CHARACTERISTICS OF SUBSTANCE ABUSE

- Abrupt changes in school or work attendance, quality of work, grades, discipline, work output
- Unusual flare-ups or outbreaks of temper
- Withdrawal from responsibility
- General changes in overall attitude
- Deterioration of physical appearance and grooming
- Furtive behavior regarding actions and possessions
- Wearing of sunglasses at inappropriate times (to hide dilated or constricted pupils)
- Continual wearing of long-sleeved garments (to hide injection marks)
- Association with known users of drugging substances
- Unusual borrowing of money from parents or friends
- Stealing small items from home, school, or employer
- Attempts to appear inconspicuous in manner and appearance (to avoid attention and suspicion)
- Frequenting odd places without cause, such as storage rooms, closets, basements (to take drugs)

From Signs of use of substances for drugging effects, Washington, D.C., 1978, Pharmaceutical Manufacturers Association.

constitute a high risk group for acquired immune deficiency syndrome (AIDS). According to Ginsburg (1984, p. 206)

> Not only is the heroin user at increased risk of contracting AIDS, but also the occasional recreational drug user who shares a needle and syringe when he or she self-administers cocaine or amphetamines at a party on a weekend. It is the sharing of the needle rather than the drug injected that places the intravenous drug user at risk for AIDS.

◆   ◆   ◆

It is not possible to describe in detail each substance that may be abused; attention is focused on the abuse of alcohol, tobacco, and selected other drugs, including marijuana, cocaine, and heroin. The restriction of drugs to these categories by no means negates the importance of abuse of other substances, such as barbiturates, hallucinogens, and amphetamines. These merely serve as prototype substances.

ALCOHOL ABUSE

Alcoholism is a chronic disease characterized by repetitive and often compulsive drinking that produces injury to the drinker's health and other aspects of life, including marital status, career, interpersonal relationships, or other required societal adaptations. Over the years, alcoholism has been considered a social problem, a medical problem, and an illegal condition. The effects of alcoholism are widespread and cost individuals, families, communities, and employers considerably in terms of direct costs, lost revenues, pain, and human suffering.

Scope of Alcohol Abuse

Approximately 10 million Americans, or 7% of those over 18 years, can be considered problem drinkers. There are an estimated 3 million drinkers between the ages of 14 and

17, comprising 19% of this age group (Public Health Reports, 1983). The average consumption of alcohol, about 2.75 gallons per person annually, represents a 10% increase in the past 10 years. Ten percent of all deaths in the United States are alcohol-related.

The problem is compounded when one considers that between 3% and 4% of all alcoholics are homeless and rely on institutional support. Such dependence results in a substantial drain on public and private resources. Additionally, alcohol annually indirectly causes many deaths as a result of accidents, homicides, suicides, or other related events or disorders. Alcohol abuse also costs individuals, families, and communities billions of dollars annually because of lost productivity, health care costs, accidents, crime, and demands on the social welfare and judicial systems.

In addition to these economic costs, the number of social costs of alcohol-related problems are nearly impossible to estimate. The families of the estimated 10 million people who misuse alcohol suffer economic hardships, broken homes, and at times physical harm.

Increased Risk Factors

Statistically, people with alcohol-related problems have a mortality and suicide rate 2.5 times greater than the average and are 7 times more prone to become involved in accidents (Community Health Nurse, 1978b). Health problems associated with alcohol abuse include higher rates of cancer of the larynx, oral cavity, liver, and esophagus. It is unclear whether the lack of adequate nutrition often associated with alcohol abuse increases susceptibility to the effects of alcohol or whether the alcohol itself causes the damage. However, it is known that alcoholic individuals with cancer have lower survival rates and a greater susceptibility for developing another primary tumor compared to nonalcoholics with the same type of cancer.

People at greatest risk for lung and esophageal cancer are those who combine heavy alcohol intake with heavy smoking. The risk of esophageal cancer is 44 times greater for those who consume more than six drinks and one or more packs of cigarettes daily (Community Health Nurse, 1978b).

Physiological Effects of Alcohol

Although there are several kinds of alcohol, ethyl alcohol, or ethanol, is the substance contained in alcoholic beverages. The ethanol concentration in a beverage indicates the relationship between the amount of alcohol in the drink and the total volume of liquid. *Proof* when applied to distilled spirits describes the concentration of ethanol and is usually based on a 2:1 ratio. That is, an 80-proof liquor contains 40% alcohol.

Alcohol, like sugar, is a simple, incomplete food with limited nutritional value. Although it lacks vitamins, amino acids, and minerals, alcohol does provide calories for heat and energy. Ethanol is absorbed directly from the gastrointestinal tract and enters the bloodstream. If food is present in the stomach, ethanol absorption is delayed. Drinks mixed with carbonated beverages are absorbed more rapidly than those with water or juices. Peak blood levels may be obtained 30 minutes to 3 hours after ingestion of the ethanol. Because of the slow process of alcohol excretion by the lungs or kidneys and oxidation by the liver, it would take a 150-lb. man approximately 1 hour to metabolize the alcohol in 12 oz. of beer (Halpern and Davis, 1983).

Soon after consumption, alcohol moves into the bloodstream and small intestine, where it is absorbed at variable rates by the organ's tissues. The *brain* is highly sensitive to alcohol, where it initially serves as a stimulant and later becomes a depressant. Extensive use of alcohol can result in premature aging of the brain. A well-known central nervous system effect of excessive alcohol is "blacking out." This episode is different from "passing out" in that it is a period of total amnesia during which the person may or may not appear to others to be under the influence of alcohol (Gitlow, and Peyes, 1980). After coming out of a blackout, the person is usually aware of a void during which memory does not fill in the details of what occurred. People may spend vast amounts of money during these episodes with no recall of doing so.

Alcohol consumption affects *emotions* by decreasing cognitive functions, thereby giving the emotions free reign. With inhibitions released, people may display emotions previously held back and become hostile, tearful, or "the life of the party." Some people drink to dull emotions. Drinking provides temporary relief, and the underlying emotions reappear when the effects of the alcohol wear off.

Small amounts of alcohol induce *sleep,* whereas larger amounts interfere with sleep by shortening the period of rapid eye movement (REM) sleep. Alcohol consumption does not affect tactile responses but does decrease *sensitivity to pain,* resulting in an increased incidence of burns, cuts, scrapes, and bruises among problem drinkers.

Nutritional deficiencies, especially deficits of the B vitamins, lead to a variety of *alcohol-related neurological disorders.* These deficiencies are the result of decreased taste for food, decreased appetite (since alcohol is high in calories), and faulty absorption of nutrients because of irritation to the lining of the stomach and small intestine. Peripheral polyneuropathy subsequent to nutritional deficiency is characterized by weakness, numbness, partial paralysis of extremities, pain in the legs, and impaired sensory reactions and motor reflexes (Community Health Nurse, 1978a). This condition is reversible with adequate diet and supplemental B vitamins. However, if untreated, polyneuropathy can progress to Wernicke's encephalopathy, which is more serious although reversible. Wernicke's encephalopathy is characterized by ophthalmoplegia, nystagmus, ataxia, apathy, drowsiness, and confusion, as well as the inability to concentrate. Without treatment this disease can be fatal.

Another disease often manifested after improvement from Wernicke's encephalopathy is Korsakoff's psychosis. This condition is characterized by disorientation and memory defect, whereby clients usually fill in the gaps in their memory (confabulation). Many people with Korsakoff's psychosis show limited improvement with treatment.

Alcohol is an irritant to the *gastrointestinal system;* it can damage the mucosa and result in esophagitis and gastritis. Increased capillary fragility can result in gastric bleeding, and ulcers often result. Excessive alcohol intake can cause weight gain because of the concentrated sugar and calorie content.

Alcohol also significantly affects the *cardiovascular system.* By causing vasodilation of peripheral vessels, alcohol produces flushing, heat loss, and a sense of warmth, while simultaneously causing vasoconstriction of the great vessels, producing resistance and increasing the work of the heart.

Prolonged alcohol use has been associated with enlargement of the *liver,* probably because of an accumulation of triglycerides in the hepatic cells (Community Health Nurse, 1978a). This fatty liver condition tends to be reversible with abstinence from alcohol and the assumption of a nutritious diet. Two serious alcohol-related hepatic diseases are hepatitis and cirrhosis. *Hepatitis* is an inflammation of the liver, resulting either from a virus or from a toxic reaction. Similarly, *cirrhosis,* a chronic liver disease ranking among the 10 leading causes of death, often leads to severe liver degeneration.

Both of these ailments are thought to result largely from the direct effects of alcohol on liver tissue, and they may occur even in the presence of adequate diet. Lack of an adequate diet in the presence of heavy alcohol consumption increases the likelihood that cirrhosis will occur.

Pancreatitis is another condition resulting from prolonged alcohol consumption, with symptoms ranging from gastritis-like sensations to severe pain with nausea, vomiting, and rigidity of the abdomen. Usually abstinence from alcohol and consumption of adequate food and fluids relieve the symptoms.

Alcohol-dependent people frequently have decreased immunity and are thus highly susceptible to infections. Because of the depression of white blood cells, they have decreased ability to fight diseases and are highly susceptible to upper respiratory infections. Alcohol use is also associated with cancer of the liver, pancreas, esophagus, and mouth.

Alcohol in Medications

Alcohol is used in some medications to increase the drug's solubility and in others to produce a sedative effect. In general, alcohol is a common component of antitussive-decongestant, cough, cold, and vitamin solutions, as well as elixirs and tonics. Alcohol content of selected pharmaceuticals is shown in Table 35-1.

Development and Effects of Addiction

Large doses of alcohol consumed over an extended time lead to decreased sensitivity to alcohol's effects. This phenomenon, *tolerance,* or the need to continually increase the dosage to achieve the desired effect, is common to all potentially addictive drugs. The withdrawal reaction, or *acute abstinence syndrome,* occurs when the addicted person suddenly stops or markedly decreases the intake of the addicting drug. Withdrawal symptoms are usually not seen unless a person has consumed the equivalent of a pint of distilled spirits for at least 10 consecutive days (Butz, 1981).

Withdrawal signs include hyperexcitability, anxiety, anorexia, insomnia, and tremor. Vital signs are usually elevated, and the person may feel irritated and shaky inside.

This stage develops a few hours after alcohol intake is stopped, peaks in 24 to 36 hours, and may end abruptly with no further problems.

More severe withdrawal problems include hallucinosis and delirium tremens. In hallucinosis, the alcohol-dependent person maintains clarity of consciousness but typically experiences vivid auditory hallucinations, usually within 48 hours after the cessation or reduction of heavy alcohol intake. The most severe reaction to alcohol withdrawal, delirium tremens, is characterized by disorientation, paranoia, and outbursts of irrational behavior, leading to threat of self-harm. Tachycardia is common and may be accompanied by fever, rapid breathing, sweating, vomiting, and diarrhea (Community health nurse, 1978a). Unless vigorous treatment is initiated, death can ensue because of shock; malignant hyperthermia; or secondary to complicating illness, infection, or injury. The delirium condition peaks usually the third day after cessation of drinking and persists 2 to 3 days, often ending abruptly and dramatically (Butz, 1981). During withdrawal some people experience grand mal seizures, usually during the first 48 hours. Because of the potentially severe physiological component of delirium tremens, treatment should be carried out in an inpatient facility.

Signs that indicate a person has been drinking considerably include tremulousness, nervous sweating, and tachycardia. Also, small bruises are often found, especially on the alcoholic housewife; these are the result of running into things and falling. There may be cigarette burns on fingers, chest, and legs. Alcoholics are especially susceptible to severe periodontal disease. As a group they do not neglect their physical or oral hygiene; however, they are for some unexplained reason particularly susceptible to acute necrotizing ulcerative gingivitis (Vincent's disease) and pyorrhea (Gitlow and Peyes, 1980).

Groups at Risk

People with a family history of alcoholism, those experiencing grave personal problems or stressful life events, or

TABLE 35-1

Alcohol content of selected pharmaceuticals

Preparation	Alcohol content (%)
Benadryl elixir	14.0
Broncho-Tussin	40.0
Digoxin elixir	9.0-11.5
Dimetapp elixir	2.3
Dristan cough formula syrup	12.0
Isuprel compound elixir	19.0
Nyquil	25.0
Robitussin	3.5
Secobarbital elixir	10.0-14.0
Tempra	10.0
Vicks Formula 44	10.0

From Halpern, J.S. and Davis, J.W.: Use and abuse of alcohol: further perspectives. Journal of Emergency Nursing 9(1):49-52, 1983, p. 50.

people with a history of other addictions are most likely to develop an alcohol-related problem. It is unclear whether the drinking patterns that seem to "run in families" result from hereditary predisposition or attitudes and patterns learned during the early formative years. Drinking problems occur less frequently in families where drinking occurred in association with meals or special occasions than where drinking was strictly prohibited. In the latter instances, a strong aura seems to surround drinking, and often during adolescence this behavior is thoroughly explored.

People with emotional problems or those beset with numerous life changes are particularly susceptible to alcohol abuse. Conditions such as desertion, divorce, separation, parental rejection, aging, role change, or role conflict comprise prime events for the onset of problem drinking. Alcohol becomes an "easy" answer for the complexities of coping with life's problems.

The elderly are at risk because of mandatory retirement and the necessity for living on a fixed income, which may restrict choices. Older people are often lonely and unhealthy and lack feelings of worth and purpose. Drinking fills in the voids in their lives. However, it should be noted that most elderly alcoholics drank before they reached old age.

Adolescents are also at risk. As discussed in Chapter 23, developmentally this is a stage of searching, testing, and defining oneself. As adolescents try to be like others, they often incorporate alcohol abuse into their repertoire of skills. Substance abuse in general has been steadily increasing among young people. In each of the 5 years between 1977 and 1982, when high school students were surveyed about alcohol use, 93% said that they had used alcohol one or more times. When asked if they were daily users who used alcohol 20 or more times in the month before the survey, 6.1% of the high school seniors surveyed in 1977 and 5.7% of the seniors surveyed in 1982 acknowledged this consumption (Durell and Bukoski, 1984). Twenty percent of the 12- to 13-year-olds in the United States are current drinkers (Cretcher, 1982).

Also, adolescents commonly mix drugs. The term "polydrug" refers to the use of two or more drugs in combination. The most common mixture is alcohol and marijuana. Many drugs are lethal at lower levels when combined with alcohol (Cretcher, 1982).

Although young people tend to drink less frequently than adults, they seem to consume larger quantities and are more likely to become intoxicated. It is not difficult to see why the leading cause of death in the 15- to 24-age group is attributed to alcohol-related accidents and 60% of all alcohol-related traffic fatalities are among young people.

Women and Alcohol

The drinking patterns of women are changing. Forty years ago it was virtually unheard of for women to drink, while today over 60% of all American women and almost 90% of all college-age women drink. Estimates of the ratio of women alcoholics to men alcoholics vary from 1:4 to 1:2 (Hennecke and Fox, 1980).

There do seem to be several differences between men and women in regard to alcohol and related problems. For example, with alcohol, as with many other behaviors, a double standard prevails. Men who drink heavily tend to be more readily accepted than women. Hence, women are more likely to try to hide their drinking; less likely to seek help, they tend to become seriously ill before the disease is detected.

Although women drink less than men, the effects are greater. Since women have a higher percentage of body fat, their tissue concentrations of alcohol are much higher than that of a man of equal weight. Similarly, fewer women become alcohol dependent than men, but they experience greater morbidity and mortality. One theory is that as a result of estrogen production, women's livers are more vulnerable to disease than men. An alcoholic woman's life expectancy is 15 years less than her nondrinking counterpart.

Women who become alcohol abusers often begin as social drinkers. Finding that a couple of drinks helps them deal with feelings of anxiety and shyness and allows them to more comfortably "be themselves" in unfamiliar situations, they accelerate their drinking to avoid painful feelings and difficult situations (Sandmaier, 1977). Before they realize it, these women are daily relying on alcohol. Why don't they seek help? Partly because they do not recognize the warning signals of problem drinking and also because they are ashamed to admit they may be drinking to excess. Rather than bear the stigma of being a "fallen woman," they hide their drinking habits from people who might offer help.

Alcoholic women can usually identify a particular life crisis that set off their drinking pattern. Examples include family or marital stresses such as separation, divorce, financial pressures, children, loss of a significant person, blow to self-esteem, health crisis, feeling of lack of meaning and fulfillment in life, and sexual problems. All women experience some of these problems; however, some cope more effectively than others.

An added problem in alcohol abuse among women is the potential for alcohol-induced birth defects. *Fetal alcohol syndrome* (FAS) occurs in about 2 per 1,000 live births. Infants suffering from this defect can demonstrate low birth weight; be mentally retarded; or have behavioral, facial, limb, genital, cardiac, or neurological abnormalities (Healthy People, 1979). Alcohol use during pregnancy is considered the third leading cause of mental retardation in the Western world. The consumption of only two drinks per day is associated with low birth weight (Women's Health, 1985).

FAS seems to be caused by ethanol intake rather than by caloric insufficiency. A high blood alcohol level during critical periods of embryonic development leads to FAS. The average alcohol intake may not be as important as the amount consumed during episodes of heavy drinking. Malformations are most likely to occur as a result of heavy drinking during the first trimester, and growth retardation caused by heavy drinking occurs during the third trimester of pregnancy. Table 35-2 presents the effects of drug use, including alcohol, during pregnancy.

TABLE 35-2

Drug use during pregnancy

Drug	Effect on fetus	Safe use of drug
Nicotine	Heavy smoking can lead to low birth weight babies, which means that the baby may have more health problems. Especially harmful during second half of pregnancy.	Should be avoided.
Alcohol	Daily drinking of more than two glasses of wine, or a mixed drink, can cause fetal alcohol syndrome. Babies tend to low birth weight, mental retardation, physical deformity, and behavioral problems, including hyperactivity, restlessness, and poor attention span.	Should be avoided.
Aspirin	During last 3 months of pregnancy frequent use may cause excessive bleeding at delivery and may prolong pregnancy and labor.	Under physician's supervision.
Tranquilizers	Taken during the first 3 months of pregnancy may cause cleft lip or palate or other congenital malformations.	Avoid if possibility of pregnancy and during early pregnancy. Use only under physician's supervision.
Barbiturates	Mothers who have taken large doses may have babies who are addicted. Babies may have tremors, restlessness, and irritability.	Only under physician's supervision.
Amphetamines	May cause birth defects.	Only under physician's supervision.

From Deciding about drugs: a woman's choice. DHEW Pub. No (ADM) 80-820. Rockville, Md., 1979, National Institute on Drug Abuse, Department of Health, Education, and Welfare.

Effects of Alcohol on the Family

The effects of alcohol are by no means limited to the drinker. In many instances families suffer multiple and long-lasting problems because of an alcoholic member. In dealing with the alcoholic relative, families often use denial to cope with the overwhelming implications of their problem. Feeling embarrassed, humiliated, and helpless, family members may simply ignore the existence of the problem. Family members struggle to avoid conflicts and try to control the environment so alcohol is not present; when these efforts fail, they often plead with, threaten, or attempt to punish the alcoholic.

As family members become more ashamed of the behavior of their alcoholic relative, many avoid contact with friends and relatives. With increasing social isolation, the family has fewer resources on which to draw for their own support.

As described in the section on chemical dependency, families frequently blame themselves for the drinking habits of their relatives and feel acute guilt for the role they may have played in the development or continuation of this problem. The family typically lives in a state of continuous anxiety about what will happen next—an accident, loss of income, or loss of esteem and status in the community. Alcoholics typically create ongoing crises for themselves and their families through unpaid bills, loss of job, and embarrassing social situations (Community Health Nurse, 1978a).

Although most alcoholics behave as though they were quite independent, many are heavily dependent on those around them. When their drinking propels them into a crisis, their usual response is to do nothing until someone comes along to bail them out. Each time the alcoholic is bailed out, the cycle of drinking—crisis—dependency is rewarded. Additionally, once the crisis is over it is easy to deny the existence of a problem, and the rescuers are often regarded with hostility for interfering.

Families of alcoholics are usually angry. Their rage may be repressed; if so, however, it is ultimately expressed in a more covert fashion, such as via ulcers or inappropriate outbursts toward strangers. The anger also may be suppressed and perceived as boredom, depression, chronic fatigue, and disinterest.

Nonalcoholic family members often make great efforts to maintain some semblance of family stability. The nonalcoholic parent may become an overachiever, trying to be sure the children are well fed and involved in age-related activities and that the home is clean and comfortable. To maintain family order, the alcoholic member is often unconsciously excluded. Order, however, is rarely maintained for lengthy periods because of the disruptive behavior brought on by the drinking. When drinking, alcoholics are often hostile, belligerent, irresponsible, self-centered, and violent; sober, these same people can be remorseful, kind, generous, affectionate, and solicitous. The startling contrast between drinking and nondrinking behavior and the lack of predictability keep families confused as to what to expect.

Children have difficulty understanding how a parent can seem like a cruel, overbearing monster one day and come home all smiles and bearing gifts the next. Also, the longer families go without seeking help, the greater the likelihood that the family will disintegrate. The divorce rate among couples in which one partner is alcoholic is four times the national average (Community Health Nurse, 1978a).

Children are particularly susceptible to the effects of alcoholism in the family. These youngsters are frequently the victims of child abuse because of poor parental control of emotions. They fear the unpredictability of their parent's behavior and may avoid bringing friends to their home. Children often assume many of the adult responsibilities of their alcoholic parent and must work at home or care for siblings when they would prefer to play with peers.

Children cope with alcoholism by fleeing, fighting, or being either "super good" or a "super coper" (Community Health Nurse, 1978a). They flee by literally escaping physically—hiding under the bed, hiding in closets, or staying away from home as much as possible—or by fleeing mentally—emotionally insulating themselves from the family.

Other children react to adult alcoholism by physical and/or verbal aggression. They strike out at other children or act out in school or at home. In contrast, some children try either to be perfect or to rescue and help the family cope, thereby increasing their level of stress by this added responsibility.

Role of the Community Health Nurse

Community health nurses are responsible for coordinating client care both via appropriate referrals and through careful monitoring, coordination of services and resources, and follow-up. Because of their lowered level of tolerance, many alcoholics (and other substance abusers) become lost in the health care system. For example, if care is not provided satisfactorily in agency A, the abuser may give up rather than seek alternative sources of care. Community health nurses can guide clients from one agency to another and offset feelings of "no one will (or can) help me."

Community health nurses also assess the potential for and/or presence of alcohol-related problems and provide direct intervention, including counseling and health education. In assessment, the guide by Heinemann and Estes (1976) provides a thorough tool. Alcoholics are generally poor historians, especially about their drinking habits, since they often deny the extent of the problem. Specific questions are suggested, including what, when, where and who. Questions asking how and why tend to increase defensiveness and are less desirable (Heinemann and Estes, 1976). During the assessment, the client should stay focused on the topic; digressions into lengthy descriptions of past drinking episodes are discouraged.

Information derived from the assessment may lead to nursing interventions directed toward maintaining adequate nutrition and hydration, providing a safe environment in the home, promoting rest and sleep, and teaching new ways to handle stress and to cope with conflict and other possible problems.

In addition, children of alcoholics are often recognized in school because of their many absences, signs of physical or emotional abuse, or behavior problems in the classroom. Often the nonalcoholic parent can be contacted via the school-age child and referrals made for all or several family members. For teens, Alateen, a nation-wide program addressing the needs of adolescent children of alcoholics, has

been helpful. This type of support is sponsored by Al-Anon, a self-help group for adult relatives and close friends of alcoholics, and is based on the principles of *Alcoholics Anonymous.* The purpose of Al-Anon is to facilitate discussion and resolution of common problems related to being closely associated with an alcoholic.

In both industries and the community, nurses are in key positions to design prevention programs, detect alcohol-related problems, and make appropriate referrals. The first step is to know the available community resources for the treatment of alcohol-related problems. Community resource directories and telephone books are resources to identify facilities for acute care of alcohol-related problems. Questions to ask include the following: Which hospitals or clinics run detoxification units? Does the community mental health center have a special program or unit for alcohol addiction? What resources are available in both the public and the private sector? Who is eligible for the various resources?

Not only should the health-related resources be assessed but the availability of lay support and self-help groups is vitally important. It is generally recognized that Alcoholics Anonymous (AA) has done more for the treatment of this disease than have health care providers. Basically, AA treatment consists of 12 steps leading toward recovery. In the first three the alcoholic acknowledges the crux of the problem and makes a commitment to work toward resolution. During the next four steps the person takes an honest look at self, shares this information with a special person, and begins to modify behavioral deficiencies. In the succeeding four steps the alcoholic continues self-scrutiny. Finally in the last step the alcoholic reaches out to help others. The fellowship, support, and encouragement among AA members, all of whom are abstaining alcoholics, is tremendous. Members are available to one another day and night to aid in crisis intervention and to respond to other calls for support and aid.

Al-Anon and Alateen are similar self-help programs for spouses, parents, children, or others involved in a painful relationship with an alcoholic. *Al-Anon* family groups are available to anyone who has been affected by their involvement with an alcoholic. Local groups meet regularly to help members learn the facts about alcoholism as an illness, the types of treatment available, ways that can help the alcoholic, and how to reduce their own tension. In addition, many cities have *Alateen* groups for youth between 12 and 20 years who live in an alcoholic family situation. These groups are of vital importance, since children who live in alcoholic families are at risk for emotional problems. The purposes of Alateen include providing a forum for discussing family stressors, learning coping skills from one another, and gaining support and encouragement from knowledgeable peers.

Alcohol-Drug Interactions

Many frequently prescribed drugs contain at least one ingredient known to interact adversely with alcohol. Most adverse effects resulting from such combinations are accidental, yet the death and morbidity tolls are high.

It is important to carefully assess clients' present and

previous drinking patterns and determine if they are impulsive drinkers or have a chronic dependence on alcohol. In addition, even when not drinking, chronic alcoholics may have altered drug effects because of liver damage. For example, among chronic heavy drinkers there is an increased metabolism rate for *phenytoin* (Dilantin), which necessitates larger than normal doses to achieve the desired effect.

Specific drugs to be aware of include analgesics, anesthetics, antialcohol preparations, antianginal and antihypertensive agents, anticoagulants, anticonvulsants, antidepressants, stimulants, antihistamines, antidiabetic agents, anti-infectives, barbiturates, tranquilizers, and narcotics. Clients taking any of these medications should be queried as to their alcohol consumption patterns. Although great detail cannot be provided here, several examples of drug-alcohol interaction are cited to focus attention on the magnitude of this problem. Table 35-3 presents selected interaction effects of alcohol with several commonly used drugs.

TABLE 35-3

Interaction effects of alcohol with other drugs

Type of drug	Generic name	Trade name	Interaction effect with alcohol
Analgesics Nonnarcotic	Salicylates	Products containing aspirin Bayer Aspirin Bufferin Alka-Seltzer	Heavy concurrent use of alcohol with analgesics can increase the potential for gastrointestinal bleeding. Special caution should be exercised by individuals with ulcers. Buffering of salicylates reduces possibility of this interaction.
Narcotic	Codeine Morphine Opium	Pantopan Paregoric	Narcotic analgesics and alcohol interact to reduce functioning of the central nervous system (CNS) and can lead to loss of effective breathing function or respiratory arrest: death may result.
	Oxycodone Propoxyphene	Percodan Darvon Darvon-N	
	Pentazocine Meperidine	Talwin Demerol	
Antianginal	Nitroglycerin Isosorbide dinitrite	Nitrostat Isordil, Sorbitrate	Alcohol in combination with antianginal drugs will cause the blood pressure to lower, creating a potentially dangerous situation.
Antibiotics Anti-infective agents	Furazolidone Metronidazole Nitrofurantoin	Furoxone Flagyl Cyantin Macrodantin	Certain antibiotics, especially those taken for urinary tract infections, have been known to produce disulfiram-like reactions (nausea, vomiting, headaches, hypotension) when combined with alcohol.
Anticoagulants	Sodium warfarin Acenocoumarol Coumarin derivatives	Coumadin, Panwarfin Sintrom Dicumarol	With chronic alcohol use, the anticoagulant effect of these drugs is inhibited. With acute intoxication the anticoagulant effect is enhanced; hemorrhaging could result.
Anticonvulsants	Phenytoin	Dilantin	Chronic heavy drinking can reduce the effectiveness of anticonvulsant drugs to the extent that seizures previously controlled by these drugs can reoccur if the dosage is not adjustable appropriately. Enhanced CNS depression may occur with concurrent use of alcohol.
Antidiabetic agents, hypoglycemics	Chlorpropamide Acetohexamide Tolbutamide Tolazamide Insulin	Diabinese Dymelor Orinase Tolinase Iletin	The interaction of alcohol and either insulin or oral antidiabetic agents may be severe and unpredictable. The interaction may induce hypoglycemia or hyperglycemia; also disulfiram-like reactions may occur.
Antidepressants	Nortriptyline Amitriptyline Desipramine Doxepin Imipramine	Aventyl Elavil, Endep Pertofrane Sinequan Tofranil	Enhanced CNS depression may occur with concurrent use of alcohol and antidepressant drugs.

Continued.

TABLE 35-3

Interaction effects of alcohol with other drugs—cont'd

Type of drug	Generic name	Trade name	Interaction effect with alcohol
Antihistamines	For example, chlorpheniramine	Many cold & allergy remedies Coricidin Allerest	The interaction of alcohol and these drugs enhances CNS depression
Antihypertensive agents	Rauwolfia preparations Resperine Guanethidine Hydralazine Pargyline Methyldopa	Rauwiloid Serpasil Ismelin Apresoline Eutonyl Aldomet	Alcohol, in moderate dosage, will increase the blood pressure-lowering effects of these drugs and can produce postural hypotension. Additionally, an increased CNS depressant effect may be seen with the rauwolfia alkaloids and methyldopa.
Antimalarials	Quinacrine	Atabrine	A disulfiram-like reaction and severe CNS toxicity will result if antimalarial drugs are combined with alcohol.
CNS depressants Barbiturate hypnotics	Phenobarbital Pentobarbital Secobarbital Butabarbital Amobarbital	Luminal Nembutal Seconal Butisol Amytal	Since alcohol is a depressant, the combination of alcohol and other depressants interact to further reduce CNS functioning. It is extremely dangerous to mix barbiturates with alcohol. What would be a nondangerous dosage of either drug by itself can interact in the body to the point of coma or fatal respiratory arrest. Many accidental deaths of this nature have been reported. A similar danger exists in mixing the nonbarbiturate hypnotics with alcohol.
Nonbarbiturate hypnotics	Methaqualone Glutethimide Bromides Flurazepam Chloral Hydrate	Quaalude Doriden Neurosine Dalmane Noctec	Disulfiram-like reactions have been reported with alcohol use in the presence of chloral hydrates.
Tranquilizers (major)	Thioridazine Chlorpromazine Trifluoperazine Haloperidol	Mellaril Thorazine Stelazine Haldol	The major tranquilizers interact with alcohol to enhance CNS depression, resulting in impairment of voluntary movement, such as walking or hand coordination; larger doses can be fatal.
Tranquilizers (minor)	Diazepam Meprobamate Chlordiazepoxide-HCL Oxazepam	Valium Equanil Miltown Librium Serax	The minor tranquilizers depress CNS functioning. Serious interactions can occur when using these drugs and alcohol.
CNS stimulants	Caffeine Amphetamines Dextroamphetamine Methamphetamine	In coffee and cola Vanquish Benzedrine Dexedrine Desoxyn	The stimulant effect of these drugs can reverse the depressant effect of alcohol on the CNS, resulting in a false sense of security. They do not help the intoxicated person gain control over coordination or psychomotor activity.
Disulfiram (antialcohol preparation)	Disulfiram	Antabuse	Severe CNS toxicity follows ingestion of even small amounts of alcohol. Effects can include headache, nausea, vomiting, convulsions, rapid fall in blood pressure, unconsciousness, and—with sufficiently high doses—death.
Diuretics (also antihypertensive)	Hydrochlorthiazide Chlorothiazide Furosemide Quinethazone	Hydrodiuril Esidrix Diuril Lasix Hydromax	Interaction of diuretics and alcohol enhances the blood pressure-lowering effects of the diuretic; could possibly precipitate postural hypotension.
Monoamine oxidase inhibitors (MAOI)	Pargyline Isocarboxazid Phenelzine Tranylcypromine	Eutonyl Marplan Nardil Parnate	Alcoholic beverages (such as beer and wines) contain tyramine, which will interact with MAOI to produce a hypertensive, hyperpyrexic crisis. Frequent use of alcohol with MAOIs may result in enhanced CNS depression.

From Blum, S., and Kreblein, K.: Interaction effect of alcohol with other drugs, Lincoln, Neb., 1977. Nebraska Division on Alcoholism: compiled from Lipman, A.G.: Drug interactions with alcohol, Mod. Med. 44(4):67-69, Feb. 15, 1976; Fact sheet—Drug interactions with alcohol, National Clearinghouse for Alcohol Information (Feb. 1976); It's dangerous to mix alcohol and drugs, National Clearinghouse for Alcohol Information; and The whole college catalog about drinking, U.S. Department of Health, Education, and Welfare, NIAAA.

DRUG ABUSE

Americans continue to use drugs, both legal and illicit, to cope with life stressors. Several commonly used drugs are discussed in some detail to highlight the problem. Table 35-4 lists signs of drug use.

Abuse of Illicit Drugs
Marijuana

Typical *marijuana* smokers are practically indistinguishable from their nonsmoking peers. The use of this substance cuts across all demographic lines, with a higher incidence among college students and college graduates than the general population. Professional and higher income adults rank among the highest occupational groups involved in the experimental use of marijuana (Carr and Meyers, 1980). Use is more frequent among males, in cities, and in the western part of the United States, followed by states in the Northeast, North Central, and South. There are currently 16 million marijuana users; the first experience with this substance tends to occur between the ages of 11 and 14 years with exposure from friends, siblings, or other family members (Wagner, 1984). The use of marijuana can produce sinusitis, pharyngitis, bronchitis, and emphysema in 1 year or less compared to 10 to 20 years with cigarette smoking (Wagner, 1984).

Tolerance, the need for increasingly large doses to achieve the same effect, and dependence are not usually associated with marijuana use. However, this substance does temporarily affect psychomotor skills, although to a lesser extent than alcohol.

Marijuana has been used for centuries as a therapeutic substance. References to cannabis use date back to the fifteenth century, and cannabis was included in the *U.S. Pharmacopoeia* until 1941. It has recently been used to help reduce intraocular pressure in the eyes of glaucoma patients; to relieve the pain of cancer patients; to reduce or eliminate loss of appetite, nausea, and vomiting following chemotherapy; to relieve asthmatic distress by temporarily dilating the bronchial passages; and to facilitate sleep as a sedative-hypnotic (Carr and Meyers, 1980).

Cocaine

The use of *cocaine* has increased dramatically in the United States in recent years. It is now estimated that 20 million Americans have used cocaine once; 4 to 5 million use it monthly, and perhaps 1 million are regular compulsive users.

Cocaine, referred to as "coke," "blow" or "snow" is a white, odorless alkaloid powder taken from the leaves of the South American coca plant (not the cocoa plant from which chocolate is derived). The street-level purity of cocaine in the United States is about 13% by the time it has been cut with substances such as lactose, glucose, and mannitol. Also, one never knows what else has been mixed with the cocaine; hence, the risk in using such a drug is great.

In recent years the street costs of cocaine have decreased, making it increasingly affordable. It is estimated that 45 tons of illegal cocaine come into the United States annually leading to a 25 to 35 billion dollar industry. Users range from junior high students to middle-aged executives; the most prevalent group are 20- to 30-year-old "achievers."

Cocaine is used in three ways: The most popular mode is to "snort" it like snuff. Prolonged or heavy snorting can erode the mucous membranes of the nose until they no longer absorb the drug. Snorters then move to freebasing or intravenous injections. *Freebasing* refers to a homemade refining process that extracts a concentrated form of cocaine from its chemical base; the user then smokes it through a water pipe usually filled with liquor. The latter method brings on a "high" effect in about 8 seconds. The high from cocaine usually lasts 15 to 30 minutes and is an intensely euphoric experience, whereby users talk a lot and feel energized as though they can do anything. When the effects of cocaine wear off, users are typically nervous, impatient, irritable, tired, and pessimistic (Drugs and Dosages, 1984).

Cocaine can be fatal when ingested in large doses or taken by people with a particular sensitivity to this drug. Besides the direct hazards associated with cocaine use, indirect effects relate to poor eating and sleeping habits. Likewise, because of the expense involved, substance abuse is often related to theft and other types of crime. Withdrawal symptoms include depression, lassitude, headache, excessive sleeping, convulsions, and seizures. It is estimated that cocaine use alone or in combination with other drugs leads to 350 deaths annually, with the greatest hazard coming from drug interactions.

Heroin

Heroin addiction, although less prevalent than in the past, is still a major health problem. There are an estimated 240,000 drug treatment "slots" in the United States, with 60% devoted to heroin users. Nearly 85% of those receiving drug treatment do so on an outpatient basis, 8% are in residential programs, and the remaining 7% are in hospitals, prisons, or day-care settings (Lewis and Sessler, 1980).

Over the decades, a variety of techniques have been developed to treat heroin addiction. The therapeutic communities of the late 1950s took a variety of forms. A forerunner of this treatment approach, Synanon, was "the first organized efforts by addicts themselves to solve their problems through self-help techniques" (Lewis and Sessler, 1980, p. 99). This program, while controversial because of its approach and some of its leaders, required total immersion into a thoroughly prescribed and disciplined lifestyle, including indefinite residence in a Synanon facility.

The greatest effort in treating heroin addiction has been the development of methadone, a synthetic opiate for use in the maintenance of heroin addicts. Although used since the 1940s as a drug to aid withdrawal at the Lexington, Kentucky, Public Health Service Hospital, it was not used as a maintenance drug until the 1960s. In 1964 researchers Vincent Dole, an internist and biochemist, and Marie Nyswander, a psychiatrist, noticed a difference in the behavior of chronic heroin addicts maintained on methadone compared to those on heroin. Those maintained on methadone seemed more alert, energetic, and interested in constructive social activities compared to those on heroin, who became lethargic after an injection and underwent withdrawal as it

Substances	Signs
Glue, vapor-producing solvents, propellants	Odor of substance on breath and clothes Excess nasal secretions, watering of eyes Poor muscular control Drowsiness or unconsciousness Increased preference for being with a group, rather than being alone Plastic or paper bags or rags containing dry plastic cement or other solvent found at home or in lockers at school or at work
Depressants (barbiturates, tranquilizers, "downs")	Symptoms of alcohol intoxication with one important exception: no odor of alcohol on breath Staggering or stumbling Falling asleep unexplainably Drowsiness; may appear disoriented Lack of interest in school and family activities
Stimulants (amphetamines, cocaine, "speed," "bennies," "ups")	Pupils may be dilated (when large amounts have been taken) Mouth and nose dry; bad breath; user licks his lips frequently Goes long periods without eating or sleeping Excess activity; user is irritable, argumentative, nervous; has difficulty sitting still Chain smoking If injecting drug, user may have hidden eyedroppers and needles among possessions
Narcotics (heroin, morphine)	Lethargic, drowsy Pupils are constricted and fail to respond to light Inhaling heroin in powder form leaves traces of white powder around nostrils, causing redness and rawness Injecting heroin leaves scars, usually on the inner surface of the arms and elbows, although user may inject drugs in body where needle marks will not be seen as readily Users often leave syringes, bent spoons, bottle caps, eyedroppers, cotton, and needles in lockers at school or at work, or hidden at home
Marijuana	In the early stages of intoxication, may appear animated with rapid, loud talking and bursts of laughter In the later stages, may be sleepy or stuporous Whites of eyes may appear inflamed; pupils may be dilated Odor (similar to burnt rope) on clothing or breath Remnants of marijuana, either loose or in partially smoked "joints," in clothing or possessions NOTE: Unless under the influence of the drug at a time of observation, marijuana users are difficult to recognize; infrequent users may not show any of the general symptoms. Marijuana is greener than tobacco. Cigarettes made of it (called "joints," "sticks," or "reefers") are rolled in a double thickness of brown or off-white cigarette paper. Smaller than a regular cigarette, with the paper twisted or tucked in at both ends, the butts (called "roaches") are not discarded but saved for later smoking if not consumed at initial usage. Marijuana also may be smoked in a pipe (very small bowl, long stem) or cooked in brownies and cookies.
Hallucinogens (LSD, PCP, mescaline)	Senses of sight, hearing, touch, body image, and time are distorted Mood and behavior are affected, the manner depending on emotional and environmental condition of the user Users may become fearful and experience a degree of terror Users of LSD may have unpredictable flashback episodes without use of the drug NOTE: It is unlikely that persons using hallucinogens will do so in school, at work, or at home at a time when they might be observed. At least in the early stages of usage, these drugs generally are taken in a group situation under special conditions designed to enhance their effect. LSD is odorless, tasteless and colorless. It usually is taken orally in tablets, capsules, or a wide variety of substances (impregnated with liquid LSD). PCP is most frequently found in tablets, powder, or mixed with leaf mixtures for smoking. Even though declared to be different chemicals, many illicit drugs may contain PCP.

From Signs of use of substances for drugging effects, Washington, D.C., 1978, Pharmaceutical Manufacturers Association.

wore off (Lewis and Sessler, 1980). A treatment program was devised to offer methadone maintenance, counseling, job training, and other forms of support.

From a social perspective, many inner-city heroin users have been raised in broken homes, live in inadequate housing, are poorly educated, and often are unemployed. It is frequently difficult to determine which comes first—the poor social conditions or the addiction. The key factor is that treatment programs must include social rehabilitation components. Community health nurses are in key positions to coordinate the needs of clients with available and accessible services. Many of these people are unskilled, unemployed, and undereducated.

Treatment of Illicit Substance Abuse

Historically "drug epidemics" have occurred during periods of job shortages and high labor surpluses (Lewis and Sessler, 1980). Many of the federal programs that previously have aided these people have recently been reduced, thereby decreasing the rehabilitation options. In the future, industry may be called on to take a more active role in social rehabilitation as the federal government's involvement diminishes in this arena.

Widely varying types of treatments have been attempted for substance abuse. The most severe event associated with substance abuse is overdose. Often this is a life-threatening situation requiring immediate emergency care. Community health nurses are not usually involved in the acute stages of drug overdose, but they are often involved in coordinating care when the person returns to the community.

Likewise, *detoxification* usually takes place in a controlled hospital setting where withdrawal from the drug can be accomplished on a regular schedule and where staff members are trained to recognize and deal with the physical and emotional problems faced during withdrawal. However, detoxification from opiates often takes place in outpatient programs (Milby, 1981). The dose schedule may be reduced over a 6-week period, providing less disruption of life routines than hospitalization. Detoxification, or gradual withdrawal, allows for a less painful method of abstinence than going "cold turkey."

Currently there are four major heroin treatment methods: maintenance programs using methadone and L-alpha acetyl methadol (LAAM, a long-acting form of methadone), detoxification programs, outpatient drug-free programs, and drug-free therapeutic communities. The first three are generally outpatient programs and the fourth is residential. There are also inpatient hospital programs and programs for those in prisons.

MAINTENANCE PROGRAMS. As mentioned, *methadone* is a synthetic opiate used as a maintenance drug for heroin addicts. Its effect lasts approximately 24 hours, compared with 3 to 4 hours for heroin. Additionally, the effect of LAAM lasts 2 to 3 days, but LAAM does not produce the same subjective effects as methadone and is thus less desired by clients. The Federal Drug Administration has set criteria for admission to methadone maintenance programs that carefully define eligible patients. The criteria require objective evidence of 2 consecutive years of opiate addiction,

evidence of current addiction, and a minimum age of 18 years (Milby, 1981).

DETOXIFICATION PROGRAMS. Detoxification programs are used to relieve withdrawal symptoms and to enable addicts to achieve temporary freedom from their addiction. The ordinary course of treatment is 21 days, although some programs have reported success in 7 to 14 days (Lewis and Sessler, 1980). The primary goals of these programs are to withdraw addicts from drugs and engage them and their families in follow-up treatment. These programs seem to have a good short-term effect but the rate of relapse is high. Programs are increasingly structuring their efforts to provide maximal amounts of supportive care and follow-up. For example, some addicts become depressed after detoxification and can be effectively treated with antidepressants. Other drugs currently being tested (naltrexone) are narcotic antagonists that block the effects of heroin.

OUTPATIENT DRUG-FREE PROGRAMS. Outpatient abstinence programs seek to help people via counseling, group therapy, employment assistance, job training, and other supportive services (Lewis and Sessler, 1980). These clinics seem more effective in treating persons using illicit drugs other than heroin. Many of these programs are offered in association with community mental health centers and other forms of comprehensive care. The nursing role in these programs is multifaceted and often includes counseling, observation, and referral.

THERAPEUTIC COMMUNITIES. "Therapeutic community (TC) is a generic term for an institution that treats and rehabilitates individuals with relatively severe behavioral problems like drug addiction and alcoholism" (Milby, 1981, p. 205). Most therapeutic communities assume that addiction results from long-term psychological problems, and the community becomes the main source for meeting the physical and emotional needs of residents.

Abuse of Legal Drugs

Substance abuse includes the use of both illicit and legally sanctioned drugs. It is becoming increasingly common in responding to the rush and stresses of life for people to rely on tranquilizers, pain relievers, antidepressants, and sedatives. Community health nurses have multifaceted goals in dealing with this problem. First, careful assessment is essential to accurately determine a person's pattern and mix of substances and the symptoms that prompt their use. People do not always tell health care providers about all of the medications they are taking; thus it is possible for a physician to prescribe adversely related combinations.

Rather than relying on drugs to relieve tension, clients may need to be referred to an agency or source providing psychological counseling, stress reduction, exercise, and so forth. The community health nurse must know what resources are available, as well as who is eligible and the specific type of assistance offered by each. Two of the most frequently abused categories of legal drugs are stimulants and benzodiazepines.

The abuse of stimulants is not a new problem; however, the substances abused tend to change over time. In the 1960s amphetamines were regulated by prescriptions, and abuse of these drugs led to manufacturing quotas in 1973. The demand for stimulants remained high while the legal production decreased. Not surprisingly, street drugs began to proliferate to meet the market's demand for stimulants. However, the quality and purity in street drugs varied greatly, and users began to lose interest.

The 1980s ushered in a new generation of stimulant users. Drug manufacturers began combining several legal over-the-counter preparations into a single-dose unit. These products, known as "street speed" produce mood elevations and altered states of consciousness (Halpern, 1983). These preparations are available in pharmacies, grocery stores, and drug paraphernalia shops. The preparation often resembles amphetamines in its effect. The most common ingredients are caffeine, ephedrine, and phenylpropanolamine (PPA); each ingredient can produce central nervous system stimulation.

Benzodiazepines are among the most frequently prescribed drugs and include such familiar names as diazepam (Valium); flurazepam (Dalmane); and chlordiazepoxide (Librium). Abuse of these drugs falls into four categories: (1) taking the drug after the medical or psychological need has abetted due to physical or psychological dependence, (2) taking the drug in larger amounts than prescribed, (3) taking the drug to obtain euphoric effects, and (4) using the drug to further psychological regression and to decrease self-awareness and reduce the ability to change (Dietch, 1983).

Community health nurses should be particularly alert to signs of benzodiazepine abuse since clients often take these drugs over long periods of time and may borrow them from friends or relatives. Although safe over a short period of time, benzodiazepines can lead to dependence when taken over 4 months in high doses. Abrupt withdrawal of benzodiazepines can lead to anxiety, insomnia, dizziness, nausea and vomiting, muscular weakness, tremor, confusion, convulsions, and psychosis.

Drug Abuse Among Nurses

While drug abuse among nurses and other health care providers is not new, it is currently receiving considerable attention. There is no way to accurately identify the number of chemically dependent nurses. However, the box at right lists several "clues" to chemical dependency among nurses. Between September, 1980, and August, 1981, 67% of 971 actions against nurses' licenses were for chemical dependency (Green, 1984). Factors that place the nurse at risk include (1) stress in the workplace, (2) family history of substance abuse, (3) social accessibility to drugs, (4) inadequate employee assistance programs, (5) ambivalence toward recreational drug use by women, and (6) consequences of alcohol use by women (Finley, 1982). Also, nurses frequently work changing shifts, thereby affecting sleep patterns and increasing the likelihood of drug use (Green, 1984).

No clinical area is immune to the possibility of drug abuse among employees. Stepter (1982, p. 43) reminds nurses to keep some basic facts in mind regarding dealing with colleagues who exhibit signs of chemical dependency:

1. Drug abuse is an illness...
2. You are helping, not harming the person abusing drugs by bringing his problem to the attention of someone qualified to help.
3. The person abusing drugs cannot "cure" himself.
4. The person abusing drugs cannot be cured by "the help of a friend" unless that friend is qualified in counseling persons abusing drugs.

SMOKING AND HEALTH

Each of the reports of the U.S. Surgeon General since 1964 has identified smoking as the single most preventable cause of morbidity and premature mortality (Fielding, 1985a). The estimated annual mortality from smoking of over 350,000 exceeds the number of lives lost in World War II, Korea, and Vietnam combined. An estimated average of 5½ minutes of life is lost for each cigarette smoked. Despite extensive documentation of the health consequences of smoking almost one third of all American adults smoked in 1982 (Remington et al., 1985). Since 1965, the rate of decline of smoking in women has not equaled that for men. Currently, over 40% of young white women smoke.

It is estimated that more than $16 billion is spent annually in direct health care costs related to smoking. An additional $37 billion in annual indirect costs due to lost productivity and earnings from excess morbidity, disability, and premature deaths is attributed to smoking (Fielding, 1985a). Smoking is the cause of one fourth of the mortality involving fires, with such fires claiming 1,500 lives and causing 4,000 injuries annually. An often hidden cost of smoking is that associated with increased health insurance premiums, disability payments, and other private and tax payer–supported programs. The adverse health effects of smoking vary considerably in their nature and severity, depending on duration and frequency of smoking, presence or absence of concurrent illness, environmental exposures to other toxic substances, age, and sex (Smoking and Health, 1979).

CLUES TO CHEMICAL DEPENDENCY IN NURSES
GENERAL GUIDELINES

1. Nurse is late or absent from work especially after several days off
2. Odor of alcohol on nurse's breath; frequent use of mouthwash
3. Fine tremor of hands
4. Emotional lability
5. Excessive drowsiness
6. Speech slurred
7. Unable to translate thoughts into words
8. Deterioration in grooming
9. Change in interactions with colleagues
10. Disturbances in memory, judgment
11. Hyperactivity: restless, talkative, irritable
12. Frequent injuries: i.e., bruises, burns from falling

Cigarette smoking is a costly and preventable hazard to health. Smoking is a primary factor in lung cancer, and other lung disease, as well as cancer of the larynx, pharynx, oral cavity, esophagus, pancreas, and bladder. In addition, cigarette smoke interacts with certain substances involved in occupational exposure, such as asbestos and uranium, to aggravate the risk that might accrue from occupational exposure or smoking alone (Disease Prevention and Health Promotion, 1979). Smoking is also associated with varying cardiovascular diseases.

Short-Term Effects

The lungs retain more than 85% of the compounds actually inhaled through the nose, mouth, and trachea. Cigarette smoke and the 2,000 known chemicals in it escape the body's first lines of defense—the mouth and nose—because of the way it is inhaled. As the smoke travels through the mouth, it affects the taste buds on the tongue so that foods can taste different.

As the smoke continues down the throat through the trachea, the mucosa becomes inflamed. The outer layer of cells along the trachea are damaged and transformed over time into types of cells not effective in protecting the body.

Smoke changes the elasticity of the bronchioles and causes them to constrict. Smoke also impairs the cilia, considerably reducing efficient washing of the tracheobronchial tree. The cilia are paralyzed, and mucus cannot be cleared from the lungs. Excessive amounts of mucus are also produced and begin to clog airways. People who smoke are much more likely to be able to cough up some of the mucus than are people who do not smoke.

Changing Cigarettes

Between 1954 and 1983 consumer demand for filtered and low tar cigarettes led to a decline in the average tar content of a U.S. cigarette from 38 mg to 12 mg, and nicotine content declined from 2.3 to 1.2 mg. In 1984, low-tar cigarettes captured 62% of the market (Fielding, 1985b). Smokers have turned to these reduced tar and nicotine cigarettes out of concern for health, yet new hazards have arisen. To make cigarettes palatable when tar and nicotine are reduced, manufacturers have introduced a variety of flavorings and other chemical additives. Since manufacturers do not have to reveal what additives they use, it is impossible to assess the current risks of cigarettes (Health Consequences of Smoking, 1981).

Involuntary Smoking

Involuntary or passive smoking is defined as "the exposure of nonsmokers to tobacco-combustion products in the indoor environment" (Fielding, 1985a, p. 494). Tobacco smoke in the environment originates from two sources: mainstream or *sidestream smoke. Mainstream smoke* is exhaled by the smoker and sidestream is generated from the burning end of the cigarette. The latter is more toxic in that it contains a higher concentration of potentially dangerous gas-components and accounts for as much as 85% of the smoke in a room occupied by cigarette smokers.

Over 90% of mainstream smoke is in the form of a gas. Seventy percent of this gas is oxygen and nitrogen, which are normally inhaled; the remaining 20% is a combination of toxic chemicals. Examples of chemicals in this collection of gas include formaldehyde, hydrogen cyanide, ammonia, and carbon monoxide.

Carbon monoxide is particularly dangerous to health, since it bumps oxygen molecules out of the red blood cells and forms a new compound—carboxyhemoglobin. As the level of this new compound increases in the blood, body cells become starved for oxygen. Nonsmokers, on inhaling carbon monoxide, evidence impairments in performing visual, auditory, and manual tasks.

Pipe and Cigar Smoke

Pipe and cigar smokers do not tend to inhale as vigorously as cigarette smokers; thus, they are at less risk of developing lung cancer. However, the risk equals that of cigarette smoking when inhaling occurs. Smoke exposure in the upper respiratory tract is approximately equal for all smokers and comprises a major health risk. This means that all smokers have about the same chance of developing cancer of the esophagus, pharynx, larynx, and oral cavity. Additionally, pipe and cigar smokers are at higher risk for developing chronic obstructive pulmonary disease (COPD) than are nonsmokers.

Smokeless Tobacco

Smokeless tobacco is not a new creation. This habit was especially popular in the 1800s and early 1900s as a form of tobacco consumption. Over the years, the habit of spitting came to be viewed as unsanitary. However, in recent years the tobacco industry has recognized that chewing could become equated with a macho image and yield lucrative returns for them. Numerous television and movie personalities have publicly endorsed this habit, and it is being promoted as the ideal habit for active people who use their hands in their work or in pursuing hobbies or leisure activities (Christen, 1981).

Approximately 22 million Americans now use smokeless tobacco, and a portrait of the typical "chewer" ranges from the young to the old and includes students, athletes, and professional and blue collar workers in urban and rural settings. It is not uncommon for young males to start dipping or chewing by the age of 10 years. Young people consider a worn imprint of a circular can on the hip pocket a symbol of virility, maturity, and toughness.

Like other forms of tobacco use, chewing and dipping have addictive properties. About 5 minutes after putting chewing tobacco or snuff in their mouths, users begin to feel a "buzz" as the nicotine gets into their systems. Most regular users chew or dip every 20 to 30 minutes during their working hours to maintain the desired nicotine level. People who dip or chew become nicotine dependent; as with cigarettes, pipes, and cigars, nicotine and other chemicals are absorbed through the lungs as well as the mucus areas of the mouth and nose.

The mechanical effects of smokeless tobacco on the

mouth and teeth make this habit especially harmful. Tobacco is generally grown in sandy soil, and after several years of its use, people who chew and dip often wear down the tips of their teeth because of the continuous association with grit. Frequent use of tobacco increases the risk of cancer of the mouth and oral leukoplakia, or lesions of the soft tissues of the mouth characterized by a white patch or plaque. These lesions are not easily differentiated from other mouth diseases, since their texture varies from a "smooth, somewhat translucent white area to a thickened, cracked, and hardened lesion" (Christen, 1981, p. 10). Currently, leukoplakia is considered precancerous and does lead to cancer in about 5% of cases. Even though the incidence is low, this is a serious condition.

In addition, like other forms of tobacco, smokeless tobacco contains a substance called N-nitroso-nornicotine (NNN), which is a proven cancer-causing agent in animals. The amount of NNN is higher in snuff and chewing tobacco than in cigarette smoke.

Interaction Between Smoking and Substances Involved in Occupational Exposures

Although many studies have examined the effects of either smoking or occupational hazards on health, few have looked at the cumulative effects of these agents. Six ways in which smoking may act with physical and chemical agents to produce or increase adverse health effects are as follows:

1. Tobacco products may serve as vectors.
2. Work place chemicals may be transformed into more harmful agents by smoking.
3. Certain toxic agents in tobacco products and/or smoke may also occur in the work place, thus increasing exposure to the agent.
4. Smoking may contribute to an effect comparable to that resulting from exposure to toxic agents found in the work place, thus causing an additive biological effect. Coal dust and cigarette smoke appear to have an additive effect in the production of obstructive airway disease.
5. Smoking may act synergistically with toxic agents found in the work place to cause a much more profound effect than that anticipated simply from the separate influences of the agent and smoking added together. Asbestos insulation workers who smoke are at a far greater risk of developing bronchogenic carcinoma than their nonsmoking counterparts (Smoking and Health, 1979).
6. Smoking may contribute to accidents in the work place as a result of lack of attention and irritation of the eyes.

Health Consequences of Smoking for Women

Cigarette smoking is causally associated with cancer of the lung, larynx, oral cavity, esophagus, and kidney in women. It is estimated that cigarette smoking accounts for 18% of all newly diagnosed cancers and 25% of all female cancer deaths. These women have 2.5 to 5 times as great a likelihood of developing lung cancer as nonsmoking women. Lung cancer death rates of all histological types are highest in industrialized countries where there has been a higher prevalence of smoking for a longer time.

Women cigarette smokers have more than three times the risk of dying of stroke resulting from subarachnoid hemorrhage and twice the risk of having a heart attack as nonsmoking women. Of critical importance is recognition among women of the synergistic effect of smoking and the use of oral contraceptives. Their combination causes a 22-fold increase in the risk of subarachnoid hemorrhage stroke and a 20-fold increase in heart attacks in heavy smokers (Health Consequences of Smoking for Women, 1980).

Spontaneous abortions are increased, and there is a greater incidence of bleeding during pregnancy and premature rupture of membranes for women who smoke. This association is independent of socioeconomic and racial factors as well as parity. There is also a greater incidence of premature and prolonged rupture of amniotic membranes, abruptio placentae, and placenta previa. In addition, women who smoke during pregnancy have more fetal and neonatal deaths than nonsmoking pregnant women, and a relationship has been established between sudden infant death syndrome and smoking (Health Consequences of Smoking for Women, 1980). Additionally, fetal growth is directly retarded by smoking. Babies born to women smokers are, on the average, 200 g lighter than those born to comparable nonsmokers (Health Consequences of Smoking for Women, 1980). If a woman gives up smoking early in the pregnancy, her risk of delivering a low birth weight baby approaches the nonsmoker's rate.

The direct effects of maternal smoking on children extend beyond the fetal and neonatal stage. Children of mothers who smoked during pregnancy lag measurably in physical growth, and some evidence points to behavioral and cognitive effects. Nicotine, which is a known poison, has been found in the breastmilk of smoking mothers. Also, children whose parents smoke have more respiratory infections and hospitalizations during the first year of life.

Smoking Cessation

Information from public opinion and attitude polls indicates that 90% of smokers have either tried to quit smoking or would like to do so if they could find an effective method. These people need help! Smoking cessation is a difficult and painful process because of the often agonizing effects of physical and psychological withdrawal.

The vast majority of people who quit smoking do so without help from any organized program. The stimuli motivating them to quit are health problems, pressure from spouse, children, friends, co-workers, costs, and fear for their health or the health of their family (Fielding, 1985b).

People seem to continue smoking for one or more of the following reasons (Smoking Digest, 1977):

1. A sense of increased energy or stimulation
2. The satisfaction of handling or manipulating things
3. The accentuation of pleasure and relaxation
4. The reduction of negative feelings (anger, anxiety, fear, etc.)
5. "Craving" or psychological addiction
6. Habit

Helping people quit smoking requires an understanding of their motivation for smoking as well as knowledge of a variety of potentially succcessful programs. In addition, various characteristics have been identified to describe people who successfully quit smoking.

Specifically, higher levels of education are associated with greater success in quitting. "Among those with a college education or higher, 52.1% of the men and 48.1% of the women who have ever smoked have quit" (Health Consequences of Smoking for Women, 1980, p. 304). For all other educational levels, 40.5% of men and 31.3% of women have quit. As might be expected from the advanced education statistics, smoking cessation is also associated with higher levels of income and professional rather than technical work.

Men are more likely than women to remain successful abstainers. Light smokers have the greatest success in stopping, as do those with a great commitment to change, those who use behavioral techniques, and those who have access to a social support system. Regardless of the approach, the success rate varies and depends on the nature of the program, the content, instructor, setting, costs, and degree of motivation (Fielding, 1985b).

Ockene and Ockene (1982) describe nine strategies physicians can use to help their patients stop smoking. They identify five objectives toward which the strategies can be targeted.

1. Immediate cessation
2. Support and reinforcement of cessation programs in which the smoker is already involved
3. Maintenance of cessation
4. Reduction of smoking if the patient is not ready or able to stop
5. Preparation of the patient for a future time when cessation will be possible

Nurses likewise can use the strategies in the box at right to accomplish the five objectives.

Smoking cessation strategies can be divided into three broad, though not mutually exclusive, categories; aversion, self-control, and pharmacological. Aversion strategies typically use laboratory sessions and minimize homework. Self-control strategies involve high participant involvement, considerable homework, and minimal aversive techniques, and pharmacological techniques use nicotine gum.

The use of *aversive techniques* is based on a behavioral modification or conditioning framework. The underlying assumption is that smokers have learned to associate certain situations with smoking in the past; positive stimulation is replaced with a negative stimulation to discourage smokers from having positive associations when they smoke. Aversive techniques pair smoking with one of the following aversive stimuli: Electric shock is received when the person smokes; rapid smoking requires the person to chain smoke and to puff every 6 seconds; the satiation strategy requires that smokers double or triple their consumption, and covert sensitization pairs an unpleasant image such as vomiting, with smoking. The person imagines something unpleasant when wishing to smoke.

Self-control strategies emphasize personal responsibility

STRATEGIES TO HELP PATIENTS QUIT SMOKING

1. Maintain a positive attitude.
2. Personalize the risk of smoking to the individual.
3. Emphasize the value of cessation.
4. Foster the smoker's belief in an ability to stop.
5. Urge the smoker to stop.
6. Use self-control strategies.
7. Forewarn the smoker about the difficulty in quitting.
8. Support the smoker in the cessation process.
9. Support the nonstopper; urge cutting down on cigarettes.

From J.K. Ockene and I.S. Ockene, 9 ways to help your patients stop smoking, Your patient and cancer. Roslyn Heights, NY: 1982, Dominus Publishing Co., pp. 55-56.

for cessation; these techniques are used in the home and can be grouped into three major categories: environmental planning rearranges the circumstances surrounding the experience of smoking; behavioral programming rewards the smoker for not smoking and punishes the smoker for smoking; cognitive controls allow the smoker to use cognition to control the smoking behavior (Benfari, Ockene, and McIntyre, 1982).

National voluntary health organizations, such as the American Cancer Society, the American Heart Association, and the American Lung Association, for several years have sponsored group smoking cessation clinics through their local community chapters. Several profit-making corporations have entered this area in recent years, including SmokEnders, the National Association on Smoking and Health, and the Schick Centers. These three programs tend to be far more expensive than the programs offered by voluntary health organizations. Additionally, the Seventh Day Adventist Church offers a 5-day program for a modest fee. This program includes lectures by a clergy-health team, films on the harmful effects of smoking, explanations of smoking cessation procedures, and group interaction.

The use of nicotine gum is the major pharmacological method currently being used. The substitution of this gum for cigarettes has a twofold benefit. First, the nicotine in the gum helps to satiate the addiction to nicotine in cigarettes. Second, chewing the gum serves as a substitute oral activity for the cigarette. The gum has been available in Sweden, England, and Canada by prescription longer than in the United States (Lichtenstein, 1982).

CLINICAL APPLICATION

Community health nurses can become actively involved in developing and implementing programs for smoking cessation. Self-control strategies offer multiple opportunities for nursing intervention. Since smoking leads to the most visible, preventable cause of morbidity and mortality, ample reasons abound for targeting this area. The following case study demonstrates nursing intervention in smoking behaviors.

In 1982, a team of professionals led by a community health nurse educator sought to evaluate the effectiveness in one state of the American Lung Association's self-help smoking cessation program *Freedom From Smoking* (Lancaster et al., 1986). This program consists of two self-help manuals designed to lead users through a series of exercises culminating in cessation on the sixteenth day of the 20-day program. One hundred one users of the program were contacted by telephone to determine the effectiveness of FFS. Data collected allowed the team to develop a profile of the person most likely to be successful with FFS. Because of the cognitive exercises and personal discipline required with FFS, it was not surprising that successful users were typically white, middle-class, middle-aged, married, white-collar workers. However, this particular state had a high blue-collar population who were at increased risk of health disruption due to their employment in settings such as mines, mills, and factories, which, when combined with smoking, are synergistically detrimental to lung health.

The team then systematically developed *Freedom From Smoking* II, which was oriented toward the needs of the population at greatest risk. The reading level was modified, the number of exercises was reduced, and the self-help format was paired with a 9-week smoking cessation clinic. Clinics were provided at employment sites and various agencies. This approach reflects a collaborative effort of nursing, a voluntary health organization, and other professionals. Such an approach could easily be replicated in other sites and used to deal with a variety of community health problems.

SUMMARY

The abuse of a variety of substances poses health problems for Americans. Alcohol, drugs, and cigarettes comprise major abusive chemicals and constitute health hazards both for those directly involved and for people indirectly involved. Prevention of substance abuse is the prevailing goal. To provide information about prevention, community health nurses must know the signs, patterns, and effects of substance abuse.

Attitudes are of critical importance in health promotion relative to substance abuse, since the way people think and feel is conveyed in verbal as well as nonverbal messages. When nurses think that people who abuse drugs are weak and could help themselves if they would only try harder, this attitude is conveyed to the client. Attitudes toward substance abuse are most helpful to clients when based on the premise that people use chemicals to deal with life. People need acceptance, understanding, and commitment to help them deal constructively with their health hazards. The health consequences of substance abuse are in many instances life threatening; most people who abuse alcohol, drugs, and cigarettes know about the consequences. What they need is consistent help in dealing with the life events leading to and encouraging this habit and support as they try to quit if that is their choice.

Numerous programs are available for dealing with the problems of substance abuse. The community health nurse needs to know what programs and resources are available in the local area, what they charge, who is eligible, and what degree of success has been reported with each one. Major roles include support, encouragement, teaching, and referral.

⩵ KEY CONCEPTS

Heavy tobacco, alcohol, and drug use have been linked to numerous forms of morbidity and mortality and present serious social and economic problems.

The necessity for community health nurses to become actively involved in the prevention and cessation of substance abuse is particularly evident when one considers the consequences of substance abuse.

Various components make up chemical dependency, including psychological, social, medical, economic, and legal aspects. Generally, more males than females are involved; the greatest incidence is among young and middle-aged adults.

The most effective way to handle chemical dependency is to prevent its onset.

Alcoholism is a chronic disease characterized by repetitive and often compulsive drinking that produces injury to the drinker's health and other aspects of life, including marital status, career, interpersonal relationships, or other required societal adaptations.

Large doses of alcohol consumed over an extended time lead to decreased sensitivity to alcohol's effects. This phenomenon, tolerance, or the need to continually increase the dosage to achieve the desired effect, is common to all potentially addictive drugs.

People with a family history of alcoholism, those experiencing grave personal problems or stressful life events, or people with a history of other addiction are most likely to develop an alcohol-related problem.

The drinking patterns of women are changing. Forty years ago it was virtually unheard of for women to drink, whereas today over 60% of all American women and almost 90% of all college-age women drink.

Many frequently prescribed drugs contain at least one ingredient known to interact adversely with alcohol. Most adverse effects resulting from such combinations are accidental, yet the death and morbidity tolls are high.

Substance abuse includes the use of both illicit and legally sanctioned drugs. It is becoming increasingly common in responding to the rush and stresses of life for people to rely on tranquilizers, pain relievers, antidepressants, and sedatives.

While drug abuse among nurses and other health care providers is not new, it is currently receiving considerable attention.

Each of the reports of the U.S. Surgeon General since 1964 has identified smoking as the single most preventable cause of morbidity and premature mortality.

Information from public opinion and attitude polls indicates that 90% of smokers have either tried to quit smoking or would like to do so if they could find an effective method.

Helping people quit smoking requires an understanding of their motivation for smoking as well as knowledge of a variety of potentially successful programs.

LEARNING ACTIVITIES

1. Read your local newspaper for four days and select stories that illustrate the effect of substance abuse on individuals, on families, and on the community.

2. For each of the stories in the newspaper related to substance abuse, describe preventive strategies that a community health nurse might have tried before the problem reached such a dire state.

3. Looking at your local community resources directory (or the telephone book), identify agencies that might serve as referral sources for individuals or families in which substance abuse is a problem.

4. Divide the students into groups of three to five and ask them to discuss their personal attitudes toward drinking, smoking, and drug abuse. Discuss each category of substance abuse separately. They may want to consider the following areas: sex, age, amount, time, occasion where substance abuse occurs, place, companions, motivation, and incentives.

5. Divide the students into groups of four to five and ask them to develop a list of examples, incidents, regulations, or practices in U.S. society that illustrate conflicting attitudes about drinking (for example, alcoholism is an illness yet people are arrested for public intoxication; drunken driving is illegal yet bars line many roads as do billboards advertising alcoholic beverages).

BIBLIOGRAPHY

Abelson, H.I., Fishburne, P.M., and Cisin, I.: National survey on drug abuse: 1977. A nationwide study—youth, young adults and older people. DHEW Pub. No. (ADM) 78-618, Washington, D.C., 1977, Public Health Service, Department of Health, Education, and Welfare.

Alcohol and drug misuse prevention, Public Health Rep. (suppl)98:116-132, 1983.

Allegrante, J.P., O'Rourke, T.W., and Tuncalp, S.: A multivariate analysis of selected variables on the development of subsequent youth smoking behavior, J. Drug Educ. 7(3):237-248, 1977-1978.

Benfari, R.C., Ockene, J.K., and McIntyre, K.M.: Control of cigarette smoking from a psychological perspective, Annu. Rev. Public Health 3:101-128, 1982.

Borland, B.R., and Rulolph, J.R.: Relative effects of low socioeconomic status, parent smoking and poor scholastic performance among high school students, Soc. Sci. Med. 9:27-30, 1975.

Butz, R.H.: Intoxication and withdrawal. In Estes, N.J., and Heinemann, M.E., editors: Alcoholism: development, consequences, and interventions, ed. 2, St. Louis, 1981, The C.V. Mosby Co.

Carr, R.R., and Meyers, E.J.: Marijuana and cocaine: the process of change in drug policy. In Drug Abuse Council: The facts about drug abuse, New York, 1980, The Free Press.

Christen, A.G.: The facts about smokeless tobacco, Listen 34:7-11, 1981.

Chychula, N.M.: Screening for substance abuse in a primary care setting, Nurse Practitioner 9:15-23, 1984.

The community health nurse and alcohol-related problems, Pub. No. 017-024-00753-6, Rockville, Md., 1978a, National Institute on Alcohol Abuse and Alcoholism, Public Health Service, Department of Health, Education, and Welfare.

The community health nurse and alcohol-related problems. instructor's curriculum planning guide, Pub. No. 017-024-00754-4, Rockville, Md., 1978b, National Institute on Alcohol Abuse and Alcoholism, Public Health Service, Department of Health, Education, and Welfare.

Cretcher, D.: Steering clear: helping your child through the high-risk drug years, Minneapolis, MN, 1982, Winston Press.

Deciding about drugs: a woman's choice. DHEW Pub. No. (ADM) 80-820, Rockville, Md., 1979, National Institute on Drug Abuse, Department of Health, Education, and Welfare.

Dietch, J.: The nature and extent of benzodiazepine abuse: an overview of recent literature, Hosp. Community Psychiatry 34(12):1139-1145, 1983.

Disease prevention and health promotion. Federal programs and prospects, Washington, D.C., 1979, DHEW Pub. No. (PHS) 79-55071 B, Department of Health, Education, and Welfare.

Drugs and dosages: Cocaine abuse spreads, Occup. Health Nurs. 32(1):50-51, 1984.

Durell, J., and Bukoski, W.: Preventing substance abuse: the state of the art, Public Health Rep. 99(1):23-31, 1984.

Fielding, J.E.: Smoking: health effects and control. I., N. Engl. J. Med. 313(8):491-498, 1985a.

Fielding, J.E.: Smoking: health effects and control. II. N. Eng. J. Med. 313(9):555-561, 1985b.

Finley, B.: Primary and secondary prevention of substance abuse in nurses, Occup. Health Nurs. 11(11):14-18, 1982.

Fisher, E.B.: Progress in reducing adolescent smoking, Am. J. Public Health. 70(7):678-679, 1980.

Ginsburg, H.M.: Intravenous drug users and the acquired immune deficiency syndrome, Public Health Rep. 99(2):206-212, 1984.

Gitlow, S.E., and Peyes, J.S.: Alcoholism: a practical treatment guide, New York, 1980, Grune & Stratton, Inc.

Goldberg, P.: The federal government's response to illicit drugs, 1969-1978. In Drug Abuse Council: The facts about drug abuse, New York, 1980, The Free Press.

Green, P.L.: The impaired nurse: chemical dependency, J. Emergency Nursing 10(1):23-26, 1984.

Halpern, J.S.: Street speed, J. Emerg. Nurs. 9(4):224-227, 1983.

Halpern, J.S., and Davis, J.W.: Use and abuse of alcohol: further perspectives, J. Emerg. Nurs. 9(1):49-52, 1983.

The health consequences of smoking. The changing cigarette. A report of the Surgeon General, DHHS (PHS) Pub. No. 81-50156, Washington, D.C., 1981, Department of Health and Human Services.

The health consequences of smoking for women. A report of the Surgeon General. Pub. No. 326-003, Washington, D.C., 1980, Office of Smoking and Health, Department of Health and Human Services.

Healthy people: the Surgeon General's report on health promotion and disease prevention. PHS Pub. No. 79-55071, Washington, D.C., Dec. 1979, Department of Health, Education and Welfare.

Heinemann, E., and Estes, H.J.: Assessing alcoholic patients, Am. J. Nurs. 76:786-794, 1976.

Hennecke, L., and Fox, V.: The woman with alcoholism. In Gitlow, S.E., and Peyser, H.S.: Alcoholism: a practical treatment guide. New York, 1980, Grune & Stratton, Inc.

Interaction effect of alcohol with other drugs, Lincoln, Neb., 1977, Nebraska Division on Alcoholism.

Johnston, L.D., Backman, J.C., and O'Malley, P.M.: Drug use among American high school students, 1975-77, DHEW Pub. No. (ADM) 78-619, Washington, D.C., 1977, Alcohol, Drug Abuse and Mental Health Administration, Public Health Service, Department of Health, Education, and Welfare.

Lancaster, J., Ellison, K.J., Myers, G.C., and Van Matre, J.G.: Evaluation of freedom from smoking among Alabama residents. Family Community Health 8(4):36-47, 1986.

Lewis, D.C., and Sessler, J.: Heroin treatment: development, status, outlook. In Drug Abuse Council: The facts about drug abuse, New York, 1980. The Free Press.

Lichtenstein, E.: The smoking problem: a behavioral perspective, J. Consult. Clin. Psychol. 50(6):804-819, 1982.

Milby, J.: Addictive behavior and its treatment, New York, 1981, Springer Publishing Co., Inc.

Ockene, J.K., and Ockene, O.S.: 9 ways to help your patients stop smoking. In your patient and cancer, Roslyn Heights, N.Y., 1982, Dominus Publishing Co.

Reeder, L.G.: Sociocultural factors in the etiology of smoking behavior: an assessment. In Jarvik, M.E., et al.: Research on smoking behavior, NIDA Research Monograph 17, DHEW Pub. No. (ADM) 80-820, Washington, D.C., 1979, Public Health Service, Department of Health, Education and Welfare.

Remington, P.L., Forman, M.R., Gentry, E.M., et al.: Current smoking trends in the United States: The 1981-1983 Behavioral Risk Factor Surveys, JAMA 253(20):2975-2978, 1985.

Sandler, D.P., Everson, R.G., and Wilcox, A.J.: Passive smoking in adulthood and cancer risk. Am. J. Epidemiol. 121(1):37-48, 1985.

Sandmaier, M.: Alcohol abuse and women: a guide to getting help, Rockville, Md., 1977, National Clearinghouse for Alcohol Information.

Signs of use of substances for drugging effects, Washington, D.C., 1978, Pharmaceutical Manufacturers Association.

Smoking and health, DHEW Pub. No. 79-50066, Washington, D.C., 1979, Department of Health, Education and Welfare.

Smoking digest: progress report on a nation kicking the habit, Bethesda, Md., 1977, Public Health Service, Department of Health, Education, and Welfare.

Stepter, N.R.: Drug abuse among nurses. Nurs. Manag. 13(12):41-43, 1982.

Tarrant Council on Alcoholism and Drug Abuse: The family illness. Fort Worth, Tex., 1981, The Council.

Wagner, B.J.: Intervening with the adolescent involved in substance abuse, J. Sch. Health, 54(7):244-246, 1984.

Westermeyer, J.: Primer on chemical dependency, Baltimore, 1976, The Williams & Wilkins Co.

Women's Health. Report of the Public Health Service Task Force on Women's Health Issues. Public Health Rep. 100(1):73-106, 1985.

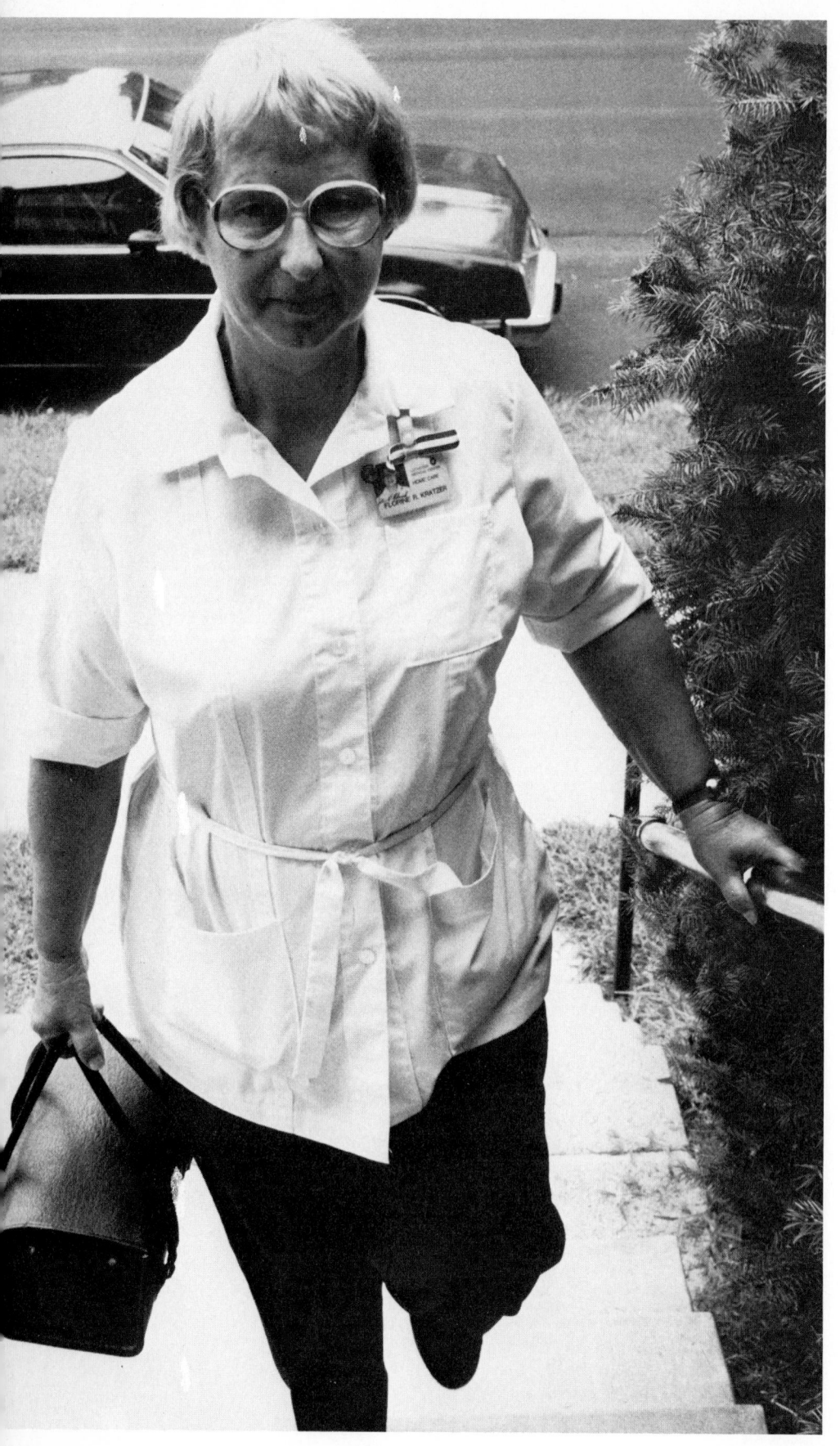

DIVERSITY IN THE COMMUNITY HEALTH NURSING ROLE

In the early beginnings of the health care delivery system in the United States, the community health nurse was primarily responsible for visiting the sick in the home and participating in communicable disease case finding. As the health care delivery system has evolved into a multidimensional industry, nursing education has expanded to embrace levels of preparation in university settings from the awarding of associate through doctoral degrees. Likewise, nursing practice has expanded and diversified to include multiple practice settings, functional roles such as educator, administrator, or consultant, and an assortment of clinical specialties.

As a result of these changes, the community health nurse's roles, functions, client population, and practice settings have diversified and expanded. Community health nurses are found in the functional roles of manager and consultant, as discussed in Chapters 36 and 37. The community health nurse is also found working with identified subpopulations, as described in Chapters 40 through 42.

In answer to the changing health care system, manpower shortages, evolving community health needs, and medically underserved rural and urban centers, a new health professional has emerged. Nursing's contribution to this category of health provider is the nurse practitioner; with a new knowledge base and set of skills, coupled with previously learned nursing principles and concepts, the nurse practitioner is able to meet primary care needs of select populations. Chapter 39 presents a discussion of the development of the family nurse practitioner role and the current status in the health care delivery system.

Regardless of the setting, the client, or the role, the community health nurse (discussed in Chapter 38) acts as advocate for the client entering and progressing through the health care delivery system.

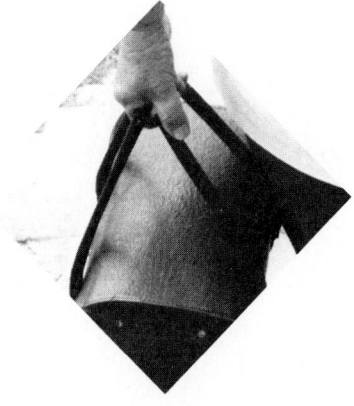

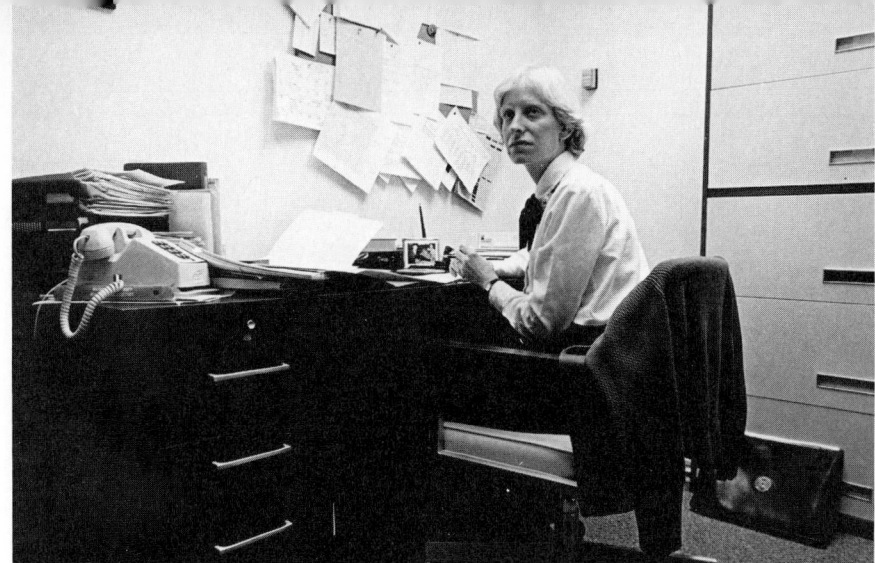

Roberta Lee

36

THE COMMUNITY HEALTH NURSE MANAGER

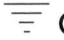 OBJECTIVES

After reading this chapter, the student should be able to:

Differentiate between the concepts of leader and manager in community health nursing.

Describe the history of management and organization theory.

Apply general systems theory to community health nursing management.

Apply concepts of the management process to community health nursing.

Apply concepts of intervention in public health to community health nursing.

Describe application of nursing care delivery models in community health nursing.

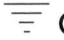 KEY TERMS

administrator

ambulatory clinics

client diagnostic category model of nursing

district nursing

financial resources planning

follower

formal structure

functional nursing

general systems theory

home visiting

human resources planning

informal structure

leader

management process

manager

mobile clinics

nursing care delivery model

organization theory

performance budgets

personal health services

primary nursing

productivity

program budgets

screening clinic

self-management

sensitive screening test

specific screening test

strategic planning

tactical planning

team nursing

The scope and complexity of the managerial role of the community health nurse varies tremendously. Factors that influence the community health nurse's management role include the size and complexity of the organization, the organization's mission and goals, and the nurse's job description. It is important to understand the relationship among the roles of *leader, follower, manager,* and *administrator* in community health nursing.

Leadership implies ability to influence the behavior of others (colleagues or clients) toward achievement of a mutually established goal or objective. The *leader* and *follower* roles are determined by the interactions of the persons in the group. In comparison, the roles of *manager* or *administrator* are jobs within an organization. Individuals are assigned to these jobs and to subordinate jobs. The role of the manager is to coordinate the efforts of the subordinates toward attainment of goals and objectives as determined by the organization.

The roles of leader and manager and follower and subordinate have parallel aspects. For example, both leaders and managers are concerned with coordinating individual efforts to achieve goals. However, the source of their power is very different. The leader's power base is *informal,* and

the role is designated by the group of followers. The manager's power base is *formalized* by the employing organization. Ideally, persons with informal leadership skills will also be selected for formal management positions in the organization. Unfortunately, this does not always occur.

Persons who are selected for managerial positions in organizations are expected to acquire skills in areas such as program development, personnel, and financial management. The degree to which the individual relies on clinical as compared with management information for problem solving is partly determined by the size and complexity of the organization.

Figure 36-1 illustrates the relationship between two types of knowledge (clinical and management) necessary to perform three management roles: staff nurse, supervisor, and executive. The relative proportions of clinical and management knowledge are represented by the slashed vertical lines on the diagram. Staff nurse's major activities are providing nursing care to many clients in an effective and efficient manner. The staff nurse is expected to manage those work responsibilities in a way that maximizes productivity. *Productivity* in community health staff nursing is usually measured by the number of clients served per unit of time

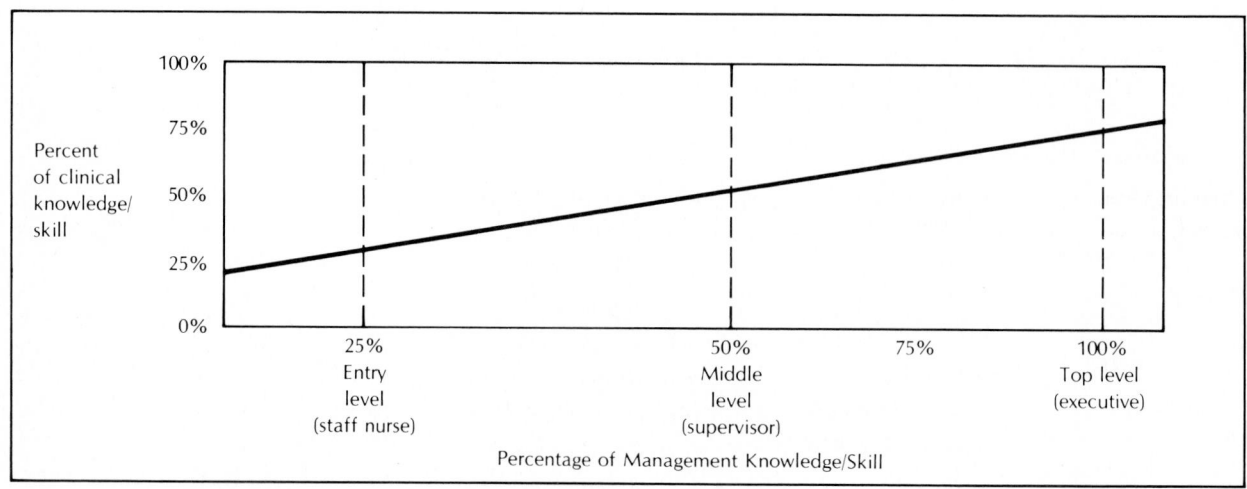

FIGURE 36-1

Clinical and management knowledge.

(such as average number of clients served per day). The supervisor's role requires additional management skills, especially in the areas of performance and program evaluation.

The executive role is predominantly administrative with respect to the knowledge and skill necessary to perform the job. This role includes preparing information to document the organization's effectiveness and efficiency to its constituents, usually represented by an elected or appointed board of directors. This conceptualization of clinical and management knowledge and skill also implies that clinical and management roles are inherent in all types of community health nursing roles and that their relative proportions change, depending on the specific job. Differentiating these three levels of management implies a relatively large community health nursing organization.

Pickett (1980) notes that although most texts on public health administration describe large, complex, "ideal" health departments, the most prevalent organizational form for health departments in the United States is the county health department. County health departments are most commonly staffed by one nurse and probably one sanitarian. The public health officer position frequently rotates among physicians residing in that county. The community health nurse in this situation not only provides all the services to all the clients but also has responsibility for management of the organization. In this situation, the community health nurse is both staff nurse and executive. The community health nurse in this situation is concurrently a clinician, manager, and administrator.

◆   ◆   ◆

To facilitate delineation of these roles, this chapter focuses on the role of the entry level or staff nurse in a moderate-to-large community nursing organization. An overview of management and organization theory focuses on application of the management process in community health nursing. Examples of executive types of goals are described and implications for the staff nurse are presented. This chapter also reviews the mission, purposes, and strategies of community health; applies these to management in community health organizations and to community nursing; and presents examples of management activities common to the staff or entry level nursing role.

HISTORY OF ORGANIZATION AND MANAGEMENT THEORY

Modern organization theory has a brief history that can be described in three phases: (1) scientific or classical period, (2) human relations period, and (3) contemporary period.

The scientific period (approximately 1900 to 1935) is typically characterized by a concern for understanding the relationships between administrative functions (described by Fayol as planning, organizing, directing, and controlling) and production. F.W. Taylor, an engineer, made major contributions to organization theory (Filley and House, 1969). During this period, workers were seen as motivated only by economic rewards, and the organization was characterized by (1) a clearly defined division of labor with highly specialized personnel, and (2) a distinct hierarchy of

authority (Etzioni, 1964). Administrative duties, according to classical or scientific thinking, include study of the work, deduction of the "best" or most efficient procedure, selection of the right person(s) for the job, and training personnel in the proper method.

The scientific period made several significant contributions to the conceptualization of organizations and administration, including the delineation of management functions and the development of concepts of authority, responsibility, accountability, and viewing the organization as one unit. Limitations, however, included an incomplete understanding of worker motivations, especially in nonsalaried areas, and a concept of one-way (administrator to employee) direction for administrative functions.

The second major phase in the development of organization theory, the human relations period, began with the writing of Barnard (1938), who described the interrelationships between the individual, the organization, and the informal organization. Barnard's work, and its extension by Simon (1947), emphasized the human dimension of organizations. This shift in the theory was strengthened by the social movement toward formal organization of labor, the emergence of labor unions (for instance, the Wagner Act of 1935), and the Hawthorne studies. These experiments suggested that productivity was affected by attitudes of individuals and the social situation in the work groups as well as mechanical efficiency in the plant (Filley and House, 1969).

The studies in organization theory that were completed following the Hawthorne findings ultimately concluded that there are limits to the belief that the happy worker and work group are necessarily productive. In the contemporary period, theoretical perspectives regarding administration reflect a blend between the research about types of organizations and research done in organizations. Behavioral science research has contributed to contemporary thinking about administration. One of the contemporary approaches to organizational theory is general systems theory, which focuses on the functions and relationships within the organization and on the interaction between the organization and its environment. Because the relationship between the environment or community and nursing is paramount in community health nursing, the general systems model is used to describe community health nursing management.

General Systems Theory

General systems theory is used extensively in contemporary organization theory. This approach states that organizations are a complex of elements in mutual interaction (Arndt and Huckabay, 1975). Systems theory and thinking represent a general (macro) rather than a specific (micro) perspective in that they demonstrate overall relationships among the components within the whole organization. According to Stevens (1979), a systems model, or framework, contains at least eight categories of information. One of these is the input–transformation–output process and is applicable to community health nursing.

In community health nursing the input component includes the personnel, financial, environmental, and other

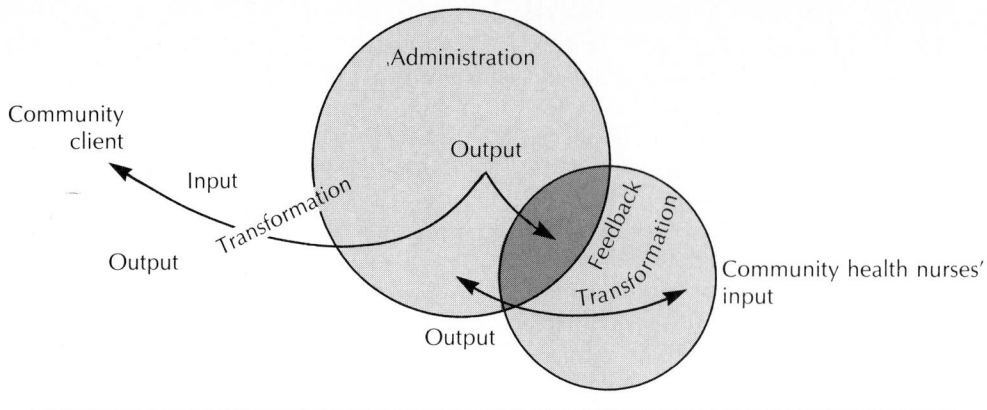

FIGURE 36-2

Transformation phase.

"raw materials" or resources needed to produce community health nursing services. In the transformation phase the organizations, personnel, information, and knowledge combine to create an output of community health nursing services (Figure 36-2). An example of the transformation of inputs to the outputs of community nursing service is illustrated by the following situation:

> There was a request for community health nursing to respond to demand for scoliosis screening in all public schools. The Board of Education had eliminated many school nurse positions and now lacked sufficient school nurse personnel to screen the large student population. A randomly selected ad hoc committee of community health staff nurses was selected and asked to make a recommendation to the nurse administrator. The committee recommended that the community health agency provide school health services (including scoliosis screening) to all of the public schools.

In this example, inputs include the request for service from the community (the environment) and the knowledge of the nursing personnel. These were transformed into a recommendation to restructure the delivery of nursing services to the school-aged population aggregate in the community.

This story, additionally, illustrates the idea of interaction between the system's subcomponents, the community health organization and the community. The community health organization considered the community's request (input) for scoliosis screening. The screening request provided input to the organization, which then requested additional information from nursing service. Nursing's information and expertise (inputs) were transformed and expressed in a recommendation. The recommendation, viewed by the nurses as a final output, was an additional input to the organization. The program for the community was the organization's output.

Whether information or other resources are an output or an input depends on the level of organization under consideration (Lancaster, 1982). The nurse administrator must deal with contingencies that are different from those considered relevant by staff nurses.

THE MANAGEMENT PROCESS

The *management process* (Figure 36-3), like the nursing process, is a systematic, cyclical method for solving problems. The management process includes four major functions: planning, organizing, leading, and evaluating (DiVincente, 1972). The major concern of management is the delivery of community health nursing services in an effective and efficient manner. In management theory, effectiveness is measured by comparing the organization's performance with its philosophy, goals, and objectives. Applied to community health nursing, effectiveness pertains to the nurse's role in reduction of risk factors, morbidity, and premature mortality in population aggregates. According to management theory, efficiency pertains to attaining goals in a way that minimize costs and maximize benefits. Costs include salaries, fringe benefits, equipment, supplies, as well as office space and maintenance, secretarial services, and so forth. Effective and efficient community health nursing services require use of the management process.

It is important for the community health nurse to appreciate that change is frequently an implied assumption underlying the management process. Often planning results in change by creating, revising, or eliminating resources available to members of a community. The community health nurse must be knowledgeable about change theory and develop skill in its application to practice.

Planning

In the past, planning was not emphasized as much as it is today. Planning involves deciding what will be done (goals and objectives) and how it will be done. Planning can be classified as either strategic and tactical (Levey and Loomba, 1973). *Strategic planning* is the process by which basic organizational goals and directions are determined. *Strategic planning is long range and encompasses ends (outcomes) as well as means (processes).* Community health nurse managers use epidemiological data and community assessment data to develop strategic plans. For example, if the data in Figure 36-4 represented the community, the community nurse executive may want to include elimination of rubella in 18-

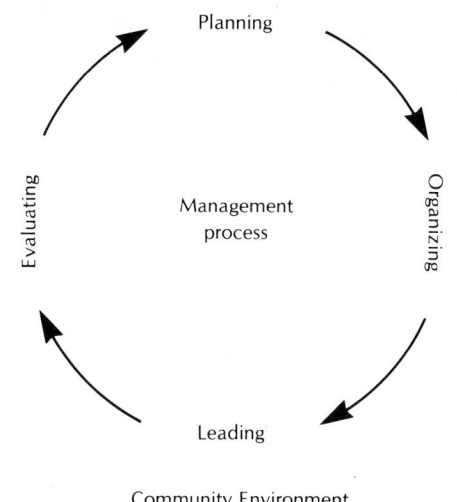

FIGURE 36-3

Management cycle.

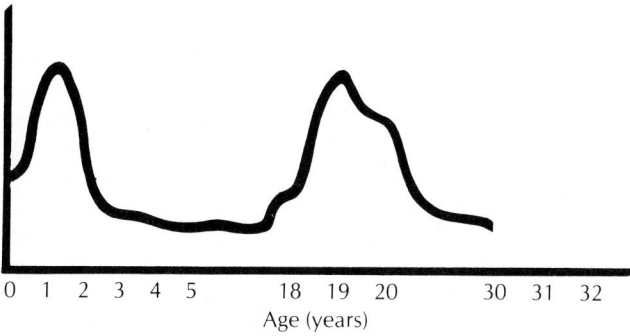

FIGURE 36-4

Incidence of rubella.

to 25-year-old persons as an objective in the strategic plan. In contrast, *tactical planning uses shorter time frames, a narrower scope, more attention to detail and is more flexible* (Arndt and Huckabay, 1975). An example of the tactical phase of planning is the work involved in establishing the rubella immunization clinics for the previously described target population (see Chapter 11).

The planning process at all levels of management requires decision-making skills. Like the nursing process, planning begins with assessment of the relevant information. In many cases, it is rapidly apparent that there are gaps between the available information and the optimal information. In some cases, it is possible to easily obtain planning information. But, that is not always true. It is common to prepare a plan based on partial information, to implement the plan, and to fall short of attaining the desired objectives. Critical review of all aspects of the plan including the objectives as well as the plan itself is a necessary part of identifying planning problems and making revisions.

An example of the importance of planning can be shown in the following situation:

A group of senior citizens, prompted by a nursing student's assessment that hypertension was prevalent in their apartment complex, requested the local health department to set up a weekly blood pressure screening clinic within its building. Assuming the student had validated all the findings, a district nursing supervisor assigned a staff nurse to set up such a clinic each Thursday and to notify the residents regarding the service. The clinic was set up and notices were sent out. After three weeks, only four residents had attended. There had been numerous phone calls from local physicians questioning this clinic. The drug store and a neighborhood center less than five blocks away notified the administrator that they did free blood pressure screening.

A plan to set up a blood pressure screening clinic had been made. Management of the clinic was delegated to the staff nurse, who was then responsible for conducting the clinic. However, evaluation of the clinic three weeks later indicated that it was a "failure." In this case, incomplete assessment of the situation led to the erroneous conclusion that an unmet need existed. Establishing a screening clinic was an inappropriate strategic plan in this situation.

The tactical plan for actual implementation of the clinic was appropriate, as in the following sample:

A community health nurse was making home visits to several elderly persons who had initially been referred to the agency for medical and nursing care problems. Over time, their medical and nursing care problems had resolved. However, the nurse was reluctant to discontinue service because these individuals were socially isolated and valued the interpersonal contact the nurse provided. The nurse discussed this problem with representatives of a local church. The church planned and implemented a "Friendly Visitor" program to socially isolated elderly and made home visits to clients of the nurse. The nurse then terminated nursing care to these families.

This example demonstrates success in planning. In the first example, the tactical plans to implement the clinic were adequate. However, it was the wrong strategic plan because the strategic plan duplicated a service that was already available. In the second example, the nurse helped plan a new and appropriate community service and the result was success.

Staff nurses in community health agencies contribute to the organization through planning. An example of day-to-day planning is managing one's own work activities. The community health nurse is frequently assigned to clinics, which operate on a regularly scheduled basis; home visiting; and other activities. Effective and efficient use of one's time is essential. For example, arriving at a family's home without essential equipment may necessitate a return trip to the office. In this situation, lack of planning results in waste of the nurse's time (salary) and excess travel costs (nurse's salary associated with travel time and actual travel expenses). Additionally, the client and family's time is wasted with nonproductive visits, and nursing care for other clients may have to be deferred.

Community health nurses also plan for comprehensive client care. The nurse may call a meeting of all agencies who are providing services to an individual or family to establish a plan of care. Planning objectives may include coordinating services and reducing interagency duplication or omissions of service. Interagency conferences are especially common with multiproblem families.

Another aspect of planning includes personal planning related to meeting employment standards. If the nurse is expected to provide transportation during the work day, vehicles must be adequately maintained, detailed maps obtained, and local weather conditions must be checked. Community health nurses in Minneapolis winterize their vehicles in October to prepare for the winter's ice and snow.

Community health nurses are frequently involved in planning for recurring clinics, such as child health or antepartum services, or sporadic clinics, such as a health fair. Planning for these services involves marketing or advertising, arranging for space and equipment, and planning for staff and volunteers, record keeping, and follow-up of clients.

Financial Resources Planning

Planning is incomplete without a budget. Simply stated, a *budget* is a plan stated in financial terms. It identifies the costs associated with implementing the plan. Community health staff nurses are frequently knowledgeable about financial aspects of community health programs.

Implementing any type of program requires money. In community health funding comes from a variety of resources (see Chapters 3 and 6). The community health organization's ability to accomplish its objectives is related to its ability to obtain adequate funding for its programs.

A budget is required by law, and regardless of the organizational structure and purpose, the nurse needs to know how much money is available and required for the nursing services. Budgets may be classified as program budgets or performance budgets.

In a *program budget,* expenses and income are related to a specific service, such as the rubella immunization program described earlier. A program budget has the advantage of directly relating financial planning to the evaluation of program outcome; that is, the costs of a rubella immunization program can be directly related to the "savings" associated with reducing the incidence of congenital rubella. The major disadvantage of program-based budgeting is that a separate budget is required for each program. A multiservice agency may have 40 to 50 separate budgets, which increase the costs of managing the financial aspects of the organization.

The *performance budget* shows clearly and concisely services to be provided in return for the funds available or income generated. The advantage of performance budgeting is that it provides more exact information on the cost per unit of service relationship. The disadvantage may arise from the complexity of developing this type budget and the danger of placing value on numbers of measurable service units (for example, the cost per rubella immunization) rather than an expression of valid expected outcomes, such as the reduction in incidence of rubella.

Regardless of type of budgeting method used (and there are many more types of budgets), the manner in which the financial resources are obtained frequently dictates the method used for budgetary purposes. For example, the medicare program requires specific budgeting procedures.

Human Resources Planning

The heart of any service organization is the human resources that have been attracted to the organization—the human knowledge and skills available that lead to the ability to implement the plans for the programs that have been designed or are expected to be accomplished. First, in *human resources planning,* the type, classification, availability, and mix of the personnel needed must be identified. The staff usually includes professional and nonprofessional personnel depending on the needs of the programs.

Establishing policies and procedures and job descriptions is also part of the planning function. Job descriptions define employee work, work-role relationship, and areas for evaluation. Policies and procedures provide guidelines for employee behavior in implementing the activities that are necessary if the organization's goals and objectives are to be achieved. They are also important in setting standards of behavior in the relationship between a community and the organization.

A key to any program is the importance of knowing how to use personnel. Therefore, in a large child health clinic with technicians, volunteers, and other nonprofessional staff members, it would be poor use of professional personnel to have the community health nurse set up the clinic and be responsible for intake as well as for cleaning and reordering of the room. Another example would be the use of a community health nurse to do mass vision screening when volunteers, school health aides, or other technical personnel can be taught the procedure under the nurse's direction.

In summary, planning, whether strategic, tactical, financial, or human resources, is a managerial function that occurs at all levels within an organization and when employees interact with the organization's environment. The community health nurse is involved in planning for care of clients and families in a variety of settings. Planning is probably the most time consuming and potentially most complex of the management process functions. Careful planning anticipates organizing, leading, and evaluating problems and attempts to prevent their occurrence. Conceptually, it is similar to primary prevention.

Organization

Once one knows the plan, the amount of money available, and the type of personnel needed and available, the next step is organization. Organizing involves arranging and defining the relationships between both personnel and other resources by establishing a structure.

Formal and Informal Structure

An examination of the organizational chart of any agency will quickly reveal that it represents only the *formal structure.* There is also an *informal structure,* and the nurse must be conscious of both. The communication flow occurs not only within a given program or department but also within other units of the organization and between individuals and agencies outside the organization. The plan needs to be put into an organized system that allows for effective use of selected and trained personnel and available resources.

Nursing Care Delivery Models in Community Health

The work of community health nurses, especially in large agencies, is often organized through use of a *nursing care delivery model.* These models facilitate supervision of nursing and other employees and assignment of specific work tasks to individuals.

The type of nursing care delivery model used by an agency is related to the size and complexity of the agency. Small agencies often employ only one staff nurse; large agencies may employ over one hundred nurses. Nursing staff frequently have multiple assignments, including both clinics and home visits. The proportion of the nurse's time spent in clinic versus the home varies enormously according to Cayner (1985), depending on the focus, such as a maternal/child health service.

PRIMARY NURSING. Small agencies most often employ a variation of the *primary nursing* model. In this method, the individual nurse is responsible for individual clients and families who are referred to the agency for service and who meet the agency's admission criteria (which often include a geographic criterion). In community health, this method is called *district nursing.* The nurse may be responsible for all cases within the agency's jurisdiction. District nursing is actually very similar to primary nursing in that the client usually has only one nurse who assumes total responsibility for the client's care. If several nurses are employed and the geographic area is large, it is common to subdivide the area and assign a nurse to the cases who live in each subdivision. This nursing care delivery model reduces travel time and travel expense. It requires each nurse to be skilled in nursing care of all client–family problems that may present themselves.

FUNCTIONAL NURSING. Functional nursing care delivery assigns staff nurses and other personnel to client functions such as medications, treatments, hygiene, and client teaching. *Functional nursing* has its roots in the scientific period of management theory, which focused on identifying the most efficient "assembly line." It is used by some agencies, especially those whose focus is home care of sick individuals. The client–family may receive care from a staff nurse responsible for nursing care planning and teaching, a practical nurse who alternates with the staff nurse and provides treatment and medications, and a home health aide who assists with hygiene and homemaker services. This nursing care delivery model may be used when the additional staff travel costs can be justified by reducing the total cost of providing the client's care by using less costly personnel.

A variation of the functional approach is to assign staff according to *client diagnostic categories.* In this approach, one nurse may be assigned all clients with tuberculosis and a different nurse's assignment may be limited to antepartum clients. The intent of this model is to improve nursing care quality by employing nurses with special expertise in the major client problem categories rather than expecting each nurse to maintain competence in all categories. This approach is often combined with the case or district method.

TEAM NURSING. In the *team nursing* care delivery model, a team of staff provides nursing care to a group of clients. The staff's work is coordinated by a designated team leader. Some community health agencies, especially larger agencies, have adapted team nursing to the community setting.

One type of team approach is a combination of team nursing and district nursing. A group of staff is assigned to a geographic area to provide care to all clients in that area. A team leader, usually an experienced community health nurse, is appointed. This position is a permanent assignment similar to the position of head nurse in a hospital. Depending on the agency's policies, nurses may be assigned their own case load. The team leader may assign cases according to the interests and experience of the nurse. This approach intends to match client and family needs with nurse expertise. The team leader may assign clients with certain nursing care problems to less experienced staff to develop the staff nurse's skills. In this case, it is important that the team leader plan for time to adequately supervise the inexperienced staff nurse so that she does learn and quality assurance objectives are not compromised.

In another variation of the team approach, the team leader retains responsibility for nursing care planning and scheduling of home visits. A master schedule is developed, and team members are assigned to clients or families on a daily or weekly basis. Team members do not have permanent caseloads. This application of organizing is more commonly observed in hospital-based home care organizations where staff move from the hospital to the home environment when providing nursing care. In this situation, the team leader assumes greater responsibility for coordinating care for each client and family and determining which personnel should be assigned. This approach is similar to the case method of delivering nursing care that was popular in hospitals in the 1920s (Marriner, 1984).

These nursing care delivery models have been applied to the home visit in the past and are still in use in public health nursing. Because of the high costs of delivering services in the home, administrators have tended to urge expansion of clinics and other approaches that increase the number of client contacts per day.

Leadership

With an appropriate plan and a clearly delineated organization, the community health nurse directs implementation of the plan. Everyone whose work involves the direction and supervision of other people is in a management position. The concept of leadership is a broader concept than the concept of manager. *Managers* systematize personal behaviors by establishing and requiring adherence to policies and procedures to meet organizational goals. Managers have formal authority by nature of their position in the organization to direct and evaluate the work of other employees.

Leaders strive to develop fresh approaches to long-standing problems and to create new options to resolve problems.

These new options may or may not be congruent with organizational goals. The effective leader projects ideas into images that excite people and only then develops choices that give the projected images substance. Followers support a leader's ideas and their implementation. In the small public health organization, the nurse's leadership opportunities occur with other community key persons, groups, and organizations.

The nurse manager will see that action is taken on all referrals and that a systematic approach is developed to carry out each request. If managers are leaders and use leadership skills, they can create an environment that allows for creativity and risk taking to meet the mandates of the organization. Leaders and managers differ in their view of their work. Leaders tend to view work as an enabling process, involving some combination of people and ideas interacting to establish strategies and make decisions. In the enabling process leaders help the process along, using a range of skills, including calculating the interests in opposing situations, staging and timing the surfacing of controversial issues, and reducing tensions. The manager, on the other hand, is more concerned with the accomplishment of organizational goals.

Staff members need to understand the management style of the nurse administrator. This will allow staff members to function much more effectively and constructively.

Evaluation and Control

The community health nurse manager is responsible for making sure that there is an ongoing evaluation of the implemented plan. The agency is accountable to the community for the quality of its care, and accountability is ensured by an effective evaluation process. Evaluation includes a reexamination of the original plan and its rationale, as well as the organization, its financial and human resources, and the degree to which goals were achieved. Evaluation may determine that there is need for reorganization. Standards for evaluation of the community nursing service have been developed by the ANA, the NLN, and the APHA. Meaningful criteria have been developed to verify the quality of the nursing unit's performance.

The community health nurse has responsibility and accountability to both the employer and the profession (as well as to clients and their families). Every community health nurse should be aware of these criteria.

MANAGEMENT PROCESS IN COMMUNITY HEALTH
Community Health Values

The management process involves consideration of values, either overtly through direct consideration or covertly through examination of organizational behavior. The values that underlie the practice of public health are rarely discussed in public health literature but appear to be known primarily through a process of oral tradition or oral history. Consideration of public health values, especially as compared with medical and nursing values, is important in understanding community health nursing management.

Community Health Goals

In community health organizations, it is desirable to specify organizational goals and objectives in terms that reflect the interest in the community's health. Miller and Moos (1981) note the renewed interest in using measures of community health to define organizational objectives and outcomes of programs. An example of such measures would be the use of a specific vital statistic rate as an objective and outcome criteria. If a community has a high fertility rate among adolescents, a reduction in the rate could be stated as an objective for the public health agency. Development and implementation of a health services program for adolescents, including family planning services, might then be considered as a program strategy for achieving the objective. Because of the community-level focus and the relationship to the social policy process, selecting intervention strategies in public health has a different focus than selecting those used by clinicians, such as in medical care settings. These strategies include regulation and provision of personal health services, education, and research.

Regulations

Community health nurses may be involved in implementing a variety of regulations. Examples include communicable disease case and contact follow-up, especially for infectious hepatitis and tuberculosis. The public health concern in these situations is protection of the noninfected members of the community by adequate treatment and quarantine of diagnosed cases and efforts to identify, diagnose, and potentially treat persons who have had contact with the client during the infectious phase. All states have communicable disease regulations as part of their public health laws. These regulations list diseases which are included. When functioning as a regulator, it is essential for the community health nurse to implement the regulations legally and uniformly.

Over time, it is possible for any regulation to become outdated, not merely because the regulation is old, but because improved surveillance, prevention, and treatment have resulted in elimination of the disease from the population. In that case, the nurse may be involved in the political process of changing the laws and regulations pertaining to that problem. An example is control of smallpox. Because of the virtual elimination of smallpox, smallpox immunizations are no longer required for school children or for most travelers to foreign countries.

Community health nurses are also involved in implementing legally required screening programs and following potential or identified cases. An example would be phenylketonuria (PKU) screening. All states have enacted mandatory PKU screening. With the trend of shorter hospitalizations for childbirth, community health nurses are more frequently involved in obtaining blood tests and following-up on infants with suspicious or positive test results. Although it may appear expensive to implement this legislation, screening is less expensive than chronic, long-term medical care for persons with untreated PKU.

Community health nurses may also be employed in positions in which regulation is the major job responsibility.

Nurses are involved with regulating the hospital and nursing home industries. In collaboration with other disciplines, the nurse's role is to verify that these organizations meet or exceed established standards.

Sometimes nurses collaborate with other community health professionals to improve services in a community. For example, environmental health professionals may be involved in implementing regulations regarding day care facilities. A community health nurse working in that team may find opportunities to improve health practices in day care facilities. The nurse may find opportunities to provide education to the day care facility staff on managing ill children, identifying children who are neglected or abused, or promoting normal growth and development.

While implementing regulations, *self-management,* including interpersonal communication, is important. Although the community, through its elected representatives, has enacted laws to protect the health of its citizens, not all members may agree that such laws and regulations are appropriate. Some persons may believe that their individual rights are improperly constrained when they are requested to comply with regulations. Others may resist because they are misinformed. The community health nurse should be sensitive to these issues and provide whatever information is appropriate to gain cooperation from the concerned individuals. Adopting a collaborative, assistive approach tends to result in cooperation more frequently than does an autocratic or controlling approach. However, if the individual and family continues to refuse mandated service, the community health nurse will need to use the enforcement strategies available in the community such as referring a family that is noncompliant with PKU screening to child protective services.

The community health nurse, depending on the specific goals and objectives of the organization, may be highly involved in regulatory strategies to promote community health. If one considers assessing clients and families for signs and symptoms of neglect and abuse or assessing the environment for compliance with minimal hygiene standards, then involvement with public health laws and regulations is part of every commuity health nurse's practice. However, community health nurses tend to perceive themselves as service providers rather than regulators.

Personal Health Services

Providing *personal health services,* especially to the medically indigent or disadvantaged, has not been highly valued among public health professionals. However, as Pickett (1980) notes, most community health programs are heavily involved in this intervention strategy. Community health nurses are especially involved in managing the delivery of personal health services. Among the several methods of service delivery are ambulatory clinics, mobile clinics, screening clinics, and home-based services.

Ambulatory Clinics

In this approach, clients are scheduled for *ambulatory clinic* services at a central location. Personnel assigned may include physicians, nurses, aides, nutritionists, social workers, and

volunteers. Frequently, especially for child and adult health screening or immunizations, these clinics are managed by nurses, either alone or with clerical staff. Clinics may be located in small communities or in suburban areas. The organization arranges for space and the nurse brings the appropriate supplies. Appointments may be scheduled or may be on a drop-in basis.

Using clinics to increase nurse efficiency has advantages and disadvantages. Nurse travel time is reduced but client travel time is increased. Travel to a clinic site may be difficult or impossible for some clients who then do not receive service. It is difficult to assess the home environment during a clinic interview. If drop-in "appointments" are allowed, maintaining consistent client charts, as well as assessing the client-family history, is a problem. Some clients attend nurse-managed clinic appointments only to find they also need physician evaluation, which may require an additional trip to another location on some future date. In some areas, it is difficult to find adequate facilities to provide clinic services. Finally, immediate access to a physician (for example, in the case of an allergic reaction to immunization) may be difficult to plan. However, for many clients these concerns present no problem; for them, a clinic format functions well.

With any clinic setting, time management may present problems. In large clinics, which use a variety of health professionals, a triage system is usually necessary. The nurse may be responsible for determining whether a visit with the nutritionist is necessary for the client. In such complex clinics, priorities are frequently established to assist the nurse in triage. An example would be referring the pregnant woman for nutrition services only if her hematocrit is below 34% or if she gains more than 5 pounds in 1 month. Volunteers are also used in clinic situations and can be very helpful in facilitating efficient flow of clients through the clinic by doing nonnursing tasks such as registration, measuring height and weight, or putting clients in examination rooms. However, it can take a tremendous amount of work to organize, schedule, and supervise volunteers.

Recording data can be problematic in the clinic setting. It is essential for the nurse to complete the record before beginning to interview the next client. If you interview 20 antepartum clients or mothers of 50 children before immunizations it is not possible to complete client records accurately at the end of the clinic session.

Mobile Clinics

Specially outfitted mobile vans have been used to provide *mobile clinic* services. They decrease the problems of inadequate physical facilities and nurse transportation of supplies, and increase the opportunity to provide services in a greater variety of geographic areas. With this approach, it is essential to communicate the various scheduled locations well in advance. The costs of adequately outfitting and maintaining mobile clinics can be high.

Screening Clinics

Management of screening clinic operations is not very different from any other type of clinic. However, there are differences in planning the procedures and follow-up activities. Certainly screening is a component of all client/nurse interactions. However, screening clinics have as their purpose early detection of specific health problems. *Screening clinics* may be single purpose or multipurpose (multiphasic). The multiphasic screening clinic screens individuals for more than one health problem during one clinic encounter.

Important issues must be considered in planning screening clinics. Screening is intended to identify unrecognized or undiagnosed disease in aggregates of the population. The proportion of a population that has been diagnosed is small compared with the presumably healthy population. Therefore the target population is usually quite large. It is essential to use a screening test that can be administered quickly and at nominal expense per person screened. Both *specific screening tests* (correctly classify persons with disease as diseased) and *sensitive screening tests* (correctly classify healthy persons as healthy) are necessary. Most screening tests are imperfect to some degree. Therefore planning for screening clinics should include procedures to minimize problems associated with misclassification. An example of problems associated with misclassification would be selection of a screening test that was highly sensitive but not highly specific for pregnancy. In this example, a positive pregnancy test would reliably predict actual pregnancy. However, a negative pregnancy test would not assure nonpregnancy. If the test was negative, the client would be advised that the test could be wrong. If a determination of her condition was important to the client, additional testing or counseling would be arranged.

Other aspects of planning include establishing a method for recording, reporting, and following up on persons with positive screening tests. Marketing the screening program involves informing the target population of the availability of screening and working with others such as physicians for support for the screening clinic. Notifying the target population may only mean placing advertisements in the mass media (including radio, television, and newspapers). It may also mean personal contact with each person in the eligible population by letter or telephone.

Planning for follow-up care or definitive diagnoses is as important as any other aspect of screening. However, it is frequently minimally addressed in the planning process. Follow-up care in many screening clinics is restricted to interpreting the results of the test to the person and advising those persons with positive results to seek further evaluation. If the community health nurse feels screening is an important activity, then follow-up should be equally valued. It may be necessary to contact persons with positive tests at some future time to ascertain whether the nurse's advice was followed (to seek further evaluation) and to learn the results of the evaluation. It is also necessary to evaluate the capacity of existing community resources to conduct the recommended evaluation and to provide the necessary treatment. As an example, the Hypertension Selection and Follow-up Program's (1979) findings illustrated the benefits that could be obtained through population-based screening, referral, and follow-up.

Home Visits

Managing a *home visit* schedule, especially if it includes both health promotion and communicable disease clients, can be complex. The problems encountered in a hospital environment (the need to return to the nurse's station to obtain additional equipment or the delay in changing a dressing because the client has gone to physical therapy) are exacerbated in the community setting. For example, arriving at a family's home without essential equipment may necessitate a return trip to the office to obtain the equipment. If the one-way transportation time is 30 minutes, then an hour has been wasted due to poor planning. Additionally, that hour might have been used to visit another client, whose care is now delayed due to poor planning.

Many organizations have policies regarding prioritization of clients. The rationale underlying prioritization includes the client's physical and psychosocial condition, as well as the organization's history with the client. If the client is new to the organization, the priority for service is usually high. Once a thorough assessment has been completed and a plan of care established it is easier to predict the complexity and frequency of further home visits. The information available to the nurse on the referral form is often limited to the person's name, address, and reason for the visit. A thorough assessment is thus essential. Additionally assessment enables rapid feedback to the person who actually made the referral. Informal data suggest that prompt response to persons who refer clients including information about the client situation tends to result in future referrals. For an organization whose main income is from home care, maintaining referral networks is important. Rapid response to referrals and rapid feedback is an important management aspect of the community nurse's role.

Harris (1985) states that in planning for the home visits, the nurse would need to consider that new clients frequently require about double the average time of 30 to 45 minutes for the home visit to complete admission and data base assessments and to establish a relationship with the client and family. More time is also required when two people (e.g., mother and child) require examination.

It is also necessary for the community health nurse to be knowledgeable about other community resources. Some communities publish books about the services available in the community. Other communities have an "information and referral" service, which functions as a clearing house for information about available services. It is often more efficient to telephone the information and referral service than to telephone 10 agencies to find out if a particular client's needs can be met by that agency.

Efficiency in home visiting also applies to nonvisit time or time spent recording, completing billing records, consulting with other professionals, supervising home health aides, and telephoning. Community health nurses are frequently equipped with dictaphones so that they can tape nursing notes while driving or during other nonvisit activities. The nurse should become expert at the art of dictation and use of the equipment to avoid spending time correcting transcribed notes (and to facilitate the transcriber's work). It is common for agencies to use computers to manage billing and financial documents. In this case, the nurse's reports must be accurate. Use of computers to manage the client's care through computerized client/family data bases and reports is becoming more common. Computer literacy may soon become an entry level skill for community health nurses.

Efficiency, especially in home visiting, is also related to having a dependable, maintained vehicle. Years ago, agencies often supplied and maintained vehicles for nurses. Today, the nurse is usually expected to provide transportation. Planning for vehicular problems is part of the nurse's job.

Monitoring and improving one's effectiveness and efficiency in community health nursing is accomplished through supervision. Home visiting as an intervention strategy is generally an independent nursing activity. Many community health nurses enjoy the autonomy and opportunity to implement the independent functions of nursing. However, when confronted with novel client situations, it is difficult to know whether the assessment data are accurate and complete and whether the nursing diagnosis and intervention plans are appropriate. It is likely that no one else knows the family and thus the only set of client data is that collected by the nurse. The community health nurse should seek supervision in these situations. Supervision may include telephone conferences, office conferences, and joint home visits. Establishing a supervisor-staff nurse relationship as a continuous routine pattern of behavior facilitates obtaining assistance for nonroutine client situations.

In organizations that employ many community health nurses, it is also possible to share complex clients with another staff nurse(s). Examples of clients to be considered for sharing include: (1) families with a history of child abuse, especially if home visits have been ordered by juvenile courts; (2) families who are caring for a terminally ill family member at home; or (3) clients or families who are extremely demanding. Sharing cases like these can help reduce the nurse's frustration and potential for burnout.

Continuing education, although necessary to stay abreast of changes in nursing, can be complex in community health nursing, especially if the nurse visits clients with a wide variety of nursing care diagnoses. Agency sponsored staff development activities are only one way to maintain competence. Attending staff development programs offered by hospitals is another method. Regular reading of professional journals and active involvement in professional associations are also appropriate. Many community health nurses also identify expert nurses in the local area and develop informal consulting relationships with them. Thus, when the nurse needs help with a specific nursing care problem, expert advice may be obtained by telephone.

From the perspective of administration, home care tends to be viewed as an expensive approach to delivering nursing care. In some cases, it is the only available approach; in others, home visiting continues because it is a tradition. The community health nurse must always be alert for opportunities to deliver quality care efficiently and for opportunities to participate in well-designed research efforts to determine the true effects of home care.

Health Education

Health education, as used here, implies education of the entire community and its aggregates regarding health. It is different than teaching an individual on a one-to-one basis. Presenting information verbally is only one teaching strategy. Instructional strategies for health education include video productions for television and preparing posters and pamphlets for use with a variety or persons in a variety of settings.

Community health nurses are frequently involved as content experts in preparing mass media productions. In this situation, the nurse may work with photographers, graphic artists, and others to develop instructional materials that are relevant, accurate, and marketable. Community health nurses may also use these materials in instructing individuals and groups about health matters. It is appropriate for the nurse to maintain a file of pamphlets and other materials to use in implementing teaching plans with clients, families, and other groups. Clients as learners may find they have questions later when the nurse is not available. Instructional materials, especially those that can be given to others, are available at any time. Learning is often enhanced when multiple teaching methods and media are used.

Research

Community health nurses are frequently involved in research. This may mean participation in data collection activities (completion of communicable disease reports), or it may mean developing studies of the epidemiology of a specific disease or nursing care problem. In most communities and states, it is relatively simple to monitor age, race, and sex specific causes of mortality. However, information about morbidity is much more difficult to obtain.

The community health nurse often uses epidemiological data to identify aggregates of the population who are at risk of developing specific health problems. These data identify "target populations" for intervention. An understanding of incidence, prevalence, risk factors, and rates is essential to the development of appropriate intervention strategies and to identifying appropriate methods for evaluating interventions. For example, if you determine that the adolescent fertility rate in the community is higher than desired, it may be appropriate to intervene. The target population in this case is all adolescents. It is appropriate to identify the risk factors associated with adolescent pregnancy and to generate a list of possible intervention strategies. These strategies should be classified as primary, secondary, or tertiary prevention. Goals, objectives, and evaluation criteria can be established and budget estimates prepared. It is essential to plan for a method for collecting surveillance data. Community health nurses are frequently involved in collecting surveillance data, especially when existing data collection systems are inappropriate.

Participation in epidemiological investigations may lead to development of new community health services or other interventions. Careful consideration should be given to the ethical dilemmas associated with participation in these studies. A current example is the epidemiological research regarding acquired immune deficiency syndrome (AIDS). In studying the epidemiology of this public health problem, investigators are monitoring entire populations, usually on a voluntary basis for HTLV-III antibodies. Identifying the subpopulation and its characteristics and monitoring this group prospectively is important to full understanding of AIDS epidemiology. However, what measures should be taken to assure confidentiality for persons who volunteer to be screened? If screening is included as part of a preemployment examination, should the employer have access to the test results? Additionally, what services should be available to persons with positive tests? What services should be available to sexual partners of persons with positive tests? Dilemmas like this often reflect conflict between the values and philosophy of public health, which tends to be community-oriented, and nursing, which tends to be oriented toward individuals. Responding to these and other ethical questions before initiating research and surveillance (as well as intervention projects) is a professional responsibility.

CLINICAL APPLICATIONS

The following situation illustrates the systems theory concept of input, transformation, and output with respect to the management process as compared to the nursing process. A community health nurse analyzes the assigned caseload and travel schedule and notices that home visits to six mothers with infants who are less than 1 year of age and who all live in the same apartment building are necessary. The nurse considers establishing a mother's group within the building for the following reasons:

1. In a group, mothers could learn from and get support from each other as well as from the nurse, who would participate in the group.
2. The nurse's productivity could be increased by seeing the six mothers together versus separately, which would create more visit time, decrease travel time, and increase time for other activities.
3. Advertising the group in the apartment building may result in involvement of other mothers who are not currently receiving community health nursing service.

The nurse discusses this idea with the supervisor, who agrees to support the idea and bring it to the nurse administrator. The administrator, knowing that there is no precedent for staff members working with community groups like this, concurs that the idea is good but requests additional information:

1. If the group meets at times outside of regular business hours, how will compensation for the nurse be managed?
2. Will the agency need to consider paying rent and/or housekeeping charges for a meeting room?
3. Has the nurse had education and experience in managing group process?
4. Is it necessary to establish a procedure for this situation?

5. How will this activity be evaluated?
6. How will the recording be done on the clients' records? Will changes in the format of the nurse's daily record be needed?

In this situation the nurse's concept of inputs includes information from clients, such as feeling isolated and needing to talk with other mothers, and the nurse's time and willingness to try a group approach. The administrator's concept of inputs includes those provided by the nurse and those having to do with organizational resources, staff knowledge, insurance, space, money, supervision, and security.

In this example, both the staff nurse and the administrator are engaged in management. The scope, or number of variables, and complexity of their management activities is different. Nevertheless, each is using the same problem-solving process.

◆　◆　◆

The next example illustrates management of multiple home visits. The community health nurse plans to visit six clients. Take 20 minutes to read the case summaries. Then plan the sequence of visits including 45 minutes for lunch and returning to the office by 3:30 PM for a staff meeting. Figure 36-5 is a map showing the location of the nurses' office and the client homes, which correspond to the client numbers.

1. Miss James is a 16-year-old who delivered a 6 lb. 3 oz. son at County Hospital last night. She had no prenatal care. She lives with her parents. She signed out of the hospital 8 hours after delivery. This is your first visit.
2. Mr. Andrews has severe chronic obstructive lung disease. He is on 2 to 4 L of O_2 per nasal cannula at home. He sees no reason to quit smoking at this late date. You have been instructing his wife on home intermittent positive pressure breathing device and chest physical therapy. She has called to report that he has had a temperature of 102 degrees for 24 hours.
3. Bill McKay is a 6-year-old who was born with myelomeningocele. He is paraplegic. You are instructing his new foster mother on catheterization. She is doing well.
4. Mrs. Fristan is a 53-year-old insulin-dependent diabetic. She has a draining, gangrenous right foot. The culture report is antibiotic-resistant *Staphylococcus aureus*. You are to soak the foot and apply dressings.
5. Mr. Landers is a 70-year-old man with serious, chronic congestive heart failure who lives alone. He is an alcoholic who alternates between sobriety and beer-and-pretzel binges. When you call to arrange the appointment, you note he is short of breath and hear gurgling as he breathes. He is complaining of chest pain.
6. Mrs. Stoddard delivered her third child 4 days ago. She has been home 1 day. She has called, frantic because the two older children are both running high fevers and are very irritable. She mentions that her baby-sitter's children just got over chickenpox.

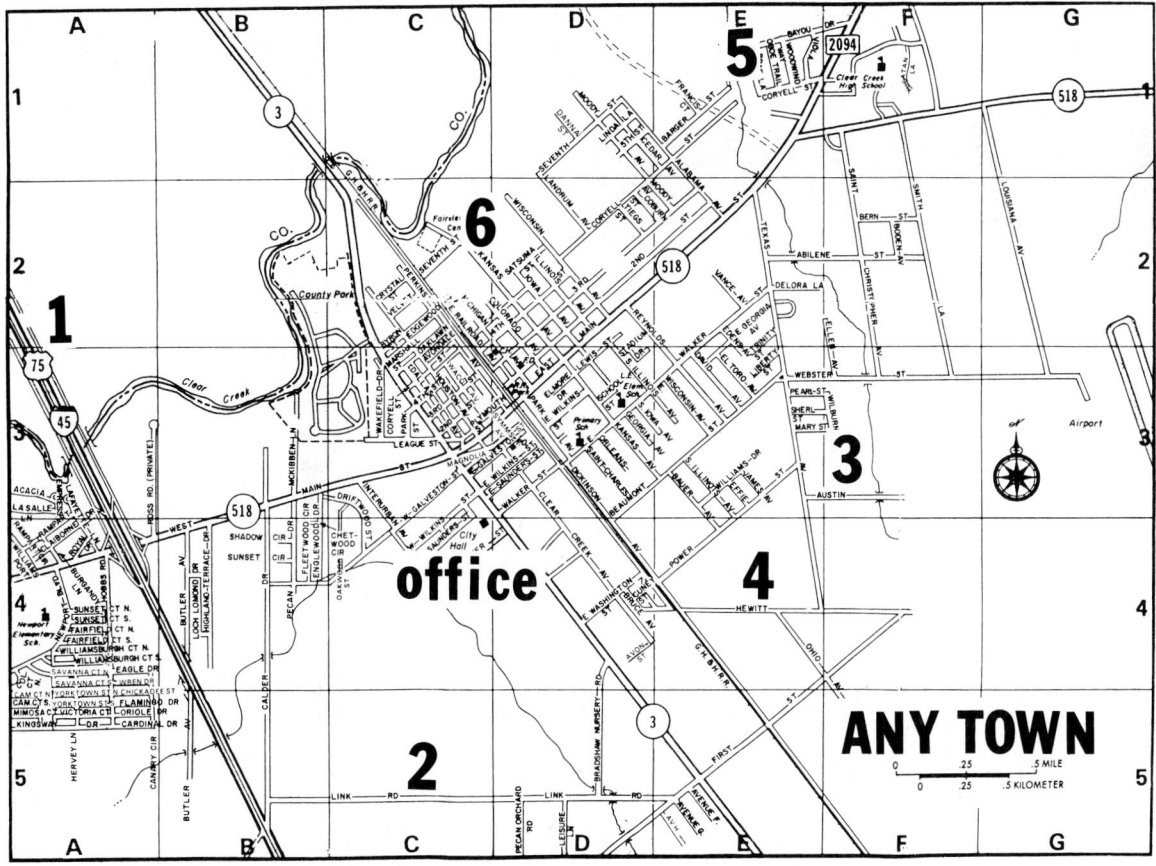

FIGURE 36-5

Anytown, USA.

After reviewing these case summaries, it may be very tempting to immediately drive to Mr. Landers or Miss James depending on your personal view about the priority needs of these clients. However, it would be wise to take a few minutes to plan your schedule for the day.

Care for clients who are experiencing life-threatening health problems should not wait until the community health nurse can arrive to assess their condition. In this situation, the nurse's most appropriate response is to telephone the physician or hospital to arrange for an ambulance. Or, the nurse should call the community's emergency medical services (EMS) team.

Three clients have high priority for visits early in the day. They are Miss James, Mr. Andrews, and Mr. Landers. The next step in setting up appointments is to consider geography and establish a visit sequence that will minimize travel time. The remaining clients, except for Mrs. Fristan, could be seen at any time, depending on travel time efficiencies. Mrs. Fristan should probably be seen last to minimize the possibility that the nurse could inadvertently infect another client. Isolation procedures in the home environment are often difficult.

Mr. Andrews and Mr. Landers may also require longer than average visits. The available information suggests that the nurse may need to refer these clients for additional services of the physician, pharmacy, and possibly the hos-

pital. Many community nurses carry notebooks with information about each client (if client records are not available in the home) so that the referral process can be expedited from the client's home rather than waiting until the nurse returns to the office.

Although the nurse plans to visit each of these clients today, the plan must be flexible. The nurse may anticipate that a home visit will last 30 minutes but, arriving at the client's home, finds that the visit will require more time. For example, let's assume that the nurse telephoned Mr. Lander's physician and anticipated arranging for hospitalization. The physician, however, orders serial doses of Lasix to be given in the home until diuresis occurs. The visit may now require additional time depending on how many doses will be needed; or, the nurse may call the office for messages and find that an additional client requires a home visit that day. It may be necessary to reschedule or work overtime, depending on the situation.

SUMMARY

Until recently, sophisticated management concepts have not been applied in community health nursing. Articles about computerization of records, development of client classification systems (including DRG's) and outcomes that may be attributed to intervention by community health nurses are relatively new in the community health nursing literature. The sophistication of community health nursing research, regarding both practice and management, will likely increase in the coming decade.

Values about community and health have determined a philosophy of public health and a set of basic intervention strategies. These intervention strategies (regulation, service, education, and research) are broader than those typically associated with nursing. Additionally, the unit of service is most commonly the individual client and family. Nurses employed in community health most frequently intervene with clients. However, these clients receive nursing service because they are target populations. Application of the nursing management process by community health nurses within public health is essential to the client, the agency, and the community.

⹀ KEY CONCEPTS

Leadership implies ability to influence the behavior of others (colleagues or clients) toward achievement of a mutually established goal or objective.

The role of the manager is to coordinate the efforts of the subordinates toward attainment of goals and objectives as determined by the organization.

Strategic planning is long range and encompasses ends (outcomes) as well as means (processes). In contrast, tactical planning uses shorter time frames, a narrower scope, more attention to detail, and more flexibility.

In the program budget expenses and income are related to a specific service. The performance budget clearly and concisely shows services to be provided in return for funds available or income generated.

The heart of any service organization is the human resources that have been attracted to the organization—the human knowledge and skills available that lead to the ability to implement the plans for the programs that have been designed or are expected to be accomplished.

Organizing involves arranging and defining the relationship between both personnel and other resources by establishing a structure.

The type of nursing care delivery model used by an agency is related to the size and complexity of the agency.

In small agencies, the nursing care delivery model most often used is a variation of primary nursing. In this method, the individual nurse is responsible for individual clients and families who are referred to the agency for service and who meet the agency's admission criteria (which often include geography).

The functional nursing care delivery model assigns staff nurses and other personnel to client functions such as medications, treatments, hygiene, and client teaching.

In the team nursing care delivery model, a team of staff provides nursing care to a group of clients.

The concept of leadership is a broader concept than the concept of manager.

Leaders strive to develop fresh approaches to long-standing problems and to create new options to resolve problems. These new options may not be congruent with organizational goals.

Evaluation includes a reexamination of the original plan and its rationale, as well as the organization and its financial and human resources, and the degree to which goals were achieved.

Public health work may be defined as an interdisciplinary activity that seeks to provide the greatest good for the greatest number at the least cost for purposes of maintaining or improving the level of health in a population.

Values about community and health have determined a philosophy of public health and a set of basic intervention strategies. These intervention strategies (regulation, service, education, and research) are broader than those typically associated with nursing.

LEARNING ACTIVITIES

1. Interview a few community health nurses and have them describe their work relationships within the organization and with other community agencies. Diagram these relationships to identify the community health nurse's work environment or system.

2. Read the job description for a community health nurse manager or administrator. Identify the types of planning which are required in that position.

3. Discuss the plan for assigning work to staff nurses in the agency where you have clinical experience. Identify the nursing care delivery model utilized by the agency.

4. Based on assessment of community needs, identify a program which needs to be developed. Prepare a brief plan for the program (goals, objectives, financial and human resources, and evaluation criteria). Describe how you visualize the management role of the community health nurse in this program.

5. Write a four paragraph paper (one paragraph each on planning, organizing, leading, and evaluation) describing how you have managed nursing care in the clinical component of your community health nursing course.

BIBLIOGRAPHY

American Nurses' Association: Standards for community health nursing practice, Kansas City, 1973, The Association.

American Nurses' Association: Standards for organized nursing services, Kansas City, 1982, The Association.

Arndt, C., and Huckabay, L.: Nursing Administration: Theory for practice with a systems approach, St. Louis, 1975, The C.V. Mosby Co.

Barnard, C.: The functions of the executive, Cambridge, 1938, Harvard University Press.

Belin, L.E.: Local health departments: a prescription against obsolesence. In Levin, A., editor: Health services: the local perspective, New York, 1977, Academy of Political Science.

Canadian Task Force on The Periodic Health Examination: The periodic health examination, J. Can. Med. Assoc., 121:1-45, 1979.

Cayner, A.: Home visiting by public health nurses: a vanishing resource for families and children, zero to three. National Center for Clinical Infant Programs, 6:1:1-7, 1985.

Clute, K.: Law and health. In McKinlay, J.B., editor: Politics and the law in health care policy, New York, 1973, Prodist.

Combs-Orme, T., Reis, J., and Ward, L.D.: Effectiveness of home visits by public health nurses: an empirical review, Public Health Rep., 100(5):490-99, 1985.

Dawson, J.: The use of computers in public health nursing: today or tomorrow, Canadian Nurse pp. 40-43, 1985.

DiVincente, M.: Administering nursing service. Boston, 1972, Little, Brown, & Co.

Etzioni, A.: Modern organizations, Englewood Cliffs, N.J., 1964, Prentice-Hall, Inc.

Filley, A., and House, R.J.: Managerial process and organizational behavior, Glenview, IL, 1969, Scott, Foresman & Co.

Freeman, Ruth B.: Community health nursing practice. Philadelphia, 1970, W.B. Saunders.

Hanlon, J.J., and Pickett, G.D.: Public health administration and practice, St. Louis, 1984, The C.V. Mosby Co.

Harris, M.D., and Santaferraro, C.: A patient classification system in home health care, Nursing Economics 3:276-282, 1985.

Hypertension Detection and Follow-up Program Cooperative Group: Five year findings of the hypertension detection and follow-up program. I and II, JAMA 23:2562-77, 1979.

Janczak, D.: Changes in a rural public health nursing program: a community profile, Home Health Care Nurse 3(5):28-34, 1985.

Knollmueller, R.N.: Community health nursing supervisor: a handbook for community/home care managers, New York, 1986, National League for Nursing.

Lancaster, J.: Systems theory and the process of change. In Lancaster, J. and Lancaster, W., editors: Concepts for advanced nursing practice: the nurse as a change agent, St. Louis, 1982, The C.V. Mosby Co.

Last, J.M., editor: Public health and preventive medicine, New York, 1980, Appleton-Century-Crofts.

Levy, S., and Loomba, N.P.: Health care administration, Philadelphia, 1973, J.B. Lippincott Co.

Marriner, A.: Guide to nursing management, St. Louis, 1984, The C.V. Mosby Co.

Miller, C.A., and Moos, M.D.: Local health departments, Washington, D.C., 1981, American Public Health Association.

Minnesota Department of Health: Outcome auditing: one component of a quality assurance program, Unpublished manuscript, 1978.

Pickett, G.: The future of health departments: the governmental presence, Annu. Rev. Public Health 1:297, 1980.

Ramsey County Public Health Nursing Service: Health-specific family coping index. Unpublished manuscript, 1983.

Sienkiewicz, J.: Patient classification in community health nursing, Nurs. Outlook 32(6):319-321, 1984.

Simon, H.: Administrative behavior, New York, 1947, Macmillan Publishing Co., Inc.

Stevens, B.: Nursing theory: analysis, application, and evaluation, Boston, 1979, Little, Brown & Co.

Suchman, E.: Evaluation research: principles and practice in public service and social action programs, New York, 1967, Russell Sage Foundation.

Wing, K.: The law and the public's health, St. Louis, 1976, The C.V. Mosby Co.

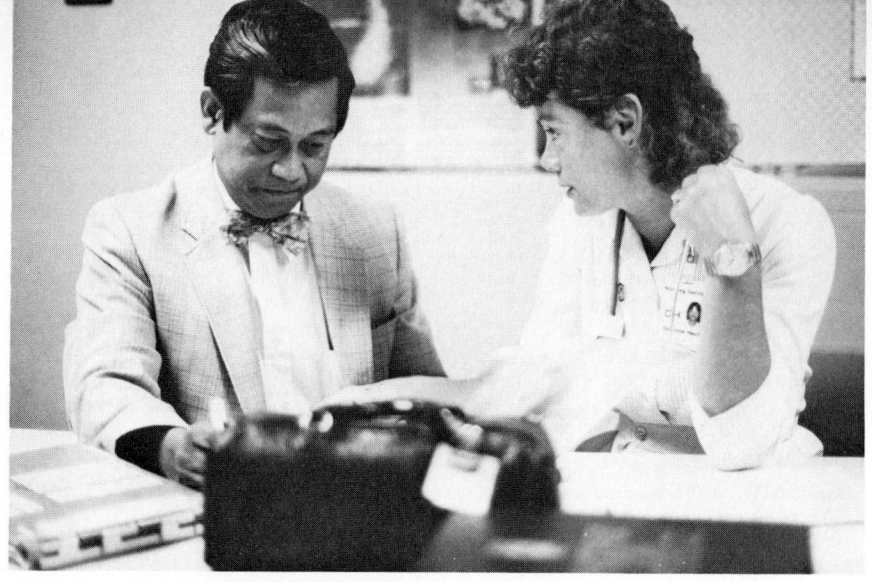

Marcia Stanhope
Rena Alford

37

THE COMMUNITY HEALTH NURSE CONSULTANT

OBJECTIVES

After reading this chapter, the student should be able to:

Describe the meaning of consultation in community health nursing practice.

State the major goals of consultation.

Discuss theories of consultation and their applicability to community health nursing practice.

Apply the principles of process consultation in community health nursing practice.

Compare and contrast the internal and the external nurse consultant role functions.

Discuss the educational requirements and select practice arenas for the nurse consultant.

KEY TERMS

acceptant intervention mode
catalytic intervention mode
client population
conflict sources
confrontation intervention mode
consultation
consultative contract
doctor—patient model
generalist
goals/objectives
morale/cohesion
norms/standards
nurse consultant
political process model
power/authority
prescriptive intervention mode
process model
purchase model
specialist
theory-principles intervention mode

Nurses bring to the community skills that allow them to be valuable contributing members in their work setting and in the community-at-large. The specific skills helpful in the community are the nurses' preparation for comprehensively assessing all factors that have an influence on individual, family, group, and community health status; the nurses' abilities to plan, implement, and evaluate goals and programs for individuals, groups, families, and communities as units of service; and the nurses' extensive knowledge of community resources and the referral process. These skills provide the nurse with the expertise and information to function as a consultant to the individual, family, group, or community client, as well as to others working with a variety of clients.

◆ ◆ ◆

This chapter focuses on the definition and goals of consultation, consultative theories pertinent to community health nursing, principles relative to process consultation, and the scope of the nurse consultant role. The purpose of the discussion is to acquaint the reader with consultation as a role function of community health nursing.

DEFINITIONS AND GOALS

Consultation, like many other concepts, has a variety of definitions. Schein (1969) described *consultation* as a process involving a set of activities on the part of the helper, which assists the client to perceive, understand, and act on events occurring in the client's environment. Caplan (1970) defined consultation as a process in which the help of a specialist is sought to identify ways to handle work problems involving either the management of clients or the planning and implementation of programs. Others refer to consultation as an interpersonal interaction between the person with expert knowledge and a client for the planned purpose of helping the client make constructive behavioral changes (Clark, 1983; Oda, 1982).

The *goal* of consultation is to stimulate clients to take more responsibility, feel more secure, deal constructively with their feelings and with others in interaction, and internalize skills of a flexible and creative nature. The functions of the consultant differ from the role functions of administrator, supervisor, coordinator, planner, educator,

researcher, and client advocate in that consultation typically is a temporary and a voluntary relationship between a professional helper and a client who has perceived a need for assistance. The relationship is a cooperative effort between consultant and client, established to share equally in the resolution of a problem.

Although consultants are commonly thought to be "outside" resource persons, that is, not part of the power system in the work setting, this statement may not apply to the community health nurse consultant. The community health nurse finds job expectations to include both internal and external consultation. For example, the community health nurse may be employed to consult with other nurses in the agency about client care problems, or the community health nurse as an employee of the health department may serve as a consultant to a local retirement center about the public health care needs of the community served by the center.

If the community health nurse is an internal consultant, the nurse is employed on a full-time salaried basis by a community agency in which the consultation takes place. If the community health nurse is an external consultant, the nurse is employed on a contractual basis within a time period by the client with whom they consult. The client of the external nurse consultant may be a colleague, another health provider, or a community group or organization. The nature of the consultative relationship, internal or external, should not change the goal of consultation.

THEORIES OF CONSULTATION

Although nursing's involvement in consultation has expanded through the decades, few data are found in the literature about the impact of the nurse consultant on health care delivery. Selected theories of consultation are discussed to provide a basic understanding of approaches for establishing the consultation relationship.

The Purchase Model

Purchase model consultation, Figure 37-1, is defined as the purchase (hiring) of a professional helper by a client for the purpose of providing expert information or expert service (Schein, 1969). Others refer to this particular model as "expert consultation" (Sedwick, 1973; Lareau, 1980; Oda, 982). Buyers may be individuals, groups, or organizations. In this model the client predetermines the need for the

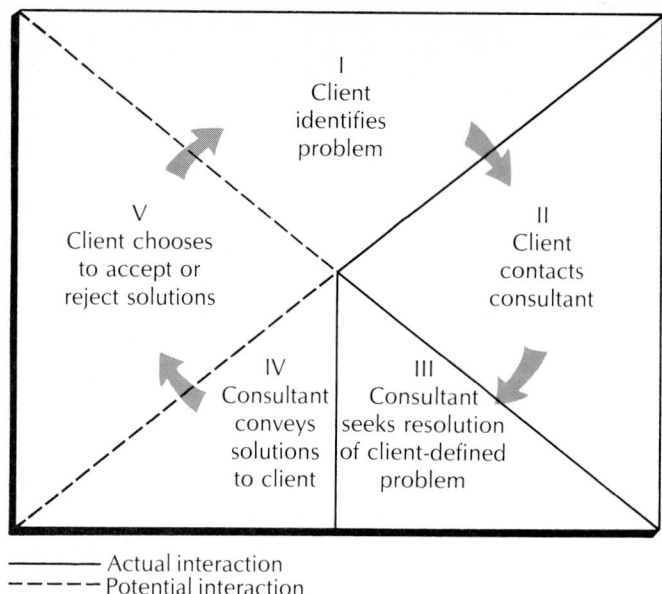

FIGURE 37-1

The purchase model.

consultant. The need is defined as something the client wants to know or some activity the client wants implemented. The purchase model assumes the following:

1. The client will correctly diagnose the problem.
2. The client will be able to correctly communicate the needs to the consultant.
3. The client will correctly assess the consultant's expertise to provide the information or perform the service.
4. The client knows the consequences of having the consultant provide the information or the consequences of implementing services suggested by the consultant.

The advantage of the popular purchase model is that the client does not have to spend time or energy in solving the identified problem because it is the responsibility of the "expert consultant" to solve the problem for the client. The disadvantage of the model is that the quality of the consultation may be questioned by the client if the client has identified the wrong problem or if the client does not like the consultant's solution to the problem.

Examples of use of the purchase model to provide information to the buyer are varied. For example, the executive director of a home health agency may employ a consultant to provide direction for a survey of client satisfaction with nursing services. The public health department supervisors may employ a consultant to instruct them in designing a method for improving nurse productivity. Similarly, a clinic administrator may request information about how to design an accounting system to highlight the costs of nursing services. In all instances, the client has defined the problem before employing the consultant and has determined that the consultant's knowledge is needed to provide a solution.

Specific examples of consultant services purchased to pro-

vide services are as follows: (1) The district nursing supervisor requests the state health department's maternal-child health nursing consultant to come to the district health department and reorganize the family planning clinic for efficient operation. The consultant may need to survey client scheduling procedures, numbers of staff available to implement the clinic, client compliance, absenteeism, and clinic demand as well as available facilities and equipment in order to make recommendations about clinic reorganization. (2) The community health nursing staff members request a consultant to analyze their caseloads to establish client mix guidelines for future client assignments. To do so, the nurse consultant may need to review records for age, sex, diagnosis, physical activity, and client service demands to arrive at a client classification system to be used for distributing equitable caseloads. The staff has determined the necessity for an expert consultant's active participation in finding and implementing a solution to the problem.

Although the purchase model is often used by consultants and clients, the consultant enters the picture at the point of implementation for problem resolution. This model may be unsatisfactory in effectively and efficiently identifying and resolving client problems. Once the consultant has implemented steps to solve the problem, the client must live with the consequences of the changes instigated by the consultants. Thus, it is not viewed as the best model to apply in community health nursing.

The Doctor–Patient Model

Another popular consultative model is the *doctor-patient model* (Figure 37-2), in which the consultant is employed by the client to find the problem and offer solutions without background data or assistance from the client (Schein, 1969). This model assumes the following:

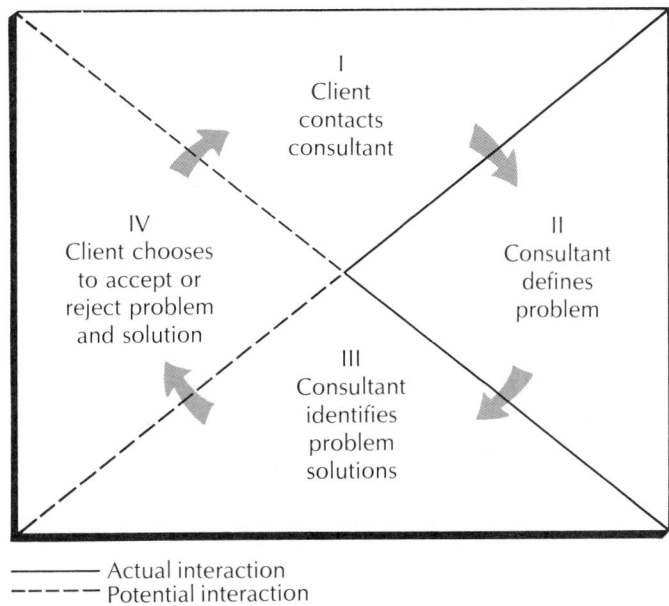

—————— Actual interaction
------- Potential interaction

FIGURE 37-2

The doctor-patient model.

1. The client is willing to reveal information needed by the consultant to make an appropriate diagnosis.
2. The consultant, through observations, will be able to get an accurate picture of the problem.
3. The client will accept the diagnosis and the prescriptions offered by the consultant.

Again, the major advantage of this model from the client's viewpoint is the limited time and energy expenditure required of the client. However, disadvantages outweigh any advantage that may exist in using this model. The patient, who is identified as the problem by the employing client, may be uncooperative and reluctant to share information the consultant needs to arrive at a fair diagnosis. Given the diagnosis, the patient and the client may be unwilling to believe and to accept suggestions for change. Also, the consultant-client-patient communication relationship is not well established, and the ensuing communication gap, resulting from lack of involvement in the diagnosis process, may make the prescriptions seem irrelevant or untenable to the client and the patient (Schein, 1969).

This model is often applied in nursing situations requiring consultative services. The director of nursing at the public health department calls in a nurse consultant from the local university. Nurse performance is poor, according to the director, and the nurse consultant is asked to diagnose what is wrong with the department. In this example the nursing director is the client and the staff nurses are the patient. The staff nurses must provide the data that will identify the problem for the consultant (doctor). If the problem is found to be poor administrative organization and direction rather than lack of quality of performance among the staff, the administrator may be reluctant to accept the diagnosis. Since the client and the patient are reluctant to be a part of the assessment of the problem, the goals of consultation cannot be met. This model, therefore,

is seen as an ineffective model to apply in community health nursing.

The Political Process Model

Consultation has been described as a political process (Baizerman and Hall, 1977; Hendrix and LaGodna, 1982). The definition offered for the *political process model* (Figure 37-3) is "consultation is a political bargaining process in which expertise, organizational position, personal and organizational reputation are the currency of the bargaining between consultant and consultee; and in which each actor attempts to maximize his currency at a minimum cost" (Baizerman and Hall, 1977, p. 143). This model assumes the following:

1. A persistent pattern of human relationships exists in consultation, which is influenced by power and authority.
2. The consultant is an agent acting on behalf of or for another.
3. Manipulation, influence, and negotiation are acceptable ways to control differences, reach settlement, and exchange expertise.
4. Participants in the bargaining system will benefit from the system.
5. Open and closed issues exist in the bargaining situation.

The political process model assumes that the consultant has four major functions:

1. *Problem creation:* defining and legitimizing the problem
2. *Priority raising:* raising the problem as a priority to get action within the consultee agency
3. *Legitimation:* legitimating or redefining the problem to arrive at problem resolution or continued bargaining

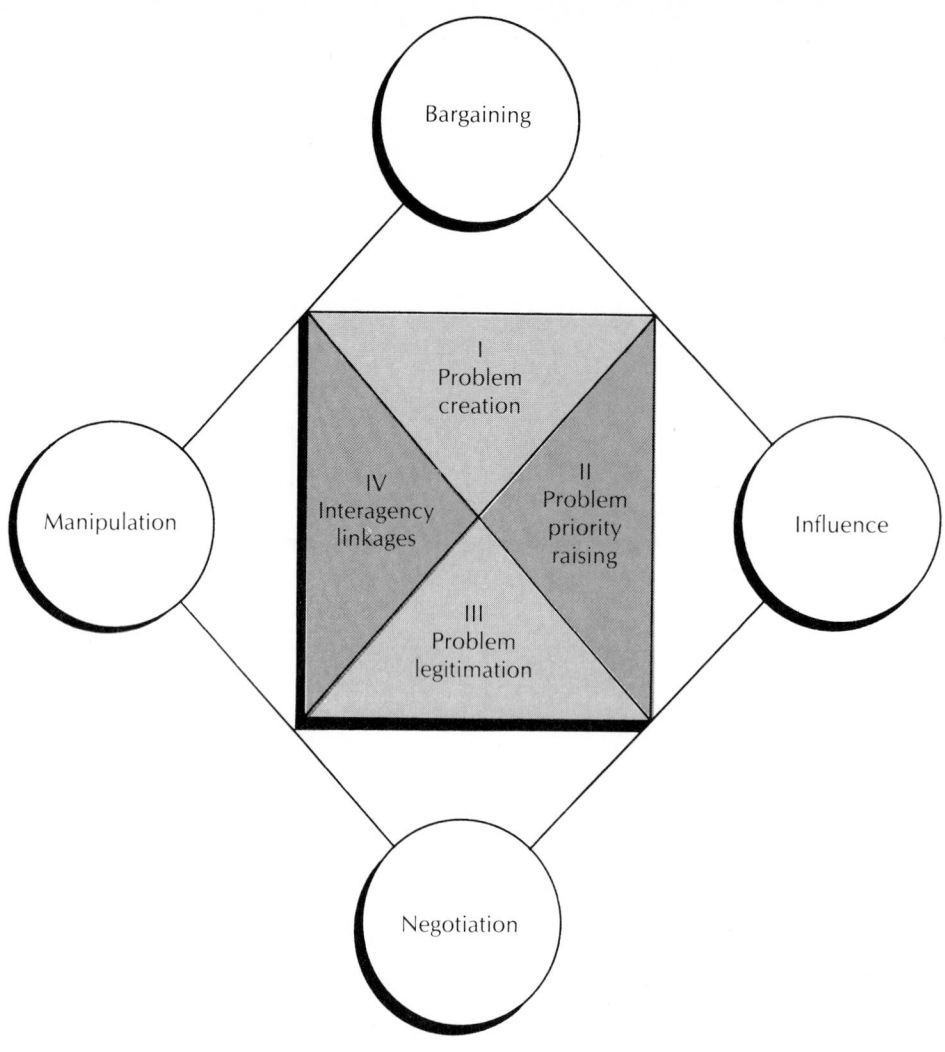

FIGURE 37-3

The political process model.

4. *Interagency linkages:* creating and sustaining interagency linkage

For example, a staff nurse in the local public health department may have noticed a number of alcoholics among the caseload. The nurse requests and is given permission to call in a member of the local alcoholism council to assist in finding data that will show alcoholism to be a major local problem *(problem creation)*. The consultant is asked by the staff nurse (consultee) to present the facts and alternative actions to the agency administration *(priority raising)*. The administration has ignored the need for an alcohol abuse program for years because the administration's philosophy is that alcoholism is a social problem and not a health problem. The consultant presents data to indicate the nature of alcoholism and the health-related problems *(legitimation)* and suggests a joint program to be sponsored by the health department and the alcoholism council *(interagency linkage)*. The political process model is viewed as a process more applicable to the community client than to the individual or family client where interagency linkage may not be an issue. The process model and the political process model are similar in scope, and each may be equally applicable in community health nursing, depending on the nature of the client.

Four models have been reviewed to offer an overview of consultation: the process consultation model, the purchase model, the doctor-patient model, and the political process model. The remaining discussion will focus on the process consultation model and its application in community health nursing.

The Process Model

Schein's definition of consultation (1969) describes process consultation. The major goals of the *process model,* as seen in Figure 37-4, are to assist the client to assess both the problem and the kind of help needed to resolve the problem. Problem solving is a key tool used in process consultation. Both the consultant and the consultee engage in the prob-

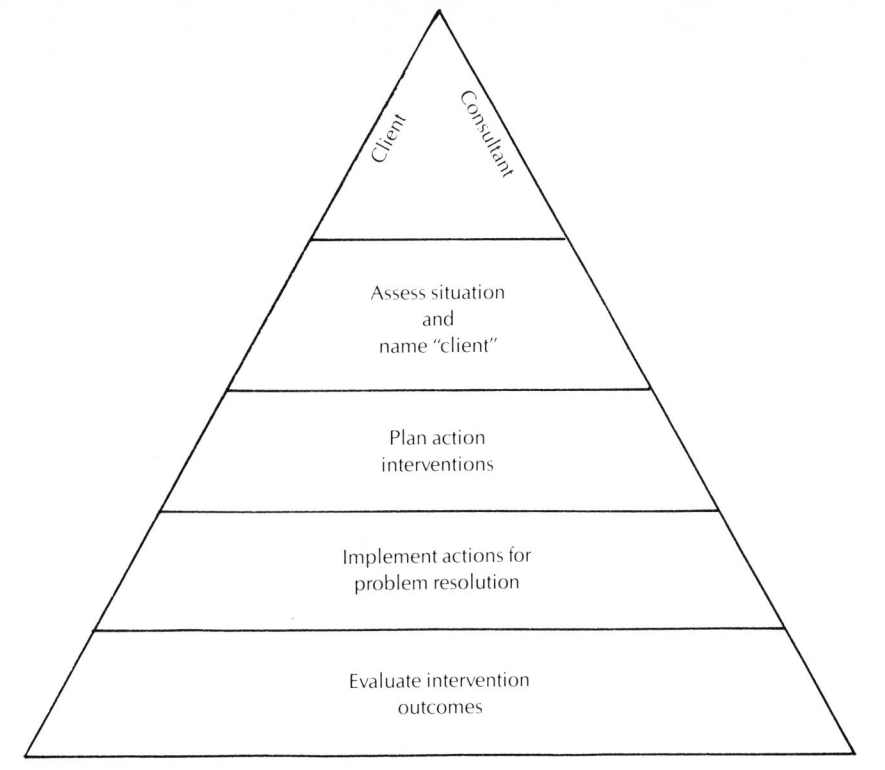

FIGURE 37-4

The process model.

lem-solving steps that lead to situation changes or to action programs for problem resolution.

In this model, the consultant is a resource person whose primary goal is to provide the consultee with choices for decision making about the indentified problem.

The assumptions underlying process consultation are as follows:

1. Clients often do not know what the problem is and need assistance in problem diagnosis.

2. Clients are not aware of the services a consultant may offer and need assistance in finding proper help.

3. Clients want to improve situations and need guidance in identifying appropriate methods to reach goals.

4. Clients can be more effective if they learn to diagnose their own strengths and limitations.

5. Consultants usually cannot spend enough time learning all variables that may help or hinder suggested courses of action, so they need to work with the client who has intimate knowledge of the effects of proposed courses of action.

6. The client who learns to diagnose situation problems and who engages in decision making about alternative courses of action will be actively involved in implementing actions for problem resolution.

7. The consultant who is an expert in problem diagnosis and in establishing an effective helping relationship will be able to pass these skills to the client.

Since process consultation emphasizes human interactions, the consultant must be an expert in individual, group, and community interaction processes (Schein, 1969). Because of the similarity among the focus of process consultation, the skills of the community health nurse, and the emphasis on problem solving, process consultation forms the basis of discussion for this chapter. However, other theories are introduced to show alternative methods used in the consultant-consultee relationship. Because process consultation closely parallels the nursing process: this model is viewed as the most appropriate model to apply in nursing.

The process of consultation is another variation of the scientific method as is the nursing process. As shown in Figure 37-4 the process consultation model embodies the same steps as the nursing process, that is nurse-client interaction for the purpose of assessing the problem, planning and implementing actions, and evaluating the outcomes of nursing interventions. Nursing interventions may be described as direct client care or as consultation activities.

PROCESS CONSULTATION—FOCUS AND PRINCIPLES

Process consultation is a helping process that involves a temporary relationship between client and consultant for the purpose of bringing about *change*. Consultation may be *proactive* or *reactive*. *Proactive consultation* is an activity directed toward the anticipation of a future problem and taking steps to prevent its occurrence. *Reactive consultation* is an activity directed toward curing an existing problem through therapeutic intervention. The board developing the new retirement center contacts the community health nurse consultant to assist with exploring options for future nursing and health care for the residents. The board wishes to be *proactive* and plan for the needs of residents before opening the center. Conversely, the administrator of the minimum security prison has been apprised by the staff that inmates are missing work for minor health problems and that health screening program costs are skyrocketing because the prison must contract with individual providers to offer these services. The community health nursing consultant is asked to help the administration explore solutions to the problem. The prison administration is *reacting* to an existing problem requiring immediate intervention.

Process consultation involves "a set of activities on the part of the consultant which assists the client (consultee) to perceive, understand, and act on events occurring in the clients' environment" (Schein, 1969, p. 9). The process consultation model parallels the nursing process by requiring the assessing, planning, implementing, and evaluating of a problem through mutual interaction between client and consultant. The application of this model requires appropriate identification of the client, definition of the problem by client and consultant, and the choice of a technique to be employed by the consultant for the attainment of problem resolution. The analysis and synthesis of the process consultation model by Blake and Mouton (1983) serves as the basis for discussion and application of this model.

Client Population

One of the most important decisions a consultant makes before accepting or writing a consultative contract is to identify the client in the situation. Clients of the community health nurse consultant may be individuals, a family, a group within the agency, a community group, or a community organization. The client is determined by identifying who in the situation has the problem and needs to change. For example, the staff nurse at the district health department is resistant to working in the clinic caring for clients with sexually transmitted diseases because of a fear of working with AIDS victims. The state community health nurse consultant may negotiate a consultative contract with the staff nurse to deal with her feelings and to arrive at alternative methods for problem resolution. It would not serve any purpose for the consultant to contract with the director of nursing or the nursing supervisor to solve a staff nurse's personal problem. Contracts with management may serve to make the staff nurse more resistant to her assigned duties.

As a second example, a school health nurse consultant receives an inquiry from the school board about ways to get parents to support the visual and hearing screening programs of the schools. The nurse consultant decides that the consultative contract needs to include representatives of the school board and representatives of the parent group to find effective answers to the issue question. The nurse consultant realizes that time would be wasted, and resistance to change would still be present if the focus is on only one group at a time. For example, if the consultant meets separately with the parent group, they may decide the school board should employ someone to do the screening. At the school board meeting the consultant may find that the school board does not have the money to employ persons to do all of the screening but may be willing to employ one person to coordinate the parents' efforts. After expending much energy meeting with both groups separately, the nurse consultant finds that by becoming a messenger between the two factions rather than a facilitator for problem resolution, the consultant role has been diluted. On the other hand, if the nurse meets with both groups together, she can serve as a resource in helping the parents and school board to explore all available alternatives for solving the problem.

Once the client has been identified, the nurse consultant must decide the best method(s) for intervening in the problem situation.

Intervention Modes

Blake and Mouton (1983) describe five basic intervention modes or techniques that can be applied to the process consultation model: acceptant, catalytic, confrontation, prescriptive, and theory-principles. The *acceptant intervention mode* is a process of catharsis intended to clear emotional blockages in order to engage in more objective problem solving. The use of this intervention mode to solve problems benefits the client by improving self-acceptance, spontaneity, emotional health, appropriate situational emotional responses, and the ability to objectively define and deal with problem situations. The disadvantages of the intervention mode are twofold. The cathartic process may assist the client in accepting the circumstances leading to the problem rather than in taking actions to correct the problem, and the emotional catharsis may be viewed by others as a hostile and aggressive act (Blake and Mouton, 1983). For example, Jane, the staff nurse, in interaction with the consultant, may realize that she is not motivated to increase her output because she never gets positive reinforcement from her supervisor. However, she may not wish to change the situation because of reluctance to discuss the problem with the supervisor. Conversely, Jane may learn to be assertive and show the supervisor evidence of quality client care during the supervisor-nurse evaluation conference. The supervisor may interpret Jane's behavior as aggressive and out of character and may penalize the nurse further with a poor evaluation.

When the acceptant intervention mode is being used, the consultant will engage in the following activities:
1. Attempt to understand the client's feelings about the situation.
2. Listen actively.
3. Encourage the client to talk.
4. Try to clarify the client's feelings and help the client to accept the feelings.
5. Refrain from agreeing or disagreeing with the client's situation.
6. Encourage the client to explore ways of dealing with the problem.
7. Listen for more data to reveal the total scope of the problem.

The *catalytic intervention mode* is a situation whereby the consultant assists clients to broaden their view of an existing situation by gaining additional information or by unifying existing data (Blake and Mouton, 1983). The consultant assists clients to (1) strengthen perceptions about problems by improving available information, (2) break down barriers to communication by identifying inadequate communication process and procedures, and (3) raise the awareness level of all involved regarding the problem issue. In the catalytic intervention mode the consultant is viewed as a facilitator moving the client toward improving information needed to solve a problem. The lack of information, however, may be the symptom and not the problem; and the resultant disadvantage of having the consultant improve information flow is that the client may rely on the facilitator for the data rather than becoming efficient in finding solutions to future problems (Caplan, 1970; Blake and Mouton, 1983).

In the local public health department the director of nurses received resignations from all of the nursing staff members on the home health care team. The director called the state health department and requested that the home health nurse consultant be sent to provide assistance in problem identification and resolution. The nurse consultant planned interviews with the staff nurses to determine the cause of the resignations. After sharing the information with the director, a staff meeting was called so the director could discuss problems with the staff and suggest solutions to the problems. The consultant served as a facilitator in the meeting to promote discussion between the staff and the director. After the meeting the consultant assisted the director in analyzing the content of the meeting. Three months later a related communication problem occurred with the same group. Rather than seek causes of the problem, the director phoned for the consultant to return to find the causes and solutions.

When the catalytic intervention mode is employed the consultant will take the following actions:

1. Set a nonauthoritarian tone for the interaction by beginning the intervention with social conversation.
2. Ask the client to describe the situation and use the description as the basis for the interaction.
3. Suggest data-gathering techniques that may provide new information of interest to the client.
4. Provide support to the client as the client attempts to accurately perceive the problem.
5. Avoid specific suggestions for problem solving or resolution.
6. Encourage the client to make decisions about problem resolution.

The *confrontation intervention mode* serves to present the client with facts that reveal the client's values and assumptions in ways that are undeniable and indisputable (Blake and Mouton, 1983). This intervention mode provides clients with an objective look at how their values and beliefs control their behavior. By looking at present behavior, the consultant can examine, with the client, alternative values to redirect behavior toward more conducive methods of problem solving. The disadvantage to this mode is that the client may not wish to participate in interactions that may be interpreted as criticism (Blake and Mouton, 1983).

In the previous example, the consultant may have found that the staff nurses were all going to resign from their positions because they viewed all of the director's decisions as autocratic and uncompromising. On the second visit to the agency, the consultant may confront the director with these observations of the director's behavior. The director may deny the existence of the behavior and point out evidence of having been democratic. As a result of the confrontation the director may either regard the consultant's observations as a personal affront or be willing to examine and analyze the discrepancies between the perceived and the actual behavior.

Activities of consultants engaged in confrontation interventions will include the following:

1. Continually question clients about their description of the situation.
2. Present data and logic to test clients' objectivity.
3. Challenge clients' chosen courses of action.
4. Probe for motives and causes of present situations.
5. Provide own thoughts about situations without personally attacking clients' values.

The *prescriptive intervention mode* requires less collaboration between consultant and client because in this mode the consultant explicitly tells the client how to solve the problem (Blake and Mouton, 1983). To adhere to the interaction goal of process consultation, the prescriptive mode is best used in conjunction with other intervention modes such as acceptant or catalytic. If clients do not participate in problem resolution, they will not be able to solve future problems and may not adhere to the prescriptions offered. The advantage of the prescriptive intervention mode is its applicability in situations where clients have lost confidence in their ability to solve problems or have given up in despair (Blake and Mouton, 1983).

The nurse consultant has decided the best method of dealing with the problems between the home health staff and the director is to present a prescription for behavioral conduct to be implemented by the director and the staff. The consultant tells the group when and how follow-up evaluation will be conducted to look at the progress of both parties in resolving their differences.

When prescriptive interventions are necessary, the consultant will take the following steps:

1. Probe for data about the client's situation.
2. Act authoritatively.
3. Control by telling the client how the problem is to be perceived.
4. Tell the client the best solutions.
5. Remind the client if the client procrastinates in implementing actions.
6. Offer praise if client does exactly what the consultant wants done.

Use of the *theory-principles intervention mode* requires the client to be taught theories, such as behavioral theory, and the application to problem solving. This intervention mode allows for the introduction of the theories after clients have shared their usual methods of problem solving. It also provides for the application of the theories to problem situations by the client and for opportunities to develop client skills in problem diagnosis and resolution through theory application. The major problem with this intervention mode is determining how to help the client internalize use of the theory for practical application, thus removing the abstract connotation that theories usually hold (Blake and Mouton, 1983).

Before using prescriptions with the home health staff and director, the consultant may present a conference on leadership theories and principles, as well as a discussion of the inherent responsibilities in administrative decision making. The consultant may be able to show both parties that leadership styles should vary with the type of decisions to be made and with the people who are to be affected by the decision.

The consultant using theory-principles intervention will proceed as follows:

1. Introduce theories for problem solving to the client.
2. Use techniques to assist the client to internalize theories.
3. Provide strategies for practical application of the theories, such as simulated problem situations or critiques of applications.
4. Offer support when the theory is applied in the actual problem situation.

The various intervention modes are summarized in Table 37-1.

Determinants of Intervention Modes

The use of a particular intervention mode is decided by two factors: (1) the client and (2) the problem. Blake and Mouton (1983) have identified four categories of problem issues: power/authority, morale/cohesion, norms/standards, and goals/objectives. Several of the intervention modes may be used with each of the problem issues.

The *power/authority* issue becomes a question of who has the right to be in charge (boss) and who has the right to make decisions. The *morale/cohesion* problem occurs when the client has lost confidence in the ability to solve problems and feels powerless to institute corrective action. The *norms/standards* problems occur when group norms, professional or organizational standards, are violated or changed. Problems related to *goals/objectives* usually involve the establishing of new goals, changing of goals, or the inability to meet goals/objectives.

Several of the intervention modes may be used with each of the problem issues. When the consultant is trying to decide which intervention mode to use, the client and the nature of the problem must be considered. Although there are exceptions, when the problem with a client is identified as a morale/cohesion problem or a power/authority issue, the most common intervention may be the acceptant mode because the issue generally elicits feelings that block action in decision making; when a norms/standards or goals/objectives problem is the issue, the catalytic mode may be the choice to strengthen the client's perceptions of the most effective decision-making methods. The theory-principles intervention mode may be helpful regardless of the problem, especially when additional insights are needed. However, the prescriptive mode may *not* be helpful unless the client is unable to cope with the situation and needs immediate direction or answers to solve the problem.

THE COMMUNITY HEALTH NURSE AND USE OF PROCESS CONSULTATION
The Consultative Contract

By nature, the consultative relationship is based on expectations. The consultant has expectations concerning time, reimbursement, resources, and the participation of the client in the process. Clients have expectations about what they will gain from the consultant relationship. Although nurses do not usually contract for their services, it is becoming commonplace for consultants to have written contracts. The discussion of the terms of the *consultative con-*

TABLE 37-1

Summary of consultative intervention modes and examples of potential problems

Intervention mode	Definition	Problem example
Acceptant	Process of sharing feelings to move to more objective problem solving.	1. Who's the boss? 2. Feeling of powerlessness to change situation.
Catalytic	Consultant broadens client's knowledge of problem by offering new data or clarifying existing data.	1. Standards are violated/changed. 2. Inability to meet goals or objectives.
Confrontation	Consultant presents clients with indisputable facts.	1. Additional insight needed. 2. Unwillingness to solve problem.
Prescriptive	Consultant tells client how to solve problem.	1. Inability to cope. 2. Needs immediate answer.
Theory-principles	Consultant teaches how to solve problem using theories or principles.	1. Additional insight needed. 2. Lack of knowledge to solve problem.

tract makes expectations more explicit, reduces the likelihood of violations of contract terms, and reduces the risk of additional demands being made on either party. Kolb and Frohmen (1970) and Sedgwick (1973) have identified areas that should be included in the written consultative contract: (1) the goals of client and consultant; (2) the identified problem; (3) the consultant's resources; (4) the time commitment; (5) limitations of the contract; (6) cost; (7) conditons under which the contract may be broken or renegotiated; (8) intervention mode to be used; (9) expected benefits for the client; (10) methods of data collection to be used; (11) client resources; (12) potential interventions; and (13) methods of evaluation of the interaction. An example of a consultation contract that may be used to establish a consultant-consultee relationship appears in the clinical application at the end of the chapter.

Writing a contract for consultative relationships has a number of advantages. The contract terms assist the consultant in determining the number of hours that must be devoted to the interaction and assist the consultant in identifying needed resources and out-of-pocket expenses required to complete the interaction. Negotiation of the contract assists the client in identifying realistic expectations of the consultant and firmly establishes what the consultant will and will not do. The client has the opportunity during the negotiation to place limits on what the consultant can do, and the contract allows for future renegotiation of terms.

Consultation Phases

Consultation involves seven basic phases:
1. Initial contact with the client
2. Definition of the relationship
3. Selection of a setting and approach
4. Collection of data and problem diagnoses
5. Intervention
6. Reduction of involvement and evaluation
7. Termination

The initial contact is made when the client or someone in a family, group, or community communicates with the consultant about a potential problem that requires intervention. The communication may be person to person during a home visit, may be written, or may occur by telephone. On initial contact, the client and the consultant have an exploratory meeting to define the problem, assess the consultant's ability to help, assess the consultant's interest, and formulate future actions.

At the initial meeting, the consultee will want to explore the consultant's expertise, personality characteristics, and interpersonal style. If the consultant has little experience with the type of problem presented, the client may wish to seek assistance elsewhere. Also, if the consultant is quick to make decisions and has a directive approach the client who has a more laissez-faire philosophy may have difficulty accepting the consultant's approach. Conversely, the consultant may conclude that the situation holds little interest or is not within the consultant's expertise and will want to recommend someone else to work with the client.

If the consultant decides at the initial meeting that the real client has been identified, the terms of the relationship will be discussed. The consultant will be interested in finding out what the client expects to gain from the relationship, and the consultant will establish terms for the interaction.

Finally, in the initial exploratory meeting the setting for the consultation will be decided on, the time schedule will be set, the goals of the interaction will be established, and the mode of intervention will be chosen.

When the terms of the contract are agreed on, the data gathering methods will be a part of the agreement. The consultant may find it essential to gather more data before finalizing the diagnosis of the problem. Data gathering methods used by consultants include direct observation, individual and group interviews, use of questionnaires or surveys, and tape recordings.

While data are being gathered as well as after the diagnosis has been finalized, the consultant will be actively engaged in the intervention mode chosen for the interaction.

Upon fulfillment of the terms of the contract, the consultant must be concerned with disengagement or reducing the amount of involvement of the consultant with the client. The disengagement process requires mutual agreement between consultant and consultee that involvement should be reduced. The amount of continuing involvement desired should be checked at varying intervals during the consultative relationship. It is at these points that contract renegotiation may take place. Determinants of continued involvement include, but are not limited to, the client's willingness to continue, value of the interaction for client and consultant, and situational changes that have resulted.

Before termination, the number of contacts between consultant and consultee should be decreased. The continued but decreased contacts will allow each party to evaluate the effectiveness of the intervention. During the disengagement period the consultant reassures the client that future interactions are possible at the client's discretion. When the agreed-on time for disengagement has passed the relationship is terminated (Blake and Mouton, 1983; Schein, 1969; Sedgwick, 1973). As a component of the disengagement and termination phases of the consultative process, the consultant typically provides the consultee with a written summary of the findings and recommendations resulting from the interaction.

As with any formal interaction, three stages of consultation encompass the several phases previously described: *trust-building,* which includes the initial contact, definition of the relationship, and selection of the setting and intervention approach; *problem solving,* which involves gathering data, formalizing the problem, and intervening; and *closure,* which involves disengagement and termination.

Examples of Consultation

Five actual examples of consultative interventions are described in the following discussion.

Intervention: prescriptive
Client: Director of Nursing
Consultant: internal
Problem: norms/standards

The client telephones the state nursing consultant and requests a meeting in the local health unit. The purpose of the meeting is to review the serious problems the local nursing staff is having in meeting program standards and requirements as identified in a recent program audit. The consultant, Elizabeth, met with the client, Maggie, and reviewed her findings, sharing her analysis of problems and causative factors. The central problem issue was defined as inconsistent supervision of staff with a need for definitive role clarification of supervisory responsibilities. Maggie was immobilized by the situation. Elizabeth directed Maggie to restructure the supervisory job descriptions to clearly reflect supervisory roles and expectations and to give supervisors written performance evaluations and guidelines for improving staff performance.

Elizabeth maintained contact with Maggie until termination of the consultation occurred as corrective action was completed.

Intervention: acceptant
Client: staff nurse
Consultant: internal
Problem: morale/cohesion

Elizabeth received a phone call from staff nurse Susan requesting a meeting to discuss problems that Susan was experiencing in her job situation. Susan was obviously under stress as evidenced by the immediacy of the requested need for the meeting. Susan talked about her perceived inability to communicate with administration, the impact of her feelings on her ability to function, and her feelings of being out of control in the job situation. Susan had decided that resignation was her only alternative. Elizabeth listened and provided a nonthreatening opportunity for Susan to verbalize freely. Elizabeth did not agree or disagree with Susan's perceptions of the job situation or respond to her direct question about resignation. Elizabeth focused on Susan's perceived problems with the job and her feelings about her performance. She then attempted to clarify events described by Susan and to keep events in perspective. Finally, Elizabeth explored with Susan ways in which she might facilitate communication with administration. Ultimately Susan decided to choose resignation as the solution.

Intervention: catalytic/theory-principles
Client: community group
Consultant: external
Problem: goals/objectives

Josie was contacted as a consultant by a representative of a local community hospital. The hospital staff and the pediatrician had expressed concern about child neglect problems the hospital was seeing and about the lack of information many mothers seemingly had about basic child care. Josie, acting as a facilitator, recognized that the problem involved not only the single community hospital but the two other community hospitals, and the county department of social services, the health department, and the county home extension office. These groups were identified by Josie as having the potential to influence the identified health issue.

Josie contacted and requested a representative from each of the involved agencies to be present at a planning meeting. At the initial meeting Josie, acting as a resource, presented the magnitude of the infant morbidity and mortality problem of the local county, presented data for 3 years regarding the causes of infant mortality, and raised the issue of preventive intervention through a hospital discharge system.

Hospitalization and discharge of the newborn were identified as prime times to provide parents with information on basic child care and local resources. The client group believed that educational materials currently provided to hospitals for use with new parents was not designed for the level of understanding of many parents in a rural multi-income-level area.

The decision was made by the group to develop a county-specific, newborn hospital discharge packet that was easily understandable and provided county-specific resource information. Through a series of five or six meetings the group reviewed and selected the most significant principles from an extensive literature review and applied them to their identified local health issue. They subsequently developed a discharge planning model with community-wide applicability. During disengagement the group renegotiated with Josie to evaluate the application of the model at the end of a 3-month period.

Intervention: confrontation
Client: departmental group
Consultant: internal
Problem: power/authority

The Director of Nursing solicited consultation for assisting the health department program supervisors to assume management-supervisory responsibility for their staff. The lack of management responsibility was having a domino effect on program standards, fiscal accountability, and nursing practice standards. In an initial meeting with the director, the consultant determined that the client was the supervisory group, not the Director of Nursing.

The consultant then met individually with supervisors to ascertain their perceptions of administration's expectations in the area of program management. The consultant, through the use of client care findings on a record audit and an audit of staff evaluations, revealed the managerial problems of each supervisor and shared these findings in the individual conferences. Reasons offered by the supervisors for lack of involvement in management functions were excessive caseload, lack of clear understanding of their management functions, the expectations of administration, and insecurity in management techniques.

The consultant met with the supervisors as a group. At this point the consultant reviewed specifically the management tasks for which the supervisors would be held responsible by administration and reviewed the organizational structure and the line authority held by each supervisor. The consultant also reviewed their caseloads and the amount of projected time they needed to perform managerial functions. The consultant-client relationship was to be continued monthly for a minimum period of 6 months at which time the contract would be renegotiated or terminated.

Intervention: catalytic
Client: community agency
Consultant: external
Problem: goals/objectives

The consultant was contacted by the Family Practice Center to discuss the issue of adolescent pregnancy problems in the county and the Family Practice Center's involvement in providing an adolescent maternity service clinic within a residency training program. A meeting was scheduled at which time the nurse consultant presented adolescent pregnancy data for the county, outlined the local health department's role in adolescent prenatal services and the current adolescent prenatal caseload, and provided data by which to project the caseload and service demands the adolescent clinic would be expected to meet. The center staff, health department staff, and consultant made a site visit to observe an adolescent prenatal clinic at another medical center.

As a result of several additional meetings the consultant was able to negotiate a collaborative arrangement between the health department and the Family Practice Center. The services to be provided included short-term nursing education, social work, and nutrition support services. The consultant assumed the facilitator role and continually clarified the ongoing developmental and agency commitments (goals) in this collaborative effort. The adolescent prenatal clinic was initiated with the aid of the short-term commitments that grew out of the interagency relationships. After the clinic was established, health department services were withdrawn and replaced by the Family Practice Center staff as scheduled. The consultant's relationship continued for approximately 6 months and was terminated after meeting a request from the center staff for evaluation.

THE NURSE CONSULTANT

As previously indicated, *nurse consultants* in the community health setting may function as internal consultants employed on a full-time basis by an organization for the purpose of facilitating the staff in problem solving; or nurses may be employed as external consultants with a contractual arrangement to assist an individual, group, or community organization to find solutions to existing problems. Nurses may provide consultation for a wide range of issues related to community health nursing, or they may narrow their scope of expertise and provide consultation only in an identified area of specialty. The following discussion focuses on the differences in the internal and external consultant, the generalist versus the specialist, the sources of conflict in the role, and the effect funding sources have on the availability of consultation.

The Internal Nurse Consultant
Generalist

The delivery system of a health agency will determine the specific framework in which a consultant functions. An agency whose delivery system is structured along the lines of an official generalized community health service will more likely employ a consultant who provides traditional or comprehensive community health nursing consultation within a broad range of community health activities.

A study of *generalist* nurse consultants by Stetler and Downs (1974) showed that official community agencies often require nurse consultants to function in dual roles, such as supervisor-consultant. The dual role functions of the consultant result in ambiguity for the staff nurse and the consultant. Role strain may result when neither the staff nurse nor the consultant knows which hat the consultant should wear in a given situation. Role stress occurs from conflict in defining role expectations and because the consultant may be experiencing role overload or may lack time to carry out all role obligations.

The generalist consultant tends to experience role conflict when the agency moves into the provision of more specialized areas of primary care. The conflict occurs when the demands of agency staff in specialized skill areas, like pediatrics, exceed the expertise of the generalized consultant. Conflicts also evolve from different role expectations between the administrator and the nurse consultant.

Specialist

A community health agency that provides a programmatic approach or specialized approach to the delivery of community health services, such as family planning, maternity, child health, crippled children services, school health, and home health, to name a few, will tend to employ *specialist* consultants who may, in addition to broad community health expertise, have skills and specialized training in a primary clinical area, for example, the clinical nurse specialist in pediatrics.

The degree to which the agency is involved in specific primary care areas influences the use of the specialized consultant. Agencies providing primary health care require a consultant with both a broad knowledge of community health practice and specialized knowledge in a clinical area. This is also a requirement in agencies involved in long-term and home health care. The specialist nurse consultant functioning within a programmatic framework, by virtue of the agency's expectations and the consultant's functional expertise, generally tends to be less involved in the administrative aspects of the program. This factor offers the potential for conflict. The consultant is expected to provide the clinical expertise to community health nursing staff and to have nursing input into administrative and programmatic development of policies, guidelines, and procedures without authority for implementation. The conflict between administration, the consultant, and the nursing staff arises when administrative priorities differ from community health nursing practice priorities.

Despite the conflict potential existing within this delivery framework, a nurse consultant with management and administrative preparation and/or background is able to function effectively while also representing community health nursing practice. The sources for role stress and strain for the specialist are similar to those of the generalist consultant. Role ambiguity and role overload are often the results of the role expectations, as defined for the consultant, by the administration and the nursing staff.

Role Functions and Expectations

The community health nurse consultant employed within an official health agency functions as an internal consultant to the employing agency and provides nursing and community health consultation to colleagues, other disciplines, agency administration, and other health and human service agencies and/or community groups as a representative of the agency.

Two primary roles of the internal consultant are resource person and facilitator (Pati, 1980). Both roles emerge from the accessibility of the consultant to all aspects of the agency and community. The degree of accessibility is enhanced or diminished by the place the consultant fits in the organizational structure of the agency. For example, the consultant may hold a line position with responsibility to the nursing director and authority over staff nurses; or the consultant may hold an advisory position to the nursing director without direct authority over the staff.

The resource role has traditionally been associated with the community health nurse consultant both within and outside of the official health agency. With the advent in the last decade of new and varied health delivery models within communities, the resource role has assumed increased significance. The community health consultant, with knowledge of available resources, can identify deficiencies and gaps in service, identify the critical components provided by the myriad of health delivery systems, and promote the interface of these systems in meeting health or social needs of the population.

With the shrinking health dollars of the 1980s, the facilitator role of the community health consultant has assumed renewed significance. The facilitator role of the consultant has been described at length throughout this chapter. The nurse consultant as a facilitator assists staff nurses, administration, groups, and organizations to solve problems relating to the needs of clients, staff, or the organization. Performing the facilitator function, the consultant will guide the staff nurse in solving problems about individual client and family health needs, health needs of a group of clients, or professional concerns and attitudes. The consultant may assist supervisors, managers, directors, and administrators to solve problems about personnel matters, program needs, organizational goals, community relationships, and client population needs. The consultant may also facilitate communications between the employing agency and facilities or other health providers in the community.

Conflict Sources

The internal consultant as a representative of the employing agency has implied authority that may present conflict between the consultant and consultee. The degree of conflict may be determined by centralization or decentralization of the health agency and the degree of autonomy of the individual units in the organizational structure. The administrative or managerial strength of the individual unit can also determine the role the consultant may assume and, to a large measure, determine the involvement of the consultant in an implementation role. One means of negating potential conflict is to clearly define the role the consultant is to assume. A consultant functioning within an agency that is strongly controlled by a central unit will tend to be more actively involved in an implementation role, such as supervisor. For example, in one state the state health department has jurisdiction over all county health departments throughout the state (centralized). The state has decided to make each county health department autonomous in their delivery of health services to the county (decentralized). The state health department will continue to provide advice to the county units about delivery of services but will not supervise the delivery of care. Nursing in the county units will have its own directors and the nursing consultants at the state level will be utilized as resource persons and facilitators offering information and advice to the county units in matters requiring problem solving. While the state health department was centralized and provided direct supervision to the counties for delivery of health care, the state family planning consultant was also responsible for supervising the county health department staff members who were responsible for delivery of family planning services. In the decentralized system, the supervisory functions are removed from the consultant's responsibilities and the consultant helps to facilitate the work of other nurses by offering advice and information that will assist them in understanding how to do their work.

Role Relationships

The consultant's role with nursing administration and staff is determined by the organizational structure. The internal consultant is generally responsible to and strongly influenced by nursing administration and agency administration. The nursing administration's framework for nursing practice, goals for nursing service, and the role the consultant is to assume should be clearly defined before employment. Who is responsible for nursing practice with commensurate authority should be clearly defined for the consultant, the supervising staff, and the staff nurses. The internal consultant, by virtue of staff level alignment, has no formal authority but informally will have inherent responsibility for making changes in nursing practice (Kohnke, 1978). The perception of the staff regarding the consultant's alignment to administration, as "eyes and ears" of administration, no doubt is a factor in the staff's relationship to the consultant. The degree to which this is true is dependent on the consultant/consultee relationship developed and established by the consultant.

The dual supervisor-consultant role with its inherent problems were described by Stetler and Downs (1975) in a research project conducted in a state public health system. Supervision denotes decision making and implementation activities in an ongoing relationship, which is the antithesis of consultation. It can be seen that the supervising role functions could usurp the consultative role parameters, and the staff could perceive the supervisor/consultant as being directly aligned with administration. Quality communication is vital in this dual role.

A plethora of allied health professionals are functioning within community health practice: clinical social workers, nutritionists, occupational therapists, physical therapists, health educators, home economists, and home health aides. The community health nurse and the allied health providers share mutual skills and commitment to community health practice and provide specific professional skills to mutual clients, to families, and to each other. The nurse consultant provides consultation to the allied health provider and serves as a resource and content person to these professionals in the areas of community health nursing practice. The nurse consultant, in a facilitator role, can enhance the efficient use of other health providers and often circumvent "turf" issues. The consultant's broad knowledge base and multidisciplinary approach to health care helps to determine the effective use of allied health providers and also promotes more efficient use of nursing manpower.

Funding Implications

Categorical funding mechanisms within the last decade have promoted in some agencies the position of specialist consultant within community health departments. Title X of the Social Security Act included provisions for funding of family planning services. This funding mechanism is one example of how a federally funded community health service promoted the use of specialist consultants within a specific area of community health care. The funding mechanism gave rise to use of the family planning nurse practitioner. To meet the agency needs, consultants with special skills and expertise in reproductive health were employed by official health agencies. Similarly, Title V of the Social Security Act provided funding that traditionally focused on more generalized services to mothers and children and has brought about use of the crippled children nurse consultant and the school health nurse consultant. The Medicare funding for home health care in 1965 gave rise to the home health services consultant with community skills in medical and surgical nursing practice.

The impact of state primary care block grant funding and the move of some health agencies from programmatic to a more integrated service delivery framework will effect the role and use of nursing consultants in official community health agencies. The competition for limited health dollars, the increasing focus on the at-risk population, the anticipated surplus of physician manpower, and the shortage of nurses are going to affect, with a potential emphasis on hiring generalist consultants, the specialist versus generalist consultant role in official health agencies.

The External Nurse Consultant
Role Functions and Expectations

When the community health nurse consultant is contacted by an agency or organization other than the employing agency, the consultant is considered an outsider to the organization and as such an external consultant. Again, the external nurse consultant acts as a facilitator or a resource person using one or a combination of the approaches described throughout the chapter. The external nurse consultant may serve as a representative of the employing agency and provide information to the consultee for the planning of interagency programs to meet population needs. The external nurse consultant may serve as a resource to health educators, health planners, school personnel, psychologists, audiologists, counselors, dentists, social workers, physicians, legislators, and probation officers providing data about individual client, group, or community needs.

The external consultant may be asked to serve as a facilitator to an official agency board, to solve problems about community health priorities. Similarly, the consultant may be asked to serve as a facilitator or resource person to a voluntary agency, such as the American Red Cross or the American Heart Association.

Consultants from federal agencies are often used in community health as external nurse consultants. The nurse consultant from the federal agency may come to the local or state agency, on request, to serve as facilitator or resource person relative to program planning, development, and implementation. The primary role function of this consultant is to serve as a resource person although the consultant may facilitate movement toward identifying actual program parameters.

Conflict Sources

The external consultant, an outsider to the client agency, has only assumed authority that may present conflict for the consultant and the consultee (Polk, 1980). Since the consultant is external to the consultee situation, upon the consultant's exit from the agency the consultee may not feel impelled to implement actions agreed on by consultant and consultee. In many instances the consultant may hold a role complementary to the consultee, such as community health nurse consultant to the school health nurse.

Although equal sharing and input should be the motto of a consultant-consultee relationship, conflict may arise if the school nurse interprets the community nurse consultant's involvement as an invasion of space. One means of preventing potential conflicts is to clearly establish the terms of the contract for the consultant-consultee interaction. For example, the community health nurse consultant is called by the school health nurse. The school nurse needs input from the consultant regarding development and implementation of a health education program for sexually transmitted diseases. The terms of the contract stipulate that the consultant will provide input on how to develop and implement the program and the school health nurse will actually do the work for the program. Thus, the consultant is not involved in the program and the school nurse's turf is protected.

The consultative relationship is also on a time-limited basis. The consultant may not have enough time to identify all variables in the situation to arrive at a diagnosis of the real problem. The consultee may be frustrated in attempts to make changes suggested by the consultant and may offer resistance because the real problem did not surface during the consultant-consultee interaction.

Role Relationships

The role relationships of the external consultant with groups or individuals are determined by the client (individual or group). The principles and process of consultation are the same for either the internal or external consultative functional framework. The external consultant was previously defined in this chapter, and the roles are the same as the roles of the internal consultant, that is, facilitator and resource.

One of the principal differences between the internal and the extenal consultant is the time constraint for the consultant to assimilate data for problem identification.

Funding Implications

As federal, state, local, and private funding becomes more competitive, fewer external nurse consultants may be used. If an external consultant is used, costs for the consulting services must be built into the consultee's budget. Such future limited funds may be reserved for program implementation rather than for the luxury of contracting with consultants. Although all external nurse consultants do not receive direct reimbursement for their services, such as the consultants acting as agency representatives, the needs of the employing agency for internal consultation may become greater and the agency may not be willing to pay, either in time or travel, for the consultant to be away from the organization.

EDUCATIONAL REQUIREMENTS

The educational requirements for the community health nurse consultant are primarily determined by two factors: the practice setting and the client population. The community health nurse with undergraduate preparation may serve as a generalist nurse consultant to individuals, families, and groups of clients with an identified health problem like hypertension or diabetes. The consultant serves either as a facilitator to seek problem resolution or as a resource to provide for community referral. This nurse may also consult with other health provider agencies involved with client groups such as the hospital, the ambulatory hypertensive clinic, the private physician, and the physical therapist.

The community health nurse consultant who has graduate preparation with a generalist or specialist clinical and functional focus has expert knowledge in the application of the theories of change, group, systems, interaction, motivation, communications, behavior, management, epidemiology, in-depth knowledge in family and individual development, advocacy, and health and nursing issues (Kohnke, 1978). This nurse may be an internal or external consultant serving as an expert resource person or as a facilitator to the client groups previously identified.

PRACTICE ARENAS

The nurse who wishes to become a consultant will find employment opportunities with governmental agencies: federal, state, and local; with private enterprise and philanthropic organizations; and with voluntary and professional organizations.

The federal government employs nurse consultants in many branches of the Public Health Service. The Division of Nursing of the Health Resources Administration employs a group of nurse consultants to serve as resource persons for education. The Health Care Financing Administration employs nurse consultants to serve as resource persons for programs such as home health. Many state health departments employ clinical specialist consultants who serve as facilitators and resource persons to local health departments regarding program needs, such as child health. State health departments also employ clinical nurse consultants to serve as resource persons to such agencies as schools and rehabilitation centers. Local city, county, or district health departments employ nurse consultants, usually generalists, who facilitate staff members in meeting client and program needs.

Private organizations use the expertise of nurses in consultation with clients (purchasers of services) of the organization. Publishing and audiovisual equipment companies often employ nurses who serve as resources and facilitators for persons who are interested in writing or developing audiovisuals for sale or for persons who require assistance in the use of goods purchased from the companies. Pharmaceutical companies and health care supply and equipment companies employ nurse consultants for similar purposes.

Private philanthropic organizations, such as the Robert Wood Johnson Foundation, may use nurse consultants to serve as resource persons for health care or education programs funded by the organizations; professional organizations, such as ANA and NLN, offer nurse consulting services to clinical agencies, for example, home health, and to educational institutions who require assistance in setting program standards or in readying themselves for accreditation review.

An employment arena that is becoming more popular to nurse consultants is the private consulting firm. The private health care consulting firms, numbering over 200 in the nation's capital alone, exist to offer assistance to individuals, groups, institutions, and government organizations in such matters as setting health care priorities; writing goals, standards, policies, and procedures; developing better managerial solutions for program efficiency; and planning health care programs. Nurses may even incorporate their own private consulting firm for the purpose of providing services directed toward nursing issues (Wright, 1981; Braddock & Sawyer, 1985).

Similarly, voluntary organizations, for example, the American Red Cross, may employ nurses to serve as resource persons in the development of local programs such as blood banks, and the World Health Organization may employ nurses to serve as resource and facilitator to third world countries in the development of health care programs. Community health nurses are prepared to meet the challenges of these employment arenas because of their expertise in comprehensive client assessment and in program development and evaluation and their extensive knowledge of the use of available resources.

CLINICAL APPLICATION

The manager of a small housing project approached the local university College of Nursing for assistance with health promotion and health monitoring activities for the project residents. Many of the residents were elderly with chronic illnesses, and were for the most part living on fixed incomes and 10 to 15 miles from medical facilities. The community health faculty member assigned a nursing student to assess this community's request for consultation.

The nursing student arranged for a meeting with the manager to discuss the problem, assess the student's ability to help with the problem, and explore the expectations the client had for the student or for the College of Nursing. As a result of these discussions the contract shown in the accompanying box was developed.

After careful consideration the student and the manager determined that a survey of resident needs and facility resources would assist them in making decisions about the

CONSULTATION CONTRACT

Client name __C. Jones, Manager__   Consultant name __S. Smith, Nursing__

Address __Housing Project__   Address __College of Nursing__

Phone __333-0000__   Phone __333-1000__

Estimated costs (external consultant only) __$500__
  (including phone, secretarial assistance, preparation, supplies, travel expenses and consultant sessions)

Client problem definition __85 unit housing project. 75% elderly residents with chronic illnesses and limited income. 10-15 miles from health facilities. Exacerbations undetected and/or chronic illnesses go unresolved until acute state of illness.__

Suggested intervention mode __Catalytic/Prescriptive__

Client goals

A healthier population through accessible and on-going health monitoring

Scope of consultation (time and no. of sessions)

3 planning and data gathering sessions in 6 weeks; 3 evaluation sessions at 2 to 3 week intervals during data collection; final evaluation session

Consultant resources (e.g., computer, secretary, library)

Computer to analyze data; library; assistance from faculty; staff to collect data (3 students)

Contract renegotiation and termination terms

Renegotiation at 2 to 3 week evaluation conferences. Termination at final evaluation conference.

Client resources (e.g., records, secretary, copy)

Project records available to collect data; secretary to type survey questionnaires; conference room for interviews; final report typed; supplies.

Anticipated client benefits

Housing project will have identified plan for meeting health needs of residents. Residents will have a permanent health monitoring program.

Contract limitations (e.g., who, what, when, how will data be shared)

Survey of resident's health, housing project staff, administration, and resources by the CNN students. Report to manager and college faculty.

Potential interventions (e.g., report shared with administration; meeting held with staff)

Meetings with staff and residents to get input about best method to solve problem. Review of resources to find housing projects potential for solving own problem.

Consultant goals

Collect data as outlined.

Assess and define problem.

Identify resources for solving problem.

Prescribe best method for meeting residents' health care needs.

Data collection methods

Interviews __staff, manager, local health care representatives__

Surveys __residents__

Questionnaires _____

Meetings __staff, residents, manager, faculty__

Phone __n/a__

Contract evaluation

At end of 12 weeks will look at potential alternatives; choose one that is satisfactory to residents, staff, and management.

alternatives they could explore for providing health monitoring to the residents.

With the approval of the community health faculty member, the community health nursing students agreed to assist with the health screening survey and to collect data about the housing project, such as the physical facilities, the available equipment and supplies, staff available to volunteer assistance with health screening and promotion activities, existing relationships with community referral sources, money available to support the program, and the attitude of staff and residents toward such a program. Anticipated outcomes for the consultation included recommending to the project management a permanent health monitoring clinic within the facility using one of several options: the development of a nursing clinic with the College of Nursing, contracting with the health department to provide the service, employing staff at the housing project to implement the clinic, or establishing a clinic staffed with volunteer nurses from the community.

At the evaluation conference, the students shared the results of their data gathering activities. After careful consideration of the data, the housing project manager decided a permanent health clinic was essential for the residents. A review of the budget revealed that money was available to employ a full-time nurse to staff the clinic at the housing project.

SUMMARY

This chapter has outlined and discussed the definition of consultation, consultation theory, principles of process consultation, intervention modes, determinants of intervention modes, client populations, various frameworks for nurse consultation, academic preparation, and practice arenas for nurse consultants. The practical application of the consultative process in community health is reflected in the varied practice situations inherent in this chapter with consultative intervention reflected in community health practice outcomes.

Kohnke (1978) described the availability of nursing consultation as a serious issue. Nursing administration's acceptance of this concept is a critical component of nursing practice. With continually diminishing health dollars and the focus on fiscal accountability, the cost effectiveness of nursing consultation will no doubt be studied and become an added dimension to the acceptance and use of nurse consultants.

KEY CONCEPTS

The goal of consultation is to stimulate clients to take responsibility, feel more secure, deal constructively with their feelings and with others in interaction, and internalize skills of a flexible and creative nature.

The major goals of the process model are to assist the client to assess both the problem and the kind of help needed to solve the problem.

Purchase model consultation involves the hiring of a professional helper to provide expert information or service.

In the doctor-patient model, the client hires the consultant to find the problem and offer solutions without background data or assistance from the client.

Consultation has also been described as a political process.

Five basic intervention modes or techniques applied to process consultation are acceptant, catalytic, confrontation, prescriptive, and theory-principles.

The use of a particular intervention mode is based on two factors: the client and the problem.

Four categories of problem issues are power/authority, morale/cohesion, norms/ standards, and goals/objectives.

The process of consultation involves seven basic phases: initial contact, definition of the relationship with the client, selection of a setting and approach, collection of data and problem diagnoses, intervention, reduction of involvement and evaluation, and termination.

Nurse consultants may function as internal consultants within an organization or external consultants from outside the client organization.

Educational requirements for the nurse consultant are primarily determined by two factors: the practice setting and the client population.

LEARNING ACTIVITIES

1. Interview one or more practicing community health staff nurses. Ask each to describe the activities of their jobs that could be categorized as consultation. During the interview attempt to determine the following:
   a. How they define consultation.
   b. The goals they are attempting to attain in the related consultative activities.
   c. The theory you perceive they most likely apply in their consultations.
   d. The intervention modes they practice.
   e. Whether their activities are of a generalist or specialist nature and an internal or external consultative nature.
   f. The strengths and limitations they perceive themselves to have in their consultative functions (may be educational, experiential, organizational, relational, economic).
2. Interview one or more community health nurse consultants. During the course of the interview, attempt to determine the answers to the aspects examined in the preceding activity.
3. After gathering data from your interviews and reading the material in this chapter, choose a definition of consultation that you perceive to be most applicable to community health nursing practice.

BIBLIOGRAPHY

Anders, R.: Program consultation by a clinical specialist, Nur. Adm. 8(11):34-38, 1978.

Baizerman, M., and Hall, W.: Consultation as a political process, Community Ment. Health J. 13(2):142-149, 1977.

Blake, R., and Mouton, J.: Consultation, ed. 2, Reading, Mass., 1983, Addison-Wesley Publishing Co., Inc.

Braddock, B., and Sawyer, D.: Becoming an independent consultant: essentials to consider, Nursing Economics, 3(6):332-335, 1985.

Caplan, G.: The theory and practice of mental health consultation, New York, 1970, Basic Books, Inc., Publishers.

Clark, M.: The nurse educator in an expanded consultant role, The Journal of Continuing Education in Nursing 14(4):5-7, 1983.

Covent, A.B.: Community mental health nursing: the role of consultant in the nursing home, J. Psychiatr. Nur. 17(7):15-19, 1979.

Emlet, C., and Froelick - Emlet, P.: Consultation in skilled nursing facilities, Nursing Homes 31:26-29, March/April, 1982.

Hendrix, M. and LaGodna, G.: Consultation: a political process aimed at change. In Lancaster, J., and Lancaster, W., Concepts for advanced nursing practice: the nurse as a change agent, St. Louis, 1982, The C.V. Mosby Co.

Koch, M.: Moving ahead, Nursing 79:72-73, July 1979.

Kohnke, M.: The case for consultation in nursing: design for professional practice, New York, 1978, John Wiley & Sons.

Kolb, D., and Frohmen A: An organization development approach to consulting. Sloan Management Review 12(1):51-65, 1970.

Lamb, H., and Peterson, C.: The new community consultation, Hosp. Community Psychiatry. 34(1):59-63, 1983.

Lange, F.: The multifaceted role of the nurse consultant, J. Nurs. Educ. 18(9):30-34, 1979.

Lareau, S.: The nurse as clinical consultant. Topic. Clin. Nurs. 2:79-84, Rockville, Md., 1980, Aspen Systems Corp.

Lippitt, R., and Lippitt, G.: Consulting process in action. In Jones, I., and Pfeiffer, J., editors: The 1977 annual handbook for group facilitators, San Diego, Calif., 1977, University Associates, Inc.

Miller, L.: Resistance to the consultation process, Nursing Leadership. 6(1):10-15, 1983.

Oda, D.: Consultation: an expectation of leadership, Nursing Leadership, 5(1):7-9, 1982.

Pati, B.: Nursing consultation: a collaborative process, J. Nurs. Adm. 10(11):33-36, Nov. 1980.

Polk, G.: The socialization and utilization of nurse consultants, J. Psychiatr. Nurs. 18(2):33-36, Feb. 1980.

Sanders, L., Chesley, D., and Kishi, A.: Curriculum consultant, would you help us out? Nurs. Outlook 11(6):315-321, June 1981.

Schein, E.: Process consultation: its role in organization development, Reading, MA, 1969, Addison-Wesley Publishing Co., Inc.

Schilling, K.: The consultant role in multidisciplinary team development, Intern. Nurs. Rev. 29(3):73-75, 96, 1982.

Sedgwick, R.: The role of the process consultant, Nurs. Outlook 21(12):773-774, Dec. 1973.

Stetler, C., and Downs, C.: The supervisor/consultant: a difficult role, Community Health Adm., Wakefield, Mass., 1975, Contemporary Publishing, Inc.

Stevens, B.: The use of consultants in nursing service, J. Nurs. Adm. 8(8):7-15, Aug. 1978.

Stickney, S., and Hall, R.: The role of the nurse on a consultation liaison team, Psychosomatics 22(3):228-235, 1981.

Stickney, S., et al.: Psychiatric nurse consultant: who calls and why, J.P.N.M.H.S. 19(10):22-26, 1981.

Stone, L.: Consultation builds success for nurses, Nursing Success Today, 1:23-29, 1984.

Wallace, S.: Some aspects of consultation and management by objectives, Occup. Health Nurs. 28:26-30, Oct. 1980.

Wright, B.L.: The nurse consultant, Can. Nurse 77(2):34-36, Feb. 1981.

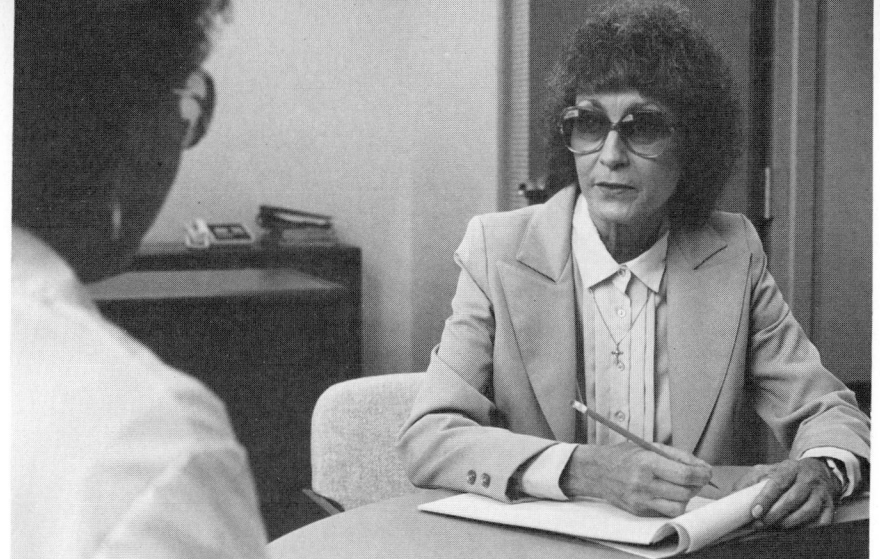

Kathleen Beckman Blomquist
Marcia Stanhope
Ellen Bailey
Sharon Sheahan

38

THE COMMUNITY HEALTH NURSE CLIENT ADVOCATE

≡ OBJECTIVES

After reading this chapter, the student should be able to:

Define coordination, collaboration, advocacy, discharge planning, and referral.

Identify the scope and limits of the nurse's coordinative and collaborative role functions as client advocate.

Analyze the concept of client advocate and its relevance to community health nursing.

Analyze the concepts of discharge planning and referral and their relevance to community health nursing.

≡ KEY TERMS

adversary relationships
aftercare programs
circle model
client advocacy
collaboration
conflicts of interest
contingency contract
continuity of care
coordination

directive change
discharge planning activities
economic barriers
functional leader
horizontal coordination
maintenance phase
orientation phase
outpatient follow-up
participative change

power
referral
resource barriers
role ambiguity
situational leader
star model
termination phase
territorialism
vertical coordination

Sue Jones, 35 years old and mother of two small children, discovered that her family had many unmet needs after their husband and father deserted them. She knew that money for food, clothing, and shelter would be her greatest priority; but how was she to work and also provide a safe environment for her children?

At the health department's Well Child Clinic, Sue had met Connie, the community health nurse. Sue called Connie and shared her problems. Being an innovative person, Connie checked her United Way Resource Guide and the local phone directory reference section and found that the community services and health services categories listed many agencies who could assist Sue in this time of need. Through these resources Connie identified social services for aid to mothers with dependent children; Medicaid, Head Start, and low-income day care services for the children; the health department for all their health care needs; and several volunteer organizations for food, clothing, and financial aid. By the end of the first year as a single parent, Sue had managed with Connie's assistance to find income plus additional assistance with food, clothing, and health care needs.

At a multiagency case management conference, Sue's family was presented by Connie. As each agency discussed their contributions to Sue's family, a new goal was identified. After discussion with Sue, the team assisted Sue in becoming involved in a career training program, whereby she could receive income while learning new skills to become self-supporting.

Sue's initiative in contacting Connie to ask for help for her family and herself is commendable, and such behavior should be rewarded by health providers. In this instance, a community health nurse was helpful and facilitated Sue's efforts to seek assistance from only the most appropriate agencies.

This case illustrates a community health nurse serving as an advocate for a family. She identified needs and problems and negotiated the bureaucracies of various community resources and health service agencies to obtain services. This example also demonstrates what can happen in a community where there is coordination of effort and collaboration among community service agencies.

Most often, examples with the opposite results are encountered. Members of a family or group have needs that community agencies can address, but the people lack knowledge of the available resources and have difficulty making the appropriate contacts to work their way through the system.

Coordination among community services and collaboration about alternative ways of providing comprehensive community services can rectify these situations. An important role of community health nurses is that of client advocate. Role functions include client care coordinator and collaborator, discharge planner, and referral manager.

◆ ◆ ◆

This chapter focuses on knowledge and skills needed for advocacy, the helping relationship, barriers and consequences related to advocacy, and advocacy issues.

DEFINITIONS AND GOALS

The community health nurse as *client advocate* acts on behalf of the client to attain two goals: health care delivery system responsiveness to clients and client independence. The conscious use of principles of coordination and collaboration to achieve health care goals makes the health care system more responsive to client needs. Discharge planning and referral are two techniques that can be used on the client's behalf to help the client move toward independence.

Coordination is the conscious activity of assembling and directing the work efforts of a group of health providers so that they function harmoniously in the attainment of the objectives of client care (Rakich, Longest, and O'Donovan, 1977). The *goal* of coordination is to maximize the collaborative effort of health providers while minimizing friction among the providers in the attainment of the client care objectives. As illustrated in the previous example, *collaboration* requires health providers working together as a team of equals toward a common goal. The community health nurse's goal in collaboration is to contribute to a comprehensive effort that provides continuity of services to clients whether they be individuals, groups, families, or communities. *Discharge planning activities* are planned events that prepare for clients' ongoing and future needs for health care resources as they move along the health–illness continuum toward their maximum potential. Referral is a significant function of the discharge planning process. *Referral* involves actions that guide clients toward and assists them to use resources available to resolve their problems. Referrals can be made for clients by the community health nurse and can be directed toward illness prevention, health promotion, health maintenance, or restoration.

CLIENT ADVOCACY

Advocacy involves defending or pleading the case of another. Advocates work on behalf of others to achieve certain rights or improve human conditions (Steinke, 1984). Advocates inform and support people so they can make the best decisions possible for themselves (Kohnke, 1980). Various professional and lay persons have assumed the advocate role, including lawyers, educators, social workers, family, and friends. Nurses too have embraced advocacy, and many consider it the cornerstone of the profession.

Community health nurses who serve as a client advocate expect their functions to include (1) facilitating of continuous client care among health care resources; (2) optimizing client use of and access to health care services; and (3) assisting health care professionals to recognize and plan for individual, group, and community client needs. The goal of these functions is to alleviate clients' anxieties about their needs.

Clients expect the community health nurse to make available and accessible the services necessary to resolve their problems, to offer assistance in the use of available services, and to avoid duplication of services so they are not subjected to unnecessary and repetitive services that tend to increase risk of harm and cost to clients. In addition, clients expect high-quality service and a reasonable effort on the part of practitioners to care for their needs with skill, knowledge, and sound judgment (Williams and Torrens, 1984).

The *community agency* for whom the nurse works expects clients' needs to be recognized, assessed, and met by the nurse; expects the nurse to follow agency policy and procedures in meeting client needs and to serve as an agency representative; expects clients to be satisfied with the services received; and expects services to be rendered at an efficient cost to the agency. The agency also expects the nurse to have expertise as an advocate of client care services.

Advocacy has been a part of nursing since the profession's inception when Florence Nightingale advocated improvements in the health care of soldiers (Freeman, 1971). A mandate for advocacy by nurses is found in the 1976 revision of the ANA Code for nurses. "In the role of client advocate the nurse must be alert to and take appropriate action regarding any instances of incompetent, unethical, or illegal practice(s) by any member of the health team or health care system itself, or any action on the part of others that is prejudicial to the client's best interest" (ANA, 1976, p. 8).

Curtin (1982) maintains that advocacy is the very philosophical foundation of nursing with the end purpose being the welfare of other human beings. She says that nursing is a moral art that acknowledges what illness does to the physical and psychological limits of a person's being. Nurses recognize that illness damages one's humanity through loss of independence, freedom of action, and interference with the ability to make choices. It is in this situation that clients need an advocate who can speak on their behalf.

CONSEQUENCES OF ADVOCACY

The history of nursing provides an interesting perspective for advocacy. Since the emergence of modern nursing in the mid-1850s, loyalty and obedience have been valued in nurses. A military metaphor describes the discipline required to produce trained nurses. Nurses were required to be loyal to the physician just as a soldier would be loyal to a superior officer. Loyalty to the physician and loyalty to the client were often interpreted as one and the same (Winslow, 1984).

As nursing entered the twentieth century and nursing education improved, there developed an awareness of potential case mismanagement, resulting in a conflict of loyalties. Nurses questioned whether greater allegiance was to the physician or to the client. Nurses were expected to follow doctors' orders without question, and under the doctrine of respondent superior were offered legal protection. This tradition was altered significantly in 1929 by the Somera case in which a nurse was found guilty of manslaughter because she failed to question a physician's order for medication. Nurses suddenly became accountable for their own actions (Winslow, 1984).

In the middle of the twentieth century, the codes of the International Council of Nurses and the American Nurses Association were revised, reflecting the increased professionalism of nursing and the impact of growing consumerism. The early codes upheld the notion of loyalty to the physician, whereas revisions completely deleted the concept. The change in language specifically delegated to nurses the responsibility to safeguard the client from unsafe or unethical practice of any individual (Winslow, 1984).

The road to advocacy is not free of difficulties. Because the advocate is not chosen by the client, the paternalistic attitude of knowing what is best should be avoided by the professional. Conflict may arise because of the nature of the nurse-client relationship and the dependency that altered health status tends to foster. Nurses are obligated to interpret their role as representative and act as a spokesperson for the client's interests (Abrams, 1978).

Nurses often put themselves in a position, either willingly or innocently, of being rescuers. Rescuers often make decisions for others and, therefore, are put in a position of jeopardy if the decision does not turn out as well as expected. The backlash of being blamed for an action, carried out for the purpose of doing good, creates an awkward position for the well-intended advocate (Kohnke, 1980).

Other consequences of the advocacy role for nurses working in the community become apparent as clients become informed and begin to assert themselves. A ripple effect is created by the client's assertion, which impinges on administrators and other health professionals. Nurses who take a position and stick to it may draw criticism and be labeled as troublemaker or informer. Nurses advocating for individuals or groups have occasionally encountered enough pressure to force them to resign their positions to prevent compromising their beliefs (Smith, 1980).

The highly publicized case of *Jolene Tuma v the Idaho Board of Nursing* is an example of the plight of one nurse who encountered legal difficulties as a result of her advocacy activities. Tuma was asked by a client about alternatives to chemotherapy for treatment of her cancer. Tuma described nutritional therapy and use of Laetrile. She was later charged with unprofessional conduct and interfering in the physician-client relationship. Her nursing license was suspended for 6 months. She appealed the ruling and after 3 years of legal battles, the Idaho Supreme Court ruled that the Board of Nursing had been wrong in their action because it had no rules and regulations that adequately indicated that Tuma's actions were prohibited (Creighton, 1984).

Those who accept the challenge of advocacy may wish to weigh that decision in light of possible consequences, and those embarking on the advocacy venture might do well to be aware of the general attitude of a few in the health care sector toward advocacy. Pitfalls of advocacy can be avoided by being aware of possible problems, clarifying one's position with the client and others, being knowledgable about the system, and planning carefully.

The community health nurse as client advocate is the facilitator of movement toward client goals. In the facilitative situation, initially the community health nurse can listen to the client's and family's description of the client situation. The community health nurse can clarify the perceptions, ideas, and feelings of the client and elaborate on the perceptions of the client. The nurse can validate and substantiate facts and feelings through observations of the client situation and can assess the reliability of the information received from the client by comparing it with previously recorded data and with family interpretations of the situation.

After gathering data from the client through interview and observation, the community health nurse may present and interpret the client situation to the multidisciplinary team. The community health nurse must be ready to listen to the team's perceptions and interpretations of the situation, to move the group toward agreement on solutions, to restate team input for accuracy, to check for goal consensus among the team, to allow all team members to evaluate new ideas introduced, and to evaluate the outcome of the team's plan of action.

The Helping Relationship

Client advocacy is practical within the framework of the helping relationship. This relationship begins before contact is made with the client as the nurse anticipates problems that might be encountered and resources and abilities of the client, considers possible alternative actions, and plans for the meeting with the client. During the introductory or *orientation phase* of the helping relationship, the nurse and client compare their expectations for the encounters, delineate limits, discuss confidentiality of communication, and develop knowledge of each other that leads to trust and commitment.

During the working or *maintenance phase* of the helping relationship, the nurse and client accomplish the tasks they planned. If the relationship is productive there should be growth, positive behavior changes and open expression of feelings. During the *termination phase,* the nurse and client review their accomplishments and discuss the ability of the client to be self-sufficient (Sundeen, Stuart, Rankin, and Cohen, 1985).

Pace (1985) described an advocacy model of helping clients reach decisions by (1) promoting and encouraging self-care, (2) providing needed health care information as it relates to the client's situation, and (3) integrating communication and human relation skills that facilitate client decision making and goal setting. Orem (1980) includes acting for or doing for another, guiding another, and teaching another as methods of helping.

Health promotion and control of chronic disease require active participation by clients. By developing methods to enlist the participation of clients in their own health care, nurses are client advocates. Nursing actions include assisting clients to adjust therapeutic regimens and to alter behaviors to increase adherence; identifying methods for coping with stresses of life; and focusing on clients' priorities, strengths, and decision-making abilities as they strive to achieve wellness. To facilitate participation by clients in their care, nurses can grasp each opportunity to systematically recognize and reinforce clients when they demonstrate well behaviors. Such well behaviors can include asking questions, keeping appointments, taking food or medication to control symptoms, and making decisions about activities to control stress. Nurses can create an environment in which clients feel they can do much to maintain their health. Nurses offer assistance in developing knowledge and techniques for control of health.

Contracting is one method of identifying desired behavior and ensuring systematic reinforcement of that behavior. A *contingency contract* is a written agreement between two parties that a reinforcement will be received in return for the performance of a specific behavior. Steckel (1982), a nurse researcher who has used contingency contracting in a variety of chronic illness and health promotion situations, described the natural alliance between the nursing process and in the use of contingency contracting. Table 38-1 compares the elements present in each process and Figure 38-1 gives an example of a contract.

Contracting requires that nurses perform thorough physical, psychosocial, and environmental assessments; develop goals with outcome measures; make specific plans and evaluate and document care and outcomes of care. Contracting clarifies the relationship between the nurse and client and specifies what each can expect of the other. It also demonstrates the contribution nurses make to increased adherence to therapeutic regimes and improved health of clients (McEnany and Tescher, 1985; Steckel, 1982). Examples of contracting with groups and families can be found in Chapters 20 and 37. As one can see, contracting is a tool the community health nurse can apply in many client situations.

There is a fine line between being a decision maker on behalf of another and being one who informs the client of

TABLE 38-1

Nursing process and contracting

Elements of the nursing process	Steps necessary in contracting	Examples for weight control program
1. Assessment of the client data (Formulation of nursing diagnosis)	1A. Collection of baseline data about the presence or absence of desired behavior.	1A. Diet history, family history, three-day log of intake, psychosocial aspects of food, ideal weight/image, exercise/activity.
	1B. Pinpointing or specifying terminal behaviors in specific measurable terms.	1B. Number of calories eaten in a day for a week.
2. Planning of goals and actions	2. Identification of successive approximations; breakdown of the terminal behavior into small, manageable steps that will lead to performance of the terminal behavior.	2. Walk 15 minutes per day, chew gum while cooking to discourage snacking.
3. Implementation of plan of care	3. Implementation of the shaping process, i.e., reinforcement of each successive approximation that approaches performance of the terminal behavior.	3. Go to movie if no snacking all week; nurse agrees to spend 15 minutes discussing client's children.
4A. Evaluation	4A. Use of written feedback in the form of recordkeeping to evaluate progress.	4A. Food intake log, activity log, weight graph, dimension chart.
4B. Revision of plan of care as necessary	4B. Alteration of successive approximations and forms of reinforcement as necessary.	4B. Goal becomes maintenance of new activity and eating habits.

Modified from Steckel, S.B.: Patient contracting, Norwalk, Conn., 1982, Appleton-Lange, pp. 49-50.

```
                          Sample Contract

I, _____ , will _____
              (client)

_____ , in return for _____
              (behavior)

_____.
              (reinforcement)


                        Signed _____Client
                        Signed _____Nurse
                        Date _____

(Note:  This part of the page is left blank so that the client
and nurse can identify bonuses or future successive approximations.
It is also used to record information the client might want, such
as blood pressure, weight, diet suggestions, telephone numbers,
or other pertinent information.)
```

FIGURE 38-1

Sample contract. (Modified from Steckel, S.B.: Patient contracting, Norwalk, Conn., 1982, Appleton-Century-Crofts, p. 44.)

available options and subsequently supports the client's decision. The nurse is a resource person who gathers information to assist clients and families in their efforts to become informed about their rights, who encourages self-help, and who contributes to the database that enhances rational decision making. This is done with an appreciation of the individual as a unique human being who is particularly vulnerable because of the stress associated with injury or illness (Gadow, 1979). The advocate supports the individual's right to fully participate in the decision making process and acts as a buffer to prevent others from undermining that process (Kohnke, 1982). Once the decision is implemented, the nurse serves as gatekeeper, maintaining responsibility for monitoring the quality and continuity of care on the client's behalf (Abrams, 1978).

Conflicts in values between the client and nurse may arise; thus, it is helpful for the nurse to try to see the situation through the client's eyes. Advocacy does not mean imposing one's values on another, even though the advocate may view the situation as being detrimental to the client's health (Mauksch, 1980).

An example of a values conflict between the client and the provider was the case of an 80-year-old woman who had diabetic complications and developed gangrene of the foot. The physician recommended amputation, but the woman wanted to die "whole." The dilemma of death versus mutilation does not offer a pleasant choice. Philosophy and values are extremely subjective, with no two people viewing a given situation from exactly the same perspective. This may be a point of conflict for nurses who feel they know what is best.

CHARACTERISTICS OF THE ADVOCATE

Individuals engaged in positive, assertive action on behalf of others share some of the following characteristics (Donahue, 1978):

1. *Understanding:* of the issues of human rights.
2. *Accountability:* thinking and acting in a rational manner, assuming the responsibility for one's actions.
3. *Risk taking:* willingness to step forward and take a chance.
4. *Ability to communicate:* presenting the client's concerns in a succinct and convincing manner.
5. *Resourcefulness:* identifying and negotiating resources to be tapped for the client's benefit.

Responsible advocacy is the hallmark for the nurse who wishes to serve the client's best interests. This is accomplished by having a concern for the client's total situation, including what effect a change in that situation will have on others (Zusman, 1982).

Initially, the nurse must perceive that a problem exists and must analyze the need to become involved before proceeding. Motivation to act is tempered with prior consideration for the various alternatives available to meet the client's needs. The nurse advocate attempts to motivate and mobilize others in working toward a common goal. The interactive process of working with colleagues, outside agencies, or family members requires the willingness to compromise when necessary. Negotiation is an art that once

learned can serve as a valuable tool in the advocate role.

Zusman (1982) outlines seven elements a health care provider should weigh in each case when making decisions about advocacy roles.

1. Analyze the need and probable results before taking the plunge.
2. Decide in advance what results are desired. Then decide what to do.
3. Consider alternative goals for the client.
4. Distinguish between honest disagreement and dishonesty, neglect, and incompetence in health care delivery before involving the client in controversy.
5. Obtain a colleague's opinion.
6. Look for ways to be unobtrusive.
7. Try asking questions.

Effective Coordination/Collaboration

Effective collaboration requires assertive persons with varied ideas and expertise, as well as a commitment to seeking goals that lead to the best alternatives to meet client needs. Collaboration involves setting mutual goals, clarifying each team member's role, identifying all possible resources, delineating alternative approaches to attain goals, selecting specific interventions, mobilizing resources, and putting a plan into operation (Friedman, 1985).

As a collaborator, the community health nurse is involved with multidisciplinary relationships with the health team to help meet client needs. The multidisciplinary team may involve nurses representing other agencies, physicians, social workers, physical therapists, nutritionists, speech therapists, attorneys, clerical personnel, environmental engineers, mental health personnel such as psychologists, other health professionals, and clients.

The nurse is also involved in intra-agency collaboration: nurse to nurse, nurse to supervisor, nurse to aide, and nurse to other health professionals. In the agency using team assignments, the nurse must collaborate with team members to assure continuity of care and must coordinate case conferences for communicating clients' health care needs. The case conference keeps health personnel and community aids informed of the progress and needs of their clients.

Coordination efforts require leadership skills, which are applied to achieve unity of effort among the group of providers to accomplish their objectives (Rakich et al., 1977).

The community health nurse as client advocate has two specific role functions relative to coordination: (1) coordination of client care and (2) coordination of resources. A third function that may be assigned to the nurse is coordination of an interagency program such as a family planning program. Additionally, there are two levels of coordination in which the nurse may engage to fulfill these role functions: (1) horizontal coordination and (2) vertical coordination. In *horizontal coordination* the nurse, a member of the health department, acts as an agent for the client in assembling and directing the work efforts of a group of resource agencies, who are external to the employing agency and who have common goals for the identified client. For example, Helen Smith, the home health nurse, has been notified by Dr. Doe that Mary Jones has had a cerebrovascular accident resulting in hemiplegia and has been hospitalized. By visiting Mary in the hospital and attending multidisciplinary staff conferences, Helen finds that Mary's prognosis is good and she is progressing rapidly. Helen describes Mary's home situation and family to the hospital staff and the staff agrees that Mary should be discharged to home care at the earliest possible date. Helen discusses plans for discharge with Mary and her family, asking for their input.

As plans develop, Helen contacts the agencies who can appropriately continue Mary's care regimen at home. Helen contacts the hospital supply house to arrange for a bed, walker, bedside commode, and essential supplies to make Mary's transition easier from hospital to home. She also arranges for a speech therapist, a physical therapist, and a home health aide for personal care.

After initial plans are made for Mary's discharge, Helen calls a meeting with Mary, the other members of the health team, and Mary's family to arrange for scheduling of activities and to discuss the group's goals for Mary's care. The meeting provides an opportunity for each person to know the roles of others in Mary's care, reduces the likelihood of duplication of services, allows Mary and the family to have input into the planned goals, and provides Helen with goal information that she can follow up and reinforce during her home visits.

In *vertical coordination,* community health nurses serve as links between their level in the organization and those above and below them. They also serve as links between the agency and the client population. The following is an example of vertical coordination within the agency. Connie Cole, the community health nurse supervisor, has been asked by the director of nursing to coordinate activities for the establishment of a prenatal clinic at the health department. Connie collects information about the need for prenatal care in the area, explores cost and funding sources, projects the number of staff needed and the staff availability, and projects client use of the clinic. Connie arranges a meeting with the nursing staff, the director of nursing, the nurse practitioners, and the medical officer to present her findings, to answer questions, to allow input into the planning of the clinic, and to assist the group to work collaboratively toward the development of the clinic.

Vertical coordination between a client group and the agency is depicted in the following example. The local consumer board for the high-rise apartment complex for the elderly has noted that a number of their residents have health needs. One day Connie is visiting a resident of the highrise complex and is approached by the manager about the health needs of these elderly residents. The consumer board is interested in developing a health screening and referral program with the health department. Connie returns to the health department to discuss the issue with her supervisor and the agency administration. After careful deliberation about costs, availability of resources, and the anticipated input from the high-rise board and residents, the administration directs Connie to implement the screening program for the client group.

In all of these examples, the community health nurse acts as advocate for a client or an aggregate of clients. The nurse is manipulating the health care system into being more responsive to client needs. In the health care delivery system, the community health nurse and the client are continually faced with several concerns: (1) the frustrations of dealing with several public agencies, each providing different and sometimes conflicting information; (2) existing rules and regulations, which often interfere with access to needed resources; and (3) communication barriers in a system that is often insensitive to providing essential services to its clients. The nurse must have the skill and expertise to perform the tasks required in advocacy; the motivation to seek the best possible care for clients; and the necessary knowledge to know how, why, where, and when to intervene for the client.

Effective Communication

Effective communication is the key ingredient in advocacy. Skill in working within a helping relationship and appropriate use of power are essential for advocacy. Knowledge of the theories of management, decision making, perception, motivation, and change are essential when guiding the work of others toward a common goal (see Chapter 7 for a brief discussion of these theories). The managerial functions of planning, organizing, and controlling are necessary tools for getting things done with and through people. As a client advocate, the community health nurse is involved in coodinating the care of clients through the *planning* of goals and objectives. Once the planning has been done, the community health nurse is responsible for *organizing* or integrating the resources—people, supplies, equipment, and facilities—in the most effective way to accomplish the goals. The community health nurse *controls* the flow of work by providing feedback (evaluation) about movement toward goals and by following the workers' accomplishments. The information is then compared with initial plans so adjustments can be made in directing future activities toward desired outcomes.

ADVOCACY AND THE NURSING PROCESS

Inherent in successfully accomplishing the managerial functions of planning, organizing, and controlling is the involvement of all concerned persons, including the client, in the decision making process. The nursing process is the framework for decision making.

First, the client situation is *assessed* and the problem is defined. The group involved in meeting the client's needs engages in problem analysis, listing all possible alternative solutions for *planning* to meet client needs. The choice of solutions for meeting client needs is made by the group, and the group organizes to *implement* the chosen solutions. A schedule of periodic *evaluation* is established during the planning phase so the group can make adjustments in its plans during implementation. When initial goals are met, the group evaluates the total plan to determine the need for continuing involvement with the client. At this point termination may occur for one or all members of the multidisciplinary team, including the community health nurse.

As client advocate, the community health nurse must

recognize and understand the motives and needs most important to the other people—client or team member. The amount of energy the players (client or team member) will expend in moving toward the established goals depends on the motivating forces directing the person. The motivating forces may be tangible and easily recognized, such as the need for food, clothing, shelter, and health care; or the forces may be intangible, such as needs for recognition, achievement, or competence. The advocate must note that commitment to attain a goal increases when individuals are involved in their own goal setting. If the community health nurse sets goals for the client or the multidisciplinary team, more frustration and less goal-directed activity will be evidenced than if a collaborative goal-setting process occurs.

Another important factor for the community health nurse to recognize is the influence of perception on goal-directed behavior. Perceptions are influenced by previous experiences with successes and failures that have occurred when engaging in goal-related activity. If a client attempting to learn to walk again after an accident is faced with persisting failure on a day-to-day basis, frustration will occur and goal-directed activity will decrease. The speech therapist who is planning activities for the aphasic client will find that past successes and failures with similar clients will influence the goals set for the new client.

All client advocate activities are change oriented. The activities of the community health nurse are directed toward changing the client's health status or changing the client's risk ratio, that is, assisting the client to change life-style habits to reduce the future risk of illness.

The community health nurse as client advocate assumes two leadership styles in achieving change (moving a group toward a common goal). The community health nurse may be a *situational leader,* one recognized by the group as the person with the leadership skills to help the group achieve its goals, or a *functional leader,* one who performs certain functions for attaining the group's goals with the client.

Throughout the discussion in this chapter the level of change promoted has been *participative change,* or involvement of all parties in helping to formalize and implement methods for attaining client goals. There may be instances where a more effective strategy is *directive change,* or forced change whereby a new behavior is practiced, new knowledge is acquired, a commitment to the change develops, and the reinforced behavior becomes voluntary (Hersey and Blanchard, 1982). For example, the client who continually fails at crutch walking is forced by the physical therapist to continue to practice. As muscles are strengthened and techniques are learned, the client voluntarily begins to walk with crutches and directive change has been effective. Similarly, when the health department administration recognizes a need for a prenatal clinic, the nursing staff is directed to operate the clinic. As client population increases and neonatal, infant, and maternal mortality decreases, nurses recognize the need for the clinic and begin to identify with and internalize the need for it. Again, directive change has been successfully used.

Communication Models

Two communication models that depict the interaction between the community health nurse and multidisciplinary team or family members are described by Hersey and Blanchard (1982) as the star and circle.

The *star model* provides a schema of the communication pattern that primarily exists when the community health nurse serves as the coordinator of client care and coordinator of resources (Figure 38-2). In this model the nurse is identified in the leadership position with responsibility for communicating with the client and other members of the team. Sometimes the community health nurse calls a meeting of members to discuss the efforts of the group in meeting the client goals or team members may interact directly on other situations as depicted in the adapted star model (Figure 38-3).

The *circle model* depicts a schema of the communication pattern that primarily exists when the community health nurse is involved in collaboration with others on behalf of the clients (Figure 38-4). For this model each person interacts with the two colleagues in either direction, and the group is free to communicate all around the circle.

The star communication model presents a picture of the

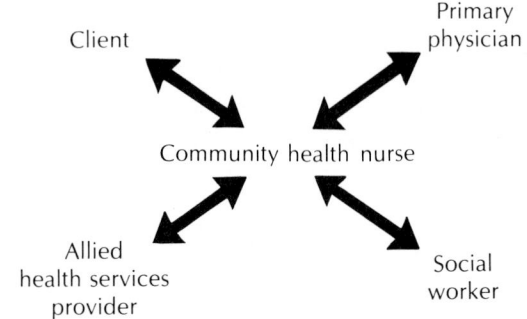

FIGURE 38-2

Star coordinative communication model. (From Hersey, P. and Blanchard, K.: Management of organization behavior: utilizing human resources, Englewood Cliffs, N.J., 1977, Prentice-Hall, Inc.)

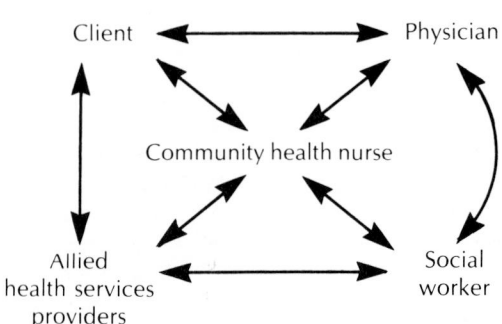

FIGURE 38-3

Interactive communication model with community health nurse as coordinator. (Modified from Hersey, P., and Blanchard, K.: Management of organization behavior: utilizing human resources, Englewood Cliffs, N.J., 1977, Prentice-Hall, Inc.)

directive change pattern, since one person is identified in the leadership role and a clear organizational network to solve problems is apparent. The adapted star and circle models show more of a participative change pattern in that all members have an opportunity for equal input in the solving of problems and in assuming leadership in the situation.

USE OF POWER IN ADVOCACY

Power is the ability to get others to achieve certain goals (Booth, 1983). Popular categorizations of power are those of French and Raven (1960) and Stevens (1983). Table 38-

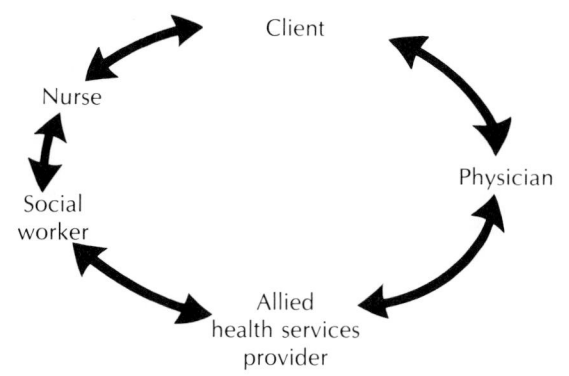

FIGURE 38-4

Circle collaborative communication model. (Modified from Hersey, P., and Blanchard, K.: Management of organization behavior: utilizing human resources, Englewood Cliffs, N.J., 1977, Prentice-Hall, Inc.)

2 lists, defines, and gives examples of these categories of power.

Nurses use power when they inspire and influence others to accomplish tasks and to create and maintain harmonious working relationships. They use it when coordinating, collaborating, and consulting with others to provide care for clients.

Nurses can exercise expert and informational power in the community by giving information and teaching self-care. These uses actually increase the power of clients over their lives. Nurses can accompany clients as they negotiate social and health service systems and use legitimate and referent power to help clients obtain services. Reward and coersive power do not help clients become independent and should be used with discretion.

Development of personal power comes with knowledge and communication abilities and perception of oneself as having influence in the health care system (Estobrook, 1986). Personal power can be developed through professional learning, developing expertise and consciousness of one's values, strengths and weaknesses, and the effects of one's actions on others. Such attributes as good health and vitality, constructive assertiveness, listening and interpersonal skills, logical thinking in problem solving rather than emotionality, and projection of a sense of self-worth through behavior and appearance are important in developing personal power (Lamar, 1985).

BARRIERS TO ADVOCACY

Some barriers to advocacy include role ambiguity, territoriality, lack of authority, adversary relationships, and conflicts of interest.

TABLE 38-2

Examples of power

Type of power	Description	Examples
Reward	Use of positive sanctions by powerful person	Employer rewards employee with recognition, money and promotions. Parents reward children with praise, love, and gifts. Nurse rewards client with praise.
Coercive	Threat of use of negative sanctions or punishment for noncompliance	Nurse refuses to visit if client doesn't comply with care regimen.
Referent (mentor)	Identification with powerful person increases power felt by another	When contacting a community resource, nurse mentions that the leader of a well respected organization suggested calling them.
Legitimate	Person believes another is in a powerful role, such as in social hierarchy, and has a right to influence actions of others	Relationships, such as teacher-student, employer-employee, parent-child, leader-member in organizations, nurse-client
Expert	Perception by others that a person possesses superior knowledge or skills, is trustworthy and credible	Physician-patient, nurse-client, plumber, electrician, carpenter and homeowner, expert witness-jurors.
Informational	Ability of a person to persuade another to behave differently by offering reasons or techniques, methods	Nurses giving information about the relationship of diet, exercise and smoking to heart disease, or diet and smoking to cancer to community groups. Professional organization providing information to legislators. Teaching a person behavior modification techniques to resist smoking or overeating.

Role ambiguity often occurs when management does not designate a primary provider who will serve as coordinator of client care. In agency team assignments, if one nurse is not designated as primary provider for a group of clients, often no nurse will assume the responsibility of coordinator; if someone attempts to assume responsibility, a problem with conflict may occur and questions of territorialism arise among the members of the team.

Problems of *territorialism* arise in the multidisciplinary team if members' roles are not clarified during the planning activities. This is a common problem, for example, in the home health arena where a person may be the client of the home health agency, the attending private physician, and the private practice physical therapists. If special efforts are not made to plan client services as a multidisciplinary team, then services may overlap, be duplicated, or not be offered because of the lack of an effective method of communication about client-related activities among the providers of service.

Traditionally, the physician has been viewed as the authority in the health care arena. Consumers do not recognize nurses as initiators of health care or client advocates, but rather as caregivers. When decisions related to participation of the client and other health care providers are involved, the authority of nurses to be effective advocates in the health care system may be questioned (Miller, Mansen, and Lee, 1983).

When nurses become advocates for clients they may put themselves and their clients in *adversary relationships* with other members of the health care team. This relationship may increase anxieties in the client rather than facilitate use of the system. Despite efforts toward clients accepting more responsibility for their own care, they may feel dependent when in health care institutions or under care of health care providers.

Conflicts of interest occur when the nurse is an employee of an agency, institution, or physician. Allegiance to employer policies can bring nurses into opposition with clients' desires and interests. Ideally, an advocate should be independent of political and financial restraints of an employer; this is seldom the case for nurses.

In the presence of these barriers, clients become dissatisfied with both providers and services offered; communication breaks down among providers and between providers and clients; referral patterns may change; and feelings of frustration, insecurity, and failure may occur in providers and clients. Client noncompliance may result, leading clients to seek health care elsewhere.

ADVOCACY IN COMMUNITY HEALTH NURSING

The discussion thus far has been directed toward defining advocacy and its role in nursing, discussing skills for the advocate, and exploring some of the conflicts associated with advocacy. The following discussion will focus on the client-consumer in the community and the problems associated with the complexity of the health care system. Attention is given to the community health nurse's planned intervention to increase consumer independence and to make the system more responsive to expressed problems.

Inexperienced health care consumers may face two problems when they need services. First, they often lack knowledge of available resources; second, they may lack a visible entry point into the health care system. With the myriad of medical specialties, agencies, and institutions, the chance of making the correct connection with the appropriate service without meeting one or more barriers is as unpredictable as a game of roulette. Consumers find themselves caught in a complex maze without knowledge of the rules of the game and consequently find many dead ends with little more than guesswork to determine which turn to take next. They may find that physicians are not taking new clients, that they do not qualify financially for a particular service, or that the hours of facility operation coincide with their hours of employment. Frustration and discouragement are inevitable outcomes and are compounded if the search for assistance is made in the urgency of a crisis situation.

There are many barriers, such as resource and economic barriers, to admittance to the health care system. *Resource barriers* are caused either by lack of specific services in the community or by insufficient services resulting from increased demand for those services by the public. *Economic barriers* affect uninsured individuals who do not qualify for medical assistance and also the insured who are hard hit by sizable deductibles and exempt services. Consumers relying on medical assistance have to search for providers who accept their form of payment.

Community health nurses may counsel clients and families on the availability of Medicaid and Medicare services. Persons may qualify for Medicaid if their income is low; if they have high medical costs in relation to their income; or if they are aged, blind, or disabled and living on a limited income. To apply for Medicaid, a client goes to a local welfare and Social Security office with proof of income level, proof of United States citizenship, and medical records proving disability or large medical bills. Aged persons may qualify for Medicare and Medicaid, and there are certain children's services that are provided by Medicaid under Early Periodic Screening, Diagnosis and Treatment programs (EPSDT). These services include screening examinations, immunizations, and diagnostic and treatment programs to prevent and correct health problems in children.

Some state Medicaid programs provide additional services not required by federal guidelines. The local Social Security or state human resource office would have information as to Medicaid benefits for that locality. Many clients think they cannot qualify for Medicaid programs if they own property or an automobile. This is not necessarily true; thus, benefit eligibility should always be explored by the community health nurse. Because the eligibility requirements and services offered by Medicare and Medicaid change frequently, the community health nurse should seek annual up-to-date information on Medicare and Medicaid from the Social Security Administration.

Use of Community Resources

The community health nurse uses a variety of community resources to aid the client. Sources of information include service directories that list agencies in the community with a brief description of each service, times of availability, terms of qualification, fees required, and the agency contact person.

When making inquiries about services, it is frustrating to deal with numerous public agencies and their conflicting information, rules, and regulations. Communications are often hampered when attempting to make connections with the appropriate person within an agency. Clients may have difficulty articulating questions to receptionists and translating them into the bureaucratic framework. The community health nurse's persistence and knowledge of the system can help to educate the client as to the nature of the resources available to meet specific needs and how to use them. For example, clients seeking information about a Medicare statement for home health services may call the Social Security general information number only to find that clients must first know whether the home health services were covered under Part A or Part B of Medicare to receive a correct phone number to call. The community health nurse can assist the client in interpreting the Medicare handbook and in seeking the correct source to contact for billing information.

When the client understands what outcomes can reasonably be expected from identified resources, the stage is set for positive planning and action. The community health nurse acts as gatekeeper during the action phase to see that the best possible services are provided in a continuous and comprehensive manner. Monitoring selected services through home visits and observation is a vital follow-up activity performed by the nurse. Important activities include discussing the client's care with the family members and collaborating with professionals to meet client care goals. The boxed material below and on p. 752 give some examples of a variety of community resources, which may be available in a mid-size community.

Nurses can participate in a number of activities associated with increasing the visibility of issues through advocacy. They can cut through red tape and make the health care delivery system more responsive to clients' needs. If one door is closed, others can be opened to achieve the same end. Writing and speaking skills come to play in building a coalition of support. Letters to the editor, articles in professional journals, and news spots on radio or television help to gain support for a cause. For example, a community

---

EXAMPLES OF COMMUNITY RESOURCES

ADVOCATES	ALCOHOL & DRUG ABUSE	CHILD CARE	CHILDREN'S SERVICES	COMMUNITY EDUCATION
Am. Civil Liberties	Alcoholics Anonymous	Dept. Soc. Serv.	Adoption Teams	American Red Cross
Long-term Care Ombudsman	Comprehensive Care	Salvation Army	Local Govt. Children's Services	Dairy & Food Nutr. Council
Local Govt. Citizen's Advocacy	Detoxification Programs	Neighborhood Organizations	Foster Care	March of Dimes
Dept. of Soc. Serv.	Nat. Council on Alcoholism		Crisis Drop-in Centers	Parents-in Training Programs
State Public Serv. Comm.	Narcotics Anonymous			Parents-Plus for Handicapped
	Rehabilitation Counseling Centers			

COUNSELING	EDUCATION	ELDERLY	EMPLOYMENT	FINANCIAL AID
Alternatives for Women	Voc./Tech. Schools	Sr. Citizen Center	Community Serv. Employ. Programs	Dept. Soc. Insurance
Comprehensive Care	Preschool for Handicapped	Alzheimer's Association	Local Govt. Employ. & Train. Centers	Salvation Army
Catholic Soc. Serv.	Hearing & Speech Center	Community Serv. Nutr. Programs	Workshops for Mentally Handicapped	Unemployment Insurance
Dept. Soc. Services		Sr. Citizen Employ. Serv.	Private Employment Agencies	
Family Counseling Services		Creative Living Center	Voc./Rehabilit. Services	
Life Educators		Public Housing		
Govt. Psychological Serv. Center		Reassurance Phone Service (Red Cross)		
Veterans Centers		Home Care		
		Nursing Homes		
		Health Dept.		
		Soc. Sec. Adm.		
		Council on Aging		

Continued.

EXAMPLES OF COMMUNITY RESOURCES—cont'd

HEALTH

Local Medical Center
American Cancer Soc.
American Lung Assoc.
Cancer Info. Services
Hospice Agencies
Diabetes Foundation
Physicians for Medical Assistance
Health Dept.
Muscular Dystrophy Assoc.
Veterans Hospitals
Home Health Agencies
Nursing Homes
Hearing & Speech Services
Child Dev. Center
Council for Blind
Mental Health Facilities
Shriner's Hospitals

HOTLINES

Adoption
Adult Abuse
American Cancer Soc.
Child Abuse
Crisis Intervention
Help Line (General)
Parental Help Line
Poison Control
Toxic Chem. Nat. Response Center
Rape Crisis Center
Spouse Abuse Crisis Center

HOUSING

Assoc. for Retarded Citizens
Community Action
Local Govt. Division of Housing Grants
Hospital Hospitality Houses
Housing Authorities
Human Rights Commission
Ronald McDonald Houses
Salvation Army

HUMAN ABUSE

Local Govt. Children's Services
Crimes Against Children
Dept. Soc. Serv.
Protective Services
Local Child Abuse Council
Rape Crisis Center
YWCA Spouse Abuse Center

LEGAL

Juvenile Service Center
Legal Aid Services

PREGNANCY/CHILDBIRTH

Pregnancy Help Center
Birthright Organizations
Florence Crittenton Homes
Planned Parenthood Assoc.
Right to Life

SELF-HELP

Al-Anon
Alternatives for Women
Alliances for Mentally Ill
Alzheimer's Societies
Compassionate Friends for Bereaved Parents
Smoking Cessation Programs
I Can Cope Ed. Programs for Cancer
Lost Chord Club
Parents Anonymous
Parents Without Partners
Parkinson's Disease Support
Prison Family Support
Reach to Recovery
United Ostomy Assoc.
Widows Helping Widows

TRANSPORTATION

Local Bus Service
Salvation Army
Wheels (Red Cross)

health nurse is concerned that the street people of Anytown, U.S.A., do not have facilities for shelter during cold winter months. The community health nurse elicits support from key community organizations, the Chamber of Commerce, and professional organizations to raise money to support the shelter concept. The nurse then speaks to the local television station and is offered a spot on the local news to plead for a location to house the shelter. The presentation is effective and the shelter coalition is offered a lease on an old nursing home site.

Working through political systems at the local, state, and even national levels helps to establish credibility. The community health nurse continues the drive for the shelter by seeking matching funds from the local government to support the shelter.

Other options for nurses include appearing at public hearings with prepared statements and arranging appointments to speak with key legislators about issues, such as the primary care block grants to see that prenatal care has continued funding in the state. Advocates should seek membership on committees and policy-making boards to influence the system through established channels. Presenting public education programs to local service organizations also spreads the message about client needs at the grass roots level. These advocacy activities are but a few of the many that can be developed to bring about greater awareness of the issues affecting consumers today (Brower, 1982).

DISCHARGE PLANNING AND CONTINUITY OF CARE

For the past few years, the health care delivery system has instituted many federal and private third-party pay policies, which focus on efforts to reduce health care costs. The institution of HMO's, Medicare deductibles, and DRG's are some examples of policies that emphasize decreased hospitalization and expenditures. Consequently, health care providers must help their clients better understand their health status and prepare them to care for themselves in their homes and communities.

The community health nurse can be the vital professional in establishing a discharge care plan whether the plan is directed toward the client's discharge from hospital to community agency or toward the client's discharge from the community agency to self-care.

Discharge planning is part of a continuum of care in which those responsible for a client's treatment collaborate in a multidisciplinary team approach to assist the client and family to move from one phase of care to the next. It incorporates the concept of holistic health planning, which includes preventive, primary, therapeutic, rehabilitative, and custodial care. Inherent in the concept of discharge planning is the need for client and family to work with the health care team in arranging a therapeutic plan of care that enhances the client's ability to return to an optimal lifestyle.

Continuity of care (client care activities rendered to the client before agency admission while under agency care and after discharge) and comprehensive health care are objectives of discharge planning. Four essential components of comprehensive health care are (1) health education, (2) personal preventive services, (3) diagnostic and therapeutic services, and (4) rehabilitative and restorative services (Bristow, Stickney, and Thompson, 1976).

Discharge planning is recognized as one of the 12 essential items in the American Hospital Association's "Statement on a Patient's Bill of Rights." The Joint Commission on Accreditation for Hospitals, PRO's, and Medicare regulations require hospitals and nursing homes to provide discharge planning.

Programs and Settings

Five basic options must be considered in the planning of care following discharge: (1) home health care programs, (2) after-care programs, (3) outpatient visits, (4) nursing home, and (5) day care centers. All options provide services outside the hospital, are considerably more economical, and strive to provide and enhance the health of the client and family. *Home health care programs* provide services of a physician, nurse, social worker, physical therapist, or occupational therapist in the client's home. Home health aides, under the supervision of the professional nurse, are also frequently used for chronically ill clients. They are used mainly to assist families in the personal care of the client. Homemakers assist families with care of the ill person and the functioning of the home (i.e., cooking, cleaning, washing). These services free up hospital beds and assist family members in the continued care of chronically ill relatives. Home health care teams may serve a particular population group. For example, an oncology team consisting of a physician, registered nurse, and social worker may assist cancer victims to maintain themselves in the home. Likewise, pediatric teams may work exclusively with high-risk parents, such as those in abused child or premature infant situations (Harvey, 1981).

Aftercare programs provide services by ensuring transportation and continuity of care for clients when they return to the hospital for treatment and then go home again. Fewer hospital visits are required if all health care needs and appointments can be coordinated in a one-day visit. This program is especially helpful for those clients who must travel long distances.

Outpatient follow-up is the most common method of providing care after hospital discharge for medical treatment of clients receiving home health care. Clients are given an appointment to a clinic or service. This is the least expensive type of care, since clients arrange their own transportation. Clients with especially troublesome illnesses, such as those having difficulty getting around or those unable to endure continuous care on an outpatient basis, find that home health care is the best option for them in reducing the number of outpatient visits.

Day-care centers for disabled or impaired children or adults who require constant supervision are innovative programs to assist families. Adult day-care centers are more economical than home or institutional care and permit family members to continue employment. Most clients are ambulatory, but some centers offer weekend services or temporary care for bedridden clients, providing weekend respites for families from the daily care of a chronically ill relative. Most adult day-care centers offer a variety of therapeutic services, such as nursing care, occupational and recreational therapy, physical and speech therapy, psychotherapy, social services, and individual or group counseling (Pomeranz and Rosenberg, 1985; Szehais, 1985).

Long-term convalescent or *nursing home care* is used for persons requiring round-the-clock supervision. Nursing homes also provide care for clients who are psychologically or physically handicapped and are unable to cope outside an institutional setting. Many elderly clients view nursing homes as the least desirable option. Nursing home care is expensive and often have rigorous admission requirements and long waiting lists (Ratliff, 1981).

THE COMMUNITY HEALTH NURSE AS DISCHARGE PLANNER

The position of a discharge planner requires an individual with (1) tact; (2) resourcefulness; (3) initiative; (4) ability to communicate effectively with agency staff, clients, and families; and (5) a knowledge of community resources. The nurse must be assertive enough to initiate the discharge process if the client's condition and resources deem it advisable. Large institutions may have a nurse to coordinate discharge planning for each major unit. These nurses are very knowledgeable regarding community resources and skilled in assisting clients and families to make the transition from one facility to another. The agency staff nurse functions in an independent and collaborative manner to ensure continuity of care for clients after discharge (Clausen, 1984).

Community health nurses are becoming discharge planners with increasing frequency. Institutions contract with the health department or Visiting Nurse Association to place nurses in their facility. The nurse remains an employee of the Visiting Nurse Association, although the hospital pays for the time the nurse spends there. The community health nurse is adept in making a home and community assessment that enhances the effectiveness of the discharge plan. In one large hospital complex, the department of community health nursing administers the extended care nursing program. This program provides an extended care nurse, who coordinates discharge planning with the primary nurses, for each major unit in the hospital. Extended care-discharge planning nurses arrange for such services as transportation; oxygen; wheelchairs; hospital beds; physical, speech or respiratory therapy; or home health (Rasmusen, 1984).

A typical day for a discharge planning nurse would include the following:

1. Meet all admissions and screen for potential discharge problems.
2. Attend morning report and rounds at the institution.
3. Give high priority to planning for clients whose discharge is imminent.
4. Complete pending referrals.
5. Contact physicians for completion of forms and contact the appropriate referral agency.
6. Interview the client and family immediately before discharge.
7. Make home visits to assess the resource and liability of the home environment.

Discharge planning nurses practice not only in the secondary or tertiary care setting but also in the primary care setting. Many outpatient clinics and emergency departments employ a nurse to coordinate discharge plans for clients and families. Basically the activities of this nurse are the same as those of the nurse practicing in the institutional setting but with minor variation. The nurse in the primary care setting does not make rounds, since the clients are usually referred to the nurse by other staff members. However, this nurse may review and screen the daily appointment schedules for potential clients. The nurse is often involved in extensive client education and referral to community agencies.

Whether the setting is an inpatient facility, such as a secondary or tertiary care hospital, a nursing home, primary care outpatient clinic, an emergency facility, a home health agency, or health department, the nurse works closely with other providers, especially social work services. Social workers have traditionally participated in discharge planning services for clients and families. In addition to having a vast knowledge of community resources, social workers can assist with financial arrangements. They usually have knowledge of private and governmental programs that offer assistance.

The nutritionist or dietician can provide information on community resources for food purchases, food substitutes, and adaptations for food preparations used in the home. Information on available programs in the community that provide nutrition education and weight loss plans are being used on a more frequent basis in the overall therapeutic plan.

The clinical pharmacist can provide information on community resources for reduced drug costs and valuable client education literature. The hospital chaplain can promote access to a community pastor for the client if contact has not been established. Chaplains also have knowledge of various church-related resources such as therapy groups, clothing, food banks, and health-related clinics. Physical therapists can assist in planning for a home care adaptation program. Many of the larger institutions providing long-term care also employ a vocational rehabilitation counselor and a recreational therapist. Counselors in school systems can assist with special educational needs of children and adults. All of these individuals are excellent resources to assist in the discharge planning process.

Referrals

All clients need some form of discharge teaching and preparation, but not all clients will need extensive discharge planning. Need may be the result of the nature of the clients' health problems, financial and family situations, or availability of existing community resources. Community health nurses who practice in an ambulatory-primary care setting must take the initiative in implementing a discharge-teaching plan for their clients. The following pediatric or maternity clients require discharge planning and follow-up:

1. Infant weighing 4½ pounds or less or weighing over 10 pounds at birth.

2. Infant with an Apgar score, at 5 minutes, of 7 or lower.
3. Infant with major congenital anomaly, such as cleft palate or spina bifida.
4. Infant with positive PKU test result.
5. New teenaged mother.
6. Mother discharged after delivery in past 48 hours.
7. Family with indication of dysfunction, parental rejection, or child abuse.
8. Baby failing to thrive and with poor feeding prognosis.
9. Family with a crisis, such as a child with a newly diagnosed serious illness (e.g. leukemia) or traumatic injuries.
10. Child of a mother with a serious medical or mental problem, such as a maternity client with depression.

The client admitted to the hospital for radical or mutilating surgery may require follow-up, especially if the surgery may produce marked changes in life-style or family relations. Examples include:
1. Nephrectomy
2. Ostomy
3. Radical neck or face reconstruction
4. Extremity amputation
5. Surgery for weight reduction
6. Cardiovascular reconstruction.

Adult or pediatric clients with an acute or chronic illness would also benefit from follow-up; for example, clients with diabetes, arthritis, heart disease, stroke, chronic renal disease, cancer, and emphysema who require the following:
1. Medication regulation or administration,
2. Special diets or treatments such as feeding tubes, I.V. therapy, or hyperalimentation,
3. Exercises or physical therapy.
4. Wound care with dressing changes.
5. Catheter care.

Because of changing third-party payer policies and DRG's, clients with more serious conditions, such as those needing respirator assistance, intravenous and hyperalimentation therapy, are being cared for by the home health nurses more often. Additionally, clients who are terminal or preterminal, comatose or semicomatose, disoriented, and confused are often cared for in the home and need more extensive discharge planning and coordination. This is especially pertinent when any medical equipment such as respirators, suction, beds, and other devices are needed. Depending on the resources in a community, it may take a few days to have the equipment delivered and set up. Home health care programs can provide many complicated therapies previously provided by the hospital setting. Not only is the cost of care reduced, but clients also experience psychological benefits that enhance the quality of life (Hughes, Cordray, and Spicher, 1984). The cost of intermittent home health care is considerably less than hospitalization regardless of the reason for referral.

Geriatric Clients

Geriatric clients present different sets of problems. Discharge planning for geriatric clients should begin on the date of admission as Medicare hospital coverages end when the client no longer requires diagnostic services or treatments that can only be provided by the acute care facility. Limits of coverage are now defined by DRG's. Many geriatric clients need long-term, restorative, recuperative care (De Young, 1982). Because of physical impairments, many clients cannot be discharged to go home alone, and special arrangements must often be made on a permanent basis. Facilities for placement of these clients are foster homes, custodial care facilities, or the client's own home with frequent periodic home visits by a community health nurse. Many communities have resources such as Meals on Wheels and home health aides, making it possible for elderly clients to stay in their homes. Special apartment complexes for the elderly may be visited by community health nurses to assist clients who are recuperating or who need special monitoring.

The discharged client with psychological illness may need food service and a resocialization program. A halfway house can meet both of these needs as well as provide a structured vocational rehabilitative program. Unfortunately, communities often have too few of these resources available.

The Process

As discharge planning begins during the admission process, the nurse solicits pertinent information about the client's resources and health information during the admission interview. Information such as the admitting problem, predicted length of hospital stay based on the DRG, type of residence, other household members and their ability to assist the client, travel resources, financial status, and client's ability to understand and carry out a treatment plan is assessed. Other essential information includes current level of care needed, projected level of care needed, projected time frame for moving client to next level of care, therapies and teaching that must be accomplished before discharge, and available resources and mechanisms for facilitating transfer from one institution to another institution or to the home.

Client (physiological, psychological, and social) readiness must be considered by a multidisciplinary team. All too often only the physiological needs are considered, and the psychological resources for the family and client are neglected. This is especially true of families who are coping with long-term debilitating or terminal problems (Shine, 1982). A visit to the home by a nurse to assess family and environmental resources will enhance discharge planning effectiveness. Dietary and nutritional resources and assets or impairments to ambulation are particularly evaluated.

Optimally, a formal discharge conference will be conducted with the primary nurse, the physician, and possibly the dietician, chaplain, and physical therapists if they are involved. As the coordinator of the team, the discharge nurse will in most cases make the necessary follow-up referrals.

A written discharge summary note is entered in the nursing notations, and some type of formal discharge instruction form is sent home with the client. The form can be tailored to a particular unit, outlining specific needs of the client, or be very general in format. All forms should contain information regarding basic needs: follow-up appointments, diet, medications, treatments, bathing, and activity instructions including when to drive and when to resume sexual relations.

The use of a discharge planning screening tool has proved effective as a teaching guide for professional personnel and it provides written reference material for the client and family (Druger and Rawling, 1984). The discharge planning screening tool will provide information about the client's activities of daily living; level of consciousness; need for dressings; wound care and other treatments, equipment, and transportation needs; medication schedules; presence of ostomies; social needs or problems; special teaching needs; and other therapies (occupational, physical, speech). To serve as a good referral mechanism, this tool should include an admission assessment, plan of care, documented client progress, and discharge summary.

A discharge planning tool can be adapted for any inpatient or ambulatory care facility client population. Instructions for problems such as wound care, head injuries, vomiting, diarrhea, fever, and special diet should be included in the discharge summary. Optimally, whenever a client seeks health care, some form of discharge teaching takes place including explicit instruction for the particular health problem and/or promotion information such as self-breast examination and mammography or colon rectal cancer screening. The nurse serves as advocate by assessing potential health problems for specific clients and providing clients with information regarding their risk factors.

The discharge planning nurse should be available if a problem does arise shortly after returning to the home. All too often the client or family will have questions that arise after discharge when the primary care provider is unavailable. These questions will go unanswered until the next day, or in desperation, the client will contact the local emergency department. All discharged clients need to have an emergency phone number and access to the discharge planning nurse or agency department. In the ambulatory care setting, many community health nurses assume responsibility for follow-up telephone inquiries of their discharged clients.

Benefits of Discharge Planning

Several rewards for clients, families, health providers, and the community can be realized when an effective discharge planning program is implemented. Money is saved to finance comprehensive service for a greater number of clients. Hospital beds are freed up. Relapses, needless hospital stays, and unnecessary emergency visits are decreased. Client and families become involved in the planning and participate actively in the education process. This involvement encourages a sense of responsibility for their own care. They develop trust in themselves to make future health care decisions and in the health provider to assist them with relevant information. Nurses in all settings can experience the rewarding feeling of observing a client and family make the transition from one phase of health status to another if they

take the opportunity to participate collaboratively and creatively in the discharge plan.

Barriers to Discharge Planning

Lack of communication and knowledge of community resources, are the two major barriers to effective discharge planning. A team approach with regularly scheduled meetings has proven successful in reviewing discharge needs of clients in an agency. As the coordinator of the team, the discharge planning nurse assures that communication lines are established among staff, client, family, and physicians. Most communities have a compiled list or book that contains available community resources. Usually eligibility criteria and contact persons are listed. Optimally the discharge planning nurse has an opportunity to meet the various agency contact persons and thus can talk to them on a more personal basis when a telephone referral is made. Some institutions have found that inviting resource agency representatives to speak with staff members facilitates the referral process.

It is desirable for the discharge planning nurse to provide feedback to the agency nurses if *written permission* to do so is obtained from the client. Information about the client's progress and receptiveness to the new environment and results of past nursing care are needed for the nurse's growth and evaluation. This information will assist the nurse to modify future nursing care where indicated. Also, administrative support is essential to provide adequate nursing staff for an agency so that quality discharge planning can be implemented. Frequently discharge planning is subordinate to maintenance of basic needs when an agency is understaffed.

CLINICAL APPLICATION

The community health nurse assumes the role of the client advocate within institutions and agencies. The nurse may be involved as a formally designated discharge planning coordinator. More frequently, the primary care or staff community health nurse is involved in the initial admission process of the client, subsequent referral, follow-up, and discharge planning. During these processes the nurse is a client advocate. This activity may also occur through participation in peer review or quality assurance committees. Additionally, most institutions, particularly those receiving federal funding, have policies protecting human rights. This policy is often reflected in the institution's Patient Bill of Rights. Institutions who engage in research activities will likewise have a policy and committee that deals with protection of human subjects in regard to research activities. Conceivably, the nurse could be involved in all of these activities as in the following example.

The nurse initially does the admitting history on Sam Brown, a 55-year-old unemployed mechanic who comes to a local health department clinic seeking treatment for episodes of chest pain that have increased in severity and frequency during the past two months. His condition is diagnosed as unstable angina and he is advised, because of his cardiac risk profile (his father died at age 50 of an acute myocardial infarction, he smokes two packages of cigarettes a day, and is 35 pounds overweight), to have a cardiology consult with an ECG stress test and possibly a heart catheterization to fully evaluate his cardiac status. As he is unemployed, he has no medical insurance to pay for these expensive tests. In fact, his economic status is very precarious. His only source of income is his wife, who is employed as a waitress. Realizing Mr. Brown is overwhelmed with the information he has received, the nurse may act as a client advocate by referring him to the social worker who can assist in securing some medical assistance. The nurse will set up appointments with the cardiologist to whom Mr. Brown has been referred and convey any special instructions to Mr. Brown regarding the appointment. Two weeks later, Mr. Brown comes into the clinic and states he does not understand what is happening. The cardiologist told him he would send a letter explaining his condition, but he has not received one. The nurse obtains the client's medical record and finds the letter was mistakenly filed in the client's chart before review by the referring physician. The cardiologist has recommended bypass graft surgery. The nurse notes that the cardiologist has referred to Mr. Brown as being disabled due to his present cardiac status. Realizing that Mr. Brown is now eligible for disability benefits, the nurse once again acts as an advocate by directing Mr. Brown to the local Social Security Insurance office where he can make a claim for disability. Before surgery, the cardiologist recommends that Mr. Brown take an experimental drug to improve the circulation to his heart. The nurse ascertains whether Mr. Brown has been informed of all the risks involved and that he does indeed understand his participation in the drug trial.

Eventually, Mr. Brown has surgery in a large tertiary care center. The nurse realizes that Mr. Brown will be discharged according to the DRG (diagnostic-related group

standards for cardiac bypass graft surgery). The community health nurse makes a telephone call to the hospital discharge planning nurse and receives all the necessary information regarding Mr. Brown's discharge plan and subsequent follow-up care. The nurse visits Mr. Brown at home to follow his progress. Client advocacy involves close surveillance of clients as they are referred to other health care providers and agencies. When the referral process involves multiple contacts, clients may become lost in the shuffle. Nurses facilitate the referral process through close contact and follow-up with clients and attempt to prevent undue delays.

SUMMARY

The community health nurse is an advocate who (1) assists clients to identify problems, needs, appropriate actions, and community resources; (2) collaborates with health care and social service professionals in planning and providing care; and (3) coordinates services for clients. Client advocacy is practiced within the frameworks of the helping relationship and the nursing process. Important advocacy functions of the community health nurse are management of interagency referrals and discharge planning from institutional settings to home care, and from home care to self-care.

Advocacy is not without problems for community health nurses. Barriers to advocacy include role ambiguity, territoriality of health and social service professionals, lack of authority, potential for adversarial relationships, conflicts of interest, and legal precedents. The nurse advocate is an assertive, accountable, resourceful risk taker. Nurse advocates use skills in communication, management, decision making, motivation, change, and appropriate use of power. The major goals of the community health nurse advocate are to make the health care system more responsive to the needs of clients and to move clients toward independence.

≡ KEY CONCEPTS

An important role of community health nurses is that of client advocate. Role functions include client care coordinator and collaborator, discharge planner, and referral manager.

The community health nurse as client advocate acts on behalf of the client to make the health care delivery system responsive to clients and to facilitate client independence.

The community health nurse as client advocate is the facilitator of movement toward client goals.

Client advocacy is done within the framework of the helping relationship. This relationship has three phases: the orientation phase, the maintenance phase, and the termination phase.

Contracting is one method of identifying desired behavior and ensuring systematic reinforcement of that behavior.

Persons engaged in client advocacy exhibit understanding, accountability, risk-taking, ability to communicate, and resourcefulness.

Responsible advocacy is the hallmark of the nurse who wishes to serve the client's best interests. This is done by understanding the client's total situation and the effect that change will have on others.

Effective communication is the most important ingredient in successful advocacy.

Skill in working with a helping relationship and appropriate use of power are essential for advocacy.

The client advocate should recognize the influence of perception on goal-directed behavior.

Power is the ability to get others to achieve certain goals.

Some barriers to advocacy include role ambiguity, territoriality, lack of authority, adversary relationships, and conflicts of interest.

Nurses can increase discussion and visibility of issues through use of writing and speaking skills and working through the political systems at the local, state, and national levels.

The community health nurse can be the vital professional establishing a discharge care plan whether the plan is directed toward discharge from hospital to community or discharge from community agency to self-care.

Five basic options to consider in planning for care after discharge are home health care programs; aftercare programs; outpatient visits; nursing home; and adult day care centers.

LEARNING ACTIVITIES

1. From your readings define the following terms: (a) coordination, (b) collaboration, (c) client advocacy, (d) discharge planning, (e) comprehensive care, (f) referral, and (g) communication.

2. In class or in a conference with a few of your peers, discuss these definitions and compare them to your own definitions. How are the definitions different or similar to your own? Give reasons why they may differ. How do these concepts relate to your perception of the role of the community health nurse?

3. In your clinical conference discuss your role functions as a client advocate. Give examples.

BIBLIOGRAPHY

Abdellah, F., Forest, H., and Chow, R.: PACE: An approach to improving care of the elderly, Am. J. Nurs. 79:1109, 1979.

Abrams, N.: A contrary view of the nurse as patient advocate, Nursing Forum 8(3):258-267, 1978.

American Nurses' Association: Standards of nursing practice, Kansas City, Mo., 1973, The Association.

American Nurses' Association: Code for nurses with interpretive statements, Kansas City, Mo., 1976, The Association.

American Nurses' Association: Human rights guidelines for nurses in clinical and other research, Kansas City, Mo., 1985, The Association.

Annas, G.: The right of hospital patients, New York, 1975, E.P. Dutton & Co., Inc. p. 35.

Aroskar, M.A.: Anatomy of an ethical dilemma. I. The theory, II. The practice, Am. J. Nurs. 80:658-663, 1980.

Bandman, E.: Protection of human subjects. Topics in Clinical Nursing 1(2):15-23, 1985.

Benne, K.D., and Birnbaum, M.: Principles of changing. In Bennis, W.G., et al., editors: Dynamics of planned change, New York, 1969, Holt, Rinehart & Winston, Inc.

Booth, R.Z.: Power: A negative or positive force in relationships? Nurs. Adm. Q. 7(4):10-20, 1983.

Bristow, O., Stickney, C., and Thompson, S.: Discharge planning for continuity of care, NLN Pub. No. 21-1604, 1976.

Brower, T.H.: Advocacy: What it is, J. Gerontol. Nurs. 8(3): 141-143, 1982.

Burston, G.R.: A holiday relief service for elderly patients normally cared for at home, Practitioner 211(263):345-350, 1973.

Channing, L.: Medicaid and you, Greenfield, Mass., 1979, Bet Co., Inc.

Clausen, C.: Staff RN: A discharge planner for every patient, Nursing Management 15(11):58-61, 1984.

Creighton, H.: RN advocate and the law, Nursing Management 15(12):14-17, 1984.

Curtin, L.L.: The nurse as advocate: a cantankerous critique, Nursing Management 14(5):9-10, 1982.

Curtin, L.L.: The nurse as advocate: a philosophical foundation for nursing, ANS Adv. Nurs. Sci. 1(3):1-10, 1979.

De Young, M.: Planning for discharge, Geriatric Nursing 4:396-399, 1982.

Donahue, P.M.: The nurse: A patient advocate?, Nursing Forum 12(2):143-151, 1978.

Estabrook, B.: More power to you, Nursing '86 16(4):89-90, 1986.

Fenwick, A.: An interdisciplinary tool for assessing patients' readiness for discharge in the rehabilitation setting, J. Adv. Nurs. 4:9-21, 1979.

Freeman, R.B.: Practice as protest, Am. J. Nurs. 71:918-921, 1971.

Friedman, M.: Family nursing theory and assessment, New York, 1985, Appleton-Century-Crofts.

French, J.R.P., Jr., and Raven, B.: The bases of social power. In Cartwright, D. and Zander, A.F., editors: Group dynamics, ed. 2, Evanston, Ill., 1960, Row, Peterson.

Gadow, S.: Advocacy nursing and new meanings of aging, Nurs. Clin. North Am. 14(1):81-91, 1979.

Harvey, B.: Your patient's discharge plan: does it include home health referral?, Nursing '81 11(7):48-51, 1981.

Hersey, P., and Blanchard, K.: Management of organization behavior: utilizing human resources, Englewood Cliffs, N.J., 1982, Prentice-Hall, Inc.

Hollingsworth, C.E., and Sokal, B.: Predischarge family conference, JAMA 239(8):740-741, 1978.

Huey, R.: Discharge planning: good planning means fewer hospitalizations for the chronically ill, Grand rounds, Nursing '81 11:70-75, 1981.

Hughes, S., Cordray, D., and Spicher, V.: Evaluation of a long term home health care program, Med. Care 22(5):460, 1984.

Hushower, G., Gamberg, D., and Smith, N.: The nursing process in discharge planning, Superv. Nurse 9:55-58, 1978.

Igoe, J.B.: Project health PACT in action, Am. J. Nurs. 80(11):2016-2021, 1980.

Inui, T., et al.: Identifying hospital patients who need early discharge planning for special dispositions: a comparison of alternative techniques, Med. Care 19(9):922-929, 1981.

Kohnke, M.F.: The nurse as advocate, Am. J. Nurs. 80(11):2038-2040, 1980.

Kohnke, M.F.: Myths and realities about advocacy-clinical research-abuse, Journal of the New York State Nursing Association 13(4):22-29, 1982.

Kruger, S., and Rawling, P.: Pediatric dismissal protocol to aid the transition from hospital care to home care, Image 16(4):120-124, 1984.

Lamar, E.K.: Communicating personal power through nonverbal behavior, J. Nurs. Adm. 15(1):41-44, 1985.

Lamb, H.R.: Securing patient's rights-responsibility, Hosp. Community Psychiatry 32(6): 393-397, 1981.

Lancaster, J., and Lancaster, W., editors: Concepts for advanced nursing practice: the nurse as a change agent, St. Louis, 1982, The C.V. Mosby Co.

Mauksch, I.G., Advocacy or control: which do we offer the elderly?, Geriatric Nursing 1(4): 278, 1980.

McDonnell, D.: An evaluation of day care center care, Int. J. Soc. Psychiatry 23(2):110-119, 1977.

McEnany, G.W., and Tescher, B.E.: Contracting for care, J. Psychosoc. Nurs. Ment. Health Serv. 23(4):11-18, 1985.

Miller, B.K., Mansen, T.J., and Lee, H.: Patient advocacy: do nurses have the power and authority to act as patient advocate?, Nursing Leadership 6(2):56-60, 1983.

Orem, D.: Nursing: concepts of practice, ed. 2, New York, 1980, McGraw-Hill.

Pace, J.C.: An advocacy model for health care professionals, Family and Community Health 7(4):77-87, 1985.

Pender, N.J.: Health promotion in nursing practice, New York, 1982, Appleton-Century-Crofts.

Pierce, S.: Peer review for clinical ladders, AORN J. 39(5):800, 1984.

Pomeranz, W., and Rosenberg, S.: Developing an adult day care center, J. Long Term Care Administration 13(1):11-22, 1985.

Previte, V.: Continuing care in a primary nursing setting role of a clinical specialist, Int. Nurs. Rev. 26(2):53-6, 1979.

Rakich, J.S., Longest, B.B., and O'Donovan, T.R.: Managing health care organizations, Philadelphia, 1977, W.B. Saunders Co.

Rasmusen, L.: A screening tool promotes early discharge planning, Nursing Management 15(5):39-43, 1984.

Ratliff, B.: Leaving the hospital: Discharge planning for total patient care, Springfield, Ill., 1981, Charles C Thomas.

Savedra, M.: Moving from hospital to home, Am. J. Maternal Child Nurs. 6:220-222, 1977.

Sheahan, S.L.: A discharge planning guide: an aid to discharge teaching, unpublished master's project, Lexington, Ky., 1974, University of Kentucky College of Nursing.

Shine, M.: Discharge planning for the elderly patient in an acute care setting, Nurs. Clin. North Am. 18(2):403-410, 1982.

Smith, C.S.: Outrageous or outraged: a nurse advocate story, Nurs. Outlook 28(10):624-625, 1980.

Sobel, D.: So that others may live, OMMI 2(3):52-58, 1979.

Steckel, S.B.: Patient contracting, Norwalk, Conn., 1982, Appleton-Century-Crofts.

Steinke, E.: Introduction to patient advocacy in nursing, The Kansas Nurse 59(1):2-3,20, 1984.

Stevens, K.R.: Power and influence: a source book for nurses, New York, 1983, John Wiley and Sons, Inc.

Stone, M.: Discharge planning guide, Am. J. Nurs. 79:1446, 1979.

Sundeen, S.J., Stuart, G.W., Rankin, E.D., and Cohen, S.A.: Nurse-client interaction: implementing the nursing process, St. Louis, 1985, The C.V. Mosby Co.

Szehais, B.: Adult day centers: geriatric day health services in the community, J. Fam. Pract. 20(10):157-161, 1985.

Thoms, F.L., and Mott, R.: A new role for the R.N.: discharge coordinator, Hosp. Prog. 59(2):38-40, 1978.

Williams, S.F., and Torrens, P.R.: Introduction to health services, New York, 1984, John Wiley and Sons, Inc.

Winslow, G.R.: From loyalty to advocacy: a new metaphor for nursing, Hastings Cent. Rep. 14:32-40, 1984.

Zusman, J.: Think twice about being a patient advocate, Nursing Life 2(6):46-50, 1982.

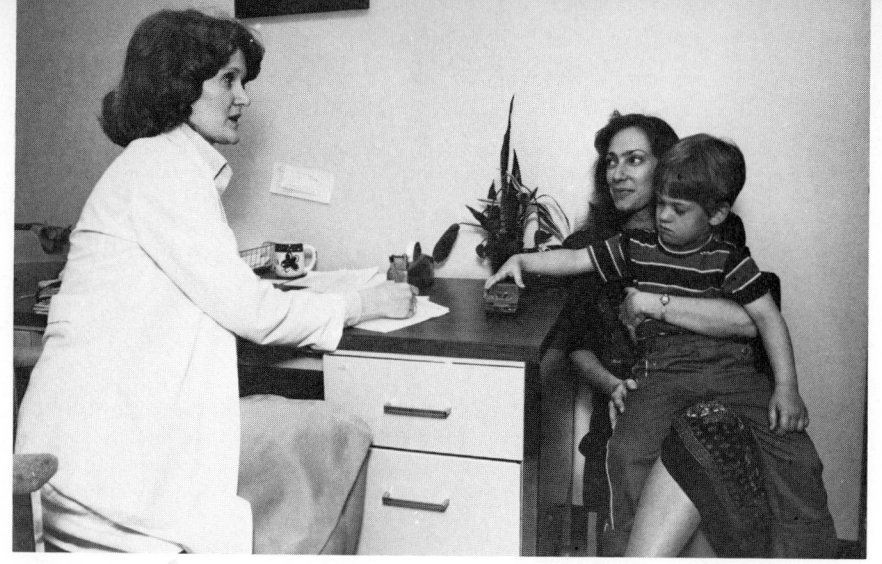

Cynthia Selleck
Ann Sirles
Rebecca Sloan

39

THE COMMUNITY HEALTH NURSE AS FAMILY NURSE PRACTITIONER IN PRIMARY/AMBULATORY CARE

OBJECTIVES

After reading this chapter, the student should be able to:

Discuss briefly the historical development of the nurse practitioner movement.

Identify members of the primary health care team.

Describe the educational requirements for family nurse practitioners.

Discuss the four credentialing mechanisms in nursing as they relate to the role of the family nurse practitioner.

Describe the various role functions of the family nurse practitioner.

Identify potential arenas for family nurse practitioner practice.

Explore current issues and concerns relative to family nurse practitioners and their practice.

Discuss the important elements of role negotiation.

Identify five stressors that have a direct bearing on the nurse in an expanded role.

Examine four practice situations for family nurse practitioners.

KEY TERMS

algorithms

collaborative practice

family nurse practitioner (FNP)

gerontology

health hazard appraisal tools

health maintenance flow sheet

health practitioner

home health agencies

independent practice

Indian Health Service

joint practice

multiphasic health screening

National Health Service Corps

nurse practitioner

peer review/quality assurance

private practice

professional isolation

protocols

Rural Health Initiative Clinics

satellite clinics

Several social phenomena and a shift in health problems over the past century have combined to redefine the pattern of health care in this country. Among these changes, and in part because of them, came the introduction of primary care. Although there have been many definitions of primary care, it is most often described as accessible, comprehensive, coordinated, and continuous care provided by accountable care givers (Institute of Medicine, 1978).

The philosophy inherent in primary care is similar to that of primary nursing, which has become a popular modality for delivering nursing care to clients in a variety of settings, particularly the hospital. The client contributes to as well as receives care, and the provider is not only available, but has authority, autonomy, and accountability.

The primary care system includes all ambulatory care. Ambulatory care is initiated when the client requests health care from a provider in a clinic or office setting within a given community.

In 1980, Andrus and Mitchell reported only 25% of physicians in the United States practiced in primary care. By 1982 the percentage of physicians in primary care had risen to 40% (American Medical Association, 1984). A growing population, escalation of medical costs, and a consumer demand for more health-related services prompted the belief that one profession alone cannot provide primary care for the combined health and illness needs of the population (Davidson and Lauver, 1984).

In looking at the demands of the primary care system and in analyzing the needs of clients who have access to this system, it became evident to health care planners that nurses, by expanding their existing skills, would be uniquely qualified to provide a major portion of primary care, using the physicians as consultants (Rogers, 1977).

◆ ◆ ◆

This chapter provides historical perspectives of the *nurse practitioner* (NP) movement as well as information regarding the current status of NPs, particularly *family nurse practitioners (FNPs)* who are primary health care providers directing their services toward all age groups. Role functions assumed by FNPs are addressed as are the arenas for FNP practice. Finally, the legal implications and areas of role stress relative to the practice of NPs are discussed.

HISTORICAL PERSPECTIVE

The evolution and the use of nonphysician providers in the primary care system are not unique to the United States. Other parts of the world have used nonphysicians in primary care who have functioned successfully with varying degrees of autonomy. Historically, the development of these roles occurred as a response to the health needs of a population and the insufficient numbers of physicians to meet these needs (Nichols, 1980).

In the United States, the 1960s witnessed not only a physician shortage but the increasing tendency among physicians to specialize. The number of physicians who might have provided medical care to communities and families across the nation was thus reduced. As this trend continued, a serious gap in primary care services developed (Bullough, 1980).

Demographic factors also influenced the evolution of nonphysician providers. Though the number of medical personnel in primary care was decreasing, the population was increasing. The lower socioeconomic groups that tended to cluster in the inner cities and rural areas were most affected by these changes. Additionally, the median age of the population was steadily rising, resulting in an increasingly higher proportion of aged persons. Many of these people live for long periods with chronic disease or the infirmities of old age coupled with dwindling financial resources and other social problems. Access to primary care for these two groups in particular was becoming a nationally recognized problem (Bullough, 1980).

Nursing and medicine responded to these inadequacies of the health care system. In 1965 at the University of Colorado School of Nursing, Loretta Ford determined that the morbidity among medically deprived children could be decreased by educating community health nurses to provide well care to children of all ages. Their scope of nursing practice included the identification, assessment, and management of common acute and chronic conditions with the appropriate referral of more complex problems (Silver, Ford, and Stearly, 1967). These nurses were referred to as pediatric nurse associates or pediatric NPs. As a profession, nursing's priorities traditionally are to care and support the well, the worried well, and the ill, from a physiological as well as a psychosocial perspective. Nurse practitioners could offer health-focused care, psychosocial supports, and a defined scope of physical care services previously provided only by physicians. Preparing nurses as primary care providers was not only consistent with traditional nursing but was also responsive to societal demands for holistic care (Davidson and Lauver, 1984). That same year the physician assistant (PA) role was initiated at Duke University. This program was intended to attract ex-military corpsmen for training as medical extenders (Fisher and Horowitz, 1977).

Nurse practitioners are often lumped together into a single category with other nonphysician providers and are erroneously portrayed as physician extenders. This misinterpretation of the intended role of nurse practitioners is addressed by the movement's founder, Loretta Ford:

> As conceptualized, the nurse practitioner was always a nursing model focused on the promotion of health in daily living, growth and development for children in families as well as the prevention of disease and disability. It evolved from such societal needs and opportunities as nursing's development as a discipline and a profession, not because there was a shortage of physicians. Nor did our early plans include preparing nurses to assume medical functions. Our interests were in health and prevention for aggregate populations in community settings including underserved groups. These were hallmarks of community health nursing (Ford, 1986, p. 178).

These innovative programs, directed at alleviating the problems of physician shortage and access to primary care for rural and other medically underserved populations, attracted the interest of the federal government. A report issued by the Department of Health, Education, and Welfare on *Extending the Scope of Nursing Practice* (1971) helped convince Congress of the value of NPs as primary care providers. The Nurse Training Act of 1971 (PL 92-150) and the comprehensive Health Manpower Act of 1971 (PL 92-157) provided educational funding for many NP and PA programs through the 1970s and into the 1980s. As the market for medical specialties became saturated, and the costs of hospital-based health care reached critical levels, primary care began attracting greater numbers of physicians. Competition among physicians in primary care is increasingly evident in the mid-1980s. Whether or not this competition for clients extends to nonphysician providers depends on factors such as role delineation and legal aspects, which are discussed in other sections of this chapter.

It is important to recognize that the NP movement has created several types of NPs. Currently, in the United States there are programs preparing adult nurse practitioners (ANP), pediatric nurse practitioners (PNP), school nurse practitioners (SNP), geriatric nurse practitioners (GNP), obstetric and gynecological nurse practitioners (OGNP), family planning nurse practitioners (FPNP), emergency nurse practitioners (ENP), and nurse midwives (NM). Whereas the FNP is prepared as a specialist in the primary care area of family practice with the ability to provide care to people of all ages and both sexes, NPs from these other programs are prepared as specialists in providing primary care to a select group of individuals (adults, children, the aged, or women). Additionally, there are hospital-based

oncology nurse practitioners who administer chemotherapy and supportive nursing care to cancer patients in the hospital and as they return for services as hospital out-patients.

It has been estimated that by 1990 the United States will actually experience a glut of physicians. It will be especially important during this time for FNPs to assert themselves as highly trained professionals capable of providing primary care in the ambulatory setting as a member of the primary health care team.

EDUCATION OF FNPs

The objectives of NP programs are to teach nurses to (1) assess normalcy, health deviations, and health risks; (2) provide anticipatory guidance, counseling about health maintenance, and disease prevention; (3) develop and implement therapeutic plans for selected health problems and clients; and (4) consult with and refer to other disciplines and collaborate with nurses in community agencies for client care beyond the NP's expertise or to meet the special needs of clients (Davidson and Lauver, 1984).

The educational trend is to make the entry level for NP practice at the Master's level (Sultz, Bullough, Sherwin, et al., 1983). This is in stark contrast to 1979 when most programs preparing FNPs were in departments of continuing education in nursing and the baccalaureate degree was not a uniform admission criterion (Golden, 1979).

CREDENTIALS FOR FNPs

Both the academic degree and accreditation are of importance to FNPs; however, it is licensure and certification that affect their practice most directly. FNPs are certified by the American Nurses' Association (ANA) through the Division of Community Health Nursing.

Since 1985 the basic qualification for certification is a baccalaureate degree in nursing and successful completion of a formal FNP program. Certification in the FNP specialty is for 5 years. To maintain certification the FNP must (1) document current licensure as an RN, (2) have practiced or provided direct supervision for a total of 1,500 hours in primary health care over the past 5 years, (3) submit a professional activities profile according to established guidelines, and (4) document 75 contact hours of continuing education relevant to the FNP's practice within the past 5 years.

ROLES OF FNPs

FNPs emerged as an answer to a population's need for primary care. To provide this primary care FNPs have practiced an expanded nursing role, taking on an array of functions, some of which had not previously been considered part of nursing's domain. Certainly FNPs continue to perform many of the same functions as staff nurses, but they are also taught to make independent judgments about their clients' conditions. Because of their nursing background, FNPs offer a valuable and unique service.

Health Practitioner

FNPs must practice as colleagues with physicians and other health care professionals. Physicians and FNPs need to continue to develop strategies for combining their expertise so that they can be integrated in a complementary fashion, which would provide a team approach in addressing the health needs of the client.

The primary health care team may consist of a variety of members. Such members usually have specialized and complementary skills that help to strengthen the team. Table 39-1 lists possible primary health care team members along with their educational backgrounds and role functions.

Physicians, NPs, and PAs may all have roles on the primary health care team. It is important to recognize that the role of the PA is defined entirely by medicine, and the role of the NP is defined entirely by nursing. Figure 39-1 illustrates the functional areas of these three roles. As is shown by the model, all three roles have overlapping functions.

The use of FNPs as primary health care providers goes beyond that of physician extender or physican substitute. The FNP facilitates access to primary care by increasing the number of qualified providers.

The FNP provides prompt screening and referral. FNPs are taught to recognize the subjective and objective signs and symptoms of potentially serious medical problems that require referral to a physician. Conversely, physicians should recognize that when clients' health problems are more amenable to care than cure, the specialized skills of self-care health counseling and guidance provided by FNPs may be the best treatment (Kweskin and Taller, 1979).

The FNP improves the health records by establishing baseline health profiles. FNPs assure through the practice of nursing that a client's record reflects the consideration of personal, family, and community health illness variables. Such records also contribute to continuity of care and health maintenance (Kweskin and Taller, 1979).

The FNP contributes to increased quality and comprehensiveness of health care, which is also cost effective (Kweskin and Taller, 1979). Family nurse practitioners contribute to a reduction in health care costs because their average earnings are only a fraction of those of physicians, and they have been found to provide care at about half the cost prevailing in the community (Tennant et al., 1980). Adding an FNP to a physician practice has been shown to increase office visits approximately 40 to 50%. Replacing a physician with an NP has been shown to save a total cost of $34,000 per year (Poirier-Elliott, 1984).

Adding the dimension of nursing to the health care team increases primary care services in diversity and quality. The use of such providers becomes cost effective when the needs of the client seeking services are matched with the provider who, by virtue of professional education and specialized skills, is best able to meet those needs.

There has been a growing concern in the United States for at least the last 25 years that the most effective way of dealing with the nation's major health problems is through prevention, and efforts have begun to move in that direction, though slowly. This means refocusing the health care system, teaching people that they control their own health, and encouraging health promotion and health maintenance activities.

Counseling people on ways to improve their health and prevent disease and assisting and supporting them in this process is a major function of FNPs in the ambulatory care setting. It is also the service that makes FNPs most valuable whether they practice independently or jointly.

FNPs use various tools in assisting people with disease prevention, health maintenance, and health promotion. History-taking and systematic physical assessment are two of these tools. Because of their psychosocial and behavioral background, nurses tend to place emphasis on the emotional, social, cultural, economic, and environmental aspects of their client's history. These are areas in which nursing can make a big difference, assisting the client toward improved health (Mundinger, 1980). FNPs are pre-

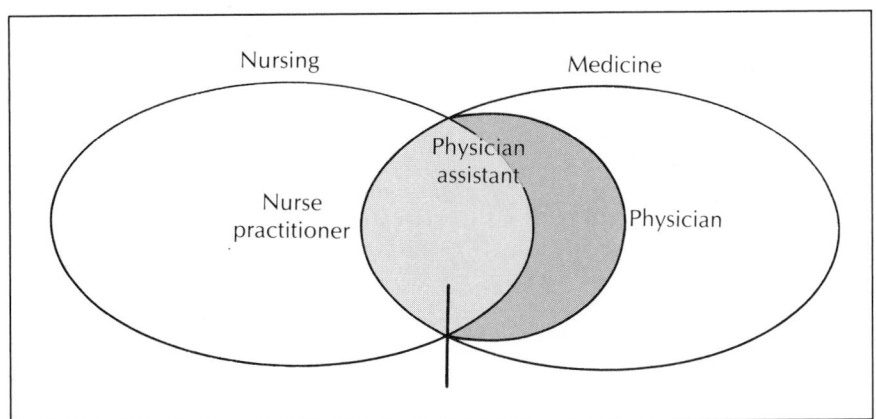

FIGURE 39-1

Nurse practitioner and physician assistant roles in relation to nursing and medicine in primary care. (Adapted from Graduate Medical Education National Advisory Committee: Nonphysician health care provider technical panel, vol. 7, DHHS, Washington, D.C., 1980, U.S. Government Printing Office.)

TABLE 39-1

Possible primary health care team members

Role	Education	Qualification	Function
Physician (MD)	Baccalaureate degree (4 years) plus graduation from medical school (4 years), plus an internship and residency of variable years, depending on specialty area	May be certified by examination in a specialty area, however, not mandatory	Elicits histories and performs physical examinations; performs appropriate diagnostic and therapeutic procedures; provides counseling and guidance; performs other procedures, including surgery, depending on specialty area
Family nurse practitioner (FNP)	Continuing education programs: must be RN with diploma, AD, or BSN preparation, granted a certificate on completion of program, usually 9-12 months Degree programs: must be RN with BSN preparation to enter master's level FNP program, usually 18-24 months	Successful completion of state board of nursing examination; licensure by state; state and/or national certification mandatory in some states; physician supervision not mandatory	Elicit histories and perform physical examinations; assess health and illness status; provide health screening, education, and counseling; assist with health maintenance and promotion activities; initiate appropriate diagnostic and therapeutic procedures with physician consultation
Physician's assistant (PA)	Baccalaureate degree preparation as PA, usually 4 years	Variable; licensure by some states; physician supervision mandatory	Elicits histories and performs physical examinations; initiates appropriate diagnostic and therapeutic procedures under physician supervision
Registered nurse (RN)	Diploma through a hospital school of nursing (3 years); associate degree through a community college (2 years) or baccalaureate degree through a college or university (4 years); master's and doctoral (DSN, PhD, EdD) preparation available	Successful completion of state board of nursing examination; licensure by state	Use the nursing process in supervising and providing total client care; carry out physician's orders for medications and therapeutic measures; carry out nursing procedures; provide health education and counseling
Licensed practical (vocational) nurse (LPN or LVN)	Course of study, usually 9-12 months through a vocational school	Variable; usually state licensed; RN or physician supervision mandatory	Assist with physical examinations; perform simple laboratory tests; carry out nursing and medically prescribed procedures; provide health education and counseling
Social worker	Master's level preparation usually required for unsupervised clinical practice; doctoral preparation (DSW, PhD) available	Variable; licensed by some states; membership in national association of social workers and academy of certified social workers and 2 years of supervised practice desirable	Provide counseling and guidance; assist client and family in locating appropriate community resources
Dietition	Baccalaureate degree plus 1-year internship or approved coordinated undergraduate program (4 years) required; master's and doctoral preparation available	Registered through the American Dietetic Association	Assess nutritional status and counsel clients and families on nutritional needs for specific situations
Medical assistant/receptionist	Course of study offered through a vocational school or community college teaches first aid and simple laboratory tests as well as office managerial skills	No registration or licensure	Serve as receptionist; make appointments; work with billing; assist with laboratory procedures

pared to listen to and counsel clients, and a good knowledge of both health and disease helps them to educate clients on the necessity of promoting and discouraging certain health behaviors.

Physical assessment techniques performed by the FNP have also proved to be quite successful. Nurse practitioners are taught to discriminate normal from abnormal findings and identify changes or conditions that may necessitate the need for medical assistance or referral to other health providers or agencies. Also, nurses can use the data gathered from the physical assessment in counseling and assisting clients with health maintenance and promotion.

Various screening procedures are performed by FNPs to detect potential problems before symptoms develop. Education of clients on the importance of health screening and responsibility for self-care is also part of the health maintenance efforts of FNPs.

It is useful for health care providers to use *health maintenance flow sheets,* such as the one shown in Appendix I5, which help to guide the practitioner in the health maintenance procedures that are recommended for different ages. A flow sheet also serves as a simple, easy-to-read summary of the client's health maintenance status (Hoole, Greenberg, and Pickard, et al., 1982).

Health hazard appraisal tools such as the one shown in Appendix C2, can be used by FNPs to determine the client's personal health risks. These health hazard appraisal tools can be brief or they can be quite lengthy and coded for computer analysis. The tool alerts the practitioner to the risk factors for that particular client and provides an environment for education and counseling regarding habits that place the client at high risk for developing future health problems (Hamm and Kitts, 1984). Additionally, the FNP can begin to screen the client for the most prominent risks. Health hazard appraisal tools provide clients with information on paper about their health risks and, therefore, are often strong motivational tools for changing behavior patterns.

Diagnosis and treatment are two functions of FNPs that were once considered to be solely the responsibility of the physician. Family nurse practitioners learn to diagnose and treat a variety of common, acute, self-limiting diseases, as well as monitor chronic, stabilized conditions. The nurse may gather the pertinent history, perform the necessary physical examination and laboratory tests, diagnose the problem, and confer with the physician for validation and to jointly decide on the plan of management. The FNP may also use *protocols* or *algorithms* (see box on p. 766) that have been previously agreed on by the physician and FNP. These documents serve as standing orders for the management of certain illnesses. Protocols enable the FNP to diagnose and treat client problems within the context of nursing management and are required by some states to regulate NP practice.

The ability of FNPs to diagnose and treat has been a boost to the provision of primary care and teaching and thus, compliance. It means that the FNP can provide total care to many individuals. Though physician input may be necessary at times, the nurse can usually carry out the treat-

ment regimen and establish the relationship of primary care giver.

Studies have shown that clients tend to be more compliant when they see the same provider regularly. Many illnesses, particularly those chronic conditions requiring a great deal of teaching and counseling, may be better managed by FNPs than physicians, with physician consultation as conditions change. When medical care is the primary need, the client is more appropriately managed by either the physician alone or jointly with the FNP providing the necessary education and counseling.

Health Educator

As the population grows more conscious of health and fitness, educating people about good health habits becomes increasingly important. FNPs are in an excellent position to provide health education to clients, and as previously discussed, this is a major function of their role. The FNP intervenes to enhance wellness and contributes to health maintenance and promotion by teaching the importance of good nutrition, physical exercise, stress management, and life-style. During illness the FNP educates the client about the disease process, what can be expected, and the importance of adhering to the treatment regimen. FNPs provide anticipatory guidance and educate clients on the use of medications, diet, birth control methods, and other therapeutic procedures. They also counsel clients and their families on the importance of assuming responsibility for their own health.

In the community, the FNP often serves as a resource for educating community groups and organizations on different aspects of health and self-care.

Health Administrator

Because of advanced knowledge and skills and often the setting where they choose to practice, FNPs may function in administrative roles. As health administrator, the FNP may be in a position to assume ultimate responsibility for all administrative matters within the setting. The FNP may be responsible and have direct or indirect authority and supervision over the clinic staff as well as client care. In this capacity the FNP serves as decision maker and problem solver and may also be involved in other business and management aspects of the organization such as policy making, finances, public relations and marketing, quality assurance, and future planning (Felton, Kelly, Renehan, & Alley, 1985; Jacox and Norris, 1977). Because of the variety of expanded roles that FNPs may encounter as institutions attempt to meet the current health care challenges, it is imperative that FNPs have a working knowledge of both business and management principles. FNPs need to be knowledgeable about the organizational structure and function of the institution supporting their clinics. FNP-initiated proposals for change within an organization should include the impact on client care as well as the overall impact on the institution's philosophy and organizational objectives. FNPs who present proposals to management without consideration of the total impact may find that they have limited roles, limited power, and, therefore, limited impact

SAMPLE PROTOCOL
OTITIS EXTERNA (PEDIATRIC AND ADULT)

I. Definition: Inflammation of the external canal and auricle caused by infectious agents that may be initiated by trauma from scratching, earplugs, bobby pins, and other foreign objects. Water from swimming or bathing may be absorbed by cerumen, forming a culture medium for infection

II. Etiology
    A. Bacteria: *Pseudomonas, Proteus,* staphylococci, streptococci
    B. Fungi

III. Clinical features
    A. Symptoms
        1. Pain in ear
        2. Occasionally, decreased hearing or sensation of obstruction
    B. Signs
        1. Pain aggravated by movement of auricle or pressure on tragus
        2. External canal partially occluded by edema or discharge
        3. External canal tender to otoscopy; erythema and exudate seen
        4. TM may be normal, injected, or covered with flecks of exudate; does *not* show signs of OM (i.e., bulging, disappearance of bony landmarks)
        5. Preauricular or postauricular lymphadenopathy may be present
        6. *No* swelling or pain over mastoid

IV. Laboratory studies: None

V. Differential diagnosis
    A. Otitis media: Pus may be present in the external canal, disappearance of bony landmarks, bulging, and exudate in middle ear
    B. Mastoiditis: Swelling and pain over mastoid area associated with an abnormal TM
    C. Chronic dermatitides: Usually not painful, may itch chronically, may be associated with cracking and scaling of auricle, and in some cases have discharge; pain may occur with secondary infection; types of chronic dermatitides include
        1. Seborrhea
        2. Eczema
        3. Psoriasis

VI. Promotion of self-care and prevention
    A. Instruments, including cotton swabs, should be kept out of ears; counsel that ear canal does not need cleaning—cleans itself
    B. Keep head out of water when bathing to avoid filling ear canals with water and irritating dirt and soap (common cause of external otitis in children)
    C. For swimmers or infection prone, use 2-3 drops of vinegar in ear canal after swimming or bathing to restore normal pH (acid)

    D. Persistent itching of the external canal should prompt consultation with health professional

VII. Specific therapy (check about any allergies)
    A. Gentle and thorough removal of debris in office to facilitate topical treatment
    B. Control of pain
        1. Heat to ear by compress, water bottle, or heating pad
        2. OTC acetaminophen (Tylenol, Datril), or aspirin
           a. Adults and children over 12 years of age
               Acetaminophen (325 mg/tab) 1 or 2 tab q 6h
               Aspirin (325 mg/tab) 1 or 2 tab q 4h
           b. Children under 12 years of age

Acetaminophen

Age	Prep	Dosage	Frequency
3 mo-1 yr	Drops	0.6 ml	
1-3 yr	Drops	1.2 ml	
3-6 yr	Elixir	1 tsp	q 6h
over 6	Elixir	2 tsp	

Aspirin (1¼ gr tab)

Kg	(lb)	Dosage	Frequency
7-11	(14-24)	1 tab	
11-16	(24-35)	2 "	
16-23	(35-50)	3 "	q 4h
23+	(50+)	4 "	

    C. Antibiotic treatment
        ℞: Neo Cort Dome otic drops or Cortisporin otic drops
        Disp.: 5 ml   Refill × 1
        Sig: 4 gtts in affected ear qid ×7d
             Lie with affected ear up for 5 min p tx
        Instruct: Keep ear dry during tx
                 Keep dropper tip out of ear
                 Reinforce method of instilling gtts

VIII. Complications—requires consultation/referral to physician
    A. Severe otitis externa associated with
        1. Swelling of canal to complete closure so that wick is required
        2. Severe pain or fever
        3. Cellulitis
        4. Failure to respond to tx in 1 wk
    B. Allergy to neomycin
    C. Recurrent otitis externa

IX. Follow-up: Return visit with physician if condition persists after 1 wk of tx on quality of care (Nettles-Carlson and McLaughlin, 1985). Remember, however, that administrative responsibilities are time-consuming. The FNP who functions in dual roles as a health practitioner and an administrator may find that certain tasks must be delegated to others for both roles to be performed effectively.

Health Consultant

Another function of the FNP is that of health consultant. Physicians can use FNPs as consultants on nursing care, such as counseling and health promotion efforts, for their clients just as FNPs use physicians as consultants on medical care. This exchange of professional expertise should be encouraged. Consultation is more common between physicians and FNPs who practice jointly. It is important that FNPs educate physicians to the fact that they have expertise in an area different from medicine but which is essential to the total care of the client.

FNPs may serve as health consultants to other nurses or NPs on a formal or informal basis, providing them with information to be used in improving client care. They may also consult with other health care providers or with organizations, schools, or programs educating FNPs.

Health Researcher

Nursing research is a necessity. Practicing FNPs are in an ideal position to identify researchable nursing problems. They are also in an ideal position to take research findings and apply them to the clinical practice setting. By virtue of their advanced education, many FNPs are trained in the research process and may use this research knowledge and skill to conduct their own investigations, answering questions relevant to nursing practice and primary care. Identifying, defining, and investigating clinical nursing problems and reporting findings foster collegial relationships with other professions and contribute to health care policy and decision making.

In reviewing the current research available on the NP it is evident that research has not been a priority. Molde and Diers (1985), after a selected literature review, suggested that future research endeavors be theory-based, coming from prudent clinical insight and meticulous design. Further, they suggested that future research be considered in a policy framework.

ARENAS FOR PRACTICE

A number of employment opportunities exist for FNPs, however it is interesting to note that the role has developed very differently from site to site. Positions for FNPs may vary greatly in their scope of practice, degree of responsibility, power and authority, working conditions, creativity, and reward structure (Edmunds, 1983).

Private Practice
Joint Practice

Because of their additional educational preparation and subsequent expansion of traditional nursing roles and responsibilities, FNPs are well suited for practice in a variety of employment settings. One setting, that of *joint practice* with a physician has aroused much interest.

In many *private practice* settings, the FNP may be the only professional nurse. When the FNP role is not clearly understood and accepted by the physician or the office staff, conflict and dissatisfaction are inevitable. There is no substitute for role negotiation before entering into an employment contract in such settings. The importance of role negotiation is discussed elsewhere in this chapter.

Joint practice is a philosophy as well as a practice model. The model will increase in popularity as research is able to document the advantages of the joint practice relationship to physicians, nurses, and clients.

Although physicians are beginning to realize the advantages of joint practice with FNPs, practice with nonphysician colleagues is still a new concept for many physicians. It is the responsibility of FNPs to clarify their services and their contributions to client care. The advantages of the FNP/physician joint practice model should be projected to show the advantages to the practice in relation to time, income, and client access to services. A Joint Practice Evaluation Project is currently being completed under the auspices of the W.K. Kellogg Foundation (1987).

Independent Practice

Another type of private practice chosen by a smaller number of FNPs is that of *independent practice*. Many reasons motivate nurses to go into independent practice, including a personal or professional desire to forge ahead and break new ground for nursing and to meet health care needs within a given community.

FNPs have a great deal to offer in an independent nursing practice, but it is important to investigate the particular state's nurse practice act to determine the limitations and legal ramifications of such an arrangement. FNPs functioning without medical back-up may perform histories, physical examinations, education, counseling, and expanded activities approved by nursing statutes or nursing board rules.

By contracting with or retaining a physician for medical back-up and referral, an FNP may expand services to a population or community. In states where it is legal for NPs to prescribe medications, the FNP may choose not to contract for physician services. The disadvantage of independent practice of FNPs from a consumer viewpoint is that the care may be less comprehensive and holistic than that received from a nurse and physician in joint practice.

Aside from the legal and philosophical issues of functioning independently in an expanded role, other areas are of concern to the FNP who sets up a private practice. These include marketing to clients and to other health care providers. Financial aspects also accompany entrepreneurial practice, including rent, utilities, furnishings, equipment, and supplies. Administrative considerations include appointment schedules, record keeping, billing, and secretarial or clerical support (Ricardi and Dayani, 1982). Additionally, if there is no insurance coverage for NP services, otherwise willing consumers may not be willing to seek services from FNPs in independent practice.

Although third party reimbursement for nursing services has been legislated in over 26 states, legislation does not include Medicare insurance. With more than 85% of the U.S. population covered by some form of health insurance, lack of third party reimbursement is a major deterrent to the practice of NPs (Cohn, 1983). Reimbursement is discussed as a separate issue elsewhere in this chapter.

It is predicted that fee-for-service health care will be extinct within 10 years. Efforts to cut costs have resulted in innovative provider systems such as Preferred Provider Organizations (PPOs) and increased competition among providers for their share of the health care market. FNPs are among nurse practitioners who are forming PPOs and marketing their services to employers, hospitals, and insurers. PPOs may be especially attractive to FNPs residing in states that have not passed third party reimbursement legislation (Griffith, 1985).

Despite the legal and financial deterrents, some FNPs find that practicing nursing independently is gratifying. As yet there are no research data to ascertain the cost effectiveness or consumer satisfaction with health care needs provided by FNPs practicing independently.

Institutional Settings
Ambulatory/Outpatient Clinics

The FNP may choose to practice in an institution such as the ambulatory center or outpatient clinic. Because of a declining number of inpatients, many institutions have developed alternative services that expand health care delivery and provide referral channels for consumers of hospital services (Lamper-Linden, Goetz-Kulas, and Lake, 1983). These ambulatory/outpatient clinics are fiscally sound and can improve the hospital's image in community service.

Generally, these clinics provide health maintenance and management for nonemergent problems, hospital referral, and hospital follow-up care. They provide acute or chronic health care. The population they serve is usually more diverse and represents a larger geographic area than populations served by private practices. The FNP in an acute care outpatient clinic typically practices jointly with physicians to provide primary care services. Hospital acute care clinics may be general medicine or family practice clinics or specialty oriented, such as pediatric, obstetric-gynecological, and ENT clinics. Outpatient clinics organized for chronic care may be problem-oriented as, for example, a hypertension or a diabetes clinic.

Although the role is well suited to both acute and chronic primary care, the FNP has had the greatest impact in chronic primary care. In chronic diseases such as hypertension the FNP's emphasis on self-care education and health promotion may be more beneficial than medical care alone in preventing complications and containing costs. Client care in hospital clinics is enhanced by the FNP's knowledge of the community and collaboration with community health nurses. Assistance from community health nurses is invaluable when serving a diverse population, many of whom need community resources, including services provided by health departments.

In developing a model for delivering client care, the FNP

may want to consider adapting the principles of primary nursing in the ambulatory setting to ensure continuity. Individualized client care, effective communication, and collaboration among staff and colleagues increases job satisfaction (Paradise & Kendall, 1985).

Emergency Departments

Because some people do not have accessible health care and because others do without health care services until illness strikes, the hospital emergency department is increasingly used for nonemergency, primary care problems. Although this may be considered inappropriate use of the emergency room, it is a reality resulting from the current system.

Some FNPs practicing in emergency rooms perform triage of clients (deciding who needs the most immediate attention and by whom), perform the initial workup (history and physical examination), assist the individual and/or family with crisis intervention, and manage the less acute problems. Emergency rooms are notorious for long waits and rapid treatment with little or no counseling and guidance given. FNPs can remedy this inadequacy by seeing clients with nonemergency problems and providing counseling. They may also help to educate clients on the importance of health care and how to gain access to the health care system.

Transients and homeless persons are more likely than others to lack a primary care provider and to thus rely on emergency departments for episodic care. Such persons are also likely to need community social services. The FNP's direct access to clients and knowledge of community health resources helps ensure that psychosocial needs are assessed and expedited.

For FNPs practicing in emergency departments, continuing education in trauma nursing is desirable. Cross training, whether learned on the job or through continuing education, is increasingly encouraged by institutions as an efficiency and cost-containment measure.

Satellite Clinics

Satellite clinics are operated under the auspices of a larger institution like a hospital or health department but are situated in a location away from the larger facility. The purpose of a *satellite clinic* is to provide accessible, high-quality health care to a population in need. These clinics often offer a range of preventive and primary care services, though some offer only skeleton services and rely heavily on referral to the larger institution.

FNPs in satellite clinics may practice alone, with physician backup from the larger institution available by telephone, or the physician may practice jointly with the FNP during some or all of the clinic hours. Practitioners may work with other support staff in the satellite clinic, or they may function alone, taking on the administrative and clerical functions as well as the health provider functions.

Long-Term Care Facilities

Currently in the United States there are approximately 20,000 long-term care facilities for the elderly. Eight percent of Americans over age 75 reside in some type of long-term care facility or nursing home for the elderly (Clemen-

Stone, Eigsti, and McGuire, 1987). Estimates have been made that by the year 2000 the United States population age 65 and older will increase by 58%. As our population ages, the number of people in long-term care facilities will undoubtedly increase.

Gerontology is becoming an increasingly popular field and numerous courses on the topic are taught. FNPs with an interest in geriatrics should avail themselves of this special education. More and more practitioners are viewing long-term care facilities as exciting arenas for practice. In this capacity the FNP may have an office within the facility where ambulatory clients are seen for health maintenance and nursing care, with off-the-premises physician backup. In less ambulatory long-term care facilities, the FNP may make regular nursing home rounds, assessing the health status of clients and providing care and counseling as appropriate. Typically, the FNP in a long-term care facility assumes maximal responsibility and functions with a great deal of independence (Edmunds, 1983). The FNP serves as a role model and consultant to the long-term care facility nursing staff, providing continuity of care; counseling with the client and family; and promoting health, activity, self-care, a positive view of aging, and when appropriate, a dignified death.

The health needs of special populations such as the institutionalized elderly are receiving much public and policy-making attention. Public policy concentration on how to provide these people services presents a specific research opportunity for FNPs to demonstrate the suitability, quality of care, and cost effectiveness of long-term care facilities (Molde & Diers, 1985).

Industry

The National Safety Council estimates that annually 4,000 deaths and 2.2 million disabling injuries can be attributed to on-the-job accidents. Similarly, the Department of Health and Human Services estimates 390,000 new cases of disease and 100,000 deaths from occupational exposures each year (Silberstein, 1981).

For decades the industrial or occupational health setting has been recognized as an area that benefits from nursing practice, but only recently has occupational health nursing been viewed as a nursing specialty. The number of continuing education and advanced educational programs in occupational health nursing is steadily increasing. The ANA recommends that nurses, and this holds true for FNPs, planning to practice in an occupational setting have previous courses in industrial and social law, industrial psychology, industrial health, statistics, research, and business management to effectively deal with the special concerns of the occupational setting (Clemen et al, 1981). Courses in toxicology, safety and ergonomics, and industrial hygiene are also quite useful.

FNPs in occupational settings generally practice independently, without direct physician supervision. As described in Chapter 41, the health and welfare of the worker is a major concern; therefore, concentration is on health maintenance, health promotion, and health education activities. The practitioner in the occupational setting is faced with the challenge of keeping the employees healthy and on the job. Responsibilities include direct nursing care for on-the-job injuries and accidents and, in some cases, care of nonoccupationally related illnesses (such as follow-up of workers with hypertension and diabetes). The FNP in this role would also function administratively in the operation and management of the occupational health service (supply ordering, record keeping, data collecting about environmental hazards, cooperating with federal and state regulations regarding occupational health and safety, planning, and evaluating). The practitioner would also be responsible for developing educational programs on health and safety for the employees and keeping abreast of the community services available for both consultation and referral.

Another potential avenue open to the FNP is the development of consultative services to provide health and safety programs. This might be considered especially valuable for small companies who vest limited time and resources on accident prevention and health promotion activities (Grove and Pruitt, 1984).

National Government
National Health Service Corps

The National Health Service Corps, a program sponsored by the Public Health Service, was established in 1970 to recruit health providers (physicians, NPs, PAs) to health manpower shortage areas. The first NPs were used by the Corps in 1972, and since that time over 450 practitioners have been placed in a variety of settings by the National Health Service Corps. Though the National Health Service Corps has employed some pediatric and adult nurse practitioners, the majority of those employed are FNPs or certified nurse midwives.

In the past the *National Health Service Corps* employed NPs who had completed their practitioner education and provided scholarships to nurses interested in becoming NPs. The latter had a 2-year commitment to the Corps following their graduation. Currently the Corps is employing only those FNPs who are in the National Health Service Corps scholarship program. These nurses are used in clinic sites in health manpower shortage areas to provide primary care services to the local population. Depending on the needs of the area, the FNP may be the only health care provider in the clinic with physician backup available by telephone, or the practitioner and a corps physician may practice jointly. It is anticipated and encouraged that at the end of the 2-year commitment the local community will be able to provide financial support for maintaining the health care provider in the clinic setting.

Armed Services

The role of the FNP in the armed services (army, navy, air force) was significant during the 1970s. Because of the physician shortage at that time, FNPs as well as other types of NPs were used in outpatient clinics to perform the bulk of duties that had previously been performed by physicians. In fact, all three branches of the armed services developed their own NP training programs to educate nurses to take on expanded functions. Currently, however, because of the increasing number of physicians, the role of the NP in the armed services has diminished. At present there is little active recruitment of NPs for the armed forces.

Indian Health Service

Many Indians still live in environments with limited health care facilities, inadequate waste disposal, and inadequate water supply systems. There is significantly higher morbidity and mortality among these people than among the general population.

The *Indian Health Service,* a bureau of the Public Health Service since 1954, is the primary health resource for approximately 800,000 Indians and Alaskan natives. It is the mission of the Indian Health Service to provide high-quality, comprehensive primary health care to Indian people. In so doing the Indian Health Service employs FNPs in hospital ambulatory clinics, health centers, and smaller outlying facilities. The FNP may practice directly with a physician or indirectly via telephone consultation (Indian Health Program, 1980).

Rural Health

The FNP is a positive and potential resource for improving primary health care in rural areas, where the availability and accessability of services is considered low. Rural consumers' attitude toward the use of the NP's services is positive (Kviz, Misener, and Vinson, 1983).

Many FNPs are employed in *Rural Health Initiative (RHI) clinics.* These clinics are situated in rural areas and were created in accordance with the Rural Health Clinic Services Act of 1977. The RHI clinics receive federal funds based on the specific needs of the area. The purpose of these clinics is to provide accessible, quality primary care health services. As with other clinics, RHIs may be staffed by FNPs alone or jointly with a physician.

Health Maintenance Organizations

Current HMO practices are aimed at holding down the increasing cost of health care by instituting incentives for providers of care to keep people well. Health maintenance and disease prevention activities are emphasized to reduce health risks and avoid expensive medical care. It is common for FNPs to be employed in HMOs for their provision of cost effective basic health care services.

Johnson and Freeborn (1986) suggest that large multi-specialty HMOs may be very favorable settings for FNPs to practice primary care.

Public Health Departments

"The majority of the nurses who consider themselves to be public health/community health nurses are those who are giving direct care in communities as a major focus of their work" (Barkauskas, 1982, p. 387). Community health nurses were among the first to expand their roles. During the 1960s and 1970s the majority of nurses entering NP programs were community health nurses. Public health departments seeking to provide preventive services and chronic care to increasing populations viewed employment of NPs as a cost effective strategy to meet the community's health needs. For example, well-child clinics, family planning clinics, and prenatal clinics have commonly and efficiently used FNPs. Home health care, another expanded area within community health nursing, has also used FNPs. Efforts to reduce health care expenditures have resulted in earlier hospital discharge with an increasing need for discharge follow-up through home health care.

Public health nursing service personnel in urban and rural areas have expressed concern as to the level of knowledge and skill nurses have entering public health positions upon graduation (Dye-White, 1984). This means that each department must evaluate the competencies individually and then, if necessary, provide continuing education, which is costly. FNPs are a viable alternative by virtue of their educational preparation. Additionally, FNPs could assist in the provision of inservice education.

An area of concern for health departments located in rural areas is the multiple problems encountered in providing health care services to the elderly. FNPs can provide *multiphasic health screening.* According to Young and Gottke (1985) the screening process serves as an entry point for other health and human services for the older adult and acts as a preventive program for many potential life crises. The extent to which a public health department uses FNPs is dependent on the community's health priorities and the fiscal restraints under which the agency functions (Ervin, 1982).

Schools

The school nurse practitioner concept evolved from the pediatric nurse practitioner model. FNP practice revolves around the concepts that relate to comprehensive assessment and management of care with particular emphasis on health education as a mechanism for changing health behavior in children and families (Igoe, 1975).

FNPs functioning in the school system assume a direct role in securing health care for the school-aged child with limited access to medical care by working collaboratively with community leaders, educators, and physicians (Oda, DeAngelis, Berman, and Meeker, 1985). In addition to health maintenance and management functions, FNPs within the school system have responsibility for planning a health education curriculum. Working with students with learning disabilities is also within the scope and practice of FNPs. Some states require that these nurses be eligible for teacher certification. Coursework relative to the assessment and management of the school-aged child is suggested. Additionally, courses in learning disabilities and psychological testing will prove advantageous.

The ANA currently offers a certification examination for school nurse practitioners. As of 1985, all applicants desiring certification as school nurse practitioners had to submit evidence that they had completed a baccalaureate in a nursing program and an additional formal program preparing them as school nurse practitioners. For further information on school nursing see Chapter 40.

Other Arenas
Home Health Agencies

The opportunities for FNP's in the home health care market are outstanding. In this arena the FNP offers advanced knowledge and skills in the following areas: (1) public/ community health principles, (2) family and individual counseling skills, (3) health education and strategies of adult learning, and (4) increased decision-making ability. Expansion of services and technology for the home care of clients is a direct result of the emphasis on cost containment seen nationwide. Job opportunities for the FNP will continue to increase as home health agencies continue to expand their services. Additionally, equipment and drug companies are developing products for home use, physicians and hospitals are exploring the development of home services, and consumers are demanding greater availability of services. Each of these changes will positively impact job availability for the FNP (Mershon and Wesolowski, 1985).

Correctional Institutions

The organizational structure of prisons and jails has long been a barrier to providing or improving health care. Research has demonstrated that the NP has had a positive effect in correctional health programs. One system reported that its primary care volume capacity doubled and that the cost of each client visit decreased by one third (Hastings, Vick, Lee, et al., 1980). Further, the technical quality of primary care continued to improve over a 3-year period, while client outcomes, satisfaction levels, and overall mortality rates remained unchanged. In this same study the suicide rate also dropped. The real challenge for future research is to evaluate the *why*.

Hospitals

Nursing within the hospital setting has changed rapidly. Hospital nurses have explored new roles through primary nursing, alternative staffing patterns, and technological skills. The Hospital Nurse Practitioner Program in Pediatrics at the University of Colorado Health Sciences Center, Denver, Colorado was a pilot project designed to prepare experienced staff nurses for a new and expanded health-care role in hospital settings (Murphy, Gitterman, and Silver, 1985). This alternative is reasonable as cost containment in health care now demands new approaches for doing more with existing resources. Preparing hospital nurse practitioners is one way of maximizing autonomy, accountability, advocacy, and responsibility in providing quality, cost-effective care. Hospital nurse practitioners may also serve to expedite institutional privileges for nonhospital-based nurse practitioners (FNPs) as the total health care team becomes more familiar with the role of the NP.

ISSUES AND CONCERNS
Legal Status

In the 1970s, increasing numbers of FNPs and other NPs began to do work that traditionally had been considered within the province of medicine. It was in diagnosis and treatment that the role of the NP assumed legal significance. It was not just that FNPs performed these acts, but rather it was the environment in which the tasks were performed. FNPs as licensed professionals functioned primarily in collaboration with physicians rather than under their supervision. Many state nursing laws were vague on the functions and responsibilities of nurses, and the legal status of NPs was being questioned.

Since 1971, when Idaho was the first state to revise its nurse practice act to accommodate the practice of NPs, states have amended their nurse practice acts or revised their definition of nursing to reflect the professional developments within nursing. Over half the states now provide for nursing specialties and an expanded scope of practice. The functions of nursing must be recognized and legally sanctioned if the health and illness needs of the public are to be met.

A legal precedent for the practice of NPs was set in 1982. The Missouri Supreme Court reversed a lower court decision ruling in favor of the Missouri medical board who charged that two nurse practitioners were practicing medicine without a license. Further, the court revoked the licenses of the five physicians with whom the NPs practiced on the grounds that the physicians aided and abetted the unauthorized practice of medicine. The Supreme Court ruled that the NPs were engaged in the legal practice of nursing. This decision was based on the court's interpretation, which held that the legislative intent of the 1975 revision of the Missouri Nurse Practice Act was to allow RNs, who had met certain educational requirements and used protocols, to expand their scope of practice (Bullough and Bullough, 1984).

Although the lack of precisely worded nursing statutes is still cited by FNPs as a barrier to practice and employment, the Missouri case provides a reassuring precedent for those states who have broad definitions of professional nursing practice without specifically naming nursing specialties with scopes of practice beyond that of ordinary RNs. It is likely that when state boards of nursing review and revise their nurse practice acts, definitions of professional nursing will allow for growth and development of practice in accordance with current nursing education.

Nursing groups scored some victories for primary care practice in 1985. Over protests of the medical board, Massachusetts legislators passed prescribing privileges for NPs (Massachusetts MDs, 1985). The Arkansas Supreme Court dismissed an attempt by the medical board to prohibit physicians from working with more than two NPs at a time. Such a prohibition would have restrained the practice and employment opportunities of NPs in Arkansas (Top Arkansas Court, 1985).

Despite the gains made in some states, legal problems and unresolved disputes still exist in others. Louisiana's medical society has sued twice since 1984 to invalidate the board of nursing's rules for NP practice (New Regs, 1985). In 1984, the Maryland Medical Society sued both the nursing and medical boards to rescind prescription privileges for NPs. There has been no resolution, although changes in Maryland's pharmacy law have already disqualified NPs as prescribers (New Regs, 1985). These attempts by medicine to exert control over the practice of nurses are attributed in part to a potential client shortage as physicians increase in number (Gardner and Fiske, 1981).

Reimbursement

The lack of third party reimbursement for nursing services has long been a concern among nurses. When FNPs provide services that are categorized as reimbursable but are unable to collect from insurers unless the claim is filed by a physician, it is viewed by the nurses as exploitation of themselves and the public. Exploitation of nurses occurs when fees are collected by one professional (physician) for services performed by another (FNP). Exploitation of the public occurs because financial constraints force clients to seek care from providers whose fees will be honored by insurers. Since over half of all personal health care services are financed by third-party payers, providers must have access to third-party reimbursement to be economically solvent. This effectively limits alternatives in health care, which could be available to the client, by discouraging independent practice by nurses (Griffith, 1982).

The Rural Health Clinic Services Act of 1977 (PL 95-210) was the first major breakthrough in third-party reimbursement for nurses in primary care roles. However, the act applies only to FNPs and PAs providing care as physician extenders in federally recognized, medically underserved areas. Under the provisions of the act, Medicare and Medicaid funds are made available for reimbursement of clinics operated or owned by qualified nonphysician providers. Under this act, a physician is not required to see the clients or be physically present for the clinic or providers to be reimbursed. A physician, however, is required to provide medical direction and be available for consultation, emergency assistance, and client referral (Silver and McAtee, 1978).

Lobbying efforts by state nurses' associations have been successful in passing reimbursement legislation that is not limited to particular sites or consumer categories. Griffith (1982) and Goldwater (1982) documented the lobbying, legislative, and negotiation efforts in Maryland where legislation was passed providing that reimbursement by any insurance company is not contingent on the NP being employed by a physician or acting according to a physician's orders. Washington state law places the requirement to reimburse nurses for services only on Blue Cross and Blue Shield (Washington Law, 1981). A prerequisite for such legislation is for nurse practice acts and rules and regulations to legally sanction nurses' diagnostic, treatment, and prescriptive authority. Both Maryland and Washington have such rules and regulations, which incorporate a requirement for a collaborative and consultative relationship with a physician in place of physician direction or supervision.

A partial victory was hailed by Arizona nurses when legislation was passed granting third-party reimbursement to nurses. However, nurses will not realize the benefits of the law until regulations are written and approved by the separate boards of nursing, medicine, and osteopathy, a process that may be laborious and consume years (Arizona Wins, 1985). New Hampshire NPs saw their reimbursement bill passed by the state legislature on the first try. The "surprising" first round success was credited to lobbying efforts by the state's 120 NPs, the N.H. Woman's Lobby, the N.H. Mental Health Association, consumers, and several physicians (NH ARNPs, 1985). North Dakota was also successful in passing reimbursement legislation on the first try.

By the end of 1985 over 26 states had enacted reimbursement legislation. However, nurses have just begun to recognize their political power and only now are learning to use that power effectively (Mason and Talbott, 1985).

Institutional Privileges

It is often difficult for FNPs to obtain hospital privileges through the department of nursing within institutions where their clients are admitted. The traditional hospital nurse is automatically responsible to and governed by the department of nursing as a condition of employment. However, if an FNP is employed, for example, in a private, joint practice with a physician, there is rarely a mechanism for clinical privileges to be granted by the department of nursing because the nurse is not employed by the hospital.

There are two purposes for providing a mechanism for community-based FNPs to gain access to their hospitalized clients. First, if people are allowed to choose or purchase direct nursing care, access to hospitalized clients is a necessity. Second, nursing must be accountable for and regulate the practice of its practitioners. No other group can knowledgeably review or set forth the standards for nursing practice (Manley, 1981). Even so, because NPs in primary care usually work to keep clients out of hospitals, staff privileges are not a high priority for most FNPs (Richards, 1984).

Many institutions do grant clinical privileges to nonphysicians, including nurses, through the department of medicine. The *Accreditation Manual for Hospitals* published in 1976 by the Joint Commission on the Accreditation of Hospitals states that hospitals will, within their bylaws and rules and regulations, have their medical staffs delineate privileges for nonphysician practitioners as well as identify the roles and responsibilities of the medical staff in relation to the nonphysician practitioners. A relaxed medical staff definition adopted by JCAH in 1984 further directed hospitals to be more permissive in granting medical staff privileges to nonphysicians (Richards, 1984).

This mechanism fails to recognize that nurses as professionals are accountable for their own actions. Such policies limit nursing's autonomy and professional responsibility within the hospital setting. Further, it leaves a gap in the institution's ability to monitor the nursing care that is provided by nurses who have been granted clinical privileges under medical authority.

Since departments of nursing should be responsible for establishing and maintaining standards of nursing care within insitutions, nurses should have the authority to grant or deny nursing privileges for all nurses within the setting whether or not they are employed by the institution (Manley, 1981).

The importance of state legislation and the role of the professional organization in expediting institutional privileges cannot be minimized. Legislative action, changes in nurse practice acts, Federal Trade Commission intervention, consumer demands, and pressure by nonphysicians will assist in breaking down barriers confronting FNPs' direct client access (Durham and Hardin, 1985).

The changing economy and health care trends are altering

the role of the traditional hospital. With competition for clients and nonhospital care on the increase, hospitals are more willing to consider alternatives to the medical model. Efforts to obtain third-party reimbursement for care provided by FNPs must continue because few hospitals will encourage admission and treatment of clients who have no means of payment.

ROLE NEGOTIATION

If the FNP is going to collaboratively provide comprehensive primary care, negotiation skills must be thoroughly understood and developed. Positive working relationships with health professionals, organizations, and clients do not happen by virtue of proximity alone.

Job opportunities for nurses traditionally have been easily identified and clearly defined. However, as nurses expand their education and responsibilities, roles become less clear. This is particularly true for FNPs who often find themselves considering pioneer positions in which few if any guidelines exist or the position is new and underdeveloped. In this instance, although it may be difficult for the FNP to informally assess the internal politics of the organization, it is a necessary skill that should be developed.

Another potential obstacle is that FNPs often seek employment rather than being sought by the employer. Assertiveness is desirable in exploring and developing potential job opportunities. It is important for FNPs to feel comfortable and confident in marketing their skills. Creative approaches and innovative ways of implementing their new role require negotiation skills.

Because of increased economic constraints and a variety of new health care legislation, job opportunities for FNPs have become less visible. It is important that FNPs be aware of a variety of marketing strategies/techniques that will allow capitalization of the less visible job market.

Informational interviewing and skills identification are two methods FNPs will find useful (Ciocci, 1984). Skills identification consists of a listing of specific skills and abilities. When skills are identified, they can then be matched with the problems identified from informational interviewing. Informational interviewing includes researching the organization of interest, identification of organizational problems, and the identification of the power structure within the organization (Ciocci, 1984).

Additionally, FNPs will find that providing copies of credential documents, samples of professional accomplishments such as audiovisual materials, client education packets or history and physical tools will enhance facilitation of the negotiation process.

The FNP should keep a folder containing examples of all professional activities that may be used for prospective employment. However, it is important to be realistic and practical in choosing examples of work and activities to be used during the interview process so as not to oversell. Names, addresses, and telephone numbers of professional and personal references should be furnished only after permission has been obtained. A business card left at the conclusion of the interview is another way of increasing visibility.

ROLE STRESS

A number of stressors have a direct bearing on the nurse in an expanded role. In addition to the legal issues that have previously been addressed, stressors include professional isolation, liability, collaborative practice, conflicting expectations, and professional responsibilities.

Professional Isolation

Professional isolation has become a source of considerable conflict for FNPs. Practicing as they do across all age groups, FNPs more than any other expanded role category are most likely to be sought for remote practice employment sites. Rural communities unable to support a physician find the FNP an affordable and logical alternative to answer their need for primary care services. The autonomy of practice in such sites attracts many FNPs who may fail to consider the liabilities of an isolated practice. Long drives, long hours, lack of social life and cultural activities, and lack of opportunity for professional development are often experienced by these rural practitioners. Such sources of stress, which lead to job dissatisfaction, can be reduced or eliminated by negotiating the employment contract at the outset to include periodic educational and personal leaves with provision of backup providers. Such anticipatory planning assures that health services are not compromised (Sirles, 1981). FNPs who choose isolated employment settings should consider their own needs as well as those of the community and negotiate accordingly.

Liability

All nurses are liable for their actions. With liability becoming more public today and more legal action specifically concerning NPs appearing in the judicial system, the importance of liability and/or malpractice insurance cannot be overemphasized. Although malpractice insurance is not a prerequisite to functioning as an FNP, most do carry their own liability insurance. It is in the best interest of FNPs to thoroughly investigate the coverage offered by different companies rather than assuming that the coverage is adequate. Particularly vulnerable are those practitioners who function without a physician on site (Daughterty and Buchanan, 1981).

NPs who have been successful in defense of illegal practice charges against them emphasize the importance of clear, objective documentation of findings, therapy, counseling, and when appropriate, physician consultation when charting client visits. Such charting should be habitual practice for nurses in expanded roles (Adler, 1979; Johnson, 1980).

Collaborative Practice

The future of FNPs depends on whether they make a recognizable difference in the health of families and communities and on their ability to practice collaboratively with physicians. Collaborative practice denotes a collegial relationship with mutual trust and respect of coprofessionals. The working out of a collaborative practice takes a considerable amount of time, and the FNP and physician may be convinced that they do not have this time available to them. However, until time and energy are spent to achieve the mutual understanding of role relationships and responsibilities, collaborative practice will continue to remain more theory than practice. Until such practice relationships evolve within joint practice situations, the quality health care that nursing and medicine collaboratively can provide will not be achieved. In addition to the professional maturity required to work together without feeling the need to be protective of one's own territory, the organizational structure and philosophy of the practice must support joint practice as a mechanism for health care delivery. The growing pains of establishing such a practice produce stress for the FNP and physician; however, the results and benefits to professionals and clients are worth the effort (Steel, 1981). Continued research aimed at demonstrating quality care and increased consumer access at significant cost savings will result in the use of FNPs (Poirier-Elliott, 1984).

Conflicting Expectations

Nursing services provided by the FNP in health promotion and maintenance are often more time-consuming and complex than the management of the client's current health problem. FNPs frequently experience conflict between their practice goals in health promotion and the need to see the number of clients required to maintain a clinic's economic goals. This is particularly true in clinics where the FNP is the sole provider. The problem is compounded when the clinic administrator or physician views the FNP as a medical extender only, and third party reimbursement is limited to medical services (Sirles, 1981).

The FNP may easily take the path of least resistance to decrease conflict and stress in such situations by adopting the medical extender role. To avoid such a situation a practice model using flexible scheduling, health maintenance flow sheets, and problem-oriented recording with nursing goals and plans prominently displayed in the client's health record assists the FNP to integrate health promotion and maintenance activities into each client visit.

Professional Responsibilities

Professional responsibilities contribute to role stress. The majority of states currently require NPs to become nationally certified and to maintain that certification for approval to practice. Recertification for FNPs requires documentation of continuing education hours in primary care topics. Considering that the practitioner role is a minority role in nursing, continuing education in primary care topics may not be locally available. Continuing education offerings may necessitate significant travel and lodging expenses in addition to time away from practice. Anticipating professional responsibilities and attendant expenses in financial planning decreases these concerns. As previously mentioned, negotiating with the employer for educational leave and expenses should be part of any FNP's contract. Certification and recertification are predictable expenses and necessitate the FNP continually identifying and meeting learning needs to maintain current knowledge and skills. Quality of client care, however, cannot be measured or assured by the hours of continuing education or the FNP's credentials. Professional responsibility includes monitoring one's own practice in relation to standards specified in advance.

A quality assurance process with peer review is becoming recognized as a professional responsibility among NPs. Such a process should evaluate need, cost, and effectiveness of care in relation to client outcomes. In 1977, a group of FNPs in Tennessee determined the need for an evaluation method that recognized the responsibility of nurses in monitoring their own practices, included characteristics of the provider that influenced care, and could be easily implemented in a rural setting. A number of factors that influenced the quality of health care were identified and developed into a peer review process that encompassed multiple components. An unexpected benefit was the sharing of knowledge and experience among NPs working in isolated, rural settings (Hiserote et al., 1980).

The difficulties encountered in the peer review/quality assurance process included the time and distance involved in traveling to widely separated clinics and planning the reviews so that there was a minimum of interference with individual schedules. Although peer review can be stressful, the Tennessee nurses came away from the review of their FNP colleagues with new ideas for their own practices and agreed that the benefits compensated for the difficulties encountered (Hiserote et al., 1980). In addition to peer review, there is self-review that can also serve as a quality assurance process. A group of nurse practitioners at the Johns Hopkins Hospital developed a performance appraisal tool that is used to reflect the practitioner's role and practice setting. This tool is divided into four large categories: clinical, leadership, education, and professional activities (Levitt, Stern, Becker, et al., 1985).

Chart audit using protocols as standards with which care can be measured is a mechanism for self-review. Many states require protocols for practicing in an expanded role. Although there are numerous published protocols to guide practice, the FNP and physician who work together must agree on the protocols' diagnostic scope and treatment regimens. This involves selecting and adapting from among published protocols or writing them to fit the particular needs of the practitioners and the practice.

Protocols may be used as quality assurance tools for peer or self-review through chart audit. Using protocols as standards of care for quality assurance through chart review requires that key elements for client history, positive and negative diagnostic findings, indications for consultation and referral, treatment regimen, and client education relative to treatment, prevention, and follow-up be clearly defined within each protocol. An example of such a protocol adapted from several sources (Hoole, Greenberg, and Pickard, et al., 1982; Komaroff, 1977; Leitch and Tinker, 1978) is shown in the box on p. 766. Such protocols take considerable time to develop, but they do provide a mechanism for establishing a standard against which client care may be objectively measured by the FNP or others.

Establishing mechanisms for quality assurance is a professional responsibility that FNPs must employ within their practice. By accepting the responsibility for monitoring their client care, FNPs assume the challenge of directing their future and defining their potential within the primary health care system.

Andreoli and Musser (1985) discuss trends that may affect the future of nursing, emphasizing that the future will belong to those nurses who develop skills and behaviors to meet health care needs. This challenge demands continuing education, adding to a scientific knowledge base through research and publication. Further, computer literacy and proficiency skills will assist FNPs in developing, implementing, and maintaining nursing care-oriented software and hardware. Home health agencies need assistance in evaluating software for management of their agencies, as they strive for cost-effective, quality health care.

CLINICAL APPLICATIONS

One FNP working for the Visiting Nurses' Association of Washington, D.C. described and discussed the research concerning use of a new type of dressing for the treatment of chronic decubitus and venous stasis ulcers (Kendrick and Sullivan, 1984). This FNP used research skills, knowledge of organizational structure, collaborative relationships, consultation contacts, and negotiation skills in developing the research proposal. This is significant because there is little clinical research being done in the home setting by nurses. In reporting these findings, Kendrick and Sullivan (1984) have identified many helpful points to assist future research endeavors.

Another clinical application can be seen in the use of relaxation therapy by the FNP in ambulatory care practice. Coslow and Steinberg (1983) report having used a variety of relaxation techniques in their ambulatory care practice. Because of the indepth preparation of FNPs in holistic approaches to health and illness, this intervention seems logical. Additionally, with the FNP's background in client teaching this approach to relieve stress-induced symptoms and disorders is worthy of exploration.

Richter and Sloan (1979) reported the effective use of progressive relaxation for a variety of problems including borderline hypertension, headaches, insomnia, and anxiety. Further, they taught the concept of relaxation to professionals and paraprofessionals and found success in both individual client sessions and group sessions.

The organization and management of ambulatory care clinics for clients with chronic health problems is another role often assumed by FNPs. An anticoagulation clinic is one such example. Safe and effective management of clients receiving oral anticoagulants requires continuous client education, skillful manipulation of therapy, careful assessment of therapeutic response at predetermined intervals, and systematic detection and immediate resolution of problems. FNPs are prepared to assess clients physically, offer psychosocial support, and develop individual client education strategies to facilitate compliance. Further, this setting challenges NPs to evaluate the quality of care they provide clients. Bulman (1985) has developed a record system for clients on anticoagulation therapy that can be used for auditing standards of care.

The multifaceted role of the FNP in joint practice is described by the following vignette. Julia Andrews is a master's level FNP who practices with two board-certified family practice physicians in an urban office. Julia has her own appointment schedule and sees 12 to 15 clients on an average day. Although she sees some acutely ill clients, most of her appointments are for routine health maintenance visits for both adults and children. The two physicians also refer clients to Julia for management of stable chronic health problems like hypertension and diabetes. Referral of these problems by the physicians did not happen until Julia had been with the practice for about a year. During the first year of her practice, Julia negotiated with the physicians to randomly assign 30 hypertensive clients to her for follow-up care. Nine months later, Julia was able to show that blood pressure measurements were lower in her group of clients than in a randomly selected group of 30 clients managed by the physicians. Additionally, her group of clients indicated a high degree of satisfaction with care from the nurse practitioner and were more knowledgeable about their medications than the physicians' group of clients. By doing the study Julia confirmed her belief that clients with chronic problems have as much or more need for nursing care as for medical care. The physicians also refer clients to Julia for weight loss, smoking cessation, and diabetes education. Because of time constraints, Julia has chosen to assess these clients for their readiness to make lifestyle changes and then assist them in choosing an appropriate program from among those offered by community agencies or private groups. One of Julia's goals as an FNP in private practice was to use her knowledge of community resources as an adjunct to her practice in serving the needs of clients in the practice. She has formally contracted with the agencies and programs to which she refers for a written assessment concerning the clients' progress. Julia is aware of the strategies used in the various community programs so that she can reinforce teaching during the clients' office visits. The practice also contracts with two local small industries to provide preemployment physicals and office visits for employees with nonemergency job-related injuries. Julia has talked with the physicians and the manager of one of the industries about conducting an on-site health screening program. The first phase, that of assessing the needs of the employees, is in the planning stage. Through the state nurses' association, Julia has had opportunity to network with other nurse practitioners, including those in occupational health nursing. One of the occupational health nurses has offered Julia consultation services as a professional courtesy.

Julia has demonstrated her value to the practice in several ways. She has increased practice income, she has formed working relationships with community health resources, she has made significant contributions to the quality and diversity of health care offered by the practice, and she is involving the practice in an outreach program to small industry—not to mention the benefits that may have accrued to the physicians in terms of time, income, and greater satisfaction in practice.

SUMMARY

The shortage of physicians that transpired during the 1960s, along with their maldistribution, created problems of access to primary care services. NPs and PAs were viewed as an answer to these medical manpower shortage and distribution problems. As nurses became knowledgeable and comfortable with the assessment and management skills of their role in primary care, it became apparent that their major contribution was not in the acute care management functions they performed but in the nursing skills that they brought to primary care.

The FNP role is one of the most comprehensive roles in primary care. FNPs specialize in the ambulatory health management of the family unit. Family dynamics, family assessment, growth and development, and management aspects of minor acute and stabilized chronic health problems provide the framework for the primary care nursing practice of FNPs. Within this framework are the components of health maintenance and management, which focus on problems in child health, women's health, adult health, and health problems of the aged.

NPs remain a controversial issue. Are they practicing medicine or nursing? Should they practice independently or jointly? How should they be educated? What is their legal relationship to the physician? Do they make a difference in the health of the people to whom they provide services? In the 22 years since the introduction of the role, these questions have yet to be fully answered. There is a limited amount of nursing research with implications relative to the roles and functions of NPs. Studies directed toward outcome as well as the process of care are greatly needed. Further, a long-range follow-up evaluation of the impact of NPs is also necessary. To remain a viable entity in the health care system, especially in this time of cost containment and physician surplus, FNPs must be perceived and valued by clients for meeting health care needs not addressed by other providers. If this can be done in an efficient, cost-effective manner FNPs will find a secure place in our health care system (Ford and Haston, 1985).

≡ KEY CONCEPTS

Several social phenomena and a shift in health problems over the past century have combined to redefine the pattern of health care in this country.

Primary care is defined as accessible, comprehensive, coordinated, and continuous care provided by accountable care givers.

The major roles of FNPs are health practitioner, health educator, health administrator, health consultant, and health researcher.

The ability of FNP to diagnose and treat has been a major benefit to the delivery of primary health care.

The major arenas of practice for FNPs are private practice, institutional settings, long-term care facilities, industry, federal government, HMOs, public health departments, and schools.

Because of the variety of expanded roles FNPs may encounter as institutions try to meet current challenges in health care delivery, it is imperative that FNPs have a working knowledge of both business and management principles.

If the FNP is going to collaboratively provide comprehensive primary care, negotiation skills must be thoroughly understood and developed.

Major stressors for FNPs include professional isolation, liability, collaborative practice, conflicting expectations, and professional responsibilities.

The FNP role is one of the most comprehensive roles in primary care. FNPs specialize in the ambulatory health management of the family.

LEARNING ACTIVITIES

1. Explore the development of the NP role locally.

2. Compare and contrast the local, state, and national NP movement.

3. Outline ways the FNP complements other team members in a specific primary care facility.

4. Investigate the FNP programs within the state or region to determine the educational requirements for admission and the type of degree or certificate conferred on graduation.

5. Review a specific state's nurse practice act as well as any rules and regulations governing expanded role practice.

6. Negotiate a clinical observation experience with an FNP.

BIBLIOGRAPHY

Adler, J.: You are charged with . . . . Nurse Pract. 4(1):6, 1979.

American Medical Association: Physician characteristics and distribution in the U.S.: 1983 edition, Survey and Data Resources, 1984.

American Nurses' Association: The study of credentialing in nursing: a new approach, vol. 1, Report of the committee, Kansas City, Mo., Jan. 1979, The Association.

Andreoli, K.G., and Musser, L. A.: Trends that may affect nursings' future, Nursing and Health Care 6(1):47-51, 1985.

Andrus, L.H., and Mitchell, F.H.: Change processes in primary care. In Renihardt, A.M., and Quinn, M.D., editors: Family-centered community nursing: a sociocultural framework, St. Louis, 1980, The C.V. Mosby Co.

Arizona wins reimbursement for NPs, Am. J. Nurs. 85:1019, 1985.

Barkauskas, V.H.: Public health nursing: an educator's view, Nurs. Outlook, 30(7):384, 1982.

Bullough, B., editor: The law and the expanding nursing role, ed. 2, New York, 1980, Appleton-Century-Crofts.

Bullough, V.L., and Bullough, B.: History, trends, and politics of nursing, Norwalk, CT, 1984, Appleton-Century-Crofts.

Bulman, T.: Ambulatory care: a practical way to quality assurance, Nursing Management 16(12):19-24, 1985.

Ciocci, G.: Capitalizing on the hidden job market, Nurse Pract. 9(12):31-33, 1984.

Clemen, S.A., Eigsti, D.G., and McGuire, S.L.: Comprehensive family and community health nursing, New York, 1981, McGraw-Hill Book Co.

Clemen-Stone, S.A., Eigsti, D.G., and McGuire, S.L.: Comprehensive family and community health nursing, ed. 2, New York, 1987, McGraw-Hill Book Co.

Cohn, S.D.: Survey of legislation on 3rd party reimbursement for nurses. Law, Medicine and Health Care, 11(6):260-263, 1983.

Coleman, J.R., and Smith, D.S.: DRGs: opportunity or crisis? Pediatric Nursing 10 (5):321, 1984.

Coslow, F., and Steinberg, M.C.: Relaxation techniques in ambulatory care practice, Nurse Pract. 9(10):26-27, 1983.

Dakota RNs win third-party reimbursement on first try, Am. J. Nurs. 85:463, 476, April 1985.

Daugherty, L.G., and Buchanan, G.J.: Nursing role in ambulatory care. In Jarvis, L.L., editor: Community health nursing: keeping the public healthy, Philadelphia, 1981, F.A. Davis Co.

Davidson, R.A., and Lauver, D.: Nurse practitioner and physician roles: delineation and complementarity of practice, Res. Nurs. Health, 7:3-9, 1984.

Draye, M.A., and Pesznecker, B.L.: Diagnostic scope and certainty: an analysis of FNP practice. Nurse Pract. 4(1):15, 1979.

Durham, J.D., and Hardin, S.B.: Nurse psychotherapists' experiences in obtaining individual practice privileges, Nurse Pract. 10(11):62-67, 1985.

Dye-White, E.E.: Public health nursing: a crisis in definition, role, and function, Home Healthcare Nurse 2(5):32-35, 1984.

Edmunds, M.: Models of clinical practice, Nurse Pract. 8(9): 59, 1983.

Ervin, N.: Public health nursing: an administrator's view, Nurs. Outlook 30(7):370, 1982.

Extending the scope of nursing practice, Department of Health, Education, and Welfare, Washington, D.C., 1971, U.S. Government Printing Office.

Felton, G., Kelly, H.D., Renehan, K., and Alley, J.: Nursing entrepreneurs: a success story, Nurs. Outlook 33(6): 276, 1985.

Fisher, D.W., and Horowitz, S.M.: The physician's assistant: profile of a new health profession. In Bliss, A.A. and Cohen, E.D., editors: The new health professionals, Germantown, Md., 1977, Aspen Systems Corp.

Ford, L.C.: Nurses, nurse practitioners: the evolution of primary care. (Book Review). Image, 18(4):177-178, 1986.

Ford, R.D., and Haston, L.: Nurse's legal handbook, Springhouse, PA, 1985, Springhouse Corporation.

Gardener, H.H., and Fishe, M.: Pluralism and competition: a possibility for primary care, Am. J. Nurs. 31:2152, 1981.

Glascock, J., Webster-Stratton, C., and McCarthy, A.M.: Infant and preschool well-child care: master's and nonmaster's prepared pediatric nurse practitioners, Nurs. Res. 34(1): 1985.

Golden, A.S.: The impact of health professionals. In National League for Nursing: health care in the 1980s: who provides? who plans? who pays? New York, 1979, National League for Nursing.

Goldwater, M.: From a legislator: views on third-party reimbursement for nurses, Am. J. Nurs. 82:411, 1982.

Graduate Medical Education National Advisory Committee: Non-physician health care provider technical panel, vol. 7, DHHS, Washington, D.C., 1980, U.S. Government Printing Office.

Griffith, H.M.: Strategies for direct third-party reimbursement for nurses. Am. J. Nurs. 82:408, 1982.

Griffith, H.: Who will become the preferred providers? Am. J. Nurs. 85:532-539, 1985.

Grove, S.K., and Pruitt, S.S.: The health needs of small company employees, Home Healthcare Nurse 2(5):32, 1984.

Hamm, R., and Kitts, J.: An approach to preventive periodic health examinations, Ala. Med. 54(2):16, 1984.

Hastings, G.E., Vick, L., Lee, G., et al.: Nurse practitioners in a jailhouse clinic, Med. Care 18(7):731-744, 1980.

Hiserote, J.L., et al.: Peer review among rural clinics, Nurse Pract. 5(1):30, 1980.

Hoole, A.J., Greenberg, R.A., and Pickard, C.G.: Patient care guidelines for nurse practitioners, ed. 2, Boston, 1982, Little, Brown, & Co.

Igoe, J.B.: The school nurse practitioner, Nurs. Outlook 23:381, 1975.

Indian health program 1955-1980, (HSA) Pub. No. 80-12005, DHHS, Washington, D.C., 1980, Indian Health Service.

Jacox, A.K., and Norris, C.M.: Organizing for independent nursing practice, New York, 1977, Appleton-Century-Crofts.

Janczak, D.F.: Changes in a rural public health nursing program: a community profile, Home Healthcare Nurse 3(5): 28-33, 1985.

Johnson, M.L.: I don't want to be a test case . . ., Nurse Pract. 5(3):7, 1980.

Johnson, R.E., and Freeborn, D.K.: Comparing HMO physicians' attitudes towards NPs and PAs, Nurse Pract. 11(1):39-49,53, 1986.

Joint Commission on Accreditation of Hospitals: Accreditation manual for hospitals, Chicago, 1976, The Commission.

W. K. Kellogg Foundation: Personal Communication, January 14, 1987.

Kendrick, V.M., and Sullivan, J.H.: Nursing research at a VNA, Home Healthcare Nurse 2(5):44-46, 1984.

Komaroff, A., editor: Common acute illnesses: a problems-oriented textbook with protocols, Boston, 1977, Little, Brown, & Co.

Kviz, F.J., Misener, T.R., and Vinson, N.: Rural health care consumers' perceptions of the nurse practitioner role, J. Commun. Health 8(4):248-262, 1983.

Kweskin, S., and Taller, S.L.: Where nurse practitioners expand good care . . ., Kaiser-Permanente Medical Center in Oakland, Calif., Patient Care 13:194-195, 1979.

Lamper-Linden, C., Goetz-Kulas, J., and Lake, R.: Developing ambulatory care clinics: nurse practitioners as primary providers, J. Nurs. Adm. 13(12):11-18, 1983.

Letich, C.J., and Tinker, R.V., editors: Primary care, Philadelphia, 1978, F.A. Davis Co.

Levitt, M.K., Stern, N.B., Becker, K.L., et al.: A performance appraisal tool for nurse practitioners, Nurse Pract. 10(8):28-33, 1985.

Mackenzie, J.A.: Order out of chaos: changes in community health and home care, Nursing and Health Care 6(1):37-38, 1985.

Manley, M.V.: Clinical privileges for nonhospital-based nurses, Am. J. Nurs. 81:1822-1825, 1981.

Mason, D.J., and Talbott, S.W., editors: Political action handbook for nurses: changing the workplace, government, organizations, and community, Reading, MA: 1985, Addison-Wesley Publishing Co.

Massachusetts MDs move to clamp limits on NPs, Am. J. Nurs. 85:315, 1985.

Mershon, K., and Wesolowski, M.: Strategic planning for the business of community health and home care, Nursing and Health Care 6(1):33-35, 1985.

Molde, S., and Diers, D.: Nurse practitioner research: selected literature review and research agenda, Nurs. Res. 34(6):362, 1985.

Mundinger, M.O.: Autonomy in nursing, Germantown, Md., 1980, Aspen Systems Corp.

Murphy, M.A., Gitterman, B.A., and Silver, H.K.: Hospital nurse practitioners: a trial approach, Pediatric Nursing 11(4): 269-291, 1985.

National Joint Practice Commission: Statement on joint practice in primary care definition and guidelines, Chicago, Sept. 1977, The Commission.

National League for Nursing: Position statement on the education of nurse practitioners, Pub. No. 11-1808, New York, 1979, The League.

Nettles-Carlson, B., and McLaughlin, C.P.: Managers and nurses: understanding both worlds, Nurse Pract. 10(10):51-54, 1985.

New regs threaten NPs, Am. J. Nurs. 85:326-327, 1985.

Newscaps. Ohio nurses battle boundaries on practice, Am. J. Nurs. 85:924, 1985.

NH ARNPs gain third-party reimbursement, Am. J. Nurs. 85:924, 1985.

Nichols, A.W.: Physician extenders: the law and the future, J. Fam. Pract. 11(1):101, 1980.

NY law allows third-party reimbursement to all RNs, Am. J. Nurs. 85:198-199, 1985.

Oda, D.S., DeAngelis, C., Berman, B., and Meeker, R.: The resolution of health problems in school children, J. Sch. Health 55(3):96-98, 1985.

Paradise, R.L., and Kendall, V.M.: Ambulatory care: primary nursing brings continuity, Nursing Management 16(12):27-30, 1985.

Poirier-Elliott, E.: Cost-effectiveness of nonphysician health care professionals, Nurse Pract. 9(10):54, 1984.

Ricardi, B.R., and Dayani, E.C.: The nurse entrepreneur, Reston, VA, 1982, Reston Publishing Co.

Richards, G.: Nonphysician practitioners make slow headway on staff privileges, Hospitals 58(24):82-86, 1984.

Richter, J., and Sloan, R.: A relaxation technique, Am. J. Nurs. 79(11):1960-1964, 1979.

Rogers, D.: The challenge of primary care. In Knowles, J.H., editor: Doing better and feeling worse, New York, 1977, W.W. Norton & Co.

Sherwood, J.J., and Glidewell, J.C.: Planned renegotiation: a norm-setting O.D. intervention. In Bennis, W.G., et al., editors: Interpersonal dynamics: essays and readings on human interaction, ed. 3, Homewood, Ill., 1973, Dorsey Press.

Silberstein, C.A.: Nursing role in occupational health. In Jarvis, L.L., editor: Community health nursing: keeping the public healthy, Philadelphia, 1981, F.A. Davis Co.

Silver, H., and McAtee, P.: The rural health clinic services act of 1977, Nurse Pract. 3(5):30, 1978.

Silver, H.K., Ford, L.C., and Stearly, S.A.: A program to increase health care for children: the pediatric nurse practitioner program, Pediatrics 39:;756-760, 1967.

Sirles, A.: The potential for the family nurse practitioner in the community, Ala. J. Med. Sci. 11(3):229, 1981.

Spicer, W.S.: Joint practice: conceptualization and implementation, part 2. In Johnson, R.W.: First annual symposium on nurse faculty fellowships in primary care, 1978.

Steel, J.E.: Putting joint practice into practice, Am. J. Nurs. 81(5):964, 1981.

Sultz, H.A., Bullough, B., Sherwin, F.S., et al.: Study of nurse practitioner programs, students, graduates, and employers of nurse practitioners, 1980-82. State University of N.Y. at Buffalo, prepared for the Bureau of Health Professions, Hyattsville, MD (HRP-0904775), Dec., 1983.

Tennant, F.S., et al.: A study of the economic viability of low-cost, fee-for-service clinics staffed by nurse practitioners, Public Health Rep. 95:321, 1980.

Top Arkansas court balks MDs' move to curb nurse practitioners, Am. J. Nurs. 85:328, 1985.

Washington law requires Blue Cross, Shield to pay RNs directly for own services, Am. J. Nurs. 81:1557, 1981.

Young, C.L., and Gottke, S.A.: Multiphasic health screening for the rural elderly, Home Healthcare Nurse 3(3):41-46, 1985.

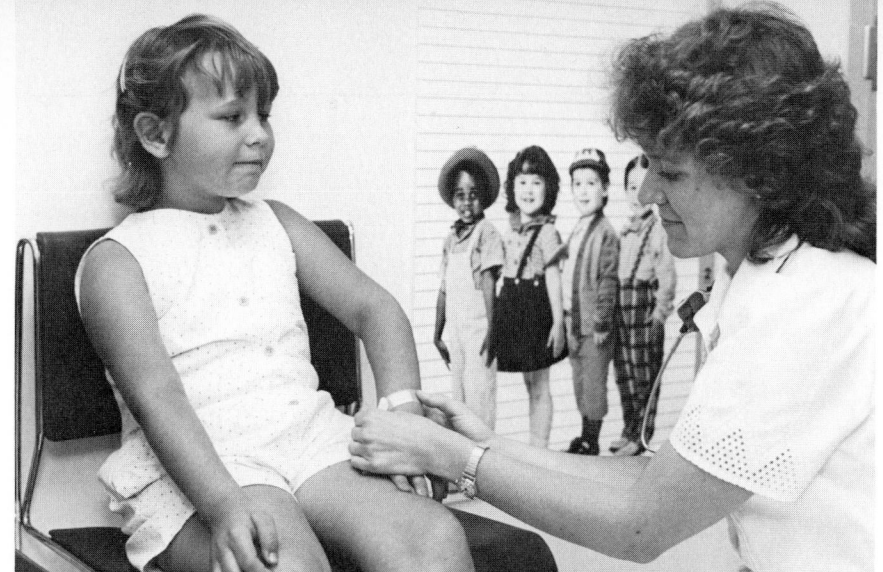

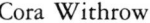

Cora Withrow

40

THE COMMUNITY HEALTH NURSE IN THE SCHOOLS

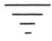 ## OBJECTIVES

After reading this chapter, the student should be able to:

Describe contemporary school nurses.

Describe the role functions of a school nurse.

Discuss disease prevention and health promotion in a school health program and describe the four domains of health.

Discuss chronic illness and special needs of children and youth in school settings.

Discuss the impact of legal influences and other issues and concerns of the school nurse.

KEY TERMS

acquired immune
  deficiency syndrome

advocate

anorexia

bulimia

case finding

consultant

counseling

domains of health

ethical issues

health education

holistic approach

Nurse Practice Acts

nurse practitioner

nurse teacher

primary prevention

referrals

screening

secondary prevention

tertiary prevention

A health panel argued in a 1981 report that the most fragile members of our society, children and youth, are the most likely to be affected by deficient or inconsistent health care. Ziegler (1976) noted that an estimated two thirds of our nation's 6.6 million children received inadequate medical attention, and an additional 25 million received little more than marginal health care. Identifying the causes of this neglect, and recognizing the need for strategies to deal with it, is of primary concern in school nursing practice.

Iverson and Kolbe (1985) hold that 30% of the nation's national health objectives could be met by health promotion programs in schools. What better place than a school for influencing the health of the nation? Most states require students to attend school until they are 16 years old, thus creating a large "captive" audience.

School nursing practice is easier to describe than to define. Wide diversities exist in education, in the role nurses play in school health programs, in the programs themselves, and in the legal and bureaucratic constraints within which school health goals are pursued. Size of the school district, local characteristics and values, availability of resources, and the abilities of the individual nurse explain, in part, this variation. But variation must also be understood by looking at trends in school health delivery.

In recent years, school health, and consequently school nursing, has become more comprehensive. In fact, the American Nursing Association (ANA) characterizes school nursing as both comprehensive and complex. This can be seen in a variety of ways. School nurses now try to work with children holistically—to help them grow emotionally and socially, as well as physically. Individuality and cultural variation are recognized and appreciated, even though health programs often involve working with large groups of children.

The promotion of these enlarged health goals has led to a more complex interpretation of school health programs and the total school system. Nurses have assumed new roles and adopted new strategies to fulfill their growing responsibilities. They are becoming more astute politically, organizing networks, using marketing concepts, and pursuing higher education, thus learning to work more effectively within the system. These new roles and strategies have also necessitated the acquisition of new skills in research, pri-

mary care, and counseling. School nursing has become as versatile as the nurses practicing and as varied as the differing school health needs.

This fluid situation, while providing challenging opportunities for professional growth, has also posed dilemmas for both the individual nurse and for the profession as a whole. At a time when important issues affecting the well-being of children are being confronted, school nurses must struggle to define their domain. They must not only cope with the demands made by their multiple roles in a changing health care field but also with the external forces that impinge on school nursing. As a result, there are calls for clarification of nursing's domain and responsibilities, more relevant research, changes in the nursing profession's organization, and increased involvement in activities that affect *health education* and health care for children and youth.

This chapter describes the range of contemporary school nursing practices. The description is not exhaustive; full descriptions of all activities engaged in by school nurses would take more than a chapter. Instead, a selection of roles school nurses fill, arenas in which they work, and important services they provide are presented to illustrate the comprehensiveness and complexity of this nursing specialty. Finally, the issues facing those who work in this arena are presented.

CONTEMPORARY SCHOOL NURSING

In the United States, approximately 30,000 professional registered nurses practice in school settings (Robert Wood Johnson, 1985). According to White (1985), school nurses can be classified into three categories based on their academic preparation and position description. Nurses with generic education, licensed registered nurses, and licensed practical nurses make up one category. School nurses who are certified fit into a second category; school nurse practitioners constitute the third category.

School nursing today, according to the American School Health Association, enhances the individual abilities of children and youth to use their intellectual potential to make worthwhile decisions affecting present and future physical, social, personal, and emotional health (ASHA, 1975). This view illustrates the increasingly comprehensive and complex nature of contemporary school nursing. Emphasis is on wellness programs, disease prevention, and health promotion from a holistic view. School health programs are viewed as ideal vehicles for transmitting health knowledge and changing and increasing the quality of health behaviors. Incorporated in these developments has been the integration of community health concepts and approaches into school health nursing (Freeman, 1970).

School Nursing Roles

School nurses have responded to changes in school health by assuming a wide variety of roles, often more than one at a time. Each nurse comes to a role with a set of expectations and an array of skills built through training, experience, and talent. On the basis of these skills, the nurse will select tools and strategies to carry out role functions. The community, school administrations, educators, families, and children also have expectations of the school nurse. The relationship between the nurse's and others' expectations may lead to conflict.

Due to factors affecting the school nurse, seven different roles have emerged, five primary roles and two secondary roles.

1. *Functional role:* Nurses in functional roles may be responsible for a group of schools to fulfill the functions of screening, follow-up, control of communicable diseases (e.g., outbreak of head lice), immunizations, and/or responding to calls from different schools.
2. *Primary role:* Primary nurses, usually generalists, are responsible for all direct health services; for example, caring for sick children, arranging screening programs, control of communicable diseases, and teaching health classes. They may also act as advocates and consultants; for example, working through others to get things done.
3. *Team member:* A school nurse with this role is a member of a multidisciplinary team, usually part of a core group consisting of the school physician, school counselors, psychologists, social workers, and teachers. Health teams in school systems are problem oriented and are activated when a need arises; for example, when mainstreamed children have problems adjusting to the school program or when children have problems interacting with mainstreamed children. The school nurse on the team may act as coordinator or advocate, conveying information to relatives about problem areas.
4. *Nurse practitioners:* School nurse practitioners are concerned with identification of children and youth at risk for specific health problems; for management of certain chronic diseases (for example, children with diabetes) and acute health concerns (for example, teenage pregnancies); and for providing a comprehensive and continuous care program to school children.
5. *Nurse teacher:* The nurse teacher's primary job is to teach health concepts and to identify ways of transmitting knowledge that supports change in health behavior (for example, teaching the relationship between nutrition and exercise).
6. *Consultant:* The role of the nurse consultant may be secondary to the primary roles of team member, primary nurse, nurse teacher, or functional nurse.
7. *Advocate:* The nurse advocate represents the interests of individual students, special need groups, or all children within the school, in the community and in the bureaucratic and political arenas.

School nurses use a variety of assessment techniques, interventions, and methodologies. Such applications include epidemiological, biostatistical data such as screening yields, absenteeism rates, self-reports, health examinations, mortality and morbidity reports that relate to the distribution of diseases (for example, Communicable Disease Centers reports on influenza and chicken pox; rates of abuse among children and youth; and immunization rates, especially for children living in the inner city and rural community). The nurse also identifies at risk populations and measures the effectiveness of health programs, services and activities (Benson and MacDevitt, 1980). School nurses are interested also in vital statistics and census data such as the number of children born to teenagers; demographics of school populations; specific screening yields to identify problems with teen pregnancies, scoliosis, etc.; risk factor analysis reports; and epidemiology of illness and health.

Functions

The school nurse's functions include health assessment and management of the school population through observation, communication, and examination; monitoring the safety of the school environment; coordinating screening programs; and providing health education, case-finding, counseling, referral, and follow-up. Other functions include liaison, leadership, management, and program planning.

Counseling

Another function of the school nurse is *counseling*. The ability to counsel students or others skillfully is an art. The counselor's responsibility is to provide information; to listen objectively; and to be supportive, caring, and trustworthy. Counselors do not make decisions; they help clients arrive at the decisions that best suit them. As such, counseling differs from both teaching and interviewing. For example, teaching is giving information; interviewing is obtaining information from someone; counseling is helping people arrive at workable solutions to their problems or conflicts.

Students usually request counseling when they are unable to make decisions about personal concerns that affect their lives, as for example, birth control methods. If the nurse lacks the ability to counsel or to recognize that counseling is needed, the student may be unable to fully comprehend the extent of the problem or to find alternatives to resolve the problem.

Student's peers can be used as counselors, especially in sensitive areas such as substance abuse and birth control. Students who act as counselors must be trained for the role. It is often effective, after providing students with technical information, to encourage them to use their personal experiences, to role play, and to be available and accessible to other students.

Health Education

Health education is another function of school nurses. These programs provide an ideal opportunity to help students develop health practices and life-style behaviors that will aid them in developing coping strategies for confronting the societal and environmental stresses specific to future developmental stages. Educational programs are central to health promotion and preparation for screening; and they aid in maintaining or restoring one's health, that is, they are useful at all levels of prevention.

School nurses are involved in educational activities in both direct and indirect ways as they teach, act as consultant, plan programs, and take advantage of every "teachable moment." Nurses are often called on to be guest speakers in the community.

School nurses are responsible for the planning, organizing, implementing, and controlling of any health problem they examine or class that they conduct. When cooperating with faculty in planning health education, the nurse is responsible for some of these activities. Whether involved only in the planning, or in both planning and teaching, knowledge of teaching techniques and curriculum design is extremely useful to the school nurse. It is also important to be able to formulate educational programs according to the developmental stages of the different age groups.

The box below gives a sample lesson plan for teaching elementary school children how to say "no." This plan illustrates some of the guidelines for this age group. In the early years of a child's school experience, special emphasis should be placed on the total approach to health, especially

as it relates to changes in behaviors. These are the formative years for attitude development; the critical period for developing health attitudes in children is 8 years of age (Palmer and Lewis, 1976). Self-motivation must be encouraged and supported, and health behaviors reinforced.

The essential elements of educational planning integrate community health, educational, and management concepts. This means that the nurse must be able to understand the topic content (e.g., the factors involved, relationships, desirable behaviors); select and use educational methods appropriate for a specific age group (e.g., use "show and tell" activities with young children, use discussion with adolescents) and target population; plan and coordinate activities, personnel, and resources; and finally, evaluate the effectiveness of the program.

Case Finding

School nurses also participate in *case finding* to alleviate problems such as those just described. Case finding identifies children who have undetected problems so that their needs can be met. Case finding techniques are designed to uncover those cases that do not surface in the screening programs. Basically, nurses practice careful, systematic observation of all children with whom they come in contact, looking for anomalies or suspect symptoms. It is also wise to check the following categories regularly:

1. Absentee list.
2. Students sent more than twice to the principal's office for illness.
3. Students sent more than twice to the principal's office for "acting out in the classroom."
4. Students who appear ill.
5. Students with subtle, as well as obvious, physical defects.
6. Students with subtle, as well as obvious, emotional problems.
7. Students who independently seek out the nurse for services.
8. Incident survey yields.

Perhaps the most likely places to begin, however, are with observations of children who are obviously physically or mentally different; children who have been bused out of their neighborhood or who have moved from rural, mountain, urban or suburban settings into a totally different social environment; and children from stressful situations where parental expectations may, at times, seem unreasonable for the child's stage of cognitive, physical, and psychosocial development. School nurses are especially concerned with detecting children who are victims of social illness (for example, neglect or abuse). The nurse's responsibility in working with children suspected of being abused is to provide them with a nonthreatening environment (i.e., providing comfort, a safe place, support, encouragement, compassion) and to report the problem to appropriate authorities such as the Children's Protective Services.

Screening

Basic *screening* tests determine whether children can hear, see, speak, and communicate. They also assess whether their

---

PERSONAL SAFETY LESSON PLAN

OBJECTIVE:

To demonstrate how to say "no."

CONTENT:

1. What does personal safety mean?
2. How can I say "no" to a stranger who seems to be nice?

MATERIALS:

Comic books, pamphlets, puppets, movies.

LEARNING ACTIVITIES:

1. Ask children to tell how they say "no."
2. Discuss the ways to say "no."
3. Demonstrate how to say "no"—use puppets for very young children.
4. Discuss the dangers of talking to strangers. Identify strangers as people who will stop them on the street to offer them candy or money.
5. Impress the children with their right to say "no" if someone tries to touch them and it makes them feel uncomfortable, even if the person is a relative.
6. Impress the children with the need to report all such incidents to parents, teachers, other relatives, or people with whom they feel safe.

development and developmental coordination, motor task development, and anthropometric measurements such as vision, hearing, speech, and DDST are appropriate for their stage of development. For example, the nurse might include scoliosis screening and instruction in self-examination of breasts and testicles in the school examination.

The nurse's responsibility in the screening process is to determine, with families and other team members, the appropriate resources for additional diagnostic workup for children with symptoms. For example, the nurse who has screened for scoliosis and found some children who are symptomatic may decide, in conjunction with the families, to refer one student to a private physician and another to a scoliosis clinic sponsored by Crippled Children's Services for confirmation and treatment.

The nurse also ensures that labeling, a problem that frequently arises because of screening, does not occur. Although it can arise for other reasons, to label is to describe, designate, or identify with a word or phrase. Frequently, the label "slow learner" is carelessly and inaccurately applied. If children are inaccurately labeled, they may be deprived of some educational opportunities and potential. Even when the label is accurate, its use as a designation is usually insensitive and a gross oversimplification of a human condition.

Referrals

Referrals are used to provide access to health care for students in need. The object of a referral service is to identify contact people within agencies and to facilitate easy movement of referred clients so that they are not lost in the system. The school nurse's responsibility is to act as liaison, dealing with the proper community or medical resources on behalf of the child. The following is an outline of some of the guidelines used in handling clients referred for special education:

1. School nurses work cooperatively with the principal, the speech teacher for the educationally handicapped, and other staff members in the school.
2. School nurses assist in appraising, both developmentally and functionally, the health status of pupils considered for admission to these classes. Nurses also interpret findings and other pertinent data.
3. Additional nursing functions include:
   a. Contact parents, after-school counselor, social worker, or school designee.
   b. Obtain developmental history.
   c. Obtain medical reports.
   d. Obtain signed authorizations.
   e. Collect data for and from source of medical care.
   f. Reevaluate pupils (if needed).
   g. Refer students (if needed).
   h. Provide nursing follow-up.

Agency conferences or meetings with representatives from agencies involved in providing service to a child are also a part of a referral service. Before a nurse can participate in an agency conference, parental consent must be obtained. Parental input is also necessary and may be obtained by parental attendance at the conference, a written statement from the parent, or a preconference meeting between parent and nurse. The family's involvement promotes compliance.

Furthermore, a referral system is evaluated in conjunction with all school health services. It is important to determine the efficiency and the cost-effectiveness of the service. For example, how quickly is the referral made? Does the referral system ease the student-patient flow and give the nurse more time for other duties? Does it lessen the cost and time spent seeking treatment for the patient?

An effective referral service is based on networking relationships built through meetings, informal gatherings, and telephone conversations. Also, it is essential that all teachers, students, principals, secretaries, and school counselors be instructed in the use of the referral system.

DISEASE PREVENTION AND HEALTH PROMOTION

Nurses practicing in schools must use community health concepts and approaches such as the three levels of prevention. Examples of *primary prevention* are promoting health and providing specific protection against disease; health education; creating healthful school environments (e.g., checking storage of chemicals, ensuring proper inspection of building materials); screening for scoliosis, hypertension, vision and hearing; and immunizations.

Secondary prevention occurs when early pathological process (disease) is identified and prompt treatment is instituted (e.g. finding ways to supplement inadequate diets, identifying a developmental delay, and providing stimulation). *Tertiary prevention* is an action(s) that assists in the restoration of individuals to their optimal level of well-being, such as teaching diabetic children about diet, and making provisions for the disabled. Behavioral changes and decision making are also essential; for example, providing supportive health services that will assist teenage mothers to avoid repeat pregnancies; helping teenage fathers to learn the parent role. The goal is to bring about long-term life-style and behavorial changes.

Unfortunately, providing information is not enough. Community health concepts must be incorporated into health instruction to help students translate what they have learned about self-imposed risks into appropriate behavior. For example, a major goal of a nutrition program might be that students not only eat appropriate foods, but also recognize that exercise is an essential component of this program (Perry, 1983). Another example is the provision of a support service for teen fathers. This service would include male role models (fathers) who are successful in their parenting role.

Four Domains of Health

The four domains of health are important to disease prevention and to health promotion behaviors of children and youth. There is a growing body of knowledge based on the multidimensional concept of the interactions and interrelationships among these health domains (Eberst, 1984; Jessor and Jessor, 1977; Langlie, 1979; Perry, 1983). The following are the four *domains of health* as described by Perry (1983):

1. *The physical domain:* the biological and organic

makeup of the individual. Important to the physical domain are the genetic process, maturation, and the aging process (Dever, 1980).

2. *The psychological domain:* the development of a sense of self (for example, identity) and inner harmony.
3. *The social domain:* the development of interpersonal relationships, the socialization process, social nurturing, and peer relationships.
4. *The personal domain:* establishing self-identity (knowing who you are and knowing what you can do in life). It is the art of becoming.

The four domains are interrelated and a breakdown in one domain affects the remaining three domains (Perry, 1983).

Figure 40-1 illustrates the interaction of the four domains. This perspective also encourages the search for the interrelated attitudes, behaviors, social relationships, physiological factors, and environmental agents underlying particular health problems. The complexity of these relationships can be appreciated when one considers that youths in junior high school are at a particularly vulnerable stage in life when body image (thinness) and self-worth are intertwined. The result can be anorexia or bulimia. Because the roots of the illness encompass each of the four domains of health, the treatment must do likewise.

Familiarity with the state of knowledge about these relationships and sensitivity to their subtle clues in a particular school population are prerequisites of effective school nursing. For example, the school nurse might assess the social relationships and the attitudes of junior high students and then consider them within the broader spectrum of the environmental, physical, psychological, and personal factors that affect the students and influence their behavior. Students' social relationships can be gauged by their response to this simple rank-in-order-of-importance question:

"My friends are:"
a. family
b. older people outside my family
c. people my age
d. no one
e. other

Other suggested questions are:
"I have a boy/girl friend." Yes_____ No_____
"I have a best friend that I hang out with." Yes____ No_____
"I belong to clubs, etc." Yes____No_____

These questions may provide clues to the depth of a student's isolation or loneliness. The following is an example of a characteristic that might be used to assess the environmental factors (influential model, i.e., a person or people providing the most influence in a student's life).

"Who do you think exerts the most influence in your life?" (Rank in order of importance)
a. Parents
b. Other relatives
c. Friends
d. Teachers
e. Television personalities
f. No one
g. Other

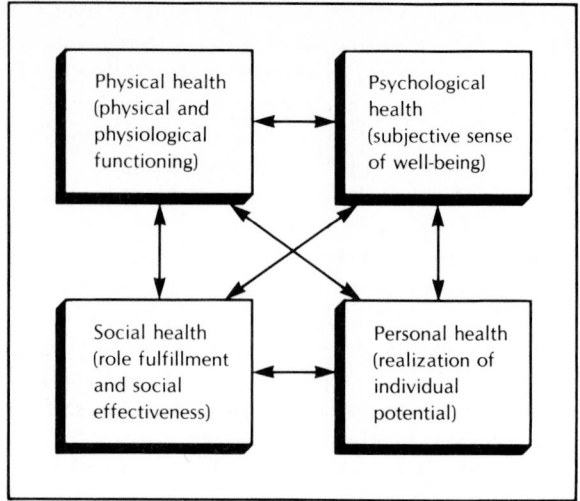

FIGURE 40-1

Domains of health. (Reprinted with permission of Cheryl Perry, 1983.)

Questions of this nature provide clues to the influencing sources. The next step is to use these sources for planned interventions. Consider, for example, an adolescent with a fractured leg. The concern is not only with the physical aspect of the injury, but also with the way the fracture will affect the student's social health (what is his role with his peers?); psychological health (how will others perceive him?); and personal health (how will this injury affect his future?). Furthermore, health promotion in schools implies the need to affect the behavior of parents as well as students. It may be sufficient to teach only the children in some aspects of health programs, such as personal hygiene, alcohol abstinence, or safety belt use, but it is always better for children and youth to have at least the support and preferably the active assistance of their families to make significant behavioral changes.

An exercise program is one example of an activity which requires the active cooperation of parents for the program to be effective. Most young people are limited by their family's socioeconomic status and by what parents practice in the way of family exercise programs and respite care. Unless parents are willing to make adjustments and are self-motivated, today's children and youth are more likely to spend their free time in front of the television rather than exercising. What does this early sedentary life-style mean to the future health of children and youth as adults? Consideration must be given now to epidemiological link-prone diseases, such as coronary heart disease. Children and youth who do not actively exercise; who smoke; and who have a strong family history of coronary heart disease, obesity, and high cholesterol are at risk.

As a consequence, school nurses can teach self-care techniques to children and youth as a part of health promotion and disease prevention. This may be accomplished with the cooperation of the physical education teacher who can teach the benefits of jumping rope for 20 minutes per day, riding a bicycle, or doing aerobic exercises for teenagers.

The awareness of the wide range of factors affecting health

problems also affects the way nurses serve and intervene in schools to achieve changes in the health behavior of children and youth.

Chronic Illness and Special Needs in Schools

Numerous chronic illnesses and special needs may be identified in a school setting; most are discussed in other chapters of this text. This section discusses three acquired long-term health problems—anorexia, bulimia, and AIDS—and a special need—juvenile delinquency—not covered elsewhere in this text.

Eating Disorders

Bulimia is a common eating disorder that involves consuming large quantities of food and then purging, either by forced vomiting or laxative abuse (Carter and Duncan, 1984). Persons with *anorexia* tend to restrict their food intake and to exercise to an extreme (Mallick, 1984). Many of the signs and symptoms of these diseases may go unrecognized in young women (and to an unknown extent in young males). Health professionals and teachers may also fail to detect these illnesses unless they are taught to recognize the symptoms.

There are several reasons that the diseases go undiagnosed. First, there may be no systematic means of monitoring weight or weight control activities in schools (Mallick, 1984). Second, school administrators and teachers may not have determined whose responsibility it is to identify and work with adolescents with these problems. Third, it is difficult to prevent either of the weight disorders because our nation is so weight conscious. Finally, there is a general lack of understanding about these health problems. Carter and Duncan (1984) found that in a study of 492 females, 38 were identified as vomiters. Of that number, 9% self-induced vomiting every time they ate, and 40% vomited only after binging. Sixty-three percent of the vomiters indicated that they would stop the practice if another effective method of weight control was available (Carter and Duncan, 1984). At this point, adolescent females with poor self-image, poor self-esteem, fear of rejection, and impulsive behaviors appear to be the most likely candidates for an eating disorder (Casper, Eckert, Halme, et al., 1980).

In bulimia the adolescent girl ingests large amounts of food secretly. She is difficult to identify because she skillfully hides her weight control behavior. Like the older woman the adolescent girl may exhibit high levels of anxiety and depression (Fairburn and Cooper, 1982). The adolescent's problem at that point is severe; once the cycle has begun, intervention is of limited value.

There are limited studies of the incidence of self-induced vomiting among middle or junior high school students. Although the exact number remains unknown in the high school population, evidence based on reports from studies of college women and the chronic nature of the problem indicates the practice of self-induced vomiting may be widespread (Maceykos and Nagleberg, 1985).

In light of an increasing incidence of self-induced vomiting, can school systems be developed as vehicles, and can epidemiological models be used to identify the problems and introduce prevention programs that will have lifetime benefits? One critic argues that approaches exist for increasing the awareness of school personnel. Although she makes several suggestions, one in particular stands out:

> Students can be weighed at the beginning of each school term and questioned about their dieting activities. Growth charts should be used and the following deviations should be watched for: no weight gain (anorexia) and weight that widely fluctuates (bulimia) (Mallick, 1984, p. 299).

It is important that the last phrase be emphasized, "no weight gain or weight that widely fluctuates." Once abuse of weight control has begun it is often extremely difficult to change behavior.

Consider this hypothetical case. Mary attempts to control her weight by self-induced vomiting. Mary has a self-image of being overweight, although she only weighs 90 pounds. Mary also has low self-esteem, anxiety, depression, and impulsive behavior, which complicates her drastic response to weight control. If people like Mary are identified in junior high or even in elementary school, and helped through peer counseling sessions, nurse-student sessions, appropriate nutrition, and exercise advice they often strengthen their self-concept and health awareness and avoid developing eating disorders in later years.

Acquired Immune Deficiency Syndrome

Since the identification of *acquired immune deficiency syndrome (AIDS)* in 1981, the Centers for Disease Control in Atlanta have recorded 70 cases of pediatric AIDS. Pediatric AIDS is defined as the diagnosis of the syndrome in infants and children to age 13 (News Briefs, 1985, p. 162). Moreover, it is not clear how many cases of AIDS have been diagnosed in older adolescents (News Briefs 1985, p. 162). In most school districts any child who contacts AIDS must be reported to school and governmental health authorities.

The American Nurses Association (ANA) is committed to assuring access to health care services for victims of AIDS and to protect the welfare and safety of health care personnel. This reaffirmation is much needed because of the growing concern among the public and health care workers as evidenced when children with AIDS attempt to enter a school system. The question is, what is the role of the school nurse? Professional school nurses are in the forefront and are approached because of their knowledge and understanding about AIDS. In addition, professional school nurses are advocates for children with AIDS and for their families. Consideration must also be given to the siblings of the victims of AIDS. How are these young people coping and how is their involuntary isolation affecting their sense of self? The nurse's role in this instance is to educate, counsel (for example, being supportive, protective, available), and teach self-care techniques.

As discussed in Chapter 17, certain population groups are at greater risk for developing AIDS. Most authorities agree that there are specific means of transmission of AIDS. Those who come into casual contact with a person with the virus are not at risk. What is needed to calm the public's overreaction is widespread education of how the disease is spread. They must be continuously reminded that they will not be infected through casual contact with an AIDS victim.

In addition, efforts must be increased to extend need-specific health education to adolescents.

Juvenile Delinquency

The federal government encourages states to place most youth status offenders in alternate facilities or programs because juveniles are often harmed when placed in jails (Kentucky Youth Advocates, 1981). A subsequent study by Kentucky Youth Advocates (1982) documented that many youths have unnecessarily been incarcerated in jails and juvenile detention centers. As a result of this incarceration, juveniles are often physically, sexually or emotionally abused by others (Mayhew, 1985).

However, depending on the laws in different states, these young men and women may be placed in temporary group homes, programs for runaways, home detention programs, and temporary foster homes. If any of these alternatives to detention are used, these young people may attend local schools. What does this mean for the school nurse? The nurse may work with young people who have received only cursory physical examinations and a minimum of referral and follow-up care (Berkman and Lippold, 1982). In addition, these young people may bring to school other unattended health problems that must be addressed by the school nurse, such as alcoholism, drug abuse, sexually transmitted diseases, pregnancy, gastrointestinal complaints, self-mutilation, injuries, nutritional deficiencies, chronic running-away, a history of sexual or physical abuse, prostitution, and emotional or mental illness. These young people need to be socialized into the school system. The problem may be exacerbated if school personnel are prejudiced and balk at including these young people in school activities such as sports and social clubs.

The nurse's role is to act as an advocate and provider of care to help socialize these young people into a school system. Nursing sevices must be comprehensive and of high quality; the status of the clients should not determine the type of services received. For example, the nurse may be working with court-appointed guardians rather than with parents. If these young people need medical care beyond the scope of the health service provided in schools, the nurse must arrange with the juvenile's legal guardian to obtain those additional services.

Finally, the school nurses may provide a comprehensive health history, which may be difficult to obtain if the juvenile is the sole source of information. Juveniles may be uninformed about their past history (this is not peculiar to this group). The nurse, via the legal guardian, must obtain all health records, such as emergency room visits, family planning services, outpatient clinic visits, and hospitalizations to develop a health composite of the individual. If at all possible, parents of these young people should be contacted. However, this may be a problem if the nurse is working with youths who have been put out of their homes by parents or placed in a temporary home by a court order.

Legal Influences

The *Nurse Practice Acts* of the 50 states define nursing practice and regulate what activities nurses are able to per-

form. The definitions of nursing vary from state to state; however, each of the 50 Nurse Practice Acts identify specific independent and dependent functions of the nurse. In most instances, nurses are instrumental in writing regulations relative to independent and dependent nursing functions.

The quality of nursing care a client population receives is determined by the professional organization's standards of nursing practice (ANA, 1983; ASHA, 1975) and the personal commitment of the school nurse.

School nurses are judged, as are other professional nurses, according to their standards of practice and what other nurses would do in the same or similar circumstances (ANA, 1973; Creighton and Squarres, 1974). On these bases, school nurses are liable for their own acts when their actions are less than prudent.

The mechanisms by which nurses obtain their credentials (licensure, registration, and certification) help to ensure that the standards for practice can be met.

There are also legal restrictions on the ways school nurses deal with their clients. Because these also vary from place to place, the school system attorney should be asked to clarify the following points:

1. What are the legal implications of having a birth control clinic in a school setting?
2. How binding is a school system's code book? (In Kentucky, for example, there is a school code book that governs what health services are to be provided.)
3. When do assent forms take precedence over consent forms?
4. What is the legal definition of a minor?
5. Are emancipated youths recognized as responsible individuals who are able to make their own decisions in school systems?

It is also recommended that school nurses evaluate both federal and state laws regarding treatment for sexually transmitted diseases and information on birth control methods, since state laws do not always conform to federal guidelines. According to the law, youths have a right to receive treatment for sexually transmitted diseases, to receive information about birth control, and to obtain birth control methods. At the federal level, however, it is now being suggested that personnel working in birth control clinics receiving federal support must inform parents when their minor children (under 18) are receiving birth control services. In addition, some state legislatures, such as Kentucky, voted to require that parental consent be obtained before minor children can receive an abortion. (Before its effective date, a restraining order was placed on the law until a court challenge is resolved.) The term "minor children" is defined by age and varies from state to state.

In 1975, Public Law 94-142, The Education For All Handicapped Children Act was passed to protect the rights of all handicapped children and to encourage all states to make public education and special services available. Encompassed in this law is the concept of "mainstreaming", which is the inclusion of handicapped children into nonhandicapped or regular school environments (Moorehead, 1982). In the 1980s, it is not unusual for a child in school to need nursing care. However, it is unusual, according to

Igoe (1980), to have nurses who are clinically prepared to meet these needs.

Issues and Concerns

Nurses are confronted with a number of serious issues and concerns that directly or indirectly affect their practice as they move toward the twenty-first century: birth control clinics in schools; social illnesses; abuse and neglect, etc.; budgetary cutbacks; mainstreaming; schools as a vehicle for meeting the nation's health objectives; AIDS; and the nationally recognized need for health education (Haro, 1974, Dagg, 1981). Other concerns center around the professional rank-and-file membership's image of school nursing, building a political base and developing an awareness of how politics impact school nursing, and improving the poor information and communications mechanisms for identifying and presenting positions and demands.

It is not known how birth control clinics in schools will affect school nursing practice directly, especially as it relates to parental and community concern and adolescent attendence. What is known is that there is a need to begin longitudinal studies to address the relationship of community attitudes, parental attitudes, and adolescent attendence in birth control clinics and to investigate the possibility of effecting a downward trend in adolescent pregnancies. There is a need to study whether the intent of birth control clinics placed in schools is to help decrease early and unwanted pregnancies or to provide sporadic birth control.

Research on risk-taking behavior among adolescents is needed to design more effective intervention programs (e.g. to reduce drug and alcohol abuse, deaths by accidents, smoking, and early pregnancies). We need to know why, at this stage in life, adolescents are willing to take risks without considering the consequences.

Other questions need to be answered, and much could be done by nurses to fill this gap. A review of the literature shows a paucity of research by school nurses, yet nurses, especially those with graduate degrees, are going into the school system with education in research methodologies. Whether or not they are equipped by education and position to direct research projects, they are often in ideal situations to help enlarge the body of nursing knowledge. They can participate in research projects, especially in the clinical setting (schools). They can direct attention to problems or situations that need attention and that may elude the less involved researcher. As the consumer of the results of research, they can provide the judgment, criticism, and feedback necessary for ongoing research in any field.

A number of researchable ideas include:

1. The long-term effects of risk factors on aggregates of children and youth, the required necessary nursing interventions, the effectiveness of external environmental influence of risk reduction factors on the families of children who have received care (Stevens, 1980).
2. The identification of the critical steps in adolescent decision making.
3. The necessary methods to assess competency levels of schools nurses.

Professional Concerns

Although there is a consensus within the nursing profession on the need for nursing services in the school, there is little agreement on the scope of those services. Primary care, for example, is supported in the literature as one mode of delivery (Dorster, 1979; Switzer and Kelly, 1981). Primary care, by definition, means continuous coverage 24 hours a day, 7 days a week, by coordinated, comprehensive services, which are accessible and acceptable to people (Dorster, 1979). If primary care is the goal for school health, can health providers in school systems live up to the definition? Many decisions about education of school nurses and program planning are contingent on some agreement about this issue.

Another issue is the need for more school nurse representation on national, state, and local committees whose decisions can facilitate nursing services in school health and health services for children. It is especially important that nurses belong to local committees since the bulk of federal funding to local areas is provided through block grants, which are federal funds not earmarked for specific programs. These grants are issued by the federal government to the states and then passed on to local governments. Local groups can influence the decision makers who decide which programs get funded. This is an arena for political involvement to assure that children and youth get their share of help.

In general, school nurses lack the organized power and influence needed to bring about change. This lack is partially a consequence of school nurses' isolation from each other and from nursing colleagues in other specialties. As an organized group, school nurses must continue to form coalitions and networks with other professional and consumer groups. Without organization and communication with others, it is difficult even to identify common concerns (Hamilton, 1982).

As leaders, school nurses must develop analytical and managerial skills to deal with organizations, program planning, and conflict of interest or goals. It is especially important to be able to analyze a situation before attempting to arrive at alternative actions (French and Bell, 1978).

There are a number of ethical issues in school nursing. One revolves around the need of nurses to understand why they are helping (Leitch, 1978). School nurses do not differ from other professionals in the range of their empathetic understanding, acceptance of clients, responsibility, and caring behaviors; but these abilities and activities need to be directed by an underlying purpose and meaning.

Another ethical issue relates to accountability. To whom and for what are school nurses accountable? The position of the school nurse in the hierarchy of health care makes answering this question difficult to answer. The nurse must respond to four interrelated publics. Which one has priority? Yura, Ozimek, and Walsh (1976) suggest that nurses are first accountable to their clients and then to the administration of the organization, their colleagues, and other members of the health team. However, according to Styles (1986), in addition to these four publics, nurses are also accountable to themselves.

Some ethical issues relate to students' rights. All children and youth have a right both to receive school health services and to refuse them. They also have a right to expect confidentiality when they share information and to know when a confidence has to be broken. These rights can conflict with some of the nurse's reporting responsibilities, however. What does the nurse do in these situations? Public Law 93-247 protects children and youth from undue harm from abusers even though they may be parents, other relatives, teachers, and nurses. Ethically and legally, school nurses are required to report suspected cases, as well as identified cases, of abuse; but cases are not always clear cut.

The nurse must also be concerned about what is being taught in the classroom and its possible effects on behavior. Subjects such as abortion, values clarification, and euthanasia must be discussed with the possible consequences carefully considered (Fulton, 1977).

CLINICAL APPLICATION

A major goal of a school nurse is to promote the health of the children and youth being served in the school. Assume you have recently accepted a position as a school nurse in a school district serving a predominantly middle income population. You have been assigned to the high school and are in your third week of employment. You have met several of the teachers, gotten to know the principal and counselors reasonably well, and have had time to observe the school and the students. You have noted that the school is particularly clean and well maintained, which leads you to assume that there is considerable pride in the school; the teachers, principal and counselors seem to enjoy a good working relationship; there is a large, clean, well-equipped cafeteria in the school; there are three snack areas in the school, which are open during the lunch periods and sell items such as carbonated beverages, candy, chips, cookies, sweet rolls, and gum; there are also two soft drink machines on the school campus; a large proportion of students leave the school either on foot or in cars during the lunch hour; there are four "fast food" establishments within two miles of the school; and a substantial portion of the students seem to be overweight and to have poor complexions.

Based on your initial assessment of several characteristics of the school, population, and area you decide that a need exists for increased nutritional awareness. Using the nursing process and considering the school as your community what would you do?

Possible interventions include:

1. Complete a thorough assessment. It is possible that you have arrived at a conclusion based on limited or inaccurate data. You would use several of the assessment techniques described in Chapter 13.

2. Remember that the role of the school nurse is multifaceted; you might serve initially as a fact finder and later as a consultant (to the principal, teachers, counselors, parents), counselor (to students, personnel), health educator, and group facilitator (see Chapter 14).

3. Nursing interventions would be planned after careful assessment of the population's health and nutrition needs; attitudes of school personnel toward health and particularly nutrition, knowledge of students' and personnel's nutrition, available resources, potential obstacles, and sources of support for developing nutritional awareness activities.

4. Implementation would be planned carefully to involve a wide range of people; an evaluation plan would be developed before starting any activity.

5. Brainstorm other ideas based on this assessment.

SUMMARY

The goal of helping young people develop into competent, coping, and healthy adults presents a challenge to the nurse whose personal philosophy is based on the belief that all people are entitled to health care. It is by working with youth that the nurse can have the greatest effect on the nation's health.

Nevertheless, the problems are dismaying. School nurses must be prepared to respond to diverse situations and work with many different kinds of people at a wide variety of tasks. Completing these tasks will demand that the nurse develop a host of new skills, some of which will be poorly related to nursing experience and training. Much of this work will be done while isolated from nursing colleagues and with little direction and no clear guidelines.

However, the nurse who does elect the role of school nurse will have an opportunity for professional development and personal growth. Each nurse who makes that choice can help to clarify the school nurse's role, define the domain of school nursing, and participate in finding solutions to the many dilemmas and issues facing those nurses who do work in schools. Having enough of these qualified nurses in schools as primary care providers will help to assure that future generations will be oriented to self-care responsibilities, will maintain high levels of wellness, and will develop into productive adult members of society.

≡ KEY CONCEPTS

School nurses can have the greatest effect on the nation's health.

School nursing practice is diverse; differences exist in education, in the role of the nurse in the school health program, in the programs themselves, and in the legal and bureaucratic restraints placed on the school health program.

School nurses must be prepared to respond to diverse situations and work with many different kinds of people at a variety of tasks.

The seven roles of the school nurse are functional, primary, team member, nurse practitioner, nurse teacher, consultant, and advocate.

School nurse functions include health assessment and management of the school population through observation, communication, and examination; monitoring the safety of the school environment; coordinating screening programs; and providing health education, case-finding, counseling and referral, and follow-up.

School nurses must adopt community health concepts and approaches. These must be incorporated into health instruction that will help students translate what they learn into appropriate behavior.

Nurse Practice Acts in various states define nursing practice and control what nurses can do. School nurses are judged according to their standards of practice and what other nurses would do in similar situations.

Nurses practicing in schools are faced with several serious issues, among them birth control clinics in schools, budgetary cutbacks, mainstreaming, increased need for health education in schools, child abuse and neglect, and prevalence of social illnesses.

Professional concerns of school nurses include delivery of care, representation, managerial and organizational skills, and ethical issues such as accountability and students' rights.

LEARNING ACTIVITIES

1. Find out from community health nursing staff in community health agencies and from school nurses hired by the board of education how school health is administered in your community. Compare your findings with your readings.

2. Talk with school nurses in your community and discuss (1) nursing roles, (2) nursing functions, (3) legal issues, and (4) issues and concerns. Compare your answers from the interview to your reading.

3. Debate with your classmates the roles and functions of school nurses.

4. Attend a meeting pertaining to the health of school children for the school health program (for example, a board of education meeting, teachers' meeting, district nurse meeting). Analyze the following: (1) the problems being discussed, (2) the needs of the school health program versus the community demand for service, (3) the interrelationships of the players, (4) the role of the school nurse at the meeting, (5) the decision (or lack thereof), (6) and the factors that influenced the decision.

BIBLIOGRAPHY

American Nurses' Association. Nursing Practice, Kansas City, Mo., 1973, The Association.

American School Health Association: Philosophy and goals for school nurse educational preparation, position paper by Subcommittee on Educational Preparation for School Nurses of the Committee on School Nursing, J. Sch. Health 45:409, 1975.

Benson, E.R., and McDevitt, J.: Community health and nursing practice, 2nd ed, Englewood Cliffs, N.J., 1980, Prentice-Hall, Inc.

Berkman, D.J., and Lippold, R.W.: Institutional neglect of juvenile health needs, New York, 1982, Haworth Press.

Carter, J.A., and Duncan, P.A.: The practice of self-induced vomiting among high-school females, J. Sch. Health 54:450-453, 1984.

Casper, R.C., Eckert, S.E., Halmi, K.A., et al: Bulimia, Arch. Gen. Psychiatry 37:1930-1935, 1980.

Creighton, H. and Squarres, G.M.: School nurses: legal aspects of their work, Clinics of Nursing Arts, 9:467-474, 1974.

Dagg, N.V.: Primary prevention: health promotion and specific protection. In Wold, S.J., editor: School nursing: a framework for practice, St. Louis, 1981, The C.V. Mosby Co.

Dever, G.E.: Community health analysis: a holistic approach, Germantown, Md., 1980, Aspen Systems Corp.

Dorster, M.: The role of the school nurse in primary care, J. Sch. Health 79:113-114, 1979.

Eberst, R.M.: Defining health: a multidimensional model, J. Sch. Health 54:99-103, 1984.

Fairburn, C.G., and Cooper, P.J.: Self-induced vomiting and bulimia nervosa: an undetected problem, Br. Med. J. (Clin Res) 254:1153-1155, 1982.

Freeman, R.B.: Community health nursing, Philadelphia, 1970, W.B. Saunders Co.

Fulton, G.B.: Bioethics and health education: some issues of biological resolution, J. Sch. Health 47:205-211, 1977.

Hamilton, P.A.: Health care consumerism, St. Louis, 1982, The C.V. Mosby Co.

Haro, M.S.: The school health revisited, J. Sch. Health 44:363-368, 1974.

Igoe, J.B.: Changing patterns in school health and school nursing, Nurs. Outlook, 28:486-492, 1980.

Iverson, D.C., and Kolbe, L.J.: School health report, Cited in The Robert Wood Johnson Special Report (1985), National School Health Services Program, New York, 1985, Institute.

Jessor, R., and Jessor, H.: Problem behavior and psychosocial development: a longitudinal study of youth, New York, 1977, Academic Press.

Kalisch, B., Kalish, P., and McHugh, M.: School nursing in the news, J. Sch. Health 83:548-553, 1983.

Kentucky Youth Advocates: A comparative study of young women and women in jails, Fourth interim report, Louisville, 1981 Kentucky Youth Advocates Inc.

Kentucky Youth Advocates: Some preliminary issues in removing juveniles from Kentucky jails, First interim report, Louisville, 1982 Kentucky Youth Advocates Inc.

Langlie, J.K.: Interrelationships among preventive health behaviors: a test of competing hypotheses, Public Health Rep 94:216-225, 1979.

Leitch, C.J.: Helping and human relationships, In Leitch, C.J., and Tinker, R.V., editors: Primary care, Philadelphia, 1978, F.A. Davis Publishing Co.

Maceykos, S.J., and Nagelberg, D.B.: The assessment of bulimia in high school students, J. Sch. Health 55:135-140, 1985.

Mallick, M.J.: Anorexia nervosa and bulimia: questions and answers for school personnel, J. Sch. Health 54:299-301, 1984.

Mayhew, B.H.: The rising cost of health care: exploring the options, Division of Health Services, 62(6):40-41, 1985.

Moorehead, Y.: The year of the disabled: everybody counts, New York, 1982, The Ivy Leaf, Inc.

News Briefs. Computer use in school doubles within one year, J. Sch. Health 54:46, 1984.

Palmer, B., and Lewis, L.: Development of health attitudes and behaviors, J. Sch. Health 46:401-405, 1976.

Perry, C.: A conceptual approach to school-based health promotion, J. Sch. Health 54:33-38, 1983.

The Robert Wood Johnson Special Report: National School Health Services Program, New York, 1985, Institute.

Stevens, B.J.: The nurse as an executive, Wakefield, Mass., 1980, Nursing Resources, Inc.

Styles, M.: Academic integrity: on candor in job shopping, Nurs. Educ. 2:49, 1986.

Switzer, K., and Kelly, J.T.: The nurse: a member of the school team, Matern. Child Nurs. 6:189-193, 1981.

White, D.: A study of current school nurse practice, J. Sch. Health 55:52-56, 1985.

Yura, H., Ozimek, D., and Walsh, M.B.: Nursing leadership theory and process, New York, 1976, Appleton-Century-Crofts.

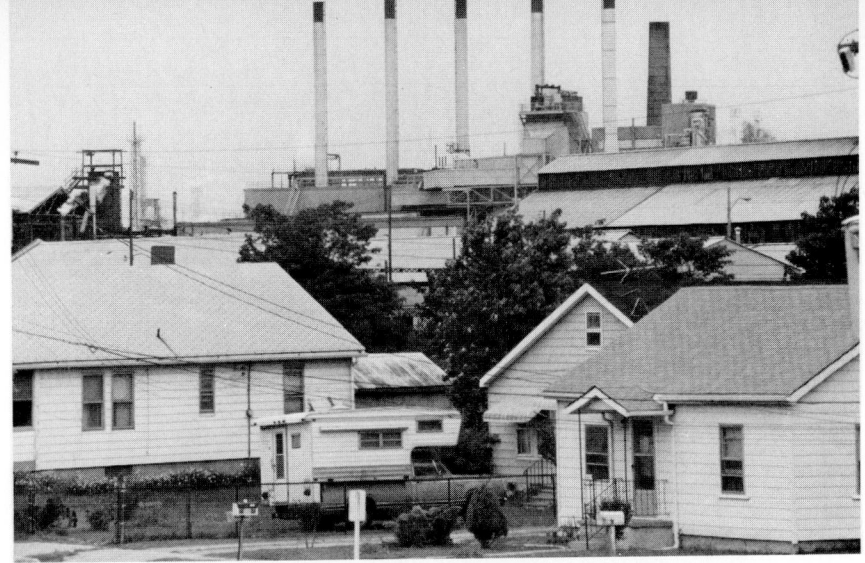

Charlene C. Ossler

41

THE COMMUNITY HEALTH NURSE IN OCCUPATIONAL HEALTH

OBJECTIVES

After reading this chapter, the student should be able to:

Describe at least three characteristics of the American work force.

Describe the extent of work-related illnesses and injuries.

Use the epidemiological model to explain work-health interactions.

Cite at least three host factors associated with increased risk from an adverse response to a hazardous workplace exposure.

Define hypersusceptible workers.

Explain one example each of biological, chemical, mechanical, physical, and psychosocial workplace hazards.

Cite at least four types of protective equipment that workers can wear to guard against the effects of hazards in the workplace.

Differentiate between health promotion programs and employee assistance programs.

Describe the functions of OSHA and NIOSH.

Complete an occupational health history.

KEY TERMS

agents
biological agents
chemical agents
employee assistance programs
environment
epidemiological triad
ergonomists
first aiders
Hazard Communication Standard
host
hypersusceptible
mechanical agents
occupational health history
physical agents
plant survey
psychosocial agents
workers' compensation acts
work-health interactions

The past two decades have witnessed revolutionary changes in the nature of work and the workplace, in the global economy, and the health care system. These numerous and complex changes are shaping future health priorities. An analysis of these trends suggests that work-health interactions will continue to grow in importance (Bezold, Carlson, and Peck, 1986). As a result of these changes, there have been impressive developments in occupational health and safety programs—those designed to control and prevent work-related illness and injury. Nurses, particularly occupational health nurses, have performed critical roles in the planning and delivery of such work site health and safety services that increasingly must be comprehensive and cost-effective.

The health impact of one's work is an important aspect of most clients for whom the community health nurse provides care. At least one third of the average adult's life is spent at work; therefore, the workplace is significant as a potential influence on individuals' health and also as a primary site for the delivery of preventive health care. According to Bezold et al. (1986, p. 168), "The dominant institutions of health—the hospital, the clinic, the laboratory, the nursing home—will steadily shrink in influence and scope in the decades ahead. They will yield to the home, the community center, and the workplace as the dominant settings in which health is pursued."

The prevalence and significance of the interactions between health and work underscore the importance of incorporating principles of occupational health and safety into general nursing practice. The nature of these interactions and the frequent use of the general health care system for the identification, treatment, and prevention of occupational illnesses and injuries require that nurses draw upon this knowledge in all practice settings.

◆ ◆ ◆

This chapter deals with the community health nurse's role with working population groups. The focus is on the knowledge and skills needed to promote the health and safety of workers through worksite occupational health programs, as well as through off-site interventions from agencies other than the employing business organizations.

The purpose of this chapter is to provide an introduction to work-related health and safety concerns and the principles for the prevention and control of adverse work-health interactions. The epidemiological triad is used as the model for understanding these interactions, risk factors, and effective nursing care for promoting health and safety among employed populations.

NURSING ROLES IN OCCUPATIONAL SETTINGS

Nurses perform a variety of roles and functions in occupational settings. The specialty of occupational health nursing in the United States began in 1898 with the employment of Ida Mayo Stewart, the first occupational health nurse (OHN), at the Vermont Marble Company (Babbitz, 1984). Although occupational health nursing has been a major force in promoting worker health since that time, rapid technological transformations, changes in the health care system, and societal expectations have demanded an increasingly complex and expanded role for occupational health nursing in the twentieth century. The primary focus of occupational health nurses' practice is the health and safety of workers with an emphasis on the prevention of illness and injury.

As American industry has shifted from agrarian to industrial to highly technological processes, the role of the occupational health nurse has continued to evolve. The focus on work-related health problems has expanded to include the entire spectrum of human responses to multiple, complex interactions of biopsychosocial factors that occur in the community and home, as well as work, environments. The customary role of the occupational health nurse has extended beyond emergency treatment and prevention of illness and injury to include the promotion and maintenance of health, overall risk management, and efforts to reduce health-related costs in businesses.

The occupational health nurse offers direct care to employees, as well as managerial skills such as program evaluation and analysis of work-related injuries and illnesses. The role changes with the mission of an organization's occupational health and safety program and therefore is diversified. The interdisciplinary nature of occupational health nursing has become more critical as occupational health and safety problems require more complex solutions. The OHN frequently collaborates closely with multiple disciplines and management.

Occupational health nurses constitute the largest group

of occupational health professionals. The most recent national survey of registered nurses indicates there are approximately 23,000 licensed occupational health nurses (U.S. Department of Health and Human Services, 1986). Nearly 70% of occupational health nurses report that they are employed as staff nurses; the majority of these manage one-nurse units in a variety of businesses. Other occupational health nurses hold positions as nurse practitioners, clinical nurse specialists, managers, supervisors, consultants, and educators (Cox, 1985). The occupational health nursing role is unique in that it adapts to an organization's needs, as well as to the needs of specific groups of workers.

The professional organization, the American Association of Occupational Health Nurses (AAOHN), describes five job titles for OHNs: solo practitioner, manager, educator, consultant, and corporate director (AAOHN, 1984). The majority of OHNs work as solo practitioners, but an increasing number of jobs have developed in the other categories over the past five years. Specialization in the field is often a requirement for the other positions. Graduate education in occupational health nursing is currently available through 14 universities as listed in the resources.

Certification in the specialty is provided by the American Board for Occupational Health Nurses (ABOHN); OHNs must meet requirements for experience, continuing education, and satisfactory recommendations before they can sit for the ABOHN certification examination. Both AAOHN and ABOHN are listed as resources in Appendix H2.

WORKERS AS A POPULATION AGGREGATE

There are approximately 107 million workers over the age of 16 in the United States who are employed in over 6 million different work sites (Bureau of Labor Statistics, 1984). This participation rate of 64% does not indicate the total number of individuals who potentially have been exposed to work-related health hazards. More than 91% of those who are able to work outside of the home do so for some portion of their lifetime (Bureau of Labor Statistics, 1980). Although some individuals may currently be unemployed or retired, they continue to bear the increased health risks of past occupational hazards. For the community health nurse, the number of individuals may be even larger, as evidence of work-related illness surfaces among the spouses, children, and neighbors of exposed workers.

Americans are employed in diverse industries that range in size from one to tens of thousands of employees. Types of industries range from traditional manufacturing (e.g., automotive and appliances) to service industries (e.g., banking, health care, and restaurants), agriculture, and the newer high technology firms such as computer chip manufacturers. Eighty-five percent of business organizations are considered small; they employ fewer than 500 people (Bureau of Labor Statistics, 1980). Although some industries are noted for the high degree of hazards associated with their work (e.g., foundries, mines, construction, and agriculture), no work site is free of occupational health and safety hazards. The larger the company, the more likely there will be an array of health and safety programs for employees. The smaller companies are more likely to rely on the external community to meet their needs for health services.

Characteristics of the Work Force

The demographic trends in the American work force picture a changing population aggregate, which has implications for the preventive services targeted to this group. Two major changes in the working population are the increasing number of women and older individuals. Due to changes in the economy, extension of lifespan, and societal acceptance of working women, forecasts are that these two groups will continue to grow as segments of the employed population. These workers tend to be married with children and dependent, aging parents for whom they are responsible. Other trends shaping the profile of the work force include increased education, mobility, and change in occupational focus among workers.

Characteristics of Work

There has been a dramatic shift in the types of jobs held by workers. In the evolution from an agrarian to a manufacturing to a highly technological workplace, the greatest proportion of paid employment is in the occupations of service (e.g., health care, banking, insurance), professional and technical (e.g., managers, computer specialists), and clerical (word processors, secretaries). These three occupational classifications account for 53% of all jobs (Didsbury, 1983). This change in the nature of work has been accompanied by a host of new occupational hazards such as complex chemicals, workstation design (the adaptation of the workplace or equipment used to do work to meet the employee's health and safety needs), and job stress.

WORK-HEALTH INTERACTIONS

The influence of work on health is evidenced by statistics on illnesses, injuries, and deaths associated with employment. In 1984, there were 5.4 million work-related illnesses and injuries that resulted in lost time from work. Of these, one third were severe enough to result in temporary or permanent disability that prevented the worker from returning to a usual job. Over the past few years, the incidence and severity of work-related injury have increased (Bureau of Labor Statistics, 1984). Approximately 4,000 deaths are attributable directly to the work environment; another 100,000 deaths occurred after work contributed or exacerbated primary illnesses. More than 390,000 cases of occupationally-induced illness are newly diagnosed annually (Office of Technology Assessment, 1985a). These figures are often described as "the tip of the iceberg" because many work-related health problems go unreported. Certainly even the recorded statistics are significant in the amount of human suffering, economic loss, and decreased productivity associated with workplace hazards.

Application of the Epidemiological Model

The epidemiological model is useful to understand the relationship between work and health. In reference to the *epidemiological triad* introduced in Chapter 8, the three elements of that model can be applied to occupational health as depicted in Figure 41-1. With a focus on the health and safety of the employed population, the *host* is described as any susceptible human being. Given the ubiquitous nature of work-related hazards, we must assume that all employed individuals and groups are potentially at risk of being exposed to occupational hazards. The *agents,* factors associated with ill health, are occupational hazards, which are classified as biological, chemical, mechanical, physical, and psychosocial. The third element, the *environment,* includes all external conditions that influence the interaction of the host and agents. These are workplace conditions such as temperature extremes, crowding, and autocratic management. The basic principle of epidemiology is that health status, and therefore interventions for restoring and promoting health, is the result of complex interactions among these three elements. To understand these interactions and to design effective nursing strategies for dealing with them, we must look at each of the three elements and how they influence each other.

Host

Workers have been described as a population group. Certain host factors are known to be associated with an increased risk of adverse response to hazardous exposures in the workplace. These include age, gender, chronic illness, work practices, immunological status, ethnicity, and life-style habits. For example, the population group at greatest risk for experiencing a work-related accident with subsequent injury

are young (18 to 30 years old) men with less than 6 months experience in their current job. The host factors of age, gender, and work experience combine to increase this group's risk of injury by virtue of characteristics such as risk taking and lessened dexterity with a new job. This population aggregate of workers is also more likely to be impaired by chronic use and abuse of drugs and alcohol.

At the other end of the age continuum, older workers may be at increased risk in the workplace because of diminished sensory abilities, the effects of chronic illnesses, and delayed reaction time (Poore, 1986). A third population group that may be more susceptible to workplace exposures is women in their childbearing years. The hormonal changes, as well as the increased stress of new roles and additional responsibilities, are host factors that may influence this group's response to potentially toxic exposures.

In addition to these host factors, there is some evidence to suggest that there are other, less well-understood individual differences in responses to occupational hazard exposures. Despite the maintenance of exposure levels below that recommended by occupational health and safety standards, 15% to 20% of the population may react to some "safe", low level exposures with health effects. This group has been termed *hypersusceptible* (Rom, 1983). A number of host factors appear to be associated with this hypersusceptibility: light skin, malnutrition, compromised immune system, glucose 6-phosphate dehydrogenase deficiency, serum alpha 1 antitrypsin deficiency, sickle cell trait, and hypertension (Stokinger, 1977). Although this

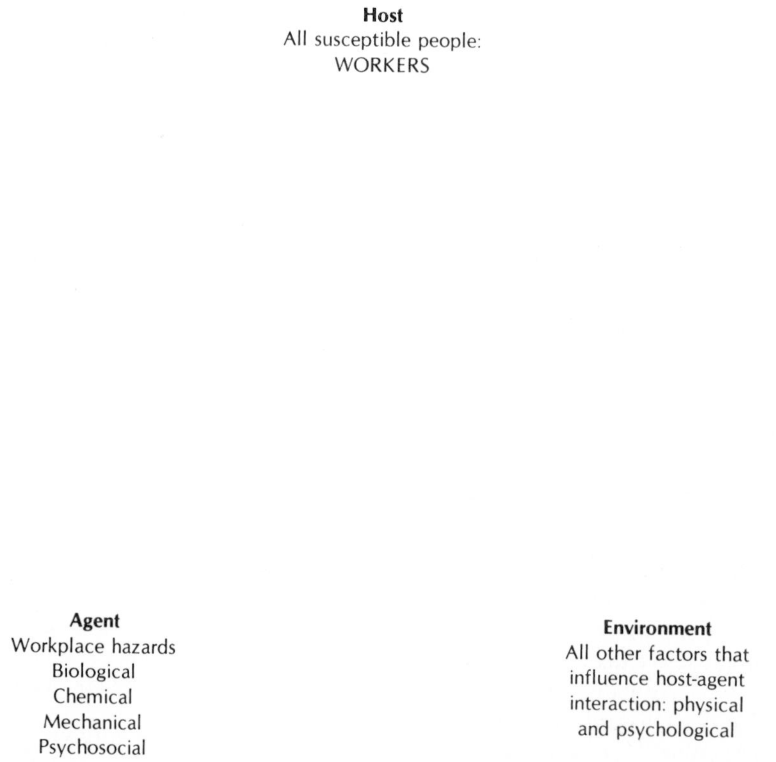

Host
All susceptible people:
WORKERS

Agent
Workplace hazards
Biological
Chemical
Mechanical
Psychosocial

Environment
All other factors that
influence host-agent
interaction: physical
and psychological

FIGURE 41-1

Elements of the epidemiological triad applied to occupational health.

has prompted some industries to consider preplacement screening for such risk factors (Severo, 1980), the associations among these individual health markers and hypersusceptible response to occupational hazards are speculative and require further research.

Agents

Work-related hazards, or agents, present potential and actual risks to the health and safety of workers in all of the 6 million different business establishments in the United States. These agents are classified into five categories: biological, chemical, physical, mechanical, and psychosocial agents. Any given work site commonly presents multiple and interacting exposures from all five categories of agents. Table 41-1 lists some of the most common workplace exposures, their known health effects, and the types of jobs associated with these hazards.

BIOLOGICAL AGENTS. Biological agents are living organisms whose excretions or parts are capable of causing human disease, usually by an infectious process (Cheremisinoff, 1984). Biological hazards are common in such workplaces as hospitals and clinical laboratories. In these work sites, employees are potentially exposed to a wide variety of infectious agents including viruses and bacteria. Health services workers are at increased risk of contracting disease from these exposures. For example, hepatitis B and tuberculosis rates are generally higher than expected among hospital personnel; a hospital employee is 41% more likely than the average worker to have lost work time attributable to a serious occupational injury or illness (Clever, 1981). Many individuals in these settings are employed as maintenance workers, security guards, aides, or cleaning people who tend not to be well protected from inadvertent exposures. Such exposures include contaminated bed linen in the laundry, soiled equipment, and trash that includes contaminated dressings and specimens.

Other occupations with exposures to biological agents include agriculture (farmer's lung) and commercial baking (baker's asthma) (Kusnetz and Hutchison, 1979). In addition, new biological agents (such as herpes and AIDS) have developed for which little is known about prevention and control.

CHEMICAL AGENTS. Over 300 billion pounds of chemicals are produced annually in this country. Of the approximately 2 million known chemicals in existence, only 6,000 have been tested for human effects. Of those that have been tested, 1,000 have carcinogenic potential, and approximately 400 are proven carcinogens (ReVelle and ReVelle, 1981). As a consequence of general environmental contamination with chemicals from work, home, and community activities, a variety of chemicals are found in the body tissues of the general population. These tissue loads may be associated with the accidental release of chemicals such as occurred in Love Canal when chemicals were leached out from buried industrial wastes. There is also significant exposure to a daily, low level dose of workplace chemicals that may be below the exposure standards but constitutes a potentially chronic, and perhaps cumulative, assault on workers' health. Predicting human responses to such exposures is further complicated because several chemicals are often combined to create a new chemical agent; human effects may be associated with the interaction of these agents rather than with a single chemical.

An evolving concern about occupational exposure to chemicals is that of reproductive health effects. Reproductive hazards in the workplace have become an important legal and scientific issue. Toxicity to both male and female reproductive systems has been demonstrated for common

---

TABLE 41-1

Common workplace exposures by job with known health effects

Workplace hazard	Health effects	Jobs with potential exposure
Carbon monoxide	Headache, angina	Firefighters, auto mechanics, drive-in bank tellers
Solvents	Dermatitis, cancer	Foundry workers, wood finishers, dry cleaners, textile workers, microelectronics
Lead	Abdominal pain, hypertension, behavioral changes	Battery makers, smelter workers, painters, shoemakers, gasoline station attendants
Asbestos, silica, coal dust	Chronic bronchitis, emphysema, lung cancer	Insulators, pipe fitters, miners, shipyard workers
Benzene	Aplastic anemia, leukemia	Furniture finishers, chemists
Hepatitis B virus	Hepatitis	Health services workers
Sunlight	Melanoma	Farmers, fishermen, highway workers
Heat	Burns, hyperthermia	Foundry and smelter workers, food services workers
Lifting heavy loads	Back pain, muscle strain, sprain	Health services workers, truckers who load and unload vehicles
Vibration	Kidney disease, bladder disease, carpal tunnel syndrome	Semitrailer truck driver, jackhammer user

occupational agents such as lead, antineoplastic drug administration, mercury, cadium, nickel, and zinc (Rao and Schwetz, 1982; Woolhandler, 1983). These concerns are addressed in a recent governmental report that calls for additional legislative intervention with occupational reproductive hazards (Office of Technology Assessment, 1985b).

Since there are inadequate data for predicting human responses to many chemical agents, workers should be assessed for all potential exposures and cautioned to work preventively with these agents. High risk or vulnerable workers should be screened carefully and monitored for optimal health protection.

MECHANICAL AGENTS. The transfer of mechanical energy can produce adverse health effects. Examples of this occupational hazard are vibration, repetitive motion, and lifting heavy loads. Vibration, which accompanies the use of power tools and certain vehicles such as trucks, affects internal organs, supportive ligaments, the upper torso, and the shoulder girdle structure. Localized effects are seen with hand-held power tools; the most common is Raynaud's phenomenon (Cheremisinoff, 1984). Carpal tunnel syndrome, tendonitis, and tendosynovitis are the most frequently seen occupational diseases observed in workers who are chronically exposed to repetitive motion. The research on these hazards, related human responses, and prevention is relatively new and incomplete. Given the recent changes in the nature of work, however, cumulative trauma from these exposures may present one of the largest categories of work-related illness and disability in the future. The most productive strategy in preventing these exposures appears to be redesign of the workplace and the work machinery.

PHYSICAL AGENTS. Physical agents are those that produce effects on humans by the transfer of physical energy. Commonly encountered *physical agents* in the workplace include extremes of temperature, noise, radiation, and lighting. The control of worker exposure to these agents is frequently dependent on the worker's compliance with preventive actions such as wearing personal protective equipment and safe work habits. Personal protective equipment includes hearing protection, eye guards, protective clothing, and devices for monitoring exposures to agents such as radiation. Examples of protective work habits are taking appropriate breaks from environments with temperature extremes and not eating or smoking in radiation contaminated areas. This class of agents is considered one of the most easily controlled. Frost bite, heat stroke, hearing loss, radiation sickness, and headaches from improper lighting can be prevented through engineering controls and appropriate education of the worker in preventive work practices.

PSYCHOSOCIAL AGENTS. Psychosocial hazards are conditions that pose a threat to the psychological and social well-being of individuals and groups of people. Psychosocial responses to the work environment occur as employees act selectively toward their environment in an attempt to achieve a harmonious relationship. When these human attempts at adaptation to the environment fail, an adverse psychosocial response may occur. Work-related "burnout" is a response to excessive and continuous occupationally induced stress. Responses to poor interpersonal relationships, particularly those with authority figures in the workplace, are often the cause of vague health symptoms and an increased absenteeism rate. Epidemiological work in the field of mental health has pointed to environmental variables such as these in the incidence of mental illness and emotional disorder (Wicker, 1979).

Environment

Environmental factors influence the occurrence of host-agent interactions and may mediate the course and outcome of those interactions. While there may be aspects of the physical environment (e.g., heat, odor, ventilation) that influence the host-agent interaction, the psychological environment can be of equal importance. To illustrate the effects of the physical environment, consider an employee who is working with a potentially toxic liquid. Providing education about safe work practices and fitting the employee with protective clothing may not be adequate if the work must occur in a very hot and humid environment. As the worker becomes uncomfortable in the hot clothing, this protection may be compromised by rolling up a sleeve, taking off a glove, or wiping the face with a contaminated piece of clothing.

The psychosocial environment includes characteristics of the work itself, as well as the interpersonal relationships required in a work setting. Job characteristics such as low autonomy, poor job satisfaction, and limited control over the pace of work have been associated with increased risk of heart disease among clerical and blue collar workers (Haynes, 1980). Interpersonal relationships between employees and co-workers or bosses and managers are often the source of conflict and stress. Another environmental aspect is that of organizational culture. This refers to the norms and patterns of behavior that are sanctioned within a particular organization (Deal and Kennedy, 1982). Such norms and rituals set guidelines for what type of work behaviors will enable the employee to succeed within a particular firm. Examples are organizational norms for working overtime, expressing dissatisfaction with management, and making work the first priority in one's life. Such factors, and the employee's response to them, must be assessed if strategies for influencing the health and safety of workers are to be effective.

The *epidemiological model* can be used as the basis for planning interventions to restore and promote the health of workers. These efforts are influenced by societal and organizational activities related to occupational health and safety.

ORGANIZATIONAL AND SOCIETAL EFFORTS TO PROMOTE WORKER HEALTH AND SAFETY

Promotion of worker health and safety is the goal of occupational health and safety programs. These programs are offered primarily by the employer at the workplace, but the range of services and the models for delivering them have changed dramatically over the past few years. In addition to specific services, legislation at the federal and state levels have had a significant impact on efforts to provide a healthy and safe environment for all workers. Whereas the initial response to this legislation was an increased use of occupational health and safety professionals, the 1980's have been a time of decreased emphasis on the enforcement of these laws. This has resulted in "down-sizing": occupational health and safety services have been decreasing in scope and more frequently are provided by paraprofessionals such as medical technicians, licensed practical nurses, or *first aiders* employed as workers in the company. Business firms are not required to provide occupational health and safety services that meet any specified standards. With few exceptions, there is no legal mandate for specific services or level of personnel provided by employers to protect worker health and safety. Therefore, the range of services offered and the qualifications of the providers of occupational health and safety vary widely across industries.

On-site Occupational Health and Safety Programs

Optimally, on-site occupational health and safety services are provided by a team of occupational health and safety professionals. The core members of this team are the occupational health nurse, occupational physician, industrial hygienist, and safety professional. The largest group of health care professionals in business settings is occupational health nurses. Therefore, the most frequently seen model is that of the one nurse unit or solo practicing occupational health nurse. This nurse collaborates with a community physician who provides consultation and accepts referrals for specific employee medical problems. This collaboration may occur primarily through telephone contact or the physician may be under contract with the company to spend a limited amount of time on-site each week. As companies become larger, they are likely to hire additional nurses, part-time or full-time physicians, safety professionals, and industrial hygienists. An increasingly popular option is to contract some health, safety, and industrial hygiene work to external providers as needed. The largest firms often have corporate occupational health and safety professionals who set policy and participate in company decision making at the corporate level. These professionals work with the nurses employed at the individual plants of the company.

Depending on the needs of the company and their workers, additional professionals may be on the occupational health and safety team. These could include, for example, employee assistance counselors or social workers, health educators, physical fitness specialists, toxicologists, and human factors engineers *(ergonomists)*. The personnel and services in an organization's occupational health and safety program differ across companies and result from decisions made by management.

The services provided by on-site occupational health programs range from those focused on only work-related health and safety problems to a wide scope of services that include primary health care. The various services are listed in the box above. For industries that have exposures regulated by law, certain programs are mandated. The ability of a company to offer additional programs is dependent on management's attitudes and understanding about health and safety, acceptance of the workers, and the economic status of the firm. There has been a significant increase in the

---

SCOPE OF SERVICES THAT CAN BE PROVIDED THROUGH AN OCCUPATIONAL HEALTH AND SAFETY PROGRAM

Health Assessments:
  Preplacement
  Periodic: mandatory, voluntary
  Transfer
  Retirement-Termination
  Executive
Preventive health screening with education
Employee assistance programs
Life-style classes: smoking cessation, weight control, stress management, physical fitness and conditioning
Rehabilitation
Treatment of illness and injury
Primary health care for workers and dependents
Fitting of protective equipment
Worker safety and health education related to occupational hazards
Prenatal and postnatal care and support groups
Medical self-help classes
Safety audits
Plant surveys and monitoring
Processing workers' compensation and OSHA claims and reports
Health-related cost containment strategies such as medical care utilization review

---

number of health promotion programs and employee assistance programs offered in industry over the past few years. Health promotion programs focus on life-style habits that pose risks to health (e.g., obesity, smoking, stress responses, and lack of exercise). Employee assistance programs are designed to address personal problems, such as marital discord, substance abuse, and financial difficulties, that affect the employee's ability to be a productive worker. Since such efforts are proving to be cost-effective for businesses, it is predicted that they will continue to multiply (Girdano, 1986).

A similar array of occupational health and safety programs are available on a contractual basis from community-based providers. These may be offered by freestanding industrial clinics, health maintenance organizations, hospitals, emergency clinics, and other health care organizations. In addition, consultants in each discipline work in the private sector—for themselves, group practice, or insurance companies—and in the public sector in local and state health departments or departments of labor and industry. These services may be brought on-site, delivered elsewhere in the community, or offered through a mobile van that visits companies. These multiple resources have increased the options for companies who need occupational health and safety services and also broadened the employment opportunities for health and safety professionals. The occupational health and safety services provided by an employer are influenced by specific legislation at the federal and state levels.

Legislation

Although the relationship between work and health has been known since the second century (Ramazzini, 1713), public policy that effectively controlled occupational hazards was not enacted until the 1960s. The Mine Safety and Health Act of 1968 was the first piece of legislation that specifically mandated certain preventive programs for workers. This was followed by the Occupational Safety and Health Act of 1970. The Occupational Safety and Health Act established two agencies, the Occupational Safety and Health Administration and the National Institute for Occupational Safety and Health, to carry out the Act's purpose of assuring "safe and healthful working conditions for working men and women" (Public Law 91-596, 1970). The functions of each of these agencies are described in the box below. The standards that regulate workers' exposure to potentially toxic substances are OSHA standards and regulations that are enforced by OSHA at the federal and state levels. The box upper right lists the major standards that have implications for occupational health and safety programs; other federal legislation with an impact on occupational health and safety is found in the box lower right.

One of the most recent and far-reaching of OSHA standards is the *Hazard Communication Standard.* Also known as the federal "right to know" law, this standard is based on the premise that we cannot rid working environments of *all* potentially toxic agents; therefore, an important line of defense is an educated work force. The Hazard Communication Standard, which took effect in May, 1986, requires that all manufacturing firms inventory their toxic agents; label them; and develop information sheets, called Material Safety Data Sheets (MSDSs), for each agent. In addition, the employer must have in place a Hazard Com-

munication Program that provides workers with education about these agents. This education must include identifying information, toxic effects, and protective measures. It is expected that this standard will be extended to all employers covered by the Occupational Safety and Health Act. Similar "right to know" legislation exists at the state and local levels in various parts of the country.

Workers' Compensation Acts are important state laws. Workers' compensation systems are developed at the state level to provide financial compensation to employees who suffer work-related health problems. These acts vary by state; each of them reimburses employees with occupational health problems for medical expenses and lost work time

---

MAJOR OCCUPATIONAL HEALTH AND SAFETY HAZARDS (U.S. DEPARTMENT OF HEALTH AND HUMAN SERVICES, NIOSH, 1986)

CHEMICAL HAZARDS

acetylene, acrylonitrile, aldrin, alkanes, ammonia, antimony, arsenic, benzene, benzoyl peroxide, beryllium, cadmium, carbaryl, carbon dioxide, carbon disulfide, carbon monoxide, carbon tetrachloride, chlorine, chloroform, chromic acid, coal tar products, cobalt, coke oven emissions, DDT, dibromochloropropane, diisocyanates, dinitrotoluenes, ethylene dibromide, ethylene oxide, fluorides, formaldehyde, glycol ethers, hexachloroethane, hydrazines, hydrogen cyanide, isopropyl alcohol, ketones, lead, malathion, mercury, methyl alcohol, nickel, nitric acid, nitriles, nitrogen oxide, parathion, phenol, phosgene, polychlorinated biphenyls (PCBs), styrene, sulfur dioxide, sulfuric acid, toluene, vanadium, vinyl chloride, xylene, zinc oxide

DUSTS, MINERAL HAZARDS

asbestos, cotton dust, nuisance dusts such as fibrous glass, silica, coal dust

OTHER HAZARDS

confined spaces, noise, elevated work stations, excavations, grain elevators, foundries

---

FUNCTIONS OF FEDERAL AGENCIES INVOLVED IN OCCUPATIONAL HEALTH AND SAFETY

OCCUPATIONAL SAFETY AND HEALTH ADMINISTRATION (OSHA)

Determine and set standards for hazardous exposures in the workplace

Enforce the occupational health and safety standards (includes the right of entry to businesses)

Educate employers about occupational health and safety

Develop and maintain a database on work-related injuries, illnesses, and deaths

Monitor compliance with occupational health and safety standards

NATIONAL INSTITUTE FOR OCCUPATIONAL SAFETY AND HEALTH (NIOSH)

Conduct research and review of research findings to recommend permissible exposure levels for occupational hazards to OSHA

Identify and research occupational health and safety hazards

Educate occupational health and safety professionals

Disseminate research findings relevant to occupational health and safety

---

LEGISLATION WITH SIGNIFICANCE FOR OCCUPATIONAL SAFETY AND HEALTH

1964 Civil Rights Act
1966 Federal Metal and Non-Metallic Safety Act
1969 Federal Coal Mine and Safety Act
1970 Occupational Safety and Health Act
1970 Environmental Protection Agency established
1970 Consumer Product Safety Commission established
1972 Equal Employment Opportunity Act
1972 Noise Control Act
1972 Clean Water Act
1976 Resource Conservation and Recovery Act
1976 Toxic Substances Control Act
1978 Quiet Communities Act

associated with the illness or injury. Workers' compensation also pays death benefits. The increased costs and frequency of workers' compensation claims and the insurance premiums paid by industry have been an important motivation for increasing the health and safety of the workplace.

NURSING INTERVENTIONS WITH WORKING POPULATIONS

Nurses are often the first health care provider seen by an individual with a work-related health problem. Consequently, nurses are in key positions to intervene with work populations at all three levels of prevention. The initial step of assessment involves the traditional history and physical assessment, with an emphasis on individual characteristics that may predispose to increased health risk at certain jobs and on occupational hazard exposures.

Assessment of Individuals and Families

The occupational health history is an indispensible component of the health assessment of individuals. Since work is a part of life for the majority of people, it is important to incorporate an occupational health history into all routine nursing assessments. Many workers in the United States do not have access to health care services in their workplace. Yet it is not unusual to encounter health care providers in the community who have little or no knowledge about workplaces or expertise in occupationally-related illnesses and injuries. Because of the large number of small businesses that do not have the resources for maintaining on-site health care, workers will be seen first in the public and private health care sector: clinics, emergency rooms, physicians' offices, hospitals, HMOs, and ambulatory care centers. Nurses often are the first line assessors of these individuals and perhaps the only contact for education about self-protection from workplace hazards. The identification of workplace exposures as sources of adverse health effects may influence the patient's course of illness and rehabilitation and also prevent similar illness among others with potential for exposure.

The incorporation of occupational health data into client assessments begins with the recognition of the possibility of a relationship between health and occupational factors. The next step is to develop routine assessment questions into history-taking that will provide the data necessary to rule out occupationally-induced symptoms. Symptoms of hazardous workplace exposures may be vague complaints involving any body system and often mimicking common medical diagnoses. Goldman and Peters (1982) suggest three points that occupational health histories should include: list of current and past jobs the client has held; questions about exposures to specific agents and relationships between the symptoms and activities at work, job titles, or history of exposures; and other factors that may enhance the client's susceptibility to occupational agents (e.g., smoking history, underlying illness, previous injury, or handicapping condition).

Questions about the client's occupational history can be woven into existing assessment tools. The more complete the data collected, the more likely the nurse is to have an influence on work-health interactions. All clients should be queried about their employment history. To describe only a current status of "retired" or "housewife" will lead to the possible omission of relevant data. The nurse should be aware that not all workers are well informed about the materials with which they work or potential hazards. For this reason, the nurse must develop basic knowledge about the types of jobs held by clients and the possible hazards associated with them. Since there is increased likelihood of multiple exposures from other environments that may interact with workplace exposures, the nurse should extend the questioning to include information on other exposures.

Identification of work-related health problems does not require an extensive knowledge of occupational agents and their effects. A systematic approach for evaluating the potential for workplace exposures is the most effective intervention for detection and prevention of occupational health risks. Figure 41-2 describes one short assessment tool that can be incorporated into routine history-taking. Similar questions can be included in the assessment of the spouses and dependents of workers who may receive secondhand or indirect exposure to occupational hazards.

During these health assessments, the nurse has the opportunity to teach about workplace hazards and the preventive measures the worker can employ. At the same time, the nurse is obtaining information that will be valuable in optimizing worker-job fit. Such assessments may be done as preplacement examinations before the client begins a job, on a periodic basis during employment, or with the onset of a work-related health problem or exposure. Work-related health assessments may also be conducted when an employee is being transferred to another job with different requirements and exposures, at termination, and at retirement.

When the health data from such assessments are considered collectively, the nurse may determine some patterns in risk factors associated with the occurrence of work-related injuries and illnesses (Ossler, 1986). For example, a nurse practitioner in a clinic noted a dramatic increase in the incidence of bladder cancer among her clients. When she looked at what these individuals had in common, she determined that they all worked at the same firm that used benzidine dyes, a known bladder carcinogen. She worked with the union and the company to assess the degree of environmental exposures to the employees. This nursing intervention led to a safer work environment and a subsequent decrease in bladder cancer among this population group. Such an approach can be used at the company, industry, and community levels; the initial collection of data and the questioning about workplace exposures are vital steps for any intervention.

Assessment of the Workplace

The nurse may conduct a similar assessment of the workplace itself. Termed a "plant survey" or walkthrough, the purpose of this assessment is to become knowledgeable about the work processes and materials, the requirements of various jobs, the presence of actual or potential hazards, and the work practices of employees (Dyal, 1982). Figure 41-3 is a brief outline that can be used to guide a plant

I.   Present Job
     A.   What do you do for a living? _____
     B.   How long have you had this job? _____
     C.   Describe the specific tasks this job involves: _____
          _____

     D.   What product or service is produced by the company where you
          work?

     E.   Are you exposed to any of the following on your present job?
          Chemicals   Vapors, gases   Radiation
          Loud noise   Vibration   Extreme heat or cold
          Infectious   Dusts   Stress
            agent   Others:

     F.   Do you feel you have any health problems related to your work?

          If yes, describe:

     G.   How would you describe your satisfaction with your job?
          Very satisfied   Satisfied   Somewhat satisfied
          Dissatisfied   Very dissatisfied

     H.   Have there been any recent changes in your job or the hours
          you work?

          Comments:

     I.   Do you use protective clothing and/or equipment on your job?

          If yes, describe:

     J.   Have any of your co-workers been complaining of illnesses or
          injuries that they associate with their jobs?

          If yes, describe:

II. All Past Work
     Starting with your first job, please provide the following
     information:

Job Title	Years Held from to	Description of work	Exposures	Injuries/ Illnesses

III. Other Exposures
     A.   Do you have any hobbies which involve exposure to chemicals,
          metals or any of the other agents mentioned before? If yes,
          describe:

     B.   Are any other members of your household exposed to any of the
          substances listed above? If yes, describe:

     C.   Do you live near any factories, dump sites, or other sources
          of pollution? If yes, describe:

FIGURE 41-2

Occupational health history.

survey. More complex surveys are performed by industrial hygienists and safety professionals when environmental monitoring or safety audits are the purpose of the survey (Lee, 1983). Some occupational health nurses have developed expertise in these areas and include such tasks as a part of their function. For any health care provider who assesses workers, this information is an important database. For the on-site health care provider, such plant surveys, or walkthroughs, assist the professional in establishing rapport and credibility among employees.

Plant surveys begin with an understanding of the type of work that occurs in the workplace. All business orga-

```
Name of company                                    Date
 Address

Parent company (if any)
 Location of corporate offices

SIC code   Major products
Major processes and operations




Raw materials used/created:


Potential health hazards:


Organizational chart that includes the occupational
health professionals:

Employees:
 Total number:          Number in production:        Others:
 % Fulltime             % Males         % Females
 First shift            Second shift    Third shift
 Age distribution
 % Unionized            Names of unions


Health Data:
 Work related illnesses, injuries, deaths per annum:
 OSHA recordable   Workers' Compensation
  Other            Most frequent complaints:
 Average number of monthly calls to the health unit:
 Absenteeism rate:
 Description of health and safety services:
 Providers:
 Examinations offered:
 Employee Assistance Programs:
 Treatment if illness/injury:
 Health education:         Preventive screening:
 Physical fitness, health promotion activities:
 Mandatory programs:
 Health and safety committee:
 Safety audits:
 Environmental monitoring:

Comments:
```

FIGURE 41-3

Guide for plant survey.

nizations are classified by a code, the Standard Industrial Classification Code (SIC code), by the U. S. Department of Commerce. This code, usually a two- to four-digit number, indicates the product of a firm and, therefore, the possible types of occupational health hazards that may accompany the processes and materials used by employees. The SIC codes are used to collect and report data on businesses. For example, to determine whether a company is experiencing an excess of illness or injury, these rates are compared with the rates of other companies of similar size in the same SIC code. All OSHA and workers' compensation data are reported by SIC code. In addition, knowing the SIC code of a company, a health care professional can access reference books that describe the usual processes, materials, and by-products of firms. A simple drawing of the work processes and work areas is used to direct the survey and to categorize information by jobs or locations in the plant. These preliminary data provide clues about what hazards may be present and an understanding of the types of jobs and health requirements that may be involved in a particular industry.

Characteristics of the employee group is the second area of important information. The nature, availability, and utilization of health and safety services also are assessed. The structure of the organization, the chain of command for occupational health professionals, and the incidence rates for work-related illnesses and injuries complete the survey

TABLE 41-2

Areas to be assessed in applying the epidemiological model to the use of VDTs in an office setting

Host: workers	Agent: VDTs	Work environment: office
Previous musculoskeletal injury	Height of workstation Lighting	Pacing of work Worker control of work Noise, other distractions
Age	Tiltable screen	Employee-supervisor relationships
Other use of VDT outside of employment	Chair with lumbar support and stability	Policies about rest breaks
	CRT shield	Adequate space for rest breaks
Underlying chronic illness Eyeglasses—other sign of visual impairment		

data. The more of this information that can be collected before the walkthrough, the more efficient the process of the survey. After the plant survey is conducted, the nurse can use this information with the aggregate health data to evaluate the effectiveness of the occupational health and safety program and to plan future programs.

CLINICAL APPLICATION: INTERACTIONS OF THE HOST, AGENT, AND ENVIRONMENT IN THE WORKPLACE

An example of how the epidemiological model can be used to assess clients and plan nursing care illustrates the usefulness of approaching occupational health problems with an epidemiological perspective. An insurance company recently renovated their claims processing office area. All typewriters were replaced with video display terminals (VDTs) and associated hardware for handling all future work by computer. The company's occupational health nurse noticed an increase in visits to the health unit for complaints of headache, stiff neck muscles, and visual disturbances. To conduct a complete investigation of this problem, the nurse assessed the workers, the new agent of VDTs as well as previously existing potential agents, and the work environment (Ossler, 1985). Table 41-2 depicts the factors for each of these areas that the nurse would assess. By collecting data for each of the three elements of the epidemiological triad, the nurse can respond most effectively to the aggregate health problem that is suggested by the increased use of the health services.

This information leads to the conclusions that certain workers may be at increased risk of adverse responses to this new agent, workstation design contributes to these unhealthy responses, and the work environment influences the host-agent interaction. Nursing interventions could include strengthening the resistance of the host by prescribing appropriate rest breaks, eye exercises, and relaxation strategies. Recognizing that previous cervical neck injury or impaired vision may increase the risk of adverse effects from VDT work, the nurse would include assessment for these factors in employees' preplacement and periodic health examinations.

Minimizing the possible hazards of the agent involves recommendations for desk, chair, and lighting design that accommodate the individual worker and shielding of the VDT. The components used to do the work comprise the workstation for the VDT operator. The nurse's recommendations about designing these components to minimize strain on the worker's comfort and health are based on principles of ergonomics—the study of adapting work and workplaces to fit humans.

For the environmental concerns, the nurse may educate the manager about the health risks of paced, externally controlled work expectations and recommend alternatives. Such an approach is likely to address most of the factors involved in this example of work-related illness and to result in interventions that are effective in promoting worker health and safety while increasing the productivity and morale of the work group.

SUMMARY

Although nurses can specialize in occupational health nursing, the principles of occupational health and safety are important to the practice of all nurses. Multiple risks to workers' health and safety in workplace settings include biological, chemical, mechanical, physical, and psychosocial agents. Basic nursing education prepares generalists who are capable of providing nursing care to individuals, families, and groups across the lifespan and along the health-illness continuum. This includes all workers, their families, and those who live in the environs of industrial areas. Incorporation of work-related exposures and health risks is a critical part of any nursing assessment. The preventive interventions for clients with workplace health and safety risks are often in the realm of nurses in occupational, as well as other, settings.

This chapter introduced the epidemiological approach to assessing and intervening with occupational health and safety problems. The key to minimizing or eliminating many of these hazards lies in the identification of the potential or actual exposures and effective education about protective measures. Two tools to assist in meeting this goal were described: the occupational health history and the plant survey. The nurse's role in this preventive approach is to incorporate occupational health data into each client assessment and to use this information to identify workplace exposures and to implement appropriate worker education.

The bibliography includes basic texts for health care providers who wish to increase their familiarity with occupational hazards and their effects on health. Appendix H2 provides information for contacting agencies involved in worker health and safety protection.

KEY CONCEPTS

The health impact of one's work is an important aspect of most clients for whom the community health nurse provides care.

Two major changes in the working population are the increasing number of women and older individuals in the workplace.

Host factors known to be associated with increased risk of adverse response to exposure to hazards in the workplace are age, gender, presence of chronic illness, work practices, immunological status, ethnicity, and life-style.

Work-related hazards or agents are classified as biological, chemical, physical, mechanical, and psychosocial.

Promotion of worker health and safety is the goal of occupational health and safety programs.

Services provided by on-site occupational health programs range from those focused on only work-related health and safety problems to a wide scope of services that include primary health care.

The ability of a company to offer health and safety programs is dependent on management's attitudes and understanding about health and safety, acceptance of the program by the workers, and the economic status of the company.

Although the relationship between work and health has been known since the second century, public policy that effectively controlled occupational hazards was not enacted until the 1960s.

Nurses are often the first health care providers seen by an individual with a work-related health problem. Consequently, nurses are in key positions to intervene in working populations at all three levels of prevention.

The occupational health history is an indispensable component of the health assessment of individuals.

A plant survey, or walkthrough, is important in assessing the workplace. It enables the nurse to gain knowledge of the requirements of various jobs, the presence of actual or potential hazards, and the work practices of employees.

The primary focus of occupational health nurses' practice is the health and safety of workers, with an emphasis on the prevention of illness and injury.

As American industry has shifted from agrarian to industrial to highly technological processes, the role of the occupational health nurse has continued to evolve.

Although nurses can specialize in occupational health nursing, the principles of occupational health and safety are important to the practice of all nurses.

LEARNING ACTIVITIES

1. Visit a small industry and describe the workers. What percentage are women? What percentage are over 40 years of age? What type of work are the workers doing? Can you detect anything about the worker's attitudes by their appearance?

2. After your visit to the small industry describe at least two real or potential occupational health hazards.

3. Select a person with either Raynaud's phenomenon or carpal tunnel syndrome and ask to trace the work history. Look for past or present employment that might precipitate these syndromes.

4. Interview a worker to evaluate the character of the psychosocial environment of the work setting. Identify hazards and possible interventions.

5. Review any work environment in which you have been employed and identify potential hazards.

6. Complete a thorough assessment of an industry and develop a model occupational health and safety plan. Include hazards, goals, resources, and deficits.

BIBLIOGRAPHY

Anderson, H.A., Lilis, R., Daum, S.M., Fischbein, A.S., et al.: Household-contact asbestos: neoplastic risk, Ann. NY Acad. Sci. 271:311-323, 1976.

American Association of Occupational Health Nurses: Job descriptions for OHNs, Atlanta, 1984, AAOHN.

Babbitz, M.A.: The practice of occupational health nursing in the United States, Occup. Health Nurs. 31(6):23-25, 1984.

Baselt, R.C.: Biological monitoring methods for industrial chemicals, Davis, Ca., 1980, Biomedical Publications.

Bezold, C., Carlson, R.J., and Peck, J.C.: The future of work and health, Dover, Mass., 1986, Auburn.

Bureau of Labor Statistics: Handbook of labor statistics, Washington, D.C., 1984, U.S. Department of Labor.

Bureau of Labor Statistics: Handbook of labor statistics, Washington, D.C., 1980, U.S. Department of Labor.

Centers for Disease Control: Legionnaire's disease, Morbidity and Mortality Weekly Report, 26:439-441, 1978.

Cheremisinoff, P.N.: Management of hazardous occupational environments, Lancaster, Pa., 1984, Technomic Publishing.

Clever, L.H.: Health hazards of hospital personnel, West. J. Med. 135:162-165, 1981.

Cox, A.R.: Profile of the occupational health nurse, Occup. Health Nurs. 33(12):591-593, 1985.

Deal, T.E., and Kennedy, A.A.: Corporate cultures: the rites and rituals of corporate life, Reading, Mass., 1982, Addison-Wesley.

Didsbury, H.F.: The world of work, Bethesda, 1983, The World Future Society.

Doull, J., Klaassen, C.D., and Amdur, M.O.: Casarett and Doull's toxicology, ed. 2, New York, 1980, Macmillan, Inc.

Dyal, L.E.: Plant profile: a contemporary interpretation of the nursing process, Occup. Health Nurs. 29(3):17-21, 1982.

Girdano, D.A.: Occupational health promotion: a practical guide to program development, New York, 1986, Macmillan Publishing Co.

Goldman, R., and Peters, J.W.: The occupational and environmental health history, JAMA 246:2831-2836, 1982.

Gosselin, R.E.: Clinical toxicology of commercial products, Baltimore, 1976, Williams & Wilkins.

Hamilton, A., and Hardy, H.: Industrial toxicology, ed. 3, Acton, Mass., 1974, Publishing Sciences Group.

Haynes, S., and Feinleib, M.: Women, work, and coronary heart disease. Am. J. Public Health 70(2):133-141, 1980.

Justice, B., and Duncan, D.F.: How do job-related problems contribute to child abuse, Occup. Health Saf. 47:42-45, 1978.

Key, M.M.: Occupational diseases—a guide to their recognition, Cincinnati, 1977, National Institute for Occupational Safety and Health.

Kustnetz, S., and Hutchison, M.: A guide to the work-relatedness of disease, Cincinnati, 1979, National Institute for Occupational Safety and Health.

Lee, J.S.: Environmental evaluation of the work place, Family and Community Health 16-23, May 1983.

Levy, B.S., and Wegman, D.H.: Occupational health: recognizing and preventing occupational disease, Boston, 1983, Little, Brown & Co.

National Safety Council: National Safety News, July, 1984.

Office of Technology Assessment, U.S. Congress: Preventing illness and injury in the workplace, Publication No. OTA-H-256, Washington, DC, 1985a, U.S. Government Printing Office.

Office of Technology Assessment, U.S. Congress: Reproductive hazards in the workplace, Publication No. GPO No. 052-003-01001-1, Washington, DC, 1985b, U.S. Government Printing Office.

Ossler, C.C.: Men's work environments and health risks, Nurs. Clin. North Am. 21(1):25-36, 1986.

Ossler, C.C.: Distributive nursing practice in occupational health and safety. In Hall, J.E., and Weaver, B.R., editors: Distributive nursing practice: a systems approach to community health, ed. 2, Philadelphia, 1985, J.B. Lippincott.

Poore, M.: Older workers, Occup. Health Saf. 55(8):12-15, 1986.

Proctor, J., and Hughes, J.: Chemical hazards of the workplace, Philadelphia, 1978, J.B. Lippincott.

Ramazzini, B.: Diseases of workers (translated by W.C. Wright From DeMorbis Artificum, 1713), New York, 1964, Hafner.

ReVelle, P., and ReVelle, C.: The environment: issues and choices for society, New York, 1981, D. Van Nostrand.

Rom, W.N.: Occupational and environmental medicine, Boston, 1983, Little, Brown and Co.

Rosenstock, L., and Cullen, M.R.: Clinical occupational medicine, Philadelphia, 1986, W.B. Saunders.

Sax, N.I.: Dangerous properties of industrial materials, ed. 5, New York, 1986, D. Van Nostrand.

Schwartz, R.M.: Injured on the job, Boston, 1979, Massachusetts Coalition for Occupational Safety and Health.

Severno, R.: The genetic barrier: job benefit or job bias? New York Times, Feb. 3-6, 1980.

Stellman, J.M., and Daum, S.M.: Work is dangerous to your health, New York, 1973, Random House Publishers, Inc.

Stokinger, H.E.: Routes of entry and modes of action. In Key, M.M., editor: Occupational diseases: a guide to their recognition, Washington, D.C., 1977, National Institute of Occupational Safety and Health.

U.S. Department of Health and Human Services: Unpublished data from The national sample survey of registered nurses, Rockville, Md., November, 1984. Bureau of Health Professions.

U.S. Department of Health and Human Services, NIOSH: NIOSH recommendations for occupational safety and health standards, Atlanta, 1986, Centers for Disease Control.

U.S. Department of Labor, Bureau of Labor Statistics: Handbook of labor statistics, Washington, DC, 1985, U.S. Government Printing Office.

U.S. Department of Labor, Bureau of Labor Statistics: Occupational injuries and illnesses in the United States by industry, 1980, Bulletin No. 2130, Washington, D.C., 1982, U.S. Government Printing Office.

Wicker, A.W.: An introduction to ecological psychology, Belmont, Calif., 1979, Wadsworth.

Williams, P.L., and Burson, J.L., editors: Industrial toxicology: safety and health implications in the workplace, New York, 1985, Van Nostrand Reinhold.

Woolhandler, S.: Toxic injury to male reproductive systems, Occup. Health Saf. 52:24-28, 1983.

Zenz, C.: Developments in occupational medicine, Chicago, 1980, Year Book Medical Publishers.

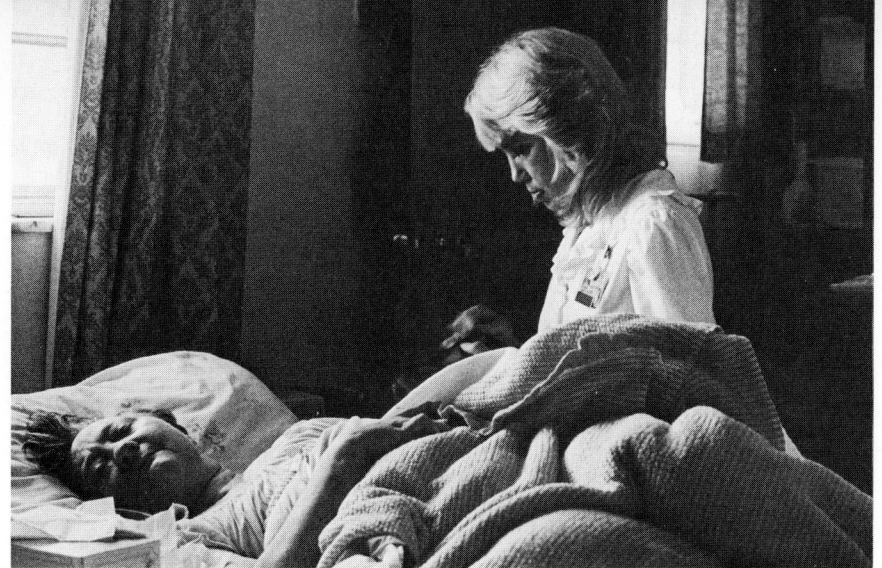

Eileen Garvey
Jacquelyne Heubel Logue

42

THE COMMUNITY HEALTH NURSE IN HOME HEALTH AND HOSPICE CARE

≡ OBJECTIVES

After reading this chapter, the student should be able to:

Define home health care.

List the types of home health agencies.

Analyze the similarities and differences in the types of home health agencies.

Discuss the educational requirements for a home health care nurse.

Relate the nursing process and the standards of community health nursing practice to the home health setting.

Identify the roles and functions of the interdisciplinary health care team.

Describe the regulatory impact on home health care and nursing practice.

Analyze the reimbursement mechanisms and issues relative to home health care.

Describe the hospice care program as a function of home health care.

Identify the impact of deregulation on future home health care programs.

≡ KEY TERMS

accreditation

combination agencies

contracting

direct care

distributive care

documentation

episodic care

facilitator

home health aide

home health care

hospital-based agencies

indirect care

interdisciplinary collaboration

medicare

occupational therapists

official agencies

patient compliance

patient education

physical therapists

professional competency

proprietary agencies

recertification

regulation

reimbursement

reimbursement system

research

self-help

speech pathologist

voluntary and nonprofit agencies

This chapter presents another aspect of community health nursing: home health care. Home health care differs from other areas of health care in that the health care providers practice in the client's environment. This unique characteristic affects several components of nursing practice. These elements are discussed to acquaint the nurse with the roles, functions, and responsibilities of this practice.

Currently, home health care is provided mainly for intermittent, short-term client needs. Cost-effectiveness, consumer preferences, technological advancements, and proven quality of service are expected to expand the parameters of home health care use in the near future.

DEFINITION OF HOME HEALTH CARE

Home health care in today's society cannot be simply defined as "care at home." It includes an arrangement of health-related services provided to people in their place of residence. A more comprehensive definition of home health care has been prepared by a Department of Health and Human Services interdepartmental work group (Warhola, 1980):

> *Home health care* is that component of a continuum of comprehensive health care whereby health services are provided to individuals and families in their places of residence for the purpose of promoting, maintaining or restoring health, or of maximizing the level of independence, while minimizing the effects of disability and illness, including terminal illness. Services appropriate to the needs of the individual patient and family are planned, coordinated, and made available by providers organized for the delivery of home care through the use of employed staff, contractual arrangements, or a combination of the two patterns.

Another definition, prepared by the American Medical Association (1979, pp. 1-3), described home health care as follows:

> The provision of nursing care, social work, therapies (such as diet, occupational, physical, psychological and speech), vocational and social services, and homemaker-home health aide services may be included as basic components of home health care. The provision of these needed services to the patient at home constitutes a logical extension of the physician's therapeutic responsibility. At the physician's request and under his medical direction, personnel who provide these home health care services operate as a team in assessing and developing the home care plan.

Home health care, as defined by Medicare, includes the following items and services (Home Health Services 1982):

1. Part-time or intermittent nursing care provided by or under the supervision of a registered professional nurse.
2. Physical, occupational, or speech therapy.
3. Medical social services under the direction of a physician.
4. Part-time or intermittent services of a home health aide as permitted by the regulations.
5. Medical supplies (other than drugs and biological such as serum and vaccinations) and the use of medical appliances.
6. Medical services provided by an intern or resident enrolled in a teaching program in hospitals affiliated or under contract with a home health agency.

Furthermore, Trager (1972, p. 5) describes *home health care* as . . . an array of services which may be brought into the home singly or in combination in order to achieve and sustain the optimum state of health, activity and independence for individuals of all ages who require such services because of acute illness, exacerbations of chronic illness, or long term permanent limitations due to chronic illness and disability.

All of these definitions integrate the components of home health care: the client, family, health care professionals (multidisciplinary) and goals to assist the client to return to an optimum level of health and independence. Their differences rest on the fact that interpretation and actual delivery of home health care vary according not only to the client, but also to the provider and reimburser of these services.

Family, which includes any caretaker or significant person who takes the responsibility to assist the client in need of care at home, is an integral part of home health care. Roles of the caretaker include supervising clients by assuring that their basic needs are being met and providing direct care such as personal hygiene, meal preparation, and administering medications. This person is valuable in providing the needed maintenance care between the skilled visits of the professional provider.

A person's *place of residence* has its own uniqueness in terms of the location for providing care, depending on what the person calls home.

The client *goals* are always related to the principles of

health promotion, maintenance, and restoration, regardless of the primary health care provider. By maximizing the level of independence, home health care nurses can help the clients function at the best possible level for preventing dependency. This assistance can take the form of teaching or linking the client with community services that provide limited assistance for enabling the client to stay at home. In addition, prevention of complications of chronically ill persons can help to minimize the effects of disability and illness. Countless complications of long-term illness seen in the form of disability are preventable with adequate home health care intervention. Terminal illness, as seen by the development of hospice home care programs, can be handled at home instead of in the hospital if the client and family accept this concept. Alleviation of pain and suffering is possible in the home care setting. Pain control through the use of medications is closely supervised by nurses in the home. They assess the client's response to the medication and report these findings to the client's physician, who then modifies the medication as needed.

Services can be tailored to any client need or problem. When the client's level of independence increases, the need for services decreases. The services are coordinated to an agency obligation to maintain quality care and provide for continuity. Thus the range of services provided in home health care is extensive. The challenge of home health care to community health nurses can be more fully appreciated by briefly tracing the history of this nursing role.

HISTORY OF HOME HEALTH CARE

Home health care began in the United States around the 1800s.* The Boston Dispensary served as one of the initial providers of home care, dating back to 1796. During this era few hospitals were available, and people did not always go to the hospital when they became ill. Public health nursing began in the United States as in England when philanthropic organizations sponsored visiting nurses, who gave care to individuals in their homes and taught families how to take care of the sick. In 1877, the New York City Mission and the New York Society for Ethical Culture had visiting nurses. The idea grew slowly, with nurses being paid by the client or by a philanthropic society. Eventually the community became more involved and developed projects and funds to support the cause of home care. In 1890 there were 21 visiting nurses associations in the United States, most of them employing only one nurse. After 1894, the use of visiting nurses grew more rapidly with the advent of growing social consciousness.

The Waltham (Massachusetts) Training School was established in 1885 by Dr. Alfred Worcester after he conferred with Florence Nightingale and designed a course to train nurses for private duty. The course included experience in the home. Later public health nursing with field experience was added to the program. The school was criticized for sending students into homes to earn money for the hospital and for overworking and not supervising the students (Dolan, 1958). In 1842, a nurse society was established in

Philadelphia to supply nurses to the independent sick and to those individuals who could pay. American communities established similar organizations primarily because visiting nursing in England had developed into a viable social service.

In the 1940s, hospitals began to take a more serious interest in home care as a result of the increased number of chronically ill clients being hospitalized. The Montefiore Hospital Home Care Program in New York began in 1947 and offered comprehensive home care services such as medical nursing and social services. Before enactment of Medicare in 1966, most agencies relied on charity and public contributions for survival.

Home care reached a turning point with the arrival of Medicare, thereby forming regulations for home care practice as well as for reimbursement mechanisms. In 1967, one year after Medicare was enacted, there were 1,753 Medicare-participating home health agencies in the United States with the majority being either visiting nursing associations or programs in public health departments. By 1974 there were 2,237 home health agencies, an increase of about 48% (Callender and Lavor, 1975). The Health Care Financing Agency (HCFA) reported 5,949 Medicare-certified home health agencies as of October, 1986, a 62% growth in 11 years (NAHC Report, 1986).

TYPES OF HOME HEALTH CARE AGENCIES

Since the beginning of organized home care, many types of organizations have established programs to meet the home care needs of people. Home health agencies are divided into the following five general types based on the administrative and organizational structure: (1) official, (2) private and voluntary, (3) combination, (4) hospital-based, and (5) proprietary. These types differ in organization and administration but are similar in terms of the standards they must meet for licensure, certification, and accreditation. Figure 42-1 shows the types of home health agencies.

Official Agencies

Official agencies (public agencies) include those agencies operated by the state or by local governments (county, city) such as health departments. They are financed primarily by tax funds and are nonprofit entities. Most official agencies, in addition to having a home care component, also provide health education and disease prevention programs to people in the community.

Community health nurses employed in this setting may provide not only general home health care, but also well-child clinics, well-child home visits, immunization, health education programs, and home visits for preventive health care. Official agencies, in addition to being funded for services with local money, are reimbursed for home care services as are the other types of home health care agencies. Medicare, Medicaid, and private insurance companies reimburse for home health care but not equally or totally in all cases. The *reimbursement system* is complicated and standardized. *Medicare* has the most standardized payment system of all third-party payers. Official agencies can offer more comprehensive types of community health services than other kinds of agencies because of their objectives of

---

*For an in-depth account of the history of public health nursing, refer to Chapter 1.

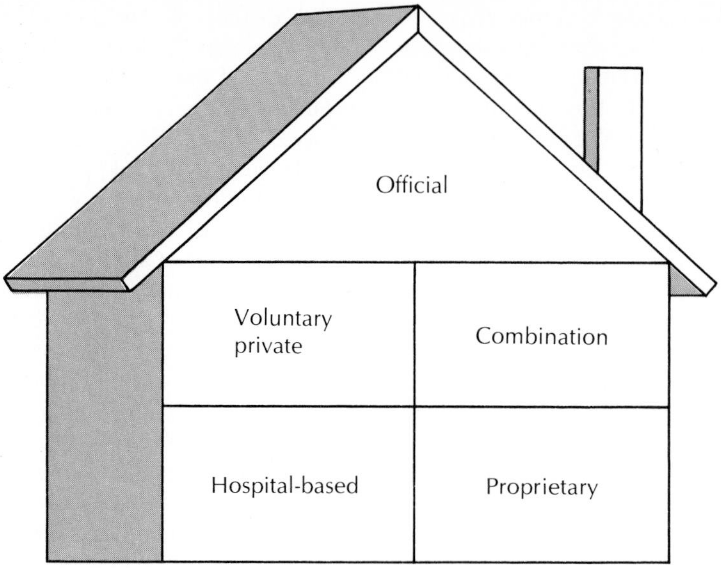

FIGURE 42-1

Types of home health care agencies.

health promotion and disease prevention and also because of the additional public funding often available.

Voluntary and Private Nonprofit Agencies

Voluntary and private agencies are grouped together as the nonprofit type of home health agency. Voluntary agencies are supported by charities such as the United Way, as well as by Medicare, Medicaid, and other third-party payers and the client payments. The amount of financial assistance the voluntary agency receives depends on the community it serves. Traditionally, visiting nurses associations were the principal voluntary type of home health agency. With the advent of Medicare in 1965, the private nonprofit agency emerged as a viable establishment.

Voluntary and private nonprofit agencies are governed by boards of directors, which represent the community they serve. These agencies are nongovernmental organizations and are exempt from federal income tax. Historically, voluntary agencies were responsible for the initial development of nursing in the home, based on the client's need for service rather than the ability to pay.

Combination Agencies

In some communities, to decrease cost and prevent duplication of services, official and voluntary home health agencies have merged into *combination agencies* to provide home health care. The services remain the same, and the administration members come from either one of the two existing agencies or a new board is formed. The nurse may serve in several community health nursing roles as does the nurse in the official type of agency.

Hospital-Based Agencies

Hospitals have long been a pivotal point for health care services. In the 1970s, *hospital-based agencies* developed in response to the need for continuity of care from the acute care setting and also in response to the high cost of institutionalization.

In 1983 implementation of the prospective payment system and DRGs by the federal government precipitated a fundamental change in the view of hospitals toward home care. Cost containment dictated earlier discharge of sicker patients to control profit margins. Concurrent increased liability risks, the desire for better patient mangement, and the potential for a diversified base of products and services affected hospital management by increasing the number of hospital-based home care agencies (Cassak, 1984). As of January 1986, hospital-based agencies outnumbered all other types of Medicare-certified agencies except for proprietary agencies (NAHC, 1986).

Hospital-based agencies differ from other home health care agencies in that the already-established hospital board of directors is responsible for governing the agency. Moreover, existing inpatient services are accessible to the recipients of hospital-based home health care. Whether the agencies are official, voluntary, private nonprofit, or proprietary depends on the hospital structure. These agencies are a source of revenue for the hospital and may compete with community-based agencies.

Proprietary Agencies

Agencies ineligible for tax exemption are called *proprietary* (profit-making) *agencies.* Proprietary agencies can be licensed and certified for Medicare by the state licensing agency. The owner of the agency is responsible for governing. Reimbursement is primarily from third-party payers and individual clients if agencies are ineligible for Medicare.

Opponents of this type of agency claim that proprietary agencies offer substandard quality of care and are involved only for monetary gains. There is little evidence to support this claim because all agencies that are Medicare-certified must comply with the same conditions. Also, as a result of the impact of prospective payment to hospitals by Medicare resulting in "quicker" discharge of "sicker" patients, the number of Medicare-certified proprietary agencies increased significantly as did hospital-based agencies (NAHC, 1986).

◆ ◆ ◆

Regardless of the type of home health agency existing in a community, the primary goal should be to provide quality home health care to the community based on the health needs of people. The development of additional agencies in a community can be an emotional issue to people working in already established home health agencies. Competition in home health care is on the rise. Traditionally, most agencies have remained noncompetitive because of the humanitarian aspect of the service. The competitive thrust is the result of the federal government's move to deregulate and deinstitutionalize areas of health care. Competition can be a positive force in developing and maintaining quality home health care programs. Nevertheless, there is profit to be made in home health care, which necessitates utilization review and quality assurance mechanisms.

Current changes in home health care have several implications for the community health nurse. Clients are being discharged at earlier stages of treatment, thereby needing a highly skilled level of care. The community health nurse must be appropriately prepared to care for these clients. Also, to survive in the competitive arena agencies must continue to provide quality care and also be cost effective without compromising accountability. These home care criteria require that community health nurses in management have highly developed administrative skills.

EDUCATIONAL REQUIREMENTS FOR PRACTICE

Demonstration of *professional competency* is the foremost requirement for home health care nurses. Home health care nurses come from a variety of educational and practice settings. Differences in both experience and educational preparation influence the contributions that nurses make to home health care.

Home health care nurses should be trained and educated to function at a high level of competency, so they can be relied on not only by their professional colleagues but also by the community. A baccalaureate degree in nursing should be the minimum requirement for entry into professional practice in the community health care setting. Nursing education has the responsibility of producing competent, skillful practitioners. A baccalaureate degree does not assure a qualified, mature professional nurse, but a quality education does lay the foundation for the development of such important characteristics. Life experience, compassion, and awareness of self are factors that are inherent in the delivery of quality client care and professionalism.

In home health care, the nurse with a baccalaureate degree usually functions in the role of a staff nurse or home health care nurse. The nurse with a master's degree is better prepared for the practitioner, administrator, or teacher role. As home care continues to develop its larger role in community health nursing, the need for specialized nurse clinicians will also increase to meet the ever-increasing, highly technological care that is transposed from the hospital into the home setting.

SCOPE OF PRACTICE
Objective in Home Health Care

A common misconception of home health care is that it is a "custodial" type of nursing. It is important to remember that home health care nursing is a *division* of community health nursing. Thus health *promotion activities are a fundamental component of practice.* Since the health promotion component of home health care is delivered in the patient's home environment and is *intermittent* care, a primary objective for the home health nurse is to facilitate self-care.

According to Johns (1985) there is not a consensus at present of a precise definition of self-care. However, there are three accepted components of the concept of self-care: *patient education, patient compliance,* and *self-help.* Patient education is provider-initiated and supervised, patient compliance is a combination of client responsibility and provider supervision, and self-help is most often demonstrated in peer groups that encourage member responsibility.

According to Orem (1985, p. 31) "Self-care is the production of actions directed to self or to the environment in order to regulate one's functioning in the interests of one's life, integrated functioning and well-being." This definition includes community health nursing activities and notably of home health care nursing. Home health care nurses use this concept for all clients, regardless of their abilities. For example, a client may be recuperating at home after suffering a stroke and unable to perform activities of daily living (ADL) without assistance. Such clients are unable to perform self-care activities but can be instructed in the performance of these activities in a modified form. In this way they have some control over their life and self-care activities, and they can be taught to prevent possible losses in other self-care areas. This example also supports another definition, which is even more specific to the home health care population. *Self-care* is "an action taken by the consumer or client, to reduce, to the degree possible, incremental debilitation resulting from chronic disease" (Funkhouser, 1976, p. 11).

A primary goal in the home setting is to help prevent the occurrence of illness and to promote the client's well-being. With the aid of basic tools such as a nursing history, physical examination, medication, and diet teaching guides, the home care nurse can use the nursing process to assess the client's needs, establish a plan of care, implement nursing actions, and then evaluate the effectiveness of nursing actions with plans for modification or resolution as needed.

In the home care setting, the clients possess more control and ability for determining their own health care needs. The client role is active because continuance of service depends a great deal on the client's understanding of plans established jointly by the client and community health nurse. The nurse serves as a *facilitator* for development of positive health behaviors for the individual who has had an episode of illness.

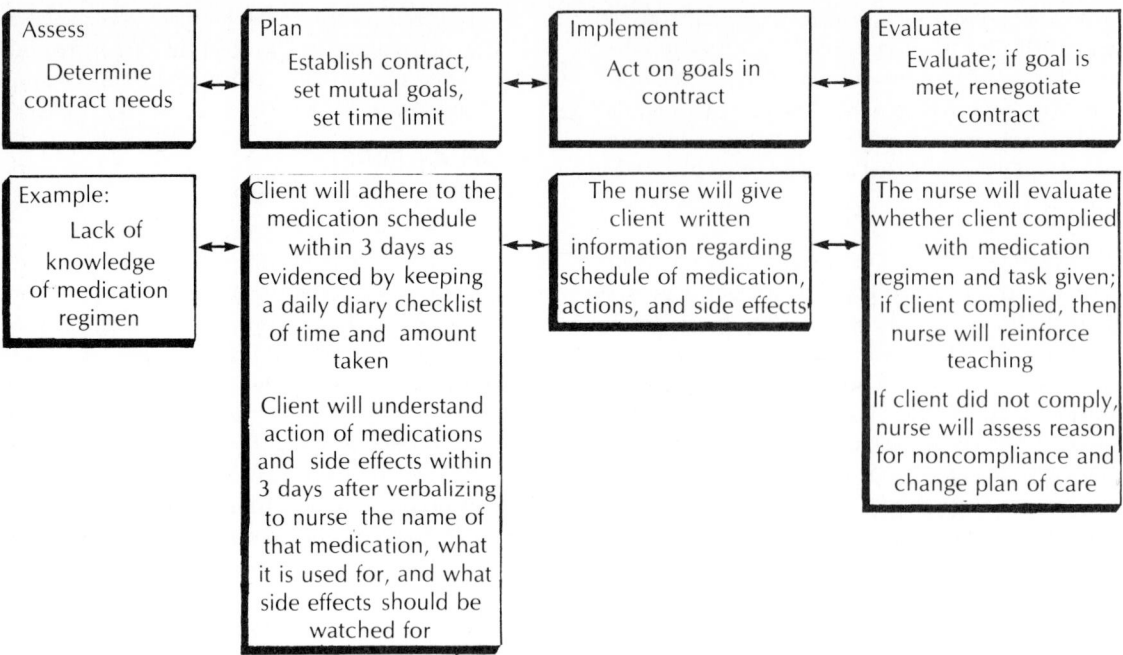

FIGURE 42-2

Contracting in relation to nursing process.

Contracting

Contracting is a vital component of all nurse/client relationships. Constantly evolving legislative guidelines, third-party payer dictates, the high risk of liability, and the intense level of nurse autonomy, require that contracting be reviewed in the home care context.

The process of contracting in home care involves not only the client and the nurse but also the family. *Contracting* refers to any working agreement, continuously renegotiable, between the nurse, client, and family (Sloan and Schummer, 1975). The process of contracting can be reflected in the client's care plan and clinical notes. Contracting allows the client and family to set their own goals and alleviates the problem of nurses who set unrealistic expectations of themselves or of the client and family.

Contracting is directly related to use of the nursing process (Figure 42-2) and can be done at each phase of the nursing process. As an example, during an initial home visit, the nurses gather data for establishing the client-home health care nurse-family contract. They determine the components of the agreement and plan for subsequent actions by establishing the contract with the client and family. During that visit, if appropriate, portions of the contract may be implemented. If not, subsequent visits will afford the opportunities.

Contracts can be formal (written) or informal (verbal), depending on the client's needs. In either case, the process is recorded in the client's chart. The most important aspect is not the type of contract, but the client's actual participation in establishing, implementing, and evaluating the process.

To avoid what Mayers (1973) refers to as the "home

visit—ritual or therapy" dilemma, the home care nurse must establish both short-term and long-term goals with the clients and families. The purpose of this is not only for continuity of care but also for evaluating the client's condition and progress toward an optimum level of self-care. Mayers found in her study of community health nurses who made home visits that half of the purposes of the visit were unknown to the clients, since the nurses in the study did not share the purposes for the visits with them. Much of the dialogue failed to show any *development* of the interrelationship between the client and nurse.

Practice Functions of the Home Health Care Nurse

Home health care nursing involves both direct and indirect functions. In performing these functions, the home health care nurse assumes a variety of roles.

Direct Care

Direct care refers to the actual "laying on of hands." In home health care, direct care activities include performing a physical assessment on the patient, dressing changes of wounds, injections, insertion of an indwelling catheter, etc. Direct care also involves teaching clients and family caretakers how to perform a certain procedure or duty. By serving as a role model, the nurse can assist the client and family to develop positive health care behaviors. Technical skill competency must be demonstrated by the nurse to receive reimbursement by Medicare and Medicaid. Nursing care is covered by Medicare and other third-party payers as long as the care being delivered is "skilled." To determine whether a service performed by the nurse is skilled, several factors are evaluated and must be adequately documented:

1. Is the service complex, thereby requiring the knowledge and skill of a registered nurse?
2. Does the client's condition warrant skilled intervention?
3. Can this service be performed by a nonmedical person?
4. Does the instruction of a service to a client involve knowledge, instructions, and demonstrations by a registered nurse?

To adequately answer these questions, the home health care nurse must have a sufficient knowledge base of regulatory mechanisms and also must be competent and experienced to know how to interpret "skilled." These interpretations can be subjective; therefore, objective data are necessary to account for the service.

Some examples of skilled nursing services include the following:
1. Observing and evaluating of client's condition, both physical and emotional.
2. Providing direct care in administering treatments, rehabilitative exercises and medications, catheter insertion, colostomy irrigation, and wound care.
3. Assisting client and family toward developing positive coping behavior.
4. Teaching client and family to give these treatments and medications when indicated.
5. Teaching client and family to carry out physician's orders such as use of a special diet, remembering to consider cultural background, financial status, and personal preferences.
6. Reporting to physician any new signs and symptoms relative to client's status and arranging for medical follow-up as indicated.
7. Assisting client and family to identify resources that will help client attain state of optimal functioning.

Indirect Care

Indirect care occurs when a client does not have personal contact with the nurse. This type of care is seen when home health care nurses serve as consultants to other health personnel who provide home care or even to those who provide in-hospital care. Clients often have their own patterns for care (such as ostomy care) and, when hospitalized, need assistance from hospital nurses to continue this program. Hospital nurses frequently contact the home health care nurse for advice on how to accomplish the client's usual method of care.

Team conferences are a means of providing indirect care in home health care. It is an ideal time for increasing coordination and continuity of services for optimal client care and use of resources and services. Advice on how to manage clients with particular problems can be shared with various members of the team. Supervision of home health aides is a direct and indirect function because the home health care nurse may not always see the home health aide performing but can evaluate the care given to the client. Regular supervision of the aide by the nurse for at least 2-week intervals is mandated. There is much indirect care in the home health

care setting. It may not be directly visible to the client, but it does exist and it does assist with ensuring quality home health care.

Although Medicare places an emphasis on episodic, or acute, care because of its limitations on benefits and requirements for skilled care, the home health care nurse cannot separate episodic and distributive nursing practice entirely because of the interrelationship. According to Hall and Weaver (1977, p. 6), distributive nursing practice is "the application of knowledge of the life process in human systems with consideration for their health maintenance requirements, contextual variables influencing their functioning, and the strategies and tactics of intervention."

Episodic Versus Distributive Care

Episodic care refers to the curative and restorative aspect of practice, and *distributive care* refers to health maintenance and disease prevention. A clinical example can best illustrate the application of these two aspects in home health care.

> Mr. Jones, a 70-year-old white man, discharged from the hospital the previous day, was admitted to home health care services for skilled nursing to assess his cardiovascular status after heart surgery for coronary artery disease. The episodic care involves teaching Mr. and Mrs. Jones about medications, exercise, and the signs and symptoms of possible heart problems postoperatively. In addition, the home health care nurse will provide direct care in assessing his cardiovascular status and helping Mr. Jones return to his optimum state of functioning.

Mr. Jones' psychosocial adaptation and needs will also be addressed in addition to assessing his level of self-care and adjustment relative to postcardiac surgery status. In regard to the distributive aspect, the home health care nurse will do additional teaching about ways Mr. Jones can prevent exacerbation of his condition by maintaining medical follow-up and adhering to the programs set up for him.

Nursing Roles

The *roles* of clinician, educator, researcher, administrator, and consultant are seen in home health care. They can be demonstrated by the experienced home health care nurse, the nursing supervisor, the director of nursing, or the administrator.

Home health care nurses in a staff position are clinicians because they provide direct nursing care to clients and families. Home health care nurses are educators because they teach clients and families the "how to's" and "why's" of self-care. Formally, they may teach classes to community groups regarding health education topics. The researcher role in home health care has been relatively dormant, even though home health care nurses often provide the data required for clinical or administrative change within their agency of employment. The home health care setting abounds with potential research areas. This role needs to take priority in the future if quality and cost effectiveness are to be maintained. A home health care administrator can be a nurse who has had advanced education with community health experience; requirements are stipulated by both federal and state rules and regulations. Consultants may provide advice and counsel to staff and clients. (Refer to Chapters 36 to 41 for discussions of specific roles in community health nursing.)

Confusion exists in some health care circles regarding role differentiation between the private duty nurse and the home health care nurse. Even registered nurses who have not been directly exposed to home health care in either their educational or clinical experiences do not know that private duty nursing and home health care are different types of nursing practice. The only similarity is that both are provided to a client in the home. Table 42-1 clarifies the different components of private duty nursing and home health care nursing.

Integration of Standards of Community Health Nursing Practice into Home Health Care

The home health care nurse practices in accordance with the Standards of Community Health Nursing Practice de-

TABLE 42-1

Components of private duty and home health care nursing

	Private duty	Home health care
Role and function	One-to-one client care assignment Maintenance Custodial Episodic	Distributive Skilled care Rehabilitative Episodic
Reimbursement	Payment to nurse Paid by some third-party insurances	Payment to agency Medicare and Medicaid Third-party insurance
Cost	Daily or hourly rate charge	Per visit charge
Frequency	Full-time and shift duty	Intermittent visits based on frequency and need of clients

TABLE 42-2

Relationship between nursing process and ANA standards of practice

Nursing process	Standard	Description
Assess	I. Theory	The nurse applies theoretical basis for decisions in practice.
	II. Data collection	The nurse systematically collects comprehensive and accurate data.
	III. Diagnosis	The nurse analyzes data collected about the community, family, and individual to determine diagnoses.
Plan	IV. Planning	At each level of prevention, the nurse develops plans that specify nursing actions unique to client needs.
Implement	V. Intervention	The nurse, guided by the plan, intervenes to promote, maintain, or restore health to prevent illness and to effect rehabilitation.
Evaluate	VI. Evaluation	The nurse evaluates responses of the community, family, and individual to interventions to determine progress toward goal achievement and to revise the database, diagnoses, and plan.
	VII. Quality assurance and professional development	The nurse participates in peer review and other means of evaluation to ensure quality of nursing practice. The nurse assumes the responsibility for professional development and contributes to the professional growth of others.
	VIII. Interdisciplinary collaboration	The nurse collaborates with other health care providers, professionals, and community representatives in assessing, planning, implementing and evaluating programs for community health.
	IX. Research	The nurse contributes to theory and practice in community health nursing through research.

veloped by the American Nurses' Association, Council of Community Health Nurses (ANA, 1986). Table 42-2 represents the relationship between the nursing process and the Standards of Practice. The use of the nursing process in the home care setting is evident by the legal requirement of documentation of all nursing action.

Standard I-III: Theory, Data Collection, Diagnosis

Theoretical concepts derived from nursing; public health; and physical, social, and behavioral sciences provide the framework for the processes of assessment, intervention, and evaluation (see Table 42-2).

The home care nurse is responsible for assessing the client and family during the initial home visit as well as during all subsequent visits. The home health nurse acquires *database* information from the client and family by obtaining subjective and objective data. Examples of *subjective* data include information that the client, family, and physicians relate to the nurse by means of verbal communication. This information is obtained from direct questioning. Information necessary to obtain a thorough data base for the information of nursing diagnoses include the following:

1. Diagnosis
2. Present health status
3. Family history
4. Review of systems (health/illness history of cardiovascular, pulmonary, musculoskeletal, gastrointestinal, genitourinary, endocrine, neurological, integumentary systems)
5. Socioeconomic status (source of income, amount, religion, education level, number of dependents, occupation, support systems, environmental safety)
6. Daily patterns (diet, meal pattern, elimination, rest and sleep, exercise, activity, recreation, interest, hygiene)

Objective data are also obtained by directly assessing the client's physical status, using a review-of-systems approach and physical assessment skills.

These data are recorded in the client's clinical home care record in the form of a flow sheet or assessment chart. From these baseline data the home health nurse develops *nursing diagnoses* for the problems identified. It is during the assessment phase that the home health nurse determines that other resources are needed (such as physical therapy, occupational therapy, speech therapy, home health aide, medical social services, Meals on Wheels, transportation assistance, or nutritional counseling). The family is included throughout the entire nursing process because it is they who will assist the implementation and evaluation of the plan of care.

Standard IV: Planning

Nursing diagnoses give the home health nurse the necessary information to develop *short-term* and *long-term* goals for the client and family in addition to formulating a *plan* for direct actions. This plan, based on nursing diagnoses, must have some indications of the expected or anticipated outcomes for each identified problem or nursing diagnosis. The information is documented on the developed client care plan,

which serves as a continuous resource for the health care providers. This not only represents accountability for actions but also serves as a means to promote continuity of care. The plan is individualized for each client and family based on their special needs. The goals focus on health promotion, maintenance, and restoration of the client's condition and prevention of complications.

Standard V: Intervention

Implementation of the plan occurs in three phases: before, during, and after the home visit, depending on plan requirements. It is the home health nurse's responsibility to assist the client to return to an optimal level of functioning and health, and ensure that the client and family are active participants in the home care. Instruction, supervision of medications, diet teaching and evaluation of diabetic management are examples of such actions.

Standard VI: Evaluation

Together the client, family, and home health nurse evaluate the client's status and progress toward goal achievement on a continual basis. During subsequent visits, previous goals may be replaced with new ones, based on the client's changing status. The home health nurse prepares the client and family for the client's discharge as early as the initial visit. She explains to the client and family the short-term nature of the services. The frequency of visits and the duration of the service are decreased when the client is able to assume self-care or the family has learned how to care for the client. Discharge must include provisions for aftercare on a periodic basis in those cases where the illness episode is not resolved.

Standard VII: Quality Assurance and Professional Development

Community health nurses as described in an earlier chapter actively participate in quality assurance including peer review, evaluation of oneself and the entire health team. Both the nurse and the employing agency are encouraged to endorse nursing participation in professional development. These areas, quality assurance and professional development, are increasingly important areas since home health care is changing rapidly in order to meet societal and health care needs.

Standard VIII: Interdisciplinary Collaboration

Collaboration about health care in the home health area is particularly important in that a multitude of health team members are needed to successfully manage the care of clients in their homes. The nurse actively collaborates with other health care providers, professionals and community representatives to assess, plan, implement and evaluate care.

Standard IX: Research

Community health nurses practicing in the home care setting have a variety of opportunities to participate in research. Although the home care nurse may not have formalized research training, she may participate in research if administrative support and adequate resources are available.

INTERDISCIPLINARY APPROACH TO HOME HEALTH CARE

Interdisciplinary collaboration is required in the home health care setting. Its use is mandated for Medicare-certified home care agencies, and it is also inherent in the definition of home health care (Warhola, 1980). Without effective collaboration there would be no continuity of care and the client's and family's understanding of the home care program would be fragmented. Each client has an individualized care plan even though the client may have problems similar to others in a specific disease category classification.

Generally, the collaborative process for home care begins in the hospital with the discharge planner and hospital nurse who identify a client's need for home care and then review their observations and plans with the physician for approval and orders. The discharge planner then calls the referral intake coordinator of the home care agency, specifying the services requested by the physician. If persons from several disciplines will be involved such as registered nurses, home health aides, and physical therapists, the director of clinical services notifies the appropriate persons and monitors the interdisciplinary collaboration.

In home care, as in other health care settings, professionals experience stress associated with changing roles and overlapping responsibilities. In collaborating, each home health care provider should carefully analyze each other's role to determine if overlapping occurs and adjust the plan of care accordingly.

In terms of legal accountability and compliance with federal regulatory mechanisms, it is the physician who must certify the plan of treatment for the client. However, in most instances, it is the health care professional who re-evaluates the client's status, reports the findings to the physician, and then with the physician modifies the plan of treatment for the client.

Medicare (see p. 817) requires that interdisciplinary services be documented. This requirement allows for accountability for each professional and fosters continuity of care. Documentation in the client's chart reflects interdisciplinary collaboration as evidenced by case conferences and contracts made between the care givers. Documentation is the evidence or means, not the end product of care. Quality assurance mechanisms (chart audits, peer review, etc.) verify the appropriateness and effectiveness of the collaboration.

Successful interdisciplinary functioning depends on numerous factors of knowledge, skills, and attitudes, with the foremost characteristic being that the team members must be competent practitioners in their own field (Kane, 1977). Factors necessary for successful interdisciplinary team functioning are shown in the box above right. These factors offer a successful approach to working in the interdisciplinary home care setting. It is unrealistic to assume that there is a clear-cut way to avoid role stress, ambiguity, or overlapping. Professionals in home care are in a unique setting in which they can truly work together to accomplish the client's care goals. Again, regulations require that appropriate resources are used with documentation of collaboration with other disciplines. Care plans and treatments by each discipline are to be built on by other health care

---

FACTORS FOR INTERDISCIPLINARY FUNCTIONING

KNOWLEDGE

1. Understand how the group process can be used to achieve group goals.
2. Understand problem-solving.
3. Understand role theory.
4. Understand what other professionals do and how they see their roles.
5. Understand the conceptual differences between home care and the practice and institutional care and practices.

SKILL

1. Use principles of group process effectively.
2. Communicate clearly and accurately.
3. Communicate without using own profession's jargon.
4. Express self clearly and concisely in writing.

ATTITUDE

1. Feel confident in role as a professional.
2. Trust and respect other professionals.
3. Share task with other professionals.
4. Work toward conflict resolution effectively.
5. Be flexible.
6. Be "research-minded."
7. Be timely.

---

providers involved. As an example, nurses must reinforce the teaching by the physical therapist of exercise regimens and gait training.

Responsibilities of the Disciplines

The responsibilities and functions of the disciplines in home health care are dictated by Medicare regulations, professional organizations, and state licensing boards. The home health care providers' roles discussed in the following sections are different from providers' roles in other health care settings. Other professional services can be provided in the home such as podiatry, pharmacology, follow-up nutrition counseling, respiratory therapy, and psychiatric or mental health nursing when indicated. Much of these contributions can be provided on a consultant basis in the form of in-service training or direct referral information.

Physician

Each client in the home care program must be under the current care of a doctor of medicine or osteopathy to certify that the client does have a medical problem. A nurse can make an *assessment* visit without physician approval but must have the physician's certification if a plan of care with follow-up is developed. The physician must *certify* a plan of treatment for the home health agency before care is provided to the client. This plan must be reviewed at least every 60 days to modify or continue the client's plan of care.

The plan of treatment must include the following information: diagnosis, functional limitations, anticipated length of care, type and frequency of services needed (nursing, physical therapy, occupational therapy, speech therapy, home health aide, medical social services), medications, diet, activities permitted, medical supplies, and appliances. Additionally, the plan of treatment needs to be reviewed by the physician in collaboration with home care professionals at least every 60 days but more often if the person's condition warrants more frequent assessment and alteration of care. This process is called *recertification.*

Physicians in the community also serve in an advisory capacity to the home health agency by assisting in the development of home care policies and procedures relative to client care. Physician involvement in and acceptance of home health care is necessary if the benefits of this form of health care are to be recognized. The American Medical Association in the early 1960s urged physicians to "participate in organized home health care programs for any patient who can benefit from the program and to promote such programs in their communities." The Physician Guide to Home Health Care (AMA, 1979, pp. 1-3) explains the important role of home health care and the benefits that clients can receive from this service. Examples cited include a more rapid client recovery, improved client emotional well-being, early discharge from the hospital, reduction in readmissions, and a savings over costs of institutional care.

Physical Therapist

Physical therapists provide maintenance, preventative, and restorative treatment for clients in the home. Physical therapists must be licensed by the state in which they practice and are graduates of a baccalaureate or master's level physical therapy program. Like home health care nurses, a physical therapist also provides direct and indirect care. Direct care activities include strengthening muscles, restoring mobility, controlling spasticity, gait training, and teaching active-passive resistive exercises. The treatment modalities used include therapeutic exercise, massage, transcutaneous electrical nerve stimulation, heat, water, ultraviolet light, ultrasound, postural drainage, and pulmonary exercises. The therapist is also responsible for teaching the client and family the treatment regimen to promote self-care and responsibility.

Indirect care activities of the physical therapist include consulting with the staff and contributing to client care conferences by sharing skills and area of expertise. Physical therapy assistants provide some therapy under the direction of a registered physical therapist. Assistants are high school graduates who have completed an approved assistants' program and have been licensed.

Occupational Therapist

Occupational therapists (OT) help clients achieve their optimal level of functioning by teaching them to develop and maintain the abilities to perform activities of daily living in their home. Occupational therapists focus most of their treatment on the client's upper extremities by assisting to restore muscle strength and mobility for functional skills. Occupational therapists earn baccalaureate degrees. When the OT becomes registered by the National Occupational

Therapy Association, they are subsequently referred to as OTRs.

Direct functions of the OTR include evaluating the client's level of function and ability by testing muscles and joints. The OTR teaches self-care activities, assesses the client's home for safety with possible modifications for removing barriers, and provides adaptive equipment when needed. Indirect care is similar to the other home care professional's roles of serving as a consultant for special client needs regarding self-care activities and adapting the home for the client. Occupational therapy has not been used to its full potential in the home because of the lack of knowledge of health care providers. This discipline is a valuable resource in assisting the client to become independent in self-care, a mutual goal of all home health care professionals.

Certified occupational therapy assistants (COTAs) are high school graduates with an approved continuing education certificate from an occupational therapy program. The COTA works under the supervision of the OTR.

Speech Pathologist

Speech pathologists or therapists are certified by the American Speech and Hearing Association and are educated at the master's level. Speech pathologists work with people with a communication problem related to speech, language, or hearing. Most clients receive direct care services, such as evaluation of speech and language ability, with specific plans being taught to the client and family for follow-up. The goal of speech therapy is to assist individuals to develop and maintain optimum speech and language ability. Speech pathologists also work with eating and swallowing problems. By serving as a consultant to other home care staff members, the speech pathologist can teach other providers of care and families how to encourage development of the best method of communication for clients.

Social Worker

The social worker in home health care holds a master's degree in social work (M.S.W.) and helps clients and families deal with social, emotional, and environmental factors that affect their well-being. Social workers assist directly in intervening or referring clients to appropriate community resources. Often after an episode in the hospital the clients return home unable to cope with their present state of functioning and need assistance in getting their lives reorganized. Many indirect care duties are performed by the social worker, since consultation and referral constitute the major focus of their practice. Other functions include resource identification and application, crisis intervention, and equipment procurement when payment is a problem.

Social work assistants are prepared at the baccalaureate level and function similar to the social worker, who directly supervises the activities of the assistant.

Homemaker Home Health Aide

With the advent of Medicare, the *home health aide,* sometimes referred to as the homemaker, became an important member of the home health care team. The home health aide (HHA) is directly supervised by the home health care nurse or physical therapist. The role of the HHA is to help clients reach their level of independence by temporarily assisting with personal hygiene. Additional duties include light housekeeping and other homemaking skills. The HHA must be experienced as an aide and be trained to provide home care services. The HHA implements the plan of care established by the nurse or other professionals to reinforce teaching. The role of the homemaker, as distinct from the HHA, emphasizes housekeeping chores.

ACCOUNTABILITY AND QUALITY ASSURANCE
Quality Control Mechanisms

Since the advent of Medicare, home health agencies have monitored the quality of care to their clients as a mandatory requirement for certification as a home health agency. All agencies are accountable to the clients and families, to their reimbursement sources, to themselves as a health care provider, and to professional standards. Quality is demonstrated through evaluations reflecting that appropriate and needed care has been given to clients in a professional manner.

Clinical records are the basis for documentation of all the care and services the client receives and of any communication between the physicians and other home health providers. It is in the clinical record that nurses must *prove* that they are delivering quality care and also identify means to *improve* the quality of care. Documentation of actions is of paramount importance in home health care because it is a legal method by which quality care can be assessed. This documentation also demonstrates the client's ongoing need for services and shows how the multiple disciplines arrange for continuity and comprehensive care.

Evaluation of the agency is required to monitor the control of cost and quality of care. Two standards serve as requirements for the evaluation in accordance with Medicare certification (Health Care Financing Administration, 1982):

1. *Policy and administrative review.* The home care program is evaluated to determine that the administrative policies and practices are appropriate, adequate, effective, and efficient in promoting patient care.
2. *Clinical record review.* An interdisciplinary quarterly review is needed of both active and closed clinical records to assure that policies are followed in the provision of patient care services. In addition, there is continuing review of clinical records for every 60-day period that the patient is under home care services. This determines the adequacy of the plan of treatment and appropriateness of the continuation of home care.

These standards are viewed as an external means of evaluating each agency because individuals from "outside" the agency evaluate the records. Representatives from appropriate disciplines such as nursing, physical therapy, occupational therapy, speech therapy, and medicine, as well as consumers objectively report the findings of the review. It is the responsibility of the agency to plan and implement goals for the revision, modification, and correction of de-

ficiencies noted. The evaluative process is valuable to the home health agency. From these reviews the agency can maintain and promote better client care for the consumers in the community. It is the responsibility of the individual agency to devise the method of implementing the process of clinical review.

Agencies also institute internal auditing processes such as peer review or nursing audit. The Phaneuf audit (1972) is used by many home health agencies and serves as a peer review mechanism. The National League for Nursing also published review methods to assist agencies to meet the Medicare requirement (NLN, 1971) and criteria to measure quality of care in home health agencies (NLN, 1980). Each publication deals with developing standards of care, outcome criteria, and the evaluation process. Two other noteworthy contributions to quality assurance are the Quality Assurance Manual (1980), developed by the Florida Association of Home Health Agency, Inc. (FAHHA) and Quality Assurance for Community Health Agencies (1980), developed by the Massachusetts Association of Community Health Agencies.

Documentation of nursing care is central to home care. It affects the home care nurse more than the nurse in any other setting. As an example, during the initial evaluation visit, the home care nurse or other health care professional assesses the client's and family's status, including a history and physical, psychological, and environmental characteristics. This information becomes a permanent part of the clinical record. Subsequent integration of health services must be noted. Besides clinical notes of all home visits, progress notes are required to be sent to the client's physician, including the assessment of the client to verify the applicability of the plan of care.

Home health care plans offer the unique opportunity to not only assess, plan, implement, and evaluate but also to document in writing. These tasks are satisfying to home health care nurses who enjoy using the nursing process in delivering client care.

Accreditation

Another means of evaluating quality assurance in home health care is *accreditation.* In 1975 the National League for Nursing and American Public Health Association developed criteria to evaluate home health agencies and community nursing services. The committee represented all personnel who delivered community and home health services. Since then, the criteria were revised and standards for measurement of quality were added.

The purpose of the accreditation process is to evaluate the administrative practices of the agency and conditions based on the major assumption that there is a relationship between the quality of administration and the quality of services delivered to the community. Components of an evaluation include (1) community assessment, (2) organization and administration, (3) program, (4) staff, (5) evaluation, and (6) future plans.

The process of self-study is an educational experience for all involved with the home health agency. The board of directors, executive director, professional advisory committee and the entire staff participate in the ongoing process of evaluation, since they make up the home care program. Refer to Appendix F2 for criteria used to measure the quality of care.

Self-study is a monitoring tool voluntarily imposed on the agency at the agency's discretion. The accreditation decision is based on the data in the self-study, the report of the site visit team, and any additional information. A noteworthy trend for the future may be the requirement of accreditation for certification for licensure of all home health agencies.

Regulatory Mechanisms

Regulation in home health care is an important concern to the home health nurse. The home health nurse is responsible on a daily basis for assuring that the clinical practice is being performed within the guidelines set up by the regulatory agencies. In view of this, the home health nurse must interpret regulations not only to colleagues but also to clients, families, and community. According to Krause (1975), the regulation is defined as "a process which is meant, in theory, to protect the public in vulnerable areas." In terms of home health care, the vulnerable areas are the target population of the elderly, the disabled, and the poor.

The Health Care Financing Administration (HCFA) is accountable for overseeing the Medicare program, federal participation in the Medicaid program, and other health care quality assurance programs. HCFA is responsible for promulgating the regulations that govern two administrative functions: health financing and quality assurance.

Home health regulation is carried out mainly at the state level, with state health departments certifying home health agencies according to the HCFA Conditions of Participation for Home Health Agencies (1982). These conditions of participation serve as the basis to evaluate each aspect of home health agencies:

1. Definitions (of home health agency terminology)
2. Compliance with federal, state and local laws
3. Organization, services and administration
4. Group of professional personnel with advisory and evaluation function
5. Acceptance of patients, plan of treatment and medical supervision
6. Services—skilled nursing, therapy, medical social work, home health aide
7. Establishment and maintenance of clinical records
8. Evaluation of the agency's total program and behavior (Krause, 1975)

The state agencies responsible for licensure and certification of home health agencies use these criteria in evaluating whether the agencies are conforming with federal regulations. Each criterion has minimum standards to which the program should adhere. Failure to meet these conditions can result in loss of licensure and the closing of the agency. Refer to Chapters 6 and 12 for further discussion of quality assurance and regulatory control.

FINANCIAL ASPECTS OF HOME HEALTH CARE
Reimbursement Mechanisms

Before federal intervention, home health care was reimbursed by clients who could pay for the service by donations, which subsidized the care provided to those who could pay only a portion or not at all. Now, Medicare and Medicaid are the principal funding sources, with third-party health insurance providing another major source.

Medicare

Reimbursement of home health services is handled through insurance companies under contract to the Social Security Administration to pay home care agencies for Medicare-covered services rendered to beneficiaries. To qualify for home health services a beneficiary must be over 65 years of age or disabled and (1) under the care of a physician; (2) confined to the home (homebound); or (3) in need of skilled nursing services, physical therapy, occupational therapy, or speech therapy on an intermittent basis.

The person's attending physician establishes the plan of treatment and also certifies the necessity of home health services. The plan must specify the (1) types of services required, (2) frequency of visits, (3) anticipated length of care, (4) diagnosis, (5) description of the client's functional limitations, (6) medications, (7) diet, (8) activities permitted, (9) medical supplies and appliances needed, and (10) safety of home environment. This plan must be reviewed at least every 60 days; continuance of care requires recertification of the plan by the physician.

A beneficiary is considered eligible for home health services provided that a physician certifies that the client is confined at home. Clients do not have to be bedridden, but they must be unable to leave their residence without assistance because of illness or injury. Feebleness and insecurity brought on by advanced age do not qualify the person to receive home health care.

Skilled services are those required by an individual that are *reasonable* and *necessary* for treatment of an illness or injury. The following factors are evaluated in determining the degree of skill: (1) complexity of service and condition of client, (2) performance or supervision of performance by a registered nurse or registered physical therapist, (3) teaching of service by skilled professional, and (4) whether the service can be accomplished by nonmedical person.

Services directed toward the prevention of illness or injury are not covered by Medicare. This does not mean, however, that these activities cannot be performed. They must be done in conjunction with a "skilled" service. The following are examples of services that are reimbursable and covered under Medicare because they require skill, knowledge, and judgment on the part of the practitioner: (1) observation and evaluation of physical status; (2) teaching and training activities to client, family, or caretaker; (3) therapeutic exercises (for restoration or loss of function); (4) insertion and irrigation of catheter; (5) administration of medications (intravenous and intramuscular injections and teaching of medication regimen), and (6) skin care (extensive decubitus ulcer).

Unlike the general population, Medicare beneficiaries usually suffer from chronic conditions with multiple disease processes. Medicare beneficiaries rely on federal reimbursement criteria that definitely influence the provision of care. Medicare places an emphasis on episodic care because of its limitations in benefits and requirements for skilled care. One of the shortcomings of Medicare is its limited protection. Medicare usually reimburses 80% of "usual, customary and reasonable charges." The remaining 20% must be "coinsured" for protection against excessive expense. The nurse should encourage the elderly client to acquire supplemental health insurance to cover the cost of charges that Medicare does not pay. The use of home health services under Medicare has increased significantly since the passage of the 1972 amendments and since the implementation of the prospective payment system for hospitals in 1983. New rules and regulations are written for Medicare and intermediaries as needed. These changes are published in bulletins sent to agencies. For example, currently Medicare does not assume the role of primary insurer in cases of accidents of liability when other insurances are available.

Medicaid

Authorized by Title XIX of the Social Security Act, Medicaid provides health services to low income persons. It is a medical assistance program for eligible people under Title XVI (Aid to Families with Dependent Children) or Title XVI (Supplemental Security Income) of the Social Security Act and also is available for those individuals whose income is insufficient to cover medical services and for disability coverage. Medicaid is administered by the states but is both state and federally subsidized. Providers are directly reimbursed by the state, which is also responsible for monitoring the operations and enforcing the regulations. Medicaid covers home health services including skilled and unskilled services such as personal care. Needy children are eligible under Medicaid, whereas the elderly usually receive Medicare.

Table 42-3 compares Medicare with Medicaid. If a client has both Medicare and Medicaid or a private insurance plan, Medicare is used as the primary payment source provided the services being delivered to the client are "skilled." When the client is no longer eligible for home care under Medicare, the Medicaid benefits can be used.

Private Insurance

Third-party payers are represented by private insurance companies in which the person subscribes individually or with a group such as an employer. Some states (e.g., Connecticut) have laws that require home health care to be a provision in health insurance coverage. Individuals under 65 years who need home care follow-up after surgery or prolonged hospitalization use this benefit the most. This benefit can decrease a client's length of stay in the hospital, thereby assisting clients to return to their former level of functioning.

Payment by Individual

Some individuals who require home health services but do not have health insurance may pay the home health agency directly. Individuals who do not meet their insurance coverage requirements and still want the services pay the established charge or may be offered the service on a sliding scale or established fee, based on their financial status. For example, clients may no longer require skilled nursing service for assessment of their condition but still need the help of a home health aide to assist with personal hygiene needs. Some persons may pay for home health services that are needed or desired above and beyond the home health services the Medicare program offers.

Nursing Visit Charges

Home health care is growing because it is assumed to be more cost-effective than hospital care. It is likely that financiers will closely scrutinize the implementation of home health services and adjustments and restrictions will evolve as needed to maintain cost containment. Several factors influence the cost and charge data: (1) type of service provided, (2) geographical location of the agency, and (3) current community staffing patterns. The term *cost* refers to the dollar amount agencies spend to provide the service. The term *charge* is the dollar amount expected or billed for rendering the service.

The Health Care Financing Administration continuously gathers data regarding use of home care services by analyzing factors such as cost, frequency, duration of services, and

TABLE 42-3

Comparison of the two major federally supported programs for home health care

Medicare (Title XVIII)	Medicaid (Title XVIX)
Federal *insurance* program administered by Social Security Administration	Federal and state *assistance* program administered by the state
Age 65 and over or disabled	Income-based eligibility
Conditions of participation	Conditions of participation
Homebound status	Not necessarily homebound status
Intermittent service	Intermittent service
Skilled service	Not necessarily skilled service
Restorative program	Custodial and maintenance program
Physician certification	Physician certification
Therapies, medical social service	State option—therapist, medical social service
Pays rental and purchase	Pays purchase
Reimbursement—"reasonable cost"	Reimbursement—maximum allowed at state level

number of visits. The federal government is interested in cost containment and also in quality of care.

Cost Effectiveness

Refer to Chapter 3 for an in-depth discussion of the economics of health care and its impact on community health nursing. Updated published data are lacking regarding the cost effectiveness of home health care. Public attention is now being focused on home health care as a cost-effective alternative to institutionalization.

Nurses are usually not exposed directly to the financial aspects of health care in their clinical setting. In home health, nurses are "cost conscious" because of their responsibility to interpret to clients what Medicare *will* or *will not* pay. It is difficult for the elderly to understand why Medicare will not pay for the nurse to make home visits to take their blood pressures if the client's condition remains stable. Medicare pays for services only if the client's condition remains unstable. The key words to remember for Medicare home health coverage are *skilled, homebound, intermittent,* and *unstable.*

Physician's case management frequently conflicts with Medicare guidelines. It should be noted that services or frequencies certified by a physician as being *necessary* for a particular home care Medicare client may not meet Medicare's guidelines of "reasonable and necessary" and, therefore, are not covered by Medicare. For example, a physician might order physical therapy for strengthening exercises for a postsurgical debilitated patient. This does not constitute a Medicare-approved physical therapy diagnosis, and therapy would not be provided. However, if skilled nursing is ordered for this same patient, and "is reasonable and necessary," during the skilled visit the nurse can instruct the family and patient regarding a plan of rehabilitation, which is developed in collaboration with the therapist.

IMPACT OF LEGISLATION ON HOME HEALTH CARE SERVICES

The federal government plays a significant role in the delivery of home health care services. The information is organized to present an overview of the historical development of the laws and their effect on home health. The student should remember that congressional activity can change federal legislation regarding home health care. For updated information concerning new amendments or bills presented in Congress, consult the *Federal Register.*

The Social Security Act of 1935 signaled the major entrance of the federal government into the area of social insurance. It significantly expanded assistance to the states and formed the foundation for the two major health programs—Medicare and Medicaid.

The Medicare program was enacted on July 30, 1965, as Title XVIII of the Social Security Act and became effective July 1, 1966. The program offers two coordinated insurance coverages—hospital insurance, referred to as Part A; and supplemental medical insurance, referred to as Part B. Each provides reimbursement for home health agency services. This legislation established requirements for client eligibility, reimbursable costs, physician participation, and agency eligibility (for specific details see pp. 917-918).

The Social Security Amendments of 1972 made the following changes in home health coverage to provide incentives for greater use of the benefit:

1. In the supplementary insurance section (Part B) the 20% co-insurance requirement was eliminated for services furnished on or after January 1, 1973.
2. The Secretary of HEW (now DHHS) was authorized to establish by diagnoses the permissible periods of coverage of home health care under Part A for clients with specified conditions.
3. Payments for services that neither the home health agency nor the beneficiary previously knew were covered.
4. Medicare coverage (including home health care) was extended to individuals receiving Social Security benefits based on disability or end-stage renal disease. This coverage began in July 1973.

The early 1980s brought substantial changes in the area of home health care services. In 1980 congress enacted legislation that modified the existing programs of Medicare and Medicaid—the Medicare and Medicaid Amendments of 1980, Title IX of the Omnibus Reconciliation Act of 1980 (Public Law 96-499). Public Law 96-499 carries provisions relating not only to home health but also to hospital services, skilled nursing facilities, intermediate care facilities, and physicians who are involved with reimbursement from Medicare and Medicaid.

The Omnibus Reconciliation Act of 1980 broadened Medicare coverage for home health services by instituting changes such as unlimited visits by home health care providers, elimination of mandatory 3-day hospital stay as a prerequisite to reimbursement, reimbursement for occupational therapy, and involvement of proprietary agencies. Other important features of the Omnibus Reconciliation Act include the establishment of regional intermediaries for home health agencies by the Department of Health and Human Services and the achievement of more effective administration of the home health benefits. (Law, Paragraph 924,097; Committee reports, Paragraph 24,347).

The Medicaid Community Care Act, Section 2176 of the Omnibus Reconciliation Act, recognizes and supports the concept of community care as a viable alternative for clients requiring long-term care. The states and providers of home health services are being afforded the opportunity to develop their own plan and implement their own ideas without the burden of excessive federal regulation. Some individuals feel, however, that the decrease in federal involvement will foster fraud and abuse in Medicare home care use by some "not-so-honest" entrepreneurs.

TRENDS AND ISSUES IN HOME HEALTH CARE
Legal and Ethical Issues Confronting the Home Health Nurse

Any health care subsystem has a potential for illegal and unethical actions. Much publicity has been given to Medicare fraud and abuse with the last decade. This avenue for exploitation has been partially caused by the increase in available federal money. Examples of such practices include overuse of home health services when the client does not need them, inaccurate billing for services, excessive administrative staff, "kickbacks" for referrals, and billing of noncovered medical supplies. In 1977, the Medicare-Medicaid Anti-Fraud and Abuse Amendments (PL 95-142) were passed to deter such practices.

Home health care nurses can be confronted with multiple issues in everyday practice. The definition of skilled care can be judgmental, and its interpretation can vary. The home health care nurse must abide by the established federal regulations when delivering care to clients. Frequency of visiting poses another issue. Home health care clients require only intermittent visits for evaluation of status. If the frequency increases, then full-time skilled services may be required. Reevaluation of the client and family needs is imperative so that overuse and inappropriate use of services can be avoided. Home health care nurses must be knowledgeable about which medical supplies are covered. This information is readily available to home health care nurses, and as professionals, nurses must work within the regulatory guideline framework and educate the community as to what home health care is and should be.

Stressors in home health care affect practicing nurses. Paperwork while often overwhelming, is necessary to document accountability. Being accountable can be stressful because the home health care nurse must demonstrate that all actions are valid and justifiable. The expanded role of the home health care nurse can be complex, since the assumption of nontraditional responsibilities can be viewed as a threat by other health team members. Physician support may be lacking, and home health care may be underused if the hospital orientation views home care as second rate and bothersome because of the excess paperwork it entails. Others view home health care as a service for the poorer classes and therefore find it unappealing.

Cost-effectiveness is another negative phrase to some health care professionals because it is difficult to link cost-effectiveness with quality in all situations. But to exist in the competitive health care arena today, home health care must be competitive. By properly organizing and using decision-making principles, home health care nurses do not have to sacrifice quality for cost-effectiveness.

Issues in the 1990s and Beyond

The 1970s brought an era of regulation, primarily since the government played an important part in financing health care. Regulations have now been accused of jeopardizing the quality of care. In the 1980s, we have seen a different trend—that of deregulation. As we approach the 1990s we will also see a more comprehensive restructuring of the health care system.

Health care providers and consumers are concerned about high quality and cost-effective alternatives to institutional care. Home health nurses can play a vital role in providing the leadership to see that this realistic dream can come true. Quality care can be provided in the home setting as evidenced by review of the literature (Hall, Baud, and Elliston,

1982). The benefit of home health care is measurable in terms of evaluating client outcomes, as described in the quality assurance section of this chapter.

The per diem cost of home health care is less than the per diem cost of hospital care (Harris, 1982). It is assumed that greater self-care is a means to cutting health care costs. Home health care encourages promotion of self-care. If home health care is to exist as a viable alternative to institutionalization, then nurses must not only continue to provide quality care but participate in research to clarify the contribution of home health care to cost effectiveness in the health care delivery system. Home health care need not be referred to only as an alternative to institutionalization. Rather, it should be the first choice, with institutionalization being an alternative when appropriate.

Gikow (1981) has developed a decision model for individuals responsible for referring clients to community resources to assist them in matching clients with the appropriate resource. The tool depends on an accurate and complete client assessment so that either skilled or supportive care can be provided appropriately and adequately.

In 1982, the National Association of Home Health Agencies (NAHHA) and the Council of Home Health Agencies/Community Health Services (CHHA/CHS) merged to form the National Association for Home Care (NAHC). The purpose and definition for the new organization was developed by a National Task Force for Home Health Services. Some of the areas that will influence home health in the 1990s include increasing political awareness of home health services, participating in legislative and regulatory processes, focusing on the positive aspects of home health care services not only with governmental but also private sector agencies, compiling data, and distributing educational information to the public regarding home health care (Rak, 1982).

Competition in home health care is on the rise. This factor is based primarily on the slant of federal programs to deinstitutionalize and deregulate areas of health care. Clients are being discharged in a more "acute" condition than previously. The level of care requires a highly skilled practitioner in community health nursing. Administrators of home health agencies are being faced with "selling" home health care to consumers. This task, although seemingly difficult, can be easy if accountability and quality assurance exist in the agencies.

Indigent Care

There is no legal right to health care in the United States, and no recognized constitutional basis exists to solicit this right. The President's Commission for the Study of Ethical Problems in Medicine showed 34 million people were uninsured during some period of 1983 and determined that clients' inability to pay was a major detriment to obtaining health care services (President's Commission, 1983). Murphy (1986) observes that health care is provided through a mutual agreement and providers can legally deny services based on an individual's ability or inability to pay for services rendered.

Inadequate health care funding, limited resources of private charitable care, and absence of legal recourse to obtain health care as a basic human right adversely affect the medically indigent and limit their access to home care. Nursing has the opportunity to ameliorate this health deficit through clinical research, public advocacy, and devising cost-reducing strategies (Murphy, 1986).

Increased Focus on Discharge Planning

The need for discharge planning was formally identified in 1972 by the American Hospital Association and legislated by Social Security (1972), JCAH (1977), and HCFA (1978). (See Chapter 6 for more details regarding legislation.) An adjunct effect of DRG implementation in hospitals has been a reevaluation and expansion of the discharge planner's role in effecting cost containment and facilitating continuity of care. The nursing student's community health curriculum ideally should include experience with this emerging specialty area. Interaction of student-discharge planner would enhance the significance of home health care and reinforce the process of collaboration in providing continuity in health care services.

High Technology Nursing

The DRG incentive for early hospital discharge has created a precipitous transfer of high-technology nursing skills from the hospital to the home care setting (Auerbach, 1985). Parenteral nutrition, chemotherapy, IV antibiotic therapy, ventilators, apnea monitors, and skeletal traction are examples of current home care technologies. Shaw (1985) envisions increased care of the organ transplant patient in the home and predicts that home surgeries and home births will be a reality in the near future. The home care nurse must be prepared to execute these high technology skills in the home to maximize professional performance, to deter inherent liability risk, to enhance patient rehabilitation, and to use research to secure nursing as a vital element of this rapidly developing component of health care.

Pediatric Home Care

Pediatric home care has changed tremendously over the past few years as children are being treated outside the institutional environment. Policymakers in the United States are beginning to appreciate the relationship between home care and pediatrics. Legislation has been proposed to require that private insurance companies cover home care in employee benefit packages. New programs, resources, and options for funding are beginning to become available for care of children at home.

The family is the key to the successful management of a child at home because children already have a built-in support system to assist with personal care, training, and developmental needs. A supportive and stable home environment for children can contribute to healing and maintenance of health.

Specialized programming for the pediatric population is mandatory. Although infants have been treated in the home for years, the focus on high technology care requires evaluation of key issues such as reimbursement, staffing, and quality assurance programs. Pediatric needs range from an infant who needs observation and treatment with home phototherapy to an infant requiring a sleep apnea monitor, to a child needing ventilator assistance and enteral feeding. Approximately 10 million children are disabled and institutionalized today because of terminal or chronic conditions. Pediatric home care in the future will continue to assist parents in the care of their children at home if resources and interventions continue to be appropriate (Pediatric Home Care 1986, p. 1398).

Family Responsibility, Roles, and Functions

The family plays an important part in the delivery of home health care. The term *family* as discussed previously, refers to a caretaker responsible for the client's well-being. An issue being discussed at this time is whether home health care services should be used as a respite, or relief, type of care. Sometimes a family member is debilitated and unable to help the client without assistance. Should supportive services be paid by the federal government? On the other hand, some family members are capable of providing the needed care but are unwilling to do so. Who should pay for the service and who should provide the needed care? Family responsibility is an issue that may not be resolved. The situations vary from one family to another. Assistance from social support systems facilitates coping with the stress of caring for an ill family member. However, the goal is to assist in maintaining the client at home for as long as possible and to provide high-quality care. To do this, resources must be used appropriately and effectively. However, determining this use poses a problem.

Population Trends and Their Effects on Home Health Care Services

The growing need for home health care services is supported by official data regarding our older American population (AARP, 1985). In 1984 there were 28 million people 65 or older representing 11.9% of the U.S. population. It is estimated that by the year 2000, the elderly population will be 13% and by 2030, 21.2%. Medicare, Medicaid, and private insurances paid 67%, or $81 billion, in health care costs for the elderly.

Hospice Home Care

Historically, the word *hospice* referred to a place of refuge for travelers. The contemporary meaning refers to "a way of caring for people nearing the end of their journey through life, faced with dying and in need of refuge" (Vines and Hartzell, 1981, p. 3). Originating in nineteenth century England, the earliest hospices first provided palliative care to terminally ill patients in hospitals and later extended the services into the homes. In 1970, the hospice movement in the United States gained momentum in response to awakened public interest generated by Dr. Elisabeth Kübler-Ross' book, *Death with Dignity*. Public-sponsored hospices, successful in meeting the special needs of the dying patient, attracted congressional attention. After evaluation of a limited trial hospice benefit, Congress enacted legislation in 1985 that provided coverage for hospice services under Medicare. Stringent controls and criteria for quality hospice care

are imposed both by the Health Care Financing Agency (HCFA) and the Joint Commission on Accreditation of Hospitals (JCAH) (McCann and Ench, 1986).

As a result of the hospice movement, people with terminal disease now are offered the opportunity to die at home, if it is their choice, with the supportive services that home care can provide. A variety of hospice care models in the United States use institutional services, home care service, or both. Those that use an existing hospital in conjunction with an established home health agency (hospital based or contracted services) are probably the most cost-efficient because each organization can contribute a portion of its resources to this concept of care (Meyer, 1980). In addition to prescribed home care services, core services unique to hospice are a medical director who actively participates as a member of the hospice team, volunteers, chaplain support, respite care, financial assistance with medicines and equipment, and bereavement support of the family after the death of the patient.

Hospice care requires a team of professionals and paraprofessionals with experience in caring for the terminally ill. Interdisciplinary coordination is imperative for a smooth transfer of clients to the home care setting from the hospital. In keeping clients at home, the primary goal is to help both the client and family in maintaining the client's integrity and comfort. Palliative rather than curative care is the objective. This goal is met by nursing actions such as alleviating symptoms and meeting the special needs of the dying client and client's family.

Health care providers who work with the dying often experience stress, which must be identified and appropriately addressed to deliver quality client care and to maintain the care provider's integrity. Employee stress factors related to hospice care differ from general job-related stressors. Understanding these differences will enable the hospice nurse to practice self-care while delivering client care.

Vachon (1979) identifies the following stress factors: (1) difficulty accepting the fact that a patient's physical and psychosocial problems cannot always be controlled, (2) frustration resulting from investing large amounts of energy for people who then die, (3) anger at being subjected to "higher-than-standard" performance expectations, (4) difficulty deciding when to set limits on involvement with patients and family, and (5) difficulty establishing realistic limitations as to what can be provided by hospice.

The hospice nurse needs a firm foundation in home care skills, knowledge of community resources, the ability to function constructively as a team member, and the mature ability to meet personal emotional needs and the emotional needs of the hospice patient and family.

One of the major issues confronting hospice care is the reimbursement structure in the health care delivery system. Initially, many hospices provided free services as a mission of ministering to the dying. Others accepted available payment from third-party payers for billable services. In November 1983, the federal government legislated a Medicare hospice benefit for reimbursement to Medicare hospice–certified agencies (Federal Register, 1983). Originally, the regulation was to be in effect through September 30, 1986;

but additional legislation changed the hospice benefit to a permanent status in April 1986 (PL 99-272, 1986).

The hospice reimbursement benefit is optional for the Medicare-eligible patient. Hospices may bill for *skilled* home care services under regular Medicare part A benefits if the patient does not want to use the hospice benefit. Responding to the perceived cost-containment potential of hospice care and the public demand for caring services during the terminal illness, third-party payors are following Medicare's lead in providing hospice service options.

Not all terminal patients choose hospice care, and of those that do, not all are eligible for Medicare or covered by private insurance. If reimbursement potential becomes an admission criterion for hospice care, it will no longer be a viable option for all terminal patients. The community health nurse choosing hospice as a specialty area must be prepared to deal with this and other potentially ethical issues. Despite the many unresolved issues, (e.g., patient choice, hospice availability, reimbursement status, admission criteria) hospice nursing is a rewarding specialty.

CLINICAL APPLICATION: INITIATION OF HOME HEALTH SERVICES

Referrals, or requests for evaluation of need for service, usually come from physicians or hospital discharge planners; but clients and family also can make direct inquiries to the agency. The agency's referral intake coordinator receives basic information on the client from the referring source, including name, diagnosis, insurance data, dates of hospital stay, and physician's specific orders for service. Many agencies schedule new admissions within 24 hours of receiving the request for service.

The nurse assigned to make the evaluation visit is given the referral information and the "admission packet." She then contacts the client by phone to clarify directions to the home and to schedule the time of the visit.

After arriving at the patient's home, the nurse explains the philosophy and purpose of the agency and verifies the insurance coverage. If the visits are to be covered by Medicare part A, the nurse ascertains that Medicare's eligibility requirements for home care are met (homebound with *skilled, intermittent* need). Medicare-approved agencies accept the amount paid by Medicare for services and do not bill patients over and above this amount. If the pay status is private insurance or private pay, the nurse will discuss charges and billing procedures with the patient and family. For the noninsured client, services can be provided either free or on a sliding-scale fee, determined by the individual agency's purpose, philosophy, and mission.

Depending on the ease in determining eligibility for home care, the client may sign the insurance release form and release of information form at this point in the interview, or the paperwork may be deferred until after the assessment. The nurse interviews the clients and caregivers and completes both a psychosocial and medical history. A physical examination is done on the first visit, incorporating information gleaned from the interview. Any treatments needed and ordered are performed at this time (e.g., catheter changes or dressing changes). The nurse focuses on teaching from the moment the interview begins until the visit is concluded. This is one major difference between home care and hospital nursing. In the hospital the nurses provide primary hands-on care; in the home the focus is on *teaching* self-care to the client and family.

At this point, the nurse reviews all medications, completes a medication schedule sheet, and teaches the purpose and side effects of the medications. Ideally, a home teaching program is completed on carbonless paper for each problem identified (e.g., catheter care). After reviewing each with the client or caregiver, the nurse has the client sign the form, leaves a copy in the home, and retains a copy for the client's record. The home teaching form, signed by the client or family, is a contract for care and a standard for measuring the client's progress and compliance. If the referral information was complete, the nurse executes the orders as received. If new problems are identified during the visit, the nurse contacts the physician for clarification and new orders. For example, the nurse may have identified a need for home health aide services that the physician had not addressed. The physician's plan of care cannot be altered without his approval.

Because third-party payer guidelines for reimbursement change frequently, the home health nurse must maintain current knowledge of the criteria. The nurse coordinates the physician's requests, the client's needs, and the reimbursement available (if applicable) to achieve maximum health services for the homebound patient. Client and family needs that exceed standard criteria are referred to the agency social worker. When available, community resources are used as needed to assure a comprehensive plan of care for the client's health care needs.

To conclude the initial visit, the nurse reviews services the physician has ordered; the assessment of the present visit; all home care programs; the plan of treatment, including frequency of visits and duration of each service to be provided; an emergency care plan, including the name and number of the agency. The nurse then establishes the date of the next visit.

An initial home visit takes about 1½ hours in the home, 1 hour for charting, contacting the physician, and arranging interdisciplinary referrals, and the remainder for travel time.

The admission visit uses all the home care nurse's professional skills, and, to the extent that a correct assessment is completed and an appropriate plan implemented, the home care program will enhance recovery in the client's own environment.

SUMMARY

Home health care is an expanding, vital component of the health care delivery system. This subsystem recently has been affected by federal interest and regulations, the expanding elderly population, and DRG implementation in the hospitals. Home care services now are viewed as both primary and secondary options to institutionalization.

The home care nurse today faces many challenges. Ethical issues (reimbursement criteria and indigent care), role development (high technology and hospice nursing), and opportunities for research (quality of care and cost-effectiveness) affect nursing practice in the home.

Home health care, the only service offered to clients in their own environment, is an ideal multidisciplinary approach to meeting the client's needs. The home care nurse is the vital coordinator, collaborator, and practitioner assuring quality care to the client in the home.

☰ KEY CONCEPTS

Home health care differs from other areas of health care in that the health care providers practice in the client's environment. This unique characteristic affects several components of nursing practice in the home care setting.

Family is an integral part of home health care, which includes any caretaker or significant person who takes the responsibility to assist the client in need of care at home.

Home care reached a turning point with the arrival of Medicare, which provided regulations for home care practice and reimbursement mechanisms.

Home health agencies are divided into the following five general types based on the administrative and organizational structures: official, private and voluntary, combination, hospital-based, and proprietary.

Regardless of the type of home health agency existing in a community, the primary goal should be to provide quality home health care to the community based on the health needs of people.

Demonstration of professional compentency is the foremost requirement for home health care nurses.

Home health care nursing is a *division* of community health nursing. Thus health *promotion activities are a fundamental component of practice.*

There are three accepted components of the concept of self-care: *patient education, patient compliance,* and *self help.*

Contracting is a vital component of all nurse-client relationships. Contracting refers to any working agreement, continuously renegotiable, between the nurse, client, and family.

The home health care nurse practices in accordance with the Standards of Community Health Nursing Practice developed by the American Nurses' Association, Council of Community Health Nurses.

Interdisciplinary collaboration is a required process in the home health care setting. Its use is mandated for Medicare-certified home care agencies, and it is also inherent in the definition of home health care.

In home care, as in other care settings, professionals experience stress associated with changing roles and overlapping responsibilities. In collaborating, home health care providers, should carefully analyze each others' roles to determine if overlapping occurs and adjust the plan of care as needed.

Since the advent of Medicare, home health agencies have monitored the quality of care to their clients as a mandatory requirement for certification as a home health agency. All agencies are accountable to clients and families, to their reimbursement sources, to themselves as a health care provider, and to professional standards.

The home care nurse today faces many challenges. Ethical issues (reimbursement criteria and indigent care), role development (high technology and hospice nursing), and opportunities for research (quality of care and cost-effectiveness) affect nursing practice in the home.

LEARNING ACTIVITIES

1. Make a joint home visit with an experienced home health care nurse to:

   a. evaluate the process and content of the nurse/patient interaction to determine if the visit was merely ritual or therapeutic, and describe the process of the visit

   b. compare actual roles and functions with the Standards of Community Health Nursing Practice.

   c. assess level of skilled care the patients receive and determine whether they are needed and appropriate. (Are they within the four criteria described in the section on roles and functions? Answer the four questions in relation to the home visit made.)

2. Make a joint home visit with another home health care professional and assess as in the preceding activity. Also attend a patient care conference meeting and write a summary of the process of the group.

BIBLIOGRAPHY

Abramson, B.J., and Klug. M.J.: Health advocacy services, Medicare/Medicaid Assistance Training Manual, January, 1985.

American Association of Retired Persons: Profile of Older Americans, Dept. D996, Washington, D.C., 1985.

American Medical Association: Physician guide to home health care, Monroe, Wis., 1979, The Association.

American Nurses Association: Standards of community health nursing practice, Kansas City, Mo., 1986, The Association.

American Nurses Association, Division of Community Health Nursing: A conceptual model of community health nursing, Pub. No. CH-102M, Kansas City, Mo., 1980, The Association.

Auerbach, M.: Changes in home health care deliver, Nurs. Outlook 33:290-291, 1985.

Callender, M., and LaVor, J.: Home health care: development, problems, and potential, Washington, D.C., 1975, Office of the Assistant Secretary for Planning and Evaluation, Social Services and Human Development, Department of Health, Education and Welfare.

Cassak, D.: Hospitals in home health care—an industry in transition, Health Industry Today 16-75, July, 1984.

Corwin, R.G.: A society of education, New York, 1965, Appleton-Century-Crofts.

Dolan, J.: Goodnow's history of nursing, Philadelphia, 1958, W.B. Saunders Co.

Funkhouser, R.: Quality of care. I, Nursing '76 16:11, 1976.

Gikow, F.F.: How to determine appropriate community services for the elderly, Nurs. Health Care 2(6):322-326, 1981.

Hall, A.D., Baud, W.R., and Elliston, E.B.: Comparing staff attitudes and patient satisfactions in a home health care agency, Home Health Rev. 4(1):4-11, 1982.

Hall, J., and Weaver, B.: Distributive nursing practice: a systems approach to community health, New York, 1977, J. B. Lippicott Co., p. 6.

Harris, M.: Evaluating home care; compare viewpoints, Nurs. Health Care 2(4):207, 1982.

Health Care Financing Administration: Conditions of participation for home health agencies, Subpart 1, Section 405.1229, Evaluation, Washington, D.C., 1982, Department of Health and Human Services.

Home Health Services: Commerce Cleaninghouse Medicare and Medicaid Guide, Paragraph 1401, Washington, D.C., 1982, Department of Health and Human Services.

Johns, J.L.: Selfcare today—in search of an identity. Nurs. Health Care 5(3):153-156, 1985.

Kane, R.: Competency for collaboration. In Reinhardt, A., and Quinn, M., editors: Current practice in family-centered community nursing, vol. 1, St. Louis, 1977, The C.V. Mosby Co.

Koren, M.J.: Home care—who cares? N. Engl. J. Med. 314(14):917-920, 1986.

Krause, F.: The political contest of health service regulation, Int. J. Health Serv. 5(4):593-607, 1975.

Medicare Program: hospice care, Federal Register, December 16, 1984; 48:560008-36.

Meyer, K.A.: Hospice concept integrated with existing community health care, Nurs. Adm. Q. 4(3):49-54, 1980.

Murphy, E.K.: Health Care: right or privilege? Nurs. Econ. 4:66-68, 1986.

National Association for Home Care Report #152, February 4, 1986.

National League for Nursing: Utilization review—guidelines for home health agencies, New York, 1971, NLN.

Orem, D.E., Nursing: concepts of practice, ed. 3, New York, 1985, McGraw-Hill Book Co.

Pediatric Home Care—Parts I and II—Caring, November, December, 1986.

Phaneuf, M.C.: The nursing audit; profile for excellence, New York, 1972, Appleton-Century-Crofts.

President's Commission: Securing access to health care. Washington, D.C., 1983, U.S. Government President's Office.

Quality assurance for community health agencies, Waltham, Mass., 1980, Massachusetts Association of Home Health and Community Health Agencies.

Quality assurance manual, 1980, Florida Association of Home Health Agencies.

Rak, K.: Home Health Line, Jan. 15, 1982.

Shaw, Stephen: A home care technology, Caring, October, 1985.

Sloan, M.R., and Schummer, B.T.: The process of contracting in community nursing. In Spradley, V.W., editor: Contemporary community nursing, Boston, 1975, Little, Brown & Co.

Tax Equity and Fiscal Responsibility Act of 1982, Section 122. Public Law 97-248.

Trager, B.: Home health services in the United States: a report to the Special Committee on Aging, 92nd Congress, 2nd Session, Washington, D.C., 1972, U.S. Government Printing Office.

Vachon, M.L.: Staff stress in care of the terminally ill, QRB 5(5):13-17, 1979.

Vines, E., and Hartzell, D.H.: The hospice movement in the United States, National Health Standards and Quality Information Clearinghouse Information Bulletin, Baltimore, March, 1981.

Warhola, C.: Planning for home health services: a resource handbook, Pub. No. (HRA) 80-14017, Washington, D.C., August, 1980, Public Health Service, Department of Health and Human Services.

INDIVIDUAL ASSESSMENT TOOLS

A1—DISCHARGED PATIENTS QUESTIONNAIRE*

We are asking patients and families who have recently received services from the agency to assist us in the evaluation of our programs. As a consumer of the services we offer, your answers to the enclosed questionnaire will help us determine if we are meeting our objectives as a provider of skilled nursing care in the home designed to meet the needs of residents of our county.

We would appreciate it if you could complete the questionnaire and return it to us in the envelope provided. It will not be necessary to sign the questionnaire as we are not interested in identifying a patient or the nurse who gave care.

Instructions: Please circle the *Yes* or *No* following each question below, as you feel it answers the question.

1. When the public health nurse visited your home, did you know why she was there? — Yes No
2. Did you and the nurse arrange a time for the visits that was convenient for both of you? — Yes No
3. Did the nurse do any of the following treatments? — Yes No
    - Change or irrigate catheter — Yes No
    - Irrigate colostomy or give an enema — Yes No
    - Change dressings — Yes No
    - Inject a medication — Yes No
    - Assist with exercise routine — Yes No
    - Suction or care for tracheotomy — Yes No
    - Insert a nasal-gastric tube — Yes No
    - If you answered *Yes* to any of the above, did you understand what the treatment was expected to do for you? — Yes No
4. Did the nurse teach you or any member of your family to do a treatment? — Yes No
    - Did you or your family learn to do the treatment yourself? — Yes No
5. Did you take medication by mouth? — Yes No
    - Did you understand how to take the medication (i.e., amount to take; number of times during the day; if taken before, after, or with meals)? — Yes No
    - Did the nurse help you understand what the medication was expected to do? — Yes No
6. Did the nurse examine you at any time (i.e., take blood pressure, pulse, listen to your chest with a stethoscope, examine your skin)? — Yes No
    - If yes, did you understand why she was making these observations? — Yes No

7. Did the nurse help you to understand your illness? — Yes No
8. Did you understand what the nurse was planning to accomplish by visiting you? — Yes No
    - Did you think it was possible to accomplish this? — Yes No
9. Did the nurse's visits make it easier for you to remain in your home and care for yourself? — Yes No
10. Did you have other problems (e.g., financial) that the public health nurse could not assist you with by herself? — Yes No
    - If yes, did the nurse assist you to contact another agency that could help you? — Yes No
11. Do you feel the nursing visits were (circle one): Too few   Too many   Right number
12. Were you aware that the nurse was going to discharge you from her service? — Yes No
13. Did you feel you could function on your own when the nurse dismissed you from the service? — Yes No
14. If you need skilled nursing service in your home at some time in the future, will you contact the agency? — Yes No
15. If you have any comments, please write them in the space below:

A2—HISTORY TAKING IN THE AMBULATORY SETTING*

The following is an outline of the specific information needed for a health history. The headings and questions are those traditionally used.

Chief Complaint

Why is the child attending clinic today? Generally the answer is a simple statement in the parent's own words (e.g., "well-child care," "cold," or "earache").

Present Illness

What signs and symptoms of illness is the child showing? It is best to list the symptoms in order of appearance. Sometimes specific questions must be asked (e.g., Is the child coughing? When? What kind? How much? Does the child have diarrhea? When? What kind? How much? For how long?). How is the child acting otherwise? (How is his or her appetite? Bowels? Fluid intake? Sleep? Activity?) Has the child been exposed to others with illness? (Anyone in the family? Relatives? Friends? School? What type of illness was it?) What kind of treatment have the

---

*From Administrator's handbook for the structure, operation, and expansion of home health agencies, Pub. No. 21-1653 (New York: National League for Nursing, 1977), pp. 409-410. Used with permission.

*From Alexander, M.M., and Brown, M.S.: Pediatric history taking and physical diagnosis for nurses, New York, 1979, McGraw-Hill Book Co., pp. 6-13. Used with permission.

parents been giving? (Have they sought medical care before? Any medications? Any procedures?)

Past History
Birth

PRENATAL. How was the mother's health during her pregnancy with this child? Where did she receive her prenatal care and for how many months of the pregnancy? Did she have any infections? During what month? Did she have any illnesses? During which month, and how were they treated? Was she taking medications during the pregnancy? What kind and why? At what point during pregnancy? What is her blood type? What is the child's father's blood type? Does she know the child's blood type? Did she have any x-rays taken during her pregnancy? Was she on any special diet during the pregnancy? How nutritional was her diet? Was she hospitalized during her pregnancy? When and for what reasons? How many living children does she have? Was either she or her doctor worried about this pregnancy for any reason? Did the pregnancy last 9 months? (A report of the baby being born less than 2 weeks early or late is usually not significant unless accompanied by a history of low birth weight or neonatal problems.)

NATAL. How long was the labor and were there any problems? What type of delivery was it? What kind of anesthesia was used and were there any problems? (Such questions as, Did the baby come headfirst? and, Did the doctor use forceps? are often helpful in eliciting this information.) Where was the baby born? What was the baby's birth weight? What was the baby's condition at birth? Did the baby cry? Was the baby blue? Did the baby need oxygen?

POSTNATAL. Did the baby have any problems while in the nursery? What was the length of the baby's hospital stay? Did the mother and infant come home together? Did the baby have jaundice? Was the baby ever cyanotic, or blue? Were there any feeding problems during the hospitalization? Did the baby develop any rashes? How much weight did the baby lose?

Allergies

Is the child allergic to any foods? To any medications? To any insects? To any animals? At any seasons? If so, describe what happens with these allergies. Does the child ever break out in rashes? Do the parents know why?

Accidents

Has the child ever had an accident? If so, was it in the car? At home? At school? At the baby-sitter's? Can the parents describe what happened? What was the treatment? Where was the child treated? What was the child's reaction? Any residual problems?

Illnesses

Has the child had any infections? When? Where? What treatment? What follow-up care? Has the child had any childhood diseases? Measles? Rubella? Roseola? Mumps? Chickenpox? Whooping cough?

Operations

Has the child ever had any operations? When? For what condition? Where? What was the outcome?

Hospitalizations

Has the child ever spent any time in a hospital? For what reason? Where? Is the condition resolved? Any residual problems?

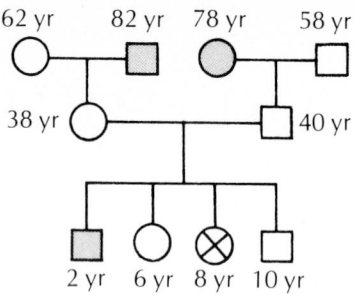

Immunizations

Has the child had any immunizations? Which kinds? Any reactions? Any boosters? (Usually a written record is the most accurate source of this information.) Has the child been tested for tuberculosis? How? When? What was the result? Has the child ever had x-rays?

Family History
Family Members

What is the mother's age and state of health? What is the father's age and state of health? Are there any siblings? What ages and what sex? State of health? A diagram is often used to show this information. A circle indicates a female, and a square indicates a male; a horizontal line indicates a marriage, and a vertical line indicates a descendant. A darkened circle or square indicates that the individual is deceased. An X indicates the child with whom this particular history is concerned. The accompanying diagram shows a maternal grandfather who died at age 82 and paternal grandmother who died at age 78; a 62-year-old maternal grandmother and a 58-year-old paternal grandfather alive; two parents, a 38-year-old mother and 40-year-old father, alive; one 10-year-old brother and one 6-year-old sister alive; and one brother who died at 2 years of age. The child about whom the history is taken is an 8-year-old girl.

Family Diseases

Within the immediate family, including both sets of grandparents and first aunts and uncles, are any of the following conditions present?

EYES, EARS, NOSE, AND THROAT. Are there any nosebleeds? Sinus problems? Glaucoma? Cataracts? Myopia? Strabismus? Any other problems with their eyes, ears, nose, or throat?

CARDIORESPIRATORY. Is there any tuberculosis? Asthma? Hay fever? Hypertension? Heart murmurs? Heart attacks? Strokes? Anemia? Rheumatic fever? Leukemia? Pneumonia? Emphysema? Any other problems with heart or lungs?

GASTROINTESTINAL. Does anyone have ulcers? Colitis? Any other problems with stomach or intestines? Does anyone have kidney infections? Bladder infections?

MUSCULOSKELETAL. Are there any congenital dislocated hips? Muscular dystrophy? Arthritis? Club feet? Any other problems with bones or muscles?

NEUROLOGICAL. Does anyone have convulsions? Mental retardation? Mental problems? Comas? Epilepsy?

SPECIAL SENSES. Is anyone deaf? Blind?

CHRONIC. Does anyone have diabetes? Congenital anomalies? Cancer? Tumors? Thyroid problems?

GENERAL. Are there any other medical problems in the family that the patient thinks are important?

SOCIAL. Where does the family live? In a house? Apartment? Room? How large? Is there a yard? Are there stairs? Does anyone live with the family? Grandparents? Aunts? Uncles? Friends? What is the financial situation of the family? Does the father work? Does the mother work? What are their occupations? If no one works, how are they living? Is there any outside help? Baby-sitters? Day-care centers? Schools? What is the general relationship of the family members? Do they seem to be a happy family? Chaotic family? Sad family? Depressed family? Violent family?

Review of Systems
Skin

Does this child have any rashes?

Eyes, Ears, Nose, and Throat

Does this child have persistent nosebleeds? Frequent streptococcal sore throats? Frequent colds (more than four a year)? Pneumonia? Frequent earaches? Do the child's eyes ever cross? Do they tear excessively?

Cardiorespiratory

Does the child have any trouble breathing? Running? Finishing a 3-ounce to 4-ounce bottle without tiring? Does the child turn blue?

Gastrointestinal

Does the child have any problems with diarrhea? Constipation? Bleeding around the rectum? Bloody stools? Pain? Vomiting?

Genitourinary

Does the child have a straight, strong urinary stream, or does the urine just dribble out? Urinary frequency? Is there any pain? Bleeding? If an older girl, does she menstruate? What was the age of onset? How often? Any problems?

Neurological

Has the child ever had a convulsion? A fainting spell? Tremors? Twitches? Blackouts? Dizzy spells? Frequent headaches?

Musculoskeletal

Has the child ever broken any bones? Had any sprains? Complained of pain in the joints, swelling, or redness around the joints?

Special Senses

Does the child see well? Hear well? Does the child seem clumsy? Can the child see the blackboard from where he or she sits in the classroom? Is the child always falling or walking into doors?

Chronic

Any long-term diseases?

General

Any other problems?

Habits
Eating

Is the child's appetite good? Poor? Varied? If on formula, what kind, how much, how is it mixed, and how frequently? How much does the child take in a 24-hour period? What kinds of foods does the child eat? Meat? Fruits? Vegetables? Cereals? Juices? Eggs? Sweets? Milk? Snacks? How often? What size portions? How many times a week or day does the child eat each of these? Does the child feed herself or himself? Does the child use a cup? Spoon? Knife? Fork? Is the child messy? Does the child sit with the rest of the family? Does the child take vitamins? What kind? How often? How much? What is the family attitude toward food? Is it used as a symbol of love? A bribe? A reward? What is the emotional climate of the meals? Relaxed? Tired? Rushed? Tense?

Bowels

What are the child's bowel patterns? Frequency? Consistency? Color? Any discomfort? Is the child toilet trained? Is toilet-training planned? When? Any problems? If the child is toilet trained, does he or she have accidents? If so, are they during the day or night? How often? Are they frequently associated with emotional upsets?

Sleep

When does the child go to bed? Wake up? Does the child awaken during the night? How often? What happens? What does the parent do? Any nightmares? Night terrors? Does the child take naps? When? For how long? Where does the child sleep? How many hours does the child sleep in a 24-hour period? When awake, is the child alert? Or does the child seem to need more sleep than he or she is getting?

Development

How does the child compare with his or her siblings? Quicker to learn? Slower to learn? When did the child first sit? Stand? Roll over? Talk? Walk? What kinds of activities does the child do now? What is the child doing that is new since the last visit? What grade is the child in? Does the child like school? Does the child have playmates? What does the child like to do in school? What games does the child like to play?

Exercise and Play

What types of play or games does the child engage in and how often? Does the older child engage in sports? Team activities? For the adolescents, do they do regular exercises? How much walking, running, or other large motor activities are involved in their daily living patterns?

Personality

What kind of personality does this child have? Is he or she quiet? Outgoing? Does the child have a temper? How does the child cope with stress? By withdrawal? By aggression? By decompensation? By symptoms of illness? How does the child handle emotions like anger, fear, jealousy, or others? Is the child able to relax well?

Family Relations

How do the members of the family get along? How do they handle disagreement within the family? How do they handle external stress? What activities do they do together? How often? Do they enjoy them?

Sexuality

How much does the younger child ask about sexuality and what is the child told about it? What is the child's attitude toward it, and what is the attitude of those around the child? Does the child masturbate? How is this handled by the rest of the family? What are the child's own feelings about it? What is the child's attitude and those of the family toward nudity in the home? What does the older child know about changes beginning in his or her body: early breast development, penile and testicular enlargement, pubic hair, axillary and facial hair, changes in body proportions, voice changes, menstruation, and nocturnal emissions?

Some of the questions asked when taking a complete history need to be modified for specific ages, and some areas need more detailed information if problems are encountered. Generally, if the nurse covers these six areas, he or she has a good idea of which topics may need more information. The nurse must also decide which of these areas need to be discussed at every visit, which must be investigated at reg-

ular intervals, and which need to be discussed only once. Certainly once the birth history has been taken and no problems appear, there is no reason to repeat that material at every visit. However, the habits of the child change from visit to visit, sometimes from day to day, and this may be an important area to include in every history. The review of systems can easily change, but usually it will take a longer period for significant change to appear. The nurse may decide to routinely take a review of systems once a year rather than monthly or weekly. The nurse must go through each category and make a decision about how frequently it will be discussed.

A3—HEALTH ASSESSMENT FOR NURSE-FAMILY ENCOUNTERS: SELECTED AGES*

Health history physical exam	Nutrition	Development	Commonly recommended laboratory procedures and immunizations
FIRST INFANT ENCOUNTER			
Prenatal concerns Prenatal history Birth history Neonatal history History of familial diseases Interval history Family and social history Length, weight, and head circumference Complete physical exam Discussion of normal variants and abnormal physical findings with parents	Assess caloric needs for optimal growth: 100-110 cal/kg/day Discuss need for iron, vitamins, fluoride Discuss current feeding methods	2 weeks: sucking and rooting reflexes, Moro reflex, and tonic neck reflex (TNR) Sensitive to light and noise One month: responds to bell, eyes follow to midline, regards face, lifts head when prone	Urine ferric chloride for PKU Discuss PKU with parents Discuss immunization schedule and its importance
HEALTH ASSESSMENT AT 5 TO 9 WEEKS			
Parental concerns Interval history to include past illnesses, eating, sleeping, elimination, behavior Family and social history Length, weight, and head circumference Complete physical exam Discussion of findings with parents	Assess caloric needs for optimal growth Discuss parental attitudes and expectations re: solids Discuss need for water	5 weeks: rooting and Moro reflexes and TNR May "smile" Fist to mouth Follows light; tracks sound 9 weeks: smiles, vocalizes, hands to midline, listens, follows light past midline, holds head up 90° in prone position	Diphtheria, tetanus, pertussis vaccine (DTP) Trivalent oral polio vaccine (TOPV)
HEALTH ASSESSMENT AT 2½ TO 4 MONTHS			
Parental concerns Interval history Family and social history Length, weight, and head circumference Complete physical exam Discussion of findings with parents	Continued need for iron-enriched formula Digestive system now mature enough to handle solids Introduction of cereal, fruits at 4 months	2½ months: holds head and chest to 90° in prone position Laughs, babbles TNR and Moro reflex diminishing	DTP and TOPV No. 2

*Adapted from Chow, M.P., et al.: Handbook of pediatric primary care, New York, 1979, John Wiley & Sons, Inc., pp. 73-110.

Health assessment for nurse-family encounters: selected ages—cont'd

Health history physical exam	Nutrition	Development	Commonly recommended laboratory procedures and immunizations
HEALTH ASSESSMENT AT 2½ TO 4 MONTHS—cont'd	Teething biscuits may be used; avoid wheat products	4 months: holds head erect and steady in sitting position Bears weight on legs May roll over, do not leave unattended	
HEALTH ASSESSMENT AT 6 MONTHS Parental concerns Interval history Family and social history Length, weight, and head circumference Complete physical exam, including eye cover test for strabismus Discussion of findings with parents	Limit milk to 24 oz/24 hr Discuss iron-containing foods, finger foods Advise waiting to wean until after 1 year Discuss fluoride, avoidance of sugared foods Discuss cleaning of teeth Avoid all bottle propping	Laughs, babbles Passes object from hand to hand and mouths objects—permit no small objects or toys Tooth eruption Turns to voice Rolls over, may get to sitting position Beginning stranger anxiety Stronger attachment to mother	DTP and TOPV No. 3
HEALTH ASSESSMENT AT 9 MONTHS Parental concerns Interval history Family and social history Length, weight, and head circumference Complete physical exam, including hearing assessment (infant should turn head at least 45° to locate sound) Discussion of findings with parents	Advise 3 meals/day May introduce cup if child ready; advise waiting to wean until after 1 year Normal drop in appetite Restriction of sugared foods, milk, and juices in bedtime bottles Advise having ipecac syrup on hand	Jabber, babbles Thumb-finger grasp Imitates speech sounds Plays pat-a-cake May pull to stand and/or crawl—secure furniture, knickknacks; cover outlets	Hematocrit, hemoglobin, and RBC indices Sickle cell and G-6 PD screening No immunizations if up to date
HEALTH ASSESSMENT AT 12 MONTHS Parental concerns Interval history Family and social history Length, weight, and head circumference Complete physical exam Discussion of findings with parents	Review basic food groups, table foods, and amounts appropriate for age Lessened appetite Milk limited to 16-20 oz/24 hr Avoidance of sugared foods and drinks Discuss weaning from bottle	Indicates wants Drinks from cup Pincer grasp May use spoon Ma-ma, da-da Crawls, walks holding on or alone—time to childproof home	Urinalysis Hemogram if not obtained sooner Tuberculin test
HEALTH ASSESSMENT AT 15 TO 18 MONTHS Parental concerns Interval history Family and social history Height and weight Complete physical exam Discussion of findings with parents	Review basic food groups Stress need for iron and avoidance of sugared foods and drinks May feed self Discuss dental care	More than 5-6 words Uses spoon Scribbles on paper Points to one or more parts of body Climbing, running	Measles, mumps, and rubella (MMR) vaccine at 15 months DTP and TOPV No. 4 at 18 months if No. 3 was given at 6 months

Continued.

Health assessment for nurse-family encounters: selected ages—cont'd

Health history physical exam	Nutrition	Development	Commonly recommended laboratory procedures and immunizations
HEALTH ASSESSMENT AT 2 YEARS			
Parental concerns Interval history Family and social history Height, weight, and head circumference Complete physical exam Discussion of findings with parents	Review basic food groups and appropriate amounts for age Reduce milk intake to 16 oz/24 hr Discuss importance of proper snacks (low sugar, high protein) Discuss teaching use of toothbrush	May talk well and follow directions Purposeful markings on paper Balances 4 blocks Performs simple household tasks Later may throw ball overhand	Urinalysis if not done earlier
HEALTH ASSESSMENT AT 3 YEARS			
Parental concerns Interval history Family and social history Height and weight; blood pressure Complete physical exam Vision screening Hearing screening Language screening (Denver Articulation Screening Examination [DASE]) Discussion of findings with parents	Review basic food groups and appropriate amounts for age Discuss proper snack foods Eating patterns are influenced by family members Discuss dental visit	Talks well, uses plurals Jumps, runs Pedals tricycle Washes and dries hands Separates from mother easily	Tuberculin skin test Urinalysis for girls Hemoglobin or hematocrit
HEALTH ASSESSMENT AT 4 YEARS			
Parental concerns Interval history Family and social history Height and weight; blood pressure Complete physical exam Vision screening Hearing screening Discussion of findings with parents Assess preschool readiness (PRESS)	Review basic food groups and appropriate amounts for age Continued need for iron-containing foods Avoidance of sugared snacks and drinks	Knows first and last names Copies circles and crosses Understands prepositions and opposites May dress self Separates from mother easily Heel-to-toe walk	Hematocrit and RBC indices Tuberculin skin test, if not done at 3 years
HEALTH ASSESSMENT AT 5 TO 10 YEARS			
Parental and client concerns Interval history: illnesses, injuries, major changes in lifestyle Review of systems Family and social history Weight, height, blood pressure, pulse, and respiration Complete physical exam Discussion of findings with parents and client Screening: visual acuity and audiogram, language (DASE)	Basic food groups: milk, 3 servings; meat (including poultry, fish, eggs, peanut butter, dried beans), 4 servings; fruits, vegetables, 4 servings; breads, cereals, 4 servings Food likes and dislikes Types of food used for snacking Sugar intake Other considerations: milk fortified with vitamin D; iodized salt; whole grain or enriched breads and cereals; evaluate calcium, fluoride, iron source	5 to 6 years: balance on one foot for 10 seconds; backward heel-to-toe walk; draws person with more than 6 parts; performs self-care activities 6 to 9 years: latency period of physical and psychological growth; questions about sex and conception 9 to 11 years: concrete thinking continues; judges thoughts only in reference to own experience, learns by trial and error	DTP and trivalent OPV boosters are given between 4 and 6 years of age Tuberculin testing every 3 years Routine urinalysis and complete blood count if not done within the last 3 years

Health assessment for nurse-family encounters: selected ages—cont'd

Health history physical exam	Nutrition	Development	Commonly recommended laboratory procedures and immunizations
HEALTH ASSESSMENT AT 5 TO 10 YEARS—cont'd	Discuss preventive dental care	Beginning growth spurt: females at approximately 9½ years and males at approximately 10½ years Females: beginning growth of pubic hair and breast budding; tomboy activities Males: male-dominated social activity	
HEALTH ASSESSMENT AT 11 TO 14 YEARS			
Past history: birth, maternal medications during pregnancy, developmental milestones, illnesses, injuries, immunizations, communicable diseases, family history Present history: client and parental concerns, history of current concern, nutrition; social: relationships with peers, school marks, social interests, future goals, sexual information and activity Review of systems Complete physical exam is done including weight, height, blood pressure, pulse, and respiration; pelvic exam if indicated Screening: visual acuity and audiogram	Eating habits: number of regular meals a day, snacking pattern and types of food; use of crash diets, fasting, food fads; source of protein and iron; knowledge of balanced food choices; availability of nutritious snacking foods Discuss need for continued dental care	Hormonal influences: as a defense mechanism against changing body image there are increased somatic complaints Males: beginning growth of pubic hair, enlargement of testicles; wet dreams Females: continued breast development, growth of axillary and pubic hair Thought process: beginning of abstract thinking to manipulate concepts outside of own experience; self-centered (egocentrism); feelings of autonomy, mood swings, antisocial behavior Family: negativism as a manifestation of rejection of parents' values and seeking own identity, testing of parental controls, beginning emancipation from family Peers: importance of peer group for psychologic support and social development	Td and TOPV boosters TB test Routine urinalysis Complete blood count (CBC) Rubella titer (females) VDRL Pap smear and gonorrhea cervical culture if sexually active (females) Sickle cell screening if indicated
HEALTH ASSESSMENT AT 15 TO 18 YEARS			
Health history Complete physical exam is done including weight, height, blood pressure, pulse, and respiration; pelvic exam if indicated	Basic food groups Eating habits Continued dental care	Hormonal influences: continued development of secondary sexual characteristics Males: increased size of penis, testes, scrotum;	Td and OPV boosters if not given within the last 10 years Routine urinalysis and CBC if not done within the last 3 years

A3—HEALTH ASSESSMENT FOR NURSE-FAMILY ENCOUNTERS: SELECTED AGES—cont'd

Health history physical exam	Nutrition	Development	Commonly recommended laboratory procedures and immunizations
HEALTH ASSESSMENT AT 15 TO 18 YEARS—cont'd Screening: visual acuity and audiogram		growth of body hair; voice and skin changes Females: enlarged breasts, broadened pelvic bones, growth of body hair, menstruation Thought process: use of formal logic in solving problems; feelings and goals directed away from self toward idealistic causes; future goals become more clear Family: movement away from family into own relationships and activities; views family's morals and culture with criticism because of idealism Peers: regular group social activity and/or individual dating	Rubella titer (females) VDRL Pap smear and gonorrhea cervical culture if sexually active (females) Sickle cell screening if indicated

A4—DIET HISTORY QUESTIONNAIRE FOR INFANTS THROUGH TEENAGERS*

Questionnaire I—Infants (Birth to 1 Year)

Date _____ Age _____

Name _____ Birth date _____

Please answer the following questions by checking the appropriate box or filling in the blank. Answer only those questions that apply to you or your child. All information is confidential.

1. Is the baby breast fed?   Yes ___ No ___
   If yes, does he/she also receive milk or formula?
   Yes ___ No ___
   If yes, what kind? _____
2. Does the baby receive formula?   Yes ___ No ___
   If yes: Ready-to-feed   ___
   Concentrated liquid ___
   Powdered   ___
   Evaporated milk   ___
   Other _____
   How is formula prepared? _____
   Is the formula iron fortified? _____
   Yes ___ No ___
   Don't know ___

3. Does the baby drink milk?   Yes ___ No ___
   If yes: Whole milk ___
   2% milk ___
   Skim milk ___
   Other _____
4. Does the baby drink any fluids other than milk or formula?
   Yes ___ No ___
   If yes, what? _____
5. How many times does the baby eat each day, including milk or formula feedings? _____
6. Does the baby usually take a bottle to bed?
   Yes ___ No ___
   If yes, what is usually in the bottle? _____
7. If the baby drinks milk or formula, what is the usual amount in a day?
   Less than 16 oz (2 cups)   ___
   16 to 32 oz   ___
   More than 32 oz (1 quart) ___
8. Does the baby take vitamin or iron drops?
   Yes ___ No ___
   If yes, how often? ___ What kind? _____
9. Is the baby on a special diet now? Yes ___ No ___
   If yes: Allergy   ___
   Weight reduction ___
   Other _____
   Who recommended the diet? _____
10. Does the baby eat clay, paint chips, dirt, paper, or anything else that is not considered food?
    Yes ___ No ___
    If yes, what? _____ How often? _____

*From Bureau of Maternal and Child Health/Nutrition: Diet history questionnaire for infants, Washington, D.C., 1978.

11. Do you think the child has a feeding problem?
Yes ___ No ___
If yes, describe _____
12. Who usually feeds the baby? _____
Does the person have the use of:
Working stove ___
Refrigerator   ___
Piped water   ___
13. Does the family participate in:
Food stamp program   Yes ___ No ___
WIC program   Yes ___ No ___
Day care food program Yes ___ No ___
14. Please check which, if any, of the following foods the baby eats and how often.

	LESS THAN ONCE A WEEK	NOT DAILY BUT AT LEAST ONCE A WEEK	EVERY DAY OR NEARLY EVERY DAY
Cheese, yogurt, ice cream, pudding	___	___	___
Milk or formula	___	___	___
Eggs	___	___	___
Dried beans, peas, peanut butter, nuts	___	___	___
Meat, fish, poultry, wild game	___	___	___
Bread, rice, grits, cereal, tortillas, noodles, spaghetti	___	___	___
Fruits or fruit juices	___	___	___
Vegetables (including potatoes)	___	___	___
Candy, desserts, sweets	___	___	___

15. If the baby eats fruits or drinks fruit juices every day or nearly every day, which ones does he/she eat or drink most often (not more than three)?

_____ _____ _____

16. If the baby eats vegetables every day or nearly every day, which ones does he/she eat most often (not more than three)?

_____ _____ _____

17. Does the baby eat:
Sticky or sweet foods? Yes ___ No ___
Salty foods?   Yes ___ No ___
If yes, what are the foods? _____
_____
Is salt added to the baby's food? Yes ___ No ___
18. Below list the foods and beverages the baby has had during the last 24 hours.

Time	Food eaten	Amount	How is this food prepared?

Questionnaire II—Preschool and Young School-Age Child (Guardian Responds)

Date _____ Age _____
Name _____ Birth date _____

Please answer the following questions by checking the appropriate box or filling in the blank. Answer only those questions that apply to you or your child. All information is confidential.

1. Does the child drink milk? Yes ___ No ___
If yes: Whole milk ___
        2% milk   ___
        Skim milk ___
        Other _____
If yes: Less than 8 oz (1 cup) ___
        8-32 oz   ___
        More than 32 oz (1 qt) ___
2. Does the child drink anything from a bottle?
Yes ___ No ___
If yes: Milk ___
        Other _____
Does the child take a bottle to bed? Yes ___ No ___
If yes, what is usually in the bottle?
_____
3. How many times a day does the child usually eat, including snacks? _____
Does the child eat anything after he/she has gone to bed?
Yes ___ No ___
If yes, what? _____
4. Does the child take vitamins or iron?
Yes ___ No ___
If yes, how often? _____
What kind? _____
5. Is the child on a special diet now? Yes ___ No ___
If yes: Allergy   ___
        Weight reduction ___
        Other _____
Who recommended the diet? _____
6. Does the child eat clay, paint chips, dirt, paper, or anything else not usually considered food?
Yes ___ No ___
If yes, what? _____ How often? _____
7. How would you describe the child's appetite?
Good ___
Fair ___
Poor ___
Other (specify) _____
8. Who usually feeds the child? _____
Does this person have use of:
Working stove ___
Refrigerator   ___
Piped water   ___
9. Does the family participate in:
Food stamp program   Yes ___ No ___
WIC program   Yes ___ No ___
Does the child participate in:
School breakfast   Yes ___ No ___
School lunch   Yes ___ No ___
Day care food program Yes ___ No ___
Summer food program   Yes ___ No ___
10. Please check which, if any, of the following foods the child eats and how often.

	LESS THAN ONCE A WEEK	NOT DAILY BUT AT LEAST ONCE A WEEK	EVERY DAY OR NEARLY EVERY DAY
Cheese, yogurt, ice cream, pudding	—	—	—
Milk	—	—	—
Eggs	—	—	—
Dried beans, peas, peanut butter, nuts	—	—	—
Meat, fish, poultry, wild game	—	—	—
Bread, rice, grits, cereal, tortillas, noodles, spaghetti	—	—	—
Fruits or fruit juices	—	—	—
Vegetables (including potatoes)	—	—	—
Candy, desserts, sweets	—	—	—

11. If the child eats fruits or drinks fruit juices every day or nearly every day, which ones does he/she eat or drink most often (not more than three)?

_____   _____   _____

12. If the child eats vegetables every day or nearly every day, which ones does he/she eat most often (not more than three)?

_____   _____   _____

13. Does the child usually eat between meals?
Yes ___ No ___
If yes, name the two or three snacks (including bedtime snacks) that the child has most often.

_____   _____   _____

14. Does the child eat:
Sticky or sweet foods?   Yes ___ No ___
Salty foods?   Yes ___ No ___
If yes, what are the foods? _____

_____
Is salt added to the child's food?   Yes ___ No ___

15. Below list the foods and beverages the child has had in the last 24 hours.

Time	Food eaten	Amount	How is this food prepared?

Questionnaire III—School-Age Child and Teenager

Date _____   Age _____
Name _____   Birth date _____

Please answer the following questions by checking the appropriate box or filling in the blank. Answer only those questions that apply to you or your child. All information is confidential.

1. Do you drink milk?   Yes ___ No ___
If yes: Whole milk ___
        2% milk   ___
        Skim milk ___
        Other _____
How often? _____
Are there other beverages you often drink?
Yes ___ No ___
If yes, what? _____

2. How many times a day do you eat, including snacks?

3. Do you take vitamins or iron?   Yes ___ No ___
If yes, how often? _____ What kind? _____

4. Are you on a special diet?   Yes ___ No ___
If yes: Allergy   ___
        Weight reduction ___
        Other _____
Who recommended the diet? _____

5. Do you eat clay, paint chips, dirt, paper, or anything else not usually considered food?   Yes ___ No ___
If yes, what? _____ How often? _____

6. Does anyone in your household participate in:
Food stamp program   Yes ___ No ___
WIC program   Yes ___ No ___
Do you participate in:
School breakfast   Yes ___ No ___
School lunch   Yes ___ No ___
Summer food program   Yes ___ No ___

7. Who usually prepares your meals? _____
Does this person have use of:
Working stove ___
Refrigerator ___
Piped water   ___

8. Do you eat any:
Sticky or sweet foods?   Yes ___ No ___
Salty foods?   Yes ___ No ___
Do you add salt to your food?   Yes ___ No ___

9. Please check which of the following foods you eat and how often:

	LESS THAN ONCE A WEEK	NOT DAILY BUT AT LEAST ONCE A WEEK	EVERY DAY OR NEARLY EVERY DAY
Cheese, yogurt, ice cream, pudding	—	—	—
Milk	—	—	—
Eggs	—	—	—
Dried beans, peas, peanut butter, nuts	—	—	—
Meat, fish, poultry, wild game	—	—	—
Bread, rice, grits, cereal, tortillas, noodles, spaghetti	—	—	—
Fruits or fruit juices	—	—	—
Vegetables (including potatoes)	—	—	—
Candy, desserts, sweets	—	—	—

10. If you eat fruits or drink fruit juices every day or nearly every day, which ones do you eat or drink most often (not more than three)?

_____   _____   _____

11. If you eat vegetables every day or nearly every day, which ones do you eat most often (not more than three)?

_____   _____   _____

12. Do you usually eat anything between meals?

Yes ___ No ___

If yes, name the two or three snacks (including bedtime snacks) that you have most often.

_____   _____   _____

13. Below list the foods and beverages you have had in the last 24 hours.

Time	Food eaten	Amount	How is this food prepared?

A5—NEEDS SATISFACTION SCALE FOR INDIVIDUALS WITH A DISABILITY

Section A: Demographic Data

Name _____
Address _____
Telephone _____
Social Security no. _____

Age _____   Birth date ____ ____ ____
           Month Day Year

Sex ___ F ___ M
Date of interview _____
Primary disability _____
Secondary disabilities _____

Marital status
___ Married
___ Separated
___ Widowed
___ Never married
___ Divorced
___ Marriage annulled

Education
___ None
___ 1-5 grade
___ 6-8 grade
___ 9-12
___ High school graduate
___ Vocational-technical without licensure/certification
___ Vocational-technical with licensure/certification
___ Attended college 1-2 years
___ Attended college 3-4 years
___ 4-year college degree
___ Graduate degree (master's)
___ Graduate degree (doctorate)

Number of dependents
___ Self only
___ 1
___ 2
___ 3
___ 4
___ 5 or more

Heritage
___ Afro-American
___ Caucasian
___ American Indian
___ Asian
___ Pacific Islander
___ Spanish
___ Other

Living arrangement
___ Living alone
___ Living with spouse
___ Living with one or both parents (including stepparents)
___ Living with nonrelatives
___ Living with other relatives
___ Other

Names and relationships of household members

_____
_____
_____
_____
_____
_____
_____

Military status
___ Previous military service
___ Currently in the military
___ Never in the military

Income sources
___ Earnings
___ Interest
___ Rent
___ Dividends
___ Private insurance, disability benefits
___ Family
___ Friends
___ Private agency
___ Annuities
___ Public assistance, state
___ Workman's Compensation
___ Social Security
___ Public assistance, federal

Income category
___ $0-3,000
___ $3,100-6,000
___ $6,100-9,000
___ $9,100-12,000
___ $12,100-15,000
___ $15,000-18,000
___ $18,100-21,000
___ $21,100-24,000
___ Above $24,000

Work status
___ Employed outside the home
 ___ Competitive labor market
 ___ Sheltered workshop
___ Employed, home
___ Unemployed
___ Self-employed, home
___ Self-employed, outside home
___ Homemaker
___ Student
___ Retired

Previous occupation
___ Professional
___ Technical
___ Laborer
___ Semiprofessional
___ Nontechnical

Currently under the services of
___ Vocational Rehabilitation Services
 ___ Regular
 ___ Homebound
___ Medicaid
___ Medicare
___ Crippled Children's Service

Source of transportation
___ Private automobile   ___ Public
___ Private van, specially   ___ None
    equipped

Main care giver
___ Self   ___ Full-time attendant
___ Family member   ___ Part-time attendant

My birth order position is _____
                                        (rank)

in a family of _____
            (total no. of children)

Sexes of children in the family are: M ___   F ___
                                         (no.)   (no.)

Functional abilities	Yes	No	N/A
Dress self			
Feed self, unassisted			
Feed self with assistance			
Brush teeth			
Comb hair			
Self-help, bowel elimination			
Self-help, bladder elimination			
Bathe self			
Walk			
Other independent mobility			

Section B: Satisfaction of Needs

Directions: Please choose the response that most nearly describes your answer to the question regarding your present needs.

Basic physiological needs
1. My current state of health is ___ Poor ___ Fair
                                        1   2

   ___ Satisfactory ___ Good ___ Excellent
     3   4   5

2. Rate each of the following health needs on a scale from 1 to 5 (1—extremely problematic, 2—somewhat problematic, 3—controlled problem, 4—inactive problem, 5—no problem).

	1	2	3	4	5
a. Vision					
b. Hearing					
c. Mobility					
d. Respirations					
e. Sleep					
f. Anxiety; depression					
g. Energy level					
h. Nutrition—food intake					
i. Nutrition—fluid intake					
j. Bowel elimination					
k. Bladder elimination					
l. Exercise					
m. Recreation, play					
n. Sexual libido					

Rate the following items on a scale from 1 to 5 (1—never, 2—hardly ever, 3—sometimes, 4—often, 5—almost all the time).

	1	2	3	4	5
3. I drink 2000-3000 cc of fluid per day.					
4. I eat a well-balanced diet.					
5. I take vitamins as prescribed.					
6. I avoid smoking cigarettes, cigars, and pipes.					
7. I drink alcoholic beverages only as prescribed.					
8. I take prescribed medicines.					
9. I take patent medicines only as directed by my physician.					
10. I have ROM or other exercises daily.					
11. I get 6-8 hours sleep minimum daily.					
12. I take rest periods during the day.					
13. I experience a high energy level.					
14. My bowel elimination habits are satisfactory.					
15. My urinary elimination habits are satisfactory.					
16. I keep my immunizations up to date.					
17. I practice regular dental care daily.					
18. I watch myself for signs of cancer.					
19. I have visual examinations as suggested by physician.					
20. I am able to relax.					
21. I take special measures to conserve my health.					
22. I do not object to having to take special measures to conserve my health.					
23. I do not object to giving up things I like for the sake of my health.					
24. I am confident I can meet my future health needs.					

Need for security

	1	2	3	4	5
25. I am secure about my physical safety in my home environment.					
26. I feel secure about special precautions I take regarding physical safety.					
27. I feel secure about my financial position.					
28. I feel secure about meeting the expenses of my routine medicine and supplies.					

	1	2	3	4	5

29. I feel satisfied about my transportation plans.
30. I am satisfied about long-term plans for my care.
31. I am satisfied with my present vocational/occupational status.

Need for love and belongingness

32. I am satisfied with the amount of love from family.
33. I am satisfied with the amount of love from friends.
34. I cope satisfactorily with stress in the home life.
35. I cope satisfactorily with stress in other aspects of life.
36. I am satisfied with my level of social effectiveness.
37. I am satisfied with my social participation.
38. I am comfortable asking for help when needed.
39. I am satisfied with the amount of religion in my life.
40. I am satisfied with family activities and traditions in which I participate.
41. I am satisfied with my role in the family.
42. I am satisfied with my level of sexual fulfillment.
43. I am satisfied with my level of knowledge about human sexuality.
44. I am satisfied with the feelings of love and belongingness I receive from others.
45. I am satisfied with the amount of love and affection I give to others.
46. I have get-togethers with friends my own age.

Need for self-esteem

47. I am satisfied with the appearance of my body.
48. I am satisfied with my intellectual functioning.
49. I am satisfied with the kind of characteristics that could be said to describe me.
50. I am satisfied with past accomplishments in my life.
51. I am satisfied with present accomplishments in my life.
52. My predominant emotional state is happy and content.
53. I am satisfied with my level of education/occupation.

Need for self-actualization

54. I am satisfied with my state of fulfillment.

	1	2	3	4	5

55. I am satisfied with the amount of enjoyment in my everyday life.
56. I make plans to increase my level of fulfillment.
57. I am optimistic about my potential to reach higher life.
58. I am satisfied with task accomplishment in my present life.
59. I am satisfied with my own motivational level.
60. I am satisfied with motivational level of family and friends to support my goals.
61. I am satisfied with amount of responsibilities I have in life.
62. I am satisfied with the amount of spontaneity in life.
63. I have a satisfactory level of hope in my life.
64. I have new interests in life.
65. I am satisfied with the amount of meaning and purpose in my life.
66. I am reconciled to the change in my life-style from the disability I have.
67. I am satisfied with my coping reaction to suffering.
68. I am satisfied with amount of strength (courage) I have now.

Needs	Client score	Possible score	Percentage
Basic physiological		185	
Security		35	
Love and belonging- ness		75	
Self-esteem		35	
Self-actualization		75	
TOTALS		405	

A6—PERSONAL INVENTORY TOOL

The reader is encouraged to respond to the following questions while reading Chapter 29.

Initial Assessment

When did you last have fun?
What do you do for fun and relaxation?
What do you do for play?
When did you last have a deep, satisfying laugh (not a giggle)?
If you had no demands nor constraints on you, how do you think you would spend a day? A week? A month? A year? The rest of your life?
Consider the amount of time you spend daily in work, in rest, and in recreation. Does each factor receive about one-third of your day on an average? If not, why not?

Were you satisfied with your responses? Do you believe that a relationship exists between your responses and your or your family's health status? Consider this question for a few minutes.

Continuing Assessment

1. How do your responses to the initial personal assessment compare with the four concepts—freedom, lack of pressure or coercion, meaning and satisfaction from an activity, and involvement—set forth by Neulinger?
2. How do you like to use your leisure time?
3. How did you enter into the spirit of last Christmas? Last Halloween? Last Fourth of July? Your local festival? Were you able to enjoy, be free, and obtain meaning and satisfaction from a change of pace? Were you able to separate the societal demands of how to celebrate from how you personally found meaning and satisfaction? How did you feel about yourself and your life after the festivities were officially over?
4. How do your responses to the initial personal assessment questions compare with the four dimensions identified by Godbey? What dimensions may need your reconsideration?
5. Identify your recreation patterns. Are you a participant or a spectator? How do you feel during and after the activity—physically, mentally, and spiritually?
6. What leisure and recreational opportunities are available in your community for all income levels? Is the potential for interaction between levels available?
7. How do you play? Do you allow yourself to engage in activities that are pleasurable, spontaneous, nonproductive? Do you have friends with whom you grew up? How did the friendship begin and how has each of each of you contributed to its maintenance?
8. If you are single, have you experienced the phenomena of being treated as an extra, an outsider, a threat? If you have a mate/family, are you aware of holding this perception of singles?
9. Reconsider your leisure and recreational patterns. What and when was your last satisfying and meaningful leisure experience?
10. How extensive is your social network? How is this reflected in your leisure and recreational patterns?
11. Into which theory (spillover, compensator, or neutrality) does your leisure and recreation pattern fit? Why? Would you want to change it?
12. Go through the Yellow Pages section of your telephone book. How many treatment sites for alcohol or drug abuse are listed in your telephone book or your social services directory?
13. If your local newspaper lists self-help groups, how many are functioning in your community?
14. In considering the psychological impact of leisure and recreation, think how you feel after playing a game of baseball, after jogging or running, after a quiet walk in the woods.
15. Consider your family as you were growing up. What is the relationship between what you experienced as a family member and your leisure and recreational philosophy and practices today?
16. In what activities do you and your family engage that are individual, joint, and parallel?

Individual _____
 _____
 _____

Joint _____
 _____
 _____

Parallel _____
 _____
 _____

17. In terms of Otto's 10 family strengths' characteristics, how do you and your family rate?
18. Considering the concepts of freedom, prevention, family, and health/wellness, how did the concepts relate to your adolescence? If you have adolescent children at home or in the neighborhood, consider your experiences with them in light of these concepts.

Your Personal Inventory Revisited

You have been given the opportunity to assess your personal beliefs and practices in leisure and recreation. As with health promotion and other activities important to a community health nurse, you must know what you do and why you do it before initiating help for others. Serving as a role model extends also into the area of leisure and recreation.

Now that you have actively participated in using the theories and concepts discussed relative to leisure and recreation, how did you rate? Are you an interested, interesting, vital, stimulating person?

Do you believe you must expand your interest areas and your recreational skills? Do you want to expand your interests and skills?

Do you have adequate knowledge and skills in a variety of leisure activities to assist an individual or family to broaden their horizons?

Can you participate in a planning and policy group for leisure and recreation?

Can you recommend good books in a variety of subjects; for example, fiction, non-fiction, gardening, travel, sports, various crafts, and self-help books?

Do you have some knowledge about the multitude of periodicals focusing on recreational interests that are readily available?

Do you know of resources in your city, town, or neighborhood that you can refer an individual or family to for learning more about their particular interests?

What are the recreational programs sponsored by the local government? Where are they held? Who leads them? How are the program topics selected? What is the cost? Who is and who is not welcome to come?

A7—HISTORY-TAKING QUESTIONS: RECREATIONAL ACTIVITIES

The following questions may be used in a health assessment to identify type and extent of recreational activity.

1. In what activities do you participate that involve a risk to you physically, emotionally, or socially? Describe the health risk.
2. In what activities do you participate that would involve no risk to you physically, emotionally, or socially?
3. In what activities do you participate that you believe promote or protect your health? Why do you believe the activity(ies) are promoting or protecting your health?
4. What activities do you enjoy alone?
5. What activities do you enjoy with other people? Who? With other living creatures?

Interpretation: Identify the active and passive involvement in leisure and recreational activities. What are detriments to the client's health? What are promotors or protectors of the client's health?

What activities should the community health nurse encourage or discourage? What is identified by the client and the community health nurse as facilitators and barriers to increased participation in recreational activities?

A8—CLASSROOM OBSERVATION SHEET*

Teacher _____ Grade ____ Date _____

Please list the names of pupils with known or suspected health problems. These problems will be discussed during the teacher-nurse conferences.

The following are conditions to record (but not limited to these):

1. Hearing problems (speaks louder than normal; turns head in direction of sound)
2. Speech problems (stuttering, lisping, difficult to understand)
3. Limited physical education
4. Dental problems (decayed teeth, missing teeth, toothache)
5. Fatigue, listlessness, inattentiveness
6. Under medical care of private physician or outpatient clinic facility
7. Vision problems (squinting, reading problems)
8. Orthopedic problems (toeing in, bowlegged, knock-kneed)
9. Allergy (hay fever), red eyes, black to bluish discoloration under eyelids
10. Extreme nervousness (constantly in motion, cries easily, irritable)
11. Known diseases such as diabetes, epilepsy, heart problems
12. Nutritional status (children who appear unusually hungry, nonbreakfast eaters)
13. Personal hygiene (more than one observation)
14. Attendance problems related to illness
15. Respiratory problems (bronchitis, asthma)

Name	Remarks	Under care of (physician, dentist, nurse practitioner)

*Modified from Bryan, D.: School nursing in transition, St. Louis, 1973, The C.V. Mosby Co.
To be used with the classroom assessment by nurse and teacher, during nurse-teacher conference (planned or unplanned), or by classroom teacher.

B1—FAMILY HEALTH CARE PLAN*

Goal: To reduce the risk of hypertension in the family

Objectives

To reduce by ⅓ to ½ the salt (sodium) intake of both family members within 5 weeks

Target activities
a. Will use only ½ as much salt in cooking at once
b. In 1 week will no longer add salt to foods at the table
c. Will increase by 50% the use of herbs, spices, and lemon in cooking in place of salt by the end of 1 week
d. Will avoid snack foods with visible salt by end of 1 week
e. Will avoid all foods prepared in brine (e.g., ham, bacon, pickles) within 2 weeks
f. Will stop drinking carbonated beverages within 3 weeks
g. Will start using salt (sodium)-free vegetables (fresh, frozen, canned) after present canned vegetable supply is depleted

Formative Evaluation

Family and community health nurse together measure progress made toward accomplishing target activities at check points.
At end of week 1 measure the following
Progress toward meeting target activities *a, b, c,* and *d*
Problems encountered meeting target activities
FINDING
Husband having difficulty meeting target activity *b*
PLAN
Objective *b* modified from 1 week to 2 weeks
Plan developed for a health counseling visit
At end of week 2 measure the following
Progress made toward meeting activity *e*
Husband's progress toward meeting activity *b*
Continuing ability to meet activities *a, b* (wife), and *d*
At end of week 3 measure the following
Progress made toward meeting activity *f*
Continuing ability to meet all other activities except *g* (because of canned vegetable supply on hand)
At end of week 4 measure the following
Continuing ability to meet activities

Summative Evaluation

Conducted by family and community health nurse at time when care plan fully implemented and executed. Measures extent to which the objective and target activities were met at end of 5 weeks. Also examine problems encountered in meeting target activities.

---

*Sample of an approach to a health care plan for a family consisting of a middle-aged husband and wife. The family health care plan is completed by adding objectives and target activities regarding stress, weight, and exercise.

B2—FAMILY–COMMUNITY HEALTH NURSE CONTRACT

Family health situation: Family members at high risk for hypertension.
Goal: To increase the family's knowledge about hypertension and low-sodium foods

FAMILY RESPONSIBILITIES (HUSBAND AND WIFE)	NURSE'S RESPONSIBILITIES
1. Demonstrate increased knowledge about hypertension Explain (from a lay perspective) the physiology of hypertension and attending risks Explain the relationship between preventive measures and reducing the risk of hypertension	1. Provide information to family about hypertension Provide reading materials about hypertension and related self-care Counsel with the family regarding the physiology and risks associated with hypertension; describe preventive measures (e.g., life-style changes)
2. Demonstrate increased knowledge about low-sodium foods Able to list common high-sodium and low-sodium foods Modifies food purchasing habits so more low-sodium foods included and more high-sodium foods excluded Uses low-sodium recipes Increasingly uses low-sodium menus	2. Provide information to family about low-sodium foods: Provide lists of high-sodium and low-sodium foods Provide low-sodium recipes and menus congruent with family's resources and life-style

Length of contract _____
Date started _____ Date concluded _____
Evaluation plan _____
_____

We mutually agree to the above goal and responsibilities. This contract may be renegotiated if it becomes necessary to do so.

Signatures:
Family members _____ Date _____
_____ Date _____
Community _____ Date _____
health nurse

B3—FAMILY HEALTH ASSESSMENT GUIDE

General instructions: Content areas of the guide should be modified and adapted as appropriate for individual families and the circumstances of the family and/or community health nurse contact(s). The factors listed for many of the major family assessment areas are examples and should be added to or omitted as necessary.

Family Unit
Family Composition (see accompanying box)

Extended family (e.g., parents, children, and other relatives outside of household)
    Relationship
    Place of residency
    Frequency of contact
Residential history
    Length of time at present address
    Frequency of residential and geographical changes
Education of family member (present and/or highest level attained)
    Educational level
    Attending school/college
    Educational goal
Vocational interests of family member
    Interest
    Goal
Avocational interests of family member (hobbies, other creative endeavors)
    Interest
    Goal
Occupation of family member
    Type of work
    Hours of work
    Satisfaction with job
    Goal(s)
Financial resources
    Sources (e.g., salaries, pension, and public assistance)
    Total income
    Distribution of income (e.g., housing, food, clothing, health/illness care, utilities, recreation, and insurance)
    Adequacy of income
Religious practices of family members
    Religious preferences
    Extent of involvement
    Relative importance of religion in everyday life (e.g., influence on activities of daily living and relationships)
Rituals
    Holidays and celebrations related to activities of daily living
Recreational interests of family members
    Interests around home (alone and with family)
    Interests outside home (alone and with family)
    Activities with relatives
    With friends
    With community groups

What does the family do for "fun" around home? Outside of home?

Family Environment
Residence

Housing
    Type of dwelling
    Number and types of rooms
    General condition
Furnishings
    Condition
    Adequacy
Living space
    Adequate for family size
    Privacy for family members
Sleeping arrangements
    Where members sleep
    Sharing of bed(s)
    Adequacy of sleeping arrangements
Bathroom facilities
    Location
    Adequacy
    Sanitation
Food preparation arrangements
    Cleanliness
    Cooking
    Refrigeration
Eating arrangements and mealtime environment
General state of cleanliness and sanitation
Adequacy of
    Water supply and source
    Waste/garbage disposal
    Lighting
    Heating and cooling
    Ventilation
    Laundry facilities
    Telephone
Condition of yard
Pets
    Number
    Kinds
    Care
Automobile
    Number
    Conditions
Provisions for emergencies
    Smoke alarm
    Emergency numbers by telephone
Environmental stressors
    Noise
    Lack of individual territory

Family member	Age	Sex	Ethnicity/race	Family position (e.g., mother, spouse)	Special status (e.g., adopted, single, divorced)
_____	__	__	_____	_____	_____
_____	__	__	_____	_____	_____
_____	__	__	_____	_____	_____

Environmental hazards
    Storage of medicines and household cleaners/poisons
    Sharp tools
    Fire dangers
    Unsafe toys
    Loose rugs
    Clutter
    Swimming pool
Family attitudes toward home, neighborhood, and community

Goals for Future
Neighborhood

Type
    Residential
    Semicommercial
    Urban/nonmetropolitan
Dwellings
    Single-family house
    Apartment
    Combination
Age of area
    Newly constructed
    Deteriorating
    Foliage (trees, shrubbery)
Sociocultural characteristics
    Age composition
    Ethnic groups
    Employment/unemployment
General condition of structures, yards, streets, alleys, etc.
Traffic patterns
Efficiency of street lighting systems
Availability of fire hydrants
Resources
    Shopping
    Transportation
    Recreational
    Educational
    Religious
    Protective services
    Health/illness
    Emergency
    Human services
    Business
    Garbage/refuse disposal
Environmental stressors
    Noise
    Crime rate
    Substance abuse
    Crowding
    Poverty
Environmental hazards
    Air pollution
    Garbage/debris
    Traffic flow
    Unsafe play areas
In-migration and out-migration of residents
Neighbors' attitude toward the family
Family's involvement in the neighborhood

Community

Leadership and government
Resources (essentially the same as those listed for neighborhood)
Occupations, industries, businesses

Family's involvement in the community
    Community memberships
    Interaction with social institutions
    Use of resources

Family Structure

Organization
    As a system
    Subsystems
Roles
    Roles being filled
    Satisfaction/dissatisfaction with role(s)
    Level of role functioning
    Perceptions about roles
    Acceptance of roles
    Flexibility of roles/interchangeable
Socialization processes for roles
Division of labor
    How is delegation of tasks determined?
    Who carries out which tasks?
    What is the flexibility of task responsibilities?
    What is the extent of satisfaction/dissatisfaction with task delegation and performance?
Authority and power
    Degree of autonomy for each family member
    Locus of authority
    Power relationships
    How authority is exercised
    How power is demonstrated
    Satisfaction/dissatisfaction with autonomy, authority, and power in family
Values, attitudes, and beliefs regarding family organization, roles, division of labor, autonomy, authority, and power
Stresses related to family organization, roles, division of labor, autonomy, authority, and power—how handled?

Family Processes
Communication

Patterns
    Ways used to communicate effectively
    Content of communications
    Interpretation of content
    Linguistic characteristics (cultural)
    Frequency of communications
    How do joy, love, anger, sadness, frustration get communicated?
    Communication patterns within family subsystems
    Effectiveness of communications—understood, clear, consistent, etc.
Satisfaction/dissatisfaction with family communication patterns
Values, attitudes and beliefs regarding family communications
Stresses related to family communications

Decision Making

How are decisions made?
    What is the process?
Who makes decisions affecting adults?
    Children?
    Entire group?
How are decisions implemented?
How are decision-making skills learned in the family?
Satisfaction/dissatisfaction with family decision-making process
Values, attitudes, and beliefs regarding family decision making
Stresses related to family decision making

Problem Solving

How are problems handled?
  What is the process?
Who is involved in the problem-solving process?
  Who provides leadership in the process?
Extent to which family can deal with problem solving and for
  what types of problems
Flexibility in approaches to problem solving
Ability to use information from outside family in problem-solving
  process
Satisfaction/dissatisfaction with family's problem-solving ability
  and process
Values, attitudes, and beliefs regarding family's problem solving
Stresses related to family problem solving

Family Functions
Physical

How are needs for food, shelter, clothing, etc., met?
Are physical needs being met satisfactorily? If not, what solutions
  have been tried by the family?
Values, attitudes, and beliefs regarding family's physical needs
  and functions
Stresses related to meeting family's physical needs

Emotional

Affectional relationships
  Between adults
  Between adults and children
  Between siblings
Ways of obtaining and giving emotional support: distribution of
  support, when given, how given, acceptance by other family
  member(s)
Ways in which family members do or do not assist each other in
  developing self-esteem
  In developing autonomy
How do family members show respect for each other?
To what extent and how is intimacy expressed?
  Physical affection and companionship?
Satisfaction/dissatisfaction regarding how family's emotional
  needs are met
Values, attitudes, and beliefs regarding family's emotional needs
  and functions
Stresses related to family's emotional functions

Social

Goals for family and individual family members
Support for individual creativity, initiative, and leadership
Process for developing and supporting family and individual lead-
  ership
Process for strengthening family members' competency regarding
  adjustment in social organizations (e.g., school)
Competency regarding appropriate use of social organizations
Seeking new experiences—kind, etc.
Discipline and limit-setting practices
Individual developmental tasks (physical, affective, intellectual,
  language, psychosocial, sexual, moral, personality)
  Level of knowledge
  Seeks information as needed
  Provides support
  Seeks support resources as needed
  Adopts socialization approaches to meet individual needs and
    tasks
Family developmental tasks
  Level of knowledge

Seeks information as needed
Intrafamily support
Uses resources as needed
Satisfaction/dissatisfaction regarding social functions
Values, attitudes, and beliefs regarding social functions
Stresses related to social functions

Coping
Conflict

To what extent and how are conflicts expressed covertly and
  overtly?
Frequency of conflicts? Kinds? Attributed causes?
How are conflicts avoided? How are conflicts resolved?
Satisfaction/dissatisfaction regarding conflict resolution process
Values, attitudes, and beliefs regarding conflict resolution
Stresses related to conflicts and conflict resolution

Life Changes

Recent, present, and anticipated life changes
Impact of change(s) on family's functioning as a unit
Impact of change(s) on family roles and functions
Ability to cope with change(s): practices, behaviors, values, at-
  titudes, beliefs
Stresses associated with change(s)

Support Systems

Resources within family—what, how used, when, effectiveness
External support systems—how used, when, effectiveness
  Significant others (e.g., extended family members and friends)
  Nonprofessional organizations
  Professional systems
  Understand how to use—seek relevant information
  Availability, accessibility, use patterns
Satisfaction/dissatisfaction with support systems
Values, attitudes, and beliefs related to using support systems

Life Satisfaction

How does family feel about its quality of life?
What influences family's quality of life?
What influences the family's feelings about life?
Would the family like to change anything about its life? What?
  What impedes change?
What can family do? Others do?

Health Behavior
Health History

Genetic or familial diseases (e.g., diabetes, heart disease)
Family history of emotional problems, suicide, etc.
Past illnesses, operations, accidents, injuries
Present illnesses and/or physical discomforts
Use of prescribed and/or over-the-counter medications
Present symptoms such as anxiety, depression, etc.
Concerns about hearing, vision, speech
Recent history regarding physical and dental examinations, im-
  munizations, Pap smear, etc.

Health Status

Family's assessment of present health status
Concerns about present health status and/or potential health prob-
  lems
Family's perceptions of vulnerability to disease/illness
What does the family perceive as a health problem?

What present and potential health problems are identified by the family? Priorities for health problems?

What is family's belief about cause of problem(s)?

What is family's belief(s) about cure/treatment for problem(s)?

Activities of Daily Living

Eating patterns and foods

Personal hygiene and daily grooming

Physical activity

Sleeping behavior

Dental practices

What are family members' daily rhythms (e.g., morning person, night person)?

How does family describe a typical weekday? A weekend?

Risk Behaviors

Inadequate nutritional behavior (overeating; undereating; irregular meals; diet high in sugar, sodium; beverages high in caffeine)

Physical inactivity

Limited sleep or irregular sleeping patterns

Smoking

Use of alcohol

Nonuse of seat belts

Excessive exposure to stress situations (family, work, social)

Health Beliefs

How does family define health? Illness?

How does family define health and illness for each family member?

What value does family assign health? Health promotion? Prevention?

What are family's perceptions about cause(s) of illness?

What are family's perceptions about control over health and illness?

What are family's perceptions about how illness/disease are cured?

What are family's health goals?

How are values, attitudes, and beliefs regarding health promotion communicated to children? What is the socialization process? How does family members' involvement in the community influence family's health values, attitudes, and beliefs?

Self-care

Knowledge

Level of knowledge regarding health promotion, preventive measures, emergency care, causes and treatment of illnesses/diseases

How is health knowledge transmitted to family members?

What are sources of health information?

How does family assess its level of health knowledge?

What would family like to know about health promotion? Prevention? Illness care?

Practices

What does family do to protect its health (physical, emotional, social, spiritual)?

What does family do to improve its health status?

What does family do to prevent illness/disease?

What does family do to generate and support health protective behaviors in family members?

What does family do to care for health problems and illnesses in the home?

How are health and illness care responsibilities distributed in the family? Is there flexibility of family roles and tasks?

What are family's perceptions regarding ability to protect family's health?

How does family care for health problems and illnesses in the home?

What are the family's values, attitudes, and beliefs regarding self-care?

Family planning

Family's values, attitudes, and beliefs regarding family planning (e.g., methods, child spacing, childlessness, and appropriateness for which family members)

Decision-making process

Practices

Health Care Resources

Utilization practices regarding formal informal health and illness care systems (e.g., what systems and frequency of use)

Availability of emergency care resources

Availability, accessibility, and attractiveness of health and illness care resources

Effectiveness and efficiency with which family uses resources

How is health/illness care financed? What are other costs for family such as transportation and work time lost?

Family's knowledge about health and illness care resources

Family's perceptions of and attitudes about experiences with health/illness care resources and health care providers (e.g., nurses and physicians)

What are the family's feelings about the kinds of health services available to them in the community?

What kinds of health services would they like to receive?

What suggestions do they have about making any necessary changes in the delivery of services?

What are the family's feelings about health care providers?

What kind of relationship would the family like to have with health care providers?

What suggestions do they have about helping the health care providers to better meet the needs of the family?

Family's values and beliefs related to health/illness care resources and health care providers

Stresses related to use of health/illness care resources and interactions with health care providers

Community Health Nursing Services

Knowledge about community health nursing

Attitudes toward community health nursing services

Expectations of community health nursing services

Family Health Assessment Summary

Family's sociodemographic profile

Family's environment—strengths and problems regarding home, neighborhood, and community

Family structure, processes, functions—strengths and limitations; existing and/or potential problems

Family's coping profile

    Conflict management—strengths and limitations

    Life changes—strengths and limitations regarding coping with changes

    Support systems—strengths and limitations

    Life satisfaction profile

Family's health behavior profile

    Health history—existing and/or potential problems

    Health status—existing and/or potential problems

    Activities of daily living—strengths and limitations/problems

    Risk profile—for family unit and family members

    Health beliefs—profile of values, attitudes, and beliefs regarding health and illness

Self-care—strengths and limitations

Health care resources—adequacy of availability, accessibility, attractiveness, and use; general practices

Community health nursing services—attitudes and expectations

B4—FAMILY PROBLEM-SOLVING GUIDE

I. Types of family problems
   A. Problems that can be resolved by the family without the community health nurse
   B. Problems that can be resolved by the family with the community health nurse's assistance
   C. Problems that should be referred to another health care professional or other human services worker

II. Problem-solving process (family and community health nurse)
   A. Assessment of the problem
      1. Who identified problem—family, community health nurse, others?
      2. Extent of problem—is the problem a threat to the health and well-being of the family? An individual family member? Others? The community?
      3. Family's assessment of the problem—seriousness? Implications of the problem for the family? If family did not identify the problem, does the family view the situation as a problem?
      4. Community health nurse's assessment of the problem (using criteria regarding extent of problem)—if the problem is of a threatening nature but not recognized as a problem by the family, the nurse will need to assist the family to recognize and understand the implications of the problem
   B. Problem solving
      1. What is the history of the problem—when started, how started, why existing, effect on family?
      2. Is family attempting to resolve or handle problem?
         If yes
         How? How successful is approach? If approach is succeeding, support should be given to the family to continue its efforts.
         If approach is not successful, assist family to explore possible reasons for limited or lack of resolution.
         What other possible approaches has family considered?
         Have any of these approaches been tried with the present situation or similar situations in the past? If so, how effective was the approach? If approach was

successful, why? If approach was unsuccessful, why?
         Would an approach used in the past be appropriate for the present situation? Would it meet with some degree of success? Explore possibilities regarding implementation and outcomes.
         If family has considered alternate approaches but has not tried them, family should be assisted to (1) think how approach could be implemented and (2) consider effectiveness of outcomes.
         If family perceives that implementation and outcomes will be successful, explore why—is the reasoning realistic? If not, explore other possibilities regarding implementation and outcomes which might be more realistic and workable.
         If family perceives that implementation and/or outcomes will be unsuccessful, use same exploratory process as preceding example.
         The family should be assisted to explore the implications for each possible approach to decide on the one most effective for the problem situation and the family.
         If it becomes necessary for the community health nurse to supplement the family's ideas with other suggested approaches, the same exploratory approach as in the previous example should be used by the family—and the final decision regarding a problem-solving approach resides with the family.
         If no (family not attempting to resolve problem)
         Must the family do something because of the nature of the problem?
         What are the family's reasons for not working on the problem? For example, is there some other family situation that must be resolved first? The problem-solving process may need to refocus unless both problems can be approached simultaneously.
         The family is provided with information about the resolution of the problem as well as the risks associated with neglecting the problem to make an informed decision about a course of action.
         The family is assisted in its problem solving in the same manner as discussed previously.
   C. Evaluation (jointly by family and community health nurse)
      1. Evaluation of problem-solving process and experience.
      2. Evaluation of the implementation and outcomes of the family's selected approach to the problem.

B5—HOME OBSERVATION FOR MEASUREMENT OF THE ENVIRONMENT

Birth to Three

Date of interview _____

Child designee _____
                              Name

Age _____ Sex _____ Ethnicity _____

Child's birthday _____   Birth order _____

Mother's name _____   Father's name _____

Address _____

Categories	Raw scores	Percentile scores
I. Emotional and verbal responsivity of mother	_____	_____
II. Avoidance of restriction and punishment	_____	_____

From Caldwell, B.: Home observation measurement of the environment, Little Rock, Ark., 1976, University of Arkansas Center for Child Development and Education.

III. Organization of physical and temporal environment	_____	_____
IV. Provision of appropriate play materials	_____	_____
V. Maternal involvement with child	_____	_____
VI. Opportunities for variety in daily stimulation	_____	_____
TOTALS	_____	_____

	Yes	No
I. Emotional and verbal responsivity of mother		
1. Mother spontaneously vocalizes to child at least twice during visit (excluding scolding).	_____	_____
2. Mother responds to child's vocalizations with a verbal response.	_____	_____
3. Mother tells child the name of some object during visit or says name of person or object in a "teaching" style.	_____	_____
4. Mother's speech is distinct, clear, and audible.	_____	_____
5. Mother initiates verbal interchanges with observer—asks questions and makes spontaneous comments.	_____	_____
6. Mother expresses ideas freely and easily and uses statements of appropriate length for conversation (e.g., gives more than brief answers).	_____	_____
* 7. Mother permits child occasionally to engage in "messy" type of play.	_____	_____
8. Mother spontaneously praises child's qualities or behavior twice during visit.	_____	_____
9. When speaking of or to child, mother's voice conveys positive feeling.	_____	_____
10. Mother caresses or kisses child at least once during visit.	_____	_____
11. Mother shows some positive emotional responses to praise of child offered by visitor.	_____	_____
SUBSCORE	_____	_____
II. Avoidance of restriction and punishment		
12. Mother does not shout at child during visit.	_____	_____
13. Mother does not express overt annoyance with or hostility toward child.	_____	_____
14. Mother neither slaps nor spanks child during visit.	_____	_____
*15. Mother reports that no more than one instance of physical punishment occurred during the past week.	_____	_____
16. Mother does not scold or derogate child during visit.	_____	_____
17. Mother does not interfere with child's actions or restrict child's movements more than three times during visit.	_____	_____
18. At least 10 books are present and visible.	_____	_____
*19. Family has a pet.	_____	_____
SUBSCORE	_____	_____
III. Organization of physical and temporal environment		
20. When mother is away, care is provided by one of three regular substitutes.	_____	_____
21. Someone takes child into grocery store at least once a week.	_____	_____
22. Child gets out of house at least four times a week.	_____	_____
23. Child is taken regularly to doctor's office or clinic.	_____	_____
*24. Child has a special place in which to keep his toys and "treasures."	_____	_____
25. Child's play environment appears safe and free of hazards.	_____	_____
SUBSCORE	_____	_____

	Yes	No
IV. Provision of appropriate play materials		
26. Child has some muscle activity toys or equipment.	_____	_____
27. Child has a push or pull toy.	_____	_____
28. Child has stroller or walker, kiddie car, scooter or tricycle.	_____	_____
29. Mother provides toys or interesting activities for child during interview.	_____	_____
30. Provides learning equipment appropriate to age—cuddly toy or role-playing toys.	_____	_____
31. Provides learning equipment appropriate to age—mobile, table and chairs, high chair, play pen.	_____	_____
32. Provides eye-hand coordination toys—items to go in and out of receptacle, fit-together toys, beads.	_____	_____
33. Provides eye-hand coordination toys that permit combinations—stacking or nesting toys, blocks or building toys.	_____	_____
34. Provides toys for literature and music.	_____	_____
SUBSCORE	_____	_____
V. Maternal involvement with child		
35. Mother tends to keep child within visual range and to look at him often.	_____	_____
36. Mother talks to child while doing her work.	_____	_____
37. Mother consciously encourages developmental advance.	_____	_____
38. Mother invests "maturing" toys with value via her attention.	_____	_____
39. Mother structures child's play periods.	_____	_____
40. Mother provides toys that challenge child to develop new skills.	_____	_____
SUBSCORE	_____	_____
VI. Opportunities for variety in daily stimulation		
41. Father provides some caretaking every day.	_____	_____
42. Mother reads stories at least three times weekly.	_____	_____
43. Child eats at least one meal per day with mother and father.	_____	_____

*Items that may require direct questions.

44. Family visits or receives visits from relatives.   _____ _____
45. Child has three or more books of his own.   _____ _____

                                                                                          SUBSCORE   _____ _____

Three to Six

Date of interview _____

Child designee _____
                                    Name   Age   Sex   Ethnicity

Child's birthday _____   Birth order _____
Mother's name _____   Father's name _____
Address _____

Categories

	Raw scores	Percentile scores
I. Provision of stimulation through equipment, toys, and experiences	_____	_____
II. Stimulation of mature behavior	_____	_____
III. Provision of stimulating physical and language environment	_____	_____
IV. Avoidance of restriction and punishment	_____	_____
V. Pride, affection, and thoughtfulness	_____	_____
VI. Masculine stimulation	_____	_____
VII. Independence from parental control	_____	_____
TOTALS	_____	_____

I. Provision of stimulation through equipment, toys, and experiences   Yes   No

1-12 The following are present in home and either belong to child subject or he is allowed to play with them:
1. Toys to learn colors, sizes, shapes (e.g., typewriter, pressouts, play school, and peg boards).   _____ _____
2. Toy or game facilitating learning letters (e.g., blocks with letters, toy typewriter, letter sticks, and books about letters).   _____ _____
3. Three or more puzzles.   _____ _____
4. Two toys necessitating some finger and whole hand movements (e.g., crayons and coloring books, paper dolls).   _____ _____
5. Record player and at least five children's records.   _____ _____
6. Real or toy musical instrument (e.g., piano, drum, toy xylophone, or guitar).   _____ _____
7. Toy or game permitting free expression (e.g., finger paints, play dough, and crayons or paint and paper).   _____ _____
8. Toys or game necessitating refined movements (paint by number, dot book, paper dolls, crayons and coloring books).   _____ _____
9. Toys to learn animals (e.g., books about animals, circus games, and animal puzzles).   _____ _____
10. Toy or game facilitating learning numbers (e.g., blocks with numbers, books about numbers, games with numbers).   _____ _____
11. Building toys (e.g., block, Tinker Toys, and Lincoln Logs).   _____ _____
12. Ten children's books.   _____ _____
13. At least 10 books are present and visible in the apartment.   _____ _____
14. Family buys a newspaper daily and reads it.   _____ _____
15. Family subscribes to at least one magazine.   _____ _____
16. Family member has taken child on one outing (picnic, shopping excursion) at least every other week.   _____ _____
17. Child has been taken out to eat in some kind of restaurant three or four times in the past year.   _____ _____
18-20 Child has been taken by a family member to the following within the past year:
18. Airport   _____ _____
19. A trip more than 50 miles from his home (50 miles radial distance, not total distance).   _____ _____
20. A scientific, historical, or art museum.   _____ _____
21. Child is taken to grocery store at least once a week.   _____ _____

                                                                                          SUBSCORE   _____ _____

II. Stimulation of mature behavior   Yes   No

22-29 Child is encouraged to learn the following:
22. Colors   _____ _____
23. Shapes   _____ _____
24. Patterned speech (e.g., nursery rhymes, prayers, songs, and TV commercials)   _____ _____
25. The alphabet   _____ _____
26. To tell time   _____ _____
27. Spatial relationships (e.g., up, down, under, big, and little)   _____ _____
28. Numbers   _____ _____
29. To read a few words   _____ _____

30. Tries to get child to pick up and put away toys after play session—without help.   ____ ____
31. Child is taught rules of social behavior that involve recognition of rights of others.   ____ ____
32. Parent teaches child some simple manners—to say, "Please," "Thank you," and "I'm sorry."   ____ ____
33. Some delay of food gratification is demanded of the child, e.g., not to whine or demand food unless within   ____ ____
    ½ hour of meal time.

SUBSCORE   ____

III. Provision of a stimulating physical and language environment   **Yes**   **No**
    (Observation items, except *45*)
    34. Building has no potentially dangerous structural or health defect (e.g., plaster coming down from ceiling,   ____ ____
        stairway with boards missing, or rodents).
    35. Child's outside play environment appears safe and free of hazards (no outside play area requires an automatic   ____ ____
        "No").
    36. The interior of the apartment is not dark or perceptibly monotonous.   ____ ____
    37. House is not overly noisy—television, shouts of children, radio, etc.   ____ ____
    38. Neighborhood has trees, grass, birds—is esthetically pleasing.   ____ ____
    39. There is at least 100 square feet of living space per person in the house.   ____ ____
    40. In terms of available floor space, the rooms are not overcrowded with furniture.   ____ ____
    41. All visible rooms of the house are reasonably clean and minimally cluttered.   ____ ____
    *42. Mother uses complex sentence structure and some long words in conversing.   ____ ____
    43. Mother uses correct grammar and pronunciation.   ____ ____
    44. Mother's speech is distinct, clear, and audible.   ____ ____
    45. Family has TV and it is used judiciously, not left on continuously (no TV requires an automatic "No"—   ____ ____
        any scheduling scores "Yes").

SUBSCORE   ____

IV. Avoidance of restriction and punishment   **Yes**   **No**
    (Observation items, except *51* and *52*)
    46. Mother does not scold or derogate child more than once during visit.   ____ ____
    47. Mother does not use physical restraint, shake, grab, or pinch child during visit.   ____ ____
    48. Mother neither slaps nor spanks child during visit.   ____ ____
    49. Mother does not express over-annoyance with or hostility toward child—complain, say child is "bad" or   ____ ____
        won't mind.
    50. Child is not punished or ridiculed for speech.   ____ ____
    51. No more than one instance of physical punishment occurred during the past week (accept parental report).   ____ ____
    52. Child does not get slapped or spanked for spilling food or drink.   ____ ____

SUBSCORE   ____

V. Pride, affection, and thoughtfulness   **Yes**   **No**
    (Observation items, except *53* through *59*)
    53. Parent turns on special TV program regarded as "good" for children (e.g., *Captain Kangaroo, Walt Disney,*   ____ ____
        Flipper, Lassie, or educational TV).
    54. Someone reads stories to child or shows and comments on pictures in magazines five times weekly.   ____ ____
    55. Parent encourages child to relate experiences or takes time to listen to him relate experiences.   ____ ____
    56. Parent holds child close 10 to 15 minutes per day (e.g., during TV, story time, or visiting).   ____ ____
    57. Parent occasionally sings to child, or sings in presence of child.   ____ ____
    58. Child has a special place in which to keep his toys and "treasures."   ____ ____
    59. Child's art work is displayed some place in house (anything that child makes).   ____ ____
    60. Mother introduces interviewer to child.   ____ ____
    61. Mother converses with child at least twice during visit (scolding and suspicious comments not counted).   ____ ____
    62. Mother answers child's questions or requests verbally.   ____ ____
    63. Mother usually responds verbally to child's taking.   ____ ____
    64. Mother provides toys or interesting activities or in other ways structures situation for child during visit   ____ ____
        when her attention will be elsewhere. (To score "Yes" mother must make an active guiding gesture or
        suggestion to structure child's play.)
    65. Mother spontaneously praises child's qualities or behavior twice during visit.   ____ ____
    66. When speaking of or to child, mother's voice conveys positive feeling.   ____ ____
    67. Mother caresses, kisses, or cuddles child at least once during visit.   ____ ____
    68. Mother sets up situation that allows child to show off during visit.   ____ ____

SUBSCORE   ____

VI. Masculine stimulation   **Yes**   **No**
    69. Child sees and spends some time with father four days a week.   ____ ____
    70. Child eats at least one meal per day, on most days, with mother (or mother figure) and father (or father   ____ ____
        figure). (One-parent families get an automatic "No.")

---

*Throughout interview this refers to mother *or* other care giver who is present for interview.

71-73 The following are present in home and either belong to child subject or he is allowed to play with them:

71. Ride toy (tricycle, scooter, wagon, bike with or without training wheels). ___ ___
72. Medium wheel toys—trucks, doll carriage, etc. ___ ___
73. Large muscle toy (e.g., jump rope, swing, ball, or climbing object). ___ ___

SUBSCORE ___ ___

	Yes	No
VII. Independence from parental control		
74. Child is encouraged to try to dress himself.	___	___
75. Child is permitted to choose some of his clothing to be worn except on very special occasions.	___	___
76. Child is permitted some choice in lunch or breakfast menu.	___	___
77. Parent lets child choose certain favorite food products or brands at grocery store.	___	___
78. Child is permitted to go to another house to play without having the caregiver accompany him.	___	___
79. Child can express negative feelings without harsh reprisal.	___	___
80. Child is permitted to hit parent without harsh reprisal.	___	___

SUBSCORE ___ ___

Total score ___ ___

B6—ASSESSMENT SURVEY: HOUSING FOR THE DISABLED

1. Entry
   ___ Ramp
      ___ 1 ft rise per 12 ft length
      ___ 4 ft wide
      ___ Nonslip surface
      ___ Handrail extended 18 inches beyond top and bottom step
      ___ 5 ft flat platform at top
      ___ 6 ft clearance at bottom
   ___ Elevator
   ___ Steps
   ___ Lighting
   ___ Sidewalks
   ___ Surface, level
   ___ Parking
   ___ Carport, 13-14 inches clearance space
2. Living area
   ___ Floors, nonslip
   ___ Floors, same level
   ___ Doorways, 36 inches wide, 5 ft square turning area
   ___ Doors, push handles
   ___ Mirrors, correct height
   ___ Telephone at bedside
   ___ Controls and electrical switches, 36 inches from floor
   ___ Cords, out of traffic pattern
   ___ Windows, 36 inches from floor
   ___ Carpet, secure—no scatter rugs
   ___ Linoleum, free of holes, dips
   ___ Furniture, sturdy; arranged for free movement
   ___ Lighting
   ___ Heating, location of vents and radiators
3. Kitchen
   ___ Stove, burner controls safe
   ___ Pots and pans, weight
   ___ Potholders, mitts; thickness
   ___ Dishes, accessibility
   ___ Counter space, height
   ___ Faucets, accessibility and ease of on/off
   ___ Table top equipment, clutter
4. Bathroom
   ___ Tub rails, 3 to 4 inches out from wall
   ___ Toilet, transfer space
   ___ Toilet, height of seat
   ___ Mirror, height
   ___ Sink, height, handles
   ___ Doorway, 36 inches wide
   ___ Floor surface, nonslip
   ___ Tub surface, nonslip
   ___ Medicine chest, height
   ___ Linen storage, height
   ___ Lighting
5. Bedroom
   ___ Space
   ___ Floor surface, nonslip
   ___ Doorway, 36 inches wide
   ___ Closet, accessibility
   ___ Lighting
   ___ Bed, ancillary equipment (e.g., side rails, trapeze)
   ___ Emergency call mechanism
   General description

   Hazards identified

   Inconveniences identified

   Recommendations

6. Family members
   Names, ages, and relationships

   Source of income

   Source for medical costs coverage/payments

   Caretaker
      Schedule of care

   Contingency plans

B7—SUMMARY CHARACTERISTICS OF NINE FAMILY ASSESSMENT TOOLS

Tools	Dimensions measured	Understandable	Ease of administration and scoring	Appropriate for all types of families	Clinical relevance
FFI*	Communication Togetherness Closeness Decision making Child orientation	Yes	15 items Quickly administered Complicated scoring	Not for families without children or those with adult children	Not sensitive to short-term change
FAD†	Problem solving Communication Roles Affective responsiveness Affective involvement Behavior control General functioning	Yes	53 items Easy to administer	Requires individual to "speak for family"	Measures areas that nurses could change through care plans
FES‡	Relationships Personal growth System maintenance and change	Yes	90 items, true/false Lengthy for clinical use (short form available) Scoring is complex Standardized scores, two categories	Universally appropriate	Useful to measure change after interventions
SFIS§	Enmeshment/disengagement Neglect/overprotection Rigidity/flexibility Conflict/avoidance Client management Triangulation of parent/child coalition Detouring	Easier to understand for those familiar with Minuchin's family functioning theory	85 items on 4-point agreement scale Easy to administer	Unknown at this time	Further testing required Useful for family counseling assessment
FFFS‖	Parent's perception of relationship and family functions	Somewhat difficult	Somewhat complicated scoring	Useful with middle-class families	Measures factors that nurses could help change through care plans
CICI:PQ¶	Perceptions of stressors Coping strategies	Yes	48 items Scoring unknown	Only for families with chronically ill children	Identifies nursing intervention areas for families with chronically ill children
Family APGAR**	Adaptability Partnership Growth Affection Resolve	Requires global assessment of five areas	Five items Quick to administer	No data reported	Measures relevant factors

From: Speer, J.J., and Sachs, B.: Selecting the appropriate family assessment tool, Pediatr. Nurs. 11:349-355, Sept./Oct. 1985. Reprinted with permission: A.J. Jannetti, Inc.
*Family Functioning Index
†The Family Assessment Device
‡Family Environment Scale
§Structural Family Interaction Scale
‖Feetham Family Functioning Survey
¶Chronicity Impact and Coping Instrument: Parent Questionnaire
**Family Adaptability, Partnership, Growth, Affection, and Resolve Test

Summary characteristics of nine family asseeement tools—cont'd

Tools	Dimensions measured	Understandable	Ease of administration and scoring	Appropriate for all types of families	Clinical relevance
IFF*	Positive/negative feelings toward each member	Yes Complicated for large families	38 items, 3-point Likertlike scale Easily scored	Unknown at this time	Limited clinical usefulness because of lack of dimension
FACES II†	Cohesion Adaptability Social desirability	Easily understood	30 items on 4-point Likertlike scale Easy to administer	Universally useful Family members may be unwilling to assess themselves	Measures relevant factors for nursing Can use as real and ideal

*The Inventory of Family Feelings
†Family Adaptability and Cohesion Evaluation Scale

C1—THE LIFETIME HEALTH-MONITORING PROGRAM: RECONCILING PUBLIC-HEALTH AND PRIVATE-PRACTICE GOALS*

Goals and Professional Services

For each of the 10 age groups, a set of distinct health goals and professional services is desirable:

Pregnancy and Perinatal Period

Health goals
1. To provide the mother a healthy, full-term pregnancy and rapid recovery after a normal delivery.
2. To facilitate the live birth of a normal baby, free of congenital or developmental damage.
3. To help both mother and father achieve the knowledge and capacity to provide for the physical, emotional, and social needs of the baby.

Professional services
1. Prior education and appropriate counseling for parents expecting their first baby in physical, emotional and social aspects of childbearing and infant care, including family planning.
2. Antenatal and postnatal care for mother and baby, education/counseling for both parents, and risk assessment through the perinatal period as needed.
3. Delivery services, including specialized perinatal care, as needed.

Infancy (First Year)

Health goals
1. To establish immunity against specified infectious diseases.
2. To detect and prevent certain other diseases and problems before irreparable damage occurs.
3. To facilitate growth and development to the infant's optimal potential.
4. To provide a basis for lifetime emotional stability, especially through a loving relation with mother, father, and other family members.

Professional services
1. Before discharge from the hospital: tests for inherited metabolic and certain other congenital disorders; parent counseling.
2. Four post-discharge professional visits with the healthy infant during the year for observation, specified immunizations and parent counseling.

Preschool Child (1 to 5 Years)

Health goals
1. To facilitate the child's optimal physical, emotional, and social growth and development.
2. To begin the process of socialization through happy and ef-

fective family relations and gradual introduction to school and other facets of the outside world.

Professional services
1. Two professional visits with the healthy child and mother (ideally, the father also) at 2 to 3 years and at school entry for compliance with immunization schedule, and for observation and counseling about nutrition, activity, vision, hearing, speech, dental health, accident prevention, and general physical, emotional, and social development.
2. For special high-risk groups, blood tests for anemia, lead poisoning, and tuberculosis.

School Child (6 to 11 Years)

Health goals
1. To facilitate the child's optimal physical, mental, emotional, and social growth and development, including a positive self-image.
2. To establish healthy behavioral patterns for nutrition, exercise, study, recreation, and family life, as a foundation for a healthy lifetime life-style.

Professional services
1. Two professional visits with the healthy child (at 6 to 7 and 9 to 10 years of age), including one complete physical, mental, behavioral, and social examination, with appropriate tests for, and follow-up observation of, any physical or mental impairment, including obesity, vision and hearing defects, muscular incoordination, and learning disabilities, and completion of any necessary immunizations.
2. Mandatory school health education and individual counseling, as needed, for physical fitness, nutrition, exercise, study, accident prevention, sexual development, and use of cigarettes, drugs, and alcohol.
3. Annual dental examination and prophylaxis.

Adolescence (12 to 17 Years)

Health goals
1. To continue optimal physical, mental, emotional, and social growth and development.
2. To reinforce healthy behavior patterns and discourage negative ones in physical fitness, nutrition, exercise, study, work, recreation, sex, individual relations, driving, smoking, alcohol, and drugs, as foundation for healthy lifetime life-style, including marriage, parenthood, and career or job.

Professional services
1. Mandatory school health education and individual counseling, as needed, for the above subjects, including a course in sex and marriage and family relations as a prerequisite to graduation from high school.
2. One professional visit with the healthy adolescent (at about 13 years of age) with attention to emotional status, vision and hearing, skin, blood pressure, blood cholesterol, and contraception.
3. Annual dental examination and prophylaxis.

---

*From Breslow, L., and Somers, A.R.: The lifetime health-monitoring program, N. Engl. J. Med. 296(11):602-604, March 1977.

Young Adulthood (18 to 24 Years)

Health goals

1. To facilitate transition from dependent adolescence to mature independent adulthood with maximum physical, mental, and emotional resources.
2. To achieve useful employment and maximum capacity for a healthy marriage, parenthood, and social relations.

Professional services

1. One professional visit with the healthy adult, including complete physical examination, tetanus booster if not received within 10 years, tests for syphilis, gonorrhea, malnutrition, cholesterol and hypertension, and medical and behavioral history. This visit may be provided upon entrance into college, the armed forces, or first full-time job, but should be before marriage.
2. Health education and individual counseling, as needed, for nutrition, exercise, study, career, job, occupational hazards and problems, sex, contraception, marriage and family relations, alcohol, drugs, smoking, and driving.
3. Dental examination and prophylaxis every 2 years.

Young Middle Age (25 to 39 Years)

Health goals

1. To prolong the period of maximum physical energy and to develop full mental, emotional, and social potential.
2. To anticipate and guard against the onset of chronic diseases through good health habits and early detection and treatment where effective.

Professional services

1. Two professional visits with the healthy person—at about 30 and 35—including tests for hypertension, anemia, cholesterol, cervical and breast cancer, and instruction in self-examination of breasts, skin, testes, neck, and mouth.
2. Professional counseling regarding nutrition, exercise, smoking, alcohol, marital, parental, and other aspects of health-related behavior and life-style.
3. Dental examination and prophylaxis every 2 years.

Older Middle Age (40 to 59 Years)

Health goals

1. To prolong the period of maximum physical energy and optimal mental and social activity, including menopausal adjustment.
2. To detect as early as possible any of the major chronic diseases, including hypertension, heart disease, diabetes, and cancer, as well as vision, hearing, and dental impairments.

Professional services

1. Four professional visits with the healthy person, once every 5 years—at about 40, 45, 50, and 55—with complete physical examination and medical history, tests for specific chronic conditions, appropriate immunizations and counseling regarding changing nutritional needs; physical activities; occupa-

tional, sex, marital, and parental problems; and use of cigarettes, alcohol, and drugs.
2. For those over 50, annual tests for hypertension, obesity, and certain cancers.
3. Annual dental prophylaxis.

The Elderly (60 to 74 Years)

Health goals

1. To prolong the period of optimum physical, mental, and social activity.
2. To minimize handicapping and discomfort from onset of chronic conditions.
3. To prepare in advance for retirement.

Professional services

1. Professional visits with the healthy adult at 60 years of age and every 2 years thereafter, including the same tests for chronic conditions as in older middle age, and professional counseling regarding changing life-style related to retirement, nutritional requirements, absence of children, possible loss of spouse, probable reduction in income, and reduced physical resources.
2. Annual immunization against influenza (unless the person is allergic to vaccine).
3. Annual dental prophylaxis.
4. Periodic podiatry treatments as needed.

Old Age (75 Years and Over)

Health goals

1. To prolong period of effective activity and ability to live independently, and to avoid institutionalization so far as possible.
2. To minimize inactivity and discomfort from chronic conditions.
3. When illness is terminal, to assure as little physical and mental distress as possible and to provide emotional support to patient and family.

Professional services

1. Professional visit at least once a year, including complete physical examination, medical and behavioral history, and professional counseling regarding changing nutritional requirements, limitations on activity and mobility, and living arrangements.
2. Annual immunization against influenza (unless the person is allergic to vaccine).
3. Periodic dental and podiatry treatments as needed.
4. For low-income and other persons not sick enough to be institutionalized but not well enough to cope entirely alone, counseling regarding sheltered housing, health visitors, home helps, day care and recreational centers, meals-on-wheels and other measures designed to help them remain in their own homes and as nearly independent as possible.
5. Professional assistance with family relations and preparations for death, if needed.

C2—HEALTH HAZARD APPRAISAL

RETURN THIS BOOKLET
FOR PROCESSING TO ⬦

prospective
medicine center

Suite 219, 3901 North Meridian Street
Indianapolis, Indiana 46208

This program
is based on the
established goals of the
Society of Prospective Medicine,
to extend useful life expectancy.
The Society's logo is the symbol
of the apothecaries' ounce.
Their motto is,
"AN OUNCE OF
PREVENTION, IS WORTH A
POUND OF CURE."

HEALTH APPRAISAL HAZARD

Please use the enclosed window envelope
and return this booklet to your provider as
instructed, or mail directly using sufficient
first class postage for one ounce.

prospective
medicine center
© 1981, Health Care Services, Inc.
Reproduction in whole or part without written permission is prohibited.

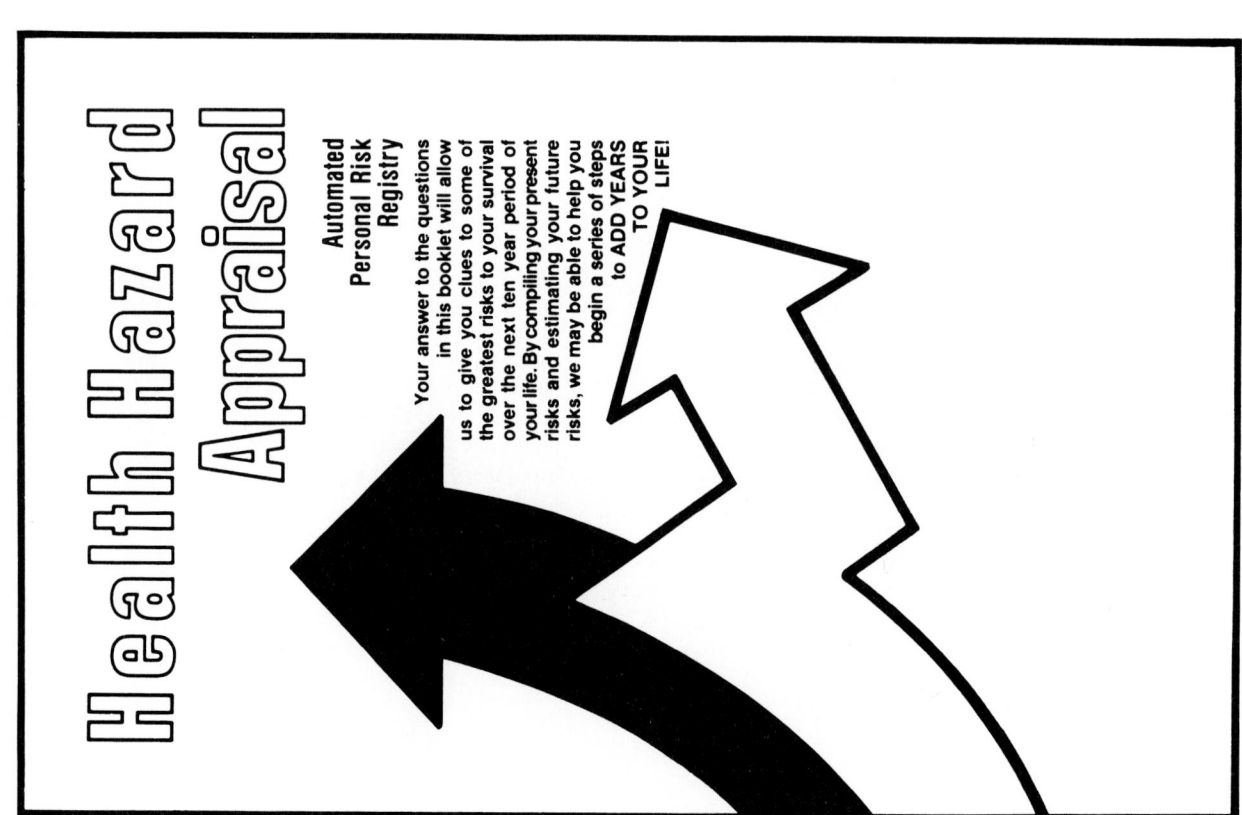

Health Hazard Appraisal

**Automated
Personal Risk
Registry**

Your answer to the questions
in this booklet will allow
us to give you clues to some of
the greatest risks to your survival
over the next ten year period of
your life. By compiling your present
risks and estimating your future
risks, we may be able to help you
begin a series of steps
to ADD YEARS
TO YOUR
LIFE!

Please answer every question. There are a few questions that inquire about race or religion. They are asked only because they are associated with different risks in certain diseases. This is your appraisal, and all answers will be completely confidential. The more honestly you answer the questions, the more accurate your appraisal will be.

PLEASE FOLLOW THESE INSTRUCTIONS:

1. Read each question thoroughly and insert the number of the most appropriate answer in the space at right. 2

   EXAMPLE: **An apple is red** ......
   1. No   2. Yes   3. Do Not Know

2. In some areas of the form you will be asked to fill-in information. In these areas we ask that you **please print**.

★ ★ ★ ★ ★ ★ ★
★ ★ ★ ★ ★ ★ ★

Social Security Number 1

Last Name 2

First Name, Middle Initial 3

Street 4

City 5

State or Province 6   Zip 7

Birth Date 8 | MONTH | DAY | YEAR | Sex 9 MALE/FEMALE   Race 10 BLACK, WHITE, OTHER

Height 11 ___ feet ___ inches   Weight 12 ___ lbs.

Systolic (upper reading) Blood Pressure (if known) 13
(120 is average)

Diastolic (lower reading) Blood Pressure (if known) 14
(80 is average)

Cholesterol level (if known) 15
(210 is average)

Please list your mileage per year as both a passenger and as a driver in an automobile or any other motor vehicle. (the national average is 10,000 miles per year.) .... 16 THOUSAND

Do you have an annual proctosigmoidoscopy? (examination of your bowel with a lighted instrument), or screening of stool specimen is negative for blood three times a year 40
1. No   2. Yes

Have you had any bleeding from your rectum? 41
1. No, have not had any bleeding   2. Yes, have had some bleeding
3. Yes, have had some bleeding, but my doctor knows about it.

Have you ever had polyps or growths in your rectum? (not piles or hemorrhoids) 42
1. No   2. Yes   3. Do Not Know

Do you have or have you had an Ulcerative Colitis? (bloody diarrhea with pus and mucous and sores inside the rectum) 43
1. No   2. Yes, 10 or more years   3. Yes, under 10 years

Have you had Bacterial Pneumonia? 44
1. No   2. Yes

Have you had or do you have Emphysema? 45
1. No   2. Yes

Have you ever had Rheumatic Fever? (inflammation of the heart and/or joints) 46
1. No   2. Yes, with treatment   3. Yes, without treatment

Have you ever been told that you have a Heart Murmur? 47
1. No   2. Yes, with treatment   3. Yes, without treatment

Please list any other significant problems which you feel may affect your life expectancy.
48 ___

Please continue on next page

Is your natural mother alive? 17
1. No   2. Yes   3. Do Not Know

Is she now over 70, or was she at the time of death? 18
1. No   2. Yes   3. Do Not Know

If she is dead, did she die of Heart Disease? 19
1. No   2. Yes   3. Do Not Know

Is your natural father alive? 20
1. No   2. Yes   3. Do Not Know

Is he now over 70, or was he at the time of death? 21
1. No   2. Yes   3. Do Not Know

If he is dead, did he die of Heart Disease? 22
1. No   2. Yes   3. Do Not Know

Has any member of your immediate family (parents, brothers, sisters, or children) ever committed or attempted Suicide? 23
1. No   2. Yes   3. Do Not Know

Has any member of your immediate family (parents, brothers, sisters, or children) had or have Diabetes? 24
1. No   2. Yes   3. Do Not Know

Have you ever been told that you have Diabetes? 25
1. No   2. Yes with treatment   3. Yes without treatment

Approximately how much of time do you wear your seatbelt? 26
1. None   2. 20%   3. 40%
4. 60%   5. 80%   6. 100%

Approximately how many alcoholic drinks do you have per week? (one drink equals 1 - 12 oz. beer, 4 oz. of wine, or 1 oz. of hard liquor) 27
1. Non Drinker   2. Have Stopped Drinking   3. 1–2 Drinks Per Week
4. 3–6 Drinks Per Week   5. 7–24 Drinks Per Week
6. 25–40 Drinks Per Week   7. 41 or More Drinks Per Week

Do you or have you ever taken any of the drugs or medications listed here before driving in your car? If your answer is YES, please indicate the type of drug or drugs you have taken or are presently taking 28
1. Do Not Take Any   2. Mood Elevators   3. Amphetamines, Diet Pills
4. Tranquilizers, Sedatives, Sleeping Pills, Nerve Pills   5. Narcotic Pain Pills
6. Antihistamines   7. Marijuana, LSD

Have you ever been arrested for a violent act or threat of a violent act? 29
1. No   2. Yes

Do you carry a weapon? (includes carrying a weapon while at work) 30
1. No   2. Yes

How much exercise do you have each day? 31
1. Walking less than 5 blocks or climbing up less than 5 flights of stairs. (Sedentary - No Sports)
2. Walking 5—15 blocks or climbing up 5—15 flights of stairs. (Little - Light Sports)
3. Walking 15—20 blocks or climbing up 15—20 flights of stairs. (Acceptable - Active Sports)
4. Walking more than 20 blocks or climbing up more than 20 flights of stairs. (Substantial - Strenuous Sports)

Do you smoke? 32
1. No   2. Yes

Did you previously smoke? 33
1. No   2. Yes

If either of the above answers were YES, please list the amount that you now smoke per day or previously smoked per day 34
1. 40 + Cigarettes   2. 20—39 Cigarettes
3. 10—19 Cigarettes   4. 1—9 Cigarettes
5. Heavy Pipe   6. Light Pipe
7. Heavy Cigar   8. Light Cigar

If you have stopped smoking, please list the number of years that you have stopped 35
1. 1 yr.   2. 2 yrs.   3. 3 yrs.   4. 4 yrs.
5. 5 yrs.   6. 6 yrs.   7. 7 yrs.   8. 8 yrs.
9. 9 yrs.   0. More than 9 years

What would you consider your economic and social status to be? 36
1. Low   2. Average   3. High

Are you often depressed? 37
1. No   2. Yes

Do you frequently have crying spells? 38
1. No   2. Yes

Do you frequently think of ending your life? 39
1. No   2. Yes

In the past 12 months, have you experienced any of the following:
(Insert appropriate number in each space at right)   1. No   2. Yes

Death of Spouse 49
Change in health of a family member 50
Death of a close family member 51
Death of a close friend 52
Trouble with your in-laws 53
Change in number of arguments with your spouse 54
Sexual difficulties 55
Marital separation 56
Marital reconciliation 57
Divorce 58
Marriage 59
Revision of personal habits 60
Change in sleeping habits 61
Change in eating habits 62
Minor violation of law 63
An outstanding personal achievement 64
Personal injury or illness 65
Change in responsibilities at work 66
Change in work hours or conditions 67
Trouble with boss 68
Fired from job 69
Change to a different line of work 70
Business readjustment 71
Change in your financial status 72
Change in residence 73
Change in living conditions 74
Change in number of family get-togethers 75
Begin or end school 76
Change in schools 77
Foreclosure of a mortgage or loan 78
Retirement 79
Spouse begins or stops work 80
Mortgage over $30,000 81
Mortgage or loan less than $30,000 82
Pregnancy 83
Son or daughter leaves home 84
Gain of a new family member 85
Change in social activities 86
Change in church activities 87
Change in recreation 88
Vacation 89
Christmas 90
Jail Term 91

THE FOLLOWING QUESTIONS ARE FOR FEMALES ONLY

Has your mother or any sisters or aunts ever had breast cancer? 92
1. None had   2. One had   3. Two or more had

Has your doctor ever told you that you had a lump or cyst in your breast that was NOT cancer? 93
1. No   2. Yes

Does your doctor examine your breasts at least once a year? 94
1. No   2. Yes

Do you examine your breasts at least once a month? 95
1. No   2. Yes

What is your current menstrual status? 96
1. Still menstruating   2. Natural menopause
3. Surgical menopause at under 35 years
4. Surgical menopause at over 35 years

How many times have you been pregnant? 97
1. None   2. 1–2 times   3. 3 or more times

If you have been pregnant, what was the age of your first pregnancy? 98
1. Under 20   2. 20–24   3. 25 or over

At what age did you begin to have regular sexual intercourse? 99
1. Never   2. Before 20   3. Between 20–25   4. After 25

Are you Jewish? 100
1. No   2. Yes

Has your cervix been removed? 101
1. No   2. Yes

Has your uterus been removed? 102
1. No   2. Yes

Have your ovaries been removed? 103
1. No.   2. Yes, one   3. Yes, both

Have you had any ABNORMAL vaginal bleeding in the past year? 104
1. No
2. Yes, between menstrual periods.
3. Yes, during or after sexual intercourse.
4. Yes, periods have stopped, but having bleeding every once in a while.
5. Yes, taking estrogens, bleed when off.
6. Yes, taking estrogens, bleed whether on them or off.

Please indicate the results of any Pap Smears, cancer smears, that you have by inserting the most appropriate answer 105
1. I have not had a Pap Smear in the past 5 years.
2. I have had one normal Pap Smear in the past year.
3. I have had one normal Pap Smear in the past 5 years.
4. I have had 3 normal Pap Smears in the past 5 years.
5. I have had 5 normal Pap Smears in the past 5 years.
6. I have had a Pap Smear in the past year, but it was abnormal.
7. I have had a Pap Smear in the past year, but I do not know the results.

C3—HEALTH 80'S QUESTIONNAIRE

HEALTH 80's QUESTIONNAIRE

Your Facility Name
Address
City, State
Zip

NOTE: *Please follow directions carefully. If you consider a question too personal, you may skip it. All information is handled confidentially.*

1-202
IDENTIFICATION

10 **Name** |___|___|___|___|___|___|___|___|___|___|___|___|___|
Last Name, First Name, Middle Name

11 **Today's Date** |__|__| |__|__| |__|__| 12 **Date of Birth** |__|__| |__|__| |__|__|
Mo.   Day   Yr.   Mo.   Day   Yr.

13 **Social Security Number** |__|__|__|—|__|__|—|__|__|__|__| 14 ___ **None**

15 ___ **Female**   16 ___ **Male**

17 **Height** ___ ft. ___ in.   18 **Weight** _____ lbs.

PERMANENT HOME ADDRESS

19 **Street** |___|___|___|___|___|___|___|___|___|___|___|___|___|

20 **City** |___|___|___|___|___|___|___|___|___|___|___|___|___|

21 **State or Province** |___|___|___|___|___|___|___|___|___|___|

22 **Zip** |__|__|__|__|__|

23 **Country** |___|___|___|___|___|___|___|___|___|___|___|___|

1-604
DEMOGRAPHIC Background
Race
10 ___ American Indian
11 ___ Black
12 ___ Caucasian
13 ___ Other

Family Income Level
16 ___ Low
17 ___ Middle
18 ___ High

Marital Status
19 ___ Single
20 ___ Married
21 ___ Widowed
22 ___ Separated
23 ___ Divorced

2-104
ILLNESSES and MEDICAL PROBLEMS
Check the problems you have or have had that have been diagnosed or treated by a physician or other health professinal.

Yes	No	Problem
10 ___	___	Alcoholism
11 ___	___	Anemia-sickle cell
12 ___	___	Bleeding trait
13 ___	___	Bronchitis, chronic
		Cancer
14 ___	___	Breast
15 ___	___	Cervix
16 ___	___	Colon
17 ___	___	Lung
18 ___	___	Uterus
19 ___	___	Other cancer
20 ___	___	Cirrhosis-liver
21 ___	___	Colitis-ulcerative
22 ___	___	Depression
23 ___	___	Diabetes
24 ___	___	Diabetes, uncontrolled
25 ___	___	Emphysema
26 ___	___	Fibrocystic breasts
		Heart problem
27 ___	___	Heart attack
28 ___	___	Coronary disease
29 ___	___	Rheumatic heart
30 ___	___	Heart valve prob.
31 ___	___	Heart murmur
32 ___	___	Enlarged heart
33 ___	___	Heart rhythm prob.
34 ___	___	Other heart prob.

Yes	No	Problem
		High blood fat (lipids).
50 ___	___	Cholesterol
51 ___	___	Triglycerides
52 ___	___	High blood pressure
53 ___	___	High blood pressure uncontrolled
54 ___	___	Obesity-more than 20 lbs. overweight
55 ___	___	Pneumonia
56 ___	___	Polyps in colon
57 ___	___	Rheumatic fever
58 ___	___	Rheumatic fever, with resultant heart murmur
59 ___	___	Stroke
60 ___	___	Suicide attempt
61 ___	___	Tuberculosis

Yes	No	In the past year, have you had -
62 ___	___	Chest pain or exertion, relieved by rest?
63 ___	___	Shortness of breath lying down, relieved by sitting up?
64 ___	___	Unexplained weight loss more than 10 lbs.?
65 ___	___	Unexplained rectal bleeding?
66 ___	___	Unexplained vaginal bleeding?

2-405
FEELINGS
Mark the frequency with which you have the feelings listed by placing a checkmark in the appropriate column.

M-Most of time   S-Some of the time   R-Rarely or none

M	S	R	
10 ___	___	___	Feel sad, depressed?
11 ___	___	___	Wish to end it all?
12 ___	___	___	Feel tense and anxious?
13 ___	___	___	Worry about things generally?
14 ___	___	___	More aggressive, hard-driving than friends
15 ___	___	___	Have an intense desire to achieve?
16 ___	___	___	Feel optimistic about the future?

FAMILY MEDICAL HISTORY (Blood Relatives)
Check items that apply for your blood relatives. Your blood relatives include your children, brothers, sisters, parents, and grandparents.

30 ___ **Do not know my family medical history.**
    (Go to next section)

Yes	No	Illness	Yes	No	Illness
31 ___	___	Anemia-sickle cell	36 ___	___	High blood press.
32 ___	___	Bleeding trait	37 ___	___	Mental illness
33 ___	___	Cancer	38 ___	___	Stroke
34 ___	___	Diabetes (sugar)	39 ___	___	Suicide
35 ___	___	Heart disease	40 ___	___	Tuberculosis

Yes	No	Check the items that apply.
50 ___	___	Father died of a heart attack before age 60?
51 ___	___	Mother died of a heart attack before age 60?
52 ___	___	Mother or sister had cancer of the breast?
53 ___	___	Did your mother take DES (diethylstilbestrol) when she was pregnant with you?

Q8020

HABITS and RISK FACTORS

Your habits influence your ability to achieve and maintain good health and long life. The questions on this page concern factors that are known to influence your health.

4-105
EATING

	Yes	No	Do you usually eat the following each day?
10	___	___	Five or more servings of dairy products or red meat?
11	___	___	Five or more servings of pastries, bread, starchy foods?

EXERCISE

Specify the amount of exercise you get each day.

12 ___ None or very little

The equivalent of-

13 ___ 10 flights of stairs, or 1 mile walking
14 ___ 20 flights of stairs, or 2 miles walking
15 ___ Over 20 flights of stairs, or over 2 miles walking

SMOKING

	Yes	No	Do you-
16	___	___	Smoke a pipe and inhale 5 or more times/day?
17	___	___	Smoke cigars and inhale 5 or more times/day?
18	___	___	Currently smoke cigarettes?
19	___	___	Have a history of cigarette smoking, but stopped?

If no longer smoking, specify number of years since you stopped.

20	___ 1 yr.	23	___ 4 yrs.	26	___ 7 yrs.
21	___ 2 yrs.	24	___ 5 yrs.	27	___ 8 yrs.
22	___ 3 yrs.	25	___ 6 yrs.	28	___ 9 or more yrs.

If you have ever smoked cigarettes, specify amount and duration.

Daily amount		**Number of years**	
29	___ 1/2 pack/day or less	33	___ Less than 1 year
30	___ 1/2 to 1 pack/day	34	___ 1 to 5 years
31	___ 1 to 2 packs/day	35	___ 5 to 10 years
32	___ Over 2 packs/day	36	___ Over 10 years

ALCOHOL

	Yes	No	
37	___	___	Do you currently drink alcohol?
38	___	___	Did you formerly drink alcohol but stopped?

If you have ever drunk alcohol, specify details.

Amount per week		**Number of years**	
39	___ Less than 2 drinks/wk.	44	___ Less than one year
40	___ 2 to 10 drinks/wk.	45	___ 1 to 5 years
41	___ 10 to 25 drinks/wk.	46	___ 5 to 10 years
42	___ 25 to 40 drinks/wk.	47	___ 10 to 20 years
43	___ Over 40 drinks/wk.	48	___ Over 20 years

TRAUMA, ACCIDENTS and OTHER HAZARDS

	Yes	No	Do you-
50	___	___	Know how to swim?
51	___	___	Drive after drinking or taking drugs?
52	___	___	Tend to exceed the speed limit?

How many miles do you travel in a car or other motor vehicle each year (average is 12,000 miles)?

53	___ Up to 10,000	55	___ 15,000 to 20,000
54	___ 10,000 to 15,000	56	___ Over 20,000

What percent of the time do you wear a seat belt?

57	___ 0 to 25%	59	___ 50% to 75%
58	___ 25% to 50%	60	___ 75% to 100%

What percent of the time do you wear a shoulder strap?

61	___ 0 to 25%	63	___ 50% to 75%
62	___ 25% to 50%	64	___ 75% to 100%

9-108
SELF-CARE

The early evaluation of symptoms, self-exams, and various professional health exams are important in detecting diseases. Regular medical follow-up is important in keeping problems under control and avoiding complications.

	Yes	No	Have you-
10	___	___	Ever had a chest x-ray?
11	___	___	Had an abnormal chest x-ray?
12	___	___	Ever had an EKG (Electrocardiogram)?
13	___	___	Had an abnormal EKG?
14	___	___	Had a TB skin test?
15	___	___	Had a positive TB skin test?
16	___	___	Had eyes checked in past two years?
17	___	___	Had hearing tested (audiometry) in past 2 years?
18	___	___	Had dental exam in the past year?
			Do you-
19	___	___	Regularly follow your physician's advice?
20	___	___	Plan annual medical symptom review with your physician or health service?
21	___	___	Plan annual rectal exam after age 30?

WOMEN *(Men go to "Tests")*

	Yes	No	Do you or have you-
30	___	___	Had a PAP test within past year?
31	___	___	Had at least three PAP tests in past 5 years?
32	___	___	Had an abnormal PAP test in past?
33	___	___	Plan annual PAP tests in the future?
34	___	___	Check your breasts once a month for lumps?
35	___	___	Have a breast exam by a doctor once yearly?

TESTS For these tests, if ever done, find out results from your physician. Check values shown that are closest to your own results. If measured more than once, use most recent value.

Blood Pressure				**Cholesterol**	
Systolic		**Diastolic**			
40 ___ 120 or less		45 ___ 82 or less		50 ___ 180 or less	
41 ___ 140		46 ___ 88		51 ___ 210	
42 ___ 160		47 ___ 94		52 ___ 240	
43 ___ 180		48 ___ 100		53 ___ 270	
44 ___ 200 or more		49 ___ 106 or more		54 ___ 300 or more	

INFORMATION

Check items for which you would like educational information.

60	___ Alcohol	68	___ Legal problems
61	___ Birth Control	69	___ Loneliness
62	___ Diet	70	___ Marital problems
63	___ Drug abuse	71	___ Medical emergencies
64	___ Emotional problems	72	___ Self-breast exam
65	___ Exercise	73	___ Sexual problems
66	___ Financial problems	74	___ Smoking
67	___ Health hazards	75	___ Venereal disease

CONCLUSION

	Yes	No	
80	___	___	Do you have any other problem not covered by this questionnaire?

Please give us your opinion of this system.

81	___ Great	83	___ Generally good, criticism minor
82	___ Good	84	___ Don't like it

Thanks for completing this questionnaire. Please review for accuracy, then mail or turn in according to instructions.

© Medical Datamation 1980

C4—LIFESTYLE ASSESSMENT QUESTIONNAIRE

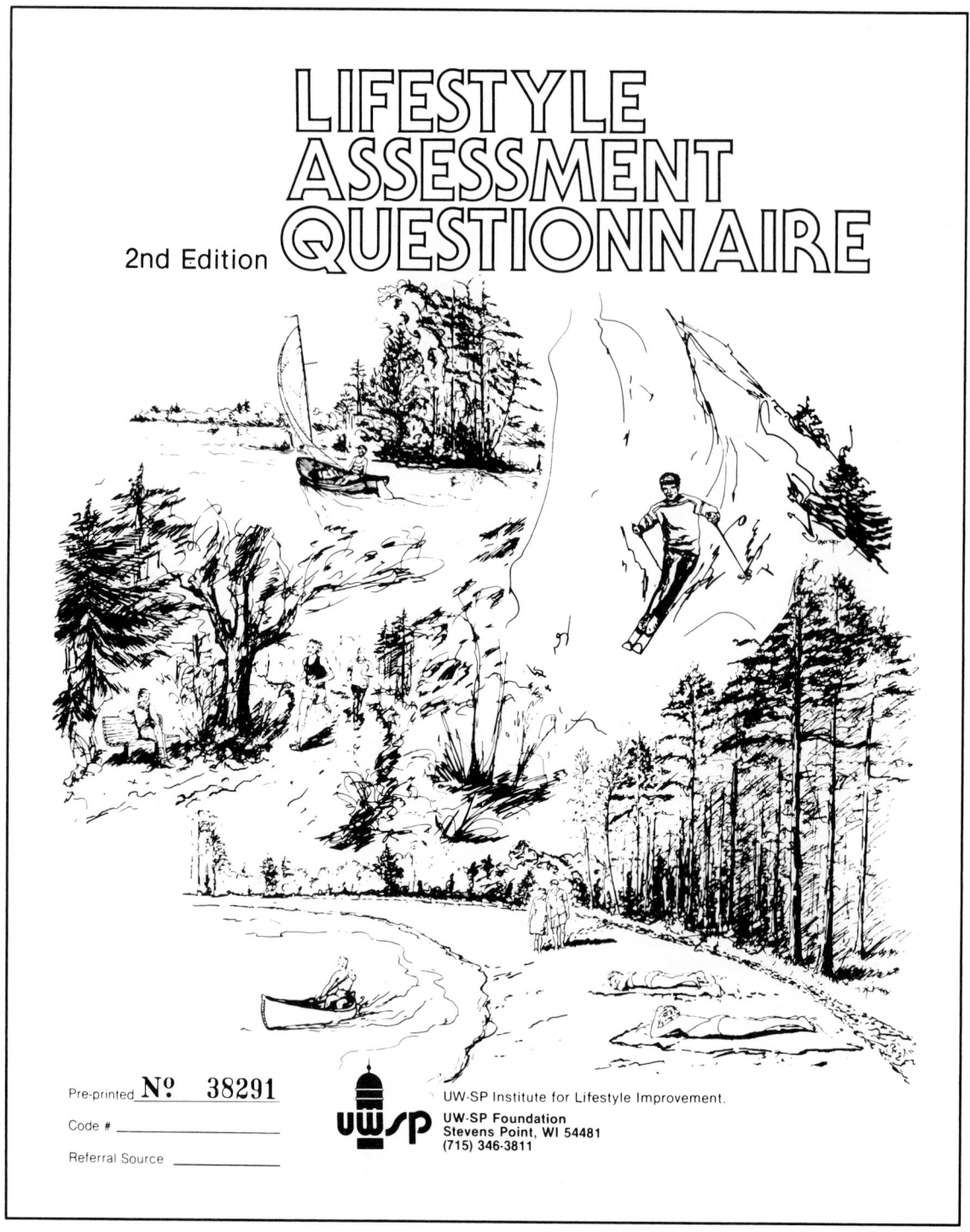

LIFESTYLE ASSESSMENT QUESTIONNAIRE
2nd Edition

Pre-printed № 38291

Code # _____

Referral Source _____

UW-SP Institute for Lifestyle Improvement.

UW-SP Foundation
Stevens Point, WI 54481
(715) 346-3811

purpose

This Lifestyle Assessment Questionnaire is designed to help you assess your current level of wellness and the potential risks or hazards that you choose to face at this point in your life. The printouts that you will receive will reflect your strengths and the possible consequences of risks that you choose to take. The questionnaire will also assess your interest in improving the quality of your life. The printout will indicate sources of information that will help you learn more about gaining higher levels of wellness.

THE MAJOR DETERMINANT FOR JOYFUL LIVING IS YOU AND YOUR LIFESTYLE

The circle graph below indicates the factors that contribute to increasing your enjoyment and quality of life. While it is true that doctors and hospitals have a significant role to play in the quality of our lives, this graph clearly indicates that it is individuals, through the choices that they make each day, that contribute the greatest percentage toward maximizing the quality of life and health. We believe this instrument can be a useful adjunct in helping individuals identify the most likely causes of death and disability, but more importantly identify the areas of self-improvement which will lead to higher levels of joy and wellness. This instrument can be used to begin a positive, wellness approach toward living. It is our belief that this instrument can help people realize that they are the most important provider of health or "illth" care. Many of the common killers in America are the direct result of individual behaviors. We all know that our behaviors can improve our chances for leading a long useful life. Collectively, all of our behaviors can be described as our lifestyle.

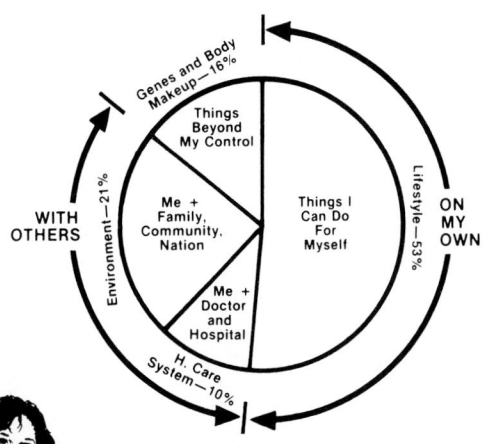

GENERAL INFORMATION CONCERNING THE LIFESTYLE ASSESSMENT QUESTIONNAIRE (LAQ)

The LAQ is organized into four sections: 1. Wellness Inventory; 2. Topics for Personal Growth; 3. Risk of Death Section, and 4. Alert Section: Medical/Behavioral/Emotional. The Wellness Inventory Section will help you identify your strengths. You will receive a printout that will indicate the percent of possible points that you gained in each topic area. The printout will also provide you with average scores for the people in your group and the total average for all people who have ever used this instrument.

The automated referral or Personal Growth section of this questionnaire will provide a printout indicating resources available for up to six topics.

The Risk of Death section will result in a printout indicating the probable number of years that you have remaining in your life, the leading causes of death for your age, race, and sex, and what behaviors could be changed to improve the chances of survival and the quality of your life.

The final section of this questionnaire entitled the Alert Section: Medical/Behavorial/Emotional will provide information which can generate a problem list for your home health record. This could also be used as part of a medical chart in a health care delivery system. We feel it will be useful for people to maintain, in their home, a current record of their immunization status and other significant problems.

It is our desire that this questionnaire be used in a positive sense to improve the understanding of self and your role in maintaining a life of high quality.

Continued.

confidentiality

The Institute for Lifestyle Improvement will maintain the confidentiality of your answers. The Institute will not permit any individually identified information from your questionnaire to be released to any person or organization other than the source from whom the LAQ was received.

Bill Hettler M.D.
Bill Hettler, M.D.

Dennis Elsenrath
Dennis Elsenrath, Ed. D.

Fred Leafgren
Fred Leafgren, Ph.D.

THE UNIVERSITY OF WISCONSIN-STEVENS POINT INSTITUTE FOR LIFESTYLE IMPROVEMENT STEVENS POINT, WISCONSIN 54481 (715) 346-3811

The Institute for Lifestyle Improvement, which exists within the structure of the UW-SP Foundation, has three broad missions: 1. To provide health promotion services to public and private agencies; 2. To conduct research on lifestyle improvement activities; and 3. To provide continuing educational and training programs for those interested in wellness promotion strategies.

The Institute offers services in four major areas:

Lifestyle Assessment Questionnaire	Consultation and Presentation	Continuing Educational and Training Programs	Audio-Visual Materials and Self-Care Modules
—Individual and group needs assessment	—Keynote speakers for local and national meetings	—Annual wellness promotion strategies conference	—Production of movies on wellness promotion topics
—Motivational tool	—Planning for community forums	—Specialized conferences for target groups	—Production of videotapes, audio-tapes and slide/tape presentations on wellness promotion
—Health planning tool to estimate current and future disease care needs	—Facilitators for health fairs	—On site training programs for corporations, universities or communities	—Written materials to support wellness promotion activities
—Self-care tool to provide home health care record	—Speakers for corporate wellness programs	—In-service training for teachers and other youth workers	—Other assessment instruments for wellness promotion
	—Corporate wellness program planning and evaluation		—Cold self-care module
	—Consultation for community health promotion		

1 lifestyle assessment questionnaire

WELLNESS INVENTORY SECTION

INSTRUCTIONS: This section will help determine the current level of wellness that you are experiencing. We hope that it will also give you ideas for areas in which you might improve. If you are uncomfortable in answering any item in this section or following sections, you may leave that item blank. Please respond to these statements using the following choices and circle your response:

A—Almost always (90% or more of the time)
B—Very frequently (approximately 75% of the time)
C—Frequently (approximately 50% of the time)
D—Occasionally (approximately 25% of the time)
E—Almost never (less than 10% of the time)
—If item does not apply to you do not mark item

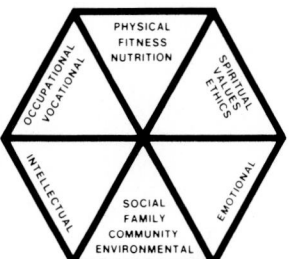

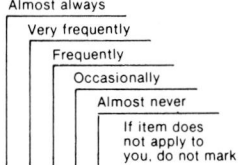

Almost always
Very frequently
Frequently
Occasionally
Almost never
If item does not apply to you, do not mark

PHYSICAL EXERCISE—Measures one's commitment to maintaining physical fitness.

1. I exercise vigorously for at least 20 minutes three or more times per week . . . .   A B C D E
2. I determine my activity level by monitoring my heart rate. . . . .   A B C D E
3. I stop exercising before I feel exhausted . . . .   A B C D E
4. I approach exercise in a relaxed manner. . . . .   A B C D E
5. I stretch before exercising. . . . .   A B C D E
6. I stretch after exercising . . . .   A B C D E
7. I walk or bike whenever possible . . . .   A B C D E
8. When feeling tired, I arrange for sufficient sleep   A B C D E
9. I participate in a strenuous sport (tennis, running, swimming, handball, basketball, etc.) . . . . .   A B C D E
10. I use foot gear of good quality, designed for the activity in which I participate . . . .   A B C D E
11. If I am not in shape, I avoid sporadic (once a week or less often) strenuous exercise. . . . .   A B C D E
12. After vigorous exercise, I "cool down" (very light exercise such as walking) for at least five minutes before sitting or lying down . . . .   A B C D E

Continued.

PHYSICAL-NUTRITIONAL—Measures the degree to which one chooses foods that are consistent with the dietary goals of the United States as published by the Senate Select Committee on Nutrition and Human Needs.

Almost always
Very frequently
Frequently
Occasionally
Almost never
If item does not apply to you, do not mark

13. When choosing non-vegetable protein, I select lean cuts of meat, poultry and fish. . . . .   A B C D E
14. I maintain an appropriate weight for my height and frame . . . .   A B C D E
15. I minimize salt intake . . . .   A B C D E
16. I eat fruits and vegetables fresh and uncooked . .   A B C D E
17. I eat breakfast . . . .   A B C D E
18. I intentionally include fiber in my diet on a daily basis . . . .   A B C D E
19. I drink enough fluid to keep my urine light yellow . . . .   A B C D E
20. I plan my diet to insure an adequate amount of vitamins and minerals. . . . .   A B C D E
21. I minimize foods in my diet that contain large amounts of refined flour (bleached white flour, typical store bread, cakes, etc.) . . . .   A B C D E
22. I minimize my intake of fats and oils including margarine and animal fats . . . .   A B C D E
23. I include items from all four basic food groups in my diet each day (fruits and vegetables; milk group; breads and cereals; meat, fowl, fish or vegetable proteins) . . . .   A B C D E
24. To avoid unnecessary calories, I choose water as one of the beverages I drink . . . .   A B C D E
25. I avoid adding sugar to my food and I minimize my intake of pre-sweetened foods such as sugar-coated cereals, syrups, chocolate milk, and most processed and fast foods.   A B C D E

PHYSICAL-SELF-CARE—Measures the behaviors that help one prevent or detect early illnesses.

26. I maintain an up-to-date immunization record . . .   A B C D E
27. I examine my breasts or testes on a monthly basis . . . .   A B C D E
28. I have my breasts or testes examined yearly by a physician . . . .   A B C D E
29. I have a Pap test annually (Males—do not mark).   A B C D E
30. I take action to minimize my exposure to tobacco smoke . . . .   A B C D E
31. When I'm experiencing illness or injury, I take necessary steps to correct the problem . . . .   A B C D E
32. I brush my teeth after eating. . . . .   A B C D E
33. I floss my teeth after eating . . . .   A B C D E
34. My resting pulse is 60 or less . . . .   A B C D E
35. I get an adequate amount of sleep. . . . .   A B C D E
36. I keep my blood pressure in a range that minimizes my chances of disease. (e.g., stroke, heart attack and kidney disease). . . . .   A B C D E
37. I keep my cholesterol level, high density lipids and triglycerides in a range that minimize my chances of disease . . . .   A B C D E
38. If I were to engage in sex and didn't want children at that time, I would use a contraceptive method . . . .   A B C D E
39. I take action to prevent contracting and/or transmitting venereal disease . . . .   A B C D E

1

Almost always
　Very frequently
　　Frequently
　　　Occasionally
　　　　Almost never
　　　　　If item does
　　　　　not apply to
　　　　　you, do not mark

PHYSICAL-VEHICLE SAFETY—Measures one's ability to minimize chances of injury or death in a vehicle accident.

40. I do not operate vehicles under the influence of alcohol or other drugs ....   A B C D E
41. I do not ride with vehicle operators who are under the influence of alcohol or other drugs .....   A B C D E
42. I stay within the speed limit ....   A B C D E
43. I use the information I learned in a driver education or defensive driving course ....   A B C D E
44. When traffic lights change from green to yellow, I prepare to stop ....   A B C D E
45. I maintain a safe driving distance between cars based on speed and road conditions...........   A B C D E
46. Vehicles which I drive are maintained to assure safety...   A B C D E
47. Because they are safer, I use radial tires on cars that I drive................................   A B C D E
48. I use caution when riding bicycles or motorcycles (e.g., helmets, adequate lights, etc.) .....   A B C D E

PHYSICAL-DRUG USAGE—Measures the degree to which one is able to function without the unnecessary use of chemicals.

49. I use drugs only when necessary ....   A B C D E
50. I avoid the use of tobacco ....   A B C D E
51. I do not consume more than two alcoholic drinks per day ....   A B C D E
52. Because of the potentially harmful effects of caffeine (e.g., coffee, tea, cola, etc.), I limit my consumption ....   A B C D E
53. I avoid using marijuana ....   A B C D E
54. I avoid the use of hallucinogens (LSD, PCP, MDA, etc.).................................   A B C D E
55. I avoid the use of stimulants ("uppers"—e.g., cocaine, amphetamines, "pep pills", etc.) .....   A B C D E
56. I avoid the use of depressants ("downers"—e.g., barbiturates, minor tranquilizers, etc.)..........   A B C D E
57. I avoid using a combination of drugs unless under medical supervision ....   A B C D E
58. I follow the instructions provided with any drug I take ....   A B C D E
59. I avoid using drugs obtained from unlicensed sources ....   A B C D E
60. I understand the expected effect of drugs I take.   A B C D E
61. I consider alternatives to drugs ....   A B C D E

SOCIAL-ENVIRONMENTAL—Measures the degree to which one contributes to the common welfare of the community. This emphasizes the interdependence with others and nature.

62. I take steps to conserve energy in my place of residence ....   A B C D E
63. I consider energy conservation when choosing a mode of transportation.....................   A B C D E
64. I offer support to members of my family when appropriate.................................   A B C D E
65. I contribute to the feeling of acceptance within my family ....   A B C D E
66. I do my part to promote clean air.............   A B C D E
67. When I see a safety hazard, I take action (warn others or correct the problem) ....   A B C D E
68. I avoid unnecessary radiation ....   A B C D E
69. I report criminal acts I observe ....   A B C D E

Continued.

```
                                              Almost always
                                               ┌ Very frequently
                                               │ ┌ Frequently
                                               │ │ ┌ Occasionally
                                               │ │ │ ┌ Almost never
                                               │ │ │ │ ┌ If item does
                                               │ │ │ │ │  not apply to
                                               │ │ │ │ │  you, do not mark
```

70. I contribute time and/or money to community
    projects . . . .   A B C D E
71. I actively seek to become acquainted with in-
    dividuals in my community . . . .   A B C D E
72. I use my creativity in constructive ways . . . .   A B C D E
73. My behavior reflects fairness and justice . . . .   A B C D E
74. When possible, I choose an environment which
    is free of noise pollution . . . .   A B C D E
75. When possible, I choose an environment which
    is free of air pollution . . . .   A B C D E
76. I participate in volunteer activities benefiting
    others . . . .   A B C D E
77. I go out of my way to help others . . . .   A B C D E
78. I beautify those parts of my environment under
    my control . . . .   A B C D E

EMOTIONAL AWARENESS & ACCEPTANCE—Meas-
    ures the degree to which one has an awareness
    and acceptance of one's feelings. This includes
    the degree to which one feels positive and en-
    thusiastic about oneself and life.

79. I have a good sense of humor . . . .   A B C D E
80. I feel positive about myself . . . .   A B C D E
81. I feel there is a satisfying amount of excitement
    in my life . . . .   A B C D E
82. My emotional life is stable . . . .   A B C D E
83. I am aware of my needs . . . .   A B C D E
84. I trust and value my own judgment . . . .   A B C D E
85. When I make mistakes, I learn from them . . . .   A B C D E
86. I feel comfortable when complimented for jobs
    well done . . . .   A B C D E
87. It is okay for me to cry . . . .   A B C D E
88. I have feelings of sensitivity for others . . . .   A B C D E
89. I feel enthusiastic about life . . . .   A B C D E
90. I find it easy to laugh . . . .   A B C D E
91. I am able to give love . . . .   A B C D E
92. I am able to receive love . . . .   A B C D E
93. I enjoy my life . . . .   A B C D E
94. I have plenty of energy . . . .   A B C D E
95. My sleep is restful . . . .   A B C D E
96. I trust others . . . .   A B C D E
97. I feel others trust me . . . .   A B C D E
98. I accept my sexual desires . . . .   A B C D E
99. I understand how I create my feelings . . . .   A B C D E
100. At times I can be both strong and sensitive . . . . .   A B C D E
101. I am aware when I feel anger . . . .   A B C D E
102. I can accept my anger . . . .   A B C D E
103. I am aware when I feel sad . . . .   A B C D E
104. I can accept my sadness . . . .   A B C D E
105. I am aware when I feel happy . . . .   A B C D E
106. I can accept my happiness . . . .   A B C D E
107. I am aware when I feel frightened . . . .   A B C D E
108. I can accept my feelings of fear . . . .   A B C D E

EMOTIONAL MANAGEMENT—Measures the cap-
    acity to appropriately control one's feelings and
    related behaviors including the realistic assess-
    ment of one's limitations.

109. I am able to be open with those with whom I
    am close . . . .   A B C D E
110. I can express my feelings of anger . . . .   A B C D E

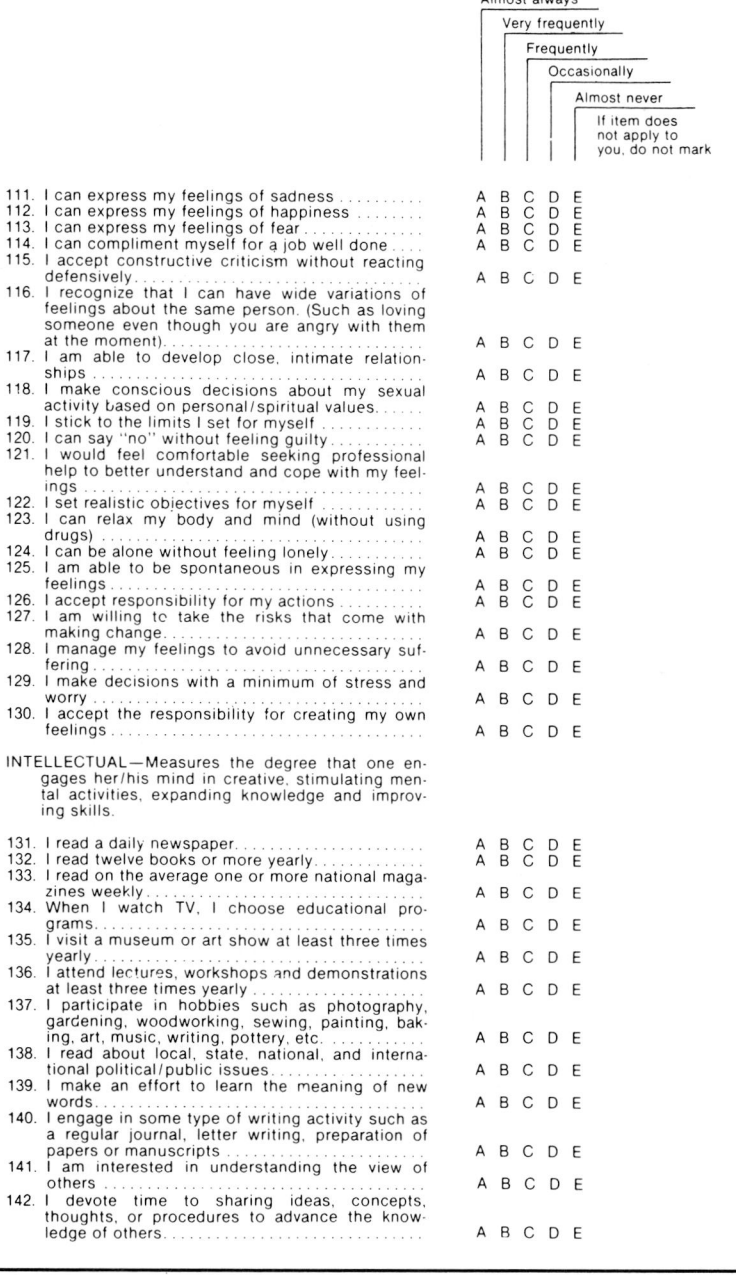

1

Almost always
Very frequently
Frequently
Occasionally
Almost never
If item does
not apply to
you, do not mark

111. I can express my feelings of sadness . . . .   A B C D E
112. I can express my feelings of happiness . . . .   A B C D E
113. I can express my feelings of fear . . . .   A B C D E
114. I can compliment myself for a job well done . . . .   A B C D E
115. I accept constructive criticism without reacting
defensively . . . .   A B C D E
116. I recognize that I can have wide variations of
feelings about the same person. (Such as loving
someone even though you are angry with them
at the moment) . . . .   A B C D E
117. I am able to develop close, intimate relation-
ships . . . .   A B C D E
118. I make conscious decisions about my sexual
activity based on personal/spiritual values . . . . . .   A B C D E
119. I stick to the limits I set for myself . . . .   A B C D E
120. I can say "no" without feeling guilty . . . .   A B C D E
121. I would feel comfortable seeking professional
help to better understand and cope with my feel-
ings . . . .   A B C D E
122. I set realistic objectives for myself . . . .   A B C D E
123. I can relax my body and mind (without using
drugs) . . . .   A B C D E
124. I can be alone without feeling lonely . . . .   A B C D E
125. I am able to be spontaneous in expressing my
feelings . . . .   A B C D E
126. I accept responsibility for my actions . . . .   A B C D E
127. I am willing to take the risks that come with
making change . . . .   A B C D E
128. I manage my feelings to avoid unnecessary suf-
fering . . . .   A B C D E
129. I make decisions with a minimum of stress and
worry . . . .   A B C D E
130. I accept the responsibility for creating my own
feelings . . . .   A B C D E

INTELLECTUAL—Measures the degree that one engages her/his mind in creative, stimulating mental activities, expanding knowledge and improving skills.

131. I read a daily newspaper.   A B C D E
132. I read twelve books or more yearly . . . .   A B C D E
133. I read on the average one or more national maga-
zines weekly . . . .   A B C D E
134. When I watch TV, I choose educational pro-
grams. . . . .   A B C D E
135. I visit a museum or art show at least three times
yearly . . . .   A B C D E
136. I attend lectures, workshops and demonstrations
at least three times yearly . . . .   A B C D E
137. I participate in hobbies such as photography,
gardening, woodworking, sewing, painting, bak-
ing, art, music, writing, pottery, etc. . . . .   A B C D E
138. I read about local, state, national, and interna-
tional political/public issues. . . . .   A B C D E
139. I make an effort to learn the meaning of new
words. . . . .   A B C D E
140. I engage in some type of writing activity such as
a regular journal, letter writing, preparation of
papers or manuscripts . . . .   A B C D E
141. I am interested in understanding the view of
others . . . .   A B C D E
142. I devote time to sharing ideas, concepts,
thoughts, or procedures to advance the know-
ledge of others. . . . .   A B C D E

Continued.

Almost always
Very frequently
Frequently
Occasionally
Almost never
If item does
not apply to
you, do not mark

143. I gather information to enable me to make in-
dependent decisions. . . . .   A B C D E
144. I listen to radio and/or TV news . . . .   A B C D E

OCCUPATIONAL—Measures the satisfaction gained
from one's work and the degree to which one is
enriched by that work.

Please answer these items from your primary frame of reference, (e.g., your
job, student, homemaker, etc.) If you are unemployed or retired, do not
mark this section.

145. I enjoy my work . . . .   A B C D E
146. My work contributes to my personal needs . . . . .   A B C D E
147. I feel that my job in some way contributes to
others and/or society . . . .   A B C D E
148. I interact cooperatively with others in my work . .   A B C D E
149. I take advantage of opportunities to learn new
skills in my work . . . .   A B C D E
150. My work is challenging. . . . .   A B C D E
151. I feel my job responsibilities are consistent with
my values . . . .   A B C D E
152. I find satisfaction from the work I do. . . . .   A B C D E
153. I find healthy ways of reducing excessive stress
when it occurs in my job . . . .   A B C D E
154. I use recommended health and safety pre-
cautions . . . .   A B C D E
155. I make recommendations for improving occupa-
tional health and safety . . . .   A B C D E
156. I am satisfied with the degree of freedom to ex-
ercise independent judgments in my job . . . .   A B C D E
157. I am satisfied with the amount of variety in my
work. . . . .   A B C D E
158. I believe I am competent in my job . . . .   A B C D E
159. My co-workers and supervisors respect me as a
competent individual . . . .   A B C D E

SPIRITUAL—Measures one's ongoing involvement
in seeking meaning and purpose in human existence. It includes an appreciation for the depth
and expanse of life and natural forces that exist
in the universe.

160. I feel good about my spiritual life. . . . .   A B C D E
161. Prayer, meditation, and/or quiet personal reflec-
tion is/are important part(s) of my life. . . . .   A B C D E
162. I contemplate my purpose in life . . . .   A B C D E
163. I reflect on the meaning of events in my life . . . .   A B C D E
164. My values guide my daily life . . . .   A B C D E
165. My values and beliefs help me to meet daily
challenges . . . .   A B C D E
166. I recognize that my spiritual growth is a lifelong
process. . . . .   A B C D E
167. I am concerned about humanitarian issues . . . . .   A B C D E
168. I enjoy participating in discussions about spirit-
ual values . . . .   A B C D E
169. I feel a sense of compassion to others in need . .   A B C D E
170. I seek spiritual knowledge . . . .   A B C D E
171. My spiritual awareness occurs other than at
times of crisis . . . .   A B C D E
172. I believe in something greater or (that I am part
of something greater) than myself . . . .   A B C D E
173. I share my spiritual values . . . .   A B C D E

2 lifestyle assessment questionnaire

TOPICS FOR PERSONAL GROWTH SECTION

INSTRUCTIONS:
This section is intended to help you identify areas in which you would like more information or sources for group activities for continued learning or confidential personal assistance. In response to your selection from the following topics we will provide you with resources or services to meet your requests.

With regard to the following list, I would like:

	Information	Group Activities	Confidential Personal Assistance
1. Responsible alcohol use	1	2	3
2. Stop smoking programs	1	2	3
3. Sexual dysfunction	1	2	3
4. Contraception	1	2	3
5. Venereal disease	1	2	3
6. Depression	1	2	3
7. Loneliness	1	2	3
8. Exercise programs	1	2	3
9. Weight reduction	1	2	3
10. Self breast exam	1	2	3
11. Medical emergencies	1	2	3
12. Vegetarian diets	1	2	3
13. Relaxation - stress reduction	1	2	3
14. Mate selection	1	2	3
15. Parenting skills	1	2	3
16. Marital (or couples) problems	1	2	3
17. Assertive training (How to say no without feeling guilty)	1	2	3
18. Biofeedback for tension headache	1	2	3
19. Overcoming phobias (ex. high places, crowded rooms, etc.)	1	2	3
20. Educational/Career goal setting/planning	1	2	3
21. Spiritual or philosophical values	1	2	3
22. Interpersonal communication skills	1	2	3
23. Automobile safety	1	2	3
24. Suicide thoughts or attempts	1	2	3
25. Drug abuse	1	2	3
26. Test anxiety reduction	1	2	3
27. Enhancing Relationships	1	2	3
28. Time Management Skills	1	2	3
29. Nutrition	1	2	3
30. Death and Dying	1	2	3
31. Learning Skills (Speed reading, comprehension, etc.)	1	2	3

Continued.

3 lifestyle assessment questionnaire

RISK OF DEATH SECTION

INSTRUCTIONS:

This section is intended to help you identify the problems most likely to interfere with the quality of your life. This will give you a statistical assessment of the most likely causes of death facing you for the next ten (10) years. This section will also indicate what impact various personal behavioral choices have on that risk of death. Although this section will give you a printout indicating a statistical measurement of your risk based on national morbidity and mortality data, the printout will be no guarantee. Pre-existing disease or chance occurrence can completely negate the recommendations or suggestions made on this printout. We do feel, however, that it is a fairly accurate assessment of your current state of risk and offers suggestions for improving the quality of life and useful longevity.

Age in years _____

Height _____ ft. _____ inches

Weight in pounds _____

1. Sex:
   1. Male
   2. Female

2. Race:
   1. White
   2. Black
   2. Other

3. How would you describe your body build?
   1. Small
   2. Medium
   3. Large

4. What is your systolic (top number) blood pressure?
   1. 190 or more
   2. 170-189
   3. 150-169
   4. 130-149
   5. Less than 130
   Note: If you don't know your blood pressure, we will use the average for your age, race, and sex.

5. What is your diastolic (lower number) blood pressure?
   1. 103 or more
   2. 97-102
   3. 91-96
   4. 85-90
   5. Less than 85

6. What is your blood cholesterol level?
   1. 270 or more
   2. 230-269
   3. 210-229
   4. 190-209
   5. Less than 190
   Note: If you don't know your cholesterol level, we will use the average for your age, race, and sex.

7. Are you
   1. An uncontrolled diabetic
   2. A controlled diabetic
   3. Not a diabetic

8. Which of the following best describes how much physical activity you get per week including work?
   1. Climb less than 5 flights of stairs or walk less than ½ mile 4 times per week (or equivalent activity)
   2. Climb 5-15 flights of stairs or walk ½-1½ miles 4 times per week (or equivalent activity)
   3. Climb 15-20 flights of stairs or walk 1½-2 miles 4 times per week (or equivalent activity)

9. Family history of heart disease:
   1. Both parents died before age 60 of heart disease
   2. One parent died before age 60 of heart disease
   3. Neither parent died before age of 60 of heart disease

10. Do you smoke tobacco?
    1. Yes
    2. No

11. If yes, how much do you smoke per day?
    1. 2 packs of cigarettes or more
    2. 1½-2 packs of cigarettes
    3. 1-1½ packs of cigarettes
    4. ½-1 pack of cigarettes or heavy pipe or cigar
    5. Less than ½ pack of cigarettes or light pipe or cigar

12. If 10 is yes, how many years have you been smoking?
    1. Less than 2
    2. 2 - 5
    3. 5 - 10
    4. 11 - 15
    5. 16 or more

13. Are you a former smoker?
    1. Yes
    2. No

14. If yes, how much did you smoke per day?
    1. 2 packs of cigarettes or more
    2. 1½-2 packs of cigarettes
    3. 1-1½ packs of cigarettes
    4. ½-1 pack of cigarettes or heavy pipe or cigar
    5. Less than ½ pack of cigarettes or light pipe or cigar

15. How many years ago did you quit?
   1. 0-2 years
   2. 3-4
   3. 5-6
   4. 7-8
   5. 9 or more

16. Do you drink alcoholic beverages?
   1. Yes
   2. No

17. If yes to the question above, how many per week?
   1. More than 40 drinks
   2. 25-40
   3. 8-24
   4. 3-7
   5. 1-2

18. When consuming alcohol, I do not consume more than one drink per hour.
   1. Yes
   2. No

19. How many miles a year do you travel in a motor vehicle as a driver or passenger?
   1. Under 10,000
   2. 10,000-20,000
   3. 20,000-30,000
   4. 30,000-40,000
   5. Over 40,000

20. While traveling in a motor vehicle how often do you use seat belts?
   1. 20% or less of the time
   2. 20%-40%
   3. 40%-60%
   4. 60%-80%
   5. 80%-100%

21. Are you depressed much of the time?
   1. Frequently
   2. Seldom
   3. Never

22. Has anyone in your immediate family (parents, brothers, sisters) committed suicide?
   1. Yes
   2. No

23. In regard to your heart, have you had:
   1. A murmur without preventive antibiotics
   2. A murmur with preventive antibiotics
   3. No murmur

24. In regard to your heart, have you had:
   1. Rheumatic fever without preventive antibiotics
   2. Rheumatic fever with preventive antibiotics
   3. No rheumatic fever

25. To the best of your knowledge, do you have any signs or symptoms of rheumatic heart disease?
   1. Yes
   2. No

26. Have you ever been arrested for burglary, robbery, or assault?
   1. Yes
   2. No

27. Do you carry a weapon with you?
   1. Yes
   2. No

28. Have you ever had bacterial pneumonia?
   1. Yes
   2. No

29. Have you ever had emphysema?
   1. Yes
   2. No

30. Has anyone in your family (parents, brothers, sisters) had diabetes?
   1. Yes
   2. No

31. Have you ever had polyps (growth in the intestines?)
   1. Yes
   2. No

32. Have you ever had undiagnosed rectal bleeding?
   1. Yes
   2. No

33. Have you ever had ulcerative colitis?
   1. Yes, 10 or more years ago
   2. Yes, less than 10 years ago
   3. No

34. Have you had a rectal examination with a lighted instrument within the last year?
   1. Yes
   2. No

IF FEMALE, ANSWER THE FOLLOWING 9 QUESTIONS:

35. Do you perform a regular monthly self-breast examination?
   1. Yes
   2. No

36. Do you have a yearly exam by your physician?
   1. Yes
   2. No

37. How many of your blood relatives (mother, sister, aunts) have had breast cancer?
   1. 2 or more
   2. 1
   3. None

38. Have you ever had fibrocystic breast disease or other noncancerous disease?
   1. Yes
   2. No

39. Are you Jewish? (Cancer of the cervix is very rare in Jewish women)
   1. Yes
   2. No

40. Age of first intercourse. (Cancer of the cervix is more common in females who have first intercourse in teens and/or have multiple partners)
   1. Under 20 years old
   2. 20-25 years old
   3. Over 25 years old or never

41. Pertaining to a Pap smear, mark the response most accurate for you (we assume none were abnormal)
   1. Haven't had one in last five (5) years
   2. Had 1 normal within the last five (5) years
   3. Had 1 normal within last year
   4. Had 3 normal within the last five (5) years
   5. Had one normal each of the last five (5) years

42. Have you experienced undiagnosed vaginal bleeding?
   1. Yes
   2. No

43. Do you now take birth control pills?
   1. Yes
   2. No

Continued.

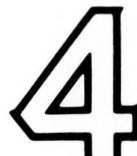

lifestyle assessment questionnaire

ALERT
SECTION

medical/behavioral/emotional

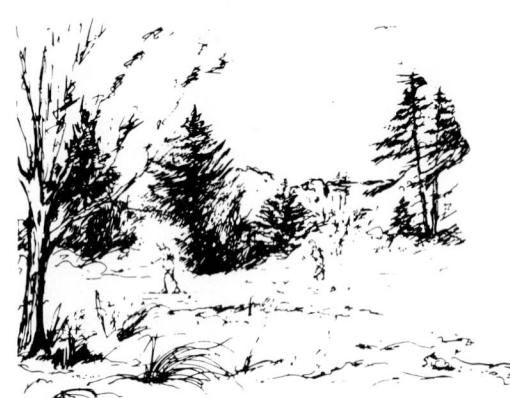

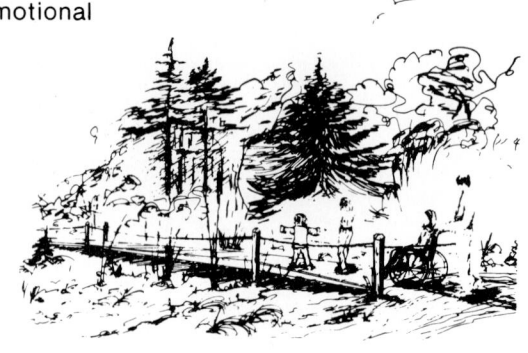

INSTRUCTIONS:

This section is intended to be used to identify high risk problems or past medical problems that we feel are important in establishing one's medical records. This can be used for a personal record by the individual or can be used by professionals as a problem list to be incorporated with the remainder of the individual's medical records. Please circle the number that is most correct in answering each question. Any question that you do not feel comfortable in answering or you think is not pertinent please leave blank.

MEDICAL

1. Do you have diabetes? .... **1. Yes 2. No**

2. Do you have a seizure disorder (epilepsy)?........................... **1. Yes 2. No**

3. Do you have known heart **trouble** (acquired or congenital)? .... **1. Yes 2. No**

4. Did any of your blood relatives die of heart disease under the age of 50?.... **1. Yes 2. No**

5. Have you had major surgery?........ **1. Yes 2. No**

6. Do you have a physical disability that interferes with routine activities including physical fitness programs? .... **1. Yes 2. No**

7. Have you had a skin test for TB in the past two (2) years?................. **1. Yes 2. No**

8. If YES to number 7, which result did you have?......................... **1. reaction**
no
2. reaction

9. Do you take any medication daily or several times per week? .... **1. Yes 2. No**

10. Do you have allergies to drugs? ...... **1. Yes 2. No**

11. Are you allergic to penicillin?........ **1. Yes 2. No**

12. Are you allergic to sulfa? .... **1. Yes 2. No**

13. Are you allergic to aspirin?.......... **1. Yes 2. No**

14. Do you have additional drug allergies not listed above? .... **1. Yes 2. No**

15. Do you have asthma? .... **1. Yes 2. No**

4

IMMUNIZATIONS

16. Did you have baby shots for DPT (diphtheria, whooping cough, and tetanus)? Ask your parents or doctor. . . . .   **1.Yes 2. No**

17. Have you had a booster for tetanus in the last five (5) years? (Recommended interval is 5-10 years.). . . . .   **1.Yes 2. No**

18. Have you had a form of polio vaccine?   **1.Yes 2. No**

19. With regard to German measles: **1.Yes 2. No**

> **1. have had a blood test showing immunity or received rubella immunization.**
>
> **2. never had a blood test or the blood test showed no immunity to rubella (German measles.)**

20. Have you had a Pap test in the last year?. . . . .   **1.Yes 2. No**

21. Have you ever had an abnormal Pap test?. . . . .   **1.Yes 2. No**

22. Were you exposed to DES (diethylstilbesterol) while your mother was pregnant with you? (Ask your mother to check with her doctor if you are not sure.). . . . .   **1.Yes 2. No**

BEHAVIORAL/EMOTIONAL

NOTE: The leading cause of death among young adults is auto accidents.

23. Do you drive a car, motorcycle, or bike after drinking alcohol?. . . . .   **1.Yes 2. No**

24. Do you ride with "drinking" drivers? . .   **1.Yes 2. No**

NOTE: The second leading cause of death among young adults is suicide.

25. Have you seriously considered killing yourself within the past year?. . . . .   **1.Yes 2. No**

26. Have you ever attempted suicide? . . . .   **1.Yes 2. No**

27. Have any of your relatives committed suicide?. . . . .   **1.Yes 2. No**

28. Do you frequently feel that life is not worth living?. . . . .   **1.Yes 2. No**

29. Does each day look so dull that you would rather not wake up in the morning?. . . . .   **1.Yes 2. No**

30. Do you feel overly tired and without motivation much of the time? . . . .   **1.Yes 2. No**

31. Do you feel you have a serious emotional problem?. . . . .   **1.Yes 2. No**

32. Do you have a history of/or have you recently experienced hallucinations? (Hearing or seeing things others don't.)   **1.Yes 2. No**

33. Do you have difficulty feeling close to people? . . . .   **1.Yes 2. No**

34. Do you worry excessively?. . . . .   **1.Yes 2. No**

35. Do you feel you've had an excessive number of illnesses in the past year?. .   **1.Yes 2. No**

36. Do impulsive behaviors cause you serious problems? . . . .   **1.Yes 2. No**

37. Are you unhappy too much of the time?. . . . .   **1.Yes 2. No**

38. Do you cry too often? . . . .   **1.Yes 2. No**

39. Do you have difficulty controlling your temper?. . . . .   **1.Yes 2. No**

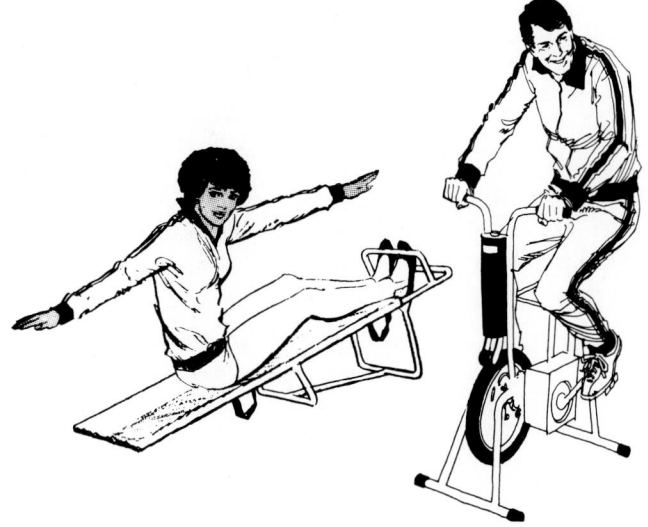

Continued.

SAMPLE PRINTOUTS

UNIVERSITY OF WISCONSIN-STEVENS POINT
LIFESTYLE ASSESSMENT RESULTS

Prepared for 9002 1 000000000

1

WELLNESS INVENTORY

The following scores indicate your wellness compared with average of people taking this survey with you, and averages of all the people who have taken the survey.

Catagory	Your Score	Group Average	Total Average
Physical Exercise	68	73	70
Physical Nutritional	52	67	52
Physical Self Care	46	60	48
Physical Vehicle Safety	47	75	49
Physical Drug Usage	72	95	75
Social Environmental	27	56	32
Emotional Awareness and Acceptance	20	50	24
Emotional Management	47	69	51
Intellectual	68	82	71
Occupational	73	79	73
Spiritual	65	68	66

2

PERSONAL GROWTH SECTION
AUTOMATED REFERRAL

EXERCISE PROGRAMS
A. Media
   1. Movies: **Coping With Life On The Run**—Sports Productions Inc.
     Run Dick, Run Jane—American Heart Association
     The Heart: An Attack—CRM
   2. Books: **Joy of Running**—Kostrubala
     Women's Running—Ullyot
     The Complete Runner—Fixx
     Stretching—Anderson
     Sheehan on Running—George Sheehan
     The Ultimate Athlete—Leonard
     Aerobics—Cooper
     Aerobics for Women—Cooper

B. Community Resources
   YMCA or YWCA programs

3

RISK OF DEATH SECTION

Age 40   Height 73
Race White   Weight 222
Sex Male

Life Expectancy Results
     1 5 10 15 20 25 30 35 40 45

Average Years of
Remaining Life in
Your Sex, Age,
Race Group   33•••••••••••••••••

Your Expected Yrs.
of Remaining Life
Based on your
Answers   25•••••••••••••

You can achieve
this expected yrs.
of remaining life
     38•••••••••••••••••••••

RISK OF DEATH SECTION (Con't.)

Major Hazards to you
     10 year deaths
Rank Hazard per 100,000   Associated risk factors
1. Cirrhosis

Average	304	Drinking Habits
Your	3800	
Achievable	61	

2. Arteriosclerotic Heart Disease

Average	1861	Systolic Blood Pressure
Your	2382	Diastolic Blood Pressure
Achievable	447	Cholesterol Level
		Smoking Habits
		Weight

3. Motor Vehicle Accidents

Average	339	Drinking Habits
Your	1763	Seat Belt Habits
Achievable	203	

4. Cancer of Lungs

Average	291	Smoking Habits
Your	582	
Achievable	58	

Suggestions For Increasing Your Expected Years Of Remaining Life
1. choosing non-drinking   will add 8.6 exp. years of life
2. choosing non-smoking   will add 2.0 exp. years of life
3. lowering cholesterol level   will add 0.7 exp. years of life
4. lowering diastolic blood pressure   will add 0.6 exp. years of life
5. lowering systolic blood pressure   will add 0.6 exp. years of life
6. losing weight   will add 0.4 exp. years of life
7. always wearing seatbelts will add 0.1 exp. years of life
8. having annual procto exam   will add 0.1 exp. years of life
Total   13

Remarks:
We have had to make the following assumptions about you:

You have an average blood cholesterol level.

Hazard Summary

Based on the Lifestyle Assessment Questionnaire you have filled out, you have a health age of 48 years. If you follow all the suggestions we have given, you can reduce your health age to 35.

4

ALERT SECTION: Medical/Behavioral/Emotional

Significant Past Illnesses	Immunizations
1. Diabetic	1. Up-to-date for DPT
2. Physical disability	2. Up-to-date for polio
	3. Rubella status unknown

Allergies	Emotions
1. Allergic to penicillin	1. History compatible with serious depression

WORDS FROM THE PAST

"To ward off disease or recover health, men as a rule find it easier to depend on the healers than to attempt the more difficult task of living wisely."

—Rene Dubos

"It's what you do hour by hour, day by day, that largely determines the state of your health; whether you get sick, what you get sick with, and perhaps when you die."

—Lester Breslow, M.D.

"For many years, while engaged in the practice of medicine, the author of this volume has been more and more impressed with the idea that the causes of the suffering, diseases, and premature deaths, which we witness around us on every hand, lie nearer our own doors . . . and that the men and women of today, are, at least, equally as responsible for existing suffering, as those who have gone before them, and often much more so. In fact, he feels satisfied that by far the greatest portion of all the suffering, disease, deformity, and premature deaths which occur, are the direct result of either the violation of, or the want of compliance with the laws of our being; calamities, which, were the requisite knowledge possessed by the community, can and should be avoided."

—taken from the Preface to **Avoidable Causes of Disease** by John Ellis, 1859.

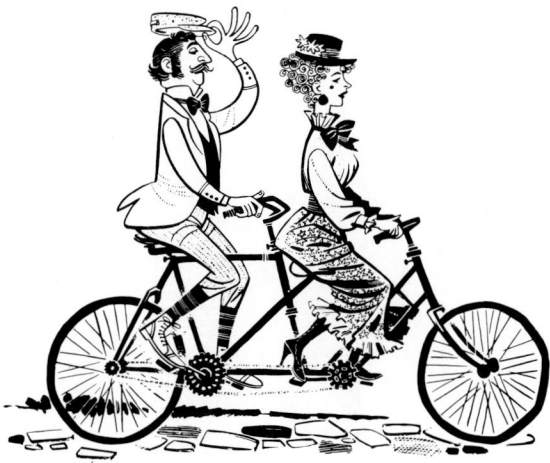

C5—HEALTH STYLE

This is a self-test that can be ordered at no charge from the United States Department of Health and Human Services, Office of Disease Prevention and Health Promotion, DHHS Pub. No. (PHS) 81-50155, Washington, D.C., 1981.

Directions: The purpose of Health Style is to tell you how well you are doing in staying healthy. The test has six sections: smoking, alcohol and drugs, nutrition, exercise and fitness, stress control, and safety. Complete one section at a time by circling the number corresponding to the answer that best describes your behavior (2 for "Almost Always," 1 for "Sometimes," and 0 for "Almost Never.") Then add the numbers you have circled to determine your score for that section. Write the score on the line provided at the end of each section. The highest score you can get for each section is 10.

HEALTH STYLE *a self test*

U.S. DEPARTMENT OF HEALTH AND HUMAN SERVICES • Public Health Service

How This Booklet Can Help You

All of us want good health. But, many of us do not know how to be as healthy as possible. Good health is not a matter of luck or fate. You have to work at it.

Good health depends on a combination of things . . . the environment in which you live and work . . . the personal traits you have inherited . . . the care you receive from doctors and hospitals . . . and the personal behaviors or habits that you perform daily, usually without much thought. All of these work together to affect your health. Many of us rely too much on doctors to keep us healthy, and we often fail to see the importance of actions we can take ourselves to look and feel healthy. You may be surprised to know that by taking action individually and collectively, you can begin to change parts of your world which may be harmful to your health.

Every day you are exposed to potential risks to good health. Pollution in the air you breathe and unsafe highways are two examples. These are risks that you, as an individual, can't do much about. Improving the quality of the environment usually requires the effort of concerned citizens working together for a healthier community.

There are, however, risks that you can control: risks stemming from your personal behaviors and habits. These behaviors are known as your lifestyle. Health experts now describe lifestyle as one of the most important factors affecting health. In fact, it is estimated that as many as seven of the ten leading causes of death in the United States could be reduced through common sense changes in lifestyle.

That's what the brief test contained in this booklet is all about. The few minutes you take to complete it may actually help you add years to your life! How? Well to start, it will enable you to identify aspects of your present lifestyle that are risky to your health. Then it will encourage you to take steps to eliminate or minimize the risks you identify. All in all, it will help you begin to change your present lifestyle into a new HEALTHSTYLE. If you do, it's possible that you may feel better, look better, and live longer too.

Before You Take the Test

This is not a pass-fail test. Its purpose is simply to tell you how well you are doing to stay healthy. The behaviors covered in the test are recommended for most Americans. Some of them may not apply to persons with certain chronic diseases or handicaps. Such persons may require special instructions from their physician or other health professional.

You will find that the test has six sections: smoking, alcohol and drugs, nutrition, exercise and fitness, stress control, and safety. Complete one section at a time by circling the number corresponding to the answer that best describes your behavior (2 for "Almost Always", 1 for "Sometimes", and 0 for "Almost Never"). Then add the numbers you have circled to determine your score for that section. Write the score on the line provided at the end of each section. The highest score you can get for each section is 10.

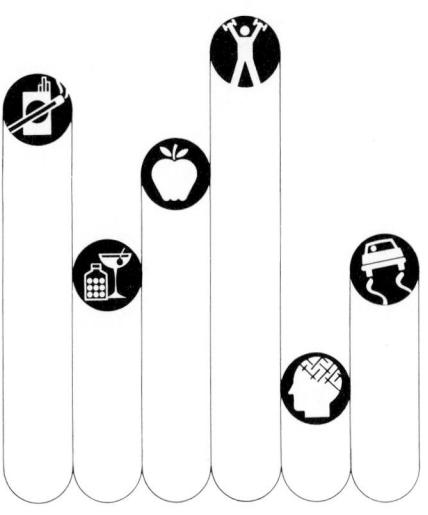

A Test for Better Health

	Almost Always	Sometimes	Almost Never
If you never smoke, enter a score of 10 for this section and go to the next section on *Alcohol and Drugs.*			
1. I avoid smoking cigarettes.	2	1	0
2. I smoke only low tar and nicotine cigarettes *or* I smoke a pipe or cigars.	2	1	0

Smoking Score: _____

	Almost Always	Sometimes	Almost Never
1. I avoid drinking alcoholic beverages *or* I drink no more than 1 or 2 drinks a day.	4	1	0
2. I avoid using alcohol or other drugs (especially illegal drugs) as a way of handling stressful situations or the problems in my life.	2	1	0
3. I am careful not to drink alcohol when taking certain medicines (for example, medicine for sleeping, pain, colds, and allergies).	2	1	0
4. I read and follow the label directions when using prescribed and over-the-counter drugs.	2	1	0

Alcohol and Drugs Score: _____

Continued.

Eating Habits

	Almost Always	Sometimes	Almost Never
1. I eat a variety of foods each day, such as fruits and vegetables, whole grain breads and cereals, lean meats, dairy products, dry peas and beans, and nuts and seeds.	4	1	0
2. I limit the amount of fat, saturated fat, and cholesterol I eat (including fat on meats, eggs, butter, cream, shortenings, and organ meats such as liver).	2	1	0
3. I limit the amount of salt I eat by cooking with only small amounts, not adding salt at the table, and avoiding salty snacks.	2	1	0
4. I avoid eating too much sugar (especially frequent snacks of sticky candy or soft drinks).	2	1	0

Eating Habits Score: _____

Exercise/Fitness

	Almost Always	Sometimes	Almost Never
1. I maintain a desired weight, avoiding overweight and underweight.	3	1	0
2. I do vigorous exercises for 15-30 minutes at least 3 times a week (examples include running, swimming, brisk walking).	3	1	0
3. I do exercises that enhance my muscle tone for 15-30 minutes at least 3 times a week (examples include yoga and calisthenics).	2	1	0
4. I use part of my leisure time participating in individual, family, or team activities that increase my level of fitness (such as gardening, bowling, golf, and baseball).	2	1	0

Exercise/Fitness Score: _____

Stress Control

	Almost Always	Sometimes	Almost Never
1. I have a job or do other work that I enjoy.	2	1	0
2. I find it easy to relax and express my feelings freely.	2	1	0
3. I recognize early, and prepare for, events or situations likely to be stressful for me.	2	1	0
4. I have close friends, relatives, or others whom I can talk to about personal matters and call on for help when needed.	2	1	0
5. I participate in group activities (such as church and community organizations) or hobbies that I enjoy.	2	1	0

Stress Control Score: _____

Safety

	Almost Always	Sometimes	Almost Never
1. I wear a seat belt while riding in a car.	2	1	0
2. I avoid driving while under the influence of alcohol and other drugs.	2	1	0
3. I obey traffic rules and the speed limit when driving.	2	1	0
4. I am careful when using potentially harmful products or substances (such as household cleaners, poisons, and electrical devices).	2	1	0
5. I avoid smoking in bed.	2	1	0

Safety Score: _____

Your HEALTHSTYLE Scores

After you have figured your scores for each of the six sections, circle the number in each column that matches your score for that section of the test.

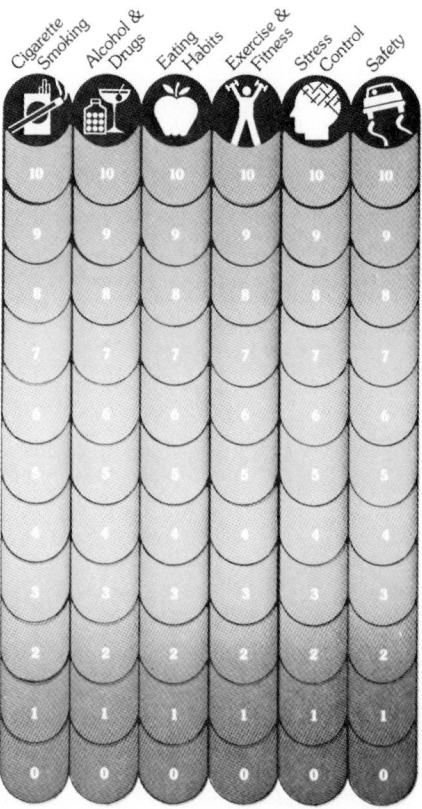

Remember, there is no total score for this test. Consider each section separately. You are trying to identify aspects of your lifestyle that you can improve in order to be healthier and to reduce the risk of illness. So let's see what your scores reveal.

What Your Scores Mean to YOU

Scores of 9 and 10

Excellent! Your answers show that you are aware of the importance of this area to your health. More importantly, you are putting your knowledge to work for you by practicing good health habits. As long as you continue to do so, this area should not pose a serious health risk. It's likely that you are setting an example for your family and friends to follow. Since you got a very high score on this part of the test, you may want to consider other areas where your scores indicate room for improvement.

Scores of 6 to 8

Your health practices in this area are good, but there is room for improvement. Look again at the items you answered with a "Sometimes" or "Almost Never". What changes can you make to improve your score? Even a small change can often help you achieve better health.

Scores of 3 to 5

Your health risks are showing! Would you like more information about the risks you are facing and about why it is important for you to change these behaviors. Perhaps you need help in deciding how to successfully make the changes you desire. In either case, help is available. See the last page of this booklet.

Scores of 0 to 2

Obviously, you were concerned enough about your health to take the test, but your answers show that you may be taking serious and unnecessary risks with your health. Perhaps you are not aware of the risks and what to do about them. You can easily get the information and help you need to improve, if you wish. A source of contact appears on the last page. The next step is up to you.

Continued.

YOU Can Start Right Now!

In the test you just completed were numerous suggestions to help you reduce your risk of disease and premature death. Here are some of the most significant:

 Avoid cigarettes. Cigarette smoking is the single most important preventable cause of illness and early death. It is especially risky for pregnant women and their unborn babies. Persons who stop smoking reduce their risk of getting heart disease and cancer. So if you're a cigarette smoker, think twice about lighting that next cigarette. If you choose to continue smoking, try decreasing the number of cigarettes you smoke and switching to a low tar and nicotine brand.

 Follow sensible drinking habits. Alcohol produces changes in mood and behavior. Most people who drink are able to control their intake of alcohol and to avoid undesired, and often harmful, effects. Heavy, regular use of alcohol can lead to cirrhosis of the liver, a leading cause of death. Also, statistics clearly show that mixing drinking and driving is often the cause of fatal or crippling accidents. So if you drink, do it wisely and in moderation.

 Use care in taking drugs. Today's greater use of drugs—both legal and illegal— is one of our most serious health risks.   Even some drugs prescribed by your doctor can be dangerous if taken when drinking alcohol or before driving. Excessive or continued use of tranquilizers (or "pep pills")can cause physical and mental problems. Using or experimenting with illicit drugs such as marijuana, heroin, cocaine, and PCP may lead to a number of damaging effects or even death.

 Eat sensibly. Overweight individuals are at greater risk for diabetes, gall bladder disease, and high blood pressure. So it makes good sense to maintain proper weight. But good eating habits also mean holding down the amount of fat (especially saturated fat), cholesterol, sugar and salt in your diet. If you must snack, try nibbling on fresh fruits and vegetables. You'll feel better—and look better, too.

 Exercise regularly. Almost everyone can benefit from exercise—and there's some form of exercise almost everyone can do. (If you have any doubt, check first with your doctor.) Usually, as little as 15-30 minutes of vigorous exercise three times a week will help you have a healthier heart, eliminate excess weight, tone up sagging muscles, and sleep better. Think how much difference all these improvements could make in the way you feel!

 Learn to handle stress. Stress is a normal part of living; everyone faces it to some degree. The causes of stress can be good or bad, desirable or undesirable (such as a promotion on the job or the loss of a spouse). Properly handled, stress need not be a problem. But unhealthy responses to stress—such as driving too fast or erratically, drinking too much, or prolonged anger or grief—can cause a variety of physical and mental problems. Even on a very busy day, find a few minutes to slow down and relax. Talking over a problem with someone you trust can often help you find a satisfactory solution. Learn to distinguish between things that are "worth fighting about" and things that are less important.

 Be safety conscious. Think "safety first" at home, at work, at school, at play, and on the highway. Buckle seat belts and obey traffic rules. Keep poisons and weapons out of the reach of children, and keep emergency numbers by your telephone. When the unexpected happens, you'll be prepared.

Where Do You Go From Here?

Start by asking yourself a few frank questions:
Am I really doing all I can to be as healthy as possible? What steps can I take to feel better? Am I willing to begin now? If you scored low in one or more sections of the test, decide what changes you want to make for improvement. You might pick that aspect of your lifestyle where you feel you have the best chance for success and tackle that one first. Once you have improved your score there, go on to other areas.

If you already have tried to change your health habits (to stop smoking or exercise regularly, for example) don't be discouraged if you haven't yet succeeded. The difficulty you have encountered may be due to influences you've never really thought about—such as advertising—or to a lack of support and encouragement. Understanding these influences is an important step toward changing the way they affect you.

There's Help Available. In addition to personal actions you can take on your own, there are community programs and groups (such as the YMCA or the local chapter of the American Heart Association) that can assist you and your family to make the changes you want to make. If you want to know more about these groups or about health risks contact your local health department or mail in the card contained in this booklet. There's a lot you can do to stay healthy or to improve your health—and there are organizations that can help you. Start a new HEALTHSTYLE today!

DRUG AND IMMUNIZATION INFORMATION

D1—DRUG INFORMATION

Psychotrophic agents: antipsychotics

Generic name	Trade name	Relative potency (mg) when compared to 100 mg of chlorpromazine	Average daily dose (mg)	Dosage range per 24 hours (mg)
PHENOTHIAZINES				
Aliphatics				
Chlorpromazine	Thorazine	100	100-1500	30-1200
Triflupromazine	Vesprin	25	25-150	60-150
Piperidines				
Thioridazine	Mellaril	100	100-800	30-800
Mesoridazine	Serentil	50	100-400	100-400
Piperacetine	Quide	10	10-160	20-160
Piperazines				
Trifluoperazine	Stelazine	5	10-50	2-20
Acetophenazine	Tindal	20	40-100	40-80
Fluphenazine	Prolixin	2	6-40	1-20
Perphenazine	Trilafon	8	8-64	6-64
Prochlorperazine	Compazine	25	30-150	15-150
Butaperazine	Repoise	10	10-100	15-100
Carphenazine	Proketazine	25	50-400	75-400
THIOXANTHENES				
Chlorprothixene	Taractan	100	75-600	
Thiothixene	Navane	4	10-60	
BUTYROPHENONES				
Haloperidol	Haldol	2	2-30	
DIHYDROINDOLONES				
Molindone	Lidone Moban	20	50-200	
DIBENZOXAPINES				
Loxapine	Loxitane Daxolin	20	20-100	

Psychotrophic agents: antidepressants

Generic name	Trade name	Usual daily dose (mg)	Maximum daily dose (mg)	Incompatible drugs
TRICYCLICS				
Imipramine	Imavate Janimine Presamine SK-Pramine Tofranil	150-200	300	MAO inhibitors Alcohol Barbiturates
Desipramine	Norpramin Pertofrane	150-200	300	Central nervous system depressants
Amitriptyline	Amitril Elavil Endep	150-200	300	Thiazide diuretics Thyroid
Nortriptyline	Aventyl Pamelor	100-150	200	Vasodilators Anticholinergic agents
Doxepin	Adapin Sinequan	150-200	300	
Protriptyline	Vivactil Triptil	15-40	60	Guanethidine
Trimipramine	Surmontil	75-150	200	
MONOAMINE OXIDASE INHIBITORS				
Isocarboxazid	Marplan	10-20	30	Combination of any MAO inhibitors
Phenelzine	Nardil	45-60	90	Phenathiazine compounds, dopamine, methyldopa, tryptophan, antihypertensive and antiparkinsonian drugs, insulin
Tranylcypromine	Parnate	20	30	Thiazide diuretics Sympathomimetics including amphetamines
TETRACYCLICS				
Maprotiline	Ludiomil	150-200	300	

Psychotrophic agents: antianxiety

Generic name	Trade name	Hypnotic dose (mg)	Sedative dose (mg)	Half-life (hrs)
BARBITURATES				
Secobarbital	Seconal	100-200	90-200	19-34
Pentobarbital	Nembutal	100-200	45-200	15-48
Amobarbital	Amytal	100-200	60-150	8-42
Butabarbital	Butisol	100-200	20-200	34-42
Phenobarbital	Barbipil and others	100-200	30-90	24-140
BENZODIAZEPINES				
Flurazepam	Dalmane	15-30		24-100
Chlordiazepoxide	Librium and others	50-100	5-40	6-30
Diazepam	Valium	20-30	2-10	20-90
Oxazepam	Serax	30-60	10-30	3-21
Clorazepam	Tranxene and others		3.25-60	40-200
Prazepam	Verstran, Centrax	20-60	10-20	10-20
Lorazepam	Ativan	2-6	2-4	5-20
NONBARBITURATES/BENZODIAZEPINES				
Propanediol				
Meprobamate	Equanil, Miltown, and others	800	200-400	10
Tybamate	Solacen, Tybatran		750-2000	
Quinazolines				
Methaqualone	Quaalude, Parest, Sopor, Optimil, and others	150-300	225-300	10-14
Acetylinic alcohols				
Ethchlorvynol	Placidyl	500-1000	200-600	10-25
Piperidinedione derivatives				
Glutethimide	Doriden	250-500		5-22
Methyprylon	Noludar	200-400	150-400	
Chloral derivatives				
Chloral Hydrate	Noctec, Somnos, and others	500-2000	750-1500	
Chloral Betaine	Beta-Chlor	870-1740		
Triclofos	Triclos	750-1500		
Monoureides				
Paraldehyde	Paral	4-15 ml		
Diphenylmethanes				
Hydroxyzine	Atarax		75-400	
Hydroxyzine pamoate	Vistaril		75-400	
Benactyzine	Suavitil		3-9	
Diphenhydramine	Benadryl		25-100	

Psychotrophic agents: predicting lithium daily dosages to achieve therapeutic blood serum levels*

24-hour lithium level (mEq/L)	Total daily dosage (mg)
0.05	1200 tid
0.05-0.09	900 tid
0.10-0.14	600 tid
0.15-0.19	300 qid
0.20-0.23	300 tid
0.24-0.30	300 bid
0.30	300 qd

*Daily lithium dosages are determined by giving a primary dose of 600 mg and measuring lithium levels in the blood 24 hours later. Dosage is administered based on the above schedule. Recommended therapeutic serum lithium levels: 1–1.5 mEq/L for acute mania; 0.6–1.2 mEq/L for maintenance therapy; and 2 mEq/L as maximum.

Psychotrophic agents: commonly used antiparkinsonian agents anticholinergic

Generic name	Trade name	Usual daily dose (mg)
ANTICHOLINERGICS		
Trihexyphenidyl	Artane, Pipanol, Antitrem, Tremin	2-15
Procyclidine	Kemadrin	5-20
Cycrimine	Pagitane	3.75-15.0
Biperiden	Akineton	2-6
ANTICHOLINERGIC-ANTIHISTAMICS		
Benztropine	Cogentin	1-6
Diphenhydramine	Benadryl	25-200
Chlorphenoxamine	Phenoxene	150-400
Orphenadrine	Disipal	50-250
Ethopropazine	Parsidol	50-600
OTHERS		
Amantadine	Symmetrel	100-400

Frequent side effects of selected antidepressants

System or organs	Effects	
	Tricyclics	MAOIs
Cardiovascular system	Hypotension, tachycardia, palpitations, arrhythmias, first-degree heart block, myocardial infarction	Orthostatic hypotension, arrhythmias, paradoxical hypertension, flushing
Central nervous system	Sedation, dizziness, fatigue, weakness, headache, disorientation, disturbed concentration, insomnia, restlessness, nightmares, ataxia, tremors, numbness, electroencephalographic changes, EPSs, mania	Restlessness, dizziness, vertigo, headache, insomnia, confusion, fatigue, paresthexias, mania
Ear, eye, nose, throat	Blurred vision, tinnitus, increased intraocular pressure, mydriasis	Blurred vision, tinnitus
Gastrointestinal system	Dry mouth, nausea, vomiting, upset stomach, constipation, diarrhea	Dry mouth, nausea, constipation, diarrhea, anorexia
Genitourinary system	Urinary retention, gynecomastia, galactorrhea, altered sexual drive	Urinary retention, altered sexual drive
Blood	Bone marrow depression (agranulocytopenia and others)	
Skin	Rash, urticaria, pruritus	Rash, flushing
Other	Cholestatic jaundice, photosensitivity, edema, weight changes, facial sweating	Hepatitis, weight changes, peripheral edema, sweating

Antipsychotic drug side effects

System or organs	Effects
Cardiovascular system	Orthostatic hypotension
	Hypertension
	Tachycardia
	Bradycardia
	Fainting
	Dizziness
	Pallor
	T wave changes, prolonged PR intervals, and QRS complex reflecting slowed conduction
Central nervous system	Drowsiness
	Sedation
	Headache
	Convulsions
	Extrapyramidal symptoms
	Electroencephalographic changes
	Cerebral edema
Ear, eye, nose, and throat	Blurred vision
	Pigmentation of eyes after sun exposure
	Nasal congestion
Gastrointestinal system	Anorexia
	Constipation
	Cholestatic jaundice
	Excessive salivation
	Weight changes
	Dyspepsia
	Diarrhea
	Paralytic ileus
	Increased appetite
	Dry mouth
Genitourinary system	Dark urine
	Incontinence
	Menstrual irregularities
	Changed libido
	Inhibited ejaculation
	Gynecomastia
	Difficult urination
	Delayed ovulation
	Impotence
	Glycosuria
	Lactation
Metabolic system	Hyperglycemia and hypoglycemia
	Hyperthermia and hypothermia
Blood	Blood dyscrasias (agranulocytosis usually)
Skin	Photosensitivity
	Excessive sweating
	Dermatoses (erythematous and eczematous)
	Pigmentation after sun exposure

Frequency (highest to lowest incidence) of antipsychotic agents causing extrapyramidal symptoms

Generic name	Trade name
Fluphenazine	Permitil, Prolixin
Trifluoperazine	Stelazine
Perphenazine	Trilafon
Prochlorperazine	Compazine
Thiopropazate	Dartalan
Acetophenazine	Tindal
Triflupromazine	Vesprin
Chlorpromazine	Thorazine
Carphenazine	Proketazine
Butaperazine	Repoise
Piperacetazine	Quide
Thiothixene	Navane
Thioridazine	Mellaril
Mesoridazine	Serentil

SYMPTOMS OF ATROPINE PSYCHOSIS

Purposeless overactivity	Tachycardia
Agitation	Sluggish dilated pupils
Confusion	Bowel hypomotility
Disorientation	Dysarthria
Dry, flushed skin	Memory impairment

Side effects of antianxiety agents

System or organ	Effects
Cardiovascular system	Hypotension, palpitations, tachycardia, swelling of the feet, arrhythmias, flushing
Central nervous system	Fatigue, drowsiness, ataxia, headache, vertigo, dizziness, slurred speech, electroencephalographic changes, sleep disturbances, hallucinations, lethargy, muscle weakness, insomnia, paradoxical rage reaction, fainting
Ear, eye, nose, throat	Blurred vision, diplopia, tinnitus
Gastrointestinal system	Nausea, vomiting, anorexia, dry mouth, constipation, diarrhea, epigastric distress, weight changes
Genitourinary system	Libido changes, urinary frequency/retention/decreased flow, minor menstrual irregularities, acute hepatic necrosis or disfunction
Blood	Decreased hematocrit, blood dyscrasias
Skin	Rash, petechiae, pruritus, urticaria, jaundice, bullous dermatitis, Stevens-Johnson syndrome

D2—IMMUNIZATION INFORMATION

Immunizing agents

Agent	Age to administer	Administration	Reaction and treatment
DPT: diphtheria toxoid, tetanus toxoid, and pertussis vaccine	2,4,6 months; 1½ years; 4-6 years (may be given through the sixth year)	a. Primary course: three 0.5 cc doses at 8-week intervals followed by fourth 0.5 cc dose 1 year after third dose. b. Booster course: one 0.5 cc dose at 4 to 6 years of age; thereafter Td 0.5 cc every 10 years. *Contraindications:* (1) any acute febrile illness; (2) delete pertussis if CNS problem present or CNS disorder/symptom(s) occurs after DPT injection; (3) exposure to disease (diphtheria and pertussis): booster dose given of appropriate single antigen unless fourth dose has been given within past year; (4) tetanus prophylaxis in wound management.	a. Local reaction: induration, redness, or nodule at injection site. Treatment: warm compress to site; rotation of injection sites. b. Systemic reaction: temperature elevation and irritability not lasting more than 24 to 48 hours. Treatment: acetaminophen for fever. If febrile or local reactions are severe, fractional doses should be considered.
DT: pediatric—diphtheria toxoid and tetanus toxoid	May be given through the sixth year	Same as DPT; indicated for use in infants and young children under 6 when pertussis vaccine is contraindicated. *Contraindications:* same as for DPT.	Same as DPT.
Td: adult type—diphtheria toxoid and tetanus toxoid	Children over 6 years; 14-16 years and every 10 years thereafter	a. Primary course: two 0.5 cc doses at 8-week interval followed by third 0.5 cc dose 6 to 12 months after second dose. b. Booster course: one 0.5 cc dose at 14 to 16 years and every 10 years thereafter. *Contraindications:* same as for DPT.	Same as DPT.

Adapted from American Academy of Pediatrics: Report of the Committee on Infectious Diseases, ed. 20, Evanston, Ill., 1986; and Committee on Infectious Disease, American Academy of Pediatrics: Hemophilus Type b polysaccharide vaccine, Pediatrics 76:322-323, Aug. 1985.

Continued.

Immunizing agents—cont'd

Agent	Age to administer	Administration	Reaction and treatment
OPV: live, oral poliovirus vaccine; vaccine must be kept frozen	2,4,6 months; 1½ years, 4-6 years (do not give to persons over 18 years) Population at risk: children not vaccinated, especially a large number in 0 to 4 age group	a. Primary course: two doses at 8 week intervals in first 6 months of life with third dose at 18 months of age. b. Booster course: one dose at 4 to 6 years. c. Course for children or adolescents under 18 years: two doses at 8-week intervals followed by third dose in 8-14 months. *Contraindications:* same as for DPT. See Chapter 23.	Risk of vaccine: live virus persists in GI tract for 4 to 6 weeks after vaccination and paralytic disease can occur. Populations with immune deficiency disorders are particularly at risk, as are those over 18 years who have had no previous polio immunization and have been exposed. Use of inactivated vaccine (Salk) is recommended for these populations.
Measles: live attenuated virus vaccine; also available in combination as (a) measles-rubella or (b) measles-mumps-rubella	15 months of age	One subcutaneous injection of total volume of reconstituted vaccine. *Contraindications.* hypersensitivity to eggs, see Chapter 23. Vaccine should be given anytime after 6 months of age if exposed to measles and repeated at 15 months. *Indications* for revaccination include children vaccinated before 13 months of age, children vaccinated with simultaneous administration of gamma globulin at any age, and children for whom doubt exists about immunization status. Tuberculin testing should be done prior to, simultaneously, or 4 to 6 weeks after measles vaccine administration.	Reaction: mild noncommunicable infection with symptoms of fever, faint rash, and minor toxicity in 15% of vaccinated population. May occur 5 to 12 days after vaccination. Treatment: symptomatic.
Rubella: live attenuated virus; in combination as (a) measles-rubella, (b) mumps-rubella, or (c) measles-mumps-rubella	15 months of age	Same as for measles *Contraindications:* pregnant women. In susceptible non-pregnant females, administer if HI titer is less than 1:10 and pregnancy is not planned for 2 months.	Reaction: rarely fever and rash. Treatment: symptomatic. In older age populations transient arthritis and arthralgia may occur 2 to 4 weeks after vaccination. Treatment: symptomatic.
Mumps: live attenuated virus. In combination as (a) mumps-rubella or (b) measles-mumps-rubella	15 months of age	Same as measles. *Contraindications:* see Chapter 23. Indicated for use in susceptible children approaching puberty, in adolescents, and in males who have no history of mumps.	Reaction: no serious side effects. Occasionally mild fever treated symptomatically.
HBPV: Haemophilus b polysaccharide vaccine; purified, capsular polysaccharide of *H. influenzae* type b	24 months of age or before 5 years	One dose given by subcutaneous injection. May be given with DTP at different site. *Contraindications:* before 18 months or after 5 years; children with chronic illness known to be associated with *H. influenzae* type b, particularly asplenia and sickle cell disease.	Reaction: mild local reactions. Treatment: warm compress to site.

D3—RECOMMENDATIONS FOR PROPHYLAXIS OF HEPATITIS A

1. *Close personal contact.* IG is recommended for all household and sexual contacts of persons with hepatitis A.

2. *Day-care centers.* Day-care facilities with children in diapers can be important settings for HAV transmission. IG should be administered to all staff and attendees of day-care centers or homes of (1) one or more hepatitis A cases are recognized among children or employees; or (2) cases are recognized in two or more households of center attendees. When an outbreak (hepatitis cases in three or more families) occurs, IG should also be considered for members of households whose diapered children attend. In centers not enrolling children in diapers, IG need only be given to classroom contacts of an index case.

3. *Schools.* Contact at elementary and secondary schools is usually not an important means of transmitting hepatitis A. Routine administration of IG is not indicated for pupils and teachers in contact with a patient. However, when epidemiological study clearly shows the existence of a school- or classroom-centered outbreak, IG may be given to those who have close personal contact with patients.

4. *Institutions for custodial care.* Living conditions in some institutions, such as prisons and facilities for the developmentally disabled, favor transmission of hepatitis A. When outbreaks occur, giving IG to residents and staff who have close contact with patients with hepatitis A may reduce spread of disease. Depending on the epidemiologic circumstances, prophylaxis can be limited or can involve the entire institution.

5. *Hospitals.* Routine IG administration is not indicated. Rather, sound hygienic practices should be emphasized. Staff education should point out the risk of exposure to hepatitis A and emphasize precautions regarding direct contact with potentially infective materials. Outbreaks of hepatitis A among hospital staff occur occasionally, usually in association with an unsuspected index patient who is fecally incontinent. Large outbreaks have occurred among staff and family contacts of infected infants in neonatal intensive-care units. In outbreaks, prophylaxis of persons exposed to feces of infected patients may be indicated.

6. *Offices and factories.* Routine IG administration is not indicated under the usual office or factory conditions for persons exposed to a fellow worker with hepatitis A. Experience shows that casual contact in the work setting does not result in virus transmission.

7. *Common-source exposure.* IG might be effective in preventing food-borne or waterborne hepatitis A if exposure is recognized in time. However, IG is not recommended for persons exposed to a common source of hepatitis infection after cases have begun to occur in those exposed, because the 2-week period during which IG is effective will have been exceeded.

If a foodhandler is diagnosed as having hepatitis A, common-source transmission is possible but uncommon. IG should be administered to other foodhandlers but is usually not recommended for patrons. However, IG administration to patrons may be considered if (1) the infected person is directly involved in handling, without gloves, foods that will not be cooked before they are eaten; (2) the hygienic practices of the foodhandler are deficient; and (3) patrons can be identified and treated within 2 weeks of exposure. Situations in which repeated exposures may have occurred, such as in institutional cafeterias, may warrant stronger consideration of IG use.

For postexposure IG prophylaxis, a single intramuscular dose of 0.02 ml/kg is recommended.

E1—COMMUNITY ORIENTED HEALTH RECORD (COHR)

Community Health Assessment Model

Definition of *community:* A locality-based entity—composed of systems of formal organizations reflecting societal institutions, informal groups, and aggregates, which are interdependent—whose function (expressed intent) is to meet a wide range of collective needs.

Definition of *community health:* The meeting of collective needs, through identifying problems and managing interactions within the community and between the community and the larger society. This requires commitment, self-other awareness and clarity of situational definitions, articulateness, effective communication, conflict containment and accommodation, participation, management of relations with the larger society, and machinery for facilitating participant interaction and decision making.

Community Health Assessment Guide Categories

A. Community
  1. Place
    a. Geopolitical boundaries of community
    b. Local or folk name for community
    c. Size in square miles/areas/blocks/census tracts
    d. Transportation avenues
    e. Physical environment
  2. People
    a. Number and density of population
    b. Demographic structure of population
    c. Informal groups
    d. Formal groups
    e. Linking structures
  3. Function
    a. Production—distribution—consumption of goods and services
    b. Socialization of new members
    c. Maintenance of social control
    d. Adapting to ongoing and unexpected change
    e. Provision of mutual aid
B. Community health
  1. Status
    a. Vital statistics
    b. Disease incidence and prevalence for leading causes of mortality and morbidity
    c. Health risk profiles
    d. Functional ability levels
  2. Structure
    a. Health facilities
    b. Health related planning groups
    c. Health manpower
    d. Health resource utilization patterns
  3. Process
    a. Commitment
    b. Self-other awareness and clarity of situational definitions
    c. Articulateness
    d. Effective communication
    e. Conflict containment and accommodation
    f. Participation
    g. Management of relations with the larger society
    h. Machinery for facilitating participant interaction and decision making

Database

This form provides a structured method for recording data. The name of the community and the assessment category and/or subcategory are noted at the top of the page. These categories correspond to those of the assessment guide. The data are collected and the source of the information and the data are recorded. Data are often entered using the SOAP format. An example of the COHR Database form is depicted on the next page.

Community Problem List

Headings of columns for the Community Problem List are Date, Number, Problem/Concern, and Supportive Data (title of appropriate section of Data Base and capsule summary of relevant data).

Community Capability List

Headings of columns for this list are Date, Number, Capability, Supportive Data (title of appropriate section of Data Base and capsule summary of relevant data).

Problem Analysis

A line labeled Problem/Statement is included at the top of the form below Name of Community. Headings of columns are Problem Correlates, Relationship of Correlates to Problem, and Data Supportive to Relationships (refer to appropriate sections of Data Base *and* relevant research findings in current literature). An example of a completed Problem Analysis is depicted on p. 263.

Problem Prioritization

Headings of columns are Criteria, Criteria Weights (1-10). Problem, Problem Rating (1-10), Rationale for Rating, Problem Significance/(Weight × Rate).

DATABASE

Name of community _____

Assessment category _____ Subcategory _____

Date	Data source	Data*

*Note with an asterisk the themes identified and meanings given.

Goals and Objectives

This form includes a line labeled Problem/Concern as well as lines for Goal Statement at the top under Name of Community. Column headings are Date, Objectives (number and statement), and By Date. An example of a completed goals and objectives statement is depicted on p. 265.

Plan

A line labeled Objective Number and Statement is included under Name of Community. Column headings are Date, Intervener Activities/Means, Value (1-10)/Probability (1-10), and Activity/Means Selected for Implementation. Sample plan sheets from the interventions related to infant malnutrition are presented on pp. 266 and 267.

Progress Notes

A line labeled Goal is included under Name of Community. Column headings are Date, Narrative, Assessment, Plan (NAP), and Budget and Time. A footnote to the second column explains the NAP procedure: Record both objective and subjective data. Interpret these data in terms of (1) whether the objectives were achieved and (2) whether the intervener activities utilized were effective. The plan is dependent on the assessment and may include both new (or revised) objectives and activities. Progress Notes reflecting evaluation of interventions aimed at assessing community health workers' educational needs are presented on p. 270.

E2—REFERRAL FORM FOR SCHOOL HEALTH PROGRAM

Name of student _____

Age _____ Sex _____ Telephone _____

Address _____

Parent(s) name _____

Reason for referral _____

_____

_____

_____

Problem interventions tried by school health program _____

_____

_____

_____

Disposition from responding agency _____

_____

_____

_____

E3—SCHOOL HEALTH RECORD

Name _____ Date of birth _____

In case of emergency call _____

Address _____ Telephone _____

Family physician _____

Family dentist _____

Family nurse practitioner _____

Existing health problem(s) _____

_____

_____

TEACHER OBSERVATIONS

Physical: Walking gait, pimples, skin rashes, etc.

Psychological: (Please state observation as it is perceived; no labeling. For example, is the student always putting himself down?)

Sociological: (Please state observation as it is perceived; no labeling. For example, describe relationships and friendships.)

What is the educational progression of this child? (No labeling.)

NURSE'S ASSESSMENT

Sex _____ Weight _____ Height _____

Immunizations:

Physical:

Objective data _____

Subjective data _____

Nursing diagnosis _____

Plan of action _____

SCHOOL HEALTH RECORD—cont'd

Psychological (developmental tasks):

Sociological (developmental tasks):

    Objective data _____

    Subjective data _____

    Nursing diagnosis _____

    Plan of action _____

History of childhood diseases:

HEALTH RISK APPRAISAL

Nutrition

Exercise

Accident and safety

Relaxation

Rest (sleep)

Self-care skills (self-examination of breasts, self-examination of
    testicles for mass)

Alcohol and drugs

Smoking

Disposition _____

_____

_____

Screening

    Blood pressure

    Dental

    Vision

    Hearing

    Scoliosis

    Coordination (musculoskeletal)

Disposition _____

_____

_____

Sexuality (to include birth control information, if allowed by
    school district)

Peer relationships

Placement of child in family

Interests (sports, hobbies, etc.)

Disposition _____

_____

_____

Referral _____

_____

_____

E4—SAMPLE NOTE TO PARENTS FROM SCHOOL NURSE

NAME OF SCHOOL (LETTERHEAD)

Date _____

Dear _____

In reviewing your child's record at school, we have found

that _____ needs:
          (name of child)

_____ Medical examination

_____ Immunizations

_____ Other

If this has already been taken care of, please send a copy of
the record to school. If you have further questions, please
call me at the school. The telephone number is 000-0000.
    Thank you,

_____
        School nurse

APPENDIX
F

CRITERIA AND STANDARDS FOR COMMUNITY HEALTH NURSING PRACTICE

F1—ANA STANDARDS OF COMMUNITY HEALTH NURSING PRACTICE*

Standard I. Theory: The nurse applies theoretical concepts as a basis for decisions in practice.

Standard II. Data collection: The nurse systematically collects data that are comprehensive and accurate.

Standard III. Diagnosis: The nurse analyzes data collected about the community, family, and individual to determine diagnoses.

Standard IV. Planning: At each level of prevention, the nurse develops plans that specify nursing actions unique to client needs.

Standard V. Intervention: The nurse, guided by the plan, intervenes to promote, maintain, or restore health, to prevent illness, and to effect rehabilitation.

Standard VI. Evaluation: The nurse evaluates responses of the community, family, and individual to interventions in order to determine progress toward goal achievement and to revise the data base, diagnoses, and plan.

Standard VII. Quality assurance and professional development: The nurse participates in peer review and other means of evaluation to assure quality of nursing practice; the nurse assumes responsibility for professional development and contributes to the professional growth of others.

Standard VIII. Interdisciplinary collaboration: The nurse collaborates with other health care providers, professionals, and community representatives in assessing, planning, implementing, and evaluating programs for community health.

Standard IX. Research: The nurse contributes to theory and practice in community health nursing through research.

F2—CRITERIA FOR DOCUMENTATION TO MEASURE THE QUALITY OF CARE IN THE HOME HEALTH AGENCY†

1. The agency assesses the community served.
2. The agency is responsive to community health needs.
3. The agency has a legally constituted body that is re-

sponsible for the effective governing of the agency. It involves consumers in broad agency affairs.

4. Administrative responsibilities and relationships are established and clearly defined.
5. The governing body delegates to a qualified individual the authority and responsibility for overall agency administration.
6. If the agency has a person (or persons) other than the chief executive officer responsible for the administration and direction of the agency's programs, this individual (or individuals) is delegated the authority and responsibility for program administration.
7. If the agency has a person other than the chief executive officer responsible for the fiscal and business affairs of the agency, this individual is delegated the authority and responsibility for fiscal and business practices.
8. Fiscal policies and practices assure effective and efficient implementation of the program(s) of the agency.
9. The agency has agreements with organizations, agencies, and/or individuals for securing or providing services.
10. Program and fiscal management activities are coordinated to promote effective planning and implementation of programs within the agency.
11. The agency coordinates its services with other health and social agencies; consumers are kept informed of services available.
12. The agency has established programs in response to community health needs.
13. For each program and service, the agency has priorities that are responsive to agency purpose and community need.
14. The agency has policies and procedures governing programs, services, and professional practices.
15. Service records are maintained for each client.
16. All agency services are coordinated.
17. The agency has the responsibility for participation, if feasible, in the education of student health personnel.
18. The staff includes professional and nonprofessional personnel commensurate with the needs of the programs of the agency. There are written job descriptions for all classifications of personnel.
19. The agency provides consultation as needed for the administrative, supervisory, and direct-service personnel.
20. The agency has written personnel policies for all personnel.
21. The agency provides ongoing professional and/or technical supervision for all personnel.

---

*From American Nurses' Association: Standards of community health nursing practice, Kansas City, MO, 1986, The Association. Reprinted with the permission of ANA.

†From National League for Nursing: Criteria and standards manual for National League for Nursing/American Public Health Association Accreditation of Home Health Agencies and Community Nursing Services. New York, 1980, Publ. No. 21-1306. Used with permission.

22. The agency provides for staff development.
23. The agency has a structure and plan for evaluation.
24. The agency evaluates its organizational structure and administrative policies and practices.
25. The agency evaluates its programs.
26. The agency evaluates its staffing patterns, policies, and practices.
27. The agency establishes goals as a result of its overall evaluation. It communicates its status to the public.
28. Long-range planning is conducted by the agency to provide for future direction and viability.

GOVERNMENTAL INFLUENCES ON HEALTH CARE DELIVERY

G1—SELECT MAJOR HISTORICAL EVENTS DEPICTING FINANCIAL INVOLVEMENT OF FEDERAL GOVERNMENT IN HEALTH CARE DELIVERY

1798 Marine Hospital Service Act was passed to provide medical care to Merchant Marines.

1878 Port Quarantine Act was passed to prevent epidemic diseases from entering the country through seaports.

1879 National Health Department was established by Congress with a budget of $500,000.

1887 Laboratory of Hygiene at Staten Island Marine Hospital marked the beginning of Public Health Service research activities. This bacteriologic research laboratory later evolved into the National Institute of Health.

1890 Marine Hospital Service was given authority to inspect all immigrants to bar "lunatics and others unable to care for self" from entering the country.

1902 National Health Department was renamed the Public Health and Marine Hospital Service.

1912 National Institute of Health functions were expanded to study and investigate diseases of persons and the conditions influencing the origin and spread of disease.

1912 The Public Health and Marine Hospital Service was renamed the United States Public Health Service.

1912 The Child Health Bureau was established within the USPHS.

1917 National leprosarium was established at Carville, Louisiana under the aegis of the USPHS.

1917 USPHS became responsible for the physical and mental examination of all aliens.

1917 Congress appropriated $25,000 to USPHS to study and provide demonstration projects sharing state and federal cooperative rural health services.

1918 Because of increased veneral disease incidence during World War I, the Division of Venereal Disease was established in USPHS providing for cooperative federal and state control and prevention programs.

1921 Shepherd-Towner Maternity Infancy Act was passed to provide for the establishment of state maternal and infant programs. The Act provided for mother-child health conferences, home delivery supplies, improved prenatal care, improved infant and child care, more public health nurses, and health education.

1929 USPHS Narcotics Division was developed to provide facilities for the confinement and treatment of drug addicts (renamed Division of Mental Hygiene in 1939).

1935 Congress passed the Social Security Act. Title VI of the Act was written for the purpose of assisting states, counties, health districts, and other political subdivisions in establishing and maintaining adequate public health service, including the training of personnel for state and local health work.

1935 The Social Security Act provided for grants-in-aid to states to finance the public's health. *Grants-in-aid* resulted in increased numbers of new health departments and the strengthening and expansion of existing health departments.

1937 National Cancer Act called for the establishment of the National Cancer Institute for research into the causes, diagnosis, and treatment of cancer; for assistance to public and private agencies; and for the promotion of the most effective prevention and treatment.

1938 The second Federal Veneral Disease Control Act was passed to promote investigation and control and to provide funds for the development and maintenance of state and local programs.

1939 The Federal Security Agency was established to bring health, welfare, and education services of the federal government together.

1940 Communicable Disease Center (National Center for Disease Control) was established in Atlanta for the purpose of conducting epidemiological studies, providing health personnel training, and establishing methods of communication and education.

1940 National Office of Vital Statistics (National Center for Health Statistics) was authorized to provide data about health, illness, injuries, and death.

1941 Nurse training appropriations provided monies to nursing programs to increase enrollment and improve programs.

Sources for this listing were Hanlon, J., and Picket, G.: *Public health administration and practice*, ed. 2, St. Louis, 1984, The C.V. Mosby Co.; Congressional Research Service: *Summary of health legislation, 1959–1981*, Library of Congress Pub. No. 82-127 EPW, Washington, D.C., May 7, 1981, U.S. Government Printing Office; Congressional Research Service: Major legislation of the 97th Congress, Library of Congress Pub. No. 9, Washington, D.C., Oct. 6, 1982 U.S. Government Printing Office; Congressional Research Service: Major Legislation of the 98th Congress, Library of Congress Pub. No. 9, Wash., D.C., Oct, 1986 U.S. Government Printing Office.

1943   Nurse Training Act established the U.S. Nurse Cadet Corps in USPHS to support nurse training.

1946   National Mental Health Act was passed for constructing and equipping hospitals and laboratories to stimulate research and training in mental health.

1946   Hill-Burton Act provided for hospital services and construction.

1947   National Institute of Health Division of Research Grants were established to administer and award grants for research projects and training.

1947   A permanent Nursing Corps in the Army and Navy was established.

1948   National Heart Institute was established (renamed Heart, Lung, and Blood Institute in 1976).

1948   Microbiological, Experimental Biology, and Medicine Institutes were established (renamed National Institute of Allergy and Infectious Diseases in 1955).

1948   National Institute of Dental Research was authorized.

1948   National Institute of Health became National Institutes of Health (NIH).

1949   National Institute of Mental Health was established (renamed Alcoholism, Drug Abuse, and Mental Health Administration in 1974).

1950   National Institute of Neurological Diseases and Blindness was established (renamed National Eye Institute in 1968 and the National Institute of Neurological and Communicative Disorders and Strokes in 1975).

1950   Health Manpower Training Acts evolved to provide for training of Health Personnel.

1953   National Clinical Center was founded to accelerate research and to confirm and apply research findings. A 600-bed research hospital evolved.

1954   Congress extended Hill-Burton Act to allow monies for construction of other types of health facilities, such as general, mental, tuberculosis, and chronic disease hospitals; public health centers; diagnostic and treatment centers; rehabilitation facilities; nursing homes; state health laboratories; and nurse training facilities.

1954   Taft Sanitary Engineering Center. was founded in Cincinnati for research and training in environmental health.

1955   National Institutes of Health Division of Biological Standards was established to oversee the growth of the pharmaceutical industry and market.

1955   Polio Vaccination Assistance Act was passed to aid state vaccination programs.

1956   U.S. Army Medical Library was transferred to USPHS, which became the Library of Medicine at the National Institutes of Health. The library provides MEDLARS, the Medical Literature Analysis and Retrieval System.

1956   CHAMPUS program was established for dependents of military personnel.

1956   National Health Survey was established for continuous monitoring of sickness and disability in U.S.

1959   National Institute of Arthritis and Metabolic Diseases was established (renamed National Institute of Arthritis, Metabolic, and Digestive Diseases in 1981).

1960   Social Security Amendments provided grants to states for medical assistance to the aged.

1962   National Institute of Child Health and Human Development was founded.

1962   Program for state assistance in preschool vaccination programs was authorized.

1963   Aid program was established for the construction of mental retardation and community mental health facilities and the development of programs to combat health problems, e.g., maternal health, crippled children, and the mentally retarded.

1965   Heart disease, cancer, and stroke legislation was provided for the establishment of Regional Medical Programs to coordinate existing services for these three health problems.

1965   Appalachian Regional Development Act was passed to provide for construction of health services facilities in economically depressed area.

1965   Social Security Act was amended to provide for Medicare and Medicaid programs.

1966   Division of Environmental Health Services was established in Public Health Service.

1966   Partnership for health legislation consolidated pre-existing projects and *formula grants* to states through a new system of grants for comprehensive health planning. The legislation allowed health planning but did not give authority to control program development, spending, or construction of health facilities.

1968   Fogarty International Center for Advanced Study in Health Sciences was founded at NIH for international collaboration, study, and research by world scholars.

1970   Occupational Health and Safety Act was passed to assure safe and healthy working conditions.

1971   Environmental Protection Agency was founded to establish an umbrella agency for all environmental programs.

1971   National Center for Toxicological Research was established at Pine Bluff, Arkansas under the aegis of the Food and Drug Administration of USPHS.

1972   National programs were established for research, screening, counseling, and treatment of sickle cell anemia and Cooley's anemia.

1972   Social Security Act amended to encourage Professional Standards Review Organizations (PSRO). PSROs were designed to review hospital services ordered by physicians to determine overuse and underuse of services for patient care.

1972   National commission was established to study and investigate causes, cures, and treatment of multiple sclerosis.

1973   Social Security Act was amended to provide for the development of health maintenance organizations (HMOs)—prepaid comprehensive health care delivery systems designed to introduce competition into the health care arena.

1973   Program of grants—contracts for establishing and operating emergency medical services systems—was authorized.

1974   National Health Planning and Resources Development Act was passed to provide a triad health planning system. The system was designed as a comprehensive planning structure to review health services and facilities and to control and limit the expenditure of federal monies by discouraging the development and continuation of unnecessary new and existing programs.

1974   National Diabetes Mellitus Research and Education Act was passed to authorize NIH to establish a National Commission on Diabetes to formulate long-range plans to combat the disease.

1974   Sudden Infant Death Syndrome Act was passed to provide a program of dissemination of research and information to the public.

1976   National Swine Flu Immunization Program was established and implemented.

1976   Toxic Substances Control Act was passed to require testing of certain chemical substances to protect human health and environment.

1977   Rural Health Clinics Services Act was passed to provide for the establishment of health clinics in rural underserved communities. The clinics were to be staffed by nurse practitioners or physician assistants. The bill marked the first national legislation passed for reimbursement of nurse practitioner and physician assistant services under Medicare and Medicaid.

1980   Civil Rights of Institutionalized Persons Act was passed to protect mentally ill, disabled, retarded, chronically ill, or handicapped persons from flagrant conditions in state-affiliated institutions.

1980   Infant Formula Act was passed to require that such formulas meet certain standards of nutrition, quality, and safety in manufacturing.

1980   Department of Health, Education, and Welfare reorganized. Department of Health and Human Services oversees the regulation of health programs.

1981   Omnibus Budget Reconciliation Act (OBRA) provided for maternal and child health block grants to states under Title V of the Social Security Act to assist the states in advancing the health of mothers and children. Legislation allows states to make decisions on how to spend monies for nine maternal-child health programs.

1981   Omnibus Budget Reconciliation Act provided preventive health services block grants to allow states to make decisions about monies spent for 10 preventive health programs like hypertensive screening, rape crisis centers, etc.

1981   Omnibus Budget Reconciliation Act provided alcohol, drug abuse, and mental health block grants for states to provide direct services through community mental health centers, and alcohol and drug abuse programs.

1981   Omnibus Budget Reconciliation Act provided primary care block grant to states for community health center funding.

1982   Defense appropriations amendments allowed for direct, independent nurse practitioner reimbursement under CHAMPUS.

1982   The Tax Equity and Fiscal Responsibility Act established reductions in Medicare and Medicaid spending, called for the development of a prospective reimbursement system, authorized Medicare payments for hospice service, and replaced PSRO with a new utilization and quality control peer review program.

1983   Public Health Emergency Act provided for a permanent revolving fund for use by the Secretary of DHHS in responding to public health emergencies.

1983   Social Security Amendments of 1983 contained provisions providing for the establishment of a prospective payment system under Medicare.

1983   Amendments to the Public Health Act; authorized grants, contracts, and loans for the development of home health agencies and training of home health personnel.

1985   Health Research Extension Act establishes a new National Center for Nursing Research.

COMMUNITY RESOURCES

H1—PARTIAL LIST OF HEALTH ORGANIZATIONS USED BY COMMUNITY HEALTH NURSES

AL-ANON Family Group Headquarters, Inc.

PO Box 182, Madison Square Station, New York, NY 10010

Founded in 1951, Al-Anon, including Alateen for teenagers, offers a self-help recovery program for relatives and friends who have been adversely affected by someone else's drinking problem. Members share experiences, strength and hope in an effort to make their own lives manageable. Membership: 15,600 groups worldwide.

Alcohol and Drug Problems Association of North America, Inc.

1101 15th Street, NW, Suite 204, Washington, DC 20005

Founded in 1949, the association serves as a focal point for action and a medium of exchange for professionals in the alcohol and drug problems field at the national, state, and local governmental levels and in the private sector.

Alcoholics Anonymous

468 Park Avenue South, New York, NY 10016

Founded in 1935. AA is a program of recovery from alcoholism.

American Association for Maternal and Child Health, Inc.

PO Box 965, Los Altos, CA 94022

Founded in 1925.

American Association for Vital Records and Public Health Statistics

c/o Utah Dept of Health, PO Box 2500, Salt Lake City, UT 84110

Founded in 1933, the AAVRPHS provides the only national forum for the study, discussion and solution of the problems related to programs of vital and health statistics by state and local representatives without undue influence of Federal government officials.

American Burn Association

c/o William Curreri, MD, New York Hospital, Cornell Medical Center, New York, NY 10021

Founded in 1967.

American Cancer Society, Inc.

777 Third Avenue, New York, NY

Founded in 1913. ACS conducts research on cause, prevention, treatment of cancer; public education programs alert Americans to protective and preventive measures; informs physicians on developments in diagnosis and treatment of cancer; provides service and rehabilitation program for patients.

American Dental Association

211 East Chicago Avenue, Chicago, IL 60611

Founded in 1859. The ADA is the national voluntary organization for the U.S. dental profession and is the second largest health profession in the country.

American Diabetes Association

600 Fifth Avenue, New York, NY 10020

Founded in 1940. ADA funds research and conducts education programs in the field of diabetes. Publishes patient magazine and two medical journals.

American Epilepsy Society

38238 Glenn Avenue, Willoughby, OH 44094

Founded in 1946. AES works to foster research and treatment of epilepsy in all of its phases—biological, clinical and social—and the promotion of better care and treatment of persons subject to seizures.

American Fertility Society

1608 13th Avenue, Suite 101, Birmingham, AL 35205

Founded in 1944. The primary objective of the Society is to disseminate that body of knowledge which encompasses all aspects of infertility, related endocrinology, conception control and reproductive biology. The greater emphasis is on those matters which are clinical in nature.

American Foundation for the Blind

15 West 16th Street, New York, NY 10011

Founded in 1921. The objective of the foundation is to stimulate, facilitate and coordinate a national effort for improving services to blind and psychological, technological/social research, gathering, preparation, publishing information to professional and general public, sponsoring workshops, seminars, conferences.

American Genetic Association

818 18th Street, NW, Washington, DC 20006

Founded in 1903.

American Geriatrics Society, Inc.

10 Columbus Circle, Suite 1470, New York, NY 10019

Founded in 1942. AGS provides dissemination of information relating to the etiology, prevention, diagnosis and treatment of diseases of the aging and aged, rehabilitation of patients and problems relating to the health care of the older patient.

American Health Foundation

320 East 43rd Street, New York, NY 10018

Founded in 1969. AHF is a unique, non-profit institution, totally committed to disease prevention and health promotion. Today, on national and community levels, AHF is achieving its goals through laboratory and clinical research, preventive health care services and public education.

American Heart Association

7320 Greenville Avenue, Dallas, TX 75231
Founded in 1948. The AHA mission is to reduce death and disability from cardiovascular diseases.

American Hepatic Foundation

PO Box 1005, Williamston, NC 27892
Founded in 1973.

American Laryngological Association

110 Irving Street, NW, Washington, DC 20010
Founded in 1878. ALA conducts annual meetings, publishes transactions in field of laryngology, rhinology, head, and neck surgery.

American Liver Foundation

30 Sunrise Terrace, Cedar Grove, NJ 07009
Founded in 1976. The ALF seeks to improve the understanding, prevention, and cure of liver diseases through professional and public education and by supporting vitally needed research training of young scientific investigators.

American Lung Association

1740 Broadway, New York, NY 10019
Founded in 1904. ALA is primarily an educational organization to fight lung disease and work for lung health. It also works against cigarette smoking and air pollution.

American Mental Health Foundation, Inc.

2 East 86th Street, New York, NY 10028
Founded in 1924. The AMHF is dedicated to extensive and intensive research in the theories of psychotherapy and to the implementation of needed reforms.

American Optometric Association

243 Lindbergh Boulevard, St. Louis, MO 63141
Founded in 1898. The objectives of the AOA as stated in its constitution are: To improve the vision care and health of the public and to promote the art and science of the profession of optometry.

American Parkinson Disease Association

147 East 50th Street, New York, NY 10022

American Pediatric Society

David Goldring, MD, PO Box 14871, St. Louis, MO 63178
Founded in 1888. APS provides an annual scientific meeting during which short papers are presented in all the pediatric subspecialties. The subspecialty sessions are preceded by a plenary session as well as a symposium on important research achievements in pediatrics.

American Physical Fitness Research Institute

824 Moraga Drive, Los Angeles, CA 90049
Founded in 1958. APFRI provides research and development of motivational and educational information on all aspects of health, fitness, and well-being directed toward personal responsibility toward one's health.

American Psychosomatic Society, Inc.

265 Nassau Road, Roosevelt, NY 11575
Founded in 1943. APS works to advance the research of psychosomatic medicine.

American Red Cross

17th and D Streets, NW, Washington, DC 20006
Founded in 1881. The aims of the Red Cross are to improve the quality of human life and enhance individual self-reliance and concern for others. It works toward these aims through national and chapter services governed and directed by volunteers.

American Venereal Disease Association

Box 385, University of Virginia Hospital, Charlottesville, VA 22908
AVDA is an association of physicians, nurses and other public health professionals concerned with research, professional education, and control of sexually transmitted diseases. Publishes a quarterly journal, *Sexually Transmitted Diseases.*

Arthritis Foundation

3400 Peachtree Road, NE, Atlanta, GA 30326
Founded in 1948.

Arthritis Society

920 Yonge Street, Suite 420, Toronto, Canada M4W 3J7
Founded in 1948. The AS is organized for the development of rheumatological manpower through associateships and fellowships; the support of research projects deemed relevant to the rheumatic diseases; and the communication about arthritis with general public and medical profession.

Association for the Care of Asthma, Inc.

Spring Valley Road, Ossining, NY 10562
Founded in 1963. ACA conducts an annual postgraduate course in allergy and clinical immunology for the advancement of the knowledge and practice of the care and treatment of asthma, by discussion at such meetings, promoting and encouraging research and study.

Association for the Care of Children in Hospitals

3615 Wisconsin Avenue, NW, Washington, DC 20016
Founded in 1965. ACCH seeks to foster and promote the health and well-being of children and families in health care settings by education, interdisciplinary interaction and planning, and research.

Association for Children with Learning Disabilities

4156 Library Road, Pittsburgh, PA 15234
Founded in 1963.

Association for Children with Retarded Mental Development, Inc.

902 Broadway, 5th Floor, New York, NY 10010
Founded in 1951. ACRMD is a nonprofit membership corporation offering services to mentally retarded adults throughout New York City. Services include rehabilitation and sheltered workshops; day training and activities centers; day treatment centers; job placement; evening and weekend social centers; various community services.

Association for Education of the Visually Handicapped

919 Walnut Street, 4th Floor, Philadelphia, PA 19107
Founded in 1853. The AEVH is a professional asso-

ciation interested in the progress and welfare of visually handicapped children.

Asthma and Allergy Foundation of America

19 West 44th Street, New York, NY 10036

Founded in 1953. The AAFA provides public education booklets and newsletters, answers inquiries on asthma and allergy; arranges for professional speakers and audio-visual materials and encourages community activities through its local chapters.

Biofeedback Society of America

4200 East Ninth, C268, Denver, CO 80262

Founded in 1969. The BSA is an interdisciplinary organization dedicated to the applied, research and educational aspects of biofeedback.

Braille Institute

741 North Vermont Avenue, Los Angeles, CA 90029

Founded in 1919. The institute provides training, education and special services for the blind of all ages.

Child Abuse Listening Mediation, Inc.

PO Box 718, Santa Barbara, CA 93102

Founded in 1971. CALM is organized for the prevention of child abuse and neglect, and provides a hot line listener, child care to reduce stress, a speakers bureau, and parent support groups.

Child Health Associate Program

4200 East Ninth Avenue, Box C219, Denver, CO 80262

Founded in 1969. The CHAP is a training program to prepare health care professionals capable of providing a wide range of diagnostic, preventive and therapeutic services to children. Working principally in ambulatory settings as colleagues and associates of physicians, child health associates have the knowledge and skill to care for a large percentage of the patients seen in a typical pediatric practice. The training program is three years in length. Prerequisites include two years of college preparation.

The Children's Foundation

1420 New York Avenue, NW, 8th Floor, Washington, DC 20005

The foundation was established in 1969 as a national, non-profit advocacy organization focusing upon the quality and availability of the federal food assistance programs for children and their families.

Committee to Combat Huntington's Disease, Inc.

250 West 57th Street, Suite 2016, New York, NY 10019

Founded in 1967. The goals of the committee are the identification of HD families, education of the lay public and professional, the promotion and support of basic and clinical research into the causes and cure of HD, and a patient services program, coordinated with various community services.

Council on Arteriosclerosis of the American Heart Assoc.

7320 Greenville Avenue, Dallas, TX 75231

Founded in 1946.

Council on Education for Public Health

1015 15th Street, NW, Washington, DC 20005

Founded in 1974. CEPH is the independent agency officially recognized by the U.S. Office of Education and the Council on Postsecondary Accreditation to accredit graduate schools of public health and certain graduate programs outside of schools of public health.

Council of World Organizations Interested in the Handicapped

432 Park Avenue, South, New York, NY 10016

Founded in 1953. The council provides a coordinating mechanism for international organizations and the UN agencies to avoid duplication of programs for disabled people.

Drug Information Association, Inc.

1050 George Street, Suite 5-L, New Brunswick, NJ 08901

Founded in 1965. The DIA is an international multidisciplinary professional association of specialists engaged in furthering modern technology of communication in medical, pharmaceutical, and allied human/animal fields. Publishes quarterly *Drug Information Journal* as proceedings of meetings and for submitted relevant papers.

Gerontological Society

1835 K Street, NW, Suite 305, Washington, DC 20006

Founded in 1945. The society is a national multidisciplinary organization of researchers, educators and professionals in aging devoted to stimulating and promoting research and its application to practice. Publishes 2 bimonthly journals: *Journal of Gerontology* and *The Gerontologist*.

Goodwill Industries of America, Inc.

9200 Wisconsin Avenue, Washington, DC 20014

Founded in 1902. Goodwill Industries provides services, materials, and information to assist member Goodwill Industries in their programs of service to handicapped people.

Gray Panthers

3635 Chestnut Street, Philadelphia, PA 19104

Founded in 1970. The Gray Panthers are people of all ages, working for social change. It tries to develop creative alternatives to the injustices in society which confront people at every phase of life.

Guide Dog Users, Inc.

Box 174, Central Station, Baldwin, NY 11510

Founded in 1969. The goals of GDU are to improve the quality of the educational, cultural, employment and rehabilitation services of all blind persons, to promote the acceptance of guide dog users by federal and state agencies, employers, educational institutions, business establishments and places of entertainment. National basis members at large; publication *Pawtracks* quarterly.

Health and Education Resources

4733 Bethesda Avenue, Suite 735, Bethesda, MD 20014

Founded in 1969. HER is a non-profit organization developing programs and communications in health, education, and social services including continuing education for clinical laboratory personnel; technical assistance for implementation of a skill-and-knowledge-based task analysis method; production of audio-visual instructional materials.

Health Sciences Communications Association

2343 North 115th Street, Wauwatosa, WI 53226
Founded in 1959. HSCA is a non-profit organization devoted to advancement of education in health sciences by means of varied contemporary educational technology.

Healthright, Inc.

41 Union Square, Room 206-8, New York, NY 10003
Founded in 1974. Healthright is a women's health education and advocacy organization which publishes a quarterly newsletter and provides a literature center with many health education pamphlets and books.

Healthy America, National Coalition for Health Promotion and Disease Prevention

1015 15th Street, NW, Suite 424, Washington, DC 20005
Founded in 1977 the coalition is a national, non-profit organization emphasizing health advocacy, disease prevention and promotion of good health habits as means to attain lasting good health. It encourages health promotion policies and programs at all levels of government and within private sector, sponsors seminars, conferences, etc. and serves as congressional liaison for membership.

International Association Cancer Victims and Friends, Inc.

7740 W. Manchester Avenue, Suite 110, Playa del Rey, CA 90291
Founded in 1963. IACVF is a non-profit (tax exempt) corporation organized under the laws of the state of California. Its purpose is the dissemination of educational materials concerning the prevention and control of cancer through the use of non-toxic therapies. Chapters have symposiums and seminars in their respective areas throughout the year.

International Childbirth Education Association, Inc.

8635 Fremont Avenue South, Minneapolis, MN 55420
Founded in 1960. The ICEA promotes family centered maternity care and helps groups and individuals promote same through classes in prepared childbirth, teacher training, publications, conferences and conventions.

International Commission for Prevention of Alcoholism

6830 Laurel Street, NW, Washington, DC 20012
Founded in 1952. The commission is a non-government organization of the UN, focusing on prevention programming through organizing of congresses, seminars, personal contacts, educational material, and other community endeavors.

International Council on Health, Physical Education and Recreation

1201 16th Street, NW, Room 417, Washington, DC 20036
Founded in 1958. The council represents and brings together teachers, administrators, leaders, national departments of physical education and related associations in health, physical education, sports, dance and recreation into one organization at the international level. It fosters international understanding, goodwill and encourages development and expansion of educationally sound programs.

The Juvenile Diabetes Foundation

23 East 26th Street, New York, NY 10010
Founded in 1970. JDF is a non-profit voluntary agency whose prime objective is to support and fund research aimed at preventing the complications and curing the disease itself. JDF chapters provide educational and counseling services in addition to fund raising.

W.K. Kellogg Foundation

400 North Avenue, Battle Creek, MI 49016
Founded in 1930. The foundation is committed to the application of existing knowledge to problems of people in the areas of health, education and agriculture. It currently assists programs of four continents, including the United States and Canada, Latin America, Europe and Australia. A grant making organization, the foundation does not operate programs.

La Leche League International, Inc.

9616 Minneapolis Avenue, Franklin Park, IL 60131
Founded in 1956. The league is a non-profit organization which provides help for breastfeeding mothers in a series of four meetings, annual seminar for physicians, biennial international conferences for parents and professionals, and a 24 hour telephone hotline.

Leukemia Society of America, Inc.

800 Second Avenue, New York, NY 10017
Founded in 1949. The LSA promotes and provides support into the causes, treatment and cure or control of the leukemias and related lymphomas. Allied programs are patient service, public and professional education and community services.

The Living Bank International

PO Box 6725, Houston, TX 77005
Founded in 1968. The LBI is an organ and body donor registry, educating the public about the importance of organ and body donations, registration, and referral of donations, at the time of death, to the appropriate medical facility closest to the point of death.

The Lupus Foundation of America, Inc.

11673 Holly Springs Drive, St. Louis, MO 63141
Founded in 1977. The corporation is organized exclusively for charitable, educational and scientific purposes to encourage development of research programs designed to discover the causes of, and to improve the methods of treating, diagnosing, curing and preventing Lupus Erythematosus.

March of Dimes Birth Defects Foundation

1275 Mamaroneck Avenue, White Plains, NY 10605
Founded in 1938. The goal of the foundation is the prevention of birth defects, our most serious child health problem, through support of research, medical services and education.

Maternity Center Association

48 East 92nd Street, New York, NY 10028

Founded in 1918. The MCA provides complete maternity service for low-risk families; childbirth education and information service; support of nurse-midwifery education; institutes on parent education and literature on childbearing and maternity care.

Medic Alert Foundation International

PO Box 1009, Turlock, CA 95380

Founded in 1956. Medic Alert provides emergency medical identification in either necklace or bracelet style which includes hidden medical condition, membership number, and emergency telephone number which can be called collect. A wallet card is provided with additional emergency information. $10 membership fee includes stainless steel emblem.

Mended Hearts, Inc.

721 Huntington Avenue, Boston, MA 02115

Founded in 1951.

Mental Health Association, National Headquarters

1800 North Kent Street, Arlington, VA 22209

Founded in 1909. The MHA is a lay, volunteer organization which provides social action and public education in the area of mental health.

Muscular Dystrophy Association

810 Seventh Avenue, 27th Floor, New York, NY 10019

The MDA is a voluntary national health agency—a dedicated partnership between scientists and concerned citizens aimed at conquering neuromuscular diseases which affect thousands of Americans.

The Myasthenia Gravis Foundation

15 East 26th Street, New York, NY 10010

Founded in 1952. The foundation fosters, coordinates, and supports research into the cause, prevention, alleviation, and cure of myasthenia gravis, and gives research grants to MG clinics, hospitals, medical schools throughout the United States and awards at least 10 medical student fellowships each year and a $20,000 post-doctoral fellowship.

National Association of Councils of Stutterers

Speech and Hearing Center, O'Boyle Hall, Room 100, Catholic Univ., Washington, DC 20064

Founded in 1965.

National Association for Down's Syndrome

PO Box 63, Oak Park, IL 60303

Founded in 1960. NADS is a not-for-profit organization comprised of parents and professionals involved with the individual with Down's Syndrome.

National Association on Drug Abuse Problems, Inc.

355 Lexington Avenue, New York, NY 10017

Founded in 1975. NADAP provides a placement service for rehabilitated drug abusers. Workshop for drug treatment counselors and corporate management.

National Association of the Physically Handicapped, Inc.

76 Elm Street, London, OH 43140

Founded in 1958. The NAPH advances the social, economic, and physical welfare of physically handicapped. It is not a resource center for information. We give no type services; nor give financial aid. We support legislation to benefit handicapped; trying to make public aware of needs of handicapped.

National Association of Retarded Citizens

2709 Avenue E East, Arlington, TX 76011

Founded in 1950.

National Association for Visually Handicapped

305 East 24th Street, New York, NY 10010

Founded in 1954. The NAVH offers guidance and counsel for all partially-seeing people and professionals and paraprofessionals working with them, informational literature. It publishes and distributes large print books, textbooks and testing material. Serves as referral agency for all services for partially seeing. Only national health agency serving only the partially-seeing (not the totally blind).

National Ataxia Foundation

6681 Country Club Drive, Minneapolis, MN 55427

Founded in 1957. NAF works to combat all types of hereditary ataxia and related disorders through four major objectives: education, service, prevention and research.

National Burn Federation

3737 Fifth Avenue, Suite 206, San Diego, CA 92103

Founded in 1975. The foundation serves as a vehicle for exchange of ideas and programs in fire safety and burn prevention; gives national focus to the burn problem, the medical resources available to treat burns, and the community prevention programs in operation which address the problem.

National Committee for the Prevention of Alcoholism and Drug Dependency

6830 Laurel Street, NW, Washington, DC 20012

Founded in 1950. The committee holds institutes and seminar-workshops throughout the U.S. periodically. It gathers and distributes information and materials concerning the effects of alcohol and other drugs on the physical, mental and moral powers of the individual citizen and promotes an educational program for prevention with visual and teaching aids throughout the country. Willing to cooperate with other organizations in holding seminar-workshops in their area.

National Council on Alcoholism, Inc.

733 Third Avenue, New York, NY 10017

Founded in 1944. The council is the only national voluntary agency founded to combat the disease of alcoholism.

National Council on Drug Abuse

571 West Jackson Boulevard, Chicago, IL 60606

Founded in 1972. NCDA is a tax-exempt not-for-profit educational and preventative organization. Our work in the fields of drug and alcohol abuse has helped thousands of professionals and laymen countrywide deter, curtail and better understand substance abuse.

National Council on Health Care Services

1200 15th Street, NW, Suite 601, Washington, DC 20005

Founded in 1969. The council is a trade association organized to foster a better understanding of the important contribution private companies make to the nation's health care delivery system and to promote standards of quality and efficiency beneficial to both the membership and the public.

National Health Council, Inc.

1740 Broadway, New York, NY 10019

Founded in 1920. NHC is a membership organization of national voluntary, professional, and related organizations interested in improving the health of all Americans in the areas of planning, coordination, and delivery of health services.

National Health Federation

PO Box 688, Monrovia, CA 91016

Founded in 1955.

National Hearing Aid Society

20361 Middlebelt Road, Livonia, MI 48152

Founded in 1951. NHAS is the professional association for those engaged in fitting and selling of hearing aids.

The National Hemophilia Foundation

25 West 39th Street, New York, NY 10018

Founded in 1948. The foundation provides information for those interested in the field, and promotes research.

National Indian Council on Aging

PO Box 2088, Albuquerque, NM 87103

Founded in 1976. The council is a national advocacy organization to bring about improved services to American Indian and Alaskan Native elders, including health-related services.

National Indian Health Board, Inc.

1602 South Parker Road, Suite 200, Denver, CO 80231

Founded in 1972. The board provides review and comment on federal legislation that affects Indian tribes and serves as an advisory board to HEW on Indian health concerns.

National Kidney Foundation

2 Park Avenue, Room 908, New York, NY 10016

Founded in 1958. NKF is a national voluntary health organization supporting research and public information on the diagnosis and treatment of diseases of the kidney.

National Lupus Erythematosus Foundation, Inc.

5430 Van Nuys Boulevard, Van Nuys, CA 91401

Founded in 1950. NLEF is a non-profit organization for the distribution of Lupus literature; compiling of information gathered from Lupus patients; funding of Lupus research, and establish Lupus City of Hope Chapters throughout the country.

National Society for Autistic Children

1234 Massachusetts Avenue, NW, Suite 1017, Washington, DC 20005

Founded in 1965. The NSAC is a non-profit organization of parents, professionals and other concerned citizens working for better education, research, treatment and legislation on behalf of autistic persons.

National Spinal Cord Injury Foundation

369 Elliot Street, Newton Upper Falls, MA 02169

Founded in 1948. The foundation addresses the needs of persons with spinal cord injuries through programs in the areas of care, cure and coping.

National Sudden Infant Death Syndrome Foundation

310 South Michigan Avenue, Chicago, IL 60604

Founded in 1962. NSIDSF provides support for SIDS research, services to families of victims of SIDS and SIDS-related disorders, and educational programs for health and emergency personnel. It also fulfills a consumer advocacy role for SIDS families.

National Tay-Sachs and Allied Disease Association

122 East 42nd Street, New York, NY 10017

Founded in 1957. The association conducts programs in support of research, family counseling, and public and professional education into the genetic disease Tay-Sachs and many other diseases due to inborn errors of metabolism.

Pediatric Pulmonary Association of America

150 North Pond Way, Roswell, GA 30076

Founded in 1975. PPAA works to combat chronic lung diseases in infants and children via the dissemination of knowledge of updated therapeutic techniques and through the promotion of advanced research. Also it provides a legislative base for permanent federal and state funding for meritorious programs. The PPAA, through its periodical publication *The Pediatric Pulmonary Digest,* circulates the field on current news. Contributions are welcomed. Send articles to the editor.

Planned Parenthood Federation of America, Inc.

810 Seventh Avenue, New York, NY 10019

PPF works to make effective means of birth control available for all.

The Salvation Army

120 West 14th Street, New York, NY 10011

Founded in 1880. The Salvation Army is an international religious and charitable organization providing health and welfare services throughout the world. In the United States a wide range of services is based upon needs of community and available local resources.

Synanon Foundation, Inc.

PO Box 786, Marshall, CA 94940

Founded in 1958. Synanon was the first community designed for the re-education of drug addicts and other character disorders, and it continues to do that work. Since 1974 Synanon has been providing re-education for children as young as 10. Facilities in Marshall, San Francisco, Los Angeles, and Badger, Calif.; Kerhonkson and New York, N.Y., Chicago, Ill., and Detroit, Mich.

United Cerebral Palsy Association, Inc.

66 East 34th Street, New York, NY 10016

Founded in 1948. UCP is the only nationwide voluntary organization targeting its services on the specific and multiple needs of persons with cerebral palsy and their families. UCPs more than 240 affiliates provide a variety of community services, support research and conduct programs of public education pertaining to cerebral palsy.

RESOURCES FOR OCCUPATIONAL HEALTH

American Association of Occupational Health Nurses, Inc.
3500 Piedmont Road, NE, Suite 400, Atlanta, GA 30305

American Board for Occupational Health Nurses, Inc.
2210 Wilshire Blvd., Suite 771, Santa Monica, CA 90403

American Conference of Governmental Industrial Hygienists
6500 Glenway Avenue, Bldg. D-5, Cincinnati, OH 45211

American Industrial Hygiene Association
475 Wolfledges Pkwy., Akron, OH 44311

American Occupational Medicine Association
AMA, 535 N. Dearborn Street, Chicago, IL 60610

American Association of Fitness Directors in Business and Industry
400 Sixth St., SW Suite 3030, Washington, DC 20201

Bureau of Labor Statistics
U.S. Department of Labor, Washington, DC 20025

Centers for Disease Control
Atlanta, GA 30333

International Labor Office
1750 New York Ave., NW Suite 311, Washington, DC 20006

NIOSH
4676 Columbia Parkway, Cincinnati, OH 45226

National Safety Council
444 N. Michigan Ave., Chicago, IL 60611

OSHA
200 Constitution Ave., NW, Washington, DC 20210

Women's Occupational Health Resource Center
School of Public Health, Columbia University, 60 Haven Ave., B-1, New York, NY 10032

H2—UNIVERSITIES WITH GRADUATE PROGRAMS IN OCCUPATIONAL HEALTH NURSING

University of Alabama at Birmingham
University of Cincinnati
University of California at San Francisco
University of California at Los Angeles
University of North Carolina at Chapel Hill
Johns Hopkins School of Public Health
Boston University with Harvard
University of Illinois
University of Utah
University of Washington
University of Wisconsin-Milwaukee
University of Minnesota
Simmons College, Boston
University of Pennsylvania

APPENDIX

I

SAMPLE GUIDES

I1—CASE PRESENTATION GUIDE FOR AGENCY COMMUNICATION

1. State the problem(s).
2. Give the following identifiable information:
   A. Family composition
   B. Occupation and/or source of income
   C. Education
   D. Ethnic group
   E. Housing
   F. Family use of health care facility(ies)
3. Community assessment (as it affects the individual or family)
   A. Nutrition
   B. Mobility
   C. Recreation
   D. Religion
   E. Politics
   F. Housing
   G. Schools
   H. Economics
   I. Sanitation and pollution
4. Family history
   A. Social and medical
   B. Current estimate of each family member's present health status
   C. Current medical diagnosis
   D. Current medical treatment plan
   E. Knowledge of diagnosis, treatment, medication
   F. Obstacles to implementation
   G. Family strengths
5. Nursing interventions as they relate to the problem (brief summary)
6. Coordination of services (brief summary)
7. Continuity of services (brief summary), including referrals, resources, strengths/supports

I2—HOME CARE OF PERSONS WITH AIDS: INFECTION CONTROL GUIDELINES

Health care providers should be familiar with current epidemiological information on AIDS, including modes of transmission of HIV.

Patient Care Precautions

Handwashing: Hands should be washed before and after direct client care and after contact with blood, body fluids, or other body excretions (Centers for Disease Control, 1982).

Gloves: Gloves should be worn when the nurse expects direct contact with clients' blood, body fluids, excretions or secretions, or direct contact with surfaces or articles contaminated with blood or body excretions (Centers for Disease Control, 1982).

Gowns: Gowns should be worn if soiling of clothing with clients' blood or body excretions is anticipated (Centers for Disease Control, 1982).

Masks: Although not routinely needed, masks have been recommended for care providers having close contact with clients with a productive cough (American Hospital Association, 1984, Conte, et al., 1983).

Needles and syringes: Needles should not be bent or recapped after they are used and the syringe and needle should be disposed of in a puncture-proof container (Centers for Disease Control, 1982). Contact the local health department for information on disposal of containers.

Treatments: Gloves should be worn and double-bagging technique used for dressing changes (Dhundale and Hubbard, 1986).

Waste disposal: Body wastes should be flushed down the toilet. Dressings or other materials contaminated with blood or body excretions should be collected in a plastic-lined trash can. Contaminated waste and other household trash may be disposed of in a garbage can lined with a plastic bag. The can should have a tight-fitting lid. Contact the local health department for further information about waste disposal (California Public Health Services, 1985; Dhundale and Hubbard, 1986).

Blood spills: Promptly clean up all blood or body fluid spills with an appropriate disinfectant solution, such as a 1:10 dilution of household bleach (5.25% sodium hypochlorite) in water (Centers for Disease Control, 1982).

Client Precautions

Sex: A variety of sexual practices have been associated with an increased risk of transmission of HTLV-III (HIV). Guidelines for safer sex practices are presented in Appendix I7. Good hygienic practices by the client and other household members, such as regular bathing and handwashing after toileting and before meal preparation, should be encouraged (California Public Health Services, 1985).

Personal hygiene items that may become contaminated with blood or body fluids, such as razors and toothbrushes, should not be shared with other household members. Towels and washcloths should not be shared between launderings (California Public Health Services, 1985; Centers for Disease Control, 1985).

Laundry: Soiled linen should be kept in a plastic bag separate from other household laundry. Clients' laundry should be washed separately in hot, soapy water. Household bleach can be added to cottons and colorfast materials. A phenolic disinfectant, such as Lysol, can be used with non-colorfast fabrics. A second wash and rinse without the phenolic assists in removing chemical residues (Dhundale and Hubbard, 1986).

Dishes: Dishes, glasses, and eating utensils may be run through the dishwasher using the hot water cycle or washed in hot, soapy water and air dried (California Public Health Services, 1985; Dhundale and Hubbard, 1986).

Food: Due to the risk of *salmonella* infection, only pasteurized milk or milk products should be eaten. Fruits and vegetables composted with manure should be peeled or cooked before being eaten (California Public Health Services, 1985).

Housecleaning: Living areas should be well-ventilated. This decreases the risk of airborne diseases (California Public Health Services, 1985; Dhundale and Hubbard, 1986). Routine housecleaning procedures in the kitchen and bathroom should be followed to prevent the growth of bacteria and fungi that may cause infections. The inside of the refrigerator should be kept clean to prevent growth of molds. The kitchen counter and sink used for food preparation should be scoured and rinsed prior to food preparation. Kitchen and bathroom floors should be mopped at least weekly, with any spills cleaned up as they occur. A 1:10 strength bleach in water solution can be used as a disinfectant in mop water and for cleaning up blood and body fluid spills. Dirty mop water should be flushed down the toilet. Mops and sponges used to clean floors or spills of blood or body fluids should not be rinsed out at the sink used for food preparation. A 1:10 bleach solution may be used to disinfect sinks. Full-strength bleach may be added to the toilet bowl as a disinfectant. Mops and sponges may be soaked in the 1:10 bleach solution for 5 minutes to disinfect them (California Public Health Services, 1985). Mops and sponges used to clean the bathroom and blood and body fluid spills should be kept separate from those used to clean other parts of the house (Dhundale and Hubbard, 1986).

Pets: Pets may pose potential infection risks. Gloves and masks should be worn when cleaning bird-cages because of the risk of psittacosis, and cat litter boxes because of risk of toxoplasmosis. Because fish tanks may harbor *Mycobacterium* species, which have caused serious infections in persons with AIDS, someone other than the client should clean the tank (California Public Health Services, 1985; Dhundale and Hubbard, 1986).

BIBLIOGRAPHY

American Hospital Association: Recommendations of the Advisory Committee on Infections Within Hospitals. In Mundeleen, I.L.: Acquired immune deficiency syndrome: an educational packet, Chicago, 1984, Educational Committee of the Association of Practitioners in Infection Control.

California Public Health Services: Public health nursing standardized care plan: acquired immune deficiency syndrome, San Francisco, 1985, CPHS.

Centers for Disease Control: Provisional public health service inter-agency recommendations for screening donated blood and plasma for antibody to the virus causing acquired immunodeficiency syndrome MMWR 34:1-5, 1985.

Centers for Disease Control: Acquired immune deficiency syndrome (AIDS): precautions for clinical and laboratory staffs, MMWR 31:577-580, 1982.

Conte, J.E., Jr., Hadley, W.K., Sande, M., and the University of California, San Francisco, Task Force on the Acquired Immunodeficiency Syndrome: Infection control guidelines for patients with the acquired immunodeficiency syndrome (AIDS). N. Engl. J. Med. 309:740-744, 1983.

Dhundale, K., and Hubbard, P.M.: Home care for the A.I.D.S. patient: safety first, Nursing 86, 16(9):34-36, 1986.

I3—GUIDE FOR EVALUATION OF GROUP EFFECTIVENESS

The following questions focus evaluation on group task accomplishment, member satisfaction, conflict management, and group purpose. Answer each question for the group, then write a descriptive summary of group effectiveness.

1. Describe the group's task goal. List the steps proposed or acted on by members relative to the goal. How well do members achieve these steps?
2. Describe leadership behavior for the group. How well do members carry out other group roles?
3. Describe comfort level for group members. Do members support each other? Is the level of tension conducive to productive behavior?
4. Is disagreement expressed clearly and openly? How do members manage and resolve conflict?
5. By what bonds are members attracted to each other and to the group?
6. Are there implicit goals for the group, and do these goals interfere with the group's work toward the explicit goal?

I4—SCHOOL AND CLASSROOM ASSESSMENT GUIDE

1. Classroom assessment for health needs
   A. People involved—classroom teacher, nurse, and student when appropriate
2. Advance preparation
   A. Health records of students in an assigned location
   B. Room and time arranged for assessment
3. Plan conference—with appropriate people
   A. When health needs are identified
   B. Include student(s), with identified health needs, in conference
4. Classroom teacher
   A. In advance, weigh and measure all children; graph results
   B. Collect all screening results and place in folder
   C. Explain to students what is about to happen
   D. Work with nurse in assessing health records
5. Nurse environmentalist
   A. Look at physical structure: Classroom—what is in it? How many students to a classroom? Cleanliness, atmosphere, arrangement of desks? Exits free from

clutter, food in proper containers, refrigeration, bathrooms (soap, towel, and hot water)?
B.   Review students records with teacher
6. Nurse appropriately arranges for the following, if needed
    A.   Health risk appraisal
    B.   Vision screening
    C.   Hearing screening
    D.   Kidney screening
    E.   Physical and dental examinations
    F.   Follow-up of all defects
    G.   Contact with parents when problems are identified
    H.   Nursing assessment
    I.   Blood pressure screening
    J.   Scoliosis screening

7. Nurse assesses teacher's attitude toward students
    A.   Use observation skills
8. School nutrition program
    A.   Review menu for week
    B.   Meet with school dietary staff
    C.   Check to see if skimmed or low fat milk is an option
    D.   Because of budget cuts, help dietary staff to make up handout to send home about nutritional brown-bag lunches
9. Nurse
    A.   Assess all children in the classroom
    B.   Compare growth and development of children with their peers
    C.   List children with health-related problems

I5—HEALTH MAINTENANCE FLOW SHEET—2 WEEKS TO 17 YEARS

Procedures and ages

Assessments: 2 wk; 2, 4, 6, 9, 12, 18 mo; 2, 3, 5, 8, 11, 13, 15, 17 yr	Date scheduled						
	Date seen						
	Age						
	Provider						
Complete history	Date						
Complete examination	Date						

Immunizations (record dates below)

DPT									
OPV									
MMR									
Td									

Rubella serology 11 yr nonvaccinated female	Titer					
Tuberculin (tine) test 1, 3, 5, 11, 15 yr	Pos/Neg					
Hematocrit 1, 5, 13 yr	Result					
Urine culture (female) 5, 8 yr	Nl/Abn					
Blood pressure 3 yr and each subsequent visit	Result					
Development 6, 18 mo; 3, 5 yr	Nl/Abn/Q					
Hearing 6 mo; 1, 3, yr; and each subsequent visit	P/F					
Vision 4 mo; 1, 3 yr; and each subsequent visit	P/F					
Language 2, 3, 5 yr	P/F					
Dental care Each visit						

From Hoole, H.A., et al.: Patient care guideline for nurse practitioners, ed. 2, Boston, 1982, Little, Brown & Co. p. 2.

Health maintenance flow sheet—2 weeks to 17 years—cont'd

Counseling: each visit					
Nutrition					
Physical care					
Behavior/psychosocial					
Sex education					
Stimulation					
Safety					
Family planning					
Other					

16—REFERRAL SERVICE GUIDE

Purpose

To provide access to health care for students in need

Procedure

Classroom teachers or any other school personnel should refer students with any of the problems listed below to the school nurse

Students

1. Any student who needs to see the nurse should come directly to the health room
2. Friends of the students may feel free to send students to the health room

Conditions and symptoms to refer

1. Chronic absenteeism (other than truancy)
2. Problems with vision, hearing, or speech
3. Headache accompanied by nausea, vomiting, or blurred vision
4. Fatigue, listlessness, inattentiveness (chronic problems)
5. Allergies (i.e., red, inflamed eyes: chronic sinusitis; constant sneezing)
7. Respiratory problems such as wheezing or shortness of breath
8. Jaundice (a yellowish tint to the skin or whites of eyes)
9. Pregnant students or ones with children
10. Suspected venereal disease cases
11. Severe acne or other skin problems
12. Suspected abuse cases

EXCEPTION: The above list is not complete and teachers should not hesitate to refer other problems that they feel need attention

17—GUIDELINES FOR SAFE SEX

Many diseases may be transmitted during sexual encounters between homosexual, bisexual, or heterosexual partners. Examples of diseases that can be transmitted sexually include syphilis, gonorrhea, herpes, hepatitis, AIDS and lesser known infections such as chlamydia. By following the "safe sex" guidelines outlined in this appendix you can greatly reduce the chances of becoming infected with any of these debilitating and sometimes fatal diseases.

1. Having fewer different partners and knowing your partner and his or her state of health and life-style reduces your risk. Avoid sex with persons who use intravenous drugs or who have multiple sex partners. From a communicable disease standpoint, the safest sexual partner is a monogamous one.

2. Engage in sex in a setting that is conducive to cleanliness. When both partners shower together as a part of foreplay, there is an opportunity to check for sores and swollen lymph glands, and bodily cleanliness is a prelude to enjoyable and safe sex. Don't share personal hygiene items such as toothbrushes and razors.

3. Kissing, so long as you or your partner have no open cuts or sores on the lips, mouth, or tongue, also has a low risk of transmitting disease (with the possible exception of mononucleosis). Sexual experience is not limited to penile penetration—be creative with other types of body contact that does not involve exchange of body fluid, such as cuddling, massaging, and mutual stimulation. Information to date indicates that AIDS is not transmitted by casual kissing.

4. Exchanging body fluids has a high risk of transmitting disease. Oral contact or swallowing semen, urine, stool particles, and menstrual flow increases the risk of transmitting disease and should be completely avoided. Oral sex should be avoided when cuts or sores are present in the mouth.

5. Some sexual practices are quite hazardous. Rimming* has a very high risk of transmitting disease, especially in nonmonogamous situations. Fisting* is extremely dangerous under any circumstance.

6. Lubricants should be water soluble (not oils or greases). Saliva is a poor lubricant, and also may be loaded with germs. The lubricant should not be in an open container nor shared with others. Use one that is packaged in a pump, squeeze, or other closed container that dispenses one application at a time. Use nonperfumed lubricants.

7. Data at this time indicate that use of quality condoms

*Rimming refers to lingual-anal contact; fisting refers to inserting the fist into the rectum.

prevents the spread of most sexually transmitted diseases when used appropriately.

8. Anal intercourse causes tiny tears through which germs from both partners can enter the body. Use of a water-soluble lubricant helps reduce friction and tears and should be used even with a condom. Anal or vaginal douching before or after sex increases the risk of acquiring some infections because it removes normal barriers to infection.

9. Urinating after sex may reduce the risk of acquiring some diseases.

10. Reduce or eliminate use of toxic substances such as alcohol, cigarettes, marijuana, poppers, and nonprescription drugs. These substances affect judgment and tend to decrease the body's ability to fight off infection.

11. Maintain your body's immune system by eating well, exercising, and getting adequate rest. Sex should not be used as your only means of stress reduction. Learn other stress reduction techniques, such as self-hypnosis.

Symptoms of sexually transmitted disease are varied, but if you experience any of the following, you should see your local health care provider for evaluation.

1. Extreme fatigue
2. Fever and night sweats
3. Unexplained weight loss
4. Enlarged lymph glands
5. Unexplained discharge from penis or vagina
6. Sores on or around genitalia
7. Painful urination or chronic diarrhea
8. Heavy, dry cough, and/or shortness of breath
9. Unexplained bruising or purplish patches

These guidelines were adapted with permission from pamphlets by the Gay Men's Health Crisis, Inc., New York City and AID Atlanta, Georgia. Copyright.

NURSING INTERVENTION TOOLS

J1—NORMAL VARIATIONS AND MINOR ABNORMALITIES IN NEWBORN PHYSICAL CHARACTERISTICS

Variant	Cause	Course	Nursing anticipatory guidance
HEAD			
Cephalhematoma	Usually caused by trauma of birth.	Soft, fluctuant, well-outlined mass of blood trapped beneath the pericranium and confined to one bone. This is a subperiosteal hematoma with no extension across suture lines.	Observe for any changes in the size or shape of the hematoma. Reassure parents.
Caput succedaneum	Caused by head pressing on the pelvic outlet in the last period of labor.	Clear fluid trapped between the scalp and bone. It is ill-defined, pits on pressure, not fluctuant. Fluid usually disappears in 1 to 2 weeks.	Explain the cause to parents and reassure them it will disappear.
Facial asymmetry	Overriding of the cranial sutures at birth caused by intrauterine molding or molding from delivery. Bones are soft and pliable.	Flattening of part of head or face. Generally disappears a few days after birth.	If the occipital area is flat because of labor and delivery, reassure parents about its disappearance in a few days. If it is caused by the "same" positioning of the child in the crib, instruct the parents to alternate the positioning of the child in the crib daily.
Asymmetry of the scalp	Usually occurs from molding during delivery or the use of forceps during delivery. Also can be caused by positioning the infant repeatedly on the same side without rotating.	Flattening of part of head.	Same as facial asymmetry.
Craniotabes	Unknown.	Softening of localized areas in the cranial bone. Sometimes found in the parietal bones at the vertex near the sagittal suture. The areas are spongelike and can be indented by the pressure of a fingertip. They resume their shape when the pressure is removed.	Usually inconsequential, but if they persist, could be indicative of a pathological cause. There is no specific treatment. It is normal for these craniotabes to persist for months. They should eventually disappear.
Fontanelle	An irregular-shaped area enclosed by a membrane which occurs where the sutures of the bone of the skull meet. These areas are called anterior fontanelle, posterior fontanelle, and temporal fontanelles.	The anterior fontanelle should be open; the posterior fontanelle may be closed.	Explain to the parents that the open fontanelle helped to protect the baby's head during the birth process. The fontanelle allows the brain to grow and will continue to do so for the next 18 months. Reassure parents that fontanelle can be touched and scalp scrubbed without ill effect.

Continued.

Normal variations and minor abnormalities in newborn physical characteristics—cont'd

Variant	Cause	Course	Nursing anticipatory guidance
MOUTH			
Bednar's aphthae (ulcers)	Unknown. May be caused by vigorous sucking.	Usually located on hard palate posteriorly; generally bilateral	Reassure and support parents. Explain to the parents that there is no specific treatment, and condition will disappear without any treatment.
Epstein's epithelial pearls	Small epithelial cysts.	Located along both sides of the middle of the hard palate or along the alveolar ridge.	Reassure parents that cysts will disappear. There is no specific treatment.
Bohn's pearls (nodules)	Small white papules.	Located on each side of the midline of the hard palate. They disappear spontaneously in several weeks.	Reassure and support parents. Parents sometimes think that these lesions look like thrush. Reassure that these lesions are not thrush and will go away without treatment.
High palatal arch		Of no significance if there are no other findings present.	Reassure, support, and explain the lack of significance.
EYES			
Chemical conjunctivitis	Irritation from silver nitrate solution instilled after birth.	Eyes red with purulent exudate. Lids swollen. Onset occurs within first 24 hours and lasts about 2 to 4 days.	Cleanse eyelids with cotton balls soaked in warm saline solution. Wipe the eyes from the inner canthus out toward the outer canthus. Reassure parents that the infant's eyesight will not be affected.
Subconjunctival hemorrhage	Caused from pressure in the birth process.	Occurs at the limbus. It may be crescent shaped or may form a red halo around the iris. The hemorrhage resolves itself without any specific treatment in a few days.	Reassure parents that no residual defects occur from the hemorrhage. The blood will reabsorb itself in a few days.
Pseudostrabismus	Poor muscle coordination of the eye.	Movements of the newborn's eyes are poorly coordinated. The eyes do not necessarily move together. Very common and usually disappears spontaneously.	Reassure parents that this generally disappears spontaneously as the eye muscles strengthen and the infant's eyes continue to develop and grow.
SKIN			
Vernix caseosa	Cheeselike material that sticks to the skin. Protective covering for infant in utero.	Skin of newborn covered with varying amounts of this substance.	Will dry and disappear within a few days. Discourage mother from trying to vigorously rub it off. Encourage good skin care.
Lanugo	Fine downy type of hair.	Usually found on the back, shoulders, and ear lobes.	Usually disappears in time as a result of the friction of the skin rubbing on the bassinet linens. Reassure parents.
Desquamation	Skin in the newborn is very tender and soft. Following birth, the skin reacts to the changed environment by becoming very red. When the redness subsides, desquamation of the skin tends to occur.	Shedding, flaking, or peeling of the skin. Usually occurs during the first week of life. Can vary from extensive to so slight it almost goes unnoticed.	Reassure, support, and explain the cause to parents. Encourage good skin care, which avoids overuse of lotions, oils, and powders.
Ecchymosis	Blood under the skin caused by superficial trauma to the skin.	Bruise—disappears as the blood is reabsorbed.	Provide reassurance.

Normal variations and minor abnormalities in newborn physical characteristics—cont'd

Variant	Cause	Course	Nursing anticipatory guidance
SKIN—cont'd			
Acrocyanosis	Venous stasis.	Blue hands and feet.	No specific treatment. Make sure the baby is warm and that the cause of the acrocyanosis is not from being cold.
Erythema toxicum	Unknown.	A rash consisting of small, red, flat or raised lesions. Looks splotchy and sometimes resembles chicken pox or flea bites. Usually occurs during the first 2 weeks.	No specific treatment. Reassure, support, and explain.
Nevi, pigmented Nevus spilus (hairless mole)	Increased pigmentation.	Range from smooth, flat, hairless pigmented areas to those with hair; some can look like warts.	No treatment unless for cosmetic reasons. Provide reassurance.
Nevi, telangiectatic	Widening of surface capillaries.	Small red areas due to widening of surface capillaries; disappear momentarily with blanching of skin, but usually do not disappear completely.	Provide reassurance.
Capillary hemangiomata (sometimes called Balmar patches)	Capillary lesions of the skin.	Irregular blotchy pink spots at the nape of the neck, eyelids, globella, or lumbosacral areas. Gradually fade; usually disappear by 2 years.	Reassurance and support. No specific treatment.
Mongolian spots	Large aggregations of melanin–rich dark cells, which give the affected area a purple or blue/black color. Occur most frequently in black children but may occur in white children.	Generally found over the sacrum and coccygeal area of a large percentage of infants of black, Chicano, and Asiatic Indian origin. They do not have any significance and most disappear with time.	Explain cause and reassure parents. The spots usually disappear within the first year of life.
Mottling	Vasoconstriction—general circulatory instability.	Overall red and white coloration of the skin. Generally occurs in fair children who become chilled. Disappears when child becomes warm.	Explain causes and reassure parents; use a blanket to warm the infant.
Milia	Retained sebum in the skin.	Yellow-white, pinpoint-size lesions located on the bridge of the nose, the chin, or the cheeks. Disappear after first few weeks of life.	No specific treatment necessary. Explain to parents that lesions will disappear.
Café au lait	Variations in pigment.	Light to dark brown pigmented spots. One or two patches considered normal. If infant has several patches, may indicate fibromas or neurofibromatosis.	Assess nature of spots. If number of spots exceeds two, refer to physician or neurologist. Reassurance and support.
Accessory nipples (supernumerary nipples)	Not adequately explained (sometimes referred to as developmental cutaneous defect).	Occurs in a unilateral or bilateral distribution along the "mammary lines" from midaxilla to the inguinal area.	Reassure parents that the nipples may be excised for cosmetic reasons.
Harlequin coloring	Thought to be caused by poorly developed vasomotor reflexes.	Half of the infant's body appears red/white, the other half is pale. Transitory condition, which usually occurs when the infant cries forcefully.	Explain to parents that this is not significant. It is apparently harmless and the cause is not adequately explained.

Continued.

Normal variations and minor abnormalities in newborn physical characteristics—cont'd

Variant	Cause	Course	Nursing anticipatory guidance
SKIN—cont'd			
Cyanosis (localized)	Inadequate oxygenation of tissues; localized cyanosis because of immature peripheral circulation and venous stasis.	Usually involves lips, hand and feet or cyanosis of the presenting parts. Usually present at birth and for variable number or days afterwards.	Keep child warm, cyanosis will decrease as peripheral circulation improves. Reassure and support parents. Explain cause.
Cyanosis (general)	Numerous causes of general cyanosis, i.e., atelectasis, congenital heart disease, central nervous system damage, obstructed airway.	Depends on the cause.	Reassurance and support. Try to determine the relationship of cyanosis to crying, i.e., if cyanosis is relieved or improved when the child cries, then the cause may be atelectasis. Crying tends to make infants with cardiac malformations worse. Refer to physician.
ABDOMEN			
Umbilical cord variations	Natural process for sloughing tissues.	Blue/white at birth. Dull and yellow/brown within 24 hours, then black/brown and dry. Usually drops off at the end of the second week.	Keep cord area clean and dry. Reassure parents. Instruct parents in cord care.
Umbilical hernia	Occurs at the defect in the musculature of the abdominal wall near the umbilicus.	Skin-covered protuberance at the umbilicus. Very common in black infants and some Italian infants. Usually disappears spontaneously at the end of one year.	Reassure parents that it will probably disappear spontaneously. If it does not, it can be treated surgically when the child is older. Discourage home remedies (e.g., coin taped to hernia, binding, etc).
OTHER			
Vaginal discharge	Physiological manifestation of increased maternal hormonal influences.	Milky white discharge, sometimes blood tinged or whole blood. Usually disappears in 2 weeks.	Reassure mother that this is nothing to worry about. It occurs quite frequently and is considered normal. Explain that it will disappear in a few weeks.
Brachial palsy	Sometimes caused when lateral traction is exerted on the head and neck during delivery of the shoulder in a vertex presentation, or in a breech presentation when the arms are extended over the head, or when there is excessive traction on the shoulders.	Should be suspected when there is asymmetric response of the upper extremities during a Moro response. The asymmetric response occurs because there is paralysis of the muscles of the upper arm or paralysis of the entire arm. Prognosis depends on the extent of damage to the nerves.	Treatment usually consists of partial immobilization and appropriate positioning. Problem needs to be evaluated and the appropriate treatment initiated. Depending on the severity of damage, there could be complete return of function within a few months or there may be permanent damage. Teach parents the importance of carrying out the immobilization-positioning treatment on a daily basis. Reassure and support parents. Observe for any changes in the movement of the upper extremities.

Home allergy-proofing techniques

Potential antigen	Proofing actions
House dust (leading cause of respiratory allergy)	1. Restrict use of bedroom to sleeping. 2. Use shades instead of blinds or curtains. 3. Place washable plastic over mattresses. 4. Use no carpeting or wool scatter rugs. 5. Damp dust daily with child out of room. 6. Allow no stuffed animals or knickknacks. 7. Have minimum furniture; if stuffed, it should be foam rubber. 8. Either close off heat ducts or cover with cheesecloth. (Wash often.) 9. Keep doors and windows closed. 10. Avoid storing wool in closets or use of wool blankets.
Mold, mildew	1. Eliminate plants and aquariums from child's bedroom and play area; keep to minimum throughout home. 2. Avoid use of cellars as play or living area. 3. Clean bathroom and tile areas with antimold agent (Lysol) regularly. 4. Cleanse vaporizers or humidifiers frequently. 5. Use dehumidifier in humid or damp areas.
Danders, feathers	1. Use Dacron or foam rubber pillows and mattresses. 2. Get rid of pets or limit to outdoors. 3. Allow no stuffed animals or furniture and no clothing stuffed or insulated with feathers (down).
Contactants	1. Buy no wool clothing. 2. Wash all new clothing and linens before using. 3. Double-rinse infant's clothing and diapers. 4. Wash baby articles in mild soap. 5. Use mild soap to bathe baby and rinse well. 6. Avoid use of perfumed lotions, powders, oils.

From Tackett, J.J., and Hunsberger, M.: Family centered care of children and adolescents, Philadelphia, 1981, W.B. Saunders Co., p. 497.

PROCEDURE FOR AN ELIMINATION DIET

The procedure is as follows:
1. A diary of each food, beverage, or medication that is ingested at meals or between meals without alteration in customary patterns is to be recorded for 7 to 10 days.
2. Constituents of all home-prepared foods must be listed as well as ingredients of all packaged foods. Concealed foods may be included in prepared products.
3. Symptoms are also recorded for 7 to 10 days. By correlating symptoms with the information in the diary, the nurse frequently can determine the elimination diet suitable for the particular case; for example, milk-free, salicylate-free, or others.
4. The elimination diet is initiated.
5. Two weeks following the start of an elimination diet, the client is interviewed, and the diet is reviewed. Improvement can be expected within 2 to 3 weeks if the correct food has been eliminated.
6. Two weeks later another interview and review are conducted.
7. If symptoms have not subsided, the program is abandoned, and another diet regimen is implemented.
8. If the diet is successful in eliminating symptoms it should be continued for at least 2 months before attempting additions of new foods to the diet.
9. New foods can then be added individually every 5 to 7 days.
10. If symptoms return, the food should be discontinued.
11. If the second attempt at introducing the food is not successful, the food should be permanently excluded from the diet.
12. This procedure is repeated with other foods, each one taken individually, until a well-balanced and varied diet is provided for the client.
13. The diet diary should be continued for a few months, if possible, in the event of a recurrence of symptoms.
14. All labels, especially of prepared foods, must be read carefully.
15. Home-prepared foods are preferable because the ingredients can be controlled.
16. Absolute adherence to the diet is imperative. If undesirable weight loss occurs, more of the prescribed carbohydrates, sugar, fats, and oils must be taken. This may require eating four to five meals a day.
17. Caution should be taken not to place a child on a nutritionally deficient diet for long periods of time when no specific results have been obtained.

From Chow, M.P., et al.: Handbook of pediatric primary care, ed. 2, New York, 1984, John Wiley & Sons, Inc., pp. 988-990.

J3—INFANT STIMULATION

BIRTH TO 1 MONTH

Babies like to
  Suck
  Listen to repeated soft sounds
  Stare at movement and light
  Be *held* and *rocked*
Give your baby
  Your *talking* and *singing*
  Lamps throwing light patterns
  Your *arms*
  Rocking

1 MONTH

Babies like to
  Listen to your voice
  Look up and to the side
  Hold things placed in their hands
Give your baby
  A lullaby *record*
  A *mobile* overhead
  Pictures on the walls
  Your *face* near his
  A *change in scenery* and *position*

2 MONTHS

Babies like to
  Listen to musical sounds
  Focus, especially on their hands
  Reach and *bat* nearby objects
  Smile
Give your baby
  A *music box* or a soft *musical toy*
  A soft security *cuddle toy* tied to crib
  Your *smile*
  Play time with you

3 MONTHS

Babies like to
  Reach and *feel* with open hands
  Grasp crudely with two hands
  Wave their fists and *watch* them
Give your baby
  Musical records
  Rattles
  Dangling toys
  Textured toys

4 MONTHS

Babies like to
  Grasp things and *let go*
  Kick
  Laugh at unexpected sights and sounds
  Make *consonant sounds*
Give your baby
  Bells
  A *crib gym*
  More *dangling toys*
  Space to kick and move

5 MONTHS

Babies like to
  Shake, feel, and *bang* things
  Sit with support
  Play peek-a-boo
  Roll over
Give your baby
  A *high chair* with a rubber *suction toy*
  A *play pen*
  A *kicking toy*
  Toys that make noise

INFANT STIMULATION—cont'd

6 MONTHS

Babies like to
  Shake, bang and throw things down
  Gum objects
  Recognize familiar *faces*
Give your baby
  Many *household objects*
  Tin *cups, spoons,* and pot *lids*
  Wire *whisks*
  A *clutch ball* and *squeaky toys*
  A *teether* and *gumming toys*
  Bouncing, swinging seat

7 MONTHS

Babies like to
  Sit alone
  Use their *fingers* and *thumb*
  Notice *cause* and *effect*
  Bite on their *first tooth*
Give your baby
  Bath tub toys
  More *'things'*
  String
  More *squeaky toys*
  Finger foods

8 MONTHS

Babies like to
  Pivot on their stomachs
  Throw, wave, and *bang* toys together
  Look for toys they have
  Make *vowel sounds*
Give your baby
  Space to pivot and creep
  2 toys at once to *bang* together
  Big *soft blocks*
  A *Jack-in-the-box*
  Nested plastic *cups*
  Your *conversation*

9 MONTHS

Babies like to
  Pull themselves up
  Creep
  Place things generally where they're wanted
  Say "da-da"
  Play pat-a-cake
Give your baby
  A *safe corner* of the room to *explore*
  Toys tied to the *high chair*
  A metal *mirror*
  Jack-in-the-box

10 MONTHS

Babies like to
  Poke and *prod* with their forefingers
  Put things in other things
  Imitate sounds
Give your baby
  A big *pegboard*
  Some *cloth books*
  Motion toys
  Textured toys

11 MONTHS TO 1 YEAR

Babies like to
  Use their *fingers*
  Lower themselves from standing
  Drink from a cup
  Mark on paper
Give your baby
  Pyramid disks
  A large *crayon*
  A baking *tin* with *clothespins*
  Personal *drinking cup*
  More *picture books*

J4—FEEDING AND NUTRITION GUIDELINES FOR INFANTS AND CHILDREN

Infants

	0-2 wk	2 wk-2 mo	2 mo	3 mo	4-5 mo	5-6
DURING THE FIRST 6 MONTHS*						
Formula						
Per feeding	2-3 oz	3-5 oz	5 oz	6-6½ oz	7-8 oz	7-8 oz
Average total	22 oz	28 oz	30 oz	32-34 oz	32 oz	28 oz
Number of feedings	6-8	5-6	5-6	5	4-5	4-5
Food texture	Liquids	Liquids	Liquids	Liquids	Baby soft	Baby soft
Food additions						
Apple juice†						3-4 oz
Baby cereal, enriched					2-2½ tb. B and S	3 tb. B and S
Strained fruits					1½-3 tb. B, L, and S	2-3 tb. B, L, and S
Strained vegetables					1-2 tb. L	2-3 tb. L
Strained meats						1-2 tb. L
Egg yolk or baby egg yolk						½ med or 1 tb.
Teething biscuit						½-1
Total calories	440	560	600	660-680	729-788	791-870
Recommended calories 117 cal/kg	410	410-608	608	667	725-784	784-878
Oral and neuromuscular development related to food intake	Rooting, sucking, swallowing	Rooting, sucking, swallowing	Rooting, sucking, swallowing	Extrusion reflex diminishes; sucking becomes voluntary	Learning to put hands to mouth; develops grasp	Chewing begins; can approximate lips to rim of cup

From Scipien, G.M., et al.: Comprehensive Pediatric Nursing, ed. 2, New York, 1979, McGraw-Hill Book Co., p. 162. Used with permission.
*Calculations based on male growing at the 50th percentile for height and weight.
†Offer small amounts (2-4 oz) when milk is presented from the cup.
NOTE: B, breakfast; L, lunch; S, supper.

	6-7 mo	7-8 mo	8-9 mo	9-10 mo	10-11 mo	11-12 mo

FOR INFANTS 6 TO 12 MONTHS OF AGE

	6-7 mo	7-8 mo	8-9 mo	9-10 mo	10-11 mo	11-12 mo
Formula						
Per feeding	8 oz†	8 oz	8 oz	8 oz	8 oz	8 oz
Average total	28 oz	28 oz	24 oz	24 oz	24 oz	24 oz
Number of feedings	3-4	3-4	3	3	3	3
Food texture	Gradual increase ———————		——Mashed at table ———————			—— Cut fine
Food items						
Orange juice	4 oz	4 oz	4 oz	4 oz	4 oz	4 oz
Fortified cereal	⅓ cup, B	⅓ cup, B	½ cup, B	½ B	½ cup, B	½ cup, B
Fruit, canned or fresh	4 tsp. B, L, and S	4 tsp. B, L, and S	2 tb. L and S	2 tb. L and S	3 tb. L and S	3 tb. L and S
Vegetables	1½ tb. L and S	2 tb. L and S	2 tb. L and S	2 tb. L and S	3 tb. L and S	3 tb. L and S
Meat, fish, poultry	1 tb. L and S	2 tb. L and S	2 tb. L and S	2 tb. L and S	2½ tb. L and S	2½ tb. L and S
Egg yolk or baby egg yolk	1 med yolk, or 2 tb.	1 med yolk, or 2 tb.	1 med yolk, or 2 tb.	1 whole egg	1 whole egg	1 whole egg
Teething biscuit or bread	1 biscuit	1 biscuit	½ slice bread	½ slice bread	½ slice bread	½ slice bread
Starch—potato, rice, macaroni				2 tb, S	2 tb, S	2 tb, S
Dessert—custard, pudding						2 tb, S
Butter			1 tsp	1 tsp	1 tsp	1 tsp
Total calories	859	876	937	974	1037	1069
Recommended calories (108 kcal/kg)	810-864	864-918	918-972	972-1015	1015-1048	1048-1083
Oral and neuromuscular development related to food intake	Begins using cup ———————————————————————————— Sits erect with support ——————— Without support ——————— Feeds himself biscuit ————————			Holds bottle	Picks up small food items and releases	Holds and licks spoon after dipped into food; self-feeding

Older children and adolescents

Food group	Servings per day	Average size of servings					
		1 year	2-3 years	4-5 years	6-9 years	10-12 years	13-15 years
MILK AND CHEESE	4	½ cup	½-¾ cup	¾ cup	¾-1 cup	1 cup	1 cup
1.5 oz cheese = 1 cup milk (1 cup = 8 oz or 240 gm)							
MEAT GROUP (PROTEIN FOODS)	3 or more						
Egg		1	1	1	1	1	1 or more
Lean meat, fish, poultry (liver once a week)		2 tb	2 tb	4 tb	2-3 oz (4-6 tb)	3-4 oz	4 oz or more
Peanut butter			1 tb	2 tb	2-3 tb	3 tb	3 tb
FRUITS AND VEGETABLES	At least 4, including:						
Vitamin C source (citrus fruits, berries, tomato, cabbage, cantaloupe	1 or more (twice as much tomato as citrus)	⅓ cup citrus	½ cup	½ cup	1 medium orange	1 medium orange	1 medium orange
Vitamin A source (green or yellow fruits and vegetables)	1 or more	2 tb	3 tb	4 tb (¼ cup)	¼ cup	⅓ cup	½ cup
Other vegetables (potato and legumes, etc.) or	2	2 tb	3 tb	4 tb (¼ cup)	⅓ cup	½ cup	¾ cup
Other fruits (apple, banana, etc.)		¼ cup	⅓ cup	½ cup	1 medium	1 medium	1 medium
CEREALS (WHOLE-GRAIN OR ENRICHED)	At least 4						
Bread		½ slice	1 slice	1½ slices	1-2 slices	2 slices	2 slices
Ready-to-eat cereal		½ oz	¾ oz	1 oz	1 oz	1 oz	1 oz
Cooked cereal (including macaroni, spaghetti, rice, etc.)		¼ cup	⅓ cup	½ cup	½ cup	¾ cup	1 cup or more
FATS AND CARBOHYDRATES	To meet caloric needs						
Butter, margarine, mayonnaise, oils: 1 tb = 100 calories (kcal)		1 tb	1 tb	1 tb	2 tb	2 tb	2-4 tb
Desserts and sweets: 100-calorie portions as follows: ⅓ cup pudding or ice cream, 2 3-inch cookies, 1 oz cake, 1⅓ oz pie, 2 tb jelly, jam, honey, sugar		1 portion	1½ portions	1½ portions	3 portions	3 portions	3-6 portions

From Behrman, R.E., and Vaughan, V.C.: Nelson textbook of pediatrics, ed. 12, 1983, W.B. Saunders Co., p. 147.
*Based on food groups and the average size of servings at different age levels.

J5—COMMON CONCERNS AND PROBLEMS OF FIRST YEAR (NEONATE AND INFANT)

Problem or concern	Assessment	Nursing intervention
Burping	Swallowed air bubbles trapped in stomach; occurs more frequently in bottle-fed infants who cry during feeding.	Burp frequently during feeding (i.e., before, during, and after, or after every 1 ounce of formula or after every 4-5 minutes at breast. Use upright position to burp (gently rub infant's back while baby sits on parent's knee and rests forward against parent's arm). Try to burp every 10-15 minutes while awake if not successful burping during and after feeding. Sit upright in infant seat for 30-45 minutes after feeding if awake or position with head elevated and on right side if sleeping.
Colic	Unexplained bouts of crying frequently occurring at same time of day (usually busiest) and often accompanied by abdominal distention, spasms, drawing up legs to stomach and/or passing gas. May be caused by feeding problems, maternal anxiety, allergy, and is aggravated by tension in household. Can last 3 months. Also see Crying.	Review basic infant needs with parents (i.e., is infant hungry, wet, have air bubble, in uncomfortable position). Review feeding method, technique and burping, review maternal diet for offending foods if breastfed. Record time when colic episodes occur. Soothe and comfort before "attack." Swaddle infant, i.e., wrap warmly and in an encompassing manner. Walk, rock, and hold infant over shoulder. Try a monotonous soothing noise (music, ticking clock) or activity (ride in a car). Change infant position from stomach to side to back to sitting position. Rest infant on abdomen on warm hard surface (i.e., parent knee, warmed crib surface). Change household routine if indicated, create a quiet environment. Try pacifier or sugar water; if bottle fed, try soy formula. Reassure parents that infant is not ill, that they are providing good care, and that colic will definitely go away. Provide support to parents, giving opportunity to discuss feelings. Explain theories about origin and cycle of colic.
Crying	Periodic crying for unexplained reason; ascertain if a pattern exists for crying spells; may be related to colic; obtain a detailed history of time and length of spell; feeding frequency, method, technique and burping; stool patterns; meeting contact and sucking needs; parental handling of crying and feelings re: crying; other household factors, i.e., siblings, relative advice, parental support of each other, presence of other symptoms and/or allergies.	See previous section on colic. Reinforce that babies cry for a reason. Best to respond to cry versus letting baby cry it out. Crying is a release and/or exercise for infant. One or two periods a day of 5-10 minutes is normal for most infants. Assist parents to develop positive, relaxed approach. Reassure and support parents in this time of stress. Suggest parents alternate infant care and meeting infant demands.

Continued.

Common concerns and problems of first year (neonate and infant)—cont'd

Problem or concern	Assessment	Nursing intervention
Constipation	Consistency of stool which is hard, pebbly, rocklike. Not related to frequency, straining, grunting or number of days between stools. Ascertain color, consistency and frequency as well as presence of blood or mucus. Review infant diet and verify parent perception of constipation and expectation of normal stool patterns.	Discuss normal elimination/stool patterns for type of feeding method (i.e., breast fed stools versus bottle fed stools). Reassure that straining, grunting, infrequent number are normal. Reinforce that each infant has individual stool pattern and educate parents re: *what* constipation actually is (i.e., consistency). Discuss parents attitude regarding toilet habits and expectations about stool patterns. If constipated, increase liquids in diet; may offer water between meals. If introduced to solids too early or in too large a quantity, discontinue use until constipation clears, then begin again with smaller amounts. Karo syrup, 1 tsp/3 oz of water may be given several times a day. If appropriate for feeding stage, add prunes (up to 3 tb.) or prune juice to diet.
Flatus	Air in stomach or intestines causing abdominal distress, distension and discomfort, frequently expelled through anus. May be caused by excess swallowing of air, overfeeding, underfeeding, or allergy. Ascertain details re: feeding, i.e., frequency and size of nipple, type bottle used, breast feeding technique, maternal diet, use of pacifier, propping of bottle, burping, etc.	Burp frequently during and after feedings. See first section. Calm infant when crying and burp after crying. Place on left side to ease expelling of gas. If suspect allergies, try soy formula or elimination diet (Appendix J, p. 917). Reassure parents.
Hiccoughs	Sudden sharp involuntary spasms of diaphragm usually occur following a meal.	Reassure patient that infant will cry if truly distressed. Offer infant something to suck (pacifier, breast, bottle with warm water).
Pacifier	Infants demonstrate a need for non-nutritional sucking.	Assist parents to understand aspects of positive and negative use of pacifier. Positive use: indicated immediately after birth before newborn can manipulate thumb into mouth; assists in developing sucking function; contributes to establishment of breast feeding; good means of satisfying sucking need especially for bottle fed infants who need extra sucking time; does not usually become a habit unless child sucks beyond infancy; most infants substitute thumb for pacifier around 3 to 4 months. Parents should look for clues to eliminate pacifier use at this time and provide stimulation suitable for the age. Negative use: pacifiers do not replace holding; stimulation, or needs satisfaction; pacifiers should not be used constantly, especially before tending to infants needs; parents should be encouraged to discontinue use by 5 months since continued use may become a habit hard to overcome. If thumb is substituted, generally it is used less frequently than pacifier.

Common concerns and problems of first year (neonate and infant)—cont'd

Problem or concern	Assessment	Nursing intervention
Spoiling	Ascertain parent definition of spoiling. Generally it is the result of basic needs not being met in early infancy leading to a demanding, undisciplined child because need for gratification continues beyond normal time. Overgratification usually occurs then. Generally it is believed that infants cannot be spoiled under 6 months of age.	Parents require counseling and education that reinforces the following: Early infant needs must be gratified. A child cannot handle frustrations well until 8 to 9 months and is unable to delay gratification of needs until this age. A gradual and gentle approach to limits and delaying gratification is best. A relaxed, positive approach is helpful. Parents often find support groups helpful in dealing with this problem.
Biting	In first year, frequently related to teething. Particularly a problem for breast-feeding mothers. In toddlerhood related to normal aggressive impulses.	If related to teething, see later section on teething for alleviation of discomfort. Breast-feeding mothers should remove infant from breast at every occurrence and may accompany with a "no", should also allow time to lapse before finishing feeding. If related to impulsivity of toddlerhood, see first section of table on p. 936.
Separation anxiety	Occurs at 9-10 months as infant is learning to differentiate self from mother. Can occur again in toddlerhood as child is learning to distance and separate self from mother in attempt to establish autonomy.	Reassure mother that this is normal developmental process. Advise parents, especially mother, to do the following: Play "peek-a-boo" games. Allow sufficient time (30-45 minutes for child to acquaint him/herself with new person (i.e., visitor, babysitter). Avoid "sneaking out." Tell child firmly that "mommy leaves, mommy comes back." Reinforce this with "peek-a-boo" or "hide and seek" games. Avoid making major changes in child's or household routines during this period (i.e., mother returning to work; changing child's room, changing regular babysitter or day care situation, etc.).
Stranger anxiety	Begins at 6 to 8 months, gradually diminishing by 18 months. Process of child development.	See preceding section on separation anxiety. Advise parents, particularly mother to hold infant in presence of strangers. If infant is to be left, mother should spend a short time with stranger.
Infant sleep patterns	Some infants have difficulty releasing into sleep or awaken easily. Separation anxiety, teething, illness are among the common causes. Ascertain history of problem to include how long infant sleeps, what feeding schedule is, bedtime and household routines, presence of illness or teething, and how problem is handled.	Counseling should be directed toward education of parents; infants need gratification and normal sleep patterns, emphasizing the following: Differences in temperament and incidence of sleep problems can be related. Infants generally sleep through the night by 3 months. Infant may need help getting to sleep by rocking, holding, pacifier, walking, etc. Environment and atmosphere conducive to sleep, e.g., quiet, dim, should be provided. If sleep problem is related to a physical problem, measures to remedy should be implemented.

Continued.

Common concerns and problems of first year (neonate and infant)—cont'd

Problem or concern	Assessment	Nursing intervention
Teething	Eruption of primary or deciduous teeth starting at about 6 months usually with lower incisors. Will continue every 2 months for first 2 years. Signs may include, but are not always present: red, swollen gums, irritable, crying and rubbing gums. Since other events in infant development are occurring simultaneously, nursing must assist parents to distinguish between these and teething as follows: Drooling, which normally occurs at 3 to 4 months and has little to do with teething, although it may persist throughout teething. Fevers do not usually accompany teething. Must be assessed separately because maternal antibody protection is diminishing and presence of fever is suspect for infectious process. Separation anxiety, sleep disturbances, or fussiness from other causes are all common developmental symptoms associated with infant age group, as is reaching for and mouthing objects.	Recommend to parents hard, clean objects for baby to chew on such as rubber teething rings, or beads, hard rubber toys, cool spoon, teething biscuits or pretzels, etc. Parents should avoid use of teething toys or rings filled with liquid because plastic covers are easily broken and liquid can be ingested.
Diaper rashes	Rashes of varying types occurring in diaper area. Persistent rashes which do not respond to home management or continue to occur in spite of preventive measures should be referred for medical evaluation.	Preventive measures to keep area clean, dry, and aerated: Frequent diaper changing. Cleansing with water (and mild soap after bowel movement) at each changing, dry area well. Thick diapers and/or absorbent pads are recommended; plastic or rubber pants are not suggested. A *thin* film of lubrication or powder may be used, such as A and D ointment, petroleum jelly, or Caldesene powder. Remove diapers for short periods every day. Wash diapers well as follows: 1. Soak soiled diapers in Borateen or borax solution (½ cup to 1 gallon of water). 2. Prerinse before washing. 3. Wash in full cycle with mild soap such as Ivory, Dreft, or Lux. 4. Avoid softeners and strong detergents. 5. Rinse diapers 2 to 3 times, and may be added ¼ to ½ cup vinegar to final rinse. 6. Dry in sun if possible. Home management of diaper rash: Follow preventive measures with emphasis on leaving diaper off more frequently, changing when wet, and cleaning area thoroughly during changes. Zinc oxide ointment often is helpful in checking early nonfungal rashes. Cornstarch is never recommended for rashes or their prevention. Seek medical help if rash worsens or does not improve.

Common concerns and problems of first year (neonate and infant)—cont'd

Problem or concern	Assessment	Nursing intervention

Cradle cap	Form of seborrheic dermatitis in neonate characterized by scalping, flaking of scalp skin especially over anterior fontanelle. May persist beyond neonate into infancy period.	Preventive measures:
		  Teach parents how to shampoo infant head and recommend shampooing every other day.
		  Reassure that vigorous scrubbing will not injure fontanelle or skull.
		Home management for mild cases:
		  Shampoo head daily with warm water and soap, using firm pressure on scalp.
		  Loosen cap by applying mineral or baby oil to scalp 15 to 20 minutes before shampooing. Remove with shampoo.
		  Comb scalp with fine comb to loosen and dislodge scaly cap.
		  Severe cases will require medical attention and are generally managed with antiseborrheic shampoos.

PROBLEMS RELATED TO FEEDING Parental concerns about overfeeding or underfeeding	Some parents find it difficult to determine appropriate amount of milk and/or solid food to give infant. Ascertain parent understanding, knowledge, and perceptions through the following: Diet history Height and weight measurement and charting on growth curve. Elimination habits and description.	Assist parents to construct a workable feeding schedule. Discuss normal feeding pattern for breast and bottle fed infants (see this chapter). Discuss infant need for nonnutrient sucking. Convey that infants will eat more than they need or require if food is offered at each cry. Offer water between feedings to postpone next feeding to reasonable time. Suggest schedule of solid food introduction (Appendix J, p. 921). Reassure parents that if infant is gaining weight he is not underfed. Explain growth and appetite spurts.

Refusal of solids	Infant may refuse new foods for a number of reasons, e.g., temperature, texture, manner presented by person feeding, or too early introduction. Ascertain through diet history which foods accepted, and likes and dislikes and parental feelings and perception regarding solid foods.	Discuss normal feeding patterns for age.
		Review indications for starting or not starting solid foods;
		  No need before 4 to 6 months.
		  Digestion begins with salivation around 4 months.
		  Feeding of solid foods is not necessarily related to sleeping through the night.
		  Tongue thrusting of solid food is normal and not a refusal.
		Discuss ways to encourage solid food acceptance:
		  Allow infant to feed self.
		  Avoid forcing infant to eat since this will only increase resistance.
		  Solids may be stopped for a while, offering only ones that infant likes.
		  Offer solid foods before milk when infant is hungriest.
		  Offer food in calm positive manner.

Refusal of food and variations in appetite	Once solid foods have been introduced and established, infants and especially toddlers will go through periods of refusal, pickiness, and preference. Obtain diet history as reviewed in preceding section (Refusal of solids).	See preceding section (Refusal of solids).
		Discuss following with parents:
		  Refusal may be due to loss of interest in food when more active or due to form of negativism and means to control.
		  Avoid use of food as substitute for attention or stimulation.

Continued.

Common concerns and problems of first year (neonate and infant)—cont'd

Problem or concern	Assessment	Nursing intervention

		Some degree of refusal and variation in appetite is normal for age.
		Try following approaches:
		  Offer small amounts of food frequently.
		  Emphasize favorite foods as much as possible.
		  Use as few nonnutritive foods as possible.
		  Allow child to feed self if child desires to and provide finger foods.
		  Be patient as child tries to master use of utensils.
		  Eating should be an enjoyable and sociable time. If hunger does not permit infant to wait until family dinner time, feed before and offer nibbles during family meal.
		  Give older infant and toddler place, chair, utensils, plate at the table.

Spitting up	Regurgitation commonly following a feeding. Usually related to air swallowed with food, inability to relax esophageal sphincter, possible overfeeding, or allergy to milk. Ascertain nature of regurgitation (frequency, amount, color, consistency, etc.) as well as diet history and data regarding weight gain. Frequently outgrown by time infant is sitting well in upright position.	Reinforce the following with parents:
		  Correct preparation of formula.
		  Use of appropriate size nipple and nipple hole.
		  Regular and frequent burping is needed.
		  Place infant in an upright position for 30 minutes after feeding.
		  Correct position of infant during feeding.
		Determine need to change method of feeding or formula.

Weaning	A transition of feeding methods. May be from bottle to cup or from breast to bottle and/or cup.
	Weaning from breast is difficult if parents (especially mother) have ambivalent feelings or if infant refuses alternative methods. Ascertain who wants baby weaned and why as well as schedule of feedings.
	Weaning from bottle should be attempted gradually, when child is ready, usually around 1 year. Ascertain who wants child weaned, what has been tried, feeding schedule and number of bottles, and ability to use cup.
		Assist parents to make decision to wean:
		  Should be discussed and decided by both parents.
		  If breast feeding, it is helpful to mother to assess every 3 months whether or not to continue nursing.
		  Positive attitude toward weaning is essential, especially for breast-feeding mothers.
		  Weaning at times of separation anxiety is not advised, especially in breast-fed infants.
		  If possible, an infant should be weaned from breast to cup. This avoids having to wean from bottle later on.
		Active weaning for breast feeding mothers:
		  Start by substituting bottle or cup for breast at one feeding and allow 5-6 days before substituting second breast feeding.
		  If resistance is encountered try giving water or juice in bottle or cup before weaning starts, using nipple similar to breast or pacifier if one is used, heating milk before offering, and having someone other than mother offer bottle or cup. Keep to a schedule and be firm, positive, and patient.
		Active weaning to cup: continue preceding steps with following additions:
		  Reinforce idea of accomplishment in using a cup to child.
		  May give one bottle a day but should contain only water to avoid incidence of dental caries.
		  Avoid forcing child to wean; forcing use of cup may increase need to suck.
		Calm, relaxed, positive approach is essential.

J6—ACCIDENT PREVENTION

Age	Development	Major accidents	Anticipatory guidance
Neonate to 1 month	Is unable to protect self; when on abdomen can lift and turn head; dependent, requires protection; little control over body and movements	Motor vehicles	Use approved car seat Do not hold infant in lap Never leave infant in car unattended For long trips, firmly secure car bed with seat belts in back seat
		Strangulation	Spacing between crib bars should be no more than 2⅜ inches apart Avoid tying anything, including pacifiers, around neck Fasten mobiles securely
		Suffocation and injuries	Crib mattress should fit firmly to sides Do not use pillows; use bumper pads Support infant's head when lifting, holding, or bathing
		Burns including sunburn	Avoid bathing near hot water faucets Test water temperature before bath Avoid handling hot liquids and do not smoke while handling infant Keep out of direct sunlight and use sun screen Use flame-resistant clothing and furniture
2-3 months	Begins gross motor movements of wiggling, squirming, thrashing, rolling	Falls	Never leave infant unattended (at any age) for any reason Keep one hand on infant while giving care Keep crib sides up Use infant seat on floor or playpen
4-5 months	Mouths objects; brings hands to mouth	Aspiration and choking	Do not prop bottles (at any age) Burp well before putting infant in crib and place on stomach with head to side or propped on side Toys should be too large for infant to swallow, nonbreakable, and free of sharp edges, strings, and detachable parts Keep diaper pins closed during changing Keep small objects (e.g., buttons, coins) out of reach Use only pacifiers with a large shield
		Suffocation	Keep all plastic bags out of reach Keep stuffed animals out of crib
		Lead poisoning	Check toys and other objects for lead-free paint
6-7 months	Sits without support; has a firm grasp; rolls and creeps	Falls and falling objects	Use safety strap in stroller or high chair Use sturdy high chair or feeding table Keep doors to stairs and outside locked; use safety gates. Avoid use of hanging table-cloths Remove knickknacks and breakables
		Ingestion	Keep small objects, medicine, and plants out of reach Keep ipecac on hand and understand use Have poison control number posted Lock up medicine, cleaning agents, insecticides, etc. Keep trashcans out of reach or use locklids
		Injuries and electric shock	Cover wall outlets Place furniture so cords are inaccessible Check furniture for sharp corners—remove or pad Inspect toys for breakage Keep sharp objects out of reach

Continued.

Accident prevention—cont'd

Age	Development	Major accidents	Anticipatory guidance
8-12 months	Pulls to stand; crawls, grabs; beginning to walk; enjoys exploring	Burns	Crawl around on floor and investigate what child could reach or get into
			Keep all hot food and drinks away from table edge; turn pot handles inward on stove
			Keep matches and lighters out of reach
			Keep kitchen closed up or gated
			Never leave child unattended near fireplace or stove
			Place guards around open hearths, registers, stoves, and fans
			Do not iron when child is crawling nearby
		Choking	Do not give child small hard foods, such as peanuts, raw vegetables, popcorn
			Inspect toys for broken parts
			Keep floors, counters, tables free of small objects
		Motor vehicle accidents	Continue use of car seat
			Keep doors locked
		Poisoning	See previous discussion
1-2 years	Walks up and down stairs; stoops and recovers; climbs; likes to take things apart	Falls and injuries	Supervise children in most activities, especially up and down stairs, out of doors, and at playgrounds
			Lock all windows; when opening, do so from top only
			Remove any objects or furniture in front of window that child could use as a ladder
			Permit climbing within child's capabilities
			Remove bumper pads or toys in crib which child could use to climb on
			Check toys, especially riding ones, for damage
			Keep small, pointed, or sharp objects out of reach
			Keep out of way of swings
		Burns	Teach child meaning of *hot*
			Avoid use of flowing clothing
		Drowning	Continue to supervise bath
			Supervise all water sport activity (e.g., swimming, boating); use floats and/or life jackets
			Teach child to respect water and seek swimming lessons
		Automobile-related accidents	Continue to use appropriate car seat
			Keep doors and windows locked
			Do not permit child to hang out of windows
			Hold onto child when crossing street or in parking lots
			Do not permit child to ride toys near street
		Poisoning and ingestion	Have ipecac in any household child frequents (babysitter, grandparents)
			Use childproof caps on medications
			Do not regard medicine as candy
			Do not give one child another's prescription

Accident prevention—cont'd

Age	Development	Major accidents	Anticipatory guidance
2-4 years	More adventuresome and curious; explores body orifices; more independent, with limited cognition; imitates	Falls and injuries	Teach child to be cautious around strange animals
			Supervise play at playground
			Keep out of reach small objects and foods (peanuts, beans) that can be inserted into orifices; check buttons on clothes and toys
			Discontinue use of crib when height of crib rail is ¾ of toddler's height
			Keep stairs well lighted and free of clutter
			Give toys a safety check
			Discourage running in house and limit outdoor running to safe places
			Teach child to respect street and cars
			Teach child to stay away from and out of old appliances
		Drowning	Continue to teach water safety
			Supervise all water activities
			Continue with swimming lessons
		Automobile-related accidents	See previous discussion
	Play increases to include rougher games and bike riding	Burns	Teach child what to do if fire breaks out; hold household drills
	Cognition improving and can identify good and bad		Teach child to roll and smother clothes if they catch on fire
		Drowning	Continue swimming lessons
			Use floats or lifejacket if child cannot swim
			Swim only where supervision is available (parent or lifeguard)
		Automobile-related accidents	Teach pedestrian safety, providing example for child
			Do not permit playing in street
			Use adult seat belt, if child is over 40 pounds
			If over 55 inches tall, use shoulder restraints
		Falls, injuries	Make periodic checks on playground or play area used frequently
			Check on child when out playing
			Instruct child in safe use of toys; keep in good condition
			Keep away from driveways and streets
			If possible, provide fenced-in play area
			Set a good example by using seat belt, looking before crossing street, etc.
		Burns	Teach child about danger of matches, lighters, stove
			Recheck radiators, space heaters, fireplaces, and protective guards
		Poisoning and ingestions	Do not become lax about keeping medication, etc., locked up
			Teach child to respect harmful objects and use a symbol to indicate "danger or harmful" to child
			Routinely check house, basement, and garage for harmful substances within reach
4-6 years	Continues to be curious, daring, and imitative; frequently plays out of sight		Involve child in safety discussions
			Continue previously described activities when using household tools and equipment

Continued.

Age	Development	Major accidents	Anticipatory guidance

School age	Increased motor coordination and cognitive ability; increased peer and group activity and involvement in sports; assumes more responsibility for self and well-being.	Motor vehicle and bicycle accidents	Involve child in safety discussion and planning
			Assign safety responsibilities, such as checking bike
			Teach child not to ride with strangers
			Teach child how to contact police and fire department and physician
			Be certain child knows address and phone number
			Discuss bicycle and pedestrian safety
			Discuss bicycle riding rules:
			    Do not hitch ride on moving vehicles
			    Do not ride on dark street
			    Use headlight or reflector light at night; wear bright clothes
			    Do not dart from behind parked cars
			    Do not carry passengers on bicycle
			    Keep bike in good repair
			Do not use street as a playground
			Use seat belts

		Injuries	Teach child to participate in sports safely using appropriate gear Permit only supervised sport activities Teach child proper use of household gadgets and equipment; supervise as necessary

		Drowning	Teach the following swimming rules:
			    Swim only where a lifeguard
			    Use buddy system
			    Know water depth before diving
			    Wear life jacket while boating or skiing or if nonswimmer
			    No horseplay or call for help jokingly

		Falls	See bicycle rules
			Discuss climbing trees:
			    Avoid slippery shoes
			    Avoid weak or dead branches
			    Keep a secure handhold

		Burns	Continue household drills Camp with supervision Teach proper campfire and barbecue care Use safe camping gear, including flame-retardant clothes
Adolescence	Seeking identity and establishment of independence; subject to strong peer pressure; rejects unsought advice; has a need for physical activity; spends most of free time away from home	Drowning	Most important to have cooperation of adolescent when discussing and implementing safety measures See previous sections Never too late to learn to swim Enroll in lifesaving classes
		Firearms accidents	Avoid having loaded guns in household Learn safety handling if involved in sport hunting Keep guns in locked closet and ammunition in separate locked area Never assume gun is not loaded Never point gun at another
		Automobile–related accidents	Take drivers education Use seat belts for self and passengers Practice pedestrian safety Do not drive under influence of drugs or alcohol Do not hitchhike or pick up hitchhikers
		Alcohol, drugs, and tobacco	Discuss effects of substance use and abuse Assist teen to identify other ways to achieve self-esteem, independence, and peer acceptance

J7—INFECTIOUS DISEASES

Disease	Presentation	Management
VIRAL INFECTIONS		
Hepatitis	See Chapters 17 and 22	Home care and supportive treatment, including rest and well-balanced diet with sufficient calories and vitamin B complex supplements Isolation: enteric precautions Prophylaxis: Gamma globulin or hepatitis B immune globulin
Herpes simplex	Seen as gingivostomatitis in young children with reinfections being localized as "cold sores" or "fever blisters"; abrupt onset with fever, irritability, anorexia, and sore mouth; red swollen gums with small vesicles appearing on palate, tongue, and mucosa	Supportive treatment, particularly mouth care of petroleum jelly for cracking and mouth washes, rinses, and analgesics for pain; secretion precautions should be observed Diet: soft, bland foods; cool liquids—avoidance of citrus juices General measures as for influenza
Herpes zoster (shingles)	Uncommon under age 10; characterized by pain and crops of vesicles confined to an area of distribution of one of spinal or cranial sensory nerves; malaise and fever may accompany vesicles	Symptomatic treatment of wet compresses, calamine lotion (for lesions), and aspirin (for pain)

Influenza	Rapid onset of chills, fever, headache, generalized aches and malaise, anorexia, and prostration; frequently young children experience vomiting and diarrhea; hacking cough and rhinitis frequently develop	Symptomatic treatment including these general measures:
		A. Fever
		  1. Antipyretic medication
		  2. Tepid sponge bath
		  3. Liberal fluid intake
		  4. Rest and limited activity
		B. Upper respiratory infections
		  1. Liberal fluid intake
		  2. Cool mist vaporizer
		  3. Decongestants
		  4. Warm gargle, saline mouth/throat irrigations
		  5. Cool liquids and soft foods for throat and mouth irritations
		  6. Petroleum jelly to protect nares and lips
		C. Aches and malaise
		  1. Rest and limited activity
		  2. Warm bath
		  3. Body massage
		  4. Cold compresses for headache
		  5. Analgesics
		D. Anorexia
		  1. Small, frequent feedings of favorite foods and liquids
		  2. Relaxed approach to oral intake
		E. Rash
		  1. Proper hygiene and bathing
		  2. Cool baths, calamine lotion, mild anesthetic ointment, or systemic antihistamines
		  3. Short, clean fingernails; gloves or mittens for young children
		  4. Saline mouthwashes if mucous membranes are involved

Continued.

Infectious diseases—cont'd

Disease	Presentation	Management
Measles (rubeola)	Malaise, fever, conjunctivitis, cough 3-4 days before appearance of red-brown or purple-red macropapular rash, first on face, hairline, and neck, proceeding to trunk and extremities; Koplek's spots appear about 12 hours before rash on buccal mucosa; rash lasts 5-7 days	General measures as for influenza; emphasis on avoiding bright lights if photophobic and using warm water to cleanse eyes Respiratory and discharge precautions Prevention: active immunization
Mononucleosis (infectious)	Mild symptoms of headache, malaise, and fatigue; fever and sore throat, tonsils enlarged, red and covered with membrane; lymph adenopathy and splenomegaly are common	General measures as for influenza; emphasis on bed rest with gradual increase in activity; no strenuous activity while spleen is enlarged; no social contact until acute phase is over
Mumps (parotitis)	Prodrome of fever, headache, anorexia, malaise, and muscle pain. Local pain around ear and jaw within 24-48 hours, followed by swelling of parotid gland.	General measures as for influenza; emphasis on avoidance of citrus foods and fluids; alleviation of pain with aspirin and warm or cold compresses; respiratory precautions. Prevention: active immunization
Roseola (exanthem subitum)	High fever and irritability for 3-4 days followed by rose-pink, maculopapular rash, beginning on chest and spreading to trunk and face; rash lasts several hours to 2 days; fever falls to normal as rash appears	General measures as for influenza; support for parents as fever may not respond or subside for 3-5 days
Rubella (german measles)	No prodrome. Pink-red maculopapular rash first on face, progressing to neck, trunk, extremities; lasts 3-5 days	General measures as for influenza; exposure of first-trimester pregnant women to be avoided. Prevention: active immunization
Varicella (chickenpox)	May have 1-2 days of fever and malaise followed by macular rash that evolves to papular to vesicles to crusts; rash appears on trunk and in crops and may progress to hairline and face; all lesions eventually dry and crust	General measures as for influenza; emphasis on skin care, alleviation of itching by cornstarch baths, systemic antipruritic medication (Benadryl) and topical lotions (calamine); general skin hygiene of bathing, changing bed linen and clothes frequently, keeping nails short and clean; isolate until vesicles dried and observe respiratory and secretion precautions
BACTERIAL INFECTIONS		
Cellulitis	Affected area is warm, tender, erythematous, swollen and indurated; fever, malaise, and lymphadenopathy are present; caused by staphylococcus aureus, group A beta-hemolytic streptococci, or hemophilus influenza	Employ general measures as described under influenza; systemic antibiotic therapy; warm compresses and immobilization of affected part

Infectious diseases—cont'd

Disease	Presentation	Management
Meningitis	Varies with age and causative organism *Neonates.* *Escherichia coli* and group B streptococci common causative agents; onset is insidious; poor tone, sucking feeding difficulties, poor cry, vomiting, irritability, drowsy or irritable, jittery; tense, full, bulging fontanelle *Infants.* Most common causative agents: hemophelus influenza, neisseria meningitides. Unexplained febrile illness preceded by respiratory or gastrointestinal infection; accompanied by irritability, fever, anorexia, vomiting, drowsiness, and high pitch cry; fontanelle may be bulging, nuchal rigidity signs may be difficult to elicit *Older children.* Causative agent as for infants; fever, chills, vomiting, severe headache, stiff neck; nuchal rigidity and positive Kernig's and Brudzinski's signs *Meningococcemia.* A medical emergency with rapidly developing petechial and purpuric rash, preceded by 24-hour period of fever, vomiting, irritability, and nuchal rigidity	Requires medical referral and antibiotic therapy that will be determined by weight of child and depends on causative agent Parent counseling regarding diagnosis and disease process is indicated as well as convalescent care and follow-up care
Scarlet fever (scarlatini)	Abrupt onset of fever, sore throat, vomiting, headache, and chills followed by bright red rash that blanches on pressure; rash has rough sandpaper texture and appears first on flexor surfaces, rapidly becoming more generalized; lasts 7 days, followed by desquamation of hands and feet.	General measures as for influenza; Penicillin is antibiotic of choice, unless allergy is present and erythromycin is indicated; prepare parents for skin desquamation; Follow-up care and throat culture is advisable as well as examination for signs of rheumatic fever and glomerulonephritis; advisable to obtain throat cultures on household contacts
Tuberculosis	Causative agents are *Mycobacterium tuberculosis* and *M. bovis;* most common portal of entry is lung where disease begins; bacilli multiply in lung parenchyma and create area of inflammatory exudate, possibly experienced as low-grade fever and productive cough; bacilli are also carried through lymphatic system to regional lymph nodes creating lymphadenopathy; hypersensitivity occurs when bacilli multiply and die as tissue reacton to bacilli changes; primary lesion becomes encapsulated and walled off; may resolve or calcify as evidenced by x-ray findings and positive tuberculin reaction	Active tuberculosis: antimicrobial therapy and general supportive measures Prevention: if positive skin test and no clinical demonstrated disease, prophylactic treatment with INH is recommended if Child is under 4 years Child has recently converted from negative to positive skin reaction Child with positive skin test has known exposure to active TB Child with inactive primary TB has never been treated All contacts with person with active tuberculosis should be skin tested, positive reactions treated and negative skin tests retested in 6 weeks and at least every 3 months for duration of contact; infants should be removed from contact with infected person until at least 6 months after all cultures are reported as negative Prevention: tuberculin testing

J8—COMMON CONCERNS AND PROBLEMS OF TODDLER AND PRESCHOOL YEARS

Problem and assessment	Nursing intervention

AGGRESSIVE AND NEGATIVE BEHAVIORS
Biting and hitting

Temporary behaviors occurring as a result of normal aggressive impulses and most frequently happening in new or difficult situations, when tired or hungry or frustrated or when expectations are too high in terms of social behaviors (ability to play with peers); used as a means of asserting control or power

Reassure parents that behaviors are normal; discuss development and tasks child is trying to accomplish
Advise parents to
  Avoid retaliation by hitting or biting back
  Cup chin or hold hand giving reminder that biting and/or hitting is unacceptable
  Anticipate circumstances in which behaviors occur and circumvent them
  Use limits such as isolation if helpful
  Limit playmates and playtime to what is reasonable for child and his age
  Allow child and playmate to work out difficulties as much as possible, redirecting their play when necessary

VERBAL NEGATIVISM

Use of the word "no" as means of control in striving for independence; often used indiscriminately and inappropriately

Advise parents to
  Offer child a choice when possible, making alternatives simple
  Avoid bargaining and arguments
  If no choice is available, do not offer one—approach with a matter-of-fact attitude
  Develop strategy for times when child will choose and then change his mind

Temper tantrums

Developmental behavior directed at gaining control; Frequently triggered by unmet needs (tired, hungry), frustration and/or overgratification and need for limits; ascertain when tantrums occur and how they are handled

Management by parents should be directed at finding cause and prevention; counseling is directed toward approaches to discipline and limit setting (see section on discipline) and the following:
  Discussion of child's needs for limits at this age
  Diary can be kept to identify pattern when tantrums occur
  Intervention is made before tantrum begins
Should tantrum occur, possible approaches include the following:
  Calm, matter-of-fact approach by parents
  Isolation of child by removal to neutral room until control is achieved
  Hold and comfort child until control is achieved, possibly offering substitute for desired object or activity that triggered tantrum
  Use of corporal punishment (spanking) to achieve control

Common concerns and problems of toddler and preschool years—cont'd

Problem and assessment	Nursing intervention

Discipline
 	
Discipline is guidance offered by parents to assist child in demonstrating correct, acceptable safe behaviors; discipline is based on the parent's concepts, feelings, and attitudes regarding desirable behaviors and rules of conduct for them; mechanisms of discipline will set limits and control undesirable behaviors
	Advise parents regarding different approaches to discipline:
	    Permissiveness
	    Overpermissiveness
	    Authoritarianism
	Advise parents that setting limits should permit self-respect and protection of parent and child integrity; parents should be aware that discipline is essential to healthy growth
	Parent techniques include the following:
	    Set examples of desirable behaviors (honesty, unselfishness, good manners)
	    Be fair, clear, and consistent
	    Agree on methods of discipline
	    Give simple clear directions; bend a little by giving warnings
	    Allow child to express feelings
	    Respect your child; be sure to praise, show approval, and encourage
	    Be realistic in behaviors expected
	    Avoid arguing, threatening, promising, sermonizing, overpermissiveness, and an overauthoritarian manner
	    Discipline (punishing the act)

PUNISHMENT
 	
A method of controlling behaviors when limits are exceeded and based on child being made to feel guilty for misdeed; guilt will eventually inhibit impulse to commit act; punishment may be verbal, restrictive, or physical and should always be appropriate to the act; most punishment is the result of parent loss of temper
	Advise parents to
	    Allow a cooling-off period
	    Direct anger at situation or act, not child
	    Avoid retaliation by hitting, belittling, sarcasm, ridicule, humiliation, or shame
	    Avoid sending to bed or going without food
	    Avoid depriving child of love to examine their feelings and experiences regarding punishment. Remind them that it can be an effective method of discipline with appropriate motivation and intent
	Review points discussed in discipline section

BREATHHOLDING
 	
A high indicator of a disturbed parent-child relationship, this symptom may be caused by overprotection, a tense rigid daily schedule, or prematurely enforced toilet training regime; it has a high familial incidence and is characterized by a preceding temper tantrum, with child holding breath and turning blue
Ascertain circumstances that trigger episodes and how handled by parents
	Counseling directed toward guidance and education regarding parent-child relationship; parents will need reassurance and support as they attempt to
	    Ignore breathholding in an attempt to prevent child satisfaction in gaining control
	    Redirect relationship with child emphasizing meeting of his needs in a positive way, reinforcing desirable behaviors
	See section on discipline

ROCKING, HEAD BANGING, BED SHAKING
 	
Forms of self-stimulation as a result of undergratification; frequently occurs at bedtime; ascertain how child's needs are met
	Counseling directed toward advising parents regarding
	    Gratification of needs
	    Avoidance of letting child "cry it out"
	    Provision of comfort and extra stimulation time
	    Provision of relaxed, calm atmosphere through holding, singing, music

Continued.

Common concerns and problems of toddler and preschool years—cont'd

Problem and assessment	Nursing intervention
MASTURBATION A normal reaction, which is an exploration of body that results in stimulation of pleasurable sexual feelings; generally occurs at bedtime and starts accidentally becoming more purposeful and frequent around 4 years Ascertain frequency, how parents handle, and their attitude and feelings	Advise parents that masturbation is normal and that censoring of open masturbation is appropriate; otherwise parents should convey to child that they are aware of and understand the behavior Avoidance of placing excessive importance on masturbation which may only encourage it; it is best to ignore it and/or set limits as appropriate to situation A punitive attitude should be avoided
PERSISTENT THUMB SUCKING A form of self-comfort occurring in times of stress and persisting beyond 3 to 4 years; generally sporadic sucking is harmless and regular sucking until 2 or 3 is considered normal	Assist parents to identify source of stress and ways to alleviate it. Reassure and support parents when thumb sucking is within normal range Suggest parents remove fingers or thumb from mouth after asleep Suggest parents avoid constant nagging and reminding; pulling thumb from mouth; use of restraints, foul-tasting medications, or bandages
FEEDING-RELATED PROBLEMS Loss of variations of appetite; refusal of food Common problems related to: "too busy to eat," development of food preferences; a normal decrease in amount of food required and/or an attempt to control and assert independence	See Chapter 22 for anticipatory guidance and Appendix J5, pp. 927-928
SLEEP-RELATED PROBLEMS Nightmares Problems may follow a tiring busy day, be associated with illness, or be the result of working things out in dreams Nightmares are frightening dreams that awaken child who feels fear and helplessness; they generally occur as a result of increased aggressive urges	Review normal sleep patterns with parents (see Chapter 23) Reassure parents that dreams and terrors are normal and tend to disappear spontaneously Parents should comfort child when awakened by dream—may attempt to explain they are not "real" Parents should avoid making a fuss over these sleep problems
Night terrors These are dreams, generally frightening in nature, from which a child does not awaken; after acting out dream and/or a period of disorientation, child returns to sleep	

TOILET TRAINING
 	
Achievement of control over bodily elimination; development of habits that make child self-sufficient in toileting; parents need to understand child's development and readiness before instituting a toilet training regime (see following); parent must ascertain attitude and expectations regarding toilet training as well as measures previously used
	Direct counseling toward parental understanding of realistic expectations, readiness of child, types of toilet training and frequent problems encountered
	Types of toilet training:
	A. Early training from ages 10 months to 15 months; Points to emphasize:
	  1. Child is not physiologically able to use toilet at this age
	  2. Parents may be ready to train child, but they will be the

Common concerns and problems of toddler and preschool years—cont'd

Problem and assessment	Nursing intervention

TOILET TRAINING—cont'd

Indicators of readiness to toilet train	Approximate age (yr)
1. Manipulates sphincter muscles	1½-2
2. Manual dexterity needed to manipulate clothing	2-2½
3. Can hold urine for up to 4 to 5 hours	2-2½
4. Can understand simple directions	1½-2
5. Can communicate needs using words or gestures	1½-2
6. Developed a sense of self	1-2
7. Demonstrates trust in mother and desire to please	1½-2
8. Demonstrates sense of independence and a desire to do for self	2-2½
9. Is proud of own accomplishments	2-2½
10. Demonstrates behavioral control	2-2½

ones who will have to pick up signals, put child on toilet, undress and redress, etc.; therefore, they should be highly motivated

3. Bowel training may be accomplished but accidents will happen and will be due to trainer (parent), not trainee (child)

4. Training should not be stressful for parent or child

B. Training at 18-30 months; points to emphasize:

1. Review readiness signs and check off which ones child has accomplished. If the majority have been achieved, probably appropriate to start training

2. Select a good time such as when

There are no major changes in household and child has shown some interest after observing others

Nursery school friends are trained

Child is aware of wet and dirty versus dry and clean

3. Select a method and stick to it

4. Training should not be stressful; if child resists it is best to forget for awhile then try again

5. Accomplishment of training is variable; it may be a few days or several weeks or months

6. Parents need to develop a relaxed, positive attitude

7. Alternative methods include

Place child on own potty chair at given intervals during the day

Place child on potty before elimination is expected

Place child on potty when parent goes

Always positively reinforce a successful attempt

C. "Natural" toilet training (children training themselves), points to emphasize:

1. Toileting is brought to child's attention when readiness is indicated

2. Child handles situation by himself

3. Child needs to know parents are willing to help

4. Although enjoying a sense of independence and accomplishment, child also needs limits set at this age

Problems are frequently encountered; reassure parents about naturalness, normalcy and transient nature of these problems:

1. Problem with sitting or standing for boys; suggest starting training with sitting progressing to standing

2. Problem using large toilet; suggest potty chair with portable seat which can be taken on excursions

3. Regression; suggest reinforcing as little as possible; depending on severity may require going back to diapers for a while

4. Need help with wiping; suggest allowing child to try if wants to clean self

5. Being able to communicate toilet needs to others; suggest parents make sure other caretakers are aware of child's progress in training, how he communicates need, what words and what degree of independence have been achieved

6. Child does not wish to flush bowel movements; suggest this point not be emphasized; flush toilet later

7. Playing with feces; suggest play with clay or fingerpaints; parent should matter-of-factly state displeasure when this occurs

J9—NURSING INTERVENTIONS FOR CHILD ABUSE PREVENTION

OBSERVATIONS OF PARENTS-TO-BE

1. Are the parents overconcerned with the baby's sex?
2. Are they overconcerned with the baby's performance? Do they worry that he will not meet the standard?
3. Is there an attempt to deny that there is a pregnancy (mother not willing to gain weight, no plans whatsoever, refusal to talk about the situation)?
4. Is this child going to be one child too many? Could he be the "last straw"?
5. Is there great depression over this pregnancy?
6. Is the mother alone and frightened, especially by the physical changes caused by the pregnancy? Do careful explanations fail to dissipate these fears?
7. Is support lacking from husband and/or family?
8. Where is the family living? Do they have a listed telephone number? Are there relatives and friends nearby?
9. Did the mother and/or father formerly want an abortion but not go through with it or waited until it was too late?
10. Have the parents considered relinquishment of their child? Why did they change their minds?

Adapted from Kempe, C.H.: Approaches to preventing child abuse, Am. J. Dis. Child. **130:**941-947, 1976; copyright 1976, American Medical Association.

OBSERVATIONS TO BE MADE AT POSTPARTUM CHECKUPS AND PEDIATRIC CHECKUPS

1. Does the mother have fun with the baby?
2. Does the mother establish eye contact (direct en face position) with the baby?
3. How does the mother talk to her baby? Is everything she expresses a demand?
4. Are most of her verbalizations about the child negative?
5. Does she remain disappointed over the child's sex?
6. What is the child's name? Where did it come from? When did they name the child?
7. Are the mother's expectations for the child's development far beyond the child's capabilities?
8. Is the mother very bothered by the baby's crying? How does she feel about the crying?
9. Does the mother see the baby as too demanding during feedings? Is she repulsed by the messiness? Does she ignore the baby's demands to be fed?
10. What is the mother's reaction to the task of changing diapers?
11. When the baby cries, does she or can she comfort him?
12. What was/is the husband's and/or family's reaction to the baby?
13. What kind of support is the mother receiving?
14. Are there sibling rivalry problems?
15. Is the husband jealous of the baby's drain on the mother's time and affection?
16. When the mother brings the child for check-ups does she get involved and take control over the baby's needs and what's going to happen (during the examination and while in the waiting room) or does she relinquish control to the physician or nurse (undressing the child, holding him, allowing him to express his fears, etc.)?
17. Can attention be focused on the child in the mother's presence? Can the mother see something positive for her in that?
18. Does the mother make nonexistent complaints about the baby? Does she describe to you a child that you don't see there at all? Does she call with strange stories that the child has, for example, stopped breathing, turned color, or is doing something "on purpose" to aggravate the parent?
19. Does the mother make emergency calls for very small things, not major things?

Adapted from Kempe, C.H.: Approaches to preventing child abuse, Am. J. Dis. Child. **130:**941-947, 1976; copyright 1976, American Medical Association.

SPECIAL WELL-CHILD CARE FOR HIGH-RISK FAMILIES

1. Promote maternal attachment to the newborn.
2. Phone the mother during the first 2 days at home.
3. Provide more frequent clinic visits.
4. Give more attention to the mother.
5. Emphasize nutrition.
6. Counsel discipline only for accident prevention.
7. Emphasize accident prevention.
8. Use compliments rather than criticism.
9. Be available during nonworking hours to provide support.
10. Arrange for regular home visits.

Adapted from Kempe, C.H.: Approaches to preventing child abuse, Am. J. Dis. Child. **130:**941-947, 1976; copyright 1976, American Medical Association.

J10—HEALTH PROBLEMS OF SCHOOL AGE CHILD

Health problem	Etiology	Incidence	Assessment	Management	Prevention
URINARY TRACT INFECTIONS	Bacteria enter urinary tract through urethra	5% to 10% of girls and 1% of boys experience a UTI before 18 years	History of signs and symptoms: urgency, frequency, burning, dribbling, foul-smelling urine, fever, irritability, GI symptoms; *may be asymptomatic*	2-week medication course based on causative organism, age, weight of child, sensitivity of organism to drug and previous occurrences	Routine urine screening, particularly for girls early in life (1-2 years)
	Predisposing factors include Short female urethra Obstruction Foreign body Poor hygiene and/or fecal contamination Incomplete bladder emptying resulting in urine stasis Chemical irritants Pinworms Indwelling catheter or catheterization Sexual intercourse Pregnancy	More frequent in girls than boys	Laboratory signs: bacteria on urine culture of greater than 100,00 colonies of a single bacteria per ml of urine confirms infection in symptomatic child.	Medication frequently used: Sulfisoxazole (Gantrisin) Ampicillin Nitrofurantoin (Furadantin) Cephalexin (Keflex)	Hygiene education: Wipe front to back Frequent voiding (3-4 hours) with complete bladder emptying Avoid bubble baths and harsh detergents Use cotton versus nylon panties Avoid tight clothing Adequate fluid intake
	Causative organisms: *Escherichia coli* accounts for 80% to 85% of cases Gram-positive organisms *(Staphylococcus aureus)* *Klebsiella, enterobacteria, Pseudomonas,* and *Proteus* sp.			Increased fluid and rest	Prompt attention for recurrent symptoms
				Symptomatic measures for generalized signs Follow-up is essential: Urine culture 48-72 hours after medication is instituted Urine culture on completion of medication	

Continued.

Health problems of school age child—cont'd

Health problem	Etiology	Incidence	Assessment	Management	Prevention

URINARY TRACT INFECTIONS—cont'd

| | | | | Further follow-up at 1 month (U/A culture); 3 months; 6 months; 12 months (physical exam); 18 months; 24 months (physical exam); annually | |

BACTERIAL INFECTIONS

Impetigo	Superficial skin lesion invaded by staphylococci or streptococci, spread by direct contact with incubation of 2-10 days	Potential risk for glomerulonephrites	Appearance of discolored spots that form vesicles or bullae; these vesicles break and form yellow, honey-colored seropurulent lesions Most frequently on hands, face, or perineum and accompanied by regional lymphadenopathy Culture fluid from lesion or at base of lesion	Topical treatment with Bacitracin or neomycin ointment after soaking with warm compresses Systemic antibiotic if numerous lesions are present Follow-up if not improved with 3 days	Teach child not to pick or scratch insect bites, healing lesions, etc. Keep nails short and clean Frequent handwashing Isolate child's washing and bed linen, drinking glass, and clothes Inspect other family members Adequate rest and nutrition
Cellulitis	Bacterial invasion of skin (both dermis and subcutaneous tissue) caused by Staphylococcus aureus, group A beta-hemolytic streptococci, or Hemophilus influenza Less communicable than impetigo but suspect throughout infection; more apt to lead to septicemia	Frequently a secondary infection to impetigo or other skin lesions	Warm tender, erythematous, swollen, and indurated area on skin Lymphangitis seen on extremities Fever, malaise, lymphadenapathy often present	Warm compresses Immobilization of affected part Rest and symptomatic measures Systemic antibiotic therapy	Prevention as for impetigo All family members should be cultured and those with positive cultures treated
Streptococcal pharyngitis	Group A-Beta hemolytic streptococcus	Increased incidence in winter and spring 30%-50% of cases appear in school-age children	Must differentiate from viral pharyngitis Obtain throat culture	10-day course of penicillin when strep confirmed by culture Repeat culture at end of medication course	Culture all symptomatic exposed family contacts Avoid contact with infected child and his eating/drinking utensils

Health problems of school age child—cont'd

Health problem	Etiology	Incidence	Assessment	Management	Prevention
BACTERIAL INFECTIONS—cont'd					
Streptococcal pharyngitis—cont'd		At risk for complications of cervical adenitis, otitis media, peritonsillar abscess, sinusitis, acute glomerulonephritis, acute rheumatic fever		Symptomatic treatment for fever reduction; normal saline gargles, hard sour candy for sore throat; hot or cold compresses for tender cervical nodes	Education regarding illness and necessity of full treatment course of medication
Tuberculosis	Communicated through sputum and cough spray of infected person Causative organism are Mycobacterium tuberculosis and M. bovis Incubation range is 2 to 10 weeks	Most at risk in first 3 years and the second year preceding puberty For children of all ages, an average of 4,000 new cases are reported annually Predisposing factors include state of health and nutrition; age; environmental and socioeconomic circumstances (crowding, poor sanitation); virulence and number of bacilli	Development of overt symptoms occurs in small percentage Demonstrated systemic hypersensitivity as evidenced by positive skin test Chest x-ray to determine presence and extent of active lesions Sputum smears	Rest, adequate diet, and gradual return to normal activity; prevention of other infection Drug therapy Counseling and support	Screening tests particularly for at risk population Identify, screen, and treat contacts Hygiene and sputum precautions/measures
PARASITIC INFECTIONS					
Scabies	Caused by parasite, female mite that burrows into stratum corneum of skin and lays eggs in the tunnel Transmitted by direct contact with infected person; can be contracted from infected bedding and clothing	Pandemic in U.S. since 1974	Vesicular or papulovesicular rash occurring typically on genitals, buttocks, between fingers and in folds of wrist, elbows, armpits, and at beltline Appear as fine wavy line; gray to pink in color Pruritus is worse at night Skin scrapings from over lesion reveal mite presence under microscope	Scabicide (Kwell) applied to affected areas; one application is generally sufficient—may be repeated Clothing and bedding should be washed	Avoid contact with infected person's bedding and clothing Family members should do self-skin inspection

Continued.

Health problems of school age child—cont'd

Health problem	Etiology	Incidence	Assessment	Management	Prevention
PARASITIC INFECTIONS—cont'd					
Tinea capitis (scalp), corporis (body), pedis (foot)	Fungal infection frequently transmitted by dogs and cats; caused by Microsporum canis or by Trichophyton transmitted by humans	Increased incidence in puberty Permanent baldness may occur with severe capitis	Capitis: bald patches with erythema, gray scaling, and crusting Corporis: macule that enlarges peripherally, healing in center to present as scaly, circular lesions found on face, upper extremities, and trunk; may have mild pruritus Pedis: vesicular eruptions with skin maceration between toes Laboratory procedures: (1) microscopic exam with KOH; (2) ultraviolet light fluoresces Microsporum infections; (3) microscopic culture	Capitis: griseofulvin—follow-up cultures should be done Corporis: tolnaftate (Tinactin) 1% solution or cream Pedis: tolnaftate (Tinactin) solution or cream and Desenex or Tinactin powder prophylactically	Capitis: avoid exchange of head gear; avoid/treat infected animal; wash scalp after haircuts; avoid use of infected person's personal care articles Corporis: preceding plus avoiding exchange of clothing and community showers or bathing places Pedis: preceding plus thoroughly dry between toes; use cotton socks and change frequently; wear well ventilated shoes; air feet; wear rubber sandals in community showers
DENTAL					
Caries	Progressive lesions of calcified dental tissue characterized by tooth structure loss Bacteria, carbohydrates, and plaque are definite factors producing tooth decay	50%-97% of children have 1 or more cavities by 6 years of age Greatest incidence occurs between 4 to 8 years and 12 to 18 years	Characterized as discolored areas or actual lesion in fissures of chewing surfaces of teeth May be visible on inspection Dental equipment and x-rays most reliable in detecting caries	Dental referral Prevention	Preventive measures: Early institution of dental care and visits Brushing and flossing after every meal Water fluoridation; oral supplemental fluoride if indicated; fluoride rinses Topical fluoride application and use of toothpaste containing fluoride Limit carbohydrate content of diet
Malocclusion	Irregularities of tooth alignment and improper fitting of teeth Causative factors: abnormal jaw alignment; abnormal muscle function; incompatibility of tooth and jaw size creating abnormal	Most frequently recognized in early school age years Not common in deciduous teeth	Variation of normal occlusion of top molars meeting firmly on opposing bottom posterior teeth with upper incisors barely overlapping and touching bottom anterior incisors	Dental referral Prevention	Preventive measures: Meeting early sucking needs Avoidance of prolonged use of bottle over 2 years Weaning to cup at 1 year to promote jaw and mouth development after sucking

Health problems of school age child—cont'd

Health problem	Etiology	Incidence	Assessment	Management	Prevention
DENTAL—cont'd					
Malocclusion—cont'd	spacing, crowding or teeth irregularities; delayed permanent teeth eruption; prolonged retention of primary teeth; neglected teeth; prolonged occurrence of lip biting, mouth breathing, tongue twisting, teeth grinding, thumb sucking				Gentle reminder about finger/thumb sucking, lip biting, etc. Remove finger, thumb from mouth when child is sleeping
Enuresis	Exact cause is not known but potential factors include: delayed development of neuromuscular control, organic causes, deep sleep and high threshold for nocturnal arousal; psychologic/emotional factors	Up to 15% of 6- to 7-year-olds and 3% of 13- to 14-year olds Males affected more than females	Primary: in children who have never achieved bladder control Secondary: in children who have achieved bladder control for 3-6 months then lose it Complete history to include: Amount and times of fluid intake Number of enuretic episodes per week/month Sleeping patterns Voiding patterns Any recent stressful events Occurrence at home and/or away from home or both Child's response to enuresis Emotional atmosphere of home Details of toilet training Family history of enuresis Past medical history Laboratory tests Routine urinalysis	**INITIAL MEASURES** Fluids are restricted after supper Child voids before bedtime Before retiring for night, parents should wake child to void A night light is provided **CONDITIONING** Enuretone, a moisture-sensitive device that rings an alarm bell upon initiation of wetting, can be used Imipramine (Tofranil), which exerts an anticholinergic effect on bladder muscle and/or an antidepressant effect on central nervous system, can be used	Preventive measures: Avoid too early toilet training Avoid negative reinforcement if accidents happen Empty bladder before bedtime Get up at night to void Decrease fluid intake from dinner time on Be supportive if accidents happen Identify stresses child may have and help resolve

Continued.

Health problems of school age child—cont'd

Health problem	Etiology	Incidence	Assessment	Management	Prevention
DENTAL—cont'd Enuresis— cont'd				**BLADDER TRAINING (A BEHAVIOR MODIFICATION PROCEDURE)** Child drinks large fluid amount during day and retains urine as long as possible When child must void, urine is measured and recorded in a daily log Dry nights are recorded Wall charts are maintained Positive reinforcers such as stars or points are maintained for advances (e.g., two dry nights, dry all day, breaking record of previous voiding volume) **COUNSELING** Family and child should be encouraged to express feelings about enuresis Parents and child should be informed that enuresis is not intentional and is no one's fault Punitive or shaming techniques should be avoided Explanation of the many variables involved in enuresis is essential for parents and child Nurse should assist parents and child to accept problem Nurse should help provide support for child parents and child to do the same	

Health problems of school age child—cont'd

Health problems of school age child—cont'd

Health problem	Etiology	Incidence	Assessment	Management	Prevention
DENTAL—cont'd					
Encopresis	Commonly caused by chronic constipation or psychogenic problems Fecal incontinence with constipated movements; frequently impactions occur	Occurs in children over 5 years Boys affected more frequently than girls	*Primary:* children have never been toilet trained. *Secondary:* children had established bowel control. Children state they are unaware of having bowel movement. Complete history focusing on patterns of occurrence, bowel habits and toilet training. Explore psychosocial development for significant factors (i.e. illness, loss, stress)	Removal of fecal impactions by use of enemas Use of stool softeners High residue diet Counseling and support to child and parents Establishment of regular bowel routine Assist parents to help child deal with anxiety Identify practical solutions (i.e. wear extra underwear) Skin care measures	Preventive measures: Avoid too early toilet training Avoid punitive techniques in toilet training Avoid negative feedback when incontinent Increase fluid intake High residue diet
OBESITY					
	Causes are related to organic problem and imbalance between caloric intake and energy expenditure Influencing factors: Genetic Activity patterns Metabolic rate Number and size of fat cells Nutritional habits Attitude about feeding Quantity of food ingested	Approximately 10% to 30% of American children are considered obese	Clinically children with weight 20% above the mean for their age and height are obese with those 10% to 20% over mean defined as overweight Organic problems must be ruled out Nutritional status and diet history (see Table 23-9 and Appendix J p. 923)	Referral if organic problem indicated Weight control or reduction plan that modifies eating habits, reduces caloric intake, increases energy expenditure, and promotes sense of well-being and self-esteem Early prevention	Preventive measures: Encourage breast feeding Avoid overfeeding in infancy/early childhood including milk Teach nutritional needs to parents Encourage healthful eating habits Avoid extra caloric foods (sweetened water, candy as reward) Delay early introduction of solids Encourage home-prepared baby foods and meals for older children Avoid commercially prepared baby dinners and meals for older children Encourage physical activity

J11—COMMON BEHAVIORS OF SCHOOL AGE CHILD AND ADOLESCENT

Behavior	Development	Guidance
SCHOOL AGE		

Cheating	Testing right and wrong; generally follow parents' rules and authority but may succumb to peer pressure to "break rules"; becoming more aware of their parents' "cheating" in different ways	Assist parents to
		  Reinforce positive "good" behaviors
		  Maintain limits and discipline standards
		  Recognize that most children confess or are caught and that disciplinary action must be immediate
		  Identify what prompted cheating

Lying	Differentiating between fantasies and realities; use of untruth to avoid the unpleasant; becoming more aware of parents not always telling the truth	Confront and assess problem with assistance from teacher and involvement of child Reassure child that a real world of absolute truthfulness does not exist Point out to child untruths that are fantasies, emphasizing the real component Use discipline for act and discuss meaning of untruths Reinforce honest behaviors positively
Stealing	Curiosity about other possessions; continue to learn and internalize concept of "mine" versus "yours"; not easy to resist temptations; limited idea of property	Act as role model; respect child's property and spouse's property; ask before use Reinforce concept of property and ownership verbally as well as behaviorally Discipline for petty acts, e.g., have child return or pay back item; use verbal disapproval Assess, help, and seek referral if problem is persistent
Fighting	More boys than girls fight; siblings usually fight; an attempt to establish position for self; may be result of frustration	Act as role model; parents who verbally and physically fight indicate behavior is acceptable Establish behaviors that are acceptable vents for frustration/and anger Emphasize the need to share, exchange, and interact in positive manner Separate siblings when fighting; then allow them to work out differences once composure is regained Avoid condoning physical assault as a means of retaliation with peers; assist child to find other solutions Discover reason for fighting if it is continual
Scatology	Uses dirty words as means of attention and testing parents; frequently has no understanding of meaning	Set an example; do not use dirty words in front of child Indicate unacceptability of dirty words; remind when child uses Avoid a struggle, argument, or excessive discipline unless profound problem exists Seek help if persistent
Fears	Often learned from parents; indicative of struggle to cope with unknown or unpleasant experience; may be result of learning right from wrong	Deal with each fear separately Avoid overemphasis of own fear Identify what specifically about situation evokes fear Reassure child; reinforce that some fears are healthy and protective in nature Seek help if fears interfere with daily life

Common behaviors of school age child and adolescent—cont'd

Behavior	Development	Guidance
ADOLESCENT		
Moodiness/non-communcative	Result of emotional conflicts of establishing an identity, developing sexually, and worries over body image and social relationships	Assist adolescent and parents to: Feel reassured about normalcy of wanting to be alone, mood swings, and fears Recognize and discuss family conflicts and possible solutions Recognize and discuss importance of communication and need to validate feelings
Preoccupation with body image and sexuality	Physical changes are dramatic; need to be the same as peers; sexual fantasies and erotic urges and behaviors are heightened with physiological changes	Recognize normalcy of feelings and preoccupation Understand normal physical growth, physiological chanes, and individual patterns Accept self; develop constructive coping behaviors (e.g., sublimate into activity; need to verbalize feelings) Identify other resources of information: courses at school, books, etc. Encourage physical activity as tension release
Rebellion	Need to establish own value and belief system	Alleviate conflicts through open communication and validation of feelings Roleplay and offer reflective feedback to each other Focus on individual needs and place value and pressure from others in perspective
Conformity	Need for allegiance and belonging; assists in challenge of authority and developingof self; serves as validation mechanism	Reinforce positive aspects of peer group and what is taught by them Recognize normalcy of need Find solutions when conformity interferes with adolescents and family's goals
Inferiority feelings	Result of feelings of loneliness and being different when unable to conform to peer group	Relate importance of social involvement to individual goals Explore interest and participation in after-school activities Recognize feelings about self (what he/or she likes/and dislikes and what are desired changes) Identify solutions to problem behaviors identified
Poor study habits	May result from disinterest, preoccupation, excessive parent expectations	Identify cause of poor habits; may need remedial help or assistance in developing constructive habits Avoid nagging or conflict over issue Identify constructive solutions Identify feelings and attitudes Discuss individual goals, methods of meeting goals as related to ability and consequences
Ambivalence	An attempt to identify dependent versus independent needs; reflects conflict between parental rules and own wishes	Identify conflict and possible solutions Maintain a system of accountability for behavior and compliance with rules of system Deal with feelings constructively (e.g., verbally, physical exercise) Recognize importance and normalcy of behavior

J12—EDUCATIONAL TOOL FOR CONTRACEPTION COUNSELING

	The pill	Minipills	Intrauterine device (IUD)	Diaphragm with spermicidal jelly or cream
Description	Pills with 2 hormones, an estrogen and progestin, similar to the hormones a woman makes in her own ovaries.	Pills with just 1 type of hormone: a progestin, similar to a hormone a woman makes in her own ovaries.	A small piece of plastic with nylon threads attached. Some have copper wire wrapped around them. One IUD gives off a hormone, progesterone.	A shallow rubber cup used with a sperm-killing jelly or cream.
Action	Prevents egg's release from woman's ovaries, makes cervical mucus thicker and changes lining of the uterus.	May prevent egg's release from woman's ovaries; makes cervical mucus thicker and changes lining of uterus, making it harder for a fertilized egg to start growing there.	The IUD is inserted into the uterus. It is not known exactly how the IUD prevents pregnancy.	Fits inside the vagina. The rubber cup forms a barrier between the uterus and the sperm. The jelly or cream kills the sperm.
Problems	Must be prescribed by a doctor. All women should have a medical exam before taking "the Pill," and some women should not take it.	Must be prescribed by a doctor. All women should have a medical exam first.	Must be inserted by a doctor after a pelvic examination. Cannot be used by all women. Sometimes the uterus "pushes" it out.	Must be fitted by a doctor after a pelvic exam. Some women find it difficult to insert, inconvenient, or messy.
Advantages	Convenient, extremely effective, does not interfere with sex, and may diminish menstrual cramps.	Convenient, effective, does not interefere with sex, and less serious side effects than with regular birth control pills.	Effective, always there when needed, but usually not felt by either partner.	Effective and safe.
Procedure	Either of two ways: 1. A pill a day for 3 wk, stop for 1 wk, then start a new pack. 2. A pill every single day with no stopping between packs.	Take 1 pill every single day as long as you want to avoid pregnancy.	Check string at least once a month right after the period ends to make sure your IUD is still properly in place.	Insert the diaphragm and jelly (or cream) before intercourse. Can be inserted up to 6 hours before intercourse. Must stay in at least 6 hours after intercourse.

Adapted from Contraception, DHEW Pub. No. (HSA) 78-5646, Washington, D.C., 1978, Public Health Services Administration, Bureau of Community Health Services, Department of Health, Education, and Welfare.

Spermicidal foam, jelly, or cream	Condom (rubber)	Condom and foam	Periodic absti- nence (natural family planning)	Sterilization
Cream and jelly come in tubes; foam comes in aerosol cans or individual applicators and is placed into the va- gina.	A sheath of rubber shaped to fit snugly over the erect penis.	Condom and foam used together.	Method to find out days each month when you are most likely to get pregnant. In- tercourse is avoided at that time.	Vasectomy (male) or tubal ligation (female). Ducts carrying sperm or the egg are tied and cut surgically.
Foam, jelly, and cream contain a chemical that kills sperm and acts as a physical barrier be- tween sperm and the uterus.	Prevents sperm from get- ting inside a woman's vagina during inter- course.	Prevents sperm from getting inside the uterus by killing the sperm and by pre- venting sperm from getting out into the vagina.	Techniques include maintaining chart of basal body tempera- ture, checking vaginal secre- tions, and keep- ing calendar of menstrual peri- ods, all of which can help predict when an egg is most likely to be released.	Closing of tubes in male prevents sperm from reaching egg; closing tubes in female pre- vents egg from reach- ing sperm.
Must be inserted just before intercourse. Some find it incon- venient or messy.	Objectionable to some men and women. In- terrupts intercourse. May be messy. Con- dom may break.	Requires more effort than some couples like. May be messy or inconvenient. Inter- rupts intercourse.	Difficult to use method if men- strual cycle is ir- regular. Sexual intercourse must be avoided for a significant part of each cycle.	Surgical operation has some risk but serious complications are rare. Sterilizations should not be done unless no more children are de- sired.
Effective, safe, a good lubricant, and can be purchased at a drugstore.	Effective, safe, and can be purchased at a drugstore; excellent protection against sex- ually transmitted in- fections.	Extremely effective, safe; both may be pur- chased at a drugstore without a doctor's prescription. Excel- lent protection against sexually trans- mitted infections.	Safe, effective if fol- lowed carefully; little if any reli- gious objection to method. Teaches women about their men- strual cycles.	The most effective method; low rate of complications; many feel that removing fear of pregnancy improves sexual relations.
Put foam, jelly, or cream into your vagina each time you have inter- course, not more than 30 min be- forehand. No douching for at least 8 hours after intercourse.	The condom should be placed on the erect penis before the penis ever comes into con- tact with the vagina. After ejaculation, the penis should be re- moved from the va- gina immediately.	Foam must be inserted within 30 min before intercourse and con- dom must be placed onto erect penis be- fore contact with va- gina.	Careful records must be main- tained of several factors: basal body tempera- ture, vaginal se- cretions, and on- set of menstrual bleeding. Careful study of these methods will dictate when in- tercourse should be avoided.	After the decision to have no more children has been well thought through, a brief surgi- cal procedure is per- formed on the man or the woman.

J13—DEVELOPMENTAL APPROACH TO SEX EDUCATION

Age	Development	Approach
Toddler	Child believes babies have always existed.	"Only people can make other people. To make a baby person, you need two grown-ups, a man and a woman to be the baby's mommy and daddy. They make the baby from an egg in mommy's body and a sperm from the daddy's body."
Preschooler	Child believes babies are manufactured.	"That's interesting. That's the way you'd make a doll. You'd buy a head and hair and put it altogether. But making a real live baby is different. Mommies and daddies have special things in their bodies to make babies. Mommies have tiny eggs and daddies have tiny sperm. When an egg from a mommy and a sperm from daddy join together, they grow into a baby."
Early school age	Child questions where the baby grows, believes tummies open up.	"Can you put your hand inside your tummy? Do you think mommies and daddies can put their hands in their tummies? There must be another way. Do you want to know how the egg and sperm come together? The daddy's sperm are in his testicles and come out through his penis. The mommy's vagina is a tunnel to where her eggs are. So if daddy puts his penis into her vagina the sperm can go through the tunnel to the egg."
School age	Child has misconceptions, apprehension, and beliefs about conception, love, and physiology. Child tries to understand how all of these relate to one another.	Provide physiological explanations. Clear up misconceptions and abate apprehension. Combine all aspects into an explanation. "It's really important for a baby that mothers and fathers love each other and love the baby, so that when the baby is born they can take good care of it. But loving is a feeling and can't start the baby all by itself. A baby is a living creature and it starts growing from living material. When the mother and father make love, a sperm from the father goes through his penis into the mother's vagina. When the sperm joins with an egg from the mother, they form a new life, which grows into a baby."
Late school age	Initial stage: Children take longer to understand why genetic material must unite to produce a baby. Later stage: Children believe whole baby exists in either sperm or egg, needing the other only to grow.	Reinforce content of previous stage. Emphasize that baby has not begun to exist until sperm and egg meet and fuse; that seeds of life come from both parents, from which baby inherits its physical characteristics. Useful explanation: "Both the sperm and egg contain coded information about the baby it will grow to be. Neither the sperm nor egg has the entire code until they unite. Together, they complete the message to develop a baby that is the child of a particular set of parents."

Adapted from Bernstein, A.C., Six stages of understanding how children learn about sex and birth, Psychology Today, Jan. 1976, pp. 31-35.

J14—RELAXATION EXERCISES

Exercise A: relaxation techniques
1. Find a comfortable place to sit.
2. Place feet flat on the floor.
3. Close eyes.
4. Breathe steadily and with purpose for about 5 minutes.
5. Take particular notice of the parts of the body that feel tense and will them to relax.

Exercise B: breathing technique for relaxation
1. Close your eyes and concentrate on your breathing; exhale comfortably pulling your abdomen in. Now inhale rapidly, taking as much air into your lungs as you can and filling your entire rib cage. Draw in your abdomen, forcing the accumulated air out through your mouth. Repeat 10 times.
2. This time inhale slowly so that the breath you draw in is held for 5 seconds. Hold for another 5 seconds and then exhale slowly until your lungs are completely empty. Repeat five times.

Exercise C: brief relaxation technique
1. Sit comfortably and close your eyes. Concentrate on bringing to mind a picture of the most peaceful setting you have experienced.
2. With each breath say to yourself, "Relax."
3. Let your mind remain free of other thoughts as you practice this for 5 minutes.

Exercise D: anxiety-reduction technique
1. Sit in a comfortable position with eyes closed.
2. Inhale a deep breath through your nose—hold—exhale through the mouth (5 times).
3. Breathe normally. Concentrate on your breathing. With each exhale say "one" silently. Breathe in . . . breathe out, with "one."
4. Open your eyes and sit quietly for 1 minute.

SCREENING TOOLS

K1—NEONATAL PERCEPTION INVENTORY*

The Neonatal Perception Inventory is easily and quickly administered by telling the mother: "We are interested in learning more about the experiences of mothers and their babies during the first few weeks after delivery. The more we can learn about mothers and their babies, the better we will be able to help other mothers with their babies. We would appreciate it if you would help us to help other mothers by answering a few questions."

The procedures are identical for administering the Average Baby form of the NPI on the first or second postpartum day and the NPI at 1 month of age. The mother is handed the Average Baby form while the individual administering the inventory says: "Although this is your first baby, you probably have some ideas of what most little babies are like. Will you please check the blank you *think* best describes what *most* little babies are like."

The tester waits until the mother has completed the Average Baby form and takes it from the mother and then hands the mother the Your Baby form.†

The procedure for administering the Your Baby forms of the NPI is the same at Time I and Time II. However, the instructions given to the mother vary slightly to take into account the time factor. At Time I the tester tells the mother: "While it is not possible to know for certain what your baby will be like, you probably have some ideas of what your baby will be like. Please check the blank you *think* best describes what *your* baby will be like."

At Time II, she says:

"You have had a chance to live with your baby for a month now. Please check the blank you think best describes your baby."

Method of Scoring

The Average Baby Perception form elicits the mother's concept of the average baby's behavior. The Your Baby Perception form elicits her rating of her own baby. Each of these instruments consists of six single item scales. Values of 1-5 are assigned to each of these scales for each of the inventories. The blank signified none is valued as 1 and a great deal has a value of 5. The lower values on the scale represent the most desirable behavior.

---

*Information regarding the NPI can be obtained from Broussard, E.R., and Hartner, S.: Further considerations regarding maternal perception of the first born. In Hellmuth, J., editor: Exceptional infant: studies in abnormalities, vol. 2, New York, 1971, Brunner/Mazel.

†The tester remains with the mother during the entire administration procedure.

The six scales are totaled with no attempt at weighing the scales for each of the inventories separately. Thus a total score is obtained for the Average Baby and a total score is obtained for the Your Baby.

The total score of Your Baby Perception form is then subtracted from the Average Baby Perception form. The discrepancy constitutes the Neonatal Perception Inventory score.

The inventories have shown both construct and criterion validity.

NEONATAL PERCEPTION INVENTORY 1
Average Baby

Although this is your first baby, you probably have some ideas of what most little babies are like. Please check the blank you think best describes the average baby.

How much crying do you think the average baby does?

| a great deal | a good bit | moderate amount | very little | none |

How much trouble do you think the average baby has in feeding?

| a great deal | a good bit | moderate amount | very little | none |

How much spitting up or vomiting do you think the average baby does?

| a great deal | a good bit | moderate amount | very little | none |

How much difficulty do you think the average baby has in sleeping?

| a great deal | a good bit | moderate amount | very little | none |

How much difficulty does the average baby have with bowel movements?

| a great deal | a good bit | moderate amount | very little | none |

How much trouble do you think the average baby has in settling down to a predictable pattern of eating and sleeping?

| a great deal | a good bit | moderate amount | very little | none |

Your Baby

While it is not possible to know for certain what your baby will be like, you probably have some ideas of what your baby will be like. Please check the blank that you think best describes what your baby will be like.

How much crying do you think your baby will do?

| a great deal | a good bit | moderate amount | very little | none |

How much trouble do you think your baby will have feeding?

| a great deal | a good bit | moderate amount | very little | none |

How much spitting up or vomiting do you think your baby will do?

_____ _____ _____ _____ _____
a great deal   a good bit   moderate amount   very little   none

How much difficulty do you think your baby will have sleeping?

_____ _____ _____ _____ _____
a great deal   a good bit   moderate amount   very little   none

How much difficulty do you expect your baby to have with bowel movements?

_____ _____ _____ _____ _____
a great deal   a good bit   moderate amount   very little   none

How much trouble do you think the average baby has in settling down to a predictable pattern of eating and sleeping?

_____ _____ _____ _____ _____
a great deal   a good bit   moderate amount   very little   none

NEONATAL PERCEPTION INVENTORY II

Note: Same inventory for average baby is given again.

Your Baby

You have had a chance to live with your baby for a month now. Please check the blank you think best describes your baby.

How much crying has your baby done?

_____ _____ _____ _____ _____
a great deal   a good bit   moderate amount   very little   none

How much trouble has your baby had feeding?

_____ _____ _____ _____ _____
a great deal   a good bit   moderate amount   very little   none

How much spitting up or vomiting has your baby done?

_____ _____ _____ _____ _____
a great deal   a good bit   moderate amount   very little   none

How much difficulty has your baby had in sleeping?

_____ _____ _____ _____ _____
a great deal   a good bit   moderate amount   very little   none

How much difficulty has your baby had with bowel movements?

_____ _____ _____ _____ _____
a great deal   a good bit   moderate amount   very little   none

How much trouble has your baby had in settling down to a predictable pattern of eating and sleeping?

_____ _____ _____ _____ _____
a great deal   a good bit   moderate amount   very little   none

Degree of Bother Inventory

Listed below are some of the things that have sometimes bothered mothers in caring for their babies. We would like to know if you were bothered about any of these. Please place a check in the blank that best describes how much you were bothered by your baby's behavior in regard to these.

Crying	a great deal	somewhat	very little	none
Spitting up or vomiting	a great deal	somewhat	very little	none
Sleeping	a great deal	somewhat	very little	none
Feeding	a great deal	somewhat	very little	none
Elimination	a great deal	somewhat	very little	none
Lack of a predict- able schedule	a great deal	somewhat	very little	none
Other (specify):	a great deal	somewhat	very little	none
_____	a great deal	somewhat	very little	none
_____	a great deal	somewhat	very little	none
_____	a great deal	somewhat	very little	none

K2—GROWTH MEASUREMENTS: BIRTH TO 18 YEARS

Height and weight measurements for boys

Age*	Height by percentiles						Weight by percentiles					
	5		50		95		5		50		95	
	cm	inches	cm	inches	cm	inches	kg	lb	kg	lb	kg	lb
Birth	46.4	18¼	50.5	20	54.4	21½	2.54	5½	3.27	7¼	4.15	9¼
3 months	56.7	22¼	61.1	24	65.4	25¾	4.43	9¾	5.98	13¼	7.37	16¼
6 months	63.4	25	67.8	26¾	72.3	28½	6.20	13¾	7.85	17¼	9.46	20¾
9 months	68.0	26¾	72.3	28½	77.1	30¼	7.52	16½	9.18	20¼	10.93	24
1	71.7	28¼	76.1	30	81.2	32	8.43	18½	10.15	22½	11.99	26½
1½	77.5	30½	82.4	32½	88.1	34¾	9.59	21¼	11.47	25¼	13.44	29½
2†	82.5	32½	86.8	34¼	94.4	37¼	10.49	23¼	12.34	27¼	15.50	34¼
2½†	85.4	33½	90.4	35½	97.8	38½	11.27	24¾	13.52	29¾	16.61	36½
3	89.0	35	94.9	37¼	102.0	40¼	12.05	26½	14.62	32¼	17.77	39¼
3½	92.5	36½	99.1	39	106.1	41¾	12.84	28¼	15.68	34½	18.98	41¾
4	95.8	37¾	102.9	40½	109.9	43¼	13.64	30	16.69	36¾	20.27	44¾
4½	98.9	39	106.6	42	113.5	44¾	14.45	31¾	17.69	39	21.63	47¾
5	102.0	40¼	109.9	43¼	117.0	46	15.27	33¾	18.67	41¼	23.09	51
6	107.7	42½	116.1	45¾	123.5	48½	16.93	37¼	20.69	45½	26.34	58
7	113.0	44½	121.7	48	129.7	51	18.64	41	22.85	50¼	30.12	66½
8	118.1	46½	127.0	50	135.7	53½	20.40	45	25.30	55¾	34.51	76
9	122.9	48½	132.2	52	141.8	55¾	22.25	49	28.13	62	39.58	87¼
10	127.7	50¼	137.5	54¼	148.1	58¼	24.33	53¾	31.44	69¼	45.27	99¾
11	132.6	52¼	143.3	56½	154.9	61	26.80	59	35.30	77¾	51.47	113½
12	137.6	54¼	149.7	59	162.3	64	29.85	65¾	39.78	87¾	58.09	128
13	142.9	56¼	156.5	61½	169.8	66¾	33.64	74¼	44.95	99	65.02	143¼
14	148.8	58½	163.1	64¼	176.7	69½	38.22	84¼	50.77	112	72.13	159
15	155.2	61	169.0	66½	181.9	71½	43.11	95	56.71	125	79.12	174½
16	161.1	63½	173.5	68¼	185.4	73	47.74	105¼	62.10	137	85.62	188¾
17	164.9	65	176.2	69¼	187.3	73¾	51.50	113½	66.31	146¼	91.31	201¼
18	165.7	65¼	176.8	69½	187.6	73¾	53.97	119	68.88	151¾	95.76	211

From: Whaley, L.F., and Wong, D.L.: Nursing care of infants and children, ed. 2, St. Louis, 1983, The C.V. Mosby Co., pp. 1598-1599 as adapted from National Center for Health Statistics, Health Resources Administration, Department of Health, Education and Welfare, Hyattsville, Md. Values correspond with NCHS percentile curves (see Figs. D-1 to D-4). Conversion of metric data to approximate inches and pounds by Ross Laboratories.

*Years unless otherwise indicated.

†Height data include some recumbent length measurements, which make values slightly higher than if all measurements had been of stature (standing height).

Height and weight measurements for girls

Age*	Height by percentiles						Weight by percentiles					
	5		50		95		5		50		95	
	cm	inches	cm	inches	cm	inches	kg	lb	kg	lb	kg	lb
Birth	45.4	17¾	49.9	19¾	52.9	20¾	2.36	5¼	3.23	7	3.81	8½
3 months	55.4	21¾	59.5	23½	63.4	25	4.18	9¼	5.4	12	6.74	14¾
6 months	61.8	24¼	65.9	26	70.2	27¾	5.79	12¾	7.21	16	8.73	19¼
9 months	66.1	26	70.4	27¾	75.0	29½	7.0	15½	8.56	18¾	10.17	22½
1	69.8	27½	74.3	29¼	79.1	31¼	7.84	17¼	9.53	21	11.24	24¾
1½	76.0	30	80.9	31¾	86.1	34	8.92	19¾	10.82	23¾	12.76	28¼
2†	81.6	32¼	86.8	34¼	93.6	36¾	9.95	22	11.8	26	14.15	31¼
2½†	84.6	33¼	90.0	35½	96.6	38	10.8	23¾	13.03	28¾	15.76	34¾
3	88.3	34¾	94.1	37	100.6	39½	11.61	25½	14.1	31	17.22	38
3½	91.7	36	97.9	38½	104.5	41¼	12.37	27¼	15.07	33¼	18.59	41
4	95.0	37½	101.6	40	108.3	42¾	13.11	29	15.96	35¼	19.91	44
4½	98.1	38½	105.0	41¼	112.0	44	13.83	30½	16.81	37	21.24	46¾
5	101.1	39¾	108.4	42¾	115.6	45½	14.55	32	17.66	39	22.62	49¾
6	106.6	42	114.6	45	122.7	48¼	16.05	35½	19.52	43	25.75	56¾
7	111.8	44	120.6	47½	129.5	51	17.71	39	21.84	48¼	29.68	65½
8	116.9	46	126.4	49¾	136.2	53½	19.62	43¼	24.84	54¾	34.71	76½
9	122.1	48	132.2	52	142.9	56¼	21.82	48	28.46	62¾	40.64	89½
10	127.5	50¼	138.3	54½	149.5	58¾	24.36	53¾	32.55	71¾	47.17	104
11	133.5	52½	144.8	57	156.2	61½	27.24	60	36.95	81½	54.0	119
12	139.8	55	151.5	59¾	162.7	64	30.52	67¼	41.53	91½	60.81	134
13	145.2	57¼	157.1	61¾	168.1	66¼	34.14	75¼	46.1	101¾	67.3	148¼
14	148.7	58½	160.4	63¼	171.3	67½	37.76	83¼	50.28	110¾	73.08	161
15	150.5	59¼	161.8	63¾	172.8	68	40.99	90¼	53.68	118¼	77.78	171½
16	151.6	59¾	162.4	64	173.3	68¼	43.41	95¾	55.89	123¼	80.99	178½
17	152.7	60	163.1	64¼	173.5	68¼	44.74	98¾	56.69	125	82.46	181¾
18	153.6	60½	163.7	64½	173.6	68¼	45.26	99¾	56.62	124¾	82.47	181¾

Adapted from National Center for Health Statistics, Health Resources Administration, Department of Health, Education and Welfare, Hyattsville, Md. Values correspond with NCHS percentile curves (see Figs. D-5 to D-8). Conversion of metric data to approximate inches and pounds by Ross Laboratories.
*Years unless otherwise indicated.
†Height data include some recumbent length measurements, which make values slightly higher than if all measurements had been of stature (standing height).

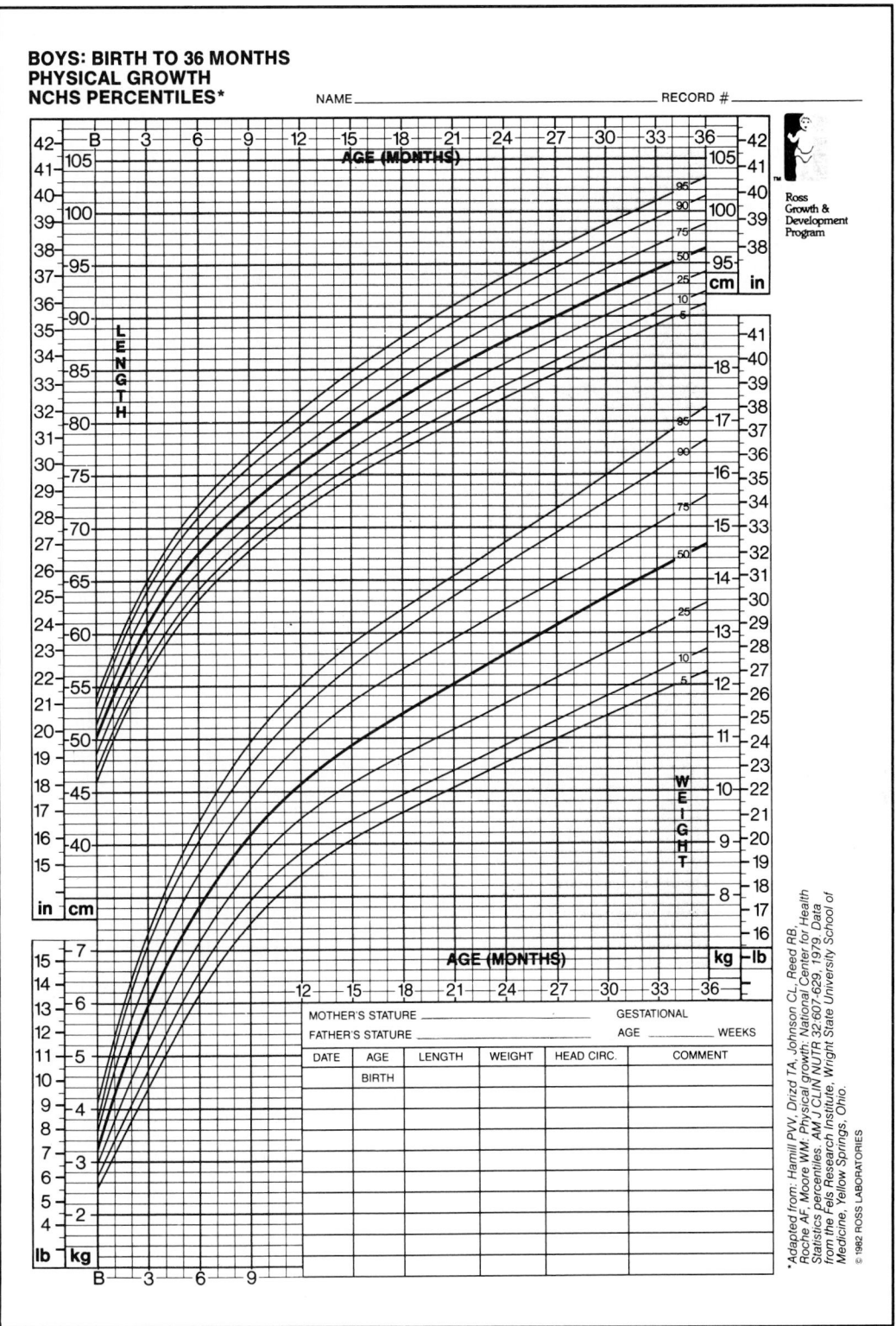

BOYS: BIRTH TO 36 MONTHS
PHYSICAL GROWTH
NCHS PERCENTILES*

NAME _____   RECORD # _____

Ross
Growth &
Development
Program

AGE (MONTHS)

LENGTH

WEIGHT

AGE (MONTHS)

MOTHER'S STATURE _____   GESTATIONAL
FATHER'S STATURE _____   AGE _____ WEEKS

DATE	AGE	LENGTH	WEIGHT	HEAD CIRC.	COMMENT
	BIRTH				

*Adapted from: Hamill PVV, Drizd TA, Johnson CL, Reed RB,
Roche AF, Moore WM: Physical growth: National Center for Health
Statistics percentiles. AM J CLIN NUTR 32:607-629, 1979. Data
from the Fels Research Institute, Wright State University School of
Medicine, Yellow Springs, Ohio.

© 1982 ROSS LABORATORIES

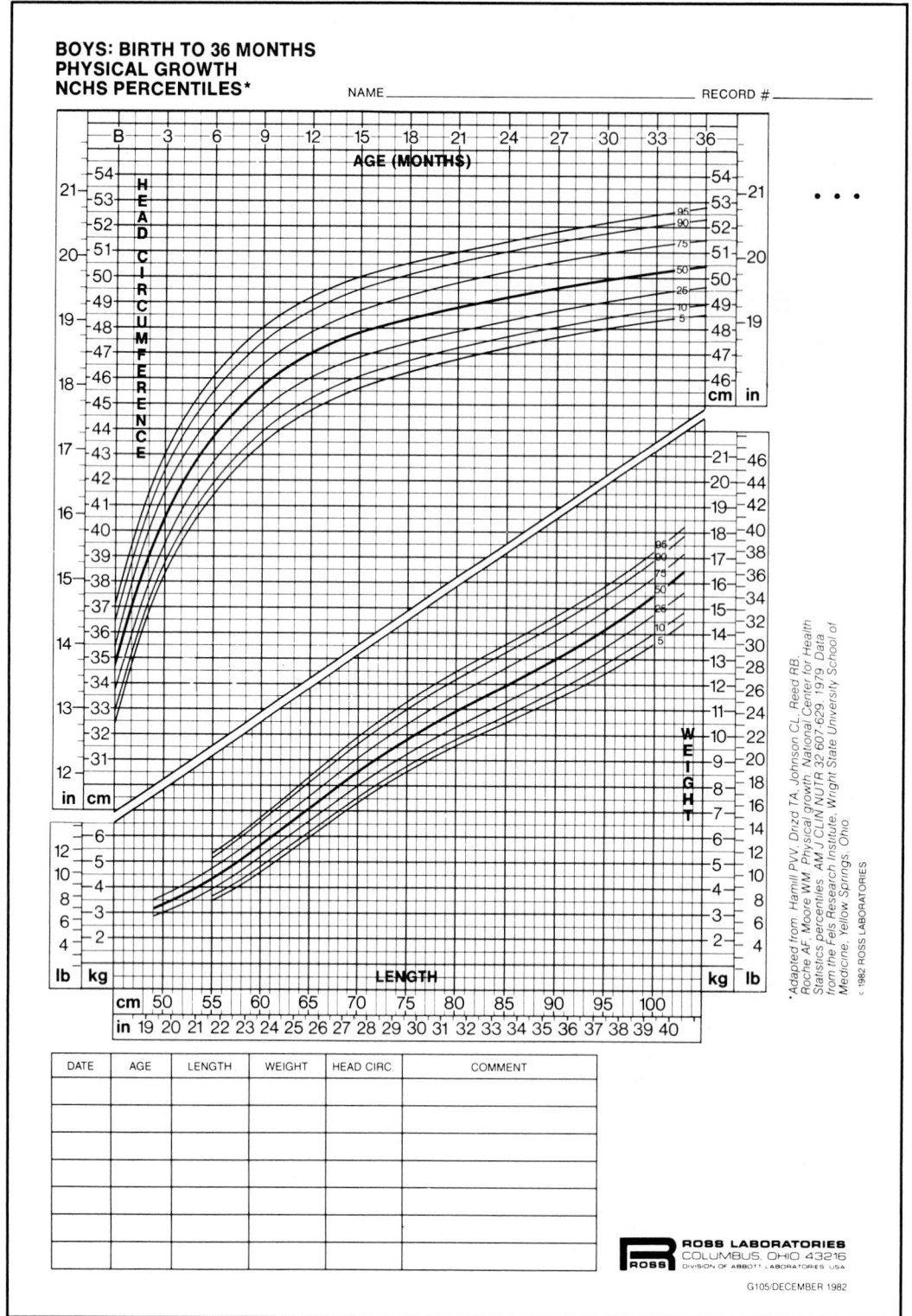

GIRLS: BIRTH TO 36 MONTHS
PHYSICAL GROWTH
NCHS PERCENTILES*

NAME _____   RECORD # _____

Ross
Growth &
Development
Program

*Adapted from: Hamill PVV, Drizd TA, Johnson CL, Reed RB,
Roche AF, Moore WM. Physical growth: National Center for Health
Statistics percentiles. AM J CLIN NUTR 32:607-629, 1979. Data
from the Fels Research Institute, Wright State University School of
Medicine, Yellow Springs, Ohio.

© 1982 ROSS LABORATORIES

DATE	AGE	LENGTH	WEIGHT	HEAD CIRC.	COMMENT
	BIRTH				

MOTHER'S STATURE
FATHER'S STATURE
GESTATIONAL
AGE: WEEKS

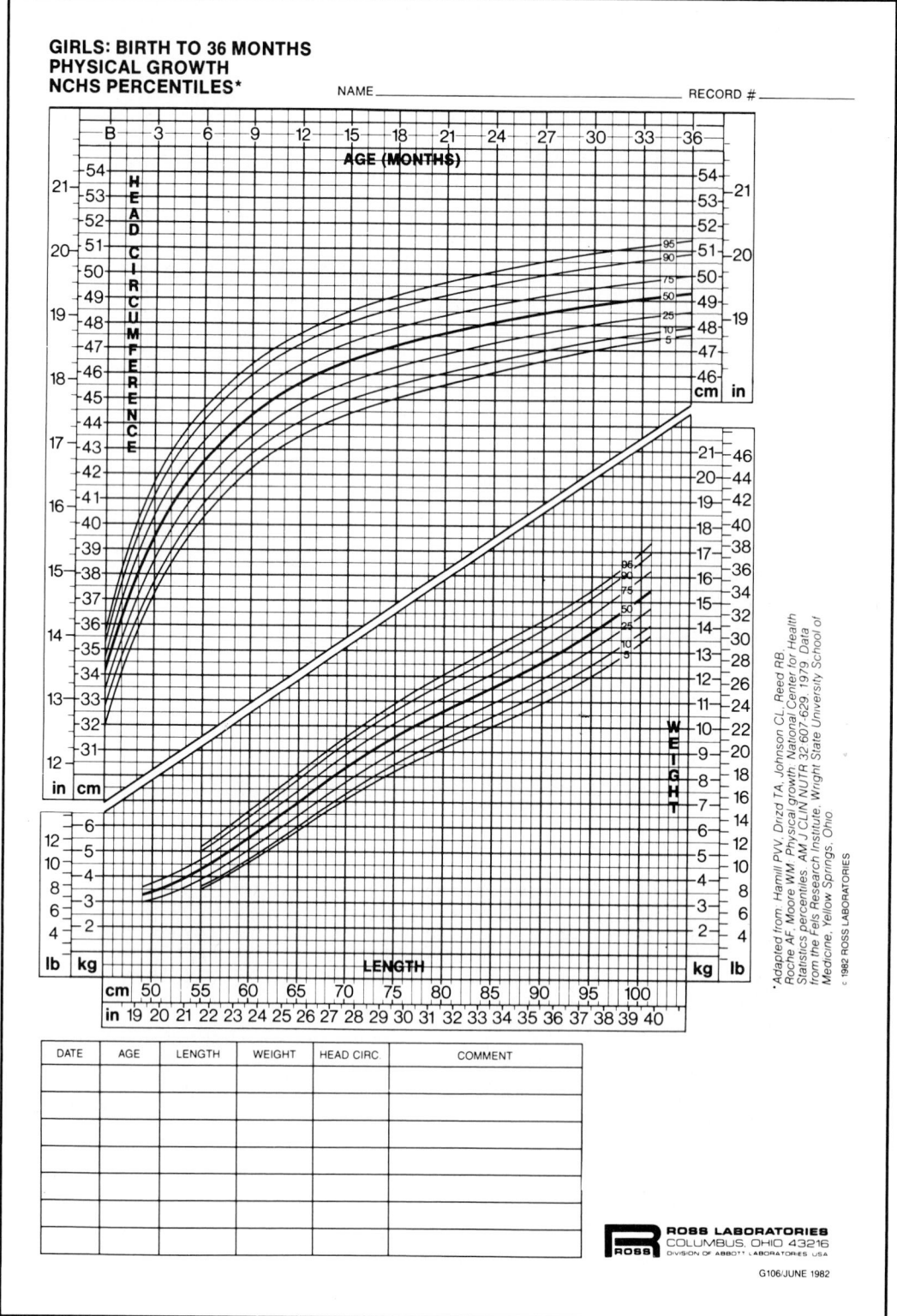

GIRLS: BIRTH TO 36 MONTHS
PHYSICAL GROWTH
NCHS PERCENTILES*

NAME _____   RECORD # _____

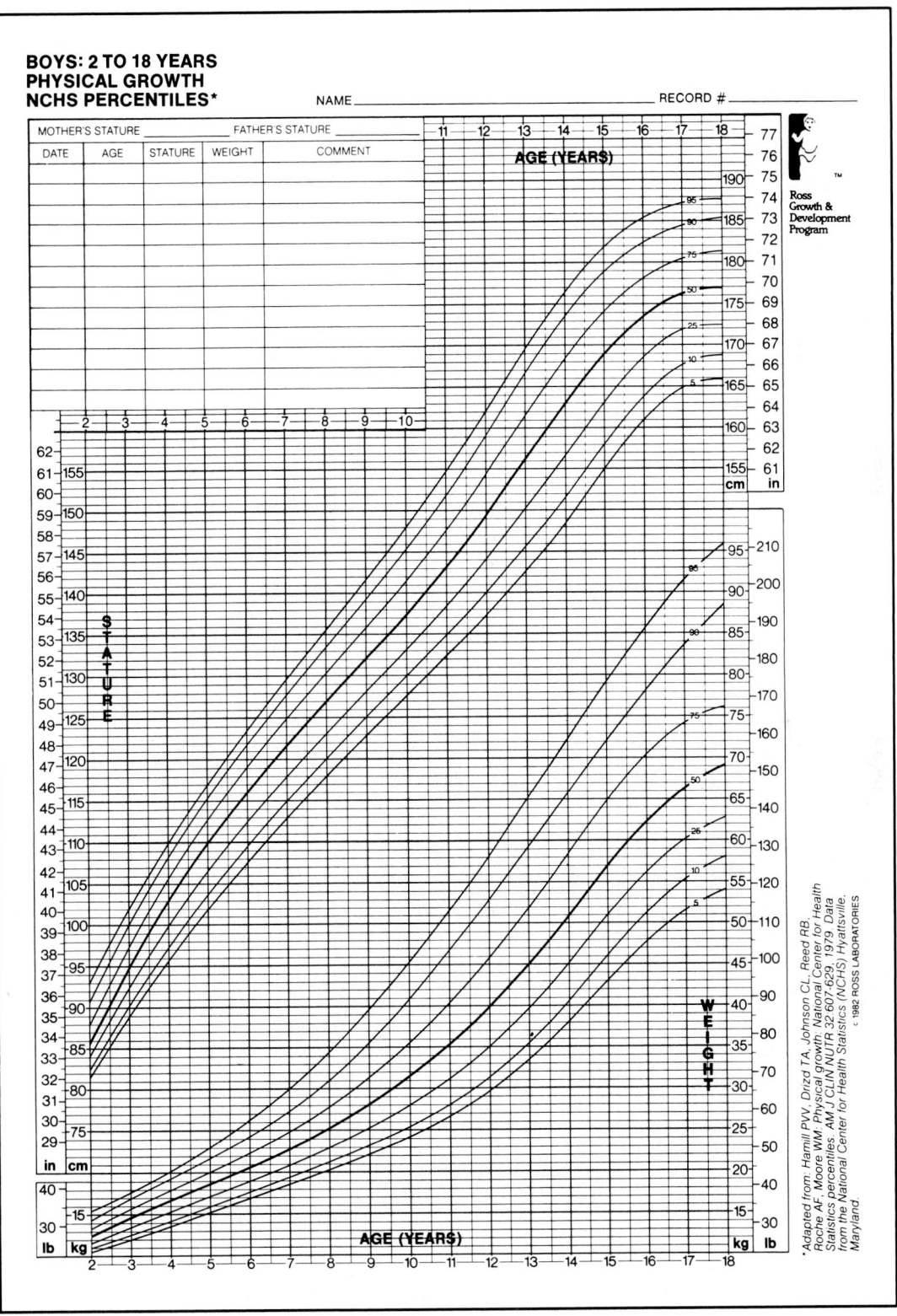

BOYS: 2 TO 18 YEARS
PHYSICAL GROWTH
NCHS PERCENTILES*

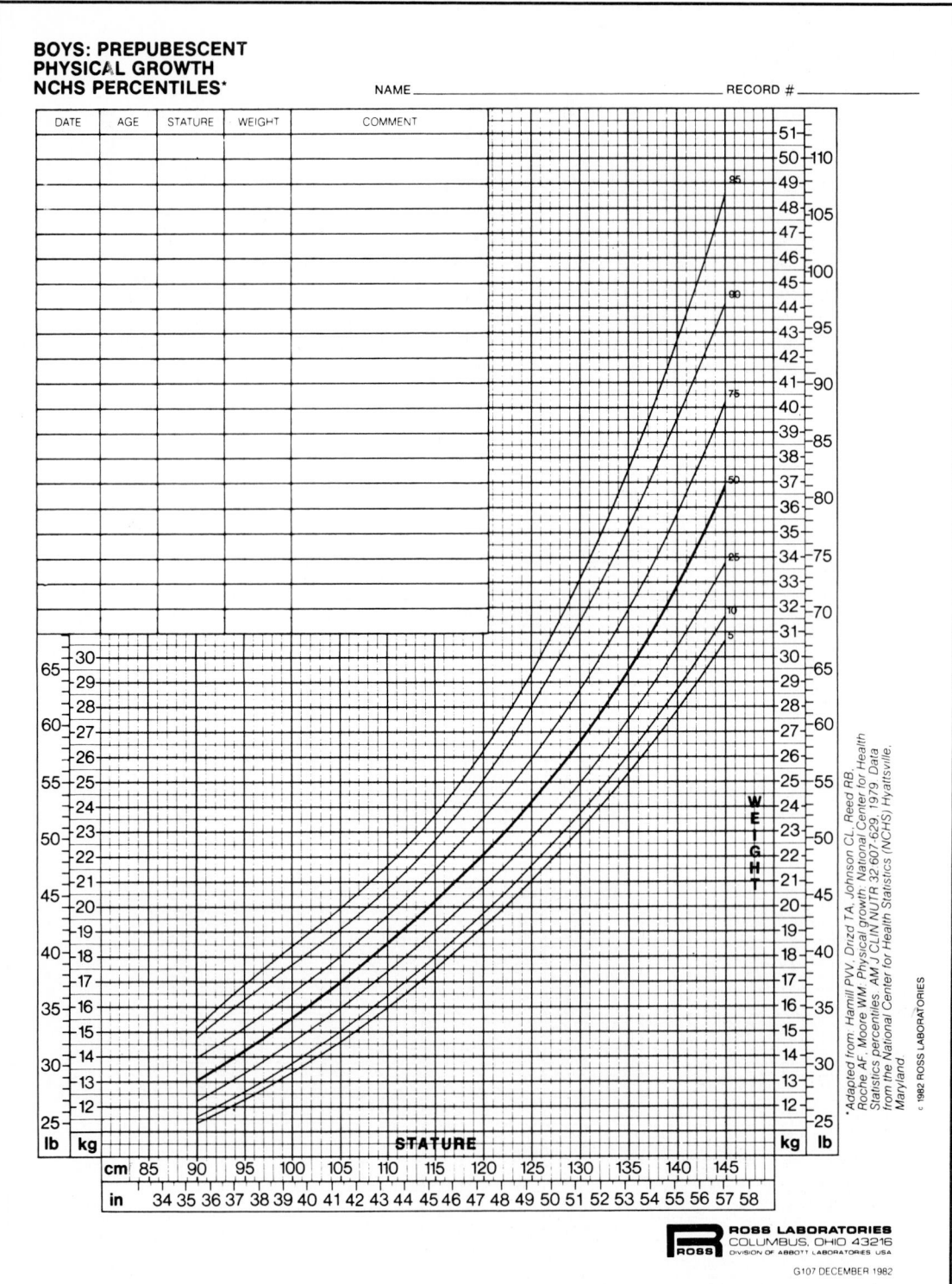

BOYS: PREPUBESCENT PHYSICAL GROWTH NCHS PERCENTILES*

NAME _____ RECORD # _____

DATE	AGE	STATURE	WEIGHT	COMMENT

STATURE

cm 85 90 95 100 105 110 115 120 125 130 135 140 145

in 34 35 36 37 38 39 40 41 42 43 44 45 46 47 48 49 50 51 52 53 54 55 56 57 58

WEIGHT

*Adapted from Hamill PVV, Drizd TA, Johnson CL, Reed RB Roche AF, Moore WM. Physical growth: National Center for Health Statistics percentiles: AM J CLIN NUTR 32:607-629, 1979. Data from the National Center for Health Statistics (NCHS) Hyattsville, Maryland.

c 1982 ROSS LABORATORIES

ROSS LABORATORIES
COLUMBUS, OHIO 43216
DIVISION OF ABBOTT LABORATORIES USA

G107 DECEMBER 1982

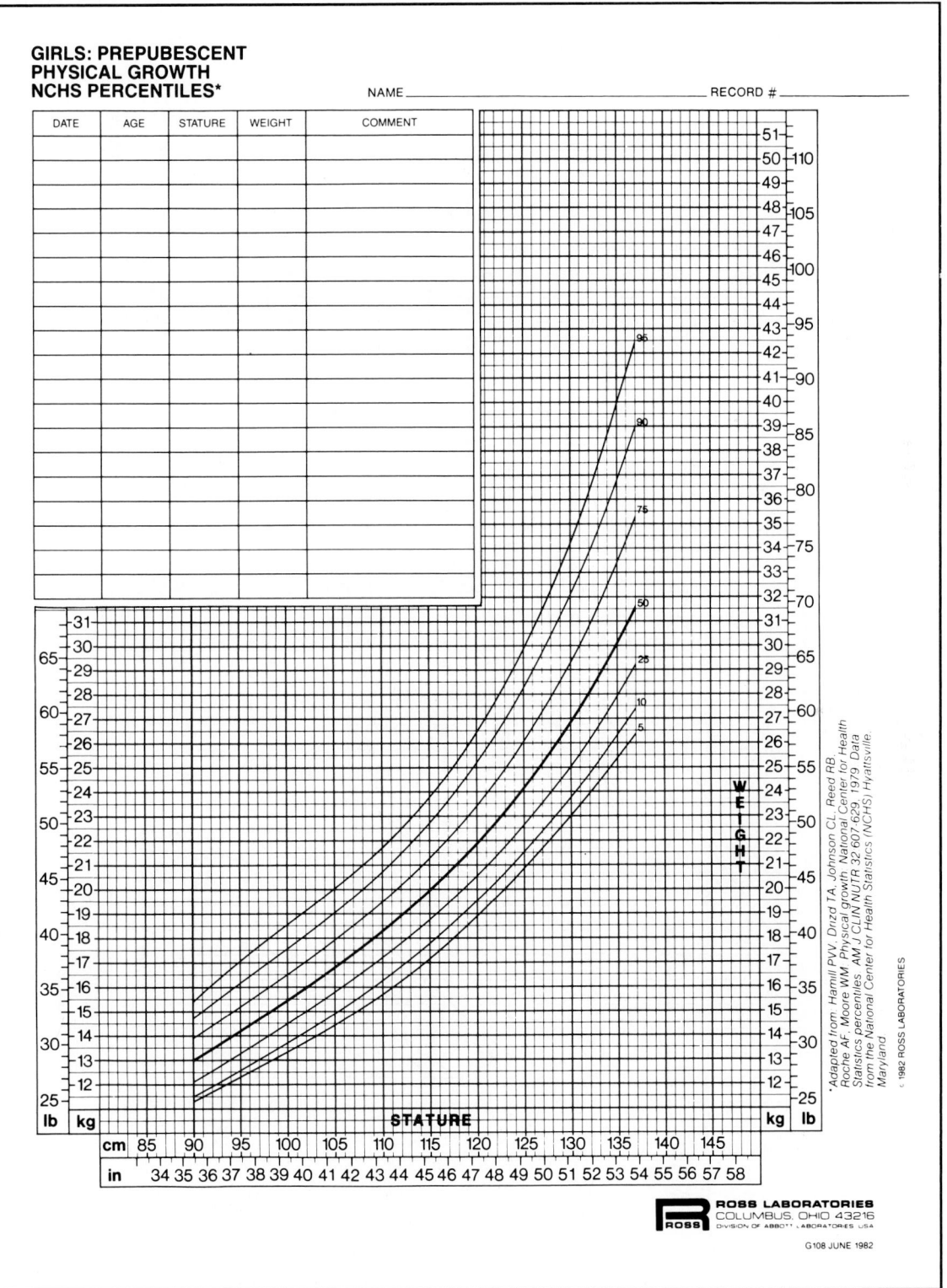

**GIRLS: PREPUBESCENT
PHYSICAL GROWTH
NCHS PERCENTILES***

NAME _____   RECORD # _____

DATE	AGE	STATURE	WEIGHT	COMMENT

*Adapted from Hamill PVV, Drizd TA, Johnson CL, Reed RB, Roche AF, Moore WM. Physical growth National Center for Health Statistics percentiles. AM J CLIN NUTR 32:607-629, 1979. Data from the National Center for Health Statistics (NCHS) Hyattsville, Maryland.

© 1982 ROSS LABORATORIES

STATURE

WEIGHT

ROSS LABORATORIES
COLUMBUS, OHIO 43216
DIVISION OF ABBOTT LABORATORIES USA

G108 JUNE 1982

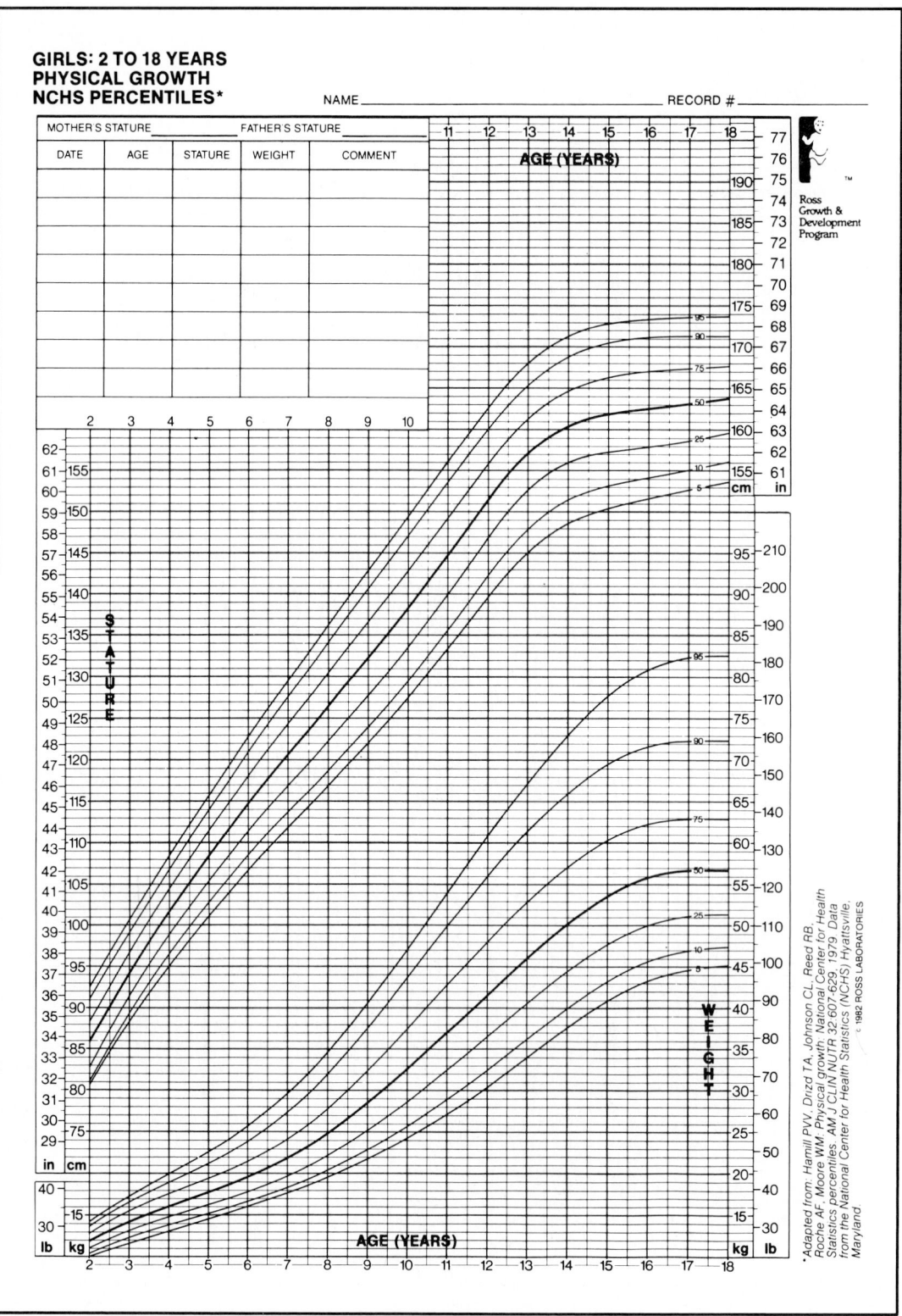

GIRLS: 2 TO 18 YEARS
PHYSICAL GROWTH
NCHS PERCENTILES*

NAME _____   RECORD # _____

K3—DENVER DEVELOPMENTAL SCREENING TEST

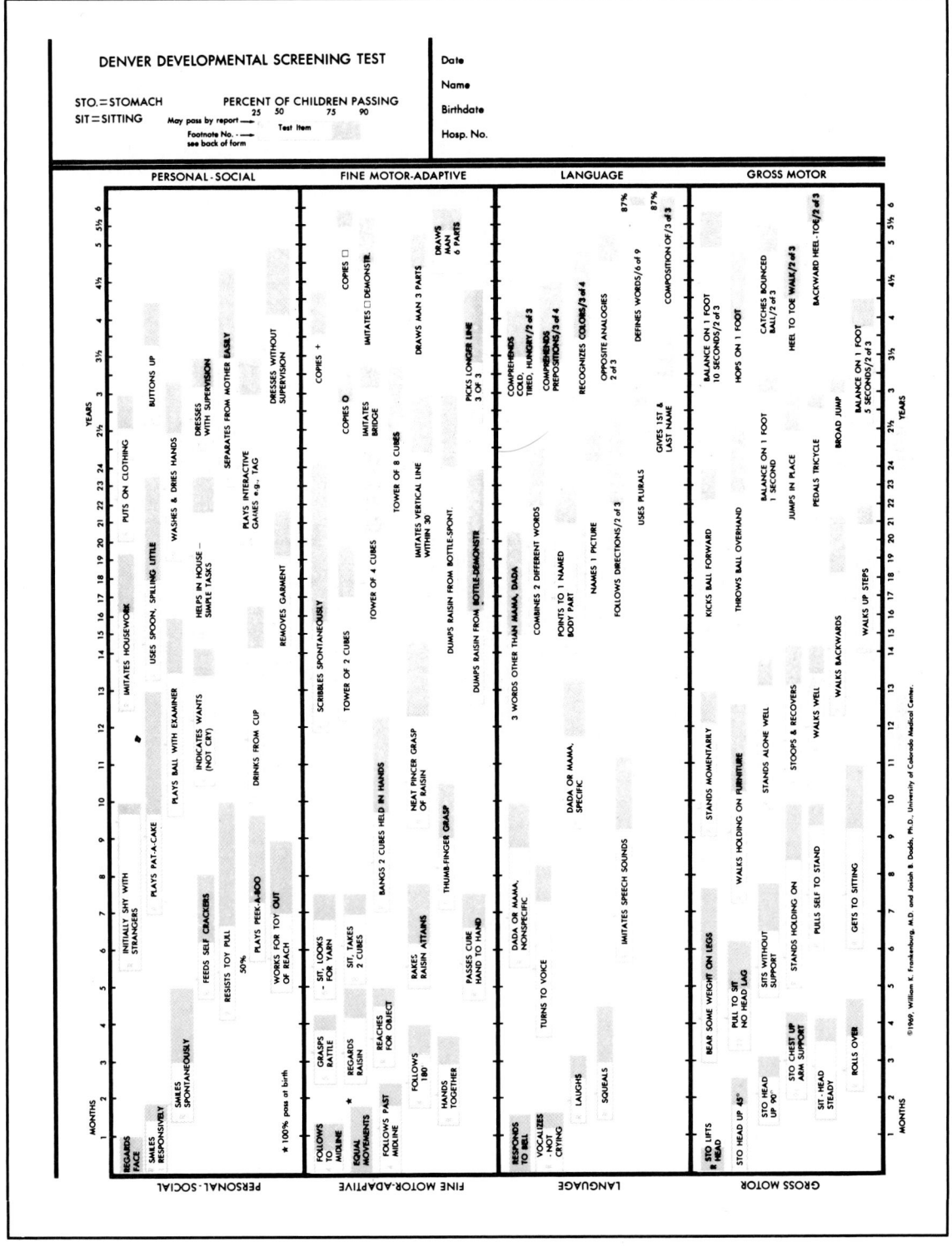

DATE

NAME

DIRECTIONS   BIRTHDATE

HOSP. NO.

1. Try to get child to smile by smiling, talking or waving to him. Do not touch him.
2. When child is playing with toy, pull it away from him. Pass if he resists.
3. Child does not have to be able to tie shoes or button in the back.
4. Move yarn slowly in an arc from one side to the other, about 6" above child's face.
   Pass if eyes follow 90° to midline. (Past midline; 180°)
5. Pass if child grasps rattle when it is touched to the backs or tips of fingers.
6. Pass if child continues to look where yarn disappeared or tries to see where it went. Yarn
   should be dropped quickly from sight from tester's hand without arm movement.
7. Pass if child picks up raisin with any part of thumb and a finger.
8. Pass if child picks up raisin with the ends of thumb and index finger using an over hand
   approach.

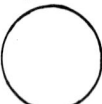 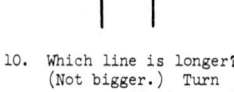 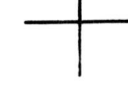 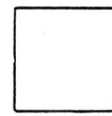

9. Pass any en-   10. Which line is longer?   11. Pass any   12. Have child copy
   closed form.   (Not bigger.) Turn   crossing   first. If failed,
   Fail continuous   paper upside down and   lines.   demonstrate
   round motions.   repeat. (3/3 or 5/6)

When giving items 9, 11 and 12, do not name the forms. Do not demonstrate 9 and 11.

13. When scoring, each pair (2 arms, 2 legs, etc.) counts as one part.
14. Point to picture and have child name it. (No credit is given for sounds only.)

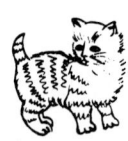 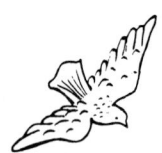 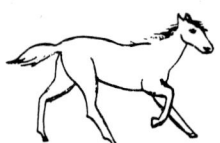 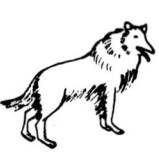 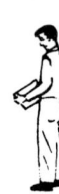

15. Tell child to: Give block to Mommie; put block on table; put block on floor. Pass 2 of 3.
    (Do not help child by pointing, moving head or eyes.)
16. Ask child: What do you do when you are cold? ..hungry? ..tired? Pass 2 of 3.
17. Tell child to: Put block on table; under table; in front of chair, behind chair.
    Pass 3 of 4. (Do not help child by pointing, moving head or eyes.)
18. Ask child: If fire is hot, ice is ?; Mother is a woman, Dad is a ?; a horse is big, a
    mouse is ?. Pass 2 of 3.
19. Ask child: What is a ball? ..lake? ..desk? ..house? ..banana? ..curtain? ..ceiling?
    ..hedge? ..pavement? Pass if defined in terms of use, shape, what it is made of or general
    category (such as banana is fruit, not just yellow). Pass 6 of 9.
20. Ask child: What is a spoon made of? ..a shoe made of? ..a door made of? (No other objects
    may be substituted.) Pass 3 of 3.
21. When placed on stomach, child lifts chest off table with support of forearms and/or hands.
22. When child is on back, grasp his hands and pull him to sitting. Pass if head does not hang back.
23. Child may use wall or rail only, not person. May not crawl.
24. Child must throw ball overhand 3 feet to within arm's reach of tester.
25. Child must perform standing broad jump over width of test sheet. (8-1/2 inches)
26. Tell child to walk forward,   heel within 1 inch of toe.
    Tester may demonstrate. Child must walk 4 consecutive steps, 2 out of 3 trials.
27. Bounce ball to child who should stand 3 feet away from tester. Child must catch ball with
    hands, not arms, 2 out of 3 trials.
28. Tell child to walk backward,   toe within 1 inch of heel.
    Tester may demonstrate. Child must walk 4 consecutive steps, 2 out of 3 trials.

DATE AND BEHAVIORAL OBSERVATIONS (how child feels at time of test, relation to tester, attention
span, verbal behavior, self-confidence, etc,):

K4—INFANT REFLEXES

Reflex	How to elicit	Response of infant	Clinical implications
Acoustic blink	Produce a sharp loud noise (a clap of the hands) about 30 cm from the head.	By second or third day of life infant blinks both eyes. Disappearance of reflex is variable.	Absence may indicate decreased hearing.
Ankle clonus	Flex the leg at the hip and knee, sharply dorsiflex the foot, and maintain pressure.	Rhythmic flexions and extensions of the foot at the ankle.	Abnormal if more than 10 beats during the first 3 months or more than 3 beats after 3 months. Sustained clonus indicates upper motor neuron disease.
Babinski	Stroke lateral aspect of the plantar surface of foot from heel to toes. Use a blunt object.	Hyperextension or fanning of toes occurs. As myelinization is completed, the normal response becomes flexion (downward curling) of all toes; the positive (pathological) sign is hyperextension (dorsiflexion) of the great toe with or without fanning of the remaining toes.	After 2 years of age, a positive sign is the most significant clinical symptom of the presence of an upper motor neuron (pyramidal tract) lesion.
Blinking	Shine a light suddenly at the infant's open eyes.	Eyelids close in response to light. Disappears after first year.	Absence may indicate poor light perception or blindness.
Landau	Suspend infant carefully in prone position by supporting infant's abdomen with examiner's hand.	By 3 months of age the expected response consists of extension of head, trunk, and hips. Head is slightly above horizontal plane. Disappears by 2 years of age.	If newborn collapses into a limp concave position, it is abnormal.
Moro	With infant in supine position gently support head and lift it a few centimeters off the surface. As soon as neck relaxes, suddenly release the head and let it drop back to the surface. *or* Produce sudden loud noise, or jar the table or crib suddenly.	Normal response is present at birth and is one in which the arms extend outward, the hands open, and then are brought together in midline. The legs flex slightly. Usually disappears by 3 to 4 months. Infant may cry.	Asymmetry indicates possible paralysis. Absence suggests severe neurological problem. Persistence beyond 4 months may indicate neurological disease. If it lasts longer than 6 months, it is definitely abnormal.
Neck righting	With infant in supine position turn head to one side.	Infant's trunk rotates in direction in which head is turned. Appears at 4 to 6 months. Disappears at 24 months.	Absent or decreased reflex may indicate spasticity.
Palmar grasp	With infant's head positioned in midline place examiner's index fingers from ulnar side into infant's palm and press against palm.	Normal response is flexion of all fingers around examiner's fingers. Present at birth and disappears by 4 months when infant is ready to reach.	Note symmetry and strength. Persistence of grasp beyond 4 months suggests cerebral dysfunction.
Parachute	Infant is held in a prone position and is quickly lowered toward the surface of the examining ftable or floor.	Normal response is extension of arms, hands, and fingers, as if to break a fall. Appears by 9 months and persists.	Asymmetry or absence of response is abnormal.

From Chow, M.P., et al.: Handbook of pediatric primary care, New York, ed. 2, 1984, John Wiley & Sons, Inc., pp. 893-894; as adapted from Erickson, M.: Assessment and management of developmental changes in children, and problems, ed. 2, St. Louis, 1981, The C.V. Mosby Co.; and Conway, B.L.: Pediatric neurological nursing, Philadelphia, 1977, J.B. Lippincott Co.

Continued.

Infant reflexes—cont'd

Reflex	How to elicit	Response of infant	Clinical implications
Perez	Infant is held in a suspended prone position in one of the examiner's hands. The thumb of the other hand is moved firmly from sacrum along entire spine.	Normal response is extension of head and spine, flexion of knees on the chest, a cry, and emptying of the bladder. Present at birth and disappears by 3 months.	Absence indicates severe neurological disease.
Placing	Infant is held erect and the dorsum of one foot touches the undersurface of the examining table top.	Infant flexes hip and knee and places stimulated foot on top of the table. Present at birth and disappears by 6 weeks or variable.	Absent in paralysis or in infants born by breech delivery.
Plantar grasp	Examiner's finger is placed firmly across base of infant's toes.	Toes curl downward. Present at birth and disappears by 10 to 12 months.	Absent in defects of lower spinal column. Infant cannot walk until this reflex disappears.
Rooting	Infant is held in supine position with head in midline and hands against chest. Examiner strokes perioral skin at corner of mouth or cheek.	Infant opens mouth and turns head toward stimulated side. Present at birth and disappears by 3 to 4 months (awake); by 7 months (asleep).	Absence indicates severe central nervous system disease or depressed infant.
Rotation test	Infant is held upright facing examiner and rotated in one direction and then the other.	Infant's head turns in the direction in which the body is being turned. If head is restrained the eyes will turn in the direction in which the infant is turned.	If head and eyes do not move, it indicates a vestibular problem.
Spontaneous crawling (Bauer's response)	Infant is lying prone and examiner presses soles of feet.	Infant makes crawling movements. Present at birth.	Crawling is absent in weak or depressed infants.
Stepping	Infant is held upright and soles of feet are put in touch with solid surface.	Infant "walks" along surface. Present at birth and disappears at 6 weeks.	Absence indicates depressed infant, breech delivery, or paralysis.
Sucking	With infant in supine position place nipple or finger 3 to 4 cm into mouth.	Vigorous sucking of finger or nipple. Present at birth and disappears by 3 to 4 months (awake) and 7 months (asleep). Tongue action should push finger up and back. Note rate of suck, amount of suction, and patterns or groupings of sucks.	Absence in term infants indicates central nervous system depression. Weak reflex may lead to feeding problems.
Tonic neck	With infant in supine position passively rotate head to one side.	Arm and leg on side to which head is turned extend, and opposite arm and leg flex (fencer's position). Present sometimes at birth but usually by 2 to 3 months. Disappears by 6 months.	Obligatory response is always abnormal. Persistence beyond 6 months is abnormal and indicates central motor lesions (e.g., cerebral palsy).
Trunk incurvation (Galant's)	Infant is held prone in examiner's hand. With the other hand the examiner moves a finger down the paravertebral portion of the spine, first on one side, then on the other.	Infant's trunk should curve to the side being stimulated. Present at birth and disappears by 2 months.	Presence of spinal cord lesions interrupts this reflex.
Vertical suspension positioning	Infant is held upright, head is maintained in midline.	Legs are flexed at the hips and knees. Present at birth and disappears after 4 months.	Scissoring or fixed extension indicates spasticity.

K5—VISION, HEARING, AND LANGUAGE SCREENING PROCEDURES

Method	Age	Procedure	Normal response
VISION			
Following	Infancy	Shine light or hold bright object directly in front of infant's line of vision; move slowly from side to side.	Follow light or bright object up to 180 degrees
Turn to light response	Infancy	Hold back of head to bright light source.	Eyes turn toward source of light
Optokinetic drum	Infancy	Twirl drum with stripes slowly in front of infant's eyes.	Nystagmus occurs.
Herschberg reflex (corneal light reflex)	Infancy through adolescence	Shine penlight into child's eyes; note where light reflex falls. For older children: have child focus and stare at point 14 inches and then 20 inches away before shining light into eyes.	Light reflex falls in same position in eye
Cover test	Toddler through adolescence	Have child focus on specified spot first 14 inches, then 20 inches away. While child is focusing, one eye is completely covered for 5 to 10 seconds. Cover is then removed and eye observed for movement. Procedure repeated for other eye.	No wandering or sharp jerky movement of eyes noted, indicating ability to focus
Snellen E	Preschool	Child is instructed to point finger in direction that the E or table legs are pointing from a distance of 20 feet. Test each eye separately, then together. Test as far down on chart as child can go.	Visual acuity of 20/30
Snellen alphabet	School age through adolescence	Child stands 20 feet from chart and reads letters. Each eye is tested separately and then together. Testing usually started at 20/30 or 20/40 line and child allowed to test as far down chart as possible. Passing score consists of reading majority of letters (or Es) on each line.	Visual acuity of 20/20
HEARING			
Startle reflex	Newborn	Loud noise or bang made near infant's ears.	Jumps at noise, blinks, cries or widen eyes
Tracks sound	3-6 months	Make noise, call name or sing.	Eyes shift toward sound; responds to mother's voice; coos to verbalization
Recognizes sound	6-8 months	As preceding, from out of line of vision.	Turns head toward sound; responds to name, babbles to verbalization
Localization of sound	8-12 months	Call name, or use tuning fork or say words.	Localizes source of sound; turns head (and body at times) toward sound, repeats words
Pure tone screening—play	Toddler to preschool	Demonstrate to child by putting headphones on and making believe you hear sound. As you say "I hear it," put a block in box or ring on holder. Put headphones on child and give block or ring to use. Sound a 50 dB tone at 1000 Hz and guide child's hand with block to box. When child can do this alone, begin screening. Set at 25 dB at 1000 Hz. If child responds, go to 2000, 4000, and 6000 Hz. Praise child and place new block in hand. Switch to other ear and test.	Should respond at 25 dB at any frequency

Continued.

Vision, hearing, and language screening procedures—cont'd

Method	Age	Procedure	Normal response
HEARING—cont'd			
Pure tone audiometry	School age through adolescence	Explain procedure to child. Place headphones on ears. Test 1 ear at a time in sequence as preceding (i.e., 25 dB at 1000, 2000, 4000 and 6000 Hz). Have child raise hand to indicate sound is heard.	Should respond at 25 dB at any frequency
Tuning fork test	Some preschoolers; school age through adolescence		
A. Weber test		Strike tuning fork to make it vibrate and place the stem in midline of scalp. Ask child if sound is same in both ears or louder in either ear.	Sound heard equally well in both ears
B. Rinne test		Strike tuning fork until it vibrates, place stem on child's mastoid until he no longer hears it. Then place vibrating fingers of fork 1 to 2 inches in front of concha. Ask child if he can still hear sound.	Sound from fingers of fork vibrating in air should be heard when child can no longer hear sound with stem against mastoid, i.e., air conduction is greater than bone conduction
LANGUAGE			
Assessment of child's language comprehension	3 to 6 years	Child points to picture named by examiner. Assesses single word vocabulary and two-word, three-word, and four-word phrases	Child able to name picture understandably
Peabody Picture Vocabulary Test	2½ to 18 years	Child looks at picture and points to one named by examiner	Child able to respond correctly by following directions
Preschool Language Scale	Birth to 3 years	Observation of child's performance	Depending on age level, child should be able to point to picture, follow direction, or manipulate objects
Expressive One Word Picture Vocabulary	2 to 12 years	Child looks at picture and names what is seen	Child able to follow directions and articulate response at age level

K6—SCREENING FOR COMMON ORTHOPEDIC PROBLEMS IN INFANCY AND CHILDHOOD

Deformity	Screening

CONGENITAL HIP DISLOCATION (CHD)

Complete or partial displacement of femoral head out of the acetabulum

Barlow's maneuver (for dislocation of femoral head): flex hip to 90 degrees; grasp symphysis in front and sacrum in back with one hand; with other hand, apply lateral pressure to medial thigh with thumb and longitudinal pressure to knee with palm; abduct flexed hip. A positive sign is sensation of abnormal movement. Reverse hands for examining other hip. See Figure K-1.

Ortolani's maneuver (for reduction of femur): abduct hip to 80 degrees, lifting proximal femur anteriorly with fingers placed on lateral thigh. A positive sign is sensation of a jerk or snap with reduction into socket. See Figure K-2.

Limited full abduction of hips: with child flat on back, abduct hips one at a time, then together. See Figure K-3 for degrees of hip abduction.

Apparent shortening of femur:

1. Allis sign: with child lying on back, pelvis flat, knees flexed and feet planted firmly, observe knees. If the knee projects further anteriorly, femur is longer; if one knee is higher, the tibia is longer.
2. With child on back, both legs are extended out with pressure on knees. Heels are matched and observed for equal or unequal length.
3. Trendelenburg sign: with child standing on one leg, observe pelvis. When child stands on abnormal leg, the pelvis drops on normal side. See Figure K-4.

METATARSUS ADDUCTUS (VARUS)

Adduction or turning in of forefoot with high longitudinal arch and wide space between first and second toes. Commonly associated with tibial torsion

Test foot for flexibility and elicit tonic foot reflexes. Rigidity is indicated by eversion or inversion when foot does not move beyond neutral position or does not respond to toe grasping or by dorsiflexing. Signs of metatarsus adductus are illustrated in Figure K-5.

PES PLANUS (FLAT FEET)

When child is weight bearing, longitudinal arch of foot appears flat on floor

(1) Pseudo flat feet: very common until ages 2 to 3; created by plantar fat pad. Feet are flexible, exhibit hypermobility of joint, and have a low arch

(2) Rigid flat feet: Uncommon; created by tightness of heel cord or tarsal coalition (a cartilaginous fibrous or bony connection between bones)

1. Observe feet in weighted and unweighted position
2. Stand child on toes. Arch disappears with weight bearing in flexible flat foot and reappears when on toes. See Figure K-6.
3. Elicit dorsal and plantar flexion to rule out tight heel cord.
4. Elicit eversion and inversion flexion to rule out tarsal coalition.

Same as for preceding No. 1 (pseudo flat feet)

GENU VALGUM (KNOCK-KNEES)

A deviant axis of thighs and calves of more than 10 to 15 degrees; (normal from ages 2-6)

1. Observe axis of thighs and calves with child standing. Normally axis are parallel with 10 to 15 degrees deviance. See Figure K-7.
2. Observe space between the knees from front to back. Normal spacing is 1½ inches.
3. Observe space between ankles from front and back. Normal spacing between medial malleoli at heel is 2 inches.

GENU VARUM (BOWLEGS)

Deviant axis of thighs and calves which is

(1) Physiological: normal until ages 2 to 3; occurs with internal tibial torsion and genu valgum

(2) Pathological

Same for genu valgum

Continued.

Screening for common orthopedic problems in infancy and childhood—cont'd

Deformity	Screening
INTERNAL TIBIAL TORSION Twisting or torsion of tibia usually accompanied by metatarsus adductus	1. Examine legs for range of motion, flexibility of ankle and elicit tonic foot reflexes. 2. Holding knee firmly with foot in neutral position, observe medial and lateral mallioli. The normal angle between them is approximately 15 to 20 degrees. See Figure K-8. 3. Have child sit on examining table and draw a circle over patellar and external mallioli. With patella facing forward only anterior edge of malleolar circle should be seen. See Figure K-9.
SCOLIOSIS S-shaped lateral curvature of spine with rotation of vertical bodies.	Screening is implemented as follows: 1. Ask the child to bend forward in a 50% flexing position with shoulders drooping forward, arms and head dangling. Observe the spine from above the head and inspect for any lateral curvature or prominent projection of the rib cage on one side (Figure K-10). 2. While the child is standing erect with weight equal on both feet, observe for Difference in levels of shoulders, scapula, and hips Differences in the size of the spaces between the arms and the trunk Prominence of either scapula or hip A curve in the vertebral spinous process alignment 3. Ask the child to walk and make observations discussed in No. 2 and observe for the presence of a waddle, limp, or tilt.

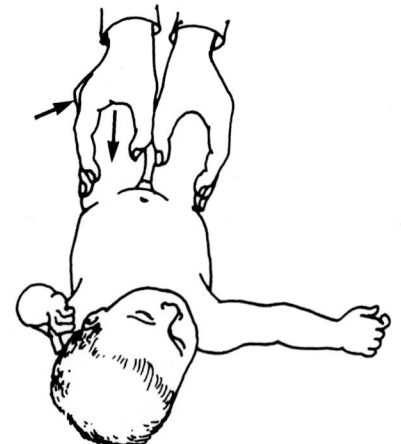

FIGURE K-1

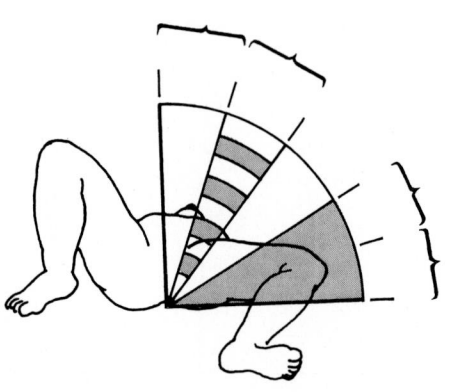

FIGURE K-2

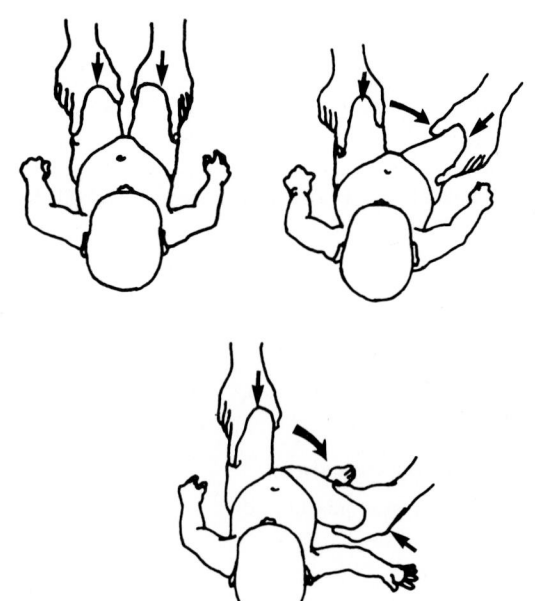

FIGURE K-3

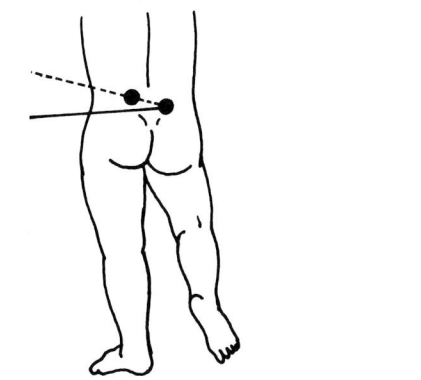

FIGURE K-4

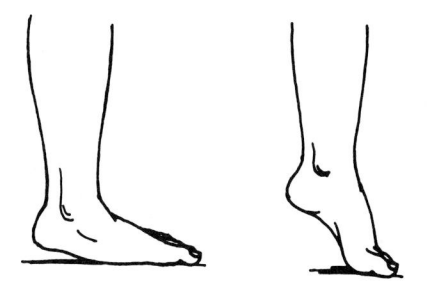

FIGURE K-5

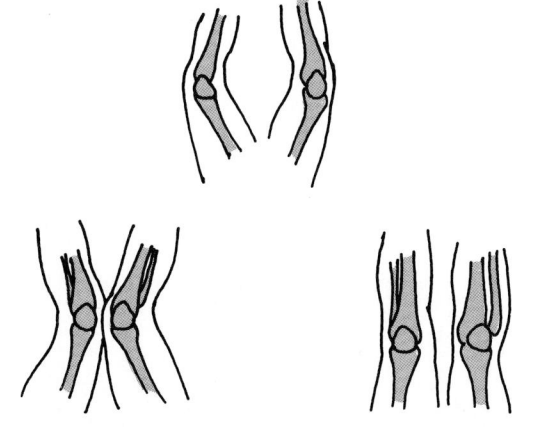

FIGURE K-7

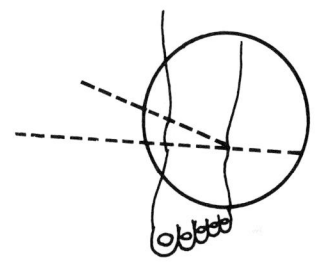

FIGURE K-6

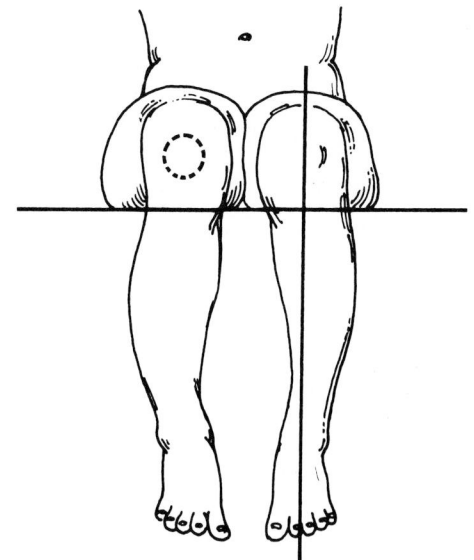

FIGURE K-8

FIGURE K-9

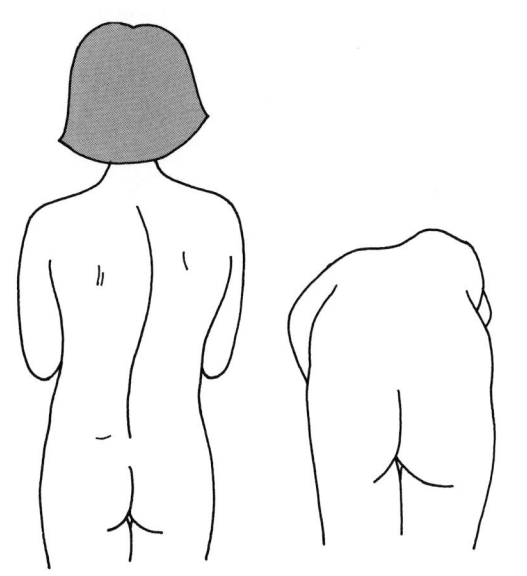

FIGURE K-10

K7—DENVER ARTICULATION SCREENING EXAMINATION

DENVER ARTICULATION SCREENING EXAM
for children 2 1/2 to 6 years of age

NAME

HOSP. NO.

Instructions: Have child repeat each word after
you. Circle the underlined sounds that he pro-
nounces correctly. Total correct sounds is the
Raw Score. Use charts on reverse side to score
results.

ADDRESS

Date: _____ Child's Age: _____ Examiner: _____ Raw Score: _____
Percentile: _____ Intelligibility: _____ Result: _____

1. table	6. zipper	11. sock	16. wagon	21. leaf
2. shirt	7. grapes	12. vacuum	17. gum	22. carrot
3. door	8. flag	13. yarn	18. house	
4. trunk	9. thumb	14. mother	19. pencil	
5. jumping	10. toothbrush	15. twinkle	20. fish	

Intelligibility: (circle one)   1. Easy to understand   3. Not understandable
                                2. Understandable 1/2   4. Can't evaluate
                                   the time.

Comments:

Date: _____ Child's Age: _____ Examiner: _____ Raw Score _____
Percentile: _____ Intelligibility: _____ Result: _____

1. table	6. zipper	11. sock	16. wagon	21. leaf
2. shirt	7. grapes	12. vacuum	17. gum	22. carrot
3. door	8. flag	13. yarn	18. house	
4. trunk	9. thumb	14. mother	19. pencil	
5. jumping	10. toothbrush	15. twinkle	20. fish	

Intelligibility: (circle one)   1. Easy to understand   3. Not understandable
                                2. Understandable 1/2   4. Can't evaluate
                                   the time.

Comments:

Date: _____ Child's Age: _____ Examiner: _____ Raw Score _____
Percentile: _____ Intelligibility: _____ Result: _____

1. table	6. zipper	11. sock	16. wagon	21. leaf
2. shirt	7. grapes	12. vacuum	17. gum	22. carrot
3. door	8. flag	13. yarn	18. house	
4. trunk	9. thumb	14. mother	19. pencil	
5. jumping	10. toothbrush	15. twinkle	20. fish	

Intelligibility: (circle one)   1. Easy to understand   3. Not understandable
                                2. Understandable 1/2   4. Can't evaluate
                                   the time.

Comments:

Copyright 1971. Amelia F. Drumwright   University of Colorado Medical Center

To score DASE words: Note Raw Score for child's performance. Match raw score line (extreme left of chart) with column representing child's age (to the closest previous age group). Where raw score line and age column meet number in that square denotes percentile rank of child's performance when compared to other children that age. Percentiles above heavy line are ABNORMAL percentiles, below heavy line are NORMAL.

PERCENTILE RANK

Raw Score	2.5 yr.	3.0	3.5	4.0	4.5	5.0	5.5	6 years
2	1							
3	2							
4	5							
5	9							
6	16							
7	23							
8	31	2						
9	37	4	1					
10	42	6	2					
11	48	7	4					
12	54	9	6	1	1			
13	58	12	9	2	3	1	1	
14	62	17	11	5	4	2	2	
15	68	23	15	9	5	3	2	
16	75	31	19	12	5	4	3	
17	79	38	25	15	6	6	4	
18	83	46	31	19	8	7	4	
19	86	51	38	24	10	9	5	1
20	89	58	45	30	12	11	7	3
21	92	65	52	36	15	15	9	4
22	94	72	58	43	18	19	12	5
23	96	77	63	50	22	24	15	7
24	97	82	70	58	29	29	20	15
25	99	87	78	66	36	34	26	17
26	99	91	84	75	46	43	34	24
27		94	89	82	57	54	44	34
28		96	94	88	70	68	59	47
29		98	98	94	84	84	77	68
30		100	100	100	100	100	100	100

To Score intelligibility:

	NORMAL	ABNORMAL
2 1/2 years	Understandable 1/2 the time, or, "easy"	Not Understandable
3 years and older	Easy to understand	Understandable 1/2 time Not understandable

Test Result: 1. NORMAL on Dase and Intelligibility = NORMAL

2. ABNORMAL on Dase and/or Intelligibility = ABNORMAL

* If abnormal on initial screening rescreen within 2 weeks. If abnormal again child should be referred for complete speech evaluation.

Copyright 1971. Amelia F. Drumwright   University of Colorado Medical Center

K8—PSYCHOSOCIAL SCREENING TESTS COMMONLY USED IN CHILDHOOD

Test name	Quality measured	Child's age	Comments
Bayley Scales of Infant Development (California First Year Mental Scale)*	Mental age	1 mo-3½ yr	Developed and used in the famous longitudinal Berkeley Growth Studies, which began in the 1930s. Heavily based on the Gesell Developmental Schedules.
The Blacky Pictures	Psychosexual adjustment; personality traits	3 or 4 yr-adult	A projective test consisting of 10 cards with cartoonish pictures of a dog (Blacky) in interactions with parents and siblings and in other everyday situations (eating, etc.) Child is asked to tell a story about each picture. Story content ostensibly reveals child's attitudes, fears, jealousies, aggressive tendencies, etc.
Cattell Infant Intelligence Scale*	Mental age, IQ	2-30 mo	Often considered the best of the infant IQ tests. Developed as a downward extension of the Stanford-Binet.
Children's Apperception Test (CAT)	Psychosexual adjustment; personality traits	3-10 yr	A projective test of 10 cards with drawings of young animals usually interacting with, watching, or being watched by adult animals (young dog being spanked by female adult dog in bathroom, young rabbit alone in crib in darkened room, baby bear and adult bear engaged in tug-of-war with another adult bear, etc.). Child is asked to tell a story about each picture. Story content ostensibly reveals child's attitudes, fears, jealousies, aggressive tendencies, etc. A supplemental form (CAT-S) includes some pictures related to health situations (young rabbit being examined by rabbit doctor, young kangaroo with bandaged leg and tail.
Gesell Developmental Schedules*	Developmental quotient (DQ)	1 mo-3 yr	One of the earliest developmental tests (devised in the 1920s), widely adapted in several subsequent tests. Includes motor, adaptive, language, and personal-social behavior. Test items much like those of Denver Developmental Screening Test. No longer in widespread use.
Goodenough-Harris Drawing Test	IQ	3-12 yr	Originally the Goodenough Draw-A-Man (1926), this revised and restandardized version asks a child to make 3 drawings—a man, a woman, and a representation of self. Test interpretation is based on the fact that children use more detail in their human figure drawings as they grow older. This revision is reportedly more accurate than the Draw-A-Man but lacks the older test's ease and simplicity of scoring. Should be used as a screening test only, not as means to diagnose retardation or acceleration.
House-Tree-Person Test (H-T-P)	Psychosexual adjustment; personality traits	4 yr-adult	Child is asked to make 3 separate drawings—a house, a tree, and a person. The tester notes the style and order of parts drawn, omissions, comments made while drawing, size, etc. The house is said to represent the home and family relationships; the tree, perceptions about oneself and relationship to the environment; and the person, either one's ideal (wished-for) self or a significant other.
Merrill-Palmer Scale	Mental age, percentile, standard score	2-6 yr	Predominantly a performance test (peg board, form board, building blocks, jigsaw puzzle, buttons and buttonhole, etc.) with some verbal tasks ("What does a doggie say?" "What flies?" . . . swims? . . . bites?" etc.) Many test items are timed. An interesting and attractive test to most children—examination goes at a fast pace and test items come packaged in individual, colored boxes.

From Barnard, M.U., et al.: Handbook of comprehensive pediatric nursing, New York, 1981, McGraw-Hill Book Co., p. 113.

*Mental age and IQ measurements of children under 4 years are poor predictors of mental age and IQ at later ages. To some extent this is because tests for young children must rely heavily upon motor skills, whereas "intelligence" as measured in older children and adults is a different highly verbal and cognitive phenomenon.

Test name	Quality measured	Child's age	Comments
Minnesota Pre-school Scale	IQ	1½-6 yr	Includes a verbal IQ test and a nonverbal test. Verbal items include naming objects, telling what is happening in a picture, pointing to pictured objects and body parts, vocabulary questions, digit span questions, problem-solving about everyday situations ("What should you do when you are hungry?", etc.). Nonverbal items include copying geometric shapes, block building, picture puzzles, spatial arrangements, etc.
Peabody Picture Vocabulary Test*	Mental age, IQ, percentile	2½ yr-adult	Vocabulary is tested against age norms as a measure of mental age and IQ. Test consists of a booklet of pictures given to the child (there are 4 drawings on each page) and a list of vocabulary words read to the child (one word to go with each page). As the word is read for each page, the child is instructed to print to (or otherwise signify) the one of the 4 drawings that best matches the word. As an IQ test for young children, should be considered a screening instrument only.
The Quick Test (QT)	Mental age, IQ after 20 years of age	1½ yr-adult	Designed to provide a rough estimate (screening) of IQ in childhood, although IQs vary from those provided by general intelligence tests. Child is asked to indicate which of 4 pictures on a page best matches a spoken vocabulary word.
Rorschach Test	Psychosexual adjustment; personality traits	3 or 4 yr-adult	The famous and controversial projective test utilizing inkblots to study personality and diagnose psychiatric disorders. Child is shown a series of 10 cards, each with a bilaterally symmetrical inkblot, and is asked to describe what the picture could represent (what he or she "sees" in it). Content of reports is analyzed, along with child's emotional responses, incidental remarks, etc.
Slosson Intelligence Test*	IQ	1 mo-adult	Largely similar to the Gesell Developmental Schedules for young children and to the Stanford-Binet for older children and adults. A convenient, brief, screening test for children from 4 years on.
Stanford-Binet Intelligence Scale*	IQ	2 yr-adult	The original (although much revised) IQ test, generally considered the most accurate and the standard by which other tests are evaluated. Test items include eye-hand coordination and manipulation tasks (blocks, form board, beads for stringing, etc.), object identification, identification of missing parts of pictures, problem solving in everyday situations ("What should you do if . . . ?"), recognition of absurdities in stories or pictures, memory tests, etc., and extend upward through the range of verbal, computational, and logical problems for older children and adults.
Vineland Social Maturity Scale	Independence (self-reliance)	Birth to adult	Information about self-help skills and responsibility for self-care is gathered either from an adult who knows the child well or from the child. Scale items include, for example, reach, grasp, large motor mobility, following instructions, chewing food, using eating utensils, dressing and undressing, toileting, using writing utensils, bathing, routine household chores, reading and letter writing, and money management. Social age and social quotient are calculated by comparing child to age norms.
Wechsler Intelligence Scale for Children (WISC)	IQ	5-15 yr	WISC has verbal and performance subtests and produces verbal, performance, and full-scale IQs. Items include digit span, vocabulary, arithmetic, general information and comprehension, mazes, picture completion, picture puzzles, etc. Scores for average and above-average children are generally a few points higher than Stanford Binet scores.
Wechsler Preschool and Primary Scale of Intelligence (WPPSI)	IQ	4-6½ yr	WPPSI is a downward extension of WISC and is of similar format. Also generally produces higher scores than the Stanford-Binet.

K9—DEVELOPMENT CHARACTERISTICS: SUMMARY FOR ALL AGES

Waechter developmental guide: the first year

Age	Physical and motor development	Intellectual development	Socialization and vocalization	Emotional development
1 month	Physiologically more stable than in new-born period Wave hands as clenched fists Objects placed in hands are dropped immediately Momentary visual fixation on objects and human face Tonic neck reflex position frequent and Moro reflex brisk Able to turn head when prone, but unable to support head Responds to sounds of bell, rattle, etc. Makes crawling motions when prone Sucking and rooting reflex present Coordinates sucking, swallowing, and breathing	Reflexive No attempt to interact with environment External stimuli do not have meaning	Cries, mews, and makes throaty noises Responds in terms of internal need states Interested in the human face	Response limited generally to tension states Panic reactions, with arching of back and extension and flexion of extremities Derives satisfaction from the feeding situation when held and pleasure from rocking, cuddling, and tactile stimulation Maximum need for sucking pleasures Quiets when picked up
2 months	Moro reflex still brisk Posture still toward tonic neck reflex position Has visual response to patterns Eye coordination to light and objects Follows objects vertically and horizontally Responds to objects placed on face Listens actively to sounds Able to lift head momentarily from prone position Turns from side to back Able to swallow pureed foods	Recognition of familiar face Indicates inspection of the environment Begins to show anticipation before feeding	Begins to vocalize; coos Beginning of social smile Actively follows movement of familiar person or object with eyes Crying becomes differentiated Vocalizes to mother's voice Visually searches to locate sounds of mother's voice	Maximum need for sucking pleasures Indicates more active satisfaction when fed, held, rocked

From Waechter, E.H., and Blake, F.G.: Nursing care of children, ed. 9, Philadelphia, 1976, J.B. Lippincott Co.

Waechter developmental guide: the first year—cont'd

Age	Physical and motor development	Intellectual development	Socialization and vocalization	Emotional development
3 months	Frequency of tonic neck reflex position and vigor of Moro response rapidly diminishing Uses arms and legs simultaneously but not separately Able to raise head from prone position; may get chest off bed Holds head in fairly good control Begins differentiation of motor responses Hands are beginning to open, and objects placed in hands are retained for brief inspection; able to carry objects to mouth Indicates preference for prone or supine position "Stepping" reflex disappears Landau reflex appears Eyes converge as objects approach face Has necessary muscular control to accept cereal and fruit	Shows active interest in environment Can recognize familiar faces and objects such as bottle; however, objects do not have permanence Recognition is indicative of recording of memory traces Begins playing with parts of body Follows objects visually Begins to be able to coordinate stimuli from various sense organs Shows awareness of a strange situation	More ready and responsive smile Facial and generalized body response to faces Preferential response to adult voices Has longer periods of wakefulness without crying Begins to use prelanguage vocalizations, babbling and cooing Laughs aloud and shows pleasure in vocalization Shows anticipatory preparation to being lifted Turns head to follow familiar person Ceases crying when mother enter the room	Maximum need for sucking pleasure Wishes to avoid unpleasant situations Not yet able to act independently to evoke response in others
4 months	Ability to carry objects to mouth Inspects and plays with hands Grasps objects with both hands Turns head to sound of bell or bottle Reaches for offered objects Eyes focus on small objects Begins to demonstrate eye-hand coordination Ability to pick up objects Rooting reflex disappears; tonic neck reflex disappearing	Recognizes bottle on sight Becomes bored when left alone for long periods of time Actively interested in environment Indicates beginnings of intentionality and interest in affecting the environment Indicates beginning anticipation of consequences of action	Vocalizes frequently and vocalizations change according to mood Begins to respond to "no, no" Enjoys being propped in a sitting position Turns head to familiar noise Chuckles socially Demands attention by fussing; enjoys attention	Interest in mother heightens Is affable and lovable Shows signs of increasing trust and security

Continued.

Waechter developmental guide: the first year—cont'd

Age	Physical and motor development	Intellectual development	Socialization and vocalization	Emotional development
4 months—cont'd	Sits with minimum support with stable head and back Turns from back to side Breathing and mouth activity coordination in relation to vocal cords Holds head up when pulled to sitting position Begins to drool			
5 months	Ability to recover near objects Reaches persistently Grasps with whole hand Ability to lift objects Begins to use thumb and finger in "pincer" movement Able to sustain visual inspection Able to sit for longer periods of time when well supported Begins to show signs of tooth eruption Ability to sleep through night without feeding Moro reflex and tonic neck reflex finally disappear	Able to discriminate strangers from family Turns head after fallen object Shows active interest in novelty Attempts to regain interesting action in environment Ability to coordinate visual impressions of an object Begins differentiation of self from environment	Enjoys play with people and objects Smiles at mirror image More exuberantly playful but also more touchy and discriminating	Other members of the family become important as the baby's emotional world expands Begins to be able to postpone gratification Awaits anticipated routines with happy expectation Begins to explore mother's body
6 months	Ability to pick up small objects directly and deftly Ability to lift cup by handle Grasps, holds, and manipulates objects Ability to pull self to sitting position Begins to "hitch" in locomotion Momentary sitting and hand support When lying in prone position, supports weight with hands Weight gain begins to decline Ability to turn completely over	Increasing awareness of self Responds with attentiveness to novel stimuli Begins to be able to recognize mother when she is dressed differently Objects begin to acquire permanence; searches for lost object for brief period	Very interested in sound production Playful response to mirror Laughs aloud when stimulated Great interest in babbling, which is self-reinforcing Begins to recognize strangers	Begins to have sense of "self" Increased growth of ego

Waechter developmental guide: the first year—cont'd

Age	Physical and motor development	Intellectual development	Socialization and vocalization	Emotional development
7 months	Ability to transfer objects from one hand to another Holds object in one hand Gums or mouths solid foods; exploratory behavior with food Ability to bang objects together Palmar grasp disappears Bears weight when held in standing position Sits alone for brief periods Rolls over adeptly	Ability to secure objects by pulling on string Repeats activities that are enjoyed Discovers and plays with own feet Drops and picks up objects in exploration Searches for lost objects outside perceptual field Has consciousness of desires Growing differentiation of self from environment Rudimentary sense of depth and space	Vocalizes four different syllables Produces vowel sounds and chained syllables Makes "talking sounds" in response to the talking of others Crows and squeals	Begins to show signs of fretfulness when mother leaves or in presence of strangers Shows beginning fear of strangers Orally aggressive in biting and mouthing
8 months	Ability to ring bell purposively Ability to feed self with finger foods Begins to experience tooth eruption Sits well alone Ability to release objects at will	Uncovers hidden toy Increased interest in feeding self Differentiation of means from end in intentionality Has lively curiosity about the world	Listens selectively to familiar words Says "da da" or equivalent Babbles to produce consonant sounds Vocalizes to toys Stretches out arms to be picked up	Plays for sheer pleasure of the activity Anxiety when confronted by strangers indicates recognition and need of mother; attachment behavior begins to be obvious and strong
9 months	Rises to sitting position Creeps and/or crawls; maybe backward at first Tries out newly developing motor capacities Ability to hold own bottle Drinks from cup or glass with assistance Begins to show regular patterns in bladder and bowel elimination Good ability to use thumb and finger in pincer grasp Pulls self to feet with help	Ability to put objects in container Examines object held in hand; explores objects by sucking, chewing, and biting	Responds to simple verbal requests Plays interactive games, such as peek-a-boo and patty cake	Mother is increasingly important for her own sake; reacts violently to threat of her loss Begins to show fears of going to bed and being left alone Increasing interest in pleasing mother Active search in play for solutions to separation anxiety

Continued.

Waechter developmental guide: the first year—cont'd

Age	Physical and motor development	Intellectual development	Socialization and vocalization	Emotional developmental
10 months	Ability to unwrap objects Pulls to standing position Uses index finger to poke and finger and thumb to hold objects Finger feeds self; controls lips around cup Plantar reflex disappears Neck-righting reflex disappears Sits without support; recovers balance easily Pulls self upright with use of furniture	Begins to imitate Looks at and follows pictures in book	Extends toy to another person without releasing Responds to own name Inhibits behavior to "no, no" or own name Begins to test reactions to parental responses during feeding and at bedtime Imitates facial expressions and sounds	Has powerful urge toward independence in locomotion, feeding; beginning to help in dressing Experiences joy when achieving a goal and mastering fear
11 months	Ability to hold crayon adaptively Ability to push toys Ability to put several objects in container; releases objects at will Stands with assistance; may be beginning attempts to walk with assistance Begins to be able to hold spoon "Cruises" around furniture	Works to get toy out of reach Growing interest in novelty Heightened curiosity and drive to explore environment	Repeats performance laughed at by others Imitates definite speech sounds Uses jargon Communicates by pointing to objects wanted	Reacts to restrictions with frustration, but has ability to master new situations with mother's help (weaning)

Waechter developmental guide: the first year—cont'd

Age	Physical and motor development	Intellectual development	Socialization and vocalization	Emotional development
12 months	Turns pages in book; can make marks on paper Babinski sign disappears Begins standing alone and toddling "Cruises" around furniture Lumbar curve develops Hand dominance becomes evident Ability to use spoon in feeding	Dogged determination to remove barriers to action Further separation of means from ends Experiments to reach goals not attained previously Concepts of space, time, and causality begin to have more objectivity	Jabbers expressively Has words that are specific to parents Few, simple words Experimentation with "pseudo-words" of great interest and pleasure	Ability to show emotions of fear, anger, affection, jealousy, anxiety Is in love with the world
15-18 months	Uses spoon and cup with little spilling; builds 2-cube tower; can undress; has refined pincer grasp	Stoops and recovers; walks well; pushes furniture to climb; walks up stairs one at a time with assistance	Rolls ball back and forth with 1 other person; imitates household chores; indicates desires without crying; drinks from a cup	Vocabulary of 10 to 20 words; understands simple questions; forms 2-word phrases; beginning to name pictures
2 years	Builds a 6-cube tower; turns pages of a book one at a time; begins to dress self; washes and dries hands	Runs; walks up and down stairs alone; walks backwards; jumps in place; throws ball overhand	Removes clothes; awareness of ownership; helps out; eats with family but cannot sit through entire meal	Points to body parts; has 300-400 word vocabulary; uses "my" pronouns and prepositions; forms 3- to 4-word phrases
3 years	Opens and closes doors using knob by self; uses fingers to hold pencil; builds 8- to 10-block tower; zips zippers; does simple buttoning	Walks up and down stairs alternating feet; rides tricycle; broad jumps; dresses with assistance	May have imaginary playmates; can put on simple garment; washes and dries hands; likes to have a choice	Uses plurals; forms 3- to 4-word sentences, using correct grammatical structures
4 years	Draws a 3-part man; buttons easily; can cut out pictures	Catches ball with hands; broad jumps; climbs up and down stairs, alternating feet; balances on one foot momentarily	Separates easily from mother; can button clothing; plays interactive and associative games, demonstrating some control; able to share	Comprehends and uses opposites; has increased vocabulary and about 90% comprehensibility; speaks in full sentences, using prepositions, pronouns, adverbs, and adjectives
5 years	Copies a square accurately; draws a 5-part man; begins to tie shoelaces	Runs with speed and agility; dresses without supervision; skips crudely	Developing attachment outside of family; engages in cooperative play; strives for independence	Vocabulary expanding to 3-syllable words; composition increasing to spoken paragraphs

K10—DEVELOPMENTAL BEHAVIORS: SCHOOL AGE CHILD

Age (years)	Physical competency	Intellectual competency	Emotional-social competency	Play	Safety
6-12 (General)	Gains an average of 2.5-3.2 kg/year (5½-7 lb/yr). Overall height gains of 5.5 cm (2 in) per year; growth occurs in spurts and is mainly in trunk and extremities. Loses deciduous teeth; most of permanent teeth erupt. Progressively more coordinated in both gross and fine motor skills. Caloric needs increase with growth spurts.	Masters concrete operations. Moves from egocentrism; learns he is not always right. Learns grammar and expression of emotions and thoughts. Vocabulary increases to 3000 words or more; handles complex sentences.	Central crisis: industry vs. inferiority; wants to do and make things. Progressive sex education needed. Wants to be like friends; competition important. Fears body mutilation, alterations in body image; earlier phobias may recur, nightmares; fears death. Nervous habits common.	Plays in groups, mostly of same sex; "gang" activities predominate. Books for all ages. Bicycles a must. Sports equipment. Cards, board, and table games. Most of play is active games requiring little or no equipment.	Enforce continued use of safety belts during car travel. Bicycle safety must be taught and enforced. Teach safety related to hobbies, handicrafts, mechanical equipment.
6-7	Depth perception developed. Vision reaches adult level of 20/20. Gross motor skill exceeds fine motor coordination. Balance and rhythm are good—runs, skips, jumps, climbs, gallops. Throws and catches ball. Dresses self with little or no help.	Vocabulary of 2500 words. Learning to read and print; beginning concrete concepts of numbers, general classification of items. Knows concepts of right and left; morning, afternoon, and evening; coinage. Intuitive thought process. Verbally aggressive, bossy, opinionated, argumentative. Likes simple games with basic rules.	Boisterous, outgoing, and know-it-all, whiney; parents should sidestep power struggles, offer choices. Becomes quiet and reflective during 7th year; very sensitive. Can use telephone. Likes to make things; starts many, finishes few. Give some responsibility for household duties.	Still enjoys dolls, cars, and trucks. Plays well alone but enjoys small groups of both sexes; begins to prefer same sex peer during seventh year. Ready to learn how to ride a bicycle. Prefers imaginary, dramatic play with real costumes. Begins collecting for quantity, not quality. Enjoys active games such as hide-and-seek, tag, jump rope, roller skating, kickball. Ready for lessons in dancing, gymnastics, music. Restrict TV time to 1-2 hours/day.	Teach and reinforce traffic safety. Still needs adult supervision of play. Teach to avoid strangers, never take anything from strangers. Teach cold prevention and reinforce continued practice of other health habits. Restrict bicycle use to home ground; no traffic areas; teach bicycle safety. Teach and set examples regarding harmful use of drugs, alcohol, smoking.

Age	Physical	Mental/Language	Social	Play/Activities	Safety
8-10	Myopia may appear. Secondary sex characteristics begin in girls. Hand-eye coordination and fine motor skills well established. Movements are graceful, coordinated. Cares for own physical needs completely. Constantly on move; plays and works hard; enforce balance in rest and activity. Vision and hearing fully developed.	Learning correct grammar and to express feelings in words. Likes books he can read by himself; will read funny papers, scan newspaper. Enjoys making detailed drawings. Mastering classification, seriation, spatial and temporal, numerical concepts. Uses language as a tool; likes riddles, jokes, chants, word games. Rules guiding force in life now. Very interested in how things work, what and how weather, seasons, etc., are made.	Strong preference for same-sex peers; antagonizes opposite-sex peers. Self-assured and pragmatic at home; questions parental values and ideas. Has a strong sense of humor. Enjoys clubs, group projects, outings, large groups, campings. Modesty about own body increases over time; sex conscious. Works diligently to perfect skills he does best. Happy, cooperative, relaxed and casual in relationships. Increasingly courteous and well-mannered with adults. Gang stage at a peak; secret codes and rituals prevail. Responds better to suggestion than dictatorial approach.	Likes hiking, sports. Enjoys cooking, woodworking, crafts. Enjoys cards and table games. Likes radio and records. Begins qualitative collecting now. Continue restriction on TV time.	Stress safety with firearms. Keep them out of reach and allow use only with adult supervision. Know who the child's friends are; parents should still have some control over friend selection. Teach water safety; swimming should be supervised by an adult.
11-12	Vital signs approximate adult norms. Growth spurt for girls; inequalities between sexes increasingly noticeable; boys attain greater physical strength. Eruption of permanent teeth complete except for third molars. Secondary sex characteristics begin in boys. Menstruation may begin.	Able to think about social problems and prejudices; sees others' points of view. Enjoys reading mysteries, love stories. Begins playing with abstract ideas. Interested in whys of health measures and understands human reproduction. Very moralistic; religious commitment often made during this time.	Intense team loyalty; boys begin teasing girls and girls flirt with boys for attention; best friend period. Wants unreasonable independence. Rebellious about routines; wide mood swings; needs some times daily for privacy. Very critical of own work. Hero worship prevails. "Facts of life" chats with friends prevail; masturbation increases. Appears under constant tension.	Enjoys projects and working with hands. Likes to do errands and jobs to earn money. Very involved in sports, dancing, talking on phone. Enjoys all aspects of acting and drama.	Continue monitoring friends; Stress bicycle safety on streets and in traffic.

Adapted from Smith, E.C.: Growth and development of school age child: maintaining wellness. In Tackett, J.J., and Hunsberger, M., editors: Family centered care of children and adolescents, Philadelphia, 1981, W.B. Saunders Co., pp. 1086-1087.

K11—ACNE ASSESSMENT QUESTIONNAIRE
History

1. How long have you had acne? _____
2. Did your parents or siblings have acne? _____
   How long? _____
3. Are there seasonal variations in your skin? _____
   What kind? _____
4. Do you find sunlight is beneficial? _____
   Do you use a sunlamp? _____
5. Do you rub your face often? _____
6. Do you use sweatbands? _____ Football helmet? ____
   Shoulderpads? _____ Tight collars or turtlenecks? ____
   Tight hats? _____
   _____
7. Describe changes, if there are any, in your skin that
   accompany your menstrual period.
8. Are there certain foods that aggravate your skin? ____
   If so, list them: _____ What happens? _____
9. Do you feel guilty when you eat certain foods? _____
10. Do your parents and/or friends say eating affects the
    skin? _____

Hygiene

1. How often do you wash your face? _____
2. What kind of soap: _____ What kind of shampoo and
   how often? _____
   _____
3. How do you wash your face? _____
4. After washing, does your face feel clean? _____ How
   long do you feel clean? _____
5. Do your parents nag you about washing? _____
6. How often do you pick your pimples? _____ With what?
   _____
7. What kind of cosmetics do you use? _____ Any mois-
   turizing cream or lotion? _____
8. Do you use pomade on your hair? _____

Medical

1. Have you ever used medication for your skin? _____ If
   so, what have you used? _____ Results? _____
   What are you currently using? _____ What is
   the dose and how often do you use it? _____ Who
   selected the present treatment? _____
2. List any other medications you take (including birth
   control pills and over-the-counter preparations). _____
   _____
3. Name any other medical problems. _____

Social

1. What is your occupation? _____
2. How many are in your family? _____ Whom do you
   live with? _____
3. How do you spend leisure time? _____ Favorite
   hobby? _____
4. If in school, are you satisfied with your performance
   there? _____

From Stone, A.C.: Facing up to acne, Pediat. Nurs. 8:229-237, July-
Aug. 1982, p. 231.

5. Whom are you emotionally closest to? _____ What do
   they say about your skin? _____
6. Describe any changes, if there are any, in your skin
   when you're upset. _____
   _____
7. Most teen-agers have acne. (True—False)
8. Masturbation has no effect on acne. (True—False)
9. Dirty thoughts cause acne. (True—False)
10. My skin makes my life harder. (True—False)
11. I believe I will be successful no matter how I look.
    (True—False)
12. Clear skin is necessary to be really happy. (True—
    False)
13. What do your parents and friends say cause acne? ____
14. What bothers you most about your body? _____ If you
    could change your body, what would you do first?
    _____
15. Do friends tease you about your skin? _____
16. Name something you are good at doing. _____

K12—SOURCES OF SCREENING AND ASSESSMENT TOOLS

AAMD Adaptive Behavior Scale for Children and Adults,
1974 Revision
AAMD Adaptive Behavior Scale Public School Version
  Source: American Association for Mental Deficiencies
           5101 Wisconsin Avenue, N.W.
           Washington, D.C. 30016
The Denver Developmental Screening Test (DDST) by
  W.K. Frankenberg, J.B. Dodds, A. Fandal, E. Kazuk,
  and M. Cohrs (birth to 6 years)
  Source: LADOCA Project and Publishing Foundation
           East 51st Avenue and Lincoln Street
           Denver, CO 80216
The Developmental Profile II by G.D. Alpern, T.J. Boll,
  and M.S. Shearer (birth to age 9)
  Source: Psychological Development Publications
           P.O. Box 3198
           Aspen, CO 81612
Education for Multi-handicapped Infants (EMI)
  Source: Department of Pediatrics
           University of Virginia
           Box 232
           Charlottesville, VA 22908
Home Observation for Measurement of the Environment
  (HOME), B. Caldwell (birth to 3 years, 3-6 years)
  Source: Center for Early Development and Education
           University of Arkansas
           814 Sherman Street
           Little Rock, AR 72202
Meeting Street School Screening Test—Early Identification
  of Children with Learning Disabilities, P.K. Hainsworth
  and M.L. Siqueland (5 years to 7 years, 6 months)
  Source: Crippled Children and Adults of Rhode Island,
           Inc.
           Meeting Street School
           333 Grotto School
           Providence, RI 02906

Nursing Child Assessment Satellite Training Developed by
K. Barnard
Source: Georgina Sumner
NCAST
WJ-10
University of Washington
Seattle, WA 98195

Peabody Individual Achievement Test (PIAT), L.M. Dunn
and F.C. Markwardt, (2 years, 6 months to 18 years)
Source: American Guidance Service, Inc.
Circle Pines, MN 55014

The Portage Guide to Early Education, S. Blumar
The Portage Project; Cooperative Educational Service—
Agency Twelve
Source: The Portage Project
412 East Slifer Street
Portage, WI 53901

Slosson Intelligence Test (SIT), R.L. Slosson (birth to adult)
Source: Western Psychological Services
Publishers and Distributors
12031 Wilshire Boulevard
Los Angeles, CA 90025

Vineland Social Maturity Scale, E.A. Doll (birth to adult)
Source: American Guidance Services, Inc.
Circle Pines, MN 55014

Washington Guide to Child Development
Source: Utah Department of Health
Family Health Services Division
Bureau of Maternal and Child Health
44 Medical Drive
Salt Lake City, UT 84113

GLOSSARY

acceptant intervention Consultative mode of client intervention that is a process of catharsis intended to clear emotional blocks in order to engage in objective problem solving.

accommodation Ways in which children modify their view of the world as they have new experiences that influence their responses.

accountability Being answerable to someone for something one has done.

  moral Being answerable to someone for how moral requirements of nursing practice have been carried out.

  legal Being answerable to someone for how legal requirements of nursing practice have been carried out.

accreditation Mechanism for assessing the quality of educational programs.

acculturation Adaptation and incorporation of ideas, values, behaviors, customs, and certain aspects of the majority culture concurrent with maintaining aspects of the traditional or primary culture. Learning one's culture through a process of acquiring knowledge and internalizing values.

achievable age Risk age, expressed in years, individuals can attain if they comply with suggested medical therapies and life-style changes. Synonymous with survival advantage and compliance age.

acid rain The precipitation of moisture, as rain, with high acidity caused by release of pollutants into the atmosphere.

acquired immune deficiency syndrome (AIDS) Disease involving a defect in cell-mediated immunity that has a long incubation period, follows a protracted and debilitating course, and has a poor prognosis; transmitted through sexual contact, exposure to contaminated blood, or possibly close personal contact.

active immunization Administration of all or part of a microorganism to stimulate active response by the host's immunological system, resulting in complete protection against a specific disease.

acupressure Form of stress reduction whereby selected metabolic and circulatory processes are stimulated by finger pressure on certain points of the body.

acupuncture Insertion of needles into selected parts of the body to control pain.

adaptation change or response to stress of any kind; may be normal, self-protective, or developmental.

adolescence A time of discovery of self, of feelings, and of the complexities of society that usually occurs between the ages of 13 and 18 years; the period of psychological maturation.

administrator One who manipulates the resources within an organization to meet the organizational goals.

administrative law Branch of law dealing with organs of government power; prescribes the manner of their activity (state board of nurse examiners, for example).

adrenocorticotropic hormone (ACTH) Hormone of the anterior pituitary gland that stimulates the growth of the adrenal gland cortex and the secretion of corticosteroids.

adult day care center Congregate facility for activities such as socialization, eating, and supervised care of older adults during specified day hours, with the person returning home for the evening hours.

adult nurse practitioner Registered nurse with additional education through a master's degree program in nursing or through a non-degree or certificate continuing education program preparing the nurse to deliver primary health care to adults.

advanced disease A stage in the natural history of a disease in which sufficient anatomical functional changes have occurred to produce recognizable signs and symptoms.

adversary relationship A situation between two or more persons or groups in which one opposes or resists the efforts of others.

affective disorder One of the most common psychiatric syndromes, essentially of three types: depressive, manic, and bipolar (manic and depressive alterations).

aftercare programs Services provided in the community after hospital discharge that ensure continuity of care and transportation for clients when they return to the hospital for treatment and go home again.

age pattern The ages of siblings, as well as the gap between the ages of the children and the parents.

agent Causative factor invading a susceptible host through a favorable environment to produce disease.

akathisia Inability to sit down because the thought of doing so causes severe anxiety. A feeling of restlessness and an urgent need of movement, with complaints of feelings of muscular quivering.

Alanon Organization of relatives of alcoholic individuals operated in many communities within the structure of Alcoholics Anonymous.

Alateen Self-help program for children of alcoholics; provides a forum for discussing family stressors, learning coping skills, and gaining support and encouragement from knowledgeable peers.

Alcoholics Anonymous Lay, self-help group that practices a 12-step approach to recovery.

algorithms See protocol.

Alzheimer's disease Presenile dementia, characterized by confusion, memory failure, disorientation, restlessness, agnosia, and speech disturbances.

analysis Fourth level of cognitive learning; requires the learner to break down communication into constituent parts to distinguish between the parts and understand the relationship among them.

analytic epidemiology Second stage of epidemiological investigation; focuses on testing etiological hypotheses using observational studies

anaphylaxis Exaggerated hypersensitivity to a previously encountered antigen; reaction ranges from a generalized itching to severe vascular collapse.

andragogy Helping people learn.

Antabuse Drug used as a deterrent to alcohol consumption; when alcohol and Antabuse are mixed, the person experiences a variety of unpleasant physiological reactions.

anthrax Illness with varying symptoms caused by a spore-forming organism. May be endemic to many agricultural areas.

anticholinergic Impeding the impulses or action of the fibers of the parasympathetic nerves; providing cholinergic blocking action.

anticipatory guidance Providing advice to clients before an event and discussing potential problems or risks so clients will be aware and may be able to prevent the occurrence of the problem.

antipsychotics Drugs effective in controlling psychotic behaviors.

anorexia nervosa Syndrome marked by severe and prolonged inability to eat, marked weight loss, amenorrhea and other symptoms resulting from emotional conflict and biological changes.

antitoxin Solution of antibodies derived from the serum of animals immunized with specific antigens (e.g., diphtheria, tetanus); used to achieve passive immunity.

Apgar scoring A tool used to score neonatal physiological functioning at birth. The newborn characteristics of appearance, pulse, grimace, activity, and respirations are observed and scored.

appeal Complaint to a superior court to reverse or correct an injustice or alleged error committed by an inferior court.

appellate court Court where judgments of trial courts are reviewed or appealed.

application Third level of cognitive learning; the learner takes the information provided and uses it in new, particular, and concrete situations.

appraised age Total health risk, expressed in years, of an individual. Determined by adjusting the average risk of death from selected causes for the individual's age, sex, and racial group to his own risk.

appropriations Actual amounts of money approved for a program authorized by law.

artificial acquired immunity Immune state that results from immunization or vaccination for a specific disease.

ascariasis (roundworm infection) Infection caused by a parasitic worm, *Ascario lumbriacoides,* that migrates through the lungs in its larval stage; symptoms are coughing, wheezing, and fever.

assertiveness training Teaching people how to honestly and directly express themselves by identifying what is blocking such behavior and by setting goals for increasing personal assertive behavior.

assessment of community resources Procedure similar to the process used on behalf of individual clients. The scope of the investigation is more detailed and includes examination of data from health planning groups, including the number of public health facilities, availability of health personnel, availability of funds, and a multitude of other statistics, such as those on mortality and morbidity.

assessment of need Verifying and mapping out the extent and location of a problem and its attendant target population.

assimilation Process of a minority group becoming absorbed into the dominant or majority culture by adopting its behaviors. Also, the process of a child's responding to the environment in accordance with his cognitive structures so that elements in the environment are incorporated into his cognitive structures.

atropine psychosis Produced by excessive anticholinergic agent usage.

attack rates Special rates expressing incidence of a disease.

attributable risk Statistical measure that estimates the reduction in the occurrence of a particular disease, which could be affected by elimination of a specific causal agent.

attribute Any physical, psychological, or social characteristic describing an individual.

audit process A six-step process used concurrently or retrospectively for nursing peer review.

authorization Process of placing a ceiling on money to be requested for a program.

autoimmunity Abnormal condition in which body reacts against parts of its own tissues.

autonomy Freedom of action as chosen by an individual.

autonomic nervous system The part of the nervous system that regulates involuntary functioning, including cardiac muscle, smooth muscle, and the glands.

aversive techniques A form of behavior therapy whereby an unpleasant stimuli, such as drugs of electric shock, are used to suppress undesirable behavior.

battered women Women who are physically and/or emotionally abused by a spouse.

battery Committing bodily harm.

BCG vaccines Several different vaccines that vary in their ability to induce active immunity and therefore prevent tuberculosis.

belief statements Statements of beliefs persons hold as true, but which may or may not be based on empirical evidence.

benefit schedule A list of services with monetary values attached by insurers that specifies the amount the insurer will pay for the services.

benzodiazepines Group of chemically related antianxiety drugs.

bicultural The straddling of two cultures, lifestyles, and sets of values.

biofeedback Process in which delicate physiological monitoring instruments serve as teaching tools by helping people become aware of and learn to consciously control many physiological variables previously thought to be automatic.

biological hazards Disease-producing agents primarily consisting of bacteria, viruses, and other microorganisms and parasites.

biological health Level of physical fitness.

biological plausibility A reasonable physiological mechanism to explain how a causal factor could operate to bring about a particular disease.

"black lung" Disease, common among coal miners, characterized by a large solid black lung mass; caused by deposits of black mining dust in the lungs.

bonding The synchronization of maternal and infant responses, which results in a unique emotional relationship.

breach of contract Unjustified failure to perform the terms of a contract as agreed on or when performance is due.

brucellosis Infectious disease of nonhuman mammals, which is contagious to humans.

botulism Often fatal form of blood poisoning caused by an endotoxin produced by the bacillus *Clostridium botulinum.*

bulimia Insatiable craving for food, often resulting in episodes of continuous eating followed by periods of depression and self-denial.

byssinosis Type of lung disease common among cotton mill workers; similar to nonoccupational bronchitis.

carbon monoxide Colorless, odorless, poisonous gas produced by the combustion of carbon or organic fuels in a limited oxygen supply.

carboxyhemoglobin Formed when carbon monoxide bumps oxygen molecules out of red blood cells.

carcinogenic agent Single cancer-inducing substance that triggers the change in behavior of cells, resulting in uncontrolled growth.

caretakers Those persons, professional and non-professional, who provide for the social and health needs of others.

case finding Careful, systematic observations of people to identify with present or potential problems.

case law Decisions by the courts; judicial opinions.

case register Systematic registration of acute, chronic, and contagious diseases.

case study A written analysis of program development and implementation throughout the life of the program. An historical depiction of the program.

catalyst A person who promotes activities of others by assisting clients in becoming involved.

catalytic intervention mode Situation whereby the consultant assists clients to broaden their view of an existing situation by gaining additional information or by unifying existing data.

catchment area Designated service area for a community mental health center, consisting of between 75,000 and 200,000 people.

causality Relating of causes to the effects they produce.

cause of action Averment of allegations or facts sufficient for defendant to respond.

census data Composite data on the population of states, local and political jurisdictions, and census tracts in organized areas provided by the federal government.

Centers for Disease Control Branch of the U.S. Public Health Service whose primary responsibility is to propose, coordinate, and evaluate changes in the surveillance of disease in the United States.

cerebral palsy Chronic nonprogressive disorders of the brain occurring in infants and young children and producing abnormalities of posture and motor function (significant developmental motor disability).

certificate of need Determination in any given community of the need for new health care facilities on the basis of the currently available resources and the anticipated demands for use.

certification One mechanism, usually by means of written examination, that provides an indication of professional competence in a specialized area of practice.

charter Mechanism by which a state government agency under state laws grants corporate status to institutions with or without rights to award degrees.

chemical additive contamination Contamination of food, either deliberately or incidentally, by chemical additives.

child abuse Active forms of maltreatment of children.

child neglect Physical or emotional. Physical neglect refers to failure to provide adequate food, clothing, shelter, hygiene, or necessary medical care, whereas emotional neglect refers to the omission of basic nurturing, acceptance, and caring essential for healthy development.

childbirth center Health facility where prenatal care and delivery services are provided to low-risk pregnant women by a team of nurse-midwives, obstetricians, pediatricians, and ancillary health personnel.

chiropractic System of manipulative treatment, which teaches that all diseases are caused by infringement on spinal nerves and can be corrected by spinal adjustments.

Chlamydia A sexually transmitted disease caused by the organism *Chlamydia trachomatis*, known to cause infection and/or inflammation of the genitals in males and females.

chlorine Toxic gas used in the chemical and paper industries.

cirrhosis Chronic degenerative liver disease, often caused by chronic alcohol abuse but can also result from nutritional deprivation, hepatitis, or other infections.

civil law Concerned with the legal rights and duties of private persons.

client-centered therapy Mode of therapy developed by Carl Rogers that emphasizes the client as the central figure in the therapy.

client population Individuals, groups, families, organizations, or communities who are the target persons of the consultant's interventions.

clients' rights Those services, programs, goods, and provider behaviors consumers are entitled to in order to maintain or achieve health, to exist as a human being.

clinical disease Stage in the natural history of a disease; begins when sufficient anatomical or functional changes have occurred to produce recognizable signs and symptoms of a disease.

clinical horizon Imaginary line dividing the point at which there are and are not detectable signs and symptoms of disease.

clinical record A system of collecting information about a client, indicating the extent and quality of services being rendered; commonly referred to as "the chart."

code of ethics Set of statements encompassing rules that apply to people in professional roles.

Code for Nurses The American Nurses Association professional statement prescribing moral behavior and actions of nurses based on moral principles.

coercive health measures Health care treatment and services required regardless of the clients wishes, choices, or life plans. Such care is usually regulated by law and is instituted to protect the public's health.

cognitive-discovery theory Learning associated with the development of thought, language, and intelligence in infants and children.

cognitive learning Acquisition of facts dealing with recall and recognition of information.

cognitive restructuring Strategy of self-modification that depends on rational self-statements and evaluations before or during a given event.

cognitive uncertainty Inability to predict the outcome of a situation because of a lack of available information.

cognitive domain Deals with the recall or recognition of knowledge and the development of intellectual skills.

cohesion Attraction between group members to one another and to the group.

cohort Group of people born during the same era, who are influenced by some of the same biological, psychological, and social factors.

collaboration Mutual sharing and working together to achieve common goals in such a way that all persons or groups are recognized and growth is enhanced.

collaborative practice Professionals working together in a collegial relationship to provide primary health care to a given population.

common fate, principle of Tendency to see objects moving in the same direction as a perceptual unit.

common law Law based on the opinion of the courts, which comes from past court decisions or opinions based on fairness, respect for individuals, autonomy, and self-determination.

communicable disease Disease that is primarily infectious in nature; requires interaction between the host and agent, direct or indirect transmission from the agent reservoir in the environment, and a host that can provide adequate living conditions for the infectious agent.

community A locality-based entity, composed of interdependent systems of formal organizations reflecting societal institutions, informal groups, and aggregates, and whose function or expressed intent is to meet a wide variety of collective needs. The target of community-oriented practice.

community attitudes Information gathered from professionals and lay people who work with health-related services in the community.

community client Target of service; that is, the population group for whom healthful change is sought.

community forum An open meeting for members of a particular community or group to address an issue of interest.

community health Meeting collective needs through problem identifying and managing interactions within the community and larger society. The goal of community-oriented practice.

community health nursing Synthesis of nursing and public health practice applied to promoting and preserving the health of populations. The practice is general and comprehensive, with the dominant responsibility to the population as a whole.

community health services Services directed to meet the needs of groups; tend to reflect a public health orientation of health promotion and maintenance of capabilities.

community health strength or capabilities Resources available to meet a community health need.

community mental health Orientation toward health care that seeks to provide a program of continuing and comprehensive mental health care to a specific population.

community resident survey A direct assessment of the population of a community to identify the need for a service, the acceptability of the service to the population and the willingness of the people to use and pay for the service.

comparative negligence, doctrine of Negligence of the plaintiff is compared with that of the defendant, and apportionment of damages is based on the acts the parties are found to have committed.

compensatory damages Amounts of money for proven loss.

compost Aerobic process whereby bacteria, and especially fungi, feed on organic material; uses a 30:1 carbon-to-nitrogen ratio.

comprehension Second level of cognitive learning; to grasp the meaning of the known information.

Comprehensive Health Planning and Public Health Services Amendments of 1966 (CHP) Emphasized regional planning and represented landmark legislation, the first time each person's "right to health care" was acknowledged.

compromise An agreement between two or more people or groups with goals that cannot be met without modification of the positions of each person or group (implies "give and take" in the negotiating process).

concept Category or class of objects or phenomena that represents either an abstract version of the real world (such as an ideal) or a concrete idea such as a chair or bench.

conceptual framework Group of concepts plus a set of propositions that spell out the relationships between them.

conceptual model Set of concepts and those assumptions that integrate them into a meaningful configuration.

concrete operation Children can think about those things they can see; a level of cognitive development.

concurrent audit A method of evaluating quality of ongoing care through appraisal of the nursing process.

concurrent resolution Document expressing the principles, opinions, and purposes of Congress on matters affecting the operation of both houses. It can originate in either chamber. Concurrent resolutions are not usually legislative in character.

conditioning Strategy for behavior modification that depends on shaping a client's behavior by rewarding changes toward the goal in the intended direction.

confidentiality Controlling the disclosure of personal information and limiting the access of others to sensitive information.

conflict of interest Situation in which there is disparity between the employer policies and the values, beliefs, or feelings of a nurse and/ or client.

conflict sources Factors that may interfere with the relationship or communication between client and nurse.

confounding variables Factors that interact in some unknown way with other factors thought to cause disease.

confrontation intervention Consultant intervention mode that provides for presentation of ideas and facts to the client and reveals the values and assumptions of the client that cannot be disputed.

congenital anomaly Any deviant organ or part existing before or at birth in an abnormal form, structure, or location, but not necessarily detected at birth.

connectionism in stimulus-response theories The connection is the neural joining between a stimulus and the response.

consistency of the association Degree to which findings of various studies investigating the relation between a particular factor and a disease outcome are consistent.

constitutional law Branch of law dealing with organization and function of government.

constraints Problems that could potentially impede the planning of programs to meet consumer needs.

constructs Conceptual components that are not directly observable; deliberately created ideas of references that cannot actually be seen but allow for explanation and analysis.

consultant One who gives professional advice, services, or information.

consultation Interactional or communication process between two or more persons, one of whom is a consultant; the other is considered a consultee. The consultant seeks to help the consultee solve a problem or improve or broaden skills.

consultative contract See contracting.

consultee Person seeking the help of an outside, usually impartial, person in problem resolution.

consumer sovereign power Consumer control in determining the behavior of products.

continuity, principles of Tendency to respond to trends and themes running through a series of objects and to perceive all corresponding to that trend or theme as being part of the same perceptual unit.

continuity of care Series of client care activities rendered to the client in three situations (before, during, and after hospitalization); a basic objective of discharge planning.

contract A promissory agreement between two or more persons that creates, modifies, or destroys a legal relation. It is a legally enforceable promise between two or more persons to do or not to do something.

contracting Any working agreement, continuously renegotiable and agreed upon by nurse and client.

contributory negligence Act or omission amounting to want of ordinary care on the part of the complaining party which, concurring with defendant's negligence, is the proximate cause of injury.

cool down The period of up to 10 minutes, after intensive exercise in which a person engages in exercises of diminishing intensity to allow the body temperature and heart rate to decrease slowly. This period reduces complications of intense exercise.

coordination Conscious activity of assembling and directing the work efforts of a group of health providers so that they can function harmoniously in the attainment of the objective of client care.

correctness of temporality Evidence that exposure to a causal factor occurs before the onset of the disease.

corroboration Strengthening or adding to credibility by adding or confirming facts or evidence.

cost-accounting studies Studies finding the actual budgetary cost of a program, procedure, or technique.

cost-benefit studies Studies assessing the desirability of a program, procedure, or technique by placing a specific quantifiable value, a dollar amount, on all costs and benefits of the variable to be evaluated.

cost-effectiveness studies Studies measuring the quality of a program, procedure, or technique as relative to cost.

cost-efficiency studies Studies analyzing the actual costs of performing a number of services at different volumes when the same standards are applied.

cost-plus reimbursement Method of payment whereby an agency receives actual costs of services delivered plus added allowable expenses, such as depreciation of facilities and equipment and administrative costs.

counselor One who helps others arrive at workable solutions to their problems.

credentialing Mechanism that seeks to produce performance of acceptable quality by individuals and programs of education and service. The four fundamental features of credentialing are quality, identity, protection, and control.

crisis intervention A short-term method of providing assistance to persons in crisis.

crude rates Statistical rates in which the events in the numerator and the denominator refer to the entire population.

cultural relativism The value of the culture as defined by its meaning to its members.

cultural values The prevailing and persistent guides influencing thinking and actions of people within a culture.

culture Standards for decisions on what is, what can be, how to feel about it, and how to do it.

culture-bound illnesses Illnesses specific to a particular culture (e.g., *mal ojo* [evil eye] in the Mexican American culture).

culture change The constant process of adding or deleting elements within a culture, such as language, customs, beliefs, attitudes, values, goals, laws, traditions, and moral codes.

culture shock Feelings of helplessness, discomfort, and disorientation experienced by a person attempting to understand or effectively adapt to a different cultural group, because of dissimilarities in practices, values, and beliefs.

data collection Process of acquiring existing information or developing new information.

data generation The development of data, frequently qualitative rather than numerical, by the data collector.

date interpretation The process of analyzing and synthesizing data, which culminates in the identification of community health problems and strengths.

decibel (dB) Unit of measure of the magnitude of noise.

deinstitutionalization Effort to move long-term psychiatric patients out of the hospital and back into their own community.

delirium tremens Severe reaction to alcohol withdrawal; characterized by disorientation, paranoia, and outbursts of irrational behavior; symptoms also may include tachycardia, fever, rapid breathing, sweating, vomiting, and diarrhea.

dementia Progressive, organic mental disorder characterized by chronic personality disintegration, confusion, and deterioration of mental functioning.

democratic leadership Cooperative structure that promotes and supports member's functioning in all aspects of decision making and planning.

demographic trends Population trends related to age at first marriage; fertility patterns; birth rates; numbers of individuals engaging in singlehood, divorce, and remarriage; number of dependent children experiencing divorce or life with a never-married parent; and the number of elderly persons.

Denver Developmental Screening Test (DDST) A simple test to evaluate childhood development in the areas of personal/social, fine motor/adaptive, language, and gross motor development.

deontology Doctrine that moral duty or obligation is binding. Also, what makes acts right are nonconsequential characteristics such as fidelity, veracity, justice, and honesty.

depression Mental state characterized by dejection, lack of hope, and absence of cheerfulness.

dereflection Logotherapeutic technique of simply taking a person's mind off the goal but a positive redirection to another goal. A technique to direct focus away from the problems at hand and to focus on assets and abilities.

descriptive epidemiology First stage of epidemiological investigation; focuses on describing disease distribution by characteristics relating to time, place, and person.

detoxification Gradual withdrawal from an abused substance; best achieved in a controlled hospital setting.

developmental crisis Disequilibrium occurring at a predictable transition in life.

Developmental Profile II Instrument to measure child development from birth to preadolescence in the areas of physical/motor, self-help, social, academic, and communication skills.

developmental disability Pathological condition that begins before 18 years of age and leads to disruption in the normal maturational process.

diagnosis-related groups A patient classification scheme that defines 468 illness categories and the corresponding health care services that are reimbursable under Medicare.

dichotomy planning Events preparing for clients' ongoing and future needs for health care resources as they move along the health/illness continuum toward their maximum potential.

dietary guidelines Simple, practical food guides developed to assist health care providers in providing good nutritional education to clients.

dietary influence A variety of factors, including biological needs, psychological variables, sociocultural issues, and environmental aspects that determine what people eat.

dioxin Ingredient in the defoliant Agent Orange, which can kill and cause birth defects, cancer, and problems of the liver, kidney, nervous system, and skin.

direct causal association Relationship in which a factor causes a disease with no other factors intervening in the process.

direct provider reimbursement Method of payment to a provider for services delivered (e.g., fee-for-service).

disability The loss, absence, or impairment of physical or mental fitness that is observable or measurable.

discharge planning Planning, by a multidisciplinary team within a given setting, that enhances the client's ability to return to an optimum life-style.

discretionary time "That portion of time that remains when work and the basic requirements for existence have been satisfied" (Murphy, 1981, p. 26). Also known as nonobligated or free time.

disengagement theory Aging theory postulated on the premise of older people withdrawing from society.

distracting A behavioral response that seems irrelevant and completely unrelated to the situation.

distress Unpleasant emotional and/or physiological response to a stressor.

distributive care Health maintenance and disease prevention.

dosage Regimen governing the size, frequency, and number of doses of a therapeutic agent to be administered to a person.

duty Moral or legal obligation, or obligation relating to one's occupation or position. Moral duty is based on moral principles and may or may not be supported by law; carrying out a moral duty may even be prohibited by law. Legal duty is that which is required by law.

absolute Cannot be overridden by any other duty; intrinsically right or wrong.

advocacy Moral obligation to speak, write, or take action in support of the client or client populations.

veracity Obligation to tell the truth and not lie or deceive people.

dysfunctional family A family unit that inhibits clear communication within family relationships and does not provide psychological support for individual members.

dystonia Impaired or disordered tonicity, especially muscle tone.

early adopters Individuals and/or groups with cosmopolitan rather than local orientations, with abilities to adopt new ideas from mass media rather than face-to-face information sources, and with specialized rather than global interests.

ecological studies Analytic studies that compare large aggregates of people, usually of a defined geographic area, with another such large population.

economic barriers Monetary factors that affect a person's ability to attain health care services.

economics Social science concerned with the problems of using or administering scarce resources in the most efficient way to attain maximum fulfillment of society's unlimited wants.

efficacy Ability of an intervention to produce desired results.

emancipated Free from parental care and control.

emergency nurse practitioner Registered nurse with additional education through a master's degree program in nursing or through a nondegree or certificate continuing education program preparing the nurse to deliver primary care within an emergency room setting.

emotional abuse Extreme debasement of a person's feelings so that he feels inept, uncared for, and worthless.

enculturation Process of acquiring knowledge and internalizing values, or learning a culture.

endemic Indigenous to an area or group.

enterobiasis Pinworm infestation.

entitlement theory People have rights to resources as determined by the natural lottery and may increase their possessions in any way possible (by purchase, gift, or legitimate exchange), as long as they do not cheat others or acquire them in an unjust manner.

environmental health Aspect of community health concerned with those forms of life, substances, forces, and conditions in the surroundings of people that may exert an influence on their health and well-being.

epidemic Occurrence of any given disease phenomenon in excess of normal expectation.

episodic care Curative and restorative aspect of nursing practice.

equalitarian theory Doctrine that takes the needs of all people into account equally.

erythema Reddened raised area on the skin produced by a tissue response to small doses of antigenic substances.

established group An existing group of persons linked by membership and group purpose.

estimation of risk Assessing the nature of a problem, size of the problem, and need for a program within a community to prevent occurrence of the problem.

ethical principles Abstract guides that serve as foundations for moral rules.

autonomy To respect people and their rights to make choices and act according to individual determinations.

beneficence To do good and prevent or avoid doing harm.

justice Equals should be treated the same, and those unequal in similar respects should be treated differently according to their similarities.

ethical theories Collection of principles and rules providing theoretical foundations for deciding what to do when moral principles or rules conflict.

ethics Science or study of moral values; also a code of principles and ideals that guide action.

ethnic collectivity Group with common origins, a sense of identity, and shared standards for behavior.

ethnocentrism Belief that one's own group or culture is superior to others.

eustress Positive form of stress; occurs when people convert negative stress into a positive form by changing their attitudes.

eutrophication Process in which nutrients in lakes promote the growth of algae, which causes cloudy, odorous water.

evaluation Collection of methods, skills, and sensitivities necessary to determine whether a human service is needed and likely to be used, is conducted as planned, and actually does help people in need. Also, provision of information through formal means, such as criteria, measurement, and statistics, for making rational judgments necessary in decision-making situations.

evaluative research A method of collecting information according to the rigors of scientific inquiry for the purpose of evaluating the long term effect of a program.

evaluative studies Systematic method for collecting information to assess the relevance, progress, effectiveness, efficiency, and impact of a program.

excess mortality Premature death; that occurring before the average life expectancy for persons of the same sex.

existential vacuum Feeling of emptiness and meaninglessness; apathy toward life; an inner void.

expansion A broadening of life experiences as a result of increasing developmental abilities.

experience insurance rate A premium rate that is based on an estimate of the risk of claims by the subscriber.

experimental epidemiology Third stage of epidemiological investigation, which uses experimental design for studies to confirm the causal nature of relationships identified through observational studies.

expert witness A witness who has special training, experience, skills, and knowledge in a relevant area, and whose testimony as to his opinion is allowed to be considered as evidence in a court of law; nonexpert opinions are usually not admissible as evidence.

expertise Mastery of developmental tasks.

expressive skills Skills one uses to respond to the environment through verbal and behavioral activities.

extrapyramidal side effects Group of side effects produced by the blockage of dopamine receptor sites in the extrapyramidal system tract.

failed expectations Beliefs and notions about marriage and family that arise from myths about marriage and lead to disappointment when family life is not healthy and happy and fair.

family Two or more individuals, coming from the same or different kinship groups, who are involved in a continuous living arrangement, usually residing in the same household, experiencing common emotional bonds, and sharing certain obligations toward each other and toward others.

family assessment Systematic collection, classification, and analysis of family data for the purpose of identifying the family's health-related strengths and problems.

family developmental framework Assumes that family development follows orderly, sequential changes throughout the family's life span.

family development task A growth responsibility that must be accomplished by a family at a specified developmental stage.

family dynamics Interactions and relationships within the family that influence the work of the family and its ability to complete its functions and tasks.

family functions Behaviors or activities performed to maintain the integrity of the family unit and to meet the family's needs, individual members' needs, and society's expectations.

family health Includes the promotion and maintenance of physical, mental, spiritual, and social health for the family unit and for individual family members.

family nurse practitioner/clinician Registered nurse with additional education through a master's degree program in nursing or a nondegree or certificate continuing education program preparing the nurse to deliver primary health care to individuals, groups, and communities of all ages.

family planning nurse practitioner (obstetric/gynecological nurse practitioner) Registered nurse with additional education through a master's degree program in nursing or a nondegree or certificate continuing education program preparing the nurse to deliver obstetrical and gynecological primary care to women.

family roles Behaviors assumed by family members to maintain the organizational structure of the family and to define the division of labor and the family processes.

family self-care Decision-making process that involves the family in self-observation, symptom perception and labeling, judgment of severity, and choice and assessment of treatment options.

family strengths Those factors or forces that contribute to family unity and solidarity and foster the development of the potentials inherent within the family.

family structure (configuration) Refers to the characteristics of the individual members (gender, age, number) who constitute the family unit.

fee-for-service benefit schedule List of physician services with monetary or unit values attached that specifies the amounts third parties must pay for specific services.

fee screen system The use of usual, customary, and reasonable charges (based on regional evaluations in all specialties) by physicians to set their own reimbursement levels for units of service.

fetal alcohol syndrome May occur when a pregnant woman has consumed alcohol regularly (about six drinks per day). Infants tend to be of low birth weight, mentally retarded, and may have behavioral, facial, limb, genital, cardiac, or neurological impairments.

field theory Belief that the environment consists of interdependent events.

figure-ground relationship Perceptual field is divided into an object of focus (figure) and a diffuse background (ground).

financial resources planning The identification of costs associated with implementing a program or project based on the essential persons, facilities, equipment and supplies to complete the project or program.

fiscal year Annual operating year of the government, October 1 to September 30 of the next calendar year.

fitness Attainment of wellness on a continuing basis. See **wellness**.

Food Exchange System Dietary guidelines that include six food groups where goods are grouped according to their similarity in calories and food values, so measured amounts of foods within the group may be traded off in meals.

formal communication Organization of channels for transmitting and receiving information within a network—social, professional, political, or economic.

formal group Persons having a defined membership and specified purpose. The group may or may not have an official or public place in the community's organization.

formal operations Level of cognitive development in which thoughts are independent of physical experience and allow children to deal with hypothetical questions.

formal structure The established power and communication relationships within an organization.

formative evaluation An evaluation instituted for the purpose of assessing the degree to which objectives are met or planned activities are conducted.

freebasing Homemade refining process that extracts a concentrated form of cocaine from its chemical base and then smokes it in a water pipe usually filled with liquor.

free radical theory Theory of aging based on the premise of an imbalance between the production and elimination of free radicals as contributory to aging.

freon Hydrocarbon gas often used as a propellant and refrigerant.

fulfillment Perception of harmony in life when the individual has found meaning and is leading a purposeful life.

function Responsibilities and tasks associated with a particular role.

functional family A family unit which provides autonomy and is responsive to the particular interests and needs of individual family members.

fungicide Chemical agent that kills or retards the growth of fungi.

general adaptation syndrome Manifestations of stress in the whole body, as they develop in time. This happens in three stages: (1) alarm reaction, (2) resistance, and (3) exhaustion.

generalist A nurse who provides a wide range of nursing services to clients.

geriatric day care facility Ambulatory health care facility for elderly people; it uses a broad range of professional and community services to maximize functional independence for this age group in the home and community.

geriatric nurse practitioner Registered nurse with additional education through a master's degree program in nursing or a nondegree or certificate continuing education program preparing the nurse to deliver primary health care to older adults.

gerontology A field of study that explores the biopsychosocial issues of aging.

gestalt German word meaning pattern or configuration.

gestational age The number of weeks spent in utero to the time of birth.

goal attainment A process for assessing the efficacy of a program by examination or measurement of predetermined goals.

goal of coordination To maximize the collaborative effort of health providers while minimizing friction among them in the attainment of the client care objectives.

goals/objectives A consultative problem that involves the inability of a group or individual to accept new goals, change goals, or meet established goals.

gross national product (GNP) The total value of all final goods and services produced in the country in one year.

group A collection of interacting individuals who have a common purpose or purposes.

group cohesion Measurement of degree of attraction between members and toward the group.

group norms Unwritten and often unspoken standards for group members that guide their behavior and influence their attitudes and perceptions.

hallucinosis Can result from alcohol withdrawal; the person remains oriented and rational but may be confused about time.

health Balanced state of well-being resulting from harmonious interaction of body, mind, and spirit.

health belief model What one believes about health based on perceptions of susceptibility, seriousness, and advantages or disadvantages of action. Useful in promoting adherence to treatment regimen.

health care Product of health services delivered through personal or public health services.

health contract Usually a written agreement between client and health care provider, which identifies and assigns priorities for health goals and includes measurable criteria to be met within a designated time frame.

health economics Branch of economics concerned with the problems of producing and distributing the health care resources of the nation in a way that provides maximum benefit to the most people.

health education Any combination of learning experiences designed to facilitate adaptations of behavior conducive to health.

health index A summary of the health features of a community that enable us to determine health care delivery needs.

health planning A continuous social process by which data about a client are collected and evaluated for the purpose of creating "a plan" to guide change in health care delivery.

health policy Public policy that affects health and health services. Delineates options from which individuals and organizations make their health-related choices. Made within a political context.

health practitioners Members of the primary health care team who as colleagues develop strategies for combining their expertise so that they can be integrated in a complementary way to address the health needs of the clients.

health risk appraisal Process of identifying and analyzing an individual's prognostic characteristics of health and comparing them with those of a standard age group, thereby providing a prediction of a person's likelihood of developing prematurely the health problems that have high morbidity and mortality in this country.

health risk/health risk factor Disease precursor whose presence is associated with higher-than-average morbidity and/or mortality. Disease precursors include demographic variables, certain individual behaviors, positive individual and/or family history, and some physiological changes.

health risk reduction Application of selected interventions to control or reduce risk factors and minimize the incidence of associated disease and premature mortality. Risk reduction is reflected in greater congruence between appraised and achievable ages.

health services Personal and public services performed by individuals or institutions for the purpose of maintaining or restoring health.

health systems agency Federally funded agency that plans and approves the development of health care facilities in a community.

health workforce shortage area An area determined by the federal government to have too few health professionals to provide adequate health care for the population.

helminth Wormlike animal.

hepatitis Inflammatory condition of the liver caused by viral or bacterial infection, parasites, alcohol, drugs, toxins, or transfusions of incompatible blood.

herbicide Chemical agent used to destroy unwanted plants.

herpes Any one of five related viruses that attack skin, genitalia, or cranial, cervical, or spinal nerves; infection is characterized by severe pain and various acute symptoms.

Hill-Burton Act First U.S. legislation to focus on planning as a major area of concern. Its primary purpose was to provide for a more equal distribution of hospitals across the nation by matching federal funds for one third to two thirds of the total cost of a facility.

HMO Act Legislation enacted in 1973 to provide a demonstration program for the development of health maintenance organizations.

holism A concept that requires that human behavior not be isolated from the context in which it occurs and that a culture be viewed and analyzed as a whole.

homeostasis Relative constancy in the internal environment of the body.

home health care An arrangement of health-related services provided to people in their place of residence.

homeopathy Belief that herbs, drugs, and chemicals, when used in small quanitities, can cure or prevent a disease ordinarily caused by a larger dose of the same substance.

homicide Any violent death that is neither a suicide nor an accident.

hospice Palliative system of health care for terminally ill people; takes place in the home with family involvment under the direction and supervision of health professionals, especially the visiting nurse. Hospice care takes place in the hospital when severe complications of terminal illness occur, there is family exhaustion, or there is loss of commitment.

host Human or animal that provides adequate living conditions for any given infectious agent.

human ecology Study of the interrelationships between individuals and their environments as well as among the individuals in the environment.

human resources planning Planning for the use of human knowledge and skills available or identified as essential to implementing the goals of a program or project.

hydrocarbons Family of compounds containing carbon and hydrogen.

hydrocephalus Increased accumulation of cerebrospinal fluid in the ventricles of the brain due to interference with the circulation and absorption of the fluid.

hyperactivity A behavior disorder with characteristic clinical manifestations resulting in non–goal-directed activity in inappropriate amounts.

hyperbilirubinemia Elevated levels of unconjugated bilirubin resulting from deficiency or inactivity of bilirubin glucuronyl transferase.

hyperintention Excess concentration on an objective, which ironically inhibits its accomplishment.

hyperreflection Compulsion to observe oneself; excess attention to oneself.

hypnosis Technique for reducing stress; a trancelike condition that may be psychically induced by another person and that is characterized by loss of consciousness and a greater or lesser degree of responsiveness to the suggestions of the hypnotist.

iatrogenesis Physician-induced illness. Clinical iatrogenesis, the most familiar, includes illnesses created as by-products of medical intervention (e.g., infections caused by antibiotics that alter the body's normal bacterial flora).

iatrogenic guilt Engendered at the time of illness because of assignment of blame for the illness by the care provider to the patient. For example, a patient with heart disease may be told by his physician, "You could have avoided this by not smoking, exercising regularly, and eating a diet low in animal fats."

identification of target market The identification of a specific geographical area and the boundaries that define the market area, constituting a selected group of residents.

imagery Creation of pictures through the use of mental processes; can be spontaneously or deliberately created and used for many purposes.

immune globulin (IG) Sterile solution containing antibodies from human blood. IG is primarily indicated for routine maintenance of certain immunodeficient individuals and for passive immunization.

immunity Natural or acquired ability to ward off disease.

immunological theory Aging theory based on the premise that normal cells are unrecognized as such, thereby setting off an immune reaction.

incidence rate The rate of newly occurring cases of a disease in a population over a defined period of time.

incidental additives Food additives resulting from the use of pesticides or herbicides, or from chemical changes brought about by processing methods.

incineration Burning of wastes.

inclusiveness, principle of Tendency to respond to objects in the environment that contain the largest number of stimuli.

incubation period Time beginning with host exposure to an infectious agent and continuing until the organism multiplies to sufficient numbers to produce a host reaction and clinical symptoms.

independent practice Private practice of a professional who works independently from other professionals.

indirect provider reimbursement Payment to an agency for services delivered by health providers, such as nurses.

Individual activities Recreation and leisure activities that are pursued by individual family members.

individual developmental task Originates during a certain period of an individual's life; successful achievement of the task leads to satisfaction and to success with later tasks; failure leads to dissatisfaction within the individual, difficulty with later tasks, and social disapproval.

infection Complex interaction between a host and a specific agent that entails the replication of organisms in the tissue of the host.

infectivity Organisms's ability to spread rapidly from one host to another.

informal structure The communication network established by the employees within an organization.

informal communication Interaction channels that arise out of the interpersonal relationships of network parts.

informal group A group of persons having no articulated membership or purpose.

informant interviewing Directed conversation with selected members of a community about community members or groups and events. A direct method of assessment.

informed consent Client has received sufficient information concerning the health care proposed, its incumbent risks, and the acceptable alternatives.

inherent resistance The ability to resist disease independently of antibodies or of specifically developed tissue response.

injunction Court order to stop a party in a contract from performing the specific promise or act under other circumstances.

insecticide Chemical pesticide used to control insects.

institutional licensure A mechanism for allowing employing agencies to be responsible for the competence of the people they employ.

integration The incorporation of development tasks and skills into a repertoire of effective behavior.

intent of law Legislative language of a law, which provides general guidelines defining the law, for the writing of specific regulations.

intentional additives Substances deliberately added in food processing to enhance or conserve nutritional value or to improve or maintain flavor, color, texture, or consistency.

interacting group A cluster of individuals who are linked by personal relationships. The links may be either primary, such as in a family, or secondary, such as in a voluntary association.

interactional framework Focuses on the family as a unit of interacting personalities and examines the symbolic communication processes by which family members relate to one another.

intervention activities Means or strategies by which objectives are achieved and change is effected.

introspection Process of an individual's inward examination of traits, habits, and qualities.

invasion of privacy Violation of the right to be left alone to live in seclusion without being subjected to unwarranted or undesired publicity.

invasiveness Agent's ability to spread within the host.

inversion Reversal of the normal atmospheric gradient.

involuntary smoking Inhaling of tobacco combustion products in a smoke-filled atmosphere by a nonsmoker.

joint activities Recreation and leisure activities that involve games and other hobbies that family members enjoy together.

joint practice Practice in which professionals work together in a complementary and consultative manner.

judicial law Law based on court or jury decisions.

jurisdiction Geographic location in which a court has the authority to hear a case.

Kawasaki disease (mucocutaneous lymph node syndrome) Acute febrile illness that occurs predominantly in children under 5 years of age. No causative agent has been identified.

kernicterus Neruological damage that occurs when unconjugated bilirubin is deposited in brain tissue.

key informants Professional experts, community leaders, politicians, and entrepreneurs who are in touch with the needs of the community and who are in a position to support new community programs.

kinesiology Study of movement that applies principles of anatomy, physiology, and physics.

Korsakoff's psychosis Results from excessive alcohol consumption and is characterized by disorientation and a memory defect whereby people fill in the gaps by making up forgotten information.

law The sum total of man-made rules and regulations by which society is governed in a formal and legally binding manner.

law witness One who testifies to what he has seen, heard, or otherwise observed.

lay advisors Individuals who are influential in approving or disapproving new ideas and who seek advice and information from others about these things.

legionnaires' disease (legionellosis) Pneumonia-like communicable disease caused by *Legionella pneumophilia*. Mode of transmission is presumed to be airborne.

legislative counsel Consultant in the House or Senate who is available to assist in the framing of ideas in suitable legislative language and form for introduction.

legislative process The process used within governments to make laws.

leveling A healthy communication style under stress in which family members are able to say what they feel and believe.

levels of prevention A three-level model of interventions based on the stages of disease, designed to halt or reverse the process of pathological change as early as possible, thereby preventing damage.

liability An obligation one has incurred or might incur through any act or failure to act, responsibility for conduct falling below a certain standard, which is the causal connection to the plaintiff's injury.

liaison Position or responsibility within an organization for maintaining communication links with external individuals or organizations.

licensure Legal sanction to practice a profession after attaining the minimum degree of competence to ensure protection of public health and safety.

life-style change Alteration in such personal behaviors and habits as diet, use of cigarettes, alcohol consumption, and exercise.

life-style-induced health problems Diseases with natural histories that include conscious exposure to certain health-compromising or risk factors. For example, heart disease is life-style-induced; that is, its onset is generally preceded by smoking, unwise eating, failing to exercise, and sustaining unbuffered stress.

litigation Trial in court to determine legal issues and the rights and duties between the parties.

logotherapy Treatment modality based on a blend of humanistic and existential psychology, which assists the client in finding meaning and purpose in life and in unique life experiences.

long-term care facility (nursing home) Typically for the older adult, where individuals can receive minimum to maximum skilled nursing care, depending on the type of facility and the need of the client.

macrolevel interventions Health-generating changes carried out at the societal level.

mainstream smoke Smoke inhaled and exhaled by the smoker.

maintenance functions Behaviors that provide physical and psychological support and therefore hold the group together.

maintenance norms Norms that create group pressures to ensure affirming actions for members and are helpful in maintaining comfort.

malpractice Professional misconduct, improper discharge of professional duties, or a failure to meet the standard of care by a professional, which results in harm to another.

malpractice litigation A lawsuit resulting from client dissatisfaction with the provider and the content or quality of care received; a quality assurance measure.

manager One who is given official power by the organization to coordinate the individual efforts of others to achieve organizational goals.

mandatory credentialing Requires statutory law (e.g., state nurse practice acts).

mandatory nurse licensure A law that requires all who practice nursing for compensation to be licensed.

markup Line-by-line review of a bill by a committee for the purpose of changing the wording or amending the intent.

maternal-infant bond See bonding.

maturational crisis Crisis resulting from an inability to accomplish tasks necessary to move to next developmental stage.

maximin theory Distribution of goods and resources to maximize the minimum position in society, while at the same time allowing free exercise of liberty on the part of all people.

mediating structures Institutions standing between the individual in private life and the larger institution of public life, such as one's neighborhood, family, church, and voluntary associations.

medically indigent A portion of the population who are usually above the recognized poverty level and have money to buy the necessities of life but who cannot afford a catastrophic illness or an acute illness crisis.

mental retardation Disorder characterized by subaverage general intelligence with impairments in the ability to learn and to fully adapt socially.

methadone A synthetic narcotic analgesic used for anesthesia or as a substitute for heroin.

microbiological food contamination Results from toxins deposited in food.

microlevel interventions Health-generating changes performed at the individual level. Examples are cognitive restructuring, self-confrontation, modeling, conditioning, and stimulus control.

middle adult Individual who is in a transitionaal stage between young adulthood and old age; person in the 36 to 64 year-old age group, whose psychosocial task is generativity versus stagnation.

middlescence Intermediate stage of life between young adulthood and old age, marked by physical, psychological, and social changes; the developmental task is generativity.

minimal brain dysfunction A descriptive term of a child of average intelligence who has difficulty learning.

modeling Strategy for self-modification that depends on the client's observing the behavior of others who have realized the goal the client has identified as his own.

moral accountability A moral obligation that directs the professional nurse to act in a particular way according to moral norms and requires the nurse to be answerable for what has been done.

morale/cohesion problem Occurs when a client has lost confidence in his ability to solve problems and feels powerless to institute corrective action.

moral obligation Duty to act in a particular way in response to moral norms.

moral virtue Ideal standard of human behavior or thinking; excellence in response to moral norms, such as goodness.

morbidity Relative disease rate; usually expressed as incidence or prevalence of a disease.

mortality Relative death rate, the proportion of deaths at a particular time and place.

mothering The process of caring for an infant.

motherliness The capacity of the mother to be gratified by the exchange between herself and her infant and to use gratification for her own growth.

motivation A conscious or unconscious need or desire to act.

multiproblem family A family unit facing a number of events within and without the family environment that does not have the ability to solve its own problems.

mycotoxin Toxic metabolite that can be produced by food molds.

National Health Planning and Resources Development Act of 1974 (P.L. 93-641) Set forth to coordinate and direct national health policy via state and regional regulatory agencies; its major goal was to establish a nationwide network of health systems agencies.

National Health Service Corps Program established in 1970 by the Public Health Service to recruit health providers to health work force shortage areas.

National Joint Practice Commission Organization established by the American Nurses' Association and the American Medical Association to promote collaborative efforts between medicine and nursing; disbanded in 1981.

National Labor Relations Act Passed in 1935 and known as the Wagner Act; protected employees' rights to organize and join unions and also provided for action against unfair labor practices of employers.

National Labor Relation Act Amendments of 1974 (P.L. 93-360) Amended the Taft Hartley Act of 1947 and extended the right to organize collectively for matters concerning wages, hours, and working conditions to all employees of nonpublic health care facilities.

National Labor Relations Board Administrative agency for implementing federal policy affecting labor relations.

natural history Process of development and progression of a disease without intervention by humans.

natural law Doctrine holding that there is a natural moral order or natural moral law inherent in the structure of the universe, which can be known by human reason.

natural radiation Radiation that comes from soil, certain rocks, body potassium, and ultraviolet sun rays.

negative assertion Open admission about oneself; acknowledging that perfection is not a goal.

negative inquiry Prompting further criticism of self or prompting more information about statements of wrongdoing in an unemotional, low-key manner.

negative right Claim to other peoples' forbearances.

negligence Failure to act as an ordinary prudent person; conduct contrary to that of a reasonable person under a specific circumstance.

nematocides Chemical pesticides used to kill worms.

neural tube defect congenital malformation involving defects in the skull and spinal column; caused primarily by failure of neural tube to close during embryonic development.

"Nightingalism" Ideology emphasizing self-sacrifice on the part of the nurse, when the primary concern of the nurse is the welfare of the client with minimum attention to personal economic and general welfare needs.

nitrogen oxide A toxic gas that comes primarily from automobile exhaust or by-products of industry.

Noise Control Act Passed by Congress in 1972 to identify major sources of noise, establish noise emission standards, and provide a mechanism for people to take civil action in their own behalf when a person or agency violates the Act.

nonassertive behavior Denial of one's own rights by failing to express thoughts, beliefs, and feelings honestly.

noncausal association Relationship in which a factor varies systematically with a causal factor and therefore with the occurrence of the disease, but the factor is not a cause of the disease.

nontraditional family Alternative family structures comprised of two or more individuals, coming from the same or different kinship groups, who are involved in a continuous living arrangement, usually residing in the same household, experiencing common emotional bonds and sharing certain obligations toward each other and toward others.

noogenic neurosis Mental health problem caused by spiritual (not religious) problems or moral conflicts; a type of mental conflict in which values are not clarified.

norms Standards that guide, control, and regulate individuals and communities.

nosocomial infection In the episodic setting an infection that is not present or incubating at the time of admission. In the distributive setting any infection that is not present or incubating at the time the client is initially admitted for care by a given agency or service.

nuclear (traditional) family A unit comprised of mother, father, and young children.

nurse practitioner Nursing role that includes a primary care component that focuses on health maintenance, disease prevention, and client counseling.

nursing centers Health care facilities in which the primary aim is to offer nursing services, including health assessment, promotion, screening, and health teaching.

obesity Weight of 20% more than the recommended normal weight for height, body structure, and sex caused by heredity, interpersonal, and/or environmental factors.

objective A precise, behavioral statement of the achievement that will accomplish partial or total realization of a goal. The date by which the achievement is expected is specified.

occupational health The state in which a worker is able to function at an optimum level of well-being (see HEALTH) at the worksite; reflected by higher employee productivity, increase in work attendance, reduction in workers' compensation claims, and increase in longevity in employment status.

occupational medicine Special field of preventive medicine concerned with the medical problems and practices relating to occupation and especially to employees of industry.

occupational socialization Orientation into a given job-related set of behaviors; that is, the set of expected behaviors that accompanies a specific job.

official agencies Agencies operated by the state or local governments to provide home health care.

Older American's Act Legislation enacted in 1965 to mandate and provide funds for services, programs, and activities deemed essential to accomplish certain goals for older Americans meeting specified criteria.

operant behavior Behavior not elicited by a known stimulus but simply emitted by the organism.

operant conditioning Form of learning used in behavior therapy, whereby person is rewarded for correct response and punished for incorrect response.

orchitis Inflammation of one or both of the testes; characterized by pain and swelling and often caused by mumps, syphilis, or tuberculosis.

osteoporosis Disorder characterized by abnormal rarefaction of bone.

outreach Finding and assisting individuals to become or remain involved in recreation and leisure activities.

ozone Unstable colorless gas with an oxidizing power surpassed only by fluorine.

pandemic An epidemic that includes widespread geographical areas of the world.

paradoxical intention Logotherapeutic technique whereby the client is encouraged to do what he fears and in fact to exaggerate it to the point of humor; useful in the treatment of phobias.

parallel activities Recreation and leisure activities that are enjoyed by family members but require minimal interaction among the participants.

parens patria Duty of state to protect its citizens.

parent-child bond The synchronization of the parents and the child as a unit, which results in a unique emotional relationship.

paternal-infant bond The development of a reciprocal relationship between a father and infant, which facilitates the development of the paternal role in the family and provides for the emotional and physical needs of the infant.

participant observation Conscious and systematic sharing in the life activities and occasionally in the interests and affects of a group of persons; observational methods of assessment; a direct method of data collection.

partnership Informed, flexible, and negotiated distribution of power among all participants in the process of change for community health. The means for improved community health.

passive immunization Administration of a preformed antibody to a susceptible host.

paternal leadership Winning respect and dependence from followers by parent-like devotion to members' needs at the leader's own expense.

pathogenicity An agent's relative ability to produce disease.

Patient Bill of Rights A document prepared by the American Hospital Association that defines the provider-client relationship within an organization.

patriarchal leadership Often controls membership through rewards and threats, keeping members in the dark about goals and rationale behind prescribed actions.

pedagogy Art and science of teaching children; based on belief that the purpose of education is the transmittal of knowledge.

pediatric nurse practitioner Registered nurse with certificate or master's level advanced education in the areas of health assessment, diagnosis, and treatment of children. The program prepares the nurse to deliver primary health care to infants and children.

pediculosis Infestation of various hairy body sites by different subspecies of *Pediculus humanus*, or lice.

perceptual constancy According to Gestalt theory, an object is seen in the same way under varying circumstances.

periodontal disease Disease of gum tissue caused by bacterial plaque, resulting in gingivitis (inflammation of the gums) and periodontitis (destruction of supporting bones and ligaments, resulting in loose or drifting teeth). The leading cause of loss of teeth after age 35.

periodontoclasia Loosening of permanent teeth.

peripheral polyneuropathy Affliction of several nerves, which usually results from nutritional deficiencies associated with excessive alcohol consumption; characterized by weakness, numbness, partial paralysis of extremities, pain in the legs, and impaired sensory reactions and motor reflexes.

performance budget A financial plan that shows clearly and concisely the services to be provided in return for the funds available or income generated.

permissive nurse licensure A law that allows a person to practice nursing without a license as long as the term *registered nurse* is not used and the practitioner does not pretend to be licensed.

personal health services Services directed toward the maintenance of the health status of individuals.

person-year Statistical measure representing one person at risk of developing a disease for one year.

phases of crisis Occurrence of a significant stressor event, onset of disequilibrium, rise in tension levels, decrease in levels of functioning, and resolution with equilibrium re-established.

phenytoin An anticonvulsant.

phi phenomenon Experience of apparent motion that is caused by lights flashing on and off at a certain frequency.

photosynthesis Formation of carbohydrates by chlorophyll-containing plants exposed to the sun.

physical abuse One or more episodes of extreme disciplining or displaced aggression or frustration, often resulting in serious physical damage to the internal organs, bones, central nervous system, or sense organs.

physical fitness A set of physiological attributes, some of which are health related, that people have or achieve, including agility, balance, coordination, speed, power, reaction time, cardiorespiratory endurance, muscular endurance, flexibility, muscular strength, and body composition.

physician assistant Health practitioner role created in the 1960s to free physician's time by completing tasks such as taking medical histories and conducting physical examinations.

physician extender Nonphysician health care provider who performs medical activities typically performed by physicians.

placating Accepting the blame for situations in which one is not at fault.

plaintiff Party who brings a civil suit seeking damages or other legal relief.

play "The behavior emitted by an individual not motivated by the end product of the behavior" (Ellis, 1973, p. 2).

plurality patterns Factors related to family size and the pairs of relationships that are a consequence of the number of members in the family.

pneumoconiosis Lung disease associated with dust.

police power States' power to act to protect the health, safety, and welfare of their citizens.

policies Guidelines within which employees of an institution must operate.

pollution Addition of something to an environment that changes its natural qualities.

position (status) Location in a social structure. Occupants of positions are collective categories of people who differ from the general public in some specified shared attribute or behavior.

position power Formal authority associated with an individual's position in the organization.

positive right Claim to other peoples' positive actions.

power/authority issue Question of who has the right to be in charge and who has the right to make a decision.

Practice Acts State laws that govern the practice of health providers.

practice setting Context and/or environment within which nursing care is given.

precedent Previous adjudged decision that serves as the authority in a similar case.

precursor or disease precursor Prognostic characteristic or feature of personal health history, health behavior or habit, physical examination, or laboratory or x-ray film findings associated with a higher or lower risk of death than the average.

prepathogenesis A stage in the natural history of a disease in which the disease has not yet developed although the groundwork has been laid through the presence of factors that favor its occurrence.

presbycusis Loss of hearing, speech intelligibility, and ability to auditory and pitch levels.

preschooler a child between the ages of three and six.

prescriptive intervention mode Requires less collaboration between consultant and client because the consultant explicitly tells the client how to solve the problem.

PRESS Acronym for preschool readiness experimental screening scale, an assessment of the maturational level of children between ages 4 and 5.

presymptomatic disease Early stages of disease when physiological changes have begun but no signs or symptoms are present.

prevalence The number of existing cases of a disease present in a defined population at a given time.

prevention, level of

primary General health promotion.

secondary Identification and prevention of disease and health problems for those who are likely to develop them.

tertiary Health restoration and maintenance.

prima facie duty Moral or legal duty that may be overridden when in conflict with other duties that are morally stronger.

primary health care team Health care providers with specialized and complementary skills who function together as a team to provide primary health care services.

primary nursing Modality for delivering nursing care in which the client contributes to and receives care, and the provider is not only available but has authority, autonomy, and accountability.

primary prevention Activities directed toward intervening in the natural history of disease before any pathological changes occur in a host; these activities seek to keep the agent away from the host or to increase host resistance.

private practice A clinical setting that is usually a single physician's office in which the nurse practitioner is employed.

private sector An individual or any part of society that is not part of the government.

probability Likelihood that an intervention activity can be implemented.

problem analysis Process of identifying problem correlates and interrelationships and substantiating them with relevant data.

problem prioritization Evaluation of problems and establishment of priorities according to predetermined criteria.

professional isolation Situation in which professionals of similar background are not employed in close proximity to each other.

professional negligence An act or failure to act when a duty is owed to another that was not reasonable and that leads to injuries compensable by law.

professional socialization Process by which a person acquires the knowledge, skills, and sense of occupational identity characteristic of members of a given profession.

program budget A financial plan that shows expenses and income related to a specific service.

program evaluation Collection of methods, skills, and sensitivities necessary to determine whether a human service is needed, likely to be used, conducted as planned, and actually helps people.

progressive relaxation Technique for combating tension and anxiety by systematically tensing and relaxing muscle groups.

proportional mortality A measure that relates the number of deaths from a particular condition to all deaths for the same period of time.

prospective medicine Early identification of pathological or potentially pathological processes and the prescription of intervention to stop the processes at this point.

prospective payment system The diagnosis-related group payment mechanism for reimbursing hospitals for inpatient health care services through Medicare.

prospective reimbursement Method of payment to an agency for services to be delivered based on predictions of what an agency's costs will be for the coming year.

protocol Outline or plan for a procedure, written and signed by a physician.

protocols (algorithms) Written, standing orders that have been mutually agreed on by the nurse practitioner and the physician. The nurse practitioner uses them as a guide to manage certain illnesses or conditions.

provider service records A written summary of the provider's work activities on a daily, weekly, or monthly basis.

proximity, principle of Objects that are close together are seen as a perceptual unit.

psittacosis Acute febrile illness that is transmitted to humans by various species of birds.

psychological health Level of emotional fitness

psychomotor domain Includes observable performance of skills that require some degree of neuromuscular coordination.

psychosis Mental disorder often characterized by delusions and hallucinations.

psychotic Pertaining to or affected by psychosis.

psychotropic drugs Drugs that affect psychic function, behavior, or experience.

puberty The biological stage of development during which physical changes occur that make reproduction possible.

quality assurance Monitoring of the activities of client care to determine the degree of excellence attained in the implementation of the activities.

quasivoluntary A form of accreditation that is linked to governmental regulations and encourages programs to participate in a voluntary accrediting process.

rape Natural or unnatural sexual intercourse forced on an unwilling person by threat of bodily injury or loss of life.

rapid eye movement (REM) Movement of the closed eyes during sleep, occurring while the subject is dreaming.

rate Statistical measure with the frequency of an event as the numerator and the number of persons among whom the event occurred as the denominator.

ratio Statistical measure in which the numerator is not included in the denominator.

reasonable care Degree of skill and knowledge customarily used by a competent health practitioner or student of similar education and experience in treating and caring for the sick and injured in the community in which the individual is practicing.

reasonably prudent person doctrine Requires a person of ordinary sense to use ordinary care and skill.

receptive skills Language skills that provide the toddler with the ability to follow simple instructions.

recertification In home health care, the review and certification performed at least every 60 days by the physician and health care team that demonstrates the client continues to need a specified plan of care.

reciprocity The recognition and acceptance of a professional's licensure between certain states.

recognition Process whereby one agency accepts the credentialing status of and the credentials conferred by another.

recommended dietary allowances The levels of intake of essential nutrients considered to be adequate to meet the known nutritional needs of practically all healthy people.

recreation "Activity indulged in voluntarily for satisfaction derived from the activity itself and leading to revitalization or re-creation of mind, body, or spirit" (Goodale and Witt, 1980, p. 25).

Red Squill Used as a poison for rodents. Since rats cannot regurgitate, Red Squill is lethal for them, whereas it acts as an enteric for humans.

referral Guiding clients toward and assisting them in using resources available to resolve their problems.

reflexology Systematic massage of the soles of the feet; uses principles similar to acupressure.

regulations Specific statements of law that relate to and clarify individual pieces of legislation.

rehabilitation Restoration to a former state of functioning or limiting of impairment and disability to the lowest possible level.

relational studies Analytic studies that relate exposure and disease in the same individuals.

relative risk ratio Statistical measure of how much the risk of acquiring a particular disease increases with exposure to a specific causal agent or risk factor.

rem (roentgen-equivalent-man) Measure of the amount of radiation absorbed in human tissues.

representative group Type of community group whose members are elected, appointed, or selected from various community sectors.

resource barriers Factors that interfere with the development of specific services needed within a community or the provision of insufficient services.

respite Relief time from responsibilities for care of a family member.

respondeat superior "Let the master answer." The employer is responsible for the legal consequences of the acts of the employee while he acts within the scope of his employment.

respondent behavior Behavior elicited by a known stimulus.

retinopathy Noninflammatory eye disorder caused by changes in the retinal blood vessels.

retrospective audit A method of evaluating quality of care through appraisal of the nursing process after the client's discharge from the health care system.

retrospective cost reimbursement Method of payment to an agency based on units of service delivered.

reversibility Once something is thought, it can be mentally undone.

right That to which a person has a just claim.

    legal Claim recognized as valid by a legal system.

    moral Claim recognized as valid by moral principles that in turn may or may not be recognized by legal rules.

right to health Right to not have one's health affected by others (a negative right).

right to health care Right to goods, resources, and services to maintain and improve one's state of health (a positive right).

risk Probability of an unfavorable event, such as developing a disease.

risk appraisal and reduction Ways of assisting individuals and groups in developing a portion of their self-health care agendas; often professionally determined and/or controlled.

risk factor Disease precursor, the presence of which is associated with higher than average mortality. Disease precursors include demographic variables, certain everyday health practices, family history of disease, and some physiological changes.

risk management Intervention designed to induce and/or sustain changes in health-compromising behaviors, such as counseling, mass media campaigns, or increased production of low-fat dairy goods.

rodenticide Chemical pesticide to kill rodents.

role Identifiable social position associated with a set of behavioral expectations.

role ambiguity Lack of clarity about what is expected.

role behavior What an actor in a position actually does in response to role expectations.

role conflict Presence of contradictory and often competing role expectations.

role overload Occurs when there is insufficient time in which to carry out all of the expected role functions.

role sequence Positions within the family and related behaviors which change over time.

role strain Results from situations requiring complex role demands and the fulfillment of multiple roles.

role structure Arrangement of group member positions according to the expected functions of members.

rubeola (measles) Acute, highly contagious, viral disease involving the respiratory tract and characterized by a rash.

rule of confidentiality Nondisclosure of personal information about others, such as clients, to those not authorized to have this information; also, a rule grounded in the principle of autonomy.

rule of utility Derived from the principle of beneficence. Includes the moral duty to weigh and balance benefits and reduce the occurrence of harms.

rules Guidelines, principles, or regulations that govern conduct.

    legal Established by legal principles.

    moral Established by moral principles.

rules and regulations Clear and concise statements mandating or prohibiting certain activity in an institution.

rural areas Areas in open country with a population less than 2,500.

Rural Health Clinic Legislation enacted in 1978 to provide for the development of rural health clinics staffed by new health professionals in existing medically underserved areas of the United States.

salmonellosis A gastroenteritis caused by ingestion of food contaminated with a species of *Salmonella*; characterized by sudden, colicky, abdominal pain, fever, and bloody, watery diarrhea.

sanitary landfill Method of solid waste disposal whereby waste is taken to canyons, swamps, and ravines; compacted by heavy machines; and covered with earth before rodent infestation occurs.

satellite clinic Health care facility generally operated under the auspices of a large institution but situated in a location away from the large facility.

schizophrenia Large group of disorders, usually of psychotic proportion, manifested by characteristic disturbances of thought, mood, and behavior.

school phobia The persistent and abnormal fear of going to school.

school nurse practitioner Registered nurse with certificate or master's level advanced education in the areas of health assessment, diagnosis, and treatment who is prepared to deliver primary health care to school-age children.

scope of practice The usual and customary practice of a profession that takes into account how legislation defines the practice of a profession within a particular jurisdiction.

screening Method of dividing people into categories on the basis of the measurement of some characteristic.

secondary analysis Method of assessment in which existing data are used.

secondary prevention Activities directed toward early detection and treatment of disease.

selected membership group A group of persons brought together for a specific purpose, such as health assessment or promotion. Some members may be linked to others through previous association, or members may be unacquainted before group formation.

selective inattention Screening out the part of the message the listener does not want to hear.

self-care Personal and medical care performed by the patient, usually in collaboration with health care providers.

self-confrontation Strategy for self-modification that depends on clients' recognition of and dissatisfaction with inconsistencies in their own values, beliefs, or behaviors or between their own personal systems and those of admired others.

self-diagnosis Lay assessment of individual health illness status.

self-esteem The degree of worth one attributes to oneself.

self-health care Continuous and episodic, volitional and unintentional activities that people can do for themselves, individually or collectively, in a variety of health and illness matters.

self-management The writing and implementation of rules and regulations that are practiced to protect the health of the community or individuals.

self-regulation An essential characteristic of a profession involving activities that have as their goals the overseeing of the rights, obligations, responsibilities, and relationships of a provider to society, to the profession, and to the client.

self-transcendence Ability to get outside oneself, to focus attention on doing something for the sake of others or for the world—as opposed to self-actualization, in which doing something for or to oneself is the end goal.

senility Mental deterioration associated with old age.

serendipity Accidental discovery.

serum sickness Reaction to various serum substances occurring hours or days after the initial injection. It consists of rash, urticaria, arthritis, adenopathy, and fever.

sex pattern Sexes represented in the family members; i.e., family with all female children, or mother with two male children.

sexual abuse Ranges from fondling to rape; robs children of the feeling of being in control of themselves; emphasizes their vulnerability.

sexually transmitted disease (STD) Contagious disease usually acquired by sexual intercourse.

shaping Altering behavior by supplying step-by-step reinforcement of actions consistent with desired behavior.

sibling relationship The interaction among brothers and sisters.

sidestream smoke Smoke generated by a smoldering cigarette.

similarity, principle of Objects that are similar to one another are organized into one perceptual unit.

situational crisis Crisis resulting from the inability to cope with an unexpected event.

social health Level of interpersonal fitness that involves networks of personal contacts established by an individual for the purposes of communication, influence, support, understanding, and prestige.

socialization Process in which people acquire the skills, knowledge, attitudes, and values necessary for performing their social roles.

somatotropin Hormone responsible for growth released by the hypotholamus.

spacing pattern Entrance of children into the family.

spastic diplegia Classification of cerebral palsy involving paresis of both legs with little or no involvement of the arms.

specialist a nurse who provides services that are specific to an area of concentration in nursing, i.e., pediatric care.

specific immune globulin Special preparation obtained from human blood preselected for its high antibody count against a specific disease (e.g., varicella zoster immune globulin).

specific protection Measures aimed at protecting individuals against specific agents, such as immunization, or attempts to remove agents from the environment.

specific rates Statistical rates in which the events in both the numerator and the denominator are restricted to a specified subgroup of the population.

specificity of the association Uniqueness of a relationship between a causal factor and occurrence of a disease.

spina bifida (neural tube defects) Disturbance in the development of the neural tube early in gestation causing defects in the formation of the spinal cord and possibly the brain. The severity of the condition varies according to the amount of central nervous system tissue involved and may range from absence of brain tissue (anencephaly) to defects anywhere along the spinal column.

staff review committees Designed to monitor client-specific aspects of care appropriate for certain levels of care.

standard of care Those acts performed or omitted that an ordinary prudent person in the defendant's position would or would not have done; a measure by which the defendant's conduct is compared to ascertain negligence.

standardized rates (adjusted rates) Artificial rates of disease that are calculated to allow comparison of rates in populations with differing distributions of characteristics such as age or race.

standards Criteria for measuring conformity to established practice.

statute of limitations Legal limit on the time one has to file suit in civil matters, usually measured from the time of the wrong or from the time a reasonable person would have discovered the wrong.

statutes Legislative enactments; acts of a legislature declaring, commanding, or prohibiting something.

statutory law Law enacted by a legislative body.

stereotypes Exaggerated beliefs and images that are generally false and serve to obscure important differences among members of a group and exaggerate the differences between groups.

stimulus control Strategy for self-modification that depends on manipulating the antecedents of behavior to increase goals and/or behaviors desired by the client and to decrease undesired ones.

stimulus-generalization Conditioning whereby the reaction to one stimulus is reinforced to allow transfer of the reaction to other occurrences.

strategic planning A process in which client needs, specific provider strength, and agency and community resources are successfully matched to offer a service to the community.

trategy Premeditated approach or method of dealing with a situation.

strengthening In stimulus response, an increase in the probability that a response will be made when the stimulus recurs.

strength of the association Degree of a relationship between a causal factor and disease occurrence, usually measured by the relative risk ratio.

structural-functional framework Views the family as a social system with members who have specific roles and functions.

structure In groups, the particular arrangement of group parts that helps to describe the group as a whole.

subpoena Court order requiring a person to come to court to give testimony; failure to appear results in punishment by the court.

substance abuse Use of chemicals having actual or potential undesirable effects.

substantive epidemiology Body of knowledge derived from epidemiological studies; for each disease it includes the natural history of the disease, patterns of occurrence, and factors associated with high risk for developing the disease.

suicide Killing oneself.

sulfur oxide Consists of bluish-white fumes and reduces visibility; generated by burning wood, coal, and petroleum products.

summative evaluation Instituted to assess program outcomes or as a follow-up of the results of program activities.

supervision Denotes line responsibility with active involvement in decision making and implementation activities in an ongoing relationship. It is the antithesis of consultation.

Supplemental Security Income Money awarded to an individual with insufficient resources for the purpose of increasing the income level to a minimum standard.

surveillance Process of monitoring a given population for the occurrence of disease.

survey Method of assessment in which data from a sample of persons are reported to the data collector.

susceptibility Potential to be affected by an agent.

synergism A condition in which factors reinforce one another.

synthesis Fifth level of cognitive learning, in which learners are required to build on the previous four by putting the parts or elements together into a unified whole.

system Complex of elements in interaction.

tabula rasa Blank state; a view of the mind.

Taft-Hartley Act Passed in 1947, it was a revision of the Wagner Act of 1935; included in the 1947 law was a provision that professional employees should not be organized in the same bargaining unit with nonprofessionals unless a majority of the professional employees voted for such an inclusion.

tardive dyskinesia Disorder characterized by slow, rhythmical, automatic, stereotyped movements, either generalized or in single muscle groups.

target heart rate A heart rate of up to 60% to 85% of age-predicted maximum heart rate during physical activity.

target of service Population group for whom healthful change is sought.

task Function with work or labor overtones assigned to or demanded of a person.

task functions Behaviors that focus or direct movement toward the main work of the group.

territory Area of expertise or space over which an individual or group exerts control.

territorialism The perceived or actual assignment of specific client groups or services to a provider group.

tertiary prevention Activities directed toward limitation of disability or restoration of function.

testimony Oral statement given by a witness under oath at a trial.

theories of justice Doctrines that indicate how to distribute goods and resources to the people.

theory-principles intervention mode Requires the client to learn theories and their application to problem solving.

therapeutic community Institution that treats and rehabilitates people with relatively severe behavioral problems, such as drug addiction and alcoholism.

therapeutic touch Method of healing that uses a meditative state to enter another person's energy field and passively visualize or free the flow of energy from practitioner to recipient to promote healing.

third-party payments Reimbursement made to health care providers by an agency other than the client for the care of the client; i.e., insurance companies, governments, or employers.

threshold limit value Maximum amount of a hazardous substance to which workers can be exposed for 8 hours per day without developing disease.

titer Measure of the concentration of a substance in a solution.

tobacco withdrawal syndrome Occurs with cessation of or reduction of nicotine intake and includes the following: changes in mood and performance as seen in temper outbursts; lack of tolerance for people, events, and things; impaired performance because of a lack of concentration; episodes of daydreaming; anxiety.

toddler A child of two or three years of age.

tolerance A state characterized by a need to continually increase the dosage of a drug to achieve the desired effects.

tort Legal or civil wrong committed by one person against the person or property of another.

toxicity Ability of a substance to cause injury to biological tissues.

toxoid Modified bacterial toxin that has been made nontoxic but retains the ability to stimulate the formation of antitoxin; used to produce active immunity.

tracer method A method of evaluating programs based on the premise that health status and care can be evaluated by observing the care and outcomes of specific health problems.

triage Deciding which individuals need the most immediate attention and by whom.

triangulation Use of multiple assessment methods.

trisomy 21 (Down syndrome) Genetic anomaly encompassing recognizable physical characteristics and limited intellectual development. The abnormal physical and central nervous system development is due to the presence of an extra 21 chromosome.

tuberculin skin test Intradermal injection of a substance in minute doses to detect or confirm mycobacterial infection.

typology Classification strategies that systematically organize concepts into dimensions of a whole or a configuration of phenomena.

unit of service Entity—individual, family, aggregate, organization, or community—to whom nursing care is given. The level at which service is delivered. The entity from which healthful changes are sought.

urban areas Areas with a population more than 50,000.

utilitarian theory Claims that the best way to distribute resources among people is to decide how expenditures or the use of resources will bring about the greatest net total of good and serve the largest number of people.

utilization review Directed toward ensuring that care is actually needed and cost is appropriate for the level of care provided.

values Beliefs about how one should or should not behave. Values are organized into value systems, and individual value systems reflect culture, reference groups, and personal needs.

variables Key characteristics of the problem under study.

vector Agent that actively carries a germ to a susceptible host.

vertical coordination Community health nurses serve as links between their level in the organization and those above and below them. They also serve as links between the agency and the client.

virulence Ability to produce severe disease.

voluntary agency An agency that relies on staff and volunteers to provide a wide range of services; must seek operating funds from a variety of sources, including gifts, dues, and fees.

warm up The period of 5 to 20 minutes before aerobic exercise in which a person engages in activities designed to increase circulation, respiration, and body temperature and gently stretch ligaments and connective tissue to prepare them for more vigorous activity and decrease the possibility of injury.

wear and tear theory Programmed process wherein cells are constantly wearing out.

web of causation Interrelationships among multiple factors that contribute to the occurrence of a disease.

wellness Dynamic state of health in which individuals progress toward a higher level of functioning, thus maximizing their potential in the environment.

Wernecke's encepholopathy Neurological disorder caused by excessive alcohol consumption; characterized by ophthalmoplegia, nystagmus atoxia, apathy, drowsiness, confusion, and inability to concentrate.

work-rest-recreation balance The relationship between the estimated percentage of time and energy put forth by an individual or family in pursuing work, rest, and leisure time.

young adult Individual in the 20- to 35-year-old age group, whose psychosocial task is intimacy versus isolation.

INDEX